LIPPINCOTT'S Textbook of Clinical Medical Assisting

Julie B. Hosley, RN, CMA
Medical Assisting Curriculum Coordinator
Carteret Community College
Morehead City, North Carolina

Elizabeth A. Molle-Matthews, RN, CEN
Clinical Research Nurse
Middlesex Hospital
Middletown, Connecticut
Formerly Director, Medical Assisting Program
Morse School of Business
Hartford, Connecticut

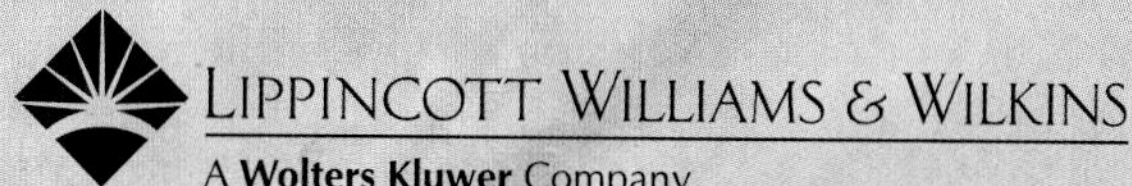

LIPPINCOTT WILLIAMS & WILKINS
A Wolters Kluwer Company
Philadelphia • Baltimore • New York • London
Buenos Aires • Hong Kong • Sydney • Tokyo

Acquisitions Editor: Margaret M. Biblis
Editorial Assistant: Amy Amico
Senior Project Editor: Erika Kors

Senior Production Manager: Helen Ewan
Production Coordinator: Patricia McCloskey
Assistant Art Director: Doug Smock

9 8 7 6 5 4 3 2 1

Library of Congress Cataloging-in-Publication Data

Lippincott's textbook of clinical medical assisting / [edited by]
Julie B. Hosley, Elizabeth A. Molle-Matthews ; with contributors.
p. cm.
Includes bibliographical references and index.
ISBN 0-7817-1457-5 (alk. paper)
1. Medical assistants. 2. Clinical medicine. I. Hosley, Julie B.
II. Molle-Matthews, Elizabeth A. III. Title: Textbook of clinical medical assisting
R728.8 .L59 1999
610.69'53 -- dc21

98-45295
CIP

Care has been taken to confirm the accuracy of the information presented and to describe generally accepted practices. However, the authors, editors, and publisher are not responsible for errors or omissions or for any consequences from application of the information in this book and make no warranty, express or implied, with respect to the contents of the publication.

The authors, editors and publisher have exerted every effort to ensure that drug selection and dosage set forth in this text are in accordance with current recommendations and practice at the time of publication. However, in view of ongoing research, changes in government regulations, and the constant flow of information relating to drug therapy and drug reactions, the reader is urged to check the package insert for each drug for any change in indications and dosage and for added warnings and precautions. This is particularly important when the recommended agent is a new or infrequently employed drug.

Some drugs and medical devices presented in this publication have Food and Drug Administration (FDA) clearance for limited use in restricted research settings. It is the responsibility of the health care provider to ascertain the FDA status of each drug or device planned for use in their clinical practice.

Selected figures (illustrations) in this text were reproduced with permission from the following Lippincott-Raven sources: Taylor C, Lillis C, LeMone P: Fundamentals of Nursing, Second Edition; Craven RF, Hirnle CJ: Fundamentals of Nursing, Second Edition; Smeltzer SC, Bare B: Brunner and Suddarth's Textbook of Medical-Surgical Nursing, Eighth Edition; Memmler RL, Cohen BJ, Wood DL: The Human Body in Health and Disease, Eighth Edition; Burton GRW, Engelkirk PG: Microbiology for the Health Sciences, Fifth Edition; Lotspeich-Steininger CA, Steine-Martin EA, Koepke JA: Clinical Hematology; Timby BK: Fundamental Skills and Concepts in Patient Care, Sixth Edition; Kurzen CR: Contemporary Practical/Vocational Nursing, Second Edition; Jones SA, Weigel A, White RD, McSwain NE, Breiter M: Advanced Emergency Care for Paramedic Practice; Bates B, Bickley LS, Hoekelman RA: A Guide to Physical Examination and History Taking, Sixth Edition; Ellis JR, Nowlis EA, Bentz PM: Modules for Basic Nursing Skills, Volume I, Sixth Edition; Bullock BL: Pathophysiology, Fourth Edition; Porth CM: Pathophysiology, Fourth Edition; Davis D: How to Quickly and Accurately Master ECG Interpretation, Second Edition; Reeder SJ, Martin LL, Griffin DK: Maternity Nursing, Eighteenth Edition; Bishop ML: Clinical Chemistry, Third Edition; Koneman EW, Allen SD, Janda WM, Schreckenberger PC, Winn WC: Color Atlas and Textbook of Diagnostic Microbiology, Fourth Edition; Harvey RA, Champe PC: Lippincott's Illustrated Reviews: Microbiology; McCall RE, Tankersley CM: Phlebotomy Exam Review; Jackson DB, Saunders RB: Child Health Nursing; Volk et al: Essentials of Medical Microbiology, Fifth Edition; Rosdahl CB: Textbook of Basic Nursing, Sixth Edition; Scott et al: Danforth's Obstetrics and Gynecology, Seventh Edition; Berman MC, Cohen HL: Diagnostic Medical Sonography, Second Edition; Cullinan AM, Cullinan JE: Producing Quality Radiographs, Second Edition; Torres LS: Basic Medical Techniques and Patient Care in Imaging Technology, Fifth Edition; Hosley JB et al: Lippincott's Textbook for Medical Assistants; Hosley JB, Molle-Matthews EA: Lippincott's Pocket Guide to Medical Assisting.

Reviewer List

Kevin Dooley, MD
Chief Resident
Middlesex Hospital
Middletown, Connecticut

Jeanne Howard, CMA, AAS
Instructor/Coordinator Medical Assisting
El Paso Community College
El Paso, Texas

Ruth E. McCall, BS, MT (ASCP), CLS (NCA)
Director of Phlebotomy and Clinical Laboratory Assistant Programs
Instructor, MLT and Healthcare Technician Programs
Albuquerque Technical-Vocational Institute
Albuquerque, New Mexico

Pat Moeck, MBA, CMA
Director, Medical Assisting Program
El Centro College
Dallas, Texas

Paulette Nitkiewicz, BNS, RN, CMA
Allied Medical Supervisor
Laurel Business Institute
Uniontown, Pennsylvania

Susanne Sniffin, CMA-C, LRT
Immediate Past President New York State Society of Medical Assistants
Great Neck, New York

Patricia Suminski, RN, BSN, CMA
Instructor, Director of Medical Assisting Program
Milwaukee Area Technical College
Milwaukee, Wisconsin

Introduction

Welcome to the profession of Clinical Medical Assisting. This is an exciting and rewarding career with a promising employment outlook.

In this profession, you will work with a variety of medical professionals as part of a multidisciplinary team. The team leaders may include physicians, nurse practitioners, or physician assistants. Other members of the team may include nurses (registered and licensed practical), physical therapists, social workers, phlebotomists, radiology technicians, paramedics and emergency medical technicians, infection control officers, dietitians, and chiropractors. Administrative members of the team may include billing clerks, administrative medical assistants, transcriptionists, risk managers, and office managers.

Settings in which you may work as a clinical medical assistant include both outpatient and inpatient centers. Examples of outpatient centers include urgent-care or walk-in centers, physicians' offices, adult day care centers, insurance companies, research centers, and clinics. Inpatient settings may include patient care units, hospital radiology and laboratory departments, skilled nursing facilities, psychiatric institutions, or drug and alcohol rehabilitation centers.

The clinical aspect of medical assisting encompasses many skills and job responsibilities, which vary greatly among individual settings. Below is a partial list of common clinical duties:

- Preparing patients for examinations and treatments
- Assisting other health care professionals with procedures
- Preparing and sterilizing instruments
- Obtaining laboratory specimens
- Performing laboratory procedures
- Completing electrocardiograms
- Applying Holter monitors
- Obtaining medical histories
- Assisting with radiographic tests (laws vary by state)
- Administering medications and immunizations
- Obtaining vital signs (blood pressure, temperature, pulse, respiration)
- Obtaining height and weight measurements
- Documenting in the medical record
- Performing eye and ear treatments
- Recognizing and treating medical emergencies
- Initiating and implementing patient education

A clinical medical assistant must perform these skills and procedures within professional, ethical, and legal boundaries. These boundaries have been developed by various professional associations, governmental organizations, and legal structures.

As a clinical medical assistant, you should always follow these professional guidelines:

- Demonstrate maturity when dealing with complex situations
- Be honest
- Be accurate and thorough
- Respect patients' feelings, fears and wishes
- Demonstrate empathy
- Use good interpersonal skills
- Project a positive self-image through a professional appearance
- Use excellent written and oral communication skills
- Participate in community services that promote good health and welfare to the general public
- Continually improve skills for the benefit of the patient and health care team

As a clinical medical assistant, you also are responsible for adhering to certain ethical and legal principles. For example, you should follow these ethical guidelines:

- Respect patient privacy
- Respect patient confidentiality
- Respect cultural diversity

You also should comply with these legal guidelines:

- Adhere to all state and federal rules and regulations, including OSHA, CLIA, and JCAHO regulations. Keep abreast of changes to the Medical Practice Act, Good Samaritan Act, Self-Determination Act (Advance Directives), Uniform Gift Act and Controlled Substance Act.
- Remain current and knowledgeable about new medical procedures, Medicare and insurance changes, and other legal updates
- Document appropriately and promptly in the medical record
- Report to the appropriate agency any health care professional who legally or ethically violates the standard of care
- Report any contagious or infectious diseases to the appropriate department of public health and/or the Centers for Disease Control and Prevention (CDC).
- Report any suspected or confirmed cases of abuse, neglect, or maltreatment
- Report all vital statistics (deaths, births)
- Report all violent injuries to the appropriate state agency
- Complete incident reports promptly and completely

In addition to obeying the legal guidelines listed above, you can decrease your potential for legal liability by:

- Keeping medical records neat and organized
- Documenting and signing the record legibly
- Completing the examination to obtain your professional credentials
- Keeping your CPR and First Aid certifications current
- Refusing to give any information over the telephone unless you are sure of the caller's identity or you have the patient's consent
- Keeping the office neat, clean and safe
- Practicing good public relations

A key to becoming a successful clinical medical assistant is your ability to communicate with patients effectively. Remember, communication involves both verbal and nonverbal exchanges. Practice active listening skills and good interviewing techniques. Follow the recommended medical care and, in addition, keep in mind that patients' cultural and religious beliefs play a key role in how they respond to your communication.

Finally, it is important to remember that when performing any skills, treatments, or procedures, your overall goal is to promote patients' health and welfare and to assist caregivers in extending proper medical care to the home setting.

We would like to thank Kevin Dooley, MD, for reviewing this textbook for clinical accuracy and for offering many suggestions for expansion and topic development.

Thanks to D. K. Minchella, CMA, for her time and effort in converting the objectives from **DACUM** *to Role Delineation to make the text more timely and topical.*

We would like to give thanks to Ruth E. McCall, BS, MT, (ASCP), CLS, (NCA) for her special assistance in coordinating the laboratory chapters and procedures to ensure their accuracy and timeliness.

Acknowledgments

The authors would like to thank the following people for their past contributions in developing the clinical and laboratory chapters and procedures to ensure that the information is accurate and current.

Beverly A. Baker, DA, CST
Program Director and Instructor, Surgical Technology
Western Iowa Technical and Community College
Sioux City, Iowa

Rita-Ann Boegel, ADN, RN, CGRN
Charge Nurse
Gastroenterology Diagnostic Center
Veterans Administration Medical Hospital
San Francisco, California

Sharon Brill, RN, BSN, PHN
Associate Instructor, Health Care Technologies
West Valley College
Saratoga, California

Harriette Cooper, LPN
Carteret Surgical Associates
Morehead City, North Carolina

Toni M. Crowell, CMA
Program Coordinator, Medical Assisting and Medical Office Administration
Sussex County Community College
Newton, New Jersey
Instructor, Medical Assisting and Medical Office Administration
Berdan Institute
Totowa, New Jersey

Laura G. Cullen, RN, CMA, AA, PARALEGAL
Nurse–Paralegal
Law Office of Kathleen C. Cresson
New Orleans, Louisiana

Theresa P. Ford, MT (ASCP), MEd
Hematology Supervisor
Craven Regional Medical Center
New Bern, North Carolina

Loretta M. Hamilton, AOS, CMA, RMLA, RPT
Paramedical Examiner
Portamedic
Metairie, Louisiana

Judy White Harris, RN, CMA-C
J.W. Harris Publications
Sarasota, Florida

Julie B. Hosley, RN, CMA
Medical Assisting Curriculum Coordinator
Carteret Community College
Morehead City, North Carolina

Shirley A. Jones, MSEd, MHA
Program director
Allied Health Education
Methodist Hospital
Indianapolis, Indiana

Lauri A. Kollross, CMA
Operations Manager, Marshfield Clinic
Advisor and Coordinator, Medical Assistant Program
Mid-State Technical College
Marshfield, Wisconsin

Pauline Leventry, ADN, CMA
Medical Assistant Department Chairman
Mount Aloysius College
Cresson, Pennsylvania

Tibby Loveman, BSN
Former Medical Assistant Instructor
Gadsden Business College
Gadsden, Alabama

Ruth E. McCall, BS, MT (ASCP), CLS (NCA)
Director of Phlebotomy and Clinical Laboratory Assistant Programs
Instructor, MLT and Healthcare Technician Programs
Albuquerque Technical-Vocational Institute
Albuquerque, New Mexico

Larry H. Miller, RT (R)
Radiography Curriculum Coordinator
Carteret Community College
Morehead City, North Carolina

Elizabeth A. Molle-Matthews, RN, CEN
Clinical Research Nurse
Middlesex Hospital
Middletown, Connecticut
Formerly Director, Medical Assisting Program
Morse School of Business
Hartford, Connecticut

Patricia M. Purscell, MT (ASCP), CMA
Laboratory Supervisor
Providence Hospital
Anchorage, Alaska

Susan Ravagni, MT (ASCP)
Medical Technologist
Hematology Laboratory
Brigham and Women's Hospital
Boston, Massachusetts

Midge Noel Ray, MSN, RN
Associate Professor, Health Information Management Program
Health Services Administration
School of Health Related Professions
University of Alabama at Birmingham
Birmingham, Alabama

Cynthia M. Reed, MT (ASCP)
School Director
Georgia Medical Institute
Atlanta, Georgia

Nora Mae Sanborn BSMT (ASCP)
Curriculum Coordinator, Phlebotomy Program
Instructor, Medical Assisting Program
Carteret Community College
Morehead City, North Carolina

Connie Stack, BSAH, ed, MLT (ASCP), CMA
Director, Medical Assisting Program
Anson Community College
Polkton, North Carolina

Kasey Coal Summer, BA, TED, RMA
Director Career Services
Ultrasound Diagnostic Schools
Atlanta, Georgia

Barbara S. Thomas, RRT, BA, BS, MPH
Curriculum Coordinator, Respiratory Care Technology
Carteret Community College
Morehead City, North Carolina

Betsy Lasarow Tozzi
Assistant Professor
Health Technology Department
University of Alaska Fairbanks
Fairbanks, Alaska

Natalie Uebele, RN, BSPA
Instructor, Nursing Department
Carteret Community College
Morehead City, North Carolina

Louise D. Yurko, MAPT
President, Carteret Physical Therapy Associates, Inc.
Morehead City, North Carolina
Adjunct Professor, School of Physical Therapy
East Carolina University
Greenville, North Carolina

Contents

Expanded Contents

Unit 1 Performing Clinical Duties

1 Asepsis and Infection Control

Chapter Outline

Microorganisms and Normal Flora
Conditions That Favor the Growth of Pathogens
The Infection Cycle
Modes of Transmission
- Direct Transmission
- Indirect Transmission
- Sources of Transmission

Isolation Precautions
Occupational Safety and Health Administration Guidelines for the Medical Office
- Exposure Risk Factors
- Personal Protective Equipment
- Hepatitis B Virus Immunization
- Postexposure Policies
- Material Safety Data Sheet
- Employee Training Requirements

Infection Control
- Levels of Infection Control
- Handling Environmental Contamination
- Cleaning and Decontaminating Biohazardous Spills
- Handling Soiled Linens
- Decontaminating and Laundering Protective Clothing
- Disposing of Infectious Waste

Medical Asepsis
Maintaining Medical Asepsis
Surgical Asepsis
Surgical Scrub

Role Delineation

CLINICAL

Fundamental Principles

- Apply principles of aseptic technique and infection control.
- Comply with quality assurance practices.

GENERAL

Legal Concepts

- Practice within the scope of education, training, and personal capabilities.
- Follow federal, state, and local legal guidelines.
- Maintain and dispose of regulated substances in compliance with government guidelines.
- Comply with established risk management and safety procedures.

Chapter Competencies

Learning Objectives

Upon successfully completing this chapter, you will be able to:

1. Spell and define the Key Terms.
2. Identify and describe conditions that promote the growth of pathogens.
3. Define the chain of infection.
4. Describe how microorganisms are transmitted.
5. Distinguish between medical and surgical asepsis.
6. Explain the difference between medical aseptic handwashing and surgical scrubbing.
7. Explain the purpose of following Standard Precautions with all patients.
8. Identify and describe the levels of infection control.
9. Properly dispose of infectious waste.

Performance Objectives

Upon successfully completing this chapter, you will be able to:

1. Perform a medical aseptic handwashing (Procedure 1-1).
2. Perform a surgical scrub (Procedure 1-2).
3. Put on sterile gloves (Procedure 1-3).

Chapter Competencies *(continued)*

4. Remove gloves after a procedure (Procedure 1-4).
5. Clean and decontaminate biohazardous spills.

Key Terms

(See Glossary for definitions.)

asepsis
carriers
centigrade (c), Celsius (C)
disease
exogenous
infection
medical asepsis
microorganisms
normal flora
OSHA
pathogens
phagocytized
spores
surgical asepsis
transient flora
vector
virulent

To prevent the spread of **disease** (a departure from wellness), proper technique must be used in every aspect of medical office practice. The term **asepsis** means freedom from **infection,** or a condition in which pathogenic organisms are absent. You will learn in this chapter that the medical aseptic handwash is the single most important factor in the prevention of disease transmission. It is the cornerstone of infection control. As a medical assistant, you will learn how important it is to adhere to strict aseptic procedures and to encourage patients and their families to practice good handwashing and disease prevention techniques in the home. In addition, you will recognize the importance of using Standard Precautions—guidelines for isolation precautions issued by the Centers for Disease Control and Prevention (CDC)—for all patients. Finally, you will learn the importance of the various levels of infection control that should be used in the medical office.

MICROORGANISMS AND NORMAL FLORA

Microorganisms—microscopic living organisms—are all around us and all through our bodies. They can be classified as bacteria, fungi, viruses, protozoa, and metazoa (see Chap. 27, Microbiology, for a more detailed discussion.) They are abundant on the skin and throughout the gastrointestinal and respiratory systems. They are even found in parts of the body not connected to the outside environment. Most microorganisms in the body are normal flora (or resident flora) and are required for the normal functioning of the various systems.

When microorganisms produce disease, they are called **pathogens.** Pathogens are easily spread from one person to another either directly or indirectly by inhalation (from contaminated air droplets from coughs and sneezes from a contaminated person), ingestion (eg, from eating contaminated foods), or injection (through a break in the sterile procedure). See "Modes of Transmission," below.

Many beneficial microorganisms reside within the body. Certain types of microorganisms are specific to special sections of the body. The presence of the normal flora in a section triggers the immune system to build and release special disease-fighting cells called antibodies, which protect the body from exogenous disease-producing microorganisms (microorganisms originating outside of the body) or from microorganisms that are normal in the body but alien to a specific system or site. For instance, *Escherichia coli* is normal for the lower gastrointestinal tract but is pathogenic in any other area of the body. For example, *E. coli* contamination from the rectal area to the genitourinary tract may cause severe infections. The relationship of normal flora to their specific system or site is so complex that when a chemical imbalance is created in the body through chemotherapy or antibiotic drugs, the resulting disruption may decrease the protection offered by the normal flora, thus allowing pathogens to grow. Certain instances of imbalance may cause normally occurring microorganisms to become a source of illness or infection.

The body is protected by many nonspecific defenses against disease. If the barriers are overpowered or breached, other backup systems are in place to protect us from the multitude of microorganisms that surround us.

- Skin. Normal flora on the skin consist mainly of *Staphylococcus aureus*. As long as the skin is kept clean and intact, the bacteria are not considered dangerous. Washing the skin frequently will flush away the microorganisms. Keeping the skin intact prevents a portal of entry.
- Eyes. Tears flush potentially dangerous bacteria from the eyes and contain a bacteria-destroying enzyme called lysozyme.
- Mouth. The greatest variety of microorganisms found in the body are in the oral cavity, which is itself the ideal host for pathogens to thrive. Good oral hygiene removes the pathogens or prevents their growth. Saliva is slightly bactericidal.
- Gastrointestinal tract. Normal hydrochloric acid in the stomach destroys many disease-producing pathogens. The normal flora of the colon and small intestines, which are vital for digestion of nutrients, are usually not disease-causing microbes as long as they remain within the gastrointestinal tract.
- Respiratory tract. Nostril hair and cilia are early defenses against airborne bacteria. If these barriers are insufficient, mucus from the membranes lining the respiratory tract constantly waves along the cilia, trapping and transporting microorganisms to the pharynx for swallowing. After swallowing, digestive enzymes usually neutralize airborne microorganisms. Those that make it to the lung fields are usually **phagocytized** (engulfed and digested) by macrophages in the alveoli and interstitial spaces.
- Genitourinary tract. The reproductive tracts and the urinary system are slightly acidic to provide a less hospitable environment for microorganisms. Frequent flushing by the urinary tract with urination removes many transient pathogens.

Any of these systems may be overpowered by a particularly **virulent** (highly pathogenic) organism, or they may be overcome if the barriers and resistance are depressed, as in old age, existing pathology, or unusual stress. **Transient flora**—organisms that do not normally reside in a particular area—are not usually pathogenic unless defenses are compromised. They are not as well adapted to the body as the normal flora and usually only become pathogenic if the disease resistance of the host is decreased for some reason.

Checkpoint Question

1. *What are normal flora and how do they protect the body from pathogens?*

CONDITIONS THAT FAVOR THE GROWTH OF PATHOGENS

As living organisms, the pathogens found in the clinical setting need certain conditions for optimum growth and reproduction. As a medical assistant, you are responsible for reducing pathogens in the clinical setting by eliminating as many of their life requirements as possible. These requirements include:

- *Moisture.* Few microbes survive well in dry places. Those that form **spores** may remain dormant until moisture is available.
- *Nutrients.* Microorganisms depend on their environment for sustenance; a nutrient-rich environment fosters growth.
- *Temperature.* Although microorganisms may survive in freezing or boiling environments, those that thrive at body temperature—98° to 100° Fahrenheit or about 37° **centigrade**—are more likely to be pathogenic to humans. (Centigrade, or **Celsius,** is a temperature scale on which 0° is the freezing point and 100° is the boiling point of water at sea level.)
- *Darkness.* Virtually no bacteria pathogenic to humans will thrive in sunlight or bright light.
- *Neutral to slightly alkaline pH environment.* The pH of the blood at 7.35 to 7.45 is preferred by those microorganisms that thrive in the human body.
- *Oxygen.* Most pathogens require free air; those that do are called aerobes. A few, however, do not live well in an oxygen-rich environment; these are called anaerobes (eg, tetanus, botulism).

If any one of these conditions is altered in any way, the result can be a change in the growth and replication of the pathogen.

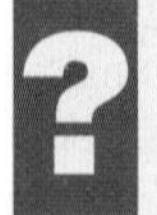

Checkpoint Question

2. *What are the six conditions that favor the growth of pathogens?*

THE INFECTION CYCLE

The infection cycle is often referred to as links of a chain around a causative agent, which is the invading microorganism (Fig. 1-1). The first link in the infection cycle is a reservoir host. If the microorganism cannot

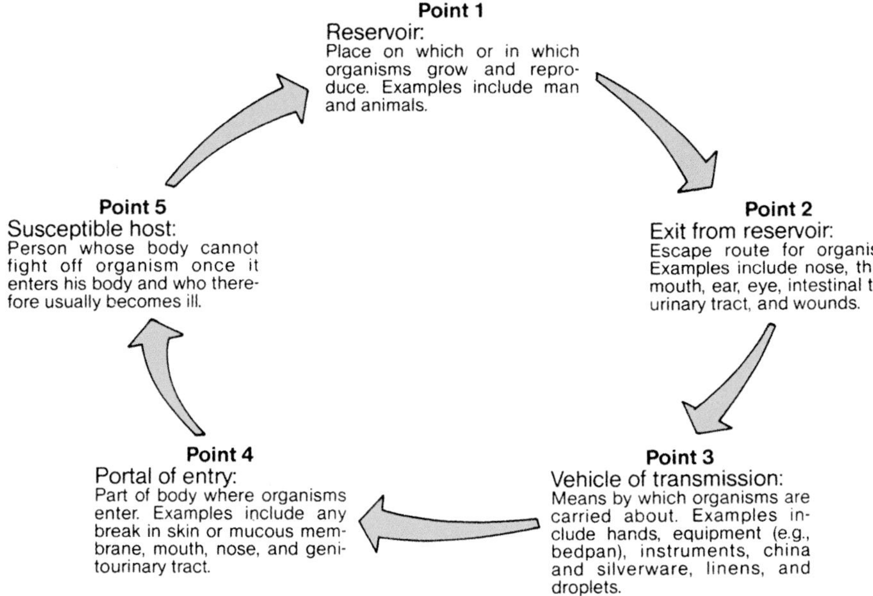
Point 1
Reservoir:
Place on which or in which organisms grow and reproduce. Examples include man and animals.
Point 2
Exit from reservoir:
Escape route for organisms. Examples include nose, throat, mouth, ear, eye, intestinal tract, urinary tract, and wounds.
Point 3
Vehicle of transmission:
Means by which organisms are carried about. Examples include hands, equipment (e.g., bedpan), instruments, china and silverware, linens, and droplets.
Point 4
Portal of entry:
Part of body where organisms enter. Examples include any break in skin or mucous membrane, mouth, nose, and genitourinary tract.
Point 5
Susceptible host:
Person whose body cannot fight off organism once it enters his body and who therefore usually becomes ill.

Figure 1-1 This sketch illustrates the infectious process cycle. Infections and infectious diseases are spread by starting from the reservoir (*Point 1*), and moving full circle to a susceptible host (*Point 5*). Microorganisms can be controlled by using methods that interfere at any point within the cycle.

find a host on which it can feed, it will die. This reservoir host provides nutrients and an incubation site for the pathogen. The pathogen may cause disease symptoms in the reservoir host, or it may asymptomatically incubate new generations there and then leave the first host to search for a second host. Persons who are infected with transmissible diseases but who are asymptomatic may be **carriers**, or reservoirs, of disease. They can still transmit those diseases simply by coming in contact with a susceptible person.

The second link in the infectious cycle is the means of exit, sometimes referred to as the portal of exit. This refers to the manner by which the pathogen leaves the host—for example, by coughing, sneezing, direct contact by shaking hands, or through an open wound as drainage.

The third link in the infection cycle is the means, or vehicle, of transmission. This includes contaminated air droplets from coughing and sneezing, pathogens on an unclean hand passing on to another by direct contact, or contact with wound drainage.

The fourth link in the infection cycle is a means of entrance, or portal of entry. This could occur by breathing in contaminated airborne droplets or ingesting contaminated food or drink. Any break in the skin or mucous membrane is a portal of entry for a pathogen. Any break in sterile procedure is a means of entrance for a pathogen.

The fifth link in the infection cycle is a susceptible host (Box 1-1). A host that permits easy entrance similar to the means of exit and allows the pathogen to grow and multiply then becomes a new reservoir host, causing the chain to repeat the cycle.

Box 1-1
The Susceptible Host

The susceptible host is unable to resist the invading pathogen for a variety of reasons:

- *Age.* As the body ages, defense mechanisms begin to lose their effectiveness. The immune system is no longer as active or as efficient. In the very young, the immune system may not be fully functional.
- *Existing pathology.* Stress of an existing illness will occupy or deplete the immune system to leave the way clear for an additional illness.
- *Poor nutrition.* A nutritionally deficient diet will not allow cells to repair and reproduce as they are weakened by disease.
- *Poor hygiene.* Although multitudes of microbes exist on our skin, keeping the numbers down will allow normal flora to maintain a proper balance with pathogens.

Checkpoint Question

3. *How are the first and fifth links of the infection cycle related?*

MODES OF TRANSMISSION

Direct Transmission

Direct transmission requires direct contact with another person. Direct transmission occurs through such means as shaking hands, sexual contact or kissing, di-

Table 1-1 **Common Communicable Diseases**

Disease	*Method of Transmission*
Acquired immunodeficiency syndrome (AIDS)	Direct contact with body fluids, sexual contact, contact with contaminated needles
Bacillary dysentery	Fecal/oral route (spread by vectors such as flies and contaminated food)
Cholera	Ingestion of contaminated food or water
Diphtheria	Airborne droplets, carriers
German measles (rubella)	Airborne droplets
Influenza	Direct contact, contaminated articles, airborne droplets
Measles (rubeola)	Airborne droplets
Mononucleosis	Airborne droplets, contamination by infected saliva
Mumps	Direct contact with materials contaminated with infected saliva, airborne droplets
Pneumonia	Airborne droplets, direct contact
Rabies	Saliva of infected animal (bites)
Tetanus	Spores or animal feces transmitted by direct contact

rect contact with blood or body fluids, or inhaling contaminated air droplets.

Indirect Transmission

Indirect transmission occurs through contact by a vehicle, either biologic or mechanical, called a **vector.** Examples include food, water, disease-carrying insects (eg, mosquitoes, ticks, lice, or fleas), or inanimate objects (eg, air, soil, instruments, wound exudate, drinking glasses).

Sources of Transmission

Most reservoir hosts are humans, animals, and insects. Human hosts include people who are ill with an infectious disease, people who are carriers of an infectious disease, and people who are in the incubation or ambulatory stage of an infectious disease. With the exception of flies and roaches, which carry many diseases, most of the insect sources are those that draw blood from an infected reservoir, such as ticks and mosquitoes, and pass the disease to their next victim. The animal sources are less abundant but include infected animals, such as those that transmit anthrax or rabies.

Table 1-1 provides some examples of common diseases and their methods of transmission.

ISOLATION PRECAUTIONS

In January 1996, the CDC and the Hospital Infection Control Practices Advisory Committee (HICPAC) issued revised guidelines for isolation precautions. These guidelines supersede previous CDC recommendations. Under this system, two tiers of precautions are recognized:

1. ***Standard Precautions*** are to be used for all patients, regardless of their known (or suspected) infection status. Standard Precautions synthesize the major features of two isolation systems: universal precautions (designed to reduce the risk of transmission of blood-borne pathogens [eg, human immunodeficiency virus, or HIV, and hepatitis B virus]) and body substance isolation (designed to reduce the risk of transmission of pathogens from moist body substances). Box 1-2 describes Standard Precautions in greater detail.
2. ***Transmission-based precautions*** are to be used for patients known (or suspected) to be infected with highly transmissible or epidemiologically important pathogens that can be transmitted by the airborne, droplet, or direct-contact routes. Transmission-based precautions are to be used in addition to Standard Precautions for specified patients. Table 1-2 describes transmission-based precautions in greater detail.

Standard Precautions are to be used for all patients in all situations and apply to:

- Blood
- All body fluids, secretions, and excretions *except sweat,* regardless of whether or not they contain visible blood
- Nonintact skin
- Mucous membranes

Box 1-2
Standard Precautions

Under Standard Precautions, you must:

- Wash your hands:
  - After touching blood, body fluids, secretions, excretions, and contaminated items whether you have worn gloves or not
  - Immediately after you remove gloves
  - Between patient contacts
  - When necessary to prevent transfer of microorganisms
- Use plain soap for routine handwashing and an antimicrobial or antiseptic agent for specified situations.
- Wear clean, nonsterile gloves when touching blood, body fluids, secretions, excretions, mucous membranes, nonintact skin, and contaminated items.
- Change gloves between procedures on the same patient after exposure to potentially infective material.
- Remove gloves immediately after patient contact, and wash your hands.
- Wear personal protective equipment (eg, mask, goggles, face shield, gown) to protect the mucous membranes of your eyes, nose, and mouth and to avoid soiling your clothing when performing procedures that may generate splashes or sprays of blood, body fluids, secretions, or excretions.
- Care for equipment and linens that are contaminated with blood, body fluids, secretions, or excretions in a way that avoids skin and mucous membrane exposures, clothing contamination, and microorganism transfer to other patients and environments. Dispose of single-use items appropriately.
- Take precautions to avoid injuries before, during, and after any procedures using needles, scalpels, or other sharp instruments.
- Ensure that used needles are not recapped, purposely bent, broken, removed from disposable syringes, or otherwise manipulated by hand. Never direct the point of a needle toward any part of your body; instead use a one-handed "scoop" technique or a device designed for holding the needle sheath.
- Place used disposable syringes and needles, scalpel blades, and all other used sharps in a puncture-resistant container that is located as close to the area of use as possible.
- Use barrier devices (eg, mouthpieces, resuscitation bags) as alternatives to mouth-to-mouth resuscitation.

(Based on information from "Guidelines for Isolation Precautions in Hospitals" developed by the Centers for Disease Control and Prevention [CDC] and the Hospital Infection Control Practices Advisory Committee [HICPAC], January 1996.)

Table 1-2 **Transmission-Based Precautions**

In addition to Standard Precautions, the following types of transmission-based precautions are to be used in specified situations.

Type	*Precautions*	*Indications and Illnesses*
Airborne precautions	• Place patient in a private room with negative airflow and appropriate ventilation. • Wear a mask when entering patient's room. • Have patient wear a mask during transport.	Use for infections that can be transmitted by airborne droplet nuclei (small particles). Examples: measles, varicella, tuberculosis
Droplet precautions	• Place patient in a private room or with another patient who has the same infection. • Wear a mask when working within 3 ft of patient. • Have patient wear mask during transport.	Use for infections that can be transmitted by droplets (large particles) during coughing, sneezing, or talking. Examples: *Haemophilus influenzae* disease, *Neisseria meningitidis* disease, streptococcal pharyngitis, mumps, rubella
Contact precautions	• Place patient in a private room or with another patient who has the same infection. • Wear gloves when entering patient's room and while providing care; change gloves after contact with infectious material. • Wear gown if clothing may have contact with patient or with infectious material.	Use for infections that can be transmitted by contact directly with patient or patient's items. Examples: multidrug-resistant infections, *Clostridium difficile, Shigella,* herpes simplex virus, impetigo, pediculosis, scabies

(Based on information from "Guidelines for Isolation Precautions in Hospitals" developed by the Centers for Disease Control and Prevention [CDC] and the Hospital Infection Control Practices Advisory Committee [HICPAC], January 1996.)

1

What If?
What if your patient is offended that you are wearing gloves when drawing blood?

Sometimes patients will become defensive and make statements to the effect that they are "disease free." If this happens, reassure the patient that wearing gloves is standard practice for all patient procedures in which there may be exposure to blood, body fluids, secretions, or excretions. Then explain that gloves are worn for the protection of the patient also. Use the occasion to educate the patient about Standard Precautions and the importance of following these guidelines.

Most transmission of infectious disease through the health care setting can be stopped by strict adherence to the Standard Precautions listed in Box 1-2. Although health care workers may take extraordinary precautions when dealing with a known carrier of disease, they may be unaware that they may treat as many as five carriers for each one they recognize as infectious or whose status is known. Therefore, Standard Precautions are mandatory for every encounter.

The prudent medical assistant understands that though visible blood or body fluid is an obvious source of infection, many diseases of concern are viable for long periods on surfaces that are not visibly contaminated.

OCCUPATIONAL SAFETY AND HEALTH ADMINISTRATION GUIDELINES FOR THE MEDICAL OFFICE

All areas of the medical office require a degree of infection control to protect staff and patients. Protective measures must be written outlining the infection control policy of each practice and incorporating the guidelines set by the Occupational Safety and Health Administration (OSHA). OSHA is a special governmental regulatory body created to oversee worker safety.

The facility's policies must be readily available to all employees, and infection control training must be part of the orientation to the site. The facility may adopt stronger policies than allowed by law, but may not set standards less strict than those mandated by OSHA. This may be part of the Policies and Procedures Manual or may be compiled and bound separately as an Infection Control Manual to be more readily available for review by either workers or OSHA representatives.

Exposure Risk Factors

Many facilities include the level of risk involved in each procedure commonly performed at the site either in the Infection Control Manual or in the Policies and Procedures Manual, with clear instructions for avoiding or reducing the danger of exposure to biohazardous materials. The exposure risk factor for each worker by job description also must be included in the

Patient Education
Basic Aseptic Technique

While performing procedures, take the opportunity to instruct your patients in basic aseptic techniques they can use at home.

- *Handwashing.* Performing this routine as part of daily hygiene is particularly important for patients who are immunosuppressed, very young or old, steroid dependent, or required to perform at-home dressing changes. Instruct patients that hands should be washed before and after eating meals; after sneezing, coughing, or nose blowing; after using the bathroom; before and after changing wound dressings; and before and after changing a child's diaper.
- *Tissue use.* Explain to patients with respiratory symptoms that using a disposable tissue to cover the mouth and nose when coughing or sneezing decreases the potential of transmitting the illness throughout the household. Immediately discard the tissue in a plastic-lined container.
- *Dressing changes.* Instruct patients regarding the differences between sterile dressings and clean bandages. Demonstrate the procedure and have patients return the demonstration to ensure comprehension.
- *Sanitation.* Explain to your patients the proper techniques for disposing of waste from members of the household with communicable diseases.

> *Box 1-3*
> **You Must Wear Gloves When . . .**
>
> - Performing any procedure that carries a high risk factor of exposure, such as minor office surgical procedures or venipuncture
> - Disposing of biohazardous waste, such as soiled dressings, test samples
> - Touching or handling surfaces that have contacted biohazardous material, such as laboratory surfaces, used surgical equipment
> - There is any chance, no matter how remote, of coming in contact with blood or body fluid

Policy Manual. For example, as the administrative assistant acting as receptionist, you would have a very low exposure risk and would require only minimal protection. However, you should be aware that patients might arrive with specimens that are not properly packaged for biohazardous protection. In such instances, exposure risk is high, and you should put on personal protective equipment (PPE), such as gloves, to receive the specimen. Other circumstances that require gloves are outlined in Box 1-3.

As the clinical assistant, you would be at frequent risk for exposure and require a full array of PPE (gloves, mask, goggles, face shield, impervious gown) in various combinations at different times depending on the practice (Fig. 1-2). If exposure occurs at any time, an incident report should be filed and a procedure established to prevent this type of exposure in the future. Box 1-4 describes biohazard and safety equipment in greater detail.

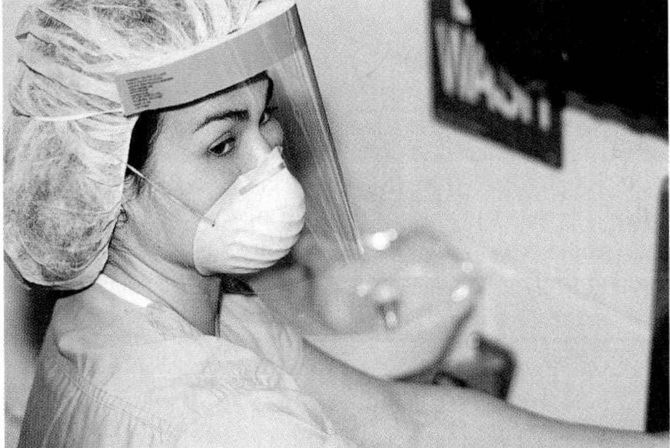

Figure 1-2 Personal protective equipment (PPE) includes a face shield and mask in situations that may result in splashes and splatters of blood or body fluids. An impervious gown also will be worn.

Personal Protective Equipment

In any area where exposure to biohazardous materials might occur, PPE must be available. For instance:

- Sharps containers for receiving items such as syringes and scalpel blades must be within easy reach of their areas of use.
- Biohazard bags must be placed near areas where soiled waste is generated.
- Gloves must be at strategic points throughout the office so employees can easily obtain them for use when receiving specimens or when assisting during procedures. Be aware that if the worker or the patient is sensitive to the latex in gloves, proper alternatives must be made available. Employers who do not make this equipment available are not in compliance with OSHA standards and may face significant fines.
- Gowns, goggles, and/or face shields must be at hand in areas where aerosolization (generation of airborne particles) or splatters may occur.

Hepatitis B Virus Immunization

Employers are responsible for ensuring that all employees have access to immunization for the hepatitis B virus, or HBV. Hepatitis B virus is spread through the health care profession by contact with infected blood or body fluid (Box 1-5). The virus may lead to cirrhosis (hardening of the liver) or severe liver dysfunction and has been associated closely with an increased risk for liver cancer. It is highly contagious and can live on inanimate objects and environmental surfaces (eg, pipettes, analyzers, counters) as a potentially infectious organism for up to a week.

The hepatitis B immunization is available in a three-dose series that is believed to offer immunity to the disease, though it is recommended that a titer be drawn at 6 months to determine if immunity has occurred. A titer detects the presence of antibodies (the body's protection against diseases to which it has been exposed) if the immune system has responded to the vaccine. The series will be repeated if no immunity is found. Employees must sign a waiver or release form stating that they are aware of the risks involved and accept those risks if they choose not to receive the vaccine.

Postexposure Policies

What if, despite using appropriate PPE, the medical assistant inadvertently sustains a stick from a contaminated sharp or experiences a splash of blood across mucous membranes? What is the procedure for assessing the risk of infection? The medical office must have a policy for postexposure follow-up.

Box 1-4
Biohazard and Safety Equipment in the Medical Setting

The items and supplies listed below are available in most health care settings. High-risk practices (eg, surgery, urgent care centers) have more varied equipment than relatively low-risk practices (eg, psychiatry, ophthalmology).

- *Biohazardous waste containers.* These properly marked, leak-proof containers have the biohazard label prominently displayed.

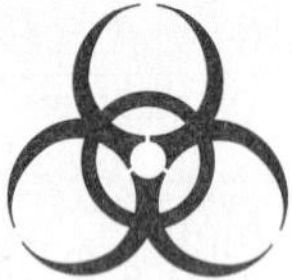

- *Sharps containers.* Puncture-proof containers are used for receiving syringes, needles, scalpel blades, and so forth.

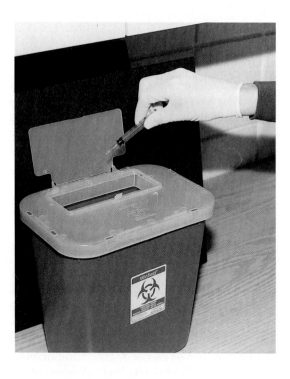

- *Latex gloves.* A suitable substitute must be made available if workers or patients are allergic to latex.
- *Safety eyewear.* Only goggles with protective side and top panels are appropriate; prescription glasses are not a substitute.
- *Mask.* Airborne contamination may require a face mask to avoid the risk of inhaled pathogens. Instructing or assisting a patient with a sputum specimen is an example of a high-risk procedure.
- *Face shield.* In the event of splash, spray, splatter, or aerosolization, goggles or a mask may not provide sufficient protection.
- *Impervious gown.* This protects the assistant's clothing from spray, splash, splatter, or aerosolization. A barrier gown prevents pathogens from migrating through to clothing or skin.
- *Fire extinguisher.* Many flammable chemicals are used and stored in the medical office, and an array of electrical equipment is available there. Every worker should be instructed in proper use of the extinguishers on premises. At least one worker, as designated in the Policies and Procedures Manual, should be responsible for ensuring that the extinguishers are serviced on schedule.
- *Eye wash station.* Facilities should have a means of flushing eyes in the event of splatters, splashes, or sprays that may contaminate unprotected eyes. In low-risk situations, a high arch faucet is sufficient; in high-risk situations, an eye wash basin is required.

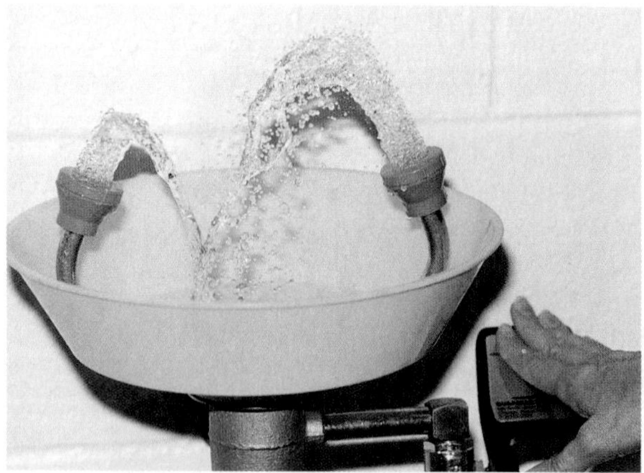

Eye wash basin. (**A**) Press the lever at the right of the basin. (**B**) The caps are forced from the water source by the stream. Lower your face and eyes into the stream and continue to wash the area until the eyes are clear.

If the exposure involved is HBV, an immediate titer level should be obtained to compare with repeat titers at intervals, usually 6 weeks, 3 months, 6 months, 9 months, and 1 year. This schedule may vary by local policy. If the worker has been immunized against HBV, usually no further treatment is required. If the worker waived the series, hepatitis B immunoglobulin (HBIG) is given for immediate, short-term protection, and the general series of standard immunization should be started. HBIG should protect the worker until the im-

Box 1-5
Focus on Hepatitis B Virus

One of our most persistent health care concerns is the transmission of hepatitis B virus, or HBV. Though HIV is the most visible public concern, HBV has been an occupational hazard for the health care profession for many years.

HBV is more viable than HIV, and may survive on laboratory equipment, clinical equipment, even pens and counter surfaces in a dried state at room temperature for as long as 1 week. It is passed through the medical setting usually by contact with contaminated hands, gloves, or other means of direct transmission. It is easily killed with a solution of 1:10 sodium hypochlorite (bleach). Its transmission is halted by proper use of Standard Precautions.

Just as HIV is passed through exposure to blood and blood-derived body fluid (serous and internal cavity fluid), HBV can be passed through the medical setting. In many instances, no parenteral inoculation or visible lesions are needed for its transmission; dry, cracked skin, dermatitis, eczema, psoriasis, and so forth will also allow its entrance into the body. Theoretically, aerosolization into the eyes or mouth may also result in transmission, though current documentation for this route of transmission is not conclusive.

Employers whose workers are at risk for HBV exposure are mandated by OSHA to provide the vaccine at no cost to the employee. The HBV vaccine follow-up has shown that immunity is consistent in as much as 85% to 90% of those immunized who also have healthy immune systems. Immunity may last as long as 9 to 10 years. Tests have shown that even if measurable antibodies decrease over time, a quick response to HBV exposure is initiated by the body. Even among those with few remaining antibodies at the time of exposure, none who were previously successfully immunized has developed the disease.

How can you protect yourself, your patient, and your coworkers? Strict adherence to Standard Precautions should stop the transmission.

- Wear PPE (eg, gloves, gowns, goggles, shields) if exposure can be reasonably anticipated.
- Wash your hands before and after each patient encounter.
- Clean the work environment with a 1:10 bleach solution made fresh daily, or use a specially prepared long-acting sodium hypochlorite agent. Low-level germicides do not work and may give a false sense of security.
- Maintain current training and continuing education for OSHA compliance.
- Label all biohazard waste and handle according to OSHA guidelines.

munization series can generate the immune system to respond to the disease.

The same schedule of evaluation is required after HIV exposure. At this time, no vaccine or treatment exists for HIV prevention, although studies are ongoing to test the efficacy of protease inhibitors and other current HIV treatments in preventing postexposure transmission.

Material Safety Data Sheet

Other medical office safety measures include information provided by manufacturers of chemicals and other hazardous materials. These manufacturers are required by law to help protect worker safety by supplying a material safety data sheet (MSDS) for each item used on site. These should be bound and stored near the site of use and should be reviewed by all workers in the office. Information listed on a MSDS includes:

- The product name and identification by generic or trade name
- Hazardous components
- The potential health danger of the substance
- The potential for flammability or explosion
- Spill or disposal procedures
- Recommended or required PPE
- Storage and handling guidelines

(MSDS is discussed in greater detail in Chap. 26, Introduction to the Clinical Laboratory.)

Employee Training Requirements

Employers whose workers are at special risk, such as those employed in medical offices, must follow specific OSHA mandates for employee training. Training must be made available, either in the form of qualified inservice or off-site continuing education, to reinforce and maintain current infection control and safety measures or to update skills to reflect new information. The qualifications of the trainer must be recorded, and records of the training must be retained in the participating employees' folders for 3 years. Records retained by the practice must include the training dates, summaries of the course content, name(s) and qualifications of the trainer(s), and the names and job titles of all employees who successfully completed the program. See Box 1-6 for more information on employee infection control training.

As a medical assistant, you are responsible for using the protective information and equipment provided by the workplace. No level of training or protec-

1

Box 1-6
Employee Infection Control Training

OSHA requires that *all* employees receive training by qualified persons in the proper use of PPE and other methods to avoid the hazards of infectious materials. Training may be conducted by the physician, by a consultant hired to train employees on-site, or by an off-site continuing education instructor.

The trainer must be qualified to present the information by virtue of completion of special courses or through documented, appropriate work experience. Trainers can include hospital infection control officers, registered nurses, nurse practitioners, or physician's assistants with additional training in infection control.

The materials and methods used for instruction must be appropriate for the level of employee and must allow time for interactive questions and answers. Following an initial training period, refresher courses must be provided and documented annually or more often when changes in procedures are initiated.

Training must include:

- An introduction to OSHA's standards. The contents must be available for study by employees.
- An explanation of blood-borne diseases and their methods of transmission
- An overview of the employer's exposure control plan and where the plan is kept for review
- An assessment of procedures that place the worker at risk and ways to avoid exposure
- A demonstration of proper use of PPE, safe work practices (eg, single-handed needle capping), and safety mechanisms (eg, eye wash stations). A discussion of when to use these safety mechanisms and their limitations must also be included.
- An explanation of signs, labels, and color coding for biohazard disposal
- A demonstration of proper biohazardous waste disposal and an explanation of local disposal guidelines
- Updated information on HBV and HIV statistics, transmission, prevention, and treatments
- Procedures to reduce the risk of transmission in an emergency situation
- Postexposure procedures and protocol
- A question-and-answer period

tion is effective when used incorrectly. Performing venipuncture without gloves, transporting used sharps great distances, handling soiled dressings improperly, and other unsafe practices put the medical assistant, the patient, and all involved in grave danger. Remember: Any pathogen transmitted may also be carried home to family members and to other persons in contact with the worker or patient.

INFECTION CONTROL

Maintaining effective infection control in the medical office will require knowledge of varying levels of sanitation and disinfection. Not all equipment needs to be sterile, but all equipment must be clean. To ensure the effectiveness of any sterilization or disinfection process, equipment and instruments must first be thoroughly cleaned or sanitized of all visible soil.

Levels of Infection Control

Sterilization

Sterilization is the highest level of infection control and destroys all forms of microorganisms, including most forms of bacterial spores. Sterilization methods include steam under pressure (autoclave), gas (ethylene oxide), dry heat, or immersion in an Environmental Protection Agency (EPA)–approved chemical sterilant for a prescribed period of time. Sterilization is used for instruments or devices that penetrate the skin or contact normally sterile areas of the body (eg, scalpels, needles, catheters). Disposable invasive equipment eliminates the need to reprocess these items and reduces the chance of cross-infections. (See Chap. 5, Instruments and Equipment, for the procedure for autoclaving.)

High-Level Disinfection

High-level disinfection is slightly less effective than sterilization, destroying all forms of microbial life except high numbers of spores. Methods of high-level disinfection are hot water pasteurization using 80° to 100°C for 30 minutes, or exposure to an EPA–approved disinfecting chemical for a shorter exposure time, such as 10 to 45 minutes. High-level disinfection is required for reusable instruments that come in contact with mucous membrane-lined body cavities that are not considered to be sterile. Such instruments include laryngoscopes or endotracheal tubes.

Intermediate-Level Disinfection

Although intermediate-level disinfection destroys *Mycobacterium tuberculosis*, vegetative bacteria, most viruses, and most fungi, it does not kill bacterial spores. Methods of intermediate-level disinfection are

EPA-approved chemical germicides with tuberculocidal properties or hard-surface germicides or solutions containing a 1:10 dilution of common household bleach (approximately ¼ cup of bleach per quart of tap water). Intermediate-level disinfection is used for surfaces that come in contact only with intact skin (eg, stethoscopes, blood pressure cuffs, splints) and have been visibly contaminated with blood or body fluids. Surfaces must be precleaned to remove contaminants before the germicidal chemical is applied for disinfection.

Low-Level Disinfection

Most bacteria and some viruses and fungi are destroyed by low-level disinfection, but *M. tuberculosis* or bacterial spores are not. Methods of low-level disinfection are EPA-approved disinfectants with no tuberculocidal properties. Low-level disinfection is used for routine cleaning or removing surface debris in the absence of visible blood or body fluid contamination.

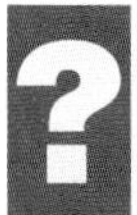

Checkpoint Question

4. *How does high-level disinfection differ from low-level disinfection?*

Handling Environmental Contamination

Any cleaner or disinfectant agent intended for environmental use can be used to clean and disinfect environmental surfaces that have become soiled. These surfaces include floors, woodwork, countertops, and so on.

Cleaning and Decontaminating Biohazardous Spills

All spills of biohazardous materials should be promptly cleaned using an EPA-approved germicide or a 1:10 solution of household bleach in the appropriate manner.

1. Put on gloves. Wear protective eyewear and an impervious apron or gown if you anticipate that splashing may occur.
2. Remove visible contaminants with disposable towels or other means that will prevent contact with the fluid.
3. Dispose of the cleaning material and contaminants in a biohazard container.
4. Decontaminate the area with an appropriate germicide, and discard the material used for wiping up the area in an appropriate biohazard container.
5. Wash your hands after removing and discarding the gloves.
6. Place soiled items in the biohazard container, and dispose of them according to facility policy. Plastic bags should be available for removing contaminated items from the site of the spill.

Note: Your shoes can become contaminated with biohazardous material as well. Where there is massive contamination on floors, the use of disposable impervious shoe coverings should be considered. Protective gloves should be worn to remove contaminated shoe coverings. The coverings and gloves should be disposed of in the biohazard containers.

Handling Soiled Linens

Although soiled linen may be contaminated with pathogenic microorganisms, the risk of actual disease transmission is small. Rather than using rigid procedures and specifications, hygienic storage and processing of clean and soiled linen are recommended. Handle soiled linen as little as possible and with minimum agitation to prevent contamination of the air and the persons handling the linen. All soiled linen should be bagged at the location where it was used. Linen soiled with biohazardous material should be placed and transported in impervious bags. Normal laundry cycles should be used according to the washer's and detergent's recommendations.

Decontaminating and Laundering Protective Clothing

Protective clothing contaminated with blood or body fluids to which Standard Precautions apply should be placed and transported in impervious bags. Anyone involved in bagging, transporting, and laundering contaminated clothing should wear gloves.

Disposing of Infectious Waste

Federal regulations on infectious waste disposal are determined at the national level by the EPA and OSHA. These agencies set the national regulatory policies and guidelines for hazardous material but require individual states to decide on specific points affecting local disposal policies. These policies vary widely and should be consulted before disposal decisions are made.

Most medical offices are considered to be small generators of waste; they generate less than 50 lb of waste per month. Hospitals and large clinics with more than 50 lb of waste per month are large generators. Large generators must obtain a certificate of registration from the EPA to maintain a record of the quantity and disposal of the waste tracked from these sources.

Box 1-7
Proper Waste Disposal

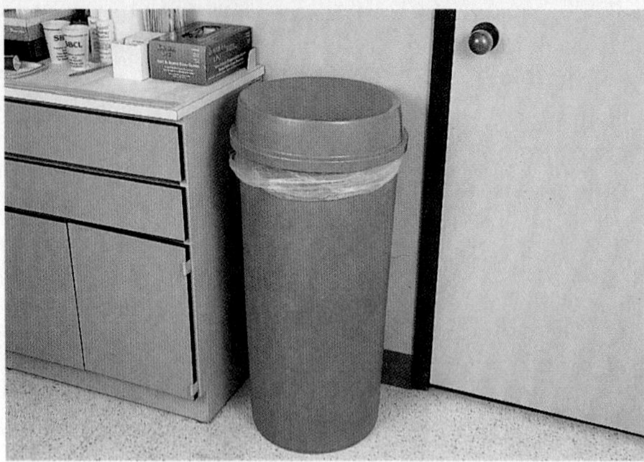

Regular waste container.

A regular waste container should be used only for disposal of "clean" waste material, such as paper, plastic, disposable tray wrapper, suture, unused gauze, or examining table paper liner. Small amounts of fluids, such as that poured off prior to adding a sterile solution to a sterile set-up, may also be disposed of here. To prevent leakage, large amounts of uncontaminated fluid should be discarded in the wash basin, not in plastic bags. NEVER discard sharps of any kind in plastic bags; these are not puncture resistant, and injury may result even from careful handling. Bags should not be filled to capacity. When the plastic bag is about two thirds full, it should be removed from its holder, the top edges brought together and secured with a twist tie. Remove the bag from the examining room and follow office procedure for disposal.

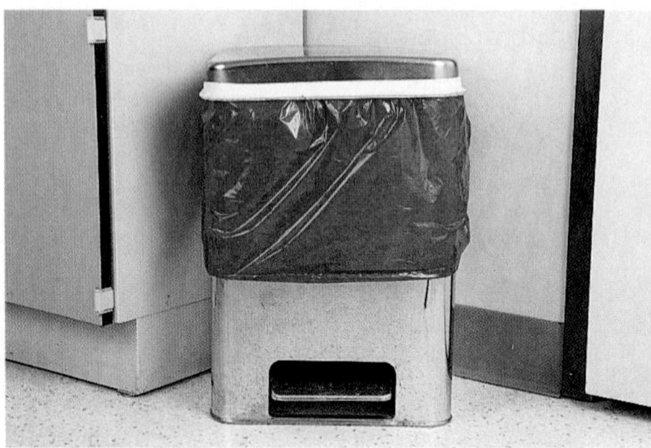

Biohazard waste container.

A biohazard waste container is reserved for the disposal of contaminated waste only. Such waste includes soiled dressings and bandages, soiled examining table paper, cotton balls, swabs, applicators, alcohol swabs, and gloves that have become soiled with, or exposed to, blood or body fluids. Other items that should be discarded in this type of container are used catheters or drains, wound packing, sutures without needles, soiled tampons and sanitary napkins, diapers, ostomy bags, and any other object contaminated with blood or body fluids of any sort.

Most large generators transfer the burden of disposal to an infectious waste service.

Medical offices that generate less than 50 lb per month may also find it more efficient to rely on an infectious waste service. These services supply the office with appropriate hazardous waste containers, such as puncture-proof biohazard bags and sharps containers. They drop off replacements and pick up filled containers on a predetermined schedule, then dispose of the material according to EPA guidelines for each state.

The service maintains a tracking record listing the type of waste, the poundage, and its disposal destination. Both the service representative and the office manager sign for the shipment as it leaves the office. When the items have been processed or destroyed, the office receives a tracking form documenting the disposal; this form must be retained in office records for 3 years and may be audited by the EPA to assess compliance with local guidelines. States impose stiff penalties for noncompliance that may include fines or imprisonment for deliberate violations of regulations.

Because the infectious waste service bases its fee on the type and amount of waste generated, medical office staff should follow the guidelines listed below to help contain costs while maintaining safety.

- Use separate containers for each type of waste. For instance, do not dispose of bandages in sharps containers; do not dispose of paper towels used for handwashing or general low-level disinfection in a biohazard bag (Box 1-7).
- Use only approved biohazard containers supplied by your waste service.
- If you must move a container (bag or sharps) for any distance or store it for pick up, secure the top by an approved closure designed for that specific container. Do not move open containers for any distance.
- When you must move a container, wear PPE appropriate for the situation.
- If the container is contaminated on the outside, secure it within another approved container marked with the appropriate biohazard logo.
- Have a secured, designated area in which to store containers awaiting pick up by the service.

Checkpoint Question

5. *What should you use to clean biohazardous spills?*

MEDICAL ASEPSIS

Medical asepsis, commonly referred to as "clean technique," means an object or area is free from infection. It requires destroying organisms after they have left the body. There will still be nonpathogens present on a clean or medically aseptic substance or surface, but pathogens have been eliminated. Medical asepsis prevents the transmission of microorganisms from one person or area to any other within the health care setting.

MAINTAINING MEDICAL ASEPSIS

Handwashing is the MOST IMPORTANT medical aseptic practice and is crucial in preventing microorganism transmission in the medical office. Hands must be washed frequently using proper technique (Procedure 1-1). For example, handwashing must be performed:

- Before and after patient contact
- Before putting on gloves
- After removing gloves
- After contact with any blood or body fluid
- After contact with contaminated material
- After handling specimens
- After coughing, sneezing, or blowing the nose
- After using the restroom

It is your responsibility to practice medical aseptic techniques in the office (Box 1-8). Patients and their families must be taught the proper medical aseptic techniques to use in the home, such as proper handwashing and proper disposal of contaminated

Box 1-8

Guidelines for Maintaining Medical Asepsis

1. Avoid touching clothing with soiled linen or instruments. Both should be held above waist level and away from the body and be kept in view at all times. Roll used linen or table paper inward with the clean surface outward. Do not allow used supplies or equipment to touch clothing.
2. Always consider the floor to be contaminated. Any item dropped must be discarded or recleaned to its former level of asepsis.
3. Clean areas immediately. Areas kept clean are less likely to harbor microorganisms or encourage their growth.
4. Always presume that blood and body fluids are contaminated. Follow guidelines published by OSHA and CDC to protect yourself and to prevent transmission of disease.

1

articles or dressings to prevent the spread of disease through the family or community. Patient education frequently will be your responsibility, so you will need to instruct and observe the patient or caregiver in proper procedures to reduce the transmission of disease.

SURGICAL ASEPSIS

The principle of **surgical asepsis** is to free an item or area from all microorganisms, both pathogens and nonpathogens (Table 1-3). The practice of surgical asepsis, also known as "sterile technique," should be used when entering any part of the body that is normally sterile. Examples include maintaining a sterile field for office surgery, handling sterile instruments to be used for incisions and excisions, or changing dressings over surgical or accidental wounds. (See Chap. 6, Assisting With Minor Office Surgery, for more information.)

Surgical asepsis prevents microorganisms from entering the patient's environment whereas medical asepsis prevents them from leaving the patient to spread to others.

You should use the principles of sterile technique when preparing for, setting up, and assisting with any surgical procedure in the medical office. This includes anything as simple and quick as ear piercing to a more lengthy and complex removal of a lesion.

The physician trusts you to use sterile technique when you set up a sterile field. If the sterile field has been contaminated by contact with an unsterile object, steps must be taken to restore sterility. The physician also expects you to be knowledgeable of sterile technique and to be able to maintain sterility throughout the procedure. Any break in sterile technique, no matter how small, can lead to infections the body cannot fight. Even mild infections delay recovery and are physically, emotionally, and financially costly to the patient.

Checkpoint Question

6. *What is surgical asepsis and when should you use it?*

SURGICAL SCRUB

If you are required to assist the physician in the performance of a procedure, it will be necessary to scrub before putting on sterile gloves (Procedures 1-2 and 1-3). It is not possible to sterilize the hands, but washing in the appropriate manner will eliminate the greatest number of pathogens possible.

After assisting with a procedure that involves blood and body fluid, as all surgical procedures will, your gloves will be more contaminated than your hands. Care must be taken to avoid contaminating the hands when removing the gloves (Procedure 1-4).

text continues on page 25

Table 1-3 **Comparing Medical and Surgical Asepsis**

	Medical Asepsis	*Surgical Asepsis*
Definition	Destroys microorganisms after they leave the body	Destroys microorganisms before they enter the body
Purpose	Prevents the transmission of microorganisms from one person to another	Maintains sterility when entering a normally sterile part of the body
When used	Used when coming in contact with a body part that is not normally sterile (eg, when performing an enema)	Used when entering a normally sterile part of the body (eg, when performing urinary catheterization)
Differences in handwashing technique	Hands and wrists are washed for 1–2 min; brush is not necessary. Hands are held down to rinse so water runs off fingertips. Paper towel is used for drying.	Hands and forearms are washed for 5–10 min; brush is used for hands, arms, and nails. Hands are held up to rinse so water runs off elbows. Sterile towel is used for drying.

1

Procedure 1-1 Handwashing for Medical Asepsis

PURPOSE:

To prevent the growth and spread of pathogens from one person to another or to instruments and equipment

EQUIPMENT

- liquid soap
- paper towels
- orangewood stick or nail instrument

STEPS

1. Remove all rings and wrist watch (or move watch above the wrist several inches).
   Rings may harbor pathogens that may not be washed away. Raising the watch protects it from water damage.
2. Stand close to but not touching the sink.
   Standing close makes it easier to perform a proper handwash without splashing, but the sink is considered contaminated, and standing too close may contaminate your clothing.
3. Turn on the faucet using a paper towel. Discard the towel. *Note:* Some facilities have faucets with knee controls, rather than hand controls. Water force is controlled by a back and forth motion and water temperature is controlled by an up and down motion. Knee controls are preferred over hand controls for surgical scrubs but may not be available in many office settings.
   The faucets are considered to be contaminated and the towel cannot be used again.
4. Wet hands and wrists under running warm water and apply liquid antibacterial soap.
   Water too warm or too cool will cause the hands to chap and crack, providing a break in the protective barriers of the hands. Antibacterial soaps help lower the number of pathogens.

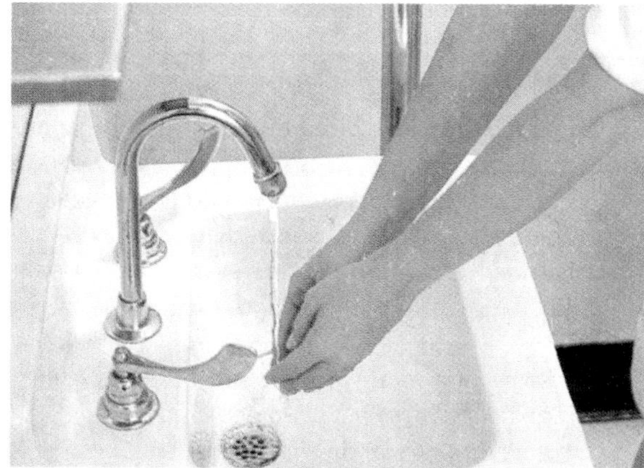

5. Work soap into a lather by rubbing the palms of the hands together, then intertwine the fingers of both hands and rub the soap between the fingers at least 10 times.
   This motion dislodges microorganisms from between the fingers and removes transient and some resident organisms.

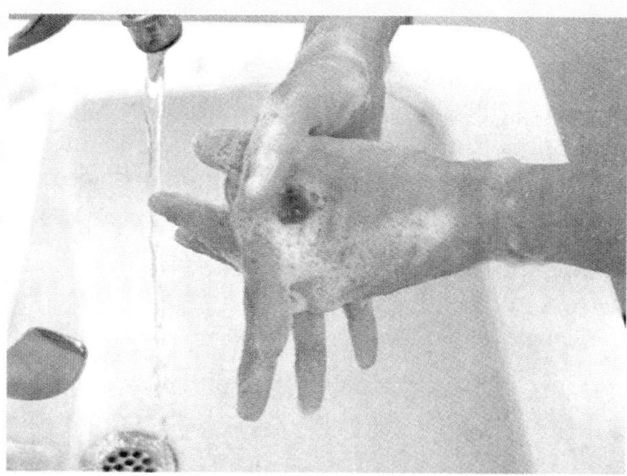

6. Scrub the palm of one hand with the fingertips of the other hand to work the soap under the nails of that hand then reverse the procedure and scrub the other hand. Scrub the wrists.
   Friction helps remove microorganisms.
7. Use an orangewood stick under the nails.
   Nails may harbor microorganisms. Metal files or pointed instruments may break the skin and cause an opening for bacteria.
8. Holding the hands in a downward position, rinse the soap from both hands, allowing the water to drip off the fingertips. Rinse well.
   Hands held lower will allow microorganisms to flow off the hands and fingers rather than back up the arms.

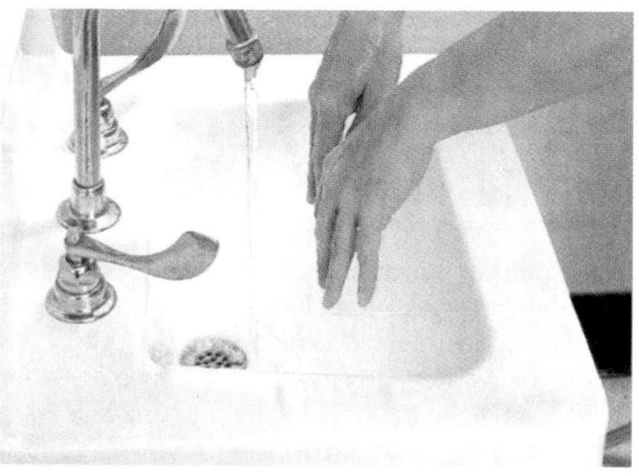

continued

1

Procedure 1-1 Continued Handwashing for Medical Asepsis

9. If hands are grossly contaminated, repeat the procedure.
10. Dry the wrists and hands gently with a paper towel and discard the towel.
    Hands must be dried completely to prevent drying and cracking. The paper is wet now and may wick contaminants back onto the clean hands.
11. Use a dry paper towel to turn off the faucets and discard the towel.
    Hands are now clean and should not touch the contaminated handles.
12. If the sink is splattered, wipe with a clean dry paper towel to reduce available moisture for pathogens and to remove as many as possible. Discard the paper towel.

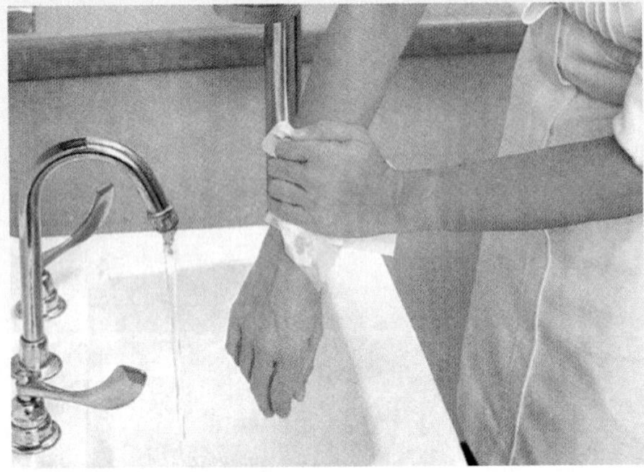

Note: This procedure should take 1–2 minutes.

Procedure 1-2 Performing a Surgical Scrub

PURPOSE

To prevent the spread of microorganisms into an area that requires a sterile or pathogen-free environment

EQUIPMENT

- paper towel
- brush
- sterile towel
- liquid bacterial soap
- orangewood stick or nail instrument

STEPS

1. Remove all jewelry.
   Jewelry may harbor microorganisms and is never worn during a sterile procedure.
2. Stand close to but not touching the sink.
   Standing close makes it easier to perform a proper handwash without splashing, but the sink is considered contaminated, and standing too close may contaminate your clothing.
3. Turn on the faucet using a paper towel. Discard the paper towel. *Note:* Some facilities have sinks equipped with knee controls rather than hand controls. Water force is controlled by a back and forth movement, temperature is controlled by an up and down movement. Knee controls are preferred for surgical scrubs but may not be available in many office settings.
   The faucets are considered to be contaminated and the towel cannot be used again.
4. Wet hands by allowing warm water to flow over them to wet completely. Keep hands above waist level.
   Warm water removes more microorganisms than cold but will not chap and crack hands as hot water will. Hands should not be allowed to drop below waist level during a surgical scrub to prevent moisture from the less clean area returning to the washed area.

continued

Procedure 1-2 Continued Performing a Surgical Scrub

5. Apply liquid bactericidal soap and work into a lather; intertwine the fingers and work the soap between the fingers and around the nails.
   Intertwining cleans surfaces between the fingers; soaping the nails dislodges particles.

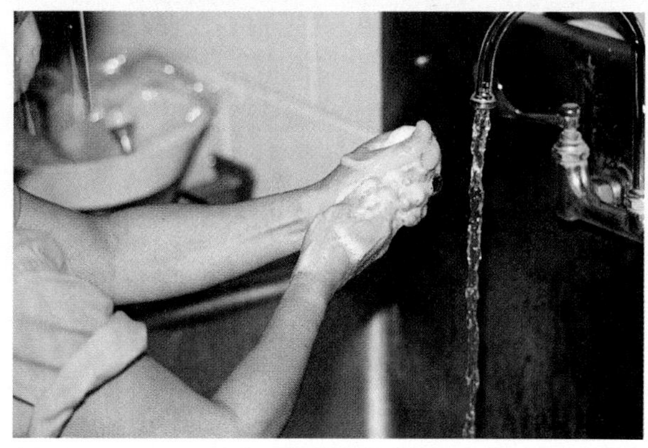

6. Using a surgical scrub brush, scrub the nails, backs, and palms of the hands and wrists and forearms.
   A brush helps dislodge and remove the maximum number of microorganisms.

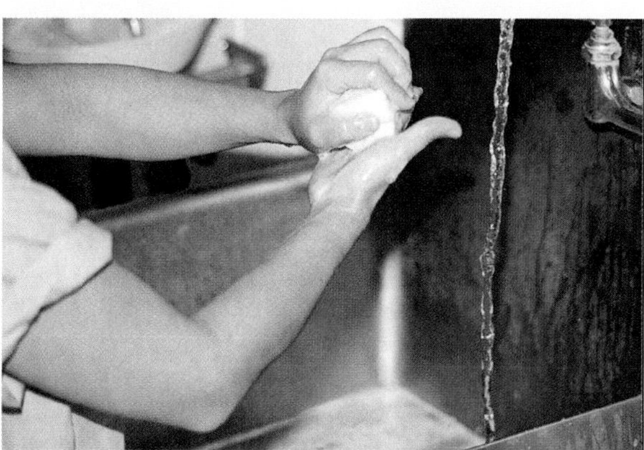

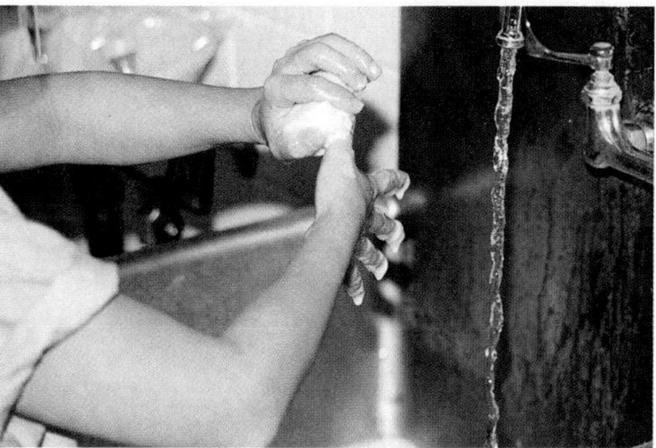

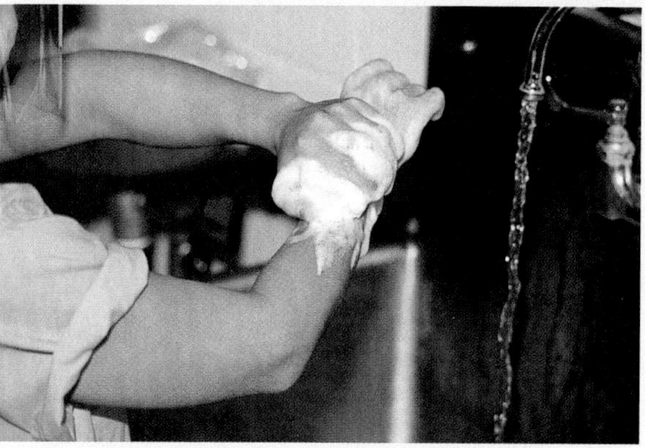

7. Using an orangewood stick or nail instrument, clean under each nail.
   Nails harbor microorganisms that must be removed by an instrument that is not likely to injure the integumentary system.

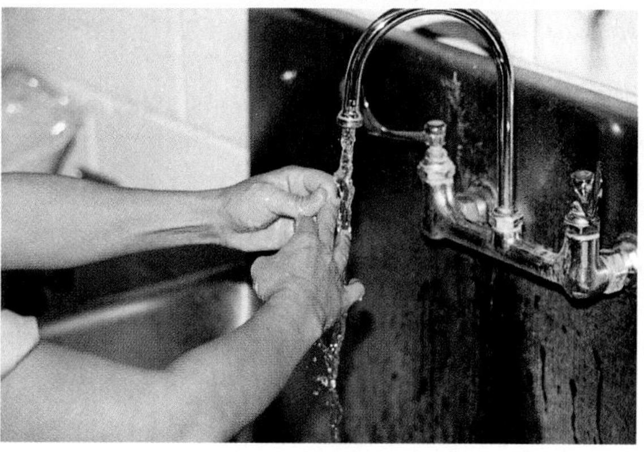

continued

1

Procedure 1-2 Continued Performing a Surgical Scrub

8. Rinse thoroughly.
a. Rinse from the fingertips to the forearms.

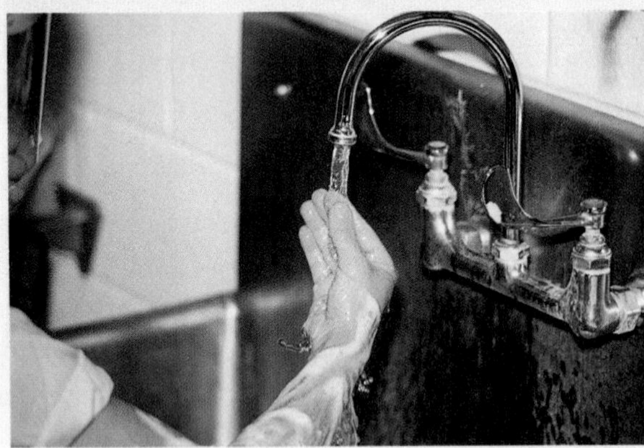

b. Keep the hands higher than the elbows so that water runs down the arms rather than off of the fingertips.
Water running back over the hands will return microorganisms to the cleaned hands.

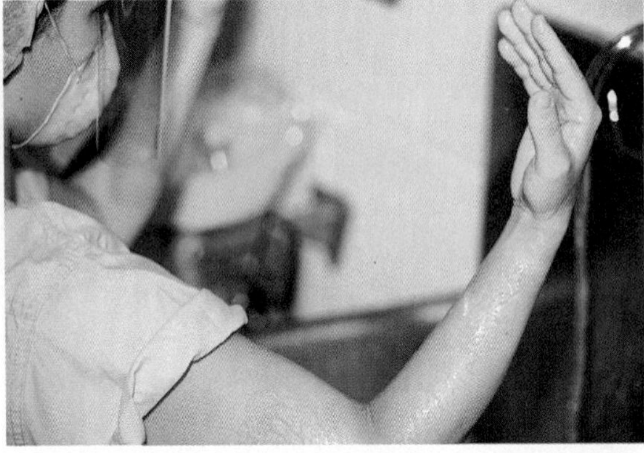

9. Dry from the hands to the forearms with a sterile towel.
Drying in this fashion prevents returning microorganisms to the cleaned hands.

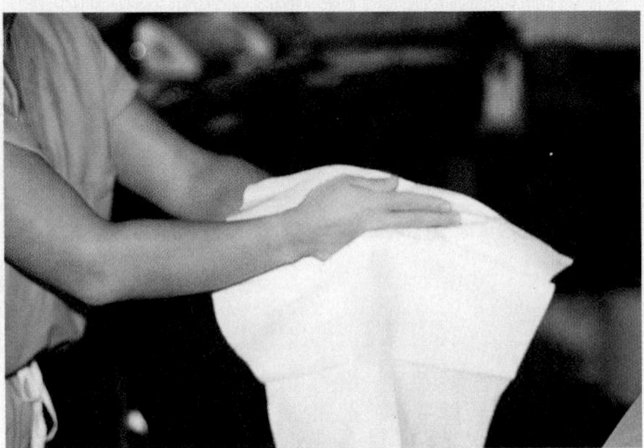

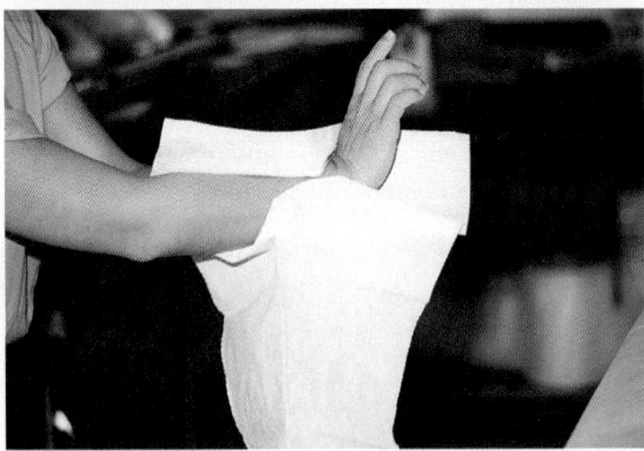

10. Turn off the faucet with the knee controls or with the forearm, or by using a dry, sterile towel.
The contaminated faucets are not to be touched by the clean hands.

Note: This procedure should take 5–10 minutes.

1

Procedure 1-3 Sterile Gloving

PURPOSE

To provide and maintain a sterile field for procedures that require an absence of pathogenic microorganisms

EQUIPMENT

- One packet of properly sized sterile gloves

STEPS

1. Remove rings and other jewelry.

Rings may pierce the gloves and contaminate the procedure.

2. Wash hands.

Gloving is not a substitute for handwashing but must be done in addition to handwashing.

3. Place the prepackaged gloves on a clean, dry, flat surface with the cuffed end toward you.

a. Pull the outer wrapping apart to expose the sterile inner wrap.

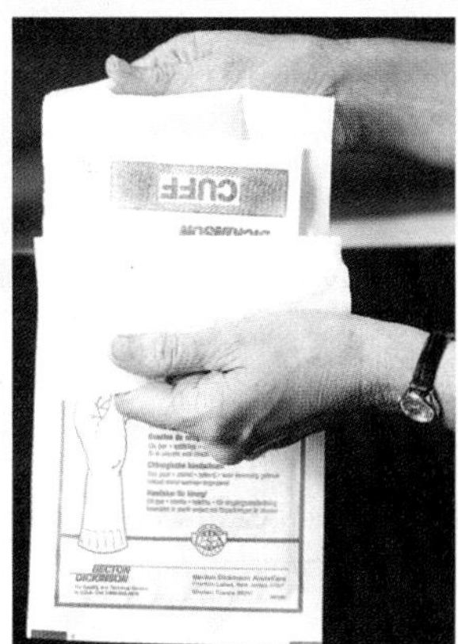

b. With the cuffs toward you, fold back the inner wrap to expose the gloves.

Gloves are packaged for ease of application in this fashion.

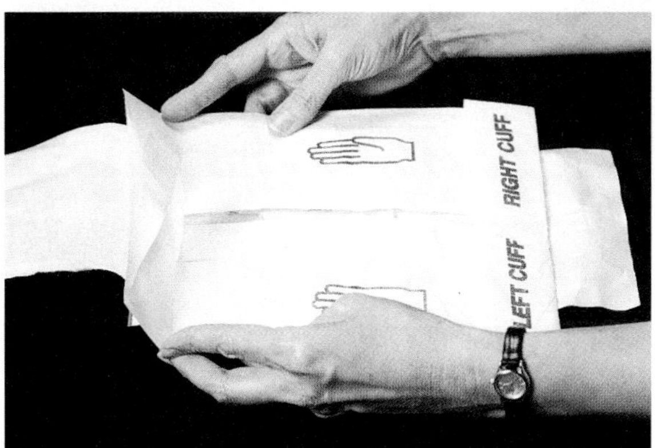

4. Grasping the edges of the outer paper, open the package out to its fullest.

The inner surface of the package is now a sterile field.

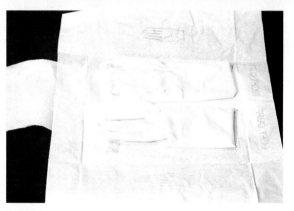

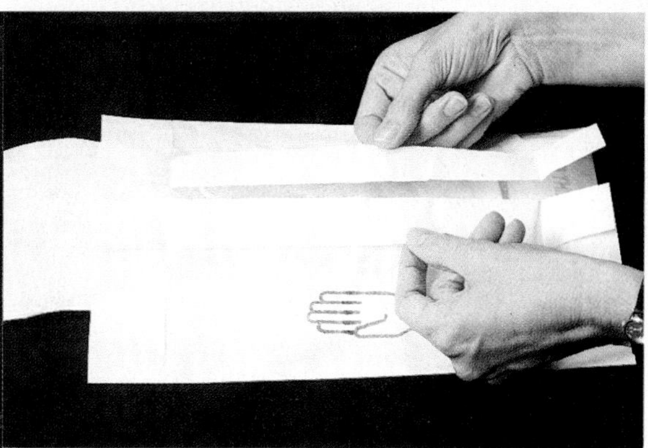

continued

1

Procedure 1-3 Continued Sterile Gloving

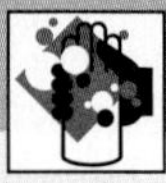

5. Using your nondominant hand, pick up the dominant hand glove by grasping the folded edge of the cuff, lifting it up and away from the paper. The folded edge of the cuff is contaminated as soon as it is touched with the ungloved hand. Be very careful not to touch the outside surface of the sterile glove with your ungloved hand.

   Lift it up and away to avoid letting the fingers of the glove brush an unsterile surface.

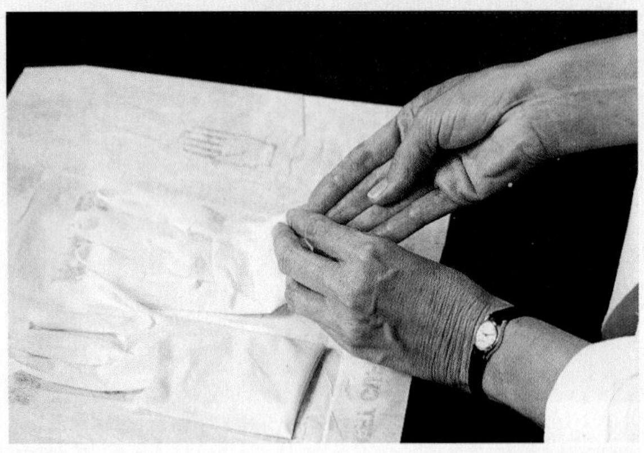

6. Curl the fingers and thumb together to insert them into the glove. Then straighten the fingers and pull the glove on with the nondominant hand still grasping the cuff.

   This prevents accidental touching of the outside surface of the glove.

7. Unfold the cuff by pinching the inside surface that will be against the wrist and pulling it toward the wrist.

   This ensures that only the unsterile portions are touched by the hands.

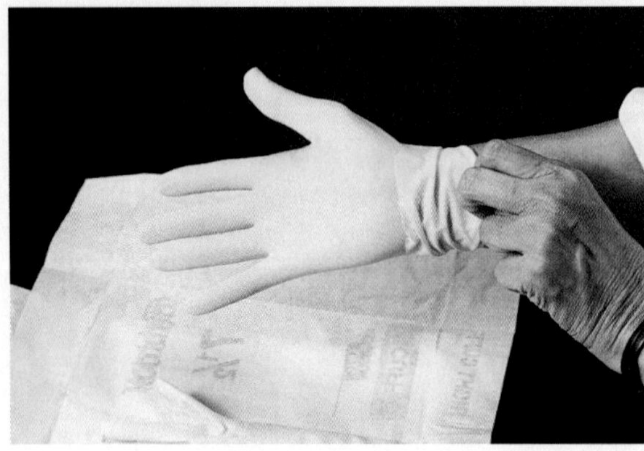

8. Place the fingers of the gloved hand under the cuff of the remaining glove, lift the glove up and away from the wrapper, and slide the ungloved hand carefully into the glove with the fingers and thumb curled together.

   This avoids letting the sterile glove accidentally touch an unsterile surface and ensures that the fingers will not brush the sterile surface of the glove.

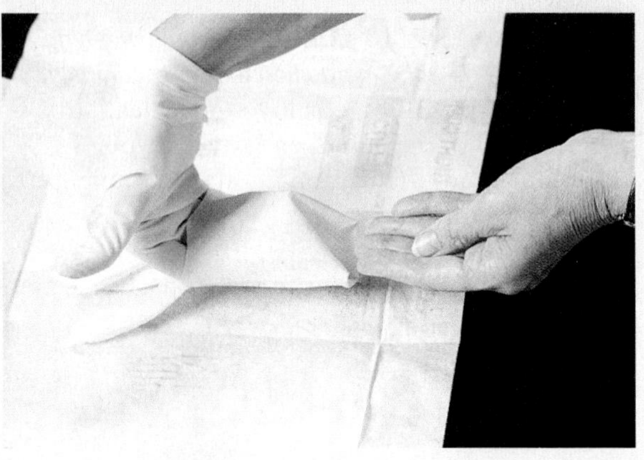

9. Straighten the fingers and pull the glove up and over the wrist by carefully unfolding the cuff.

   At all times, sterile must touch sterile only. Folding the cuffs out to their fullest allows the greatest area of sterility.

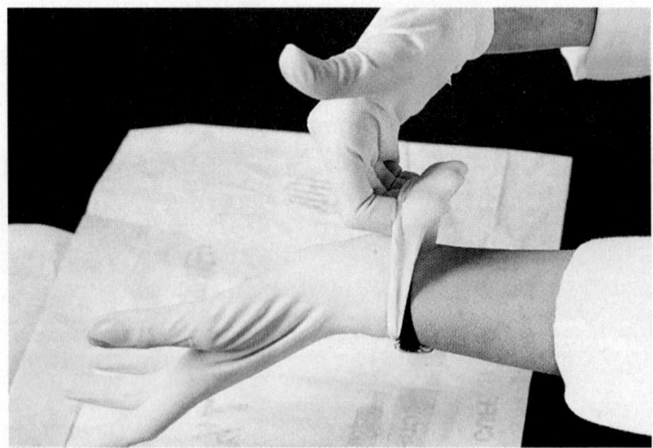

continued

Procedure 1-3 Continued Sterile Gloving

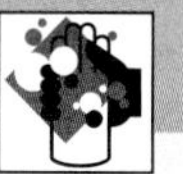

10. Settle the gloves comfortably onto the fingers by lacing the fingers together and adjusting the tension over the hands.
    The gloves should fit snugly without wrinkles or areas that bind the fingers.

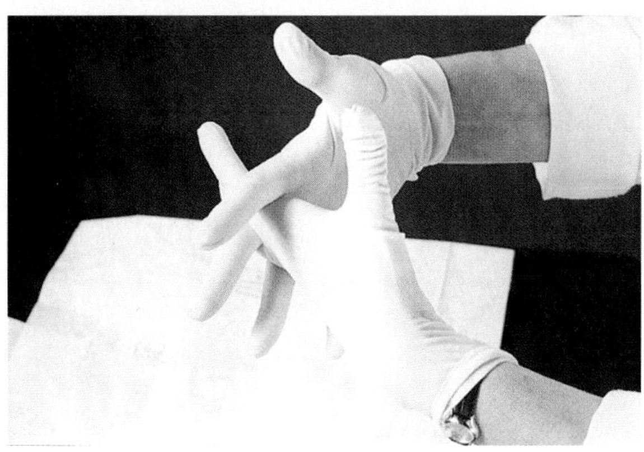

Procedure 1-4 Removing Gloves After a Procedure

PURPOSE

To prevent the spread of pathogenic microorganisms in the medical setting

EQUIPMENT

- biohazard disposal container

STEPS

1. With the gloved dominant hand, grasp the area of glove over the wrist or at the palm of the nondominant hand and pull it away from the hand.
   This avoids touching soiled glove to clean hand.

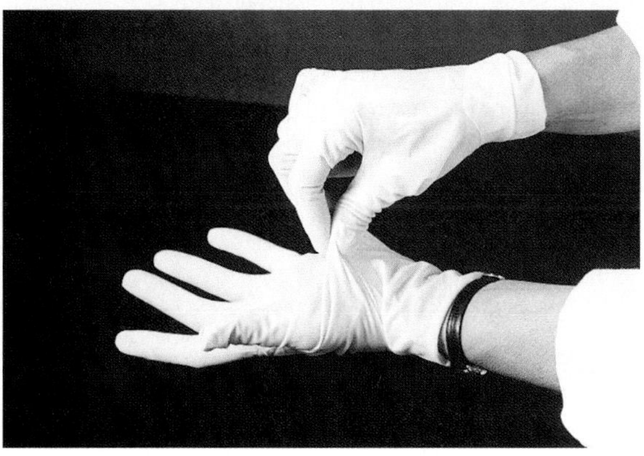

2. Stretch this soiled glove down over the fingers by pulling it away with the gloved hand.
   This frees the hand without touching the soiled surface.

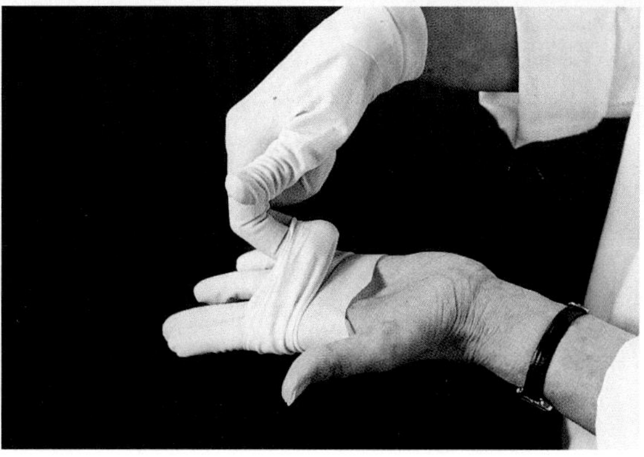

continued

1

Procedure 1-4 Continued **Removing Gloves After a Procedure**

3. As you pull the glove from the hand, ball it into the palm of the still gloved hand.

Balling it into a small area prevents the fingers of the glove from accidentally brushing a clean area.

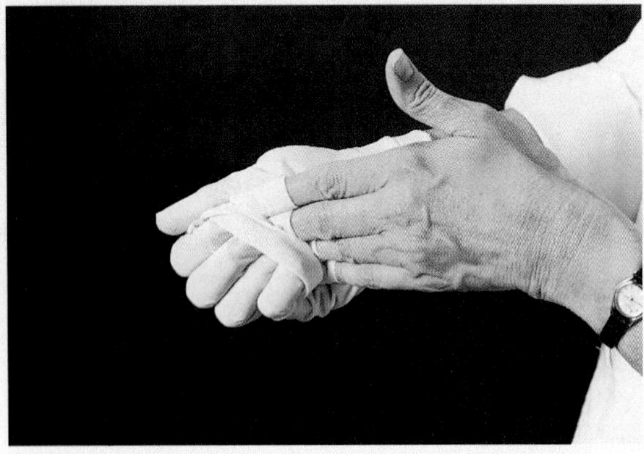

4. Holding the soiled glove in the palm of the gloved hand, slip the ungloved fingers under the cuff of the gloved hand against the skin, being careful not to touch the soiled outside of the glove.

This ensures that skin touches skin, with no opportunity to touch the soiled area of the glove.

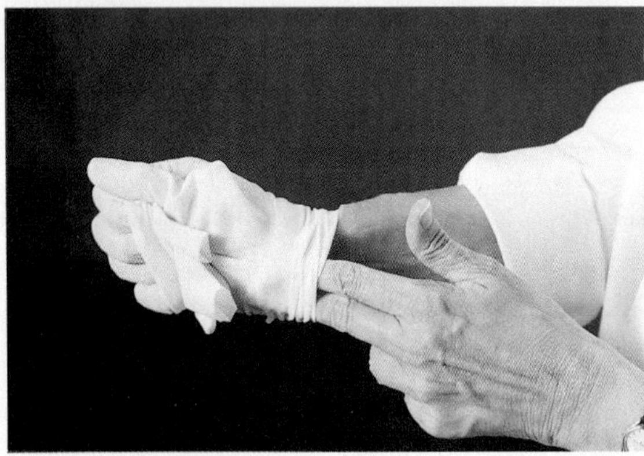

5. Stretch the glove up and away from the hand, and turn it inside out as it is pulled off over the first glove.

Turning it inside out exposes only clean surfaces. Soiled surfaces will be enclosed within.

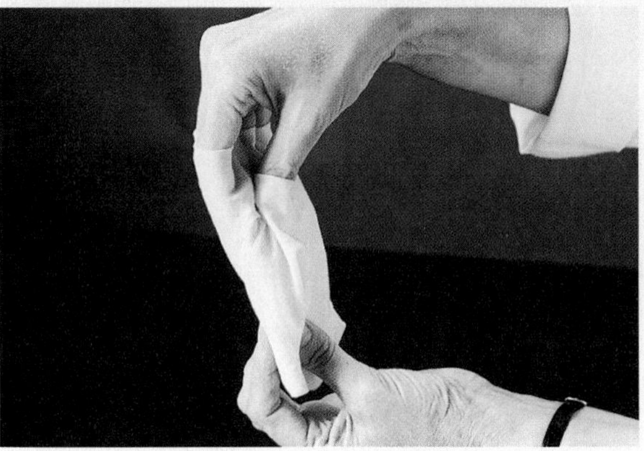

6. Both gloves should now be off with the first inside the palm of the last glove to be removed and the last glove should be inside out.

This reduces the chance of accidental contamination.

7. Discard in a biohazard waste receptacle.

If the gloves are contaminated with blood and body fluid, they are a potential source of infection by blood-borne pathogens.

8. Wash your hands well.

Gloving is not a substitute for handwashing.

Note: *This procedure is also used for removing nonsterile treatment gloves.*

Answers to Checkpoint Questions

1. *Normal flora are organisms normally found in a particular area of the body. Their presence triggers the immune system to build and release antibodies to defend against pathogens.*
2. *The six conditions that favor the growth of pathogens include moisture, nutrients, temperature, darkness, neutral to slightly alkaline pH, and oxygen.*
3. *The first link in the infection cycle, the reservoir host, provides nutrients and an incubation site for the pathogen. The fifth link, the susceptible host, allows the pathogen easy entrance and permits it to grow and multiply and thus becomes a new reservoir host, repeating the cycle.*
4. *High-level disinfection destroys all forms of bacterial life except high numbers of spores. Low-level disinfection destroys most bacteria and only some viruses and fungi.*
5. *Use an EPA-approved germicide or a 1:10 solution of household bleach to clean all biohazardous spills promptly.*
6. *Surgical asepsis, also known as sterile technique, means that an item or area is free from both pathogens and nonpathogens. It is used whenever entering any part of the body that is normally sterile.*

Critical Thinking Challenges

1. Review Table 1-1 on common communicable diseases. Compare the various modes of transmission, then create a patient education booklet that focuses on preventing the spread of these diseases.
2. Identify the conditions that favor the growth of pathogens, then formulate a list of ways to control each of these factors.
3. Your patient has a leg wound that must be cared for at home. He says he knows what to do, but you suspect that he may be confused. How would you handle this situation? What other health caregivers may be able to assist your patient at home? How would you contact them?
4. Determine which of the following procedures would require medical asepsis and which would require surgical asepsis:
   - Rectal temperature
   - Excision of cyst
   - Catheterization
   - Injection
   - Throat culture
   - Cystoscopy

Suggestions for Further Reading

Blood Borne Pathogens Regulations, OSHA Instructions 29CFR 1910.1030.

Burton, G. R. W. (1992). *Microbiology for the Health Sciences,* 4th ed. Philadelphia: J.B. Lippincott.

Centers for Disease Control. (1988). Recommendations for prevention of HIV transmission in the health care setting. *MMWR, 37*(24).

Earnest, V. V. (1993). *Clinical Skills in Nursing Practice,* 2nd ed. Philadelphia: J.B. Lippincott.

Haman, B. (1994). *Disease: Identification, Prevention and Control.* St. Louis: Mosby–Year Book.

Timby, B. K. (1996). *Fundamental Skills and Concepts in Nursing Care,* 6th ed. Philadelphia: Lippincott-Raven.

Smeltzer, S. C., & Bare, B. C. (1996). *Brunner and Suddarth's Textbook of Medical-Surgical Nursing,* 8th ed. Philadelphia: Lippincott-Raven.

Staines, N., Brostoff, J., & James, K. (1993). *Introducing Immunology.* London: C. V. Mosby.

Taylor, C., Lillis, C., & LeMone, P. (1997). *Fundamentals of Nursing: The Art and Science of Nursing Care,* 3rd ed. Philadelphia: Lippincott-Raven.

Volk, W. A., et al. (1995). *Essentials of Medical Microbiology,* 5th ed. Philadelphia: J.B. Lippincott.

2 Medical History and Patient Interview

Chapter Outline

The Medical History
- Methods of Collecting Information
- Elements of the Medical History

Conducting the Patient Interview
- Preparing for the Interview
- Introducing Yourself
- Barriers to Communication

Assessing the Patient
- Signs and Symptoms
- Chief Complaint and Present Illness

Documenting Patient Encounters
- Patient Record Contents
- Record Formats
- Documentation Formats
- Documentation Guidelines

Role Delineation

CLINICAL

Patient Care

- Obtain patient history and vital signs.
- Coordinate patient care information with other health care providers.

GENERAL

Professionalism

- Project a professional manner and image.
- Adhere to ethical principles.
- Manage time effectively.

Communication Skills

- Treat all patients with compassion and empathy.
- Recognize and respect cultural diversity.
- Adapt communications to individual's ability to understand.
- Use effective and correct verbal and written communications.
- Recognize and respond to verbal and nonverbal communications.
- Use medical terminology appropriately.
- Receive, organize, prioritize, and transmit information.
- Serve as liaison.

Legal Concepts

- Maintain confidentiality.
- Practice within the scope of education, training, and personal capabilities.
- Prepare and maintain medical records.
- Document accurately.
- Follow employer's established policies dealing with the health care contract.
- Follow federal, state, and local legal guidelines.
- Comply with established risk management and safety procedures.

Chapter Competencies

Learning Objectives

Upon successfully completing this chapter, you will be able to:

1. Spell and define the Key Terms.
2. List the different sections of the medical history and give examples of the type of information included in each.
3. Explain why certain information is included in the various sections.
4. List guidelines for conducting a patient interview.
5. Explain the difference between a sign and a symptom and give examples of each.
6. Explain chief complaint and present illness.

Performance Objectives

Upon successfully completing this chapter, you will be able to:

1. Interview a patient and correctly complete appropriate sections of the medical history form (Procedure 2-1).
2. Demonstrate effective communication techniques during the patient interview process.

Key Terms

(See Glossary for definitions.)

assessment
chief complaint
familial
hereditary
medical history
over-the-counter
signs
symptoms

Diagnosing a patient's present illness requires that the physician have access to the patient's health status, both past and current. The medical assistant is responsible for eliciting this information as part of the **medical history** and patient **assessment.** The medical history is a record containing information about all past health concerns, including those not considered pertinent to the presenting problem. Assessment is the process of gathering information to determine the patient's problem or reason for seeking treatment. To ensure consistent care, you will ask standard questions and obtain information about each patient. Responses are usually documented on preprinted forms or in a manner decided by the physician.

THE MEDICAL HISTORY

Methods of Collecting Information

In many practices, the medical assistant and the physician work cooperatively to obtain the patient's complete medical history. The medical assistant gathers initial patient information by obtaining answers to a printed list of questions and conducting a patient interview. The physician then reviews that information, using it as the basis for more extensive questioning and data gathering.

In some practices, the physician may prefer to complete the medical history. In others, the patient is responsible for filling out a standardized medical history form. The form may be mailed to the patient for completion before the initial visit, or it may be given to the patient at the first appointment.

Elements of the Medical History

Depending on the practice specialty, medical history forms will vary somewhat in content and complexity; however, the medical history is composed of these common elements: identifying

2

Professional Medical Associates – History Form

NAME: ______ DATE OF BIRTH: ______

What is the main reason for your visit to the doctor? ______

Were you referred? ______ if so, by whom? ______

PAST MEDICAL HISTORY:

Are you allergic to any medication? ______

If so, list medications: ______

List current medications, dosage, and how many times a day you take them:

Medication	**Dose**	**Times A Day**

Alcohol Consumption: What type? ______ Amount ______ How Often? ______

History of Alcoholism? ______

When was your last TB or Tine test? ______

Have you ever had a positive test for tuberculosis? ______

When was your last Tetanus shot? ______

List all surgeries you have had in the past:

Date	**Type of Surgery**

List all past hospitalizations (not involving surgeries above):

Date	**Reason For Hospital Stay**

List all past problems with trauma (broken bones, lacerations, etc.): ______

REVIEW OF SYSTEMS, PAST MEDICAL PROBLEMS:
If you have been told you have any of the problems listed below, or are having any of the problems listed below, please CIRCLE:

1. GENERAL: Weight loss, weight gain, fever, chills, night sweats, hot flashes, tire easily, problems with sleep, crying spells, history of cancer.
2. SKIN: Rash, sores that won't heal, moles that are new or changing, history of skin problems.
3. HEENT: Headache, eye problems, hearing problems, sinus problems, hay fever, dizziness, hoarseness, sores in your mouth that won't heal, dental problems.

   Do you chew tobacco or dip snuff? ______
4. METABOLIC/ENDOCRINE: Thyroid problems, diabetes or sugar problems, high cholesterol.

Figure 2-1 A sample medical history form.

data (data base), past history (PH), review of systems (ROS), family history (FH), and social history. Figure 2-1 is an example of a medical history form.

- *Identifying data or data base.* Information in this section always includes the patient's name and date of birth and will usually include the patient's address, home and work telephone numbers, insurance carrier and policy number, Social Security number, gender, and race. This information is required for administrative purposes.
- *Past history (PH).* This is a summary of the patient's prior health status. It can include allergies, immunizations, childhood diseases, current and past medications, previous illnesses, traumatic injuries, surgeries, and hospitalizations. Female patients may require an obstetric or gynecologic history. Knowing

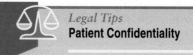

Legal Tips
Patient Confidentiality

You are responsible for ensuring that information obtained as part of the patient's medical history is kept confidential. Legally and ethically, the patient has a right to privacy concerning his or her medical records, which should be kept in a secure place. Only those health care providers directly involved in the patient's care should be allowed access to the records. Patients must sign a consent form before their medical records can be released.

5. RESPIRATORY: Cough, wheezing, breathing problems, history of asthma, history of lung problems.

Do you smoke cigarettes or pipe? ____________________

How much? ____________________ For how long? ____________________

6. BREAST (WOMEN): Breast lumps, changes in nipples, nipple discharge, breast problems, family history of breast cancer. When was your last mammogram? ____________________

7. CARDIOVASCULAR: Heart murmur, rheumatic fever, high blood pressure, angina, heart problems, heart attack, abnormal heart rhythm, chest pain, palpitations, leg swelling, history of phlebitis or blood clots.

8. GI: Problems with appetite, swallowing, heartburn, nausea, vomiting, pain in the abdomen, constipation, diarrhea, blood in stool, history of ulcers, liver problems, hepatitis, jaundice, pancreas problems, gallbladder problems, or colon problems.

9. REPRODUCTIVE (WOMEN): Problems with irregular menstrual cycles, abnormal vaginal bleeding or discharge, history of sexually transmitted diseases, sexual problems.

AGE OF FIRST MENSES (PERIOD) ____________________ AGE OF MENOPAUSE ____________________

LAST PAP SMEAR ____________________ METHOD OF CONTRACEPTION ____________________

Obstetric History (Women)

NUMBER OF PREGNANCIES ____________________ PLEASE LIST AS FOLLOWS:

Delivery Date Pregnancy Complications Type Delivery Baby's Weight

____

____

MEN: Problems with genital discharge, history of venereal diseases, sexual problems, prostate problems.

METHOD OF CONTRACEPTION ____________________

10. UROLOGIC: Problems with painful urination, urinary frequency, blood in urine, weak urinary stream, history of bladder or kidney infections, or kidney stones.

11. MUSCULOSKELETAL: Arthritis, back pain, cramps in legs.

12. NEUROLOGIC: Seizures, stroke, arm or leg weakness or numbness, black-out spells, memory or thinking problems, depression, anxiety, psychiatric problems.

13. HEMATOLOGIC: Anemia, bleeding problems, enlarged lymph nodes.

HAVE YOU EVER HAD A BLOOD TRANSFUSION? ____________________ DATE ____________________

FAMILY HISTORY:

List any medical problems that run in your family and which family members have these problems.

____

____

SOCIAL HISTORY:

MARITAL STATUS: ____________________

OCCUPATION: ____________________

EDUCATION: ____________________

HOBBIES: ____________________

WHAT DO YOU DO FOR ENJOYMENT? ____________________

Figure 2-1 *(continued)*

this information can help the physician plan appropriate care for the patient's present illness.

- *Review of systems (ROS).* A thorough review of each body system elicits information that the patient may have forgotten to mention or may have felt was irrelevant. Careful questioning can uncover potential areas of concern for the physician to explore further.
- *Family history (FH).* The health status of the patient's parents, siblings, and grandparents is summarized, including specific diseases or disorders that any immediate family member may have. This information is important because certain diseases have **familial** or **hereditary** tendencies. Familial diseases tend to occur more often in a particular family. Hereditary diseases are transmitted from parent to offspring. If any of the patient's family members are deceased, you should obtain information about the cause of death.
- *Social history.* Included in this information is the patient's life-style, such as marital status, education, hobbies, and occupational history. It may also include questions about the use of alcohol and tobacco and a sexual history. Knowing this information aids the physician in understanding how the patient's present illness and any planned treatment may affect the individual's life-style.

Checkpoint Questions

1. *What are the common elements of a medical history?*
2. *What is the difference between the past history and family history?*

CONDUCTING THE PATIENT INTERVIEW

Preparing for the Interview

An interview involves reviewing past or current medical history. As a medical assistant, your primary goal during the patient interview is to obtain accurate and pertinent information. To do this, you will need to understand the basic components of communication and to use active listening skills. You also will need to use a variety of interviewing techniques, including reflecting, paraphrasing, asking for examples, asking questions, summarizing, and allowing silence. Procedure 2-1 outlines the process for conducting a successful patient interview.

Be sure you are familiar with the medical history forms and questions before you start interviewing. Shuffling papers while the patient is talking or backtracking in your line of questioning distracts the patient and disrupts the flow of the interview. Know the order of the questions and the type of information the physician is trying to elicit. If the patient is new to the practice, review his or her new patient questionnaire before beginning. If the patient is an established one, review his or her chart.

To enhance the potential for open communication—and to safeguard patient confidentiality—find a private and comfortable place, such as an office or conference room, in which to conduct the interview. Avoid areas where distractions are likely, such as the reception area. Interview the patient alone, unless he or she wishes to have family members or significant others present (Fig. 2-2).

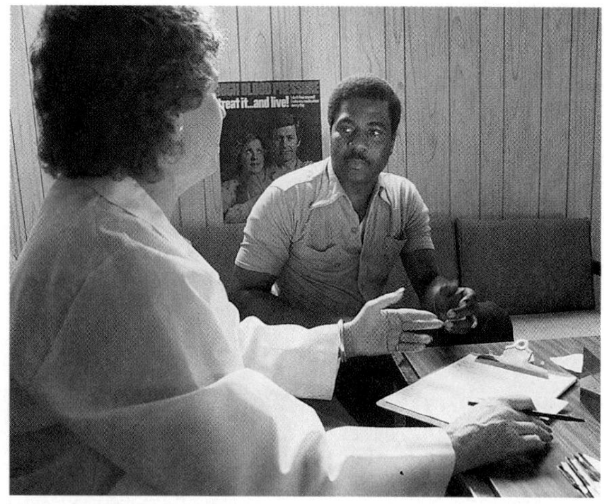

Figure 2-2 Conduct the patient interview in a private and comfortable place.

Introducing Yourself

For both new and established patients, begin by identifying yourself and stating the purpose of the interview. For example, you might say, "Good morning, Mr. Frank. My name is Angela, and I'm Dr. Martin's medical assistant. I want to ask a few questions that will help the doctor plan appropriate care for you. Please be assured that your responses will be kept strictly confidential."

The initial impression you make on the patient will be a lasting one, so be sure your demeanor and words communicate genuine respect and concern. By developing a professional rapport, you will gain the patient's confidence and trust.

Advice and Tips

Helping Patients Feel at Ease

Over time, many medical procedures will become routine for you. But for many patients, these "routine" procedures are cause for fear and intimidation during a visit to the physician's office. To help put patients at ease, follow these tips:

- Treat each patient as an individual with unique needs.
- Help elderly or disabled patients onto and off of the examining table.
- When weighing patients, do not announce their weight verbally because this may be embarrassing. Instead, ask them in the privacy of the examining room if they want to know their weight.
- Always offer a sheet or blanket to a patient who has changed into an examining gown and is waiting for the physician.
- When preparing a woman for a gynecologic examination, have her sit on the examining table until the physician is ready for the examination. Then assist her into the stirrups.
- If the physician is delayed, let the patient know. Explain that an emergency has occurred, and let the patient know the approximate length of the delay. You can further help the situation by offering the patient a magazine or a glass of water. Also invite the patient to use the telephone to alert family, friends, or employers about the delay.
- Keep the patient informed of each step of any procedure. Patients who understand the procedure and its purpose will be more at ease and will be more cooperative.

Procedure 2-1 Interviewing the Patient to Obtain a Medical History

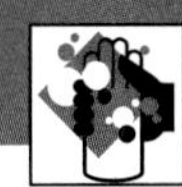

PURPOSE:

To provide a background or baseline for diagnosis of the presenting condition

EQUIPMENT/SUPPLIES

- medical history form or questionnaire
- pen
- any available previous information

2

STEPS

1. Gather the supplies.
2. Review the medical history form.
   It is important that you become familiar with the order of the questions and the type of information required.
3. Find a private and comfortable place.
   A quiet place avoids distractions and ensures patient confidentiality.
4. Sit across from the patient at eye level and maintain frequent eye contact.
   Standing above the patient may be perceived as threatening and may result in poor communication.
5. Introduce yourself and explain the purpose of the interview.
   This helps establish a professional rapport with the patient.
6. Using language the patient can understand, ask the appropriate questions and document the patient's responses. Be sure to determine the patient's chief complaint (CC) and present illness (PI).
   You must obtain accurate and complete data.
7. Listen actively, stop writing from time to time, and look at the patient while he or she is speaking.
   Patients can sense when the interviewer is not listening, so be sure you show interest in what the patient is saying.
8. Regardless of the confidences shared by the patient, avoid projecting a judgmental attitude by your words or your actions.
   You must maintain your professionalism and ensure the patient's trust in you.
9. If appropriate, explain to the patient what to expect during any examinations or procedures that may be scheduled for the day.
   It's vital to keep the patient informed of his or her care.
10. Thank the patient for cooperating during the interview and offer to answer any questions.
    Courtesy encourages the patient to have a positive attitude about the physician's office.

DOCUMENTATION GUIDELINES

- Date and time
- Height and weight
- Vital signs as required by office protocol
- All laboratory values obtained as required by office protocol
- Patient complaints/concerns
- Patient education/instructions
- Your signature

Charting Example

DATE	TIME Pt examination for insurance
	policy. Pt states he has no complaints.
	Ht - 6'1", Wt - 178, T - 98.8, P - 84, R - 16,
	BP - 128/78. Urinalysis dip essentially
	negative, pH 6.5, sp grav 1.020. Pt
	received office visit protocol brochure,
	expressed understanding. Dr. Carson in to
	examine pt. ——Your Signature

Barriers to Communication

As you begin speaking with the patient, assess any barriers to communication. Determine the patient's level of understanding and adjust your questioning accordingly—for instance, avoid using highly technical terms. Also note if the patient is hearing or vision impaired or has trouble understanding or speaking English. Again, adjust your interviewing techniques to best fit the patient's needs.

Checkpoint Question

3. *What should you do before beginning a patient interview?*

2

What If?

What if the patient is highly anxious about the interview? For example, when you ask a question, the patient speaks so quickly you have trouble understanding the answer. The patient also seems unable to focus on one topic at a time and often rambles.

Speak slowly and softly. Reassure the patient that people commonly feel nervous when talking about their health. Let the patient know that there is no rush and that you can take as much time as needed to complete the interview.

ASSESSING THE PATIENT

Signs and Symptoms

You must listen carefully as the patient describes current medical problems to identify **signs** and **symptoms.** These are also referred to as subjective and objective information. Symptoms are subjective indications of disease or changes in the body as sensed by the patient; they are not usually discernible by anyone else. Examples of symptoms a patient may describe include "leg pain," "headache," or "nausea." Signs are objective indications of disease or bodily dysfunction that can be perceived by others, such as vital signs or findings made by the physician. Signs include a rash, bleeding, cough, discharge, or blood pressure readings.

Patient Education

General Teaching Topics

While performing a patient assessment, you can initiate patient education. The teaching may consist of information about a specific disease or general care. For example, a diabetic patient may need instruction on glucose testing or diet control.

General topics for *all* patients can include:

- Blood pressure management
- Stress management techniques
- Diet or weight control tips
- The importance of exercise and sample exercises
- The effects of alcohol and the need to limit alcohol consumption
- Instructions for conducting breast or testicular self-examination
- Proper immunizations
- Cancer prevention tips
- Awareness of acquired immunodeficiency syndrome
- Prevention of sexually transmitted diseases

Chief Complaint and Present Illness

After recording the patient's medical history and reviewing the information for accuracy and clarity, you must find out exactly why the patient has come to see the physician. To do this, ask an open-ended question—a question that allows a broad response—to encourage the patient to describe the chain of events leading to this appointment. For example, you might ask, "What can we do to help you?" or "What is the reason for your appointment today?" or "Can you describe what has been going on?"

The patient's answer will reveal the **chief complaint** (CC). The CC is a description of the symptom(s) that led the patient to seek the physician's care. Examples might include "I've had a headache for the last 3 days" or "Yesterday I lifted a heavy crate and strained my back." Document the CC in the patient's record using the patient's own words in quotation marks.

Continue to probe for more details to define the patient's present illness (PI)—a more specific account of the CC. The PI includes a chronologic order of events, including dates of onset, home remedies used by the patient, and **over-the-counter** medications taken by the patient. Over-the-counter medications are those that are available without prescriptions. Questions to ask might include:

- How did this first begin?
- Can you describe the pain?
- What medications have you taken for the pain?

Avoid suggesting answers, such as, "Is the pain sharp?" or "Is the pain worse when you walk?" Many patients will agree or answer positively because they think this must be the expected answer. Anything the patient has felt or has done up to this time should be noted on the initial interview.

After asking several open-ended questions, go to closed-ended questions to obtain specific data. For example, you might ask the patient, "How long have you had this pain?" "What was your temperature?" These kinds of questions require only a short answer, not a lengthy description.

Both the CC and the PI include subjective and objective information. The medical assistant must carefully describe and correctly designate each as either subjective or objective findings.

Of course, not all patients visit the doctor because they are ill. Some patient appointments are for routine examinations or tests. You must document the reasons for these visits in the patient record as well.

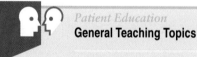

> **Checkpoint Question**
> 4. *What is the difference between a sign and a symptom? Give an example of each.*

DOCUMENTING PATIENT ENCOUNTERS

Medical record documentation primarily is used to:

- *Communicate* patient information between health care workers (eg, orders from the physician, notes from the assistant, laboratory results).
- *Assess* the patient's current versus past health status. For instance, by reviewing and comparing previous and baseline data, the physician can determine if the patient's condition is better or worse, if the medication has produced the desired response, and so forth.
- *Plan* what to do next, such as change the treatment or continue the current therapy until the condition resolves.

Other uses for the medical record include:

- *Research.* The information in a patient record can be used to evaluate the demographics of a disease and determine the answers to questions such as, "Which population is most likely to develop a certain disease?" "Which population responds best to various therapies?"
- *Reimbursement.* Health benefit carriers (eg, insurance companies, health maintenance organizations, Medicare, Medicaid) require specific documentation for reimbursement and typically supply participating offices with guidelines for submitting claims. If these guidelines are not followed to the letter, the carrier is within its rights to deny payment. Documentation must support the treatment or procedure, or payment will not be made.
- *Quality assurance.* Documentation ensures that the medical office is in compliance with quality assurance policies. These policies may include treatment follow-up to determine if patient education and compliance are leading to a resolution of the health concern. Documentation of test results and follow-up therapy shows that the medical office staff is continuing to monitor the patient's health.
- *Legal evidence.* In the event of a lawsuit, documentation may be used as evidence that procedures were performed, medication was given, therapy was explained, and findings were evaluated. It is presumed that none of the above was done if there is no supporting documentation.

Patient Record Contents

Patient records—also called files, folders, or charts—usually follow a standard organization decided by the physician and staff to offer the quickest, easiest access to the information. Information contained in the records includes (but is not limited to) the following:

2

- Patient data base (eg, name, birth date, address, Social Security number, insurance information, next of kin)
- PH
- CC (the reason for the visit) and history of the PI
- ROS
- General medical history and physical examination (PE)
- Progress notes or flow charts
- Laboratory, radiology, and other diagnostic reports
- Consultations and treatment summaries from other physicians or health care professionals

Though most office records are retained on paper in folders, many now are being entered on computer terminals in each examining and interviewing room (Fig. 2-3). Often, staff members have access to the record at points throughout the office. Many medical office software programs offer on-screen prompts to ensure that all required information is included.

With the patient's consent to release information, the appropriate contents can be transferred electronically from the physician's office to consulting practitioners, the hospital, or the insurance carrier. However, confidentiality of computerized records is an ongoing concern. Protection devices are being developed to ensure that information cannot be accessed without the patient's expressed and written permission. To safeguard patient confidentiality, never leave patient information on a computer screen when you have finished making an entry. Save the information and escape from the screen before leaving a terminal. Also, be sure to save information added at each encounter in backup files in the event of a system failure.

For traditional hard copy records, the order in which information appears and the form the folder takes will be decided by the physician with input from the staff responsible for maintaining the information. Records are arranged in reverse chronologic order—the most recent information is placed on top of previous information. As the patient is seen for various reasons, new information is added to the most recent previous information in an ongoing narrative.

Record Formats

Two record formats accepted by the medical profession include the source-oriented medical record (SOMR) and the problem-oriented medical record (POMR).

2

Patient Encounter Form

Name	Date	Medical Record #

CC:

HPI:

Elements:
Location; quality; severity; timing; context; modifying factors; associated signs & symptoms.
Brief = 1-3 elements; Extended = more than 4 elements

ROS: Reviewed and Updated from ____________

- O Constitutional
- O Eyes
- O Ears, Nose, Mouth, Throat
- O Resp.
- O GI
- O GU
- O Musculoskeletal
- O Skin
- O Neuro
- O Psych
- O Hem/Lymph
- O Cardiovascular
- O Allergic/Immune
- O Endocrine

PFSH: Reviewed and updated from ____________.
Elements:

Exam

Constitutional B.P. ______ HR ______ RR ______ Temp ______ Wt ______

General Appearance ____________

Eyes ____________

ENT ____________

Respiratory ____________

Cardiovascular ____________

Gastrointestinal ____________

Genitourinary ____________

Musculoskeletal ____________

Skin ____________

Neurologic ____________

Psychiatric ____________

Hematologic/Lymphatic/Immunologic ____________

Figure 2-3 A sample computerized medical history form. (Courtesy of Parente Consulting, Philadelphia, PA)

Source Oriented Medical Record

The SOMR groups all similar categories or *sources* of information together. Typically these include:

- Patient data base
- Physician orders
- Progress notes
- Laboratory, radiographic, or other diagnostic results
- Consultation reports

Because the SOMR is organized by the source of care—doctor, physical therapist, radiologist—this method is not used often in the medical office. Information necessary for charting or assessment may be easier for a certain specialty to find in its assigned section, but it is harder to coordinate and compare care between disciplines.

Problem-Oriented Medical Record

The POMR lists each patient problem and references each problem with a number that is used throughout the folder (Fig. 2-4). This method offers easy access to the information and virtually eliminates the possibility of missing vital data. As information is gathered

ACUTE, SELF-LIMITED, OR UNDIAGNOSED PROBLEMS

	Date	Problem
A	6/13/96	acute pharyngitis
B	10/1/97	UTI
C	12/6/98	viral enteritis
D		
E		
F		
G		
H		
I		
J		
K		
L		

Betty Q. Brown
02-14-51
123 Maple Lane
Centerville, NC
29411
#654321000

PROFESSIONAL
MEDICAL ASSOCIATES, P.A.

CUMULATIVE PROBLEM LIST

	Date	Problem Title
1	3/5/96	hypertension - BP 158/96
2	4/20/97	hypoglycemia - FBS 56
3	9/17/98	Ⓛ breast mass 1 cm ⓧ
4		
5		
6		
7		
8		
9		
10		
11		
12		
13		
14		
15		
16		
17		

Figure 2-4 A cumulative problem list is used to document a patient's chief complaint.

MEDICATION RECORD

Drug Intolerances:

Drug	Reaction	Date
Keflex	hives	5/16/90
Codeine	nausea	? mid 80s

Betty Q. Brown
02-14-51
123 Maple Lane
Centerville, NC
29411
#654321000

LONG-TERM MEDICATIONS

Date	Problem	Medication, Dose, Frequency
3/5/96	hypertension	Inderal-LA 80mg BID

Figure 2-4 *(continued)*

by members of the health care team, it is listed in the patient's folder and referenced by the appropriate number.

The patient's problem list is usually attached to the inside front of the folder. Each diagnosis made for the patient is then listed as either chronic (ongoing, long-term) or acute (short-term, self-limiting) and dated. For example, Ms. Smith presents as a new patient with a lump in her left breast and mild hypertension. These problems will be listed under chronic, cumulative, or ongoing. The breast lump may be listed as #1 and the hypertension as #2 (or vice versa) in order of occurrence rather than importance.

1/15/99 #1 L breast mass, 2 cm at R upper margin
1/15/99 #2 Hypertension, mild

All subsequent procedures, tests, medications and treatments relating to these problems will be listed in the progress notes and referenced by the appropriate problem numbers.

If Ms. Smith returns complaining of a urinary tract infection, for example, this new problem is given a number and recorded under acute problems. During this visit, the physician also will assess problems #1 and #2 and document the findings according to the problem number. When a problem is resolved, it either will be crossed off the master problem list with a single line and a date of resolution, or it will be listed in a particular column stating the date of resolution. Either method requires supporting documentation called out by number in the progress notes to prove that the problem is resolved. In this way, ongoing patient concerns can be noted immediately by checking the problem list inside the front cover of the folder.

Checkpoint Question

5. *What are the two ways in which the medical record can be organized?*

Documentation Formats

Several standard formats of charting or documentation are used to record each patient encounter in the progress notes. The most accepted formats are:

- Narrative notes
- SOAP (subjective, objective, assessment, plan)
- PIE (problem, intervention, evaluation)
- Focus (also known as DAR—data, action, response)
- CBE (charting by exception)

Entries in any of these formats include the date and time of the encounter; the patient's complaint or concern; observations and assessments made by the worker; any treatment, medication, or other action taken; and the signature and title of the worker. Other information included varies with the need for the visit.

Narrative Notes

Narrative notes are the easiest to write. This format is simply a paragraph stating the reason for the patient contact (visit or phone call). Information is entered in complete sentences or phrases and time sequenced like a journal or diary of the patient's health care (Fig. 2-5).

2-13-99	1035
	Pt presents c/o T x 3 days. Mild nausea,
	no vomiting or diarrhea, generalized joint
	and muscle discomfort. Has taken ASA at
	intervals. T-101.2, P-84, R-18,
	BP-126/74. —— Rita Day, CMA

Figure 2-5 Example of narrative notes.

3-15-99	11:10 am
	S: "I think I have the flu." Generalized
	achiness x 2 days, no NVD
	O: T-102.2, P-92, R-24, BP-110/68
	A: T elevation
	P: To see Dr. Parker —— Alison Carter, RMA

Figure 2-6 Example of SOAP notes.

Advantages: There is no format to learn. It is as simple as taking notes and may be as brief or as detailed as the situation requires.
Disadvantages: It is difficult to extract pertinent information from the narrative flow and has a tendency not to be focused on a specific problem.

SOAP Notes

SOAP notes use a standard format that outlines subjective data (information reported by the patient), objective data (information obtained from the health care worker's observation of the patient), the assessment (problem identification), and the plan (proposed treatment) (Fig. 2-6). The format may be expanded to include implementation (what care was provided), evaluation (treatment outcome), and revision (treatment changes) to give the chart a SOAPIER format.
Advantages: Entries are specific to the patient's concerns, and the information can be accessed by the whole health care team at a glance.
Disadvantages: It is a bit more difficult to master and more time-consuming than a simple narrative. Also does not easily allow for inclusion of general information not pertinent to a listed problem.

PIE Notes

PIE notes use problem, intervention, and evaluation to prompt the assistant to refer to a specific health care concern included on the problem list (Fig. 2-7). Nor-

4-20-99	0825
	P: #1 Hypertension - pt presents for Rx
	renewal. Pt states she is doing well on
	current Rx.
	I: #1 BP-142/94, P-84. Pt to see Dr. Dare
	E: #1 Pt offers no additional complaints
	—— Agnes Dale, CMA

Figure 2-7 Example of PIE notes.

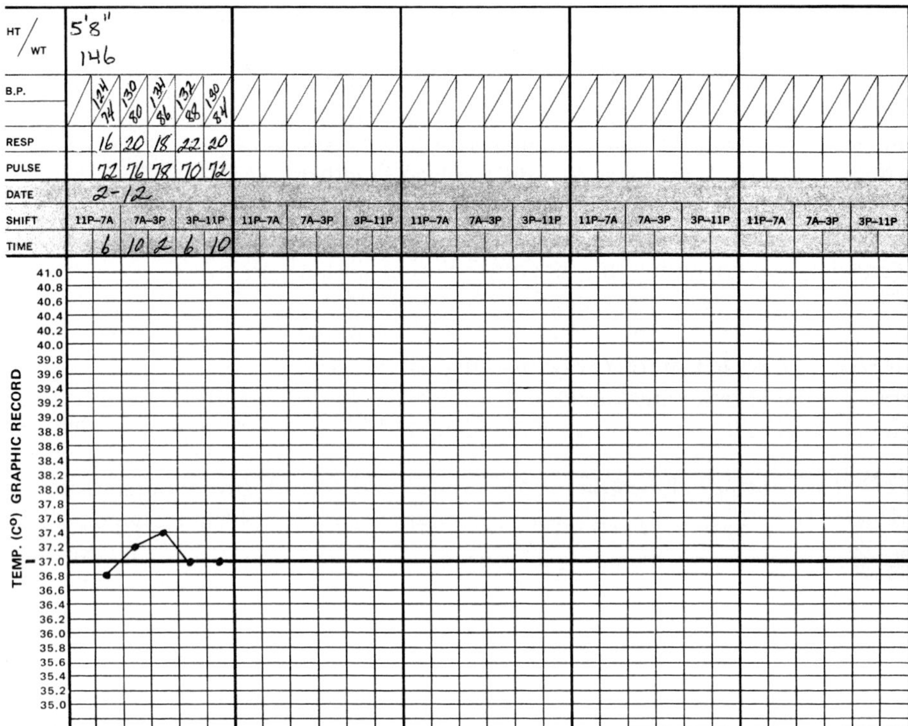

Figure 2-8 A graphic flow sheet is a preprinted checklist that is designed to document a specific task.

mal values are usually recorded or checked off on a separate flow sheet (Fig. 2-8). (A flow sheet is a graph with a preprinted checklist that usually includes such information as vital signs, patient education, and specific procedures required by the office practice.)
Advantages: This format prevents the assistant from overlooking a concern that should be evaluated, which complies with quality assurance measures. Assessment for therapy outcomes is built into the format.
Disadvantages: If the patient presents with a problem not listed, it may be more difficult to document. The need for a flow sheet makes it less adaptable for the medical office.

Focus Notes

Focus notes are somewhat similar in format to SOAPIER notes, but use data, action, and result (instead of objective, plan, and evaluation, respectively) as the organizing parameters. This format requires information to be listed in three columns: date and time, focus of the patient's visit, and patient care notes, which includes data (CC), the action taken, and the results (Fig. 2-9).
Advantages: Charting on any issue is easier without the concentration on problems. The negative connotation of "problem" is eliminated by using the term "focus," which may even be used to signify a positive event. This is a very flexible format that allows easy access to information.
Disadvantages: Long-standing problems may not be addressed with the somewhat looser format.

Charting by Exception

Using CBE eliminates the need to record normal findings, such as vital signs within normal limits for the patient, and concentrates on abnormal findings. This format requires a flow sheet to document that values were assessed for legal purposes, but progress notes are usually limited to a brief SOAP or DAR for a present concern. Because Medicare and other carriers will not pay for care that is not documented, this format is not usually used in medical offices.
Advantages: This is very time efficient and allows quick access to health care concerns.

Date/Time	Focus	Patient Care Notes
05-19-99	Hypertension	D: Pt presents for recheck to evaluate therapy.
1415		A: BP-148/76, P-92
		R: Pressure reported to Dr. Sutton. Rx renewed. —Dottie Wagner, CMA

Figure 2-9 Example of focus notes.

Disadvantages: This is generally not applicable for the medical office because of the episodic nature of office care. This format works best in hospitals or long-term care facilities, where there is constant care and monitoring.

Checkpoint Question

6. *What are five formats used for charting progress notes?*

Documentation Guidelines

No matter which documentation format you use, follow the guidelines below to help ensure that the information recorded is appropriate and the records are legally presentable.

- *Chart accurately.* Include a time frame for the presenting condition (1 week, 2 hours), sizes (2 cm, 0.5 cm), numbers (2 lesions, 3 sutures), location (RUQ, medial aspect of L forearm), and color (yellow sputum, pink-tinged fluid). Use the patient's words in quotation marks as appropriate. Be sure to use only those abbreviations that are accepted by your facility (see Appendices). If you make an error, correct it properly (Box 2-1).
- *Chart completely.* Document everything you think is important. Remember: It is better to overchart than to omit vital information. Note each patient encounter (eg, office visits, phone calls to or from the patient, and correspondence regarding the patient).
- *Chart legibly.* Print if you must. Use black ink, because it will photocopy better than other colors. Illegible or sloppy writing may cause errors in treatment (was the patient's pressure 164/94 or 104/44?) and will not hold up in court.
- *Chart immediately.* Sign the entry and note the time of the procedure right away. Another worker may presume that the ordered medication was not given, for example, or the treatment was not provided if you delay charting. Many patients are so unaware of medical protocol that they may not question the second medication or treatment.
- *Chart confidentially.* Only authorized individuals can have access to patient information. If the information is to be transmitted to someone outside the medical office staff, the patient must sign a release of information form. Though the chart belongs to the facility, the information belongs to the patient to do with as he or she sees fit.

Box 2-1

Correcting a Charting Error

Never delete, erase, scribble over, or white-out information in the medical record because this can be construed as tampering with a legal document. If you do make an error, draw a single line through it, initial it, date it, and write "error." Then document the correct information.

error 05/15/99 SB

05/15/99 0930 Patient complaining of pain in ~~right~~ eye. ——————— Sue Brown, RMA

05/15/99 1000 Correction note: Patient complaining of pain in left eye. ——— Sue Brown, RMA

When correcting a charting error, draw a single line through the error, initial it, date it, and write "error." Then document the correct information.

2

Answers to Checkpoint Questions

1. *The common elements of a medical history include identifying data, past history (PH), review of systems (ROS), family history (FH), and social history.*
2. *The past history summarizes the patient's prior health status; the family history summarizes the health status of the patient's parents, siblings, and grandparents.*
3. *Before beginning a patient interview, you should:*
   - Review the patient's past and current medical history.
   - Familiarize yourself with the medical history form and questions.
   - Choose a private and comfortable place to conduct the interview.
   - Introduce yourself and explain the purpose for the interview.
4. *A sign is an objective indication of disease or bodily dysfunction that can be perceived by others; examples include rash, bleeding, or discharge. A symptom is a subjective indication of disease or changes in the body that can be perceived only by the patient; examples include leg pain, headache, or nausea.*
5. *Medical records can be organized as either source-oriented or problem-oriented formats.*
6. *The five formats used for documenting progress notes are narrative, SOAP, PIE, focus, and charting by exception (CBE).*

Critical Thinking Challenges

1. Mrs. Jones has always been impeccably groomed. Today her hair is not combed, she is wearing no makeup, and her clothes do not match. Is this worth noting on her chart?
2. Mrs. Brown speaks English as a second language. You need to ask her about her urinary symptoms. Compare the following phrases. Which one should you use? Why?
   - "Do you have trouble voiding?"
   - "Do you have trouble passing your water?"
3. Review the following items. Determine in which section of the medical history each should be included and explain why. Identify any items that are irrelevant.
   - Sister died of breast cancer
   - Son had chickenpox last year
   - Patient has many allergies
   - Father died of heart disease
   - Mother is living and well
   - Brother works in real estate
   - Patient smokes three packs of cigarettes a day
   - Patient works in cotton mill
   - Patient is a runner and teaches aerobics
   - Patient has recently lost 60 pounds
   - Patient had angioplasty last year
4. Determine which of the following are signs and which are symptoms:
   nausea
   vomiting
   itching
   rash
   dizziness
   abdominal pain
   pallor
   tingling toes
   fever
   edema
5. Interview a fellow student regarding a made-up injury. Document the incident and what treatments you did in narrative, SOAP, PIE, and focus formats.

Suggestions for Further Reading

Bates, B., Buckley, L. S., & Hockleman, R. A. (1995). *A Guide to Physical Examination and History Taking,* 6th ed. Philadelphia: J.B. Lippincott.

Craven, R. F., & Hirnle, C. J. (1996). *Fundamentals of Nursing,* 2nd ed. Philadelphia: Lippincott-Raven.

Kerschner, V. (1992). *Health Unit Coordinating, Principles and Practices.* Albany, NY: Delmar.

Kozier, B., & Erb, G. (1993). *Techniques of Clinical Nursing,* 4th ed. Redwood City, CA: Addison and Wesley.

Smeltzer, S., & Bare, B. (1996). *Brunner and Suddarth's Textbook of Medical-Surgical Nursing,* 8th ed. Philadelphia: Lippincott-Raven.

Timby, B. K. (1996). *Fundamental Skills and Concepts in Patient Care,* 6th ed. Philadelphia: Lippincott-Raven.

3 Anthropometric Measurements and Vital Signs

Chapter Outline

Role Delineation

CLINICAL

Fundamental Principles

- Apply principles of aseptic technique and infection control.
- Comply with quality assurance practices.

Patient Care

- Obtain patient history and vital signs.

GENERAL

Legal Concepts

- Maintain confidentiality.
- Practice within the scope of education, training, and personal capabilities.
- Document accurately.
- Maintain and dispose of regulated substances in compliance with government guidelines.
- Comply with established risk management and safety practices.

Chapter Competencies

Learning Objectives

Upon successfully completing this chapter, you will be able to:

1. Spell and define the Key Terms.
2. Explain the procedures for measuring a patient's height and weight.
3. Identify and describe different types of thermometers.
4. Explain the procedure for measuring a patient's temperature using the oral, rectal, axillary, or tympanic methods.
5. Explain the procedure for measuring a patient's pulse rate.
6. Explain the procedure for counting a patient's respirations.
7. Describe Korotkoff sounds and the five phases of blood pressure.
8. Explain the procedure for measuring a patient's blood pressure.
9. State normal values and value ranges for temperature, pulse, respiration, and blood pressure in a variety of patients.

Chapter Competencies *(continued)*

Performance Objectives

Upon successfully completing this chapter, you will be able to:

1. Measure and record a patient's weight (Procedure 3-1).
2. Measure and record a patient's height (Procedure 3-2).
3. Measure and record a patient's oral temperature using a glass mercury thermometer (Procedure 3-3).
4. Measure and record a patient's rectal temperature using a glass mercury thermometer (Procedure 3-4).
5. Measure and record a patient's axillary temperature using a glass mercury thermometer (Procedure 3-5).
6. Measure and record a patient's temperature using an electronic thermometer (Procedure 3-6).
7. Measure and record a patient's temperature using a tympanic thermometer (Procedure 3-7).
8. Disinfect a glass thermometer (Procedure 3-8).
9. Measure and record a patient's radial pulse (Procedure 3-9).
10. Measure and record a patient's apical pulse (Procedure 3-10).
11. Count a patient's respirations (Procedure 3-11).
12. Measure a patient's blood pressure (Procedure 3-12).
13. Auscultate a patient's pedal pulse using a Doppler unit.

Key Terms

(See Glossary for definitions.)

anthropometric
baseline
calibrated
cardiac cycle
cardinal signs
diastole
diaphoresis
febrile
hypertension
intermittent
postural hypotension
remittent
systole

Vital signs, also called **cardinal signs,** are measurements of the functions essential to sustaining life. These include temperature (T), pulse (P), respiration (R), and blood pressure (BP). These signs are recorded at almost every visit made to the medical office.

Height and weight measurements, called **anthropometric** measurements, usually are acquired as the patient is escorted to the examining room. Height and weight are considered to be as important as any of the measurements required for diagnosis and treatment.

At the first visit, anthropometric measurements and vital signs are recorded as **baseline** data, or reference points, for comparison during all subsequent visits. These measurements are the most frequently performed procedures in the medical assistant's daily schedule.

WEIGHT

Weights are always required for prenatal patients, infants, children, and the elderly. In addition, constant weight monitoring may be required if the patient is prescribed medications that must be carefully calculated by body weight. When the physician is following a patient who is attempting to gain or lose weight, the ideal is compared to the weights in an adult desirable weight chart.

The placement of the scales in the office should be carefully considered. Many patients will be uncomfortable if weight is measured in a place that is not private. The type of scales used to measure weight include balance beam scales (Fig. 3-1), digital scales, or dial scales. Weight may be measured in pounds (lb) or kilograms (kg). (See Appendix for information about metric and U.S. equivalents for weight, length, and volume.) Procedure 3-1 describes how to measure weight.

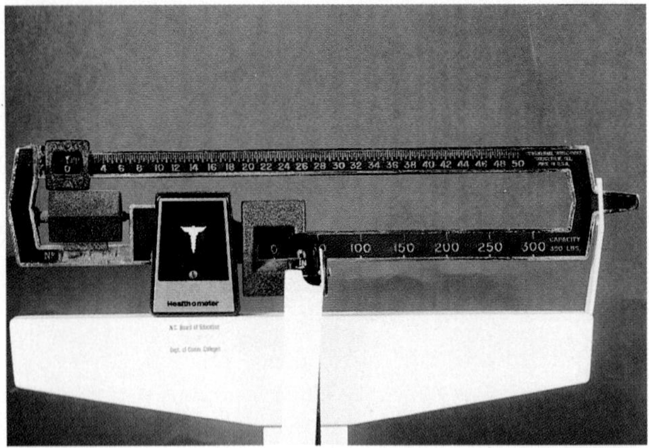

Figure 3-1 A balance beam scale. The large weight indicator is the bottom bar; measurements are in 50-lb increments. The small weight indicator is the top bar; measurements are in ¼-lb increments. On the small weight indicator bar, the even number pounds are numbered (eg, 0, 2, 4, 6) while the odd number pounds are each represented by a long line. Between the numbers and the long lines are smaller lines that represent ¼-lb measurements. A very slightly longer line is at ½-lb increments.

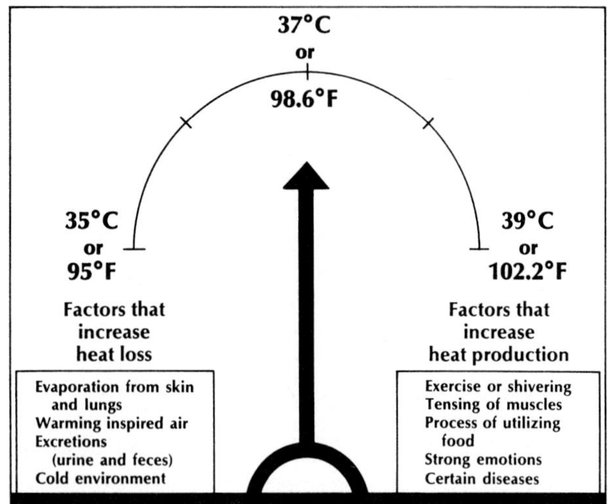

Figure 3-2 Factors affecting temperature balance. The illustration shows the balance between factors that increase heat loss and factors that increase heat production.

HEIGHT

Height may be measured using the movable ruler on the back of most scales (Procedure 3-2), or it may be measured against a graph mounted on a wall. A most accurate measure will be made by any device with a parallel bar that can be moved against the patient's head. Height can be measured in inches or centimeters (cm), depending on the physician's preference.

TEMPERATURE (T)

Temperature is defined as the balance between heat produced and heat lost by the body (Fig. 3-2). All human beings have a temperature that is produced by the energy generated during the physical and chemical changes called metabolism and lost through respiration, elimination, and conduction through the skin. Table 3-1 describes and illustrates processes by which heat is transferred.

Metabolism is the process of using stored energy for life maintenance. The heat produced by this activity can be measured in four different ways using thermometers designed for each method: oral, rectal, axillary, and tympanic. The two scales used to measure temperature are Fahrenheit (F) and centigrade (Celsius). Because thermometers may be **calibrated** (marked) in either scale (Fig. 3-3), you should be able to convert from one scale to another if the need occurs (see Appendix).

Each temperature measurement is fairly constant in relation to the others. The oral temperature is the most common with all other temperatures relating to its average of 98.6° Fahrenheit or about 37.0° centigrade. Rectal temperatures are generally 1° higher than oral because of the vascularity and tightly closed environment of the rectum. Axillary temperatures are usually 1° lower due to the lower vascularity in the area and the difficulty in keeping the axilla tightly closed. Tympanic membrane temperatures are taken with tympanic thermometers, which have been designed to produce a reading that is comparable to either the oral or rectal temperature.

A patient whose temperature is above normal is referred to as **febrile**, and one whose temperature is normal is said to be afebrile. Pyrexia refers to fevers of 102°F or higher rectally or 101°F or higher orally. An extremely high temperature, at the danger level of 105° to 106°F, may be referred to as hyperpyrexia.

Abnormal temperature is usually produced by the presence of a disease process, such as a bacterial or viral infection. Body temperature may rise during intense exercise, anxiety, passion, or dehydration unrelated to a disease process, but these elevations are not considered fevers.

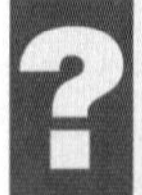

Checkpoint Question

1. *How does an oral temperature differ from a rectal temperature? Why?*

Fever Processes

The body temperature is regulated by the hypothalamus. When the hypothalamus senses that the body is

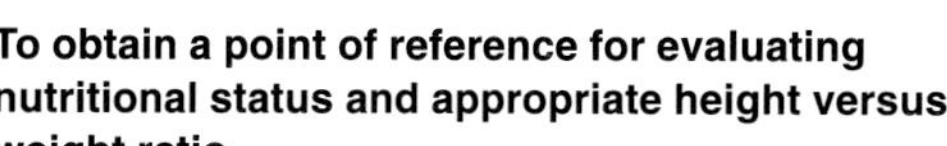

Procedure 3-1 Measuring Weight

PURPOSE:

To obtain a point of reference for evaluating nutritional status and appropriate height versus weight ratio

EQUIPMENT/SUPPLIES

- calibrated scale
- paper towel

STEPS

1. Wash your hands.

   Handwashing promotes infection control.

2. Ensure the scale is properly calibrated by observing that the balance beam hangs freely at midpoint when the counter weights are resting at zero.

   This avoids error in measurement.

3. Greet and identify the patient. Explain the procedure.

   Identifying the patient prevents errors. Explaining the procedure helps ensure cooperation.

4. Escort the patient to the scale. Place a paper towel on the scale.

   The patient will be standing barefooted or in socks or stocking feet; the paper towel helps minimize microorganism transmission and increases patient comfort.

5. Make sure the scale is balanced at zero. (A balance beam scale should always be returned to zero after each use.)

   A scale is a delicate instrument and may easily become inaccurate. Ensuring that it registers zero will eliminate one source of error.

6. Have the patient remove shoes, heavy coats or jackets, put down the purse, and step up onto the scale. *Note:* Certain circumstances require that the patient be weighed wearing only a gown. In this situation, ensure patient privacy by moving the scale to the examining room, where the gowned patient will be waiting.

   Unnecessary items must be removed for an accurate weight.

7. Assist the patient onto the scale. Have the patient stand steady without touching anything; watch closely for a loss of balance.

   Some patients may lose their balance and fall. Some may feel unsteady as the plate of the scale settles momentarily.

8. Weigh the patient.

   a. *On a balance beam scale:*
   Slide counterweights on the bottom and top bars from zero to the approximate weight and then adjust to the proper weight. Each counterweight should rest securely in its notch, with the indicator mark at the proper calibration. To obtain the measurement, the balance bar must hang freely at the exact midpoint. To calculate the weight, add the top reading to the bottom reading (Example: If the bottom counterweight reads 100 and the top one reads 16 plus three small lines, the weight is 116¾ lb.)

   b. *On a digital scale:*
   Read the weight, which will be displayed automatically on the digital screen.

   c. *On a dial scale:*
   The indicator arrow will rest at the proper weight. Read this number from directly above the dial.

   Reading at an angle will result in an incorrect measurement.

DOCUMENTATION GUIDELINES

- Date and time
- Patient's weight indicated in pounds or kilograms
- Any patient data regarding weight progression/diet
- Patient concerns/complaints
- Patient education/instructions
- Your signature

Charting Example

DATE	TIME Pt in for scheduled weight check.
	Today's weight - 230 lb; 3 lb weight loss
	since last visit. Pt has no complaints and
	states she is adhering to prescribed diet,
	has follow-up appointment with dietician in
	10 days. Dr. Persons notified.
	— Your Signature

Note: *If the physician prefers pounds to kilograms or vice versa, the preferred scale will usually be provided. If it is necessary to convert pounds to kilograms or vice versa, remember that 1 k = 2.2 lb.*

To change pounds to kilograms: Divide the number of pounds by 2.2.

To change kilograms to pounds: Multiply the number of kilograms by 2.2.

3

Procedure 3-2 Measuring Height

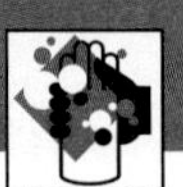

PURPOSE:

To establish a basis of comparison for height versus weight ratio in evaluating nutritional status

EQUIPMENT/SUPPLIES

- scale with ruler or standard marked or mounted on a wall

STEPS

1. Have the patient stand straight and erect on the scale, heels together, eyes straight ahead. (The patient may be measured on the scale facing the ruler, but a better measurement will be made with the patient's back to the ruler.) If the measurement is against a wall standard, the posture requirements are the same.

   The posture must be erect for an accurate measurement.

2. With the measuring bar perpendicular to the ruler, slowly lower it until it firmly touches the patient's head. Press lightly if the hair is full and high.

   Height is being measured, not hair.

3. Read the measurement at the point of movement on the ruler. If the measurements are in inches (with smaller marks for ¼, ½, and ¾), convert the inches to feet and inches. (Example: If the point of movement reads 65 plus two smaller lines, read it as 65½. Remember that 12 inches equal 1 foot; therefore, the patient is 5 feet 5½ inches tall.)
4. At the completion of the procedure, assist the patient from the scale.
5. Return the balance bar on the scale to zero and return the measuring bar to a safe position for the next procedure.

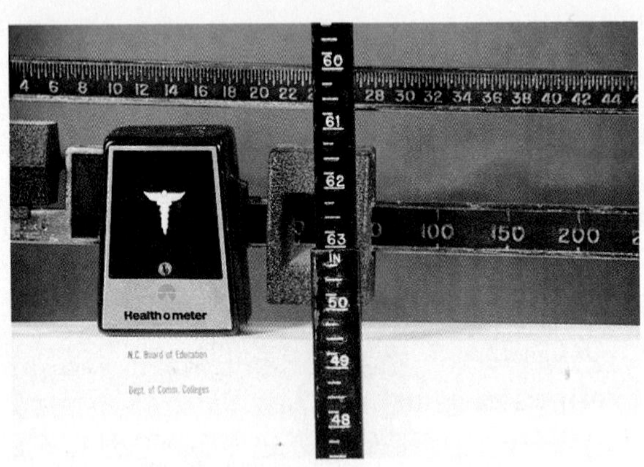

DOCUMENTATION GUIDELINES

- Date and time
- Patient's height in preferred measurement
- Patient concerns/complaints
- Your signature

Charting Example

DATE	TIME 75 y/o WF c/o increased
	cervicothoracic spinal curvature. No pain
	other than "arthritis," Rxed/c OTC meds.
	Baseline measurement 5 years ago 5′4″.
	Today's height 5′2 ½″. Dr. Nowell to see pt.
	—Your Signature

Note: If the physician prefers inches to centimeters or vice versa, the ruler will usually be in the preferred measurement. If it is necessary to convert from inches to centimeters or vice versa, remember that 1 inch = 2.5 cm.

To convert inches to centimeters: Multiply the number of inches by 2.5.

To convert centimeters to inches: Divide the number of centimeters by 2.5.

too warm, it initiates peripheral vasodilation (opening the vessels on the skin surface) to carry core heat to the body surface and increases perspiration to cool the body by evaporation. If the temperature registers as too low, vasoconstriction (narrowing the vessels) and shivering will usually maintain a fairly normal core temperature. Temperature elevations and variations are a *sign* of disease and are not a disease in themselves (Box 3-1).

Temperatures that vary from the normal are caused by:

Table 3-1 **Mechanisms of Heat Transfer**

	Radiation	*Convection*	*Evaporation*	*Conduction*
Definition	The diffusion or dissemination of heat by electromagnetic waves	The dissemination of heat by motion between areas of unequal density	The conversion of a liquid to a vapor	The transfer of heat to another object during direct contact
Example	The body gives off waves of heat from uncovered surfaces.	An oscillating fan blows currents of cool air across the surface of a warm body.	Body fluid in the form of perspiration and insensible loss is vaporized from the skin.	The body transfers heat to an ice pack, causing the ice to melt.
Illustration	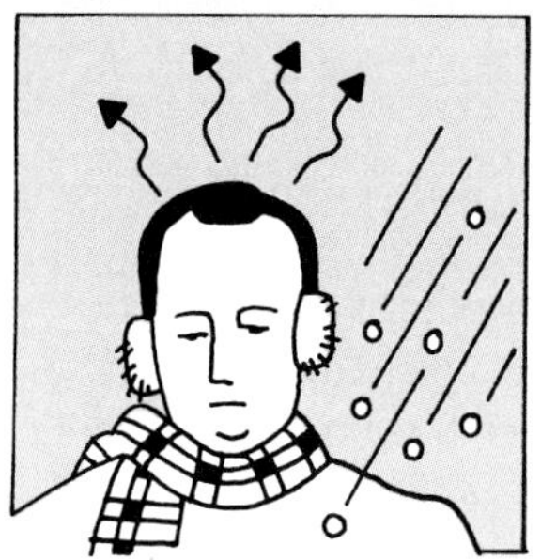	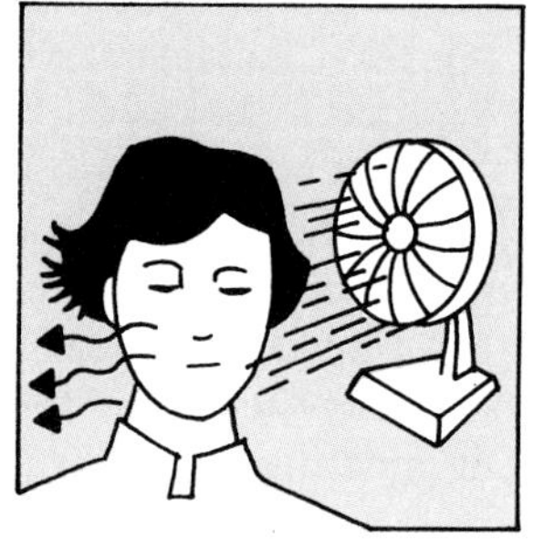	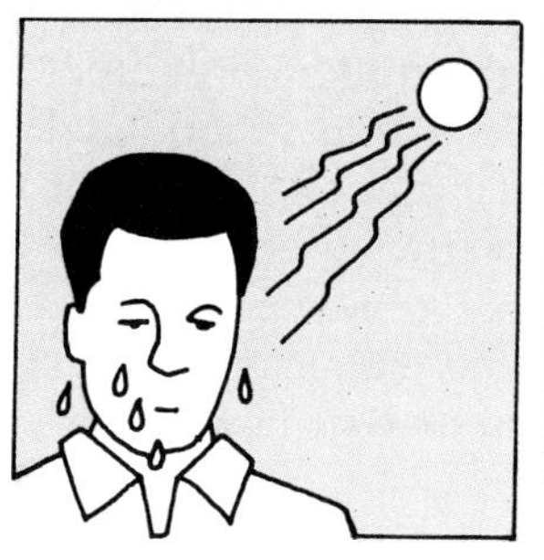	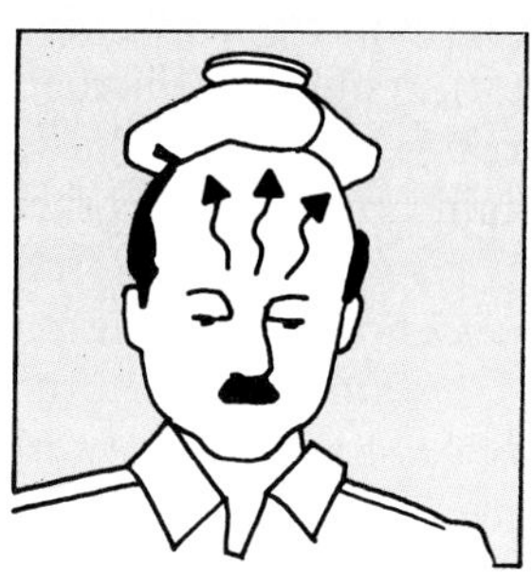

From Taylor, C., Lillis, C., & Le Mone, P. (1993). *Fundamentals of Nursing,* 2nd ed., p. 388. Philadelphia: J.B. Lippincott.

CENTIGRADE

35 37 39 41

RECTAL

35 37 39 41

ORAL

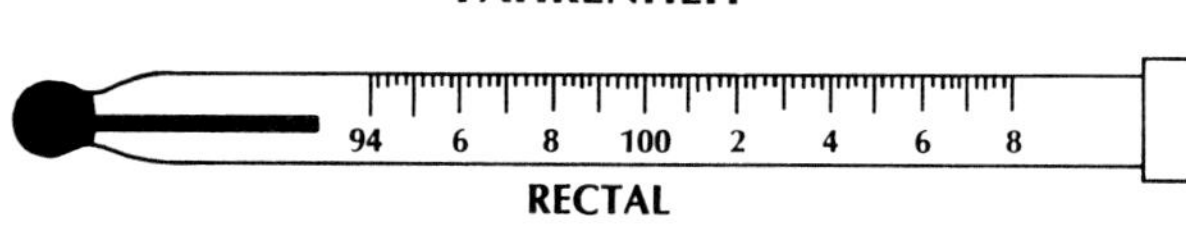

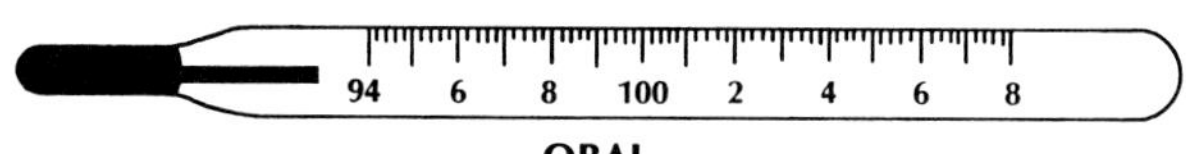

ORAL

Figure 3-3 The two glass thermometers on the top use the centigrade scale to measure temperature. The two on the bottom use the Fahrenheit scale. Note the blunt bulbs on the rectal thermometers and the long, thin bulbs on the oral thermometers.

Age—Children usually have a higher metabolism and therefore a higher body temperature than adults. The elderly, with slower metabolism, usually have lower readings than younger adults. Temperatures for both the very young and the very old are easily affected by the environment.

Gender or hormones—Women usually have a slightly higher temperature than men, especially at the time of ovulation.

Exercise—Activity raises the need for cellular metabolism, causing the body to respond by raising the temperature to burn more calories for energy.

Time of day or diurnal influences—The body temperature is usually lowest in the early morning before activity has begun.

Box 3-1
Temperature Comparisons

	Fahrenheit	*Centigrade*
Oral	98.6°	37.0°
Rectal	99.6°R	37.6°
Axillary	97.6°A	36.4°
Tympanic	98.6°T	37.0°

Emotions—Temperature tends to be higher during times of stress and lower with depression.

Illness—Most variations in temperature, either higher or lower than normal for the patient, are an indication of a disease process.

Stages of Fever

Fever has several clearly defined stages, as described below.

1. The *onset* may be abrupt or gradual.
2. The *course* or *stadium* will range from a day or so to several weeks. Fever may be *sustained* (constant), **remittent** (fluctuating), or **intermittent** (occurring at intervals). Table 3-2 describes and graphically illustrates these courses of fever. Fever may also be *relapsing* (return after an extended period of normal readings).
3. The *resolution,* or return to normal, may occur as either a crisis (abrupt return) or lysis (gradual return).

Checkpoint Question

2. *How does a child's normal body temperature differ from an adult's? Why?*

Types of Thermometers

Glass Mercury Thermometers

Oral, rectal, and axillary temperatures have traditionally been measured by the glass mercury thermometer. This thermometer is a glass tube divided into two major parts. The bulb end is filled with mercury and shaped in a long slender form for oral use, and a rounded stub form for rectal use. Heat expands the mercury, which rises in the glass column to measure degrees of temperature.

The major portion or glass stem of the Fahrenheit thermometer is calibrated with lines designating temperature in even degrees—94°, 96°, 98°, 100°, and so on. Uneven numbers are marked only with a longer line. Between these longer lines are four smaller lines designating temperature in 0.2°F increments. There-

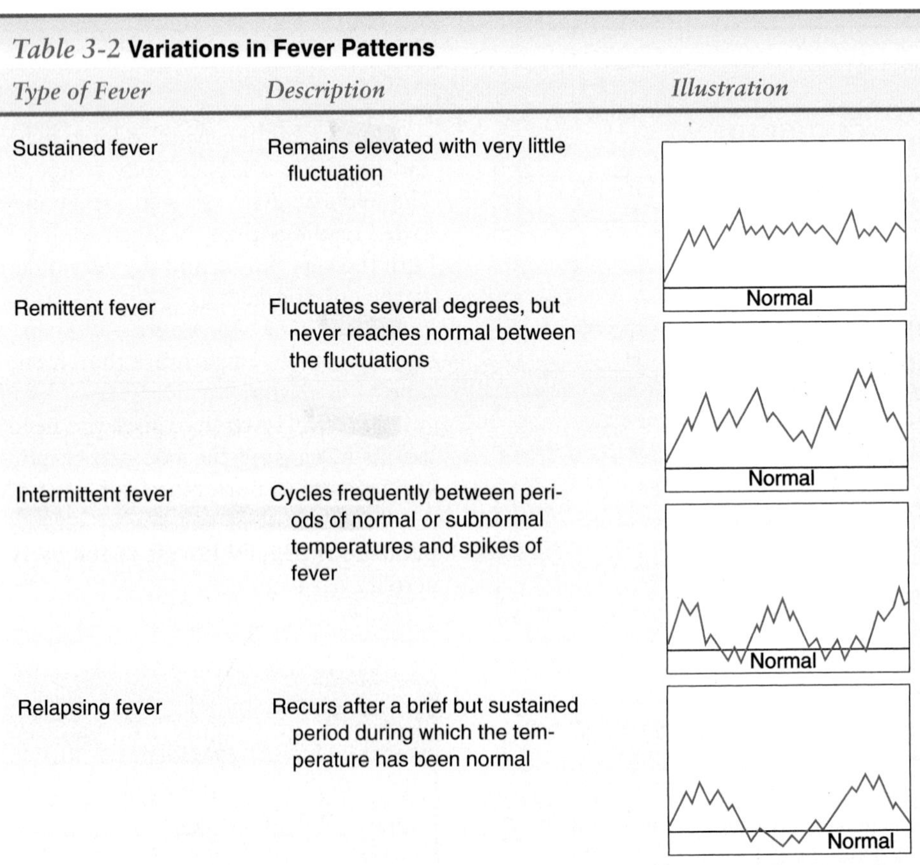

Table 3-2 **Variations in Fever Patterns**

Type of Fever	*Description*	*Illustration*
Sustained fever	Remains elevated with very little fluctuation	Normal
Remittent fever	Fluctuates several degrees, but never reaches normal between the fluctuations	Normal
Intermittent fever	Cycles frequently between periods of normal or subnormal temperatures and spikes of fever	Normal
Relapsing fever	Recurs after a brief but sustained period during which the temperature has been normal	Normal

From Timby, B. K. (1996). *Fundamental Skills and Concepts in Patient Care,* 6th ed., p. 147. Philadelphia: Lippincott-Raven.

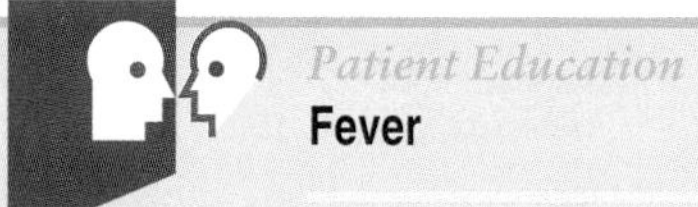

Patient Education

Fever

When instructing patients about fever, explain that current theories suggest that temperature elevations are a natural response to disease and that efforts to bring the temperature back to normal are counterproductive. However, if the patient is uncomfortable, or the temperature is abnormally high, it should be brought down to about 101°F. At 101°F, the body's natural defenses may still be able to destroy the pathogen without extreme discomfort to the patient.

After consulting with the physician, instruct all patients regarding the following comfort measures:

- Consume liquids to rehydrate the tissues. The liquids should be clear if nausea and vomiting are present.
- Keep clothing and bedding clean and dry, especially after **diaphoresis** (sweating).
- Avoid chilling. Chills bring on shivering, which raises the temperature to compensate.
- Rest and eat a light diet as tolerated.
- Use antipyretics to keep comfortable, but **do not** give aspirin to children younger than 18 years with viral fevers. Aspirin has been associated with Reye's syndrome, a potentially fatal disorder, following cases of varicella zoster (chickenpox) and viral illnesses.

fore, a large line marked 100 with the mercury falling on the second smaller line after it would read 100.4°F.

Some glass thermometers are color coded, with blue tips meaning oral use and red tips meaning rectal use. Some thermometers will have "rectal" or "oral" written on them or etched into the glass. Rectal and oral thermometers are never used interchangeably. Figure 3-4 shows oral and rectal thermometers.

Electronic Thermometers

Electronic thermometers use portable battery-operated units with sheath-covered probes (Fig. 3-5). The temperature is sensed and a digital read-out is given in the window of the hand-held base. Electronic thermometers are kept in a charging unit when not in use to ensure that the batteries are operative at all times. Most units can be used for either oral or rectal measurement but will have clearly marked probes to avoid errors.

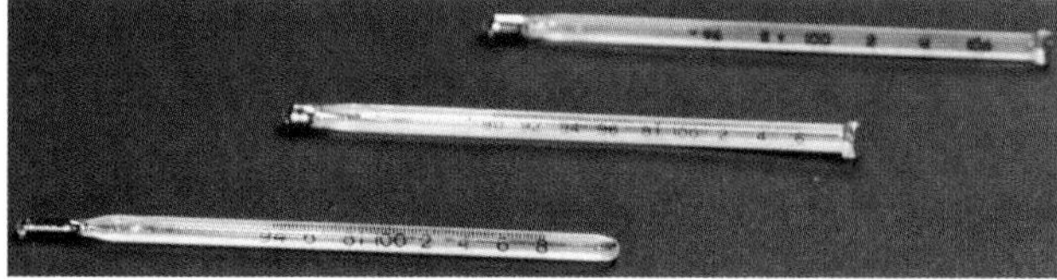

Figure 3-4 Glass mercury thermometers. Slender bulb, oral (*front*). Rounded stub, red tip, rectal (*center*). Rounded stub, blue tip, oral (*back*).

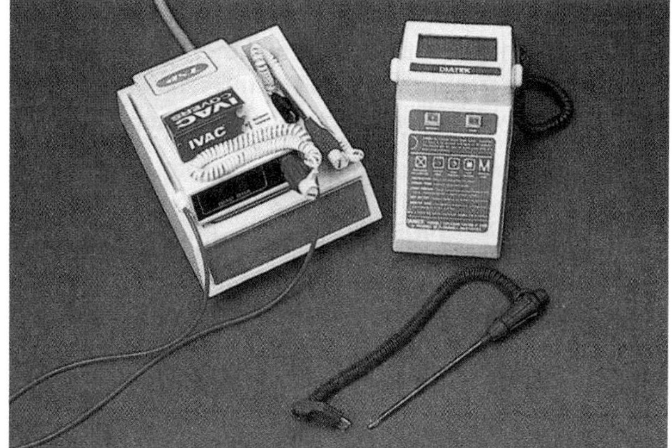

Figure 3-5 Two types of electronic thermometers and probes.

Tympanic Thermometers

The newest type of thermometer is the tympanic thermometer. This device is usually battery powered. It is fitted with a disposable cover and is inserted in the ear much like an otoscope (Fig. 3-6). A trigger is pulled or a button is pressed and an infrared light bounces off the tympanic membrane (eardrum), recording the body's temperature on the digital screen within 2 seconds. The sensor in a tympanic thermometer checks the temperature of the blood in the tympanic membrane on its way to the hypothalamus. Provided that a tight seal is formed by the thermometer against the ear canal, this is considered a highly reliable form of temperature measurement.

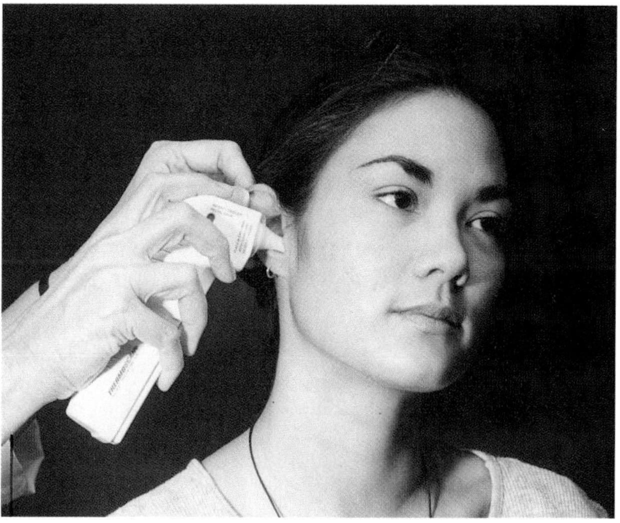

Figure 3-6 The tympanic thermometer in use.

Disposable Thermometers

Disposable, single-use thermometers register quickly with color changes on a strip (Fig. 3-7). Although many disposable thermometers are fairly accurate, they are not considered as reliable as either electronic or glass thermometers. Single-use patches or tapes are applied to the forehead or chest and register by changing colors on dots or stripes or by displaying an array of colors. They are not reliable for definitive measurement but are acceptable for screening in special circumstances, such as day-care centers or schools.

Oral Temperature

Measuring temperature orally is readily accepted by most patients. This method should not be used for patients after oral surgery, those with seizure disorders, mouth breathers, those receiving oxygen, or for small children. Some agencies provide clear plastic sheaths for glass thermometers; these are to be disposed of after the temperature has been taken. Check for integrity of the sheath before inserting the thermometer in the patient's mouth and dispose of properly after the procedure. Sheath designs vary somewhat; follow the manufacturer's directions for applying the sheath available at your facility (Fig. 3-8). Procedure 3-3 describes the steps for measuring oral temperature using a glass mercury thermometer. See Procedure 3-6 for taking an oral temperature electronically.

Rectal Temperature

The rectal temperature is thought to be more accurate than the oral temperature because of the closed, highly vascular environment of the rectal canal. This is the least acceptable method for patients and is not considered to be accurate if stool is present in the rectum. This method may never be used for patients closely following rectal surgery and is discouraged for patients with seizure disorders or cardiac disorders. The rectal method of measurement is not recommended for infants younger than 2 months to prevent potential damage to the rectal canal. Unless properly performed, there is the danger of rectal perforation. Procedure 3-4 outlines the steps for measuring rectal temperature using a glass mercury thermometer. See Procedure 3-6 for taking a rectal temperature electronically.

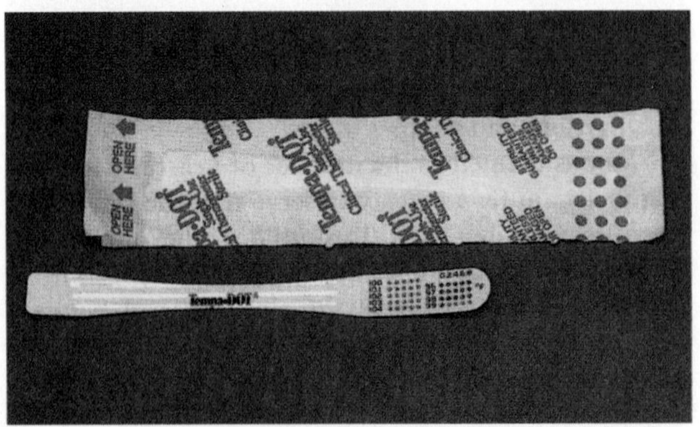

Figure 3-7 Disposable paper thermometer. The dots change color to indicate temperature.

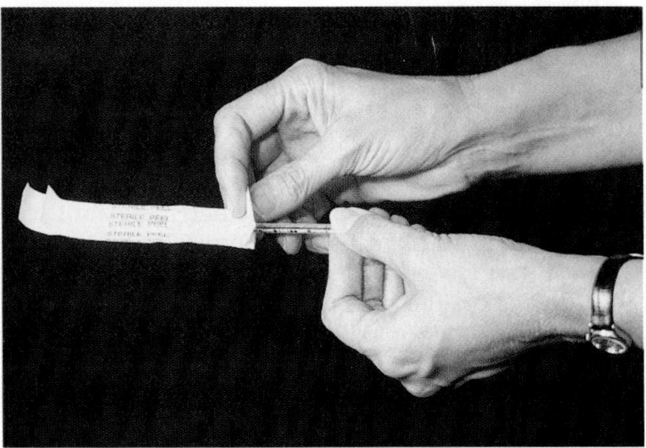

Figure 3-8 Standard thermometer sheaths are applied by inserting the bulb end into the indicated opening and removing the paper cover as directed.

Axillary Temperature

If performed properly, axillary measurements are considered to be very accurate. This method of measurement is becoming more acceptable to the medical profession and always has been preferred by patients who were unable to use the oral site. It is safe, and there is less chance of the transfer of microorganisms. It may be used for children, especially infants younger than 2 months; mouth breathers; patients receiving oxygen; postoperatively for patients who have undergone oral surgery; or in any instance where the oral route is contraindicated. Procedure 3-5 explains how to measure axillary temperature using a glass mercury thermometer. See Procedure 3-6 for measuring axillary temperature electronically.

Tympanic Temperature

Temperatures taken via the tympanic route are noninvasive and are readily acceptable to patients. In addition, the site is easily accessible. For these reasons, this route is rapidly becoming the route of choice. Procedure 3-7 outlines the steps for assessing temperature using a tympanic thermometer.

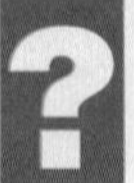

Checkpoint Question

3. *Why would a tympanic membrane temperature be more accurate than an axillary?*

Procedure 3-3 Measuring Oral Temperature Using a Glass Mercury Thermometer

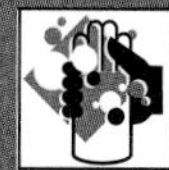
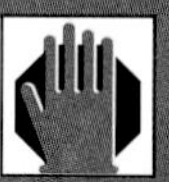

PURPOSE:

To evaluate the degree of heat produced and lost by the body as a basis for assessing the patient's health status

EQUIPMENT/SUPPLIES

- glass mercury thermometer designed for oral use
- tissues or cotton balls
- disposable plastic sheath (if used)
- gloves

3 minutes

3

STEPS

1. Wash your hands.
   Handwashing promotes infection control.
2. Assemble the equipment and supplies. Check the thermometer for chips or cracks.
   This ensures that everything you need is available. A safety check prevents patient injury.
3. Greet and identify the patient. Explain the procedure. Check for recent eating, drinking, gum chewing, or smoking.
   Identifying the patient prevents errors in treatment. Explaining the procedure helps ease anxiety and ensure compliance. Recent eating, drinking, gum chewing, or smoking may alter the reading for oral temperature.
4. Rinse and dry the thermometer if it has been stored in solution. Wipe it from bulb to stem.
   Chemical disinfectants can be irritating to the oral mucosa. Always wipe from the cleanest to the less clean area.
5. Read the thermometer by holding it by the stem horizontal to your face and turning it slowly to see the mercury column.
   It will be easier to see the column in this position. The thermometer should not be held by the bulb, which will be inserted in the patient's mouth.
6. If the mercury registers above 94°F, grasp the thermometer by the stem with the thumb and forefinger and snap the wrist quickly several times to shake the mercury down to about 94°F. Avoid hitting the thermometer against anything.
   The mercury must be below the lowest mark to register correctly. Glass thermometers are fragile and break easily.
7. If using a clear plastic sheath, cover the thermometer now.
   Sheaths reduce the number of microorganisms on the thermometer. Follow package instructions for application.
8. Put on gloves.
   Standard Precautions must be followed when there is potential exposure to body fluids.
9. Place the thermometer under the tongue to either side of the frenulum.
   This is the area of the highest vascularity and will give the most accurate reading.

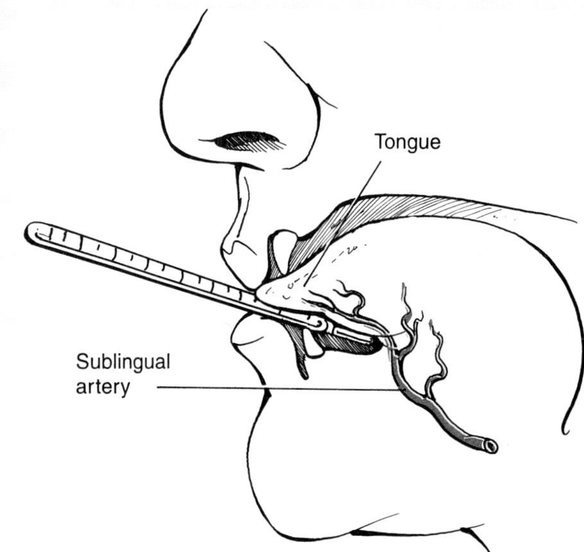

10. Tell the patient to keep his or her mouth closed but caution against biting down on the glass column.
    The reading will be inaccurate if air is entering the mouth. Biting down on the thermometer may cause it to break.

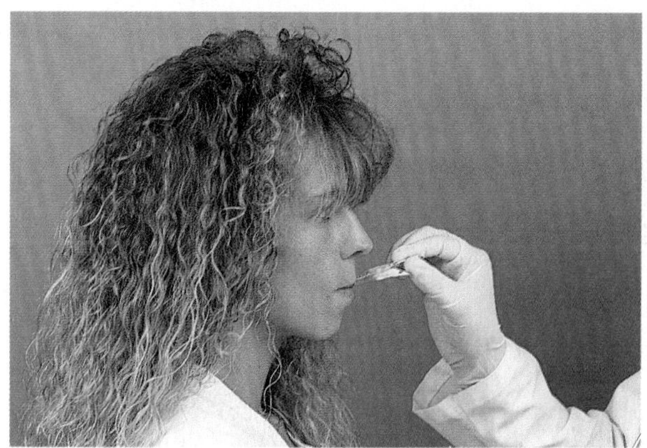

continued

Procedure 3-3 Continued — Measuring Oral Temperature Using a Glass Mercury Thermometer

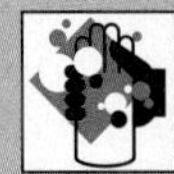
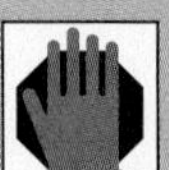

11. Leave the thermometer in place for 3–5 minutes. *Note:* The pulse and respirations may be taken at this time. (See Procedure 3-9, Procedure 3-10, and Procedure 3-11)

The thermometer may be left in place for 3 minutes if there is no evidence of fever and the patient is compliant. It should be left in for 5 minutes if the patient is febrile or noncompliant.

12. Remove the thermometer after the prescribed time. Remove and discard the sheath (if used) in an appropriate container or wipe the thermometer with a clean tissue or cotton ball from stem to bulb.

If the sheath remains on or if mucus is present, either may obscure the column. Wipe from clean to less clean.

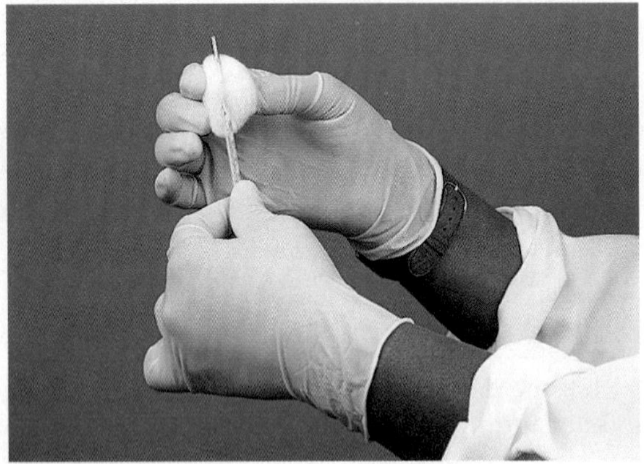

13. Hold the thermometer as before and note the reading.

14. Thank the patient and provide appropriate instructions.

Courtesy encourages the patient to have a positive attitude about the physician's office.

15. Disinfect the thermometer according to the facility's policy. Remove gloves. Wash your hands.

This prevents the spread of microorganisms.

DOCUMENTATION GUIDELINES

- Date and time
- Patient complaints/concerns
- Temperature, indicate by mouth (O), if necessary
- Other vitals as needed or required by office protocol
- Patient education/instructions
- Your signature

Charting Example

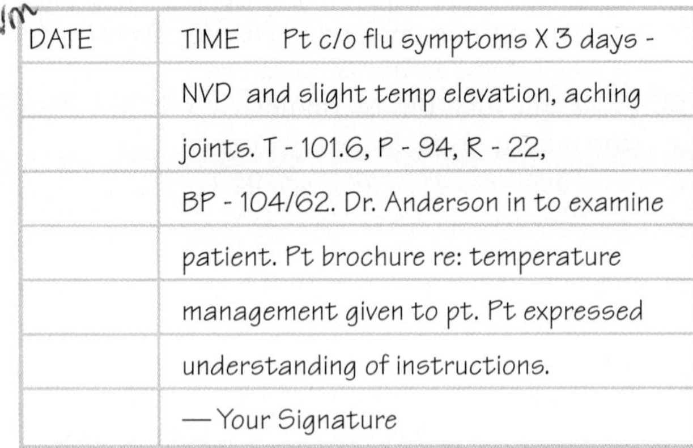

DATE	TIME Pt c/o flu symptoms X 3 days -
	NVD and slight temp elevation, aching
	joints. T - 101.6, P - 94, R - 22,
	BP - 104/62. Dr. Anderson in to examine
	patient. Pt brochure re: temperature
	management given to pt. Pt expressed
	understanding of instructions.
	— Your Signature

Note: *Thermometers are usually provided in the system of measurement preferred by the physician. If conversion from Fahrenheit to Celsius, or vice versa, is necessary, use this rule:*

Celsius to Fahrenheit: Multiply the number of degrees Celsius by 9/5 and add 32 to the result.

Fahrenheit to Celsius: Subtract 32 from the number of degrees Fahrenheit and multiply the difference by 5/9.

Cleaning Thermometers

After use, thermometers must be sanitized and disinfected for the next patient. Electronic units and tympanic thermometers only need to be wiped down with disinfectant during environmental cleaning. Glass thermometers must be thoroughly disinfected (Procedure 3-8). During the disinfecting process, check all equipment for safety and function. Check the glass thermometer for chips or cracks, for example. Check the electronic base for malfunction.

In addition to cleaning thermometers, medical assistants are often responsible for disinfecting the instrument trays used for storing thermometers or the special thermometer containers. These must be washed with hot soapy water and dried thoroughly. Some facilities will recommend daily autoclaving. The containers are then refilled with the proper freshly prepared solution or the disinfected thermometers may be stored in a dry container. It is customary to place a gauze sponge in the bottom of instrument trays to avoid damage to the glass instruments.

text continues on page 58

Procedure 3-4 Measuring Rectal Temperature Using a Glass Mercury Thermometer

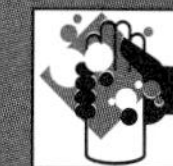
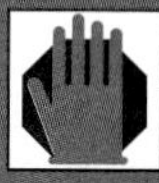

PURPOSE:

To evaluate the degree of heat produced and lost in patients for whom other methods of measurement are contraindicated

EQUIPMENT/SUPPLIES

- glass mercury thermometer designed for rectal use
- surgical lubricant
- tissues
- disposable plastic sheath
- gloves

STEPS

1–7. Follow steps 1–7 as described in Procedure 3-3.

8. Spread lubricant onto a tissue, then from the tissue to the thermometer. Put on gloves.

Never lubricate directly from the tube to avoid the spread of pathogens that might be present on the thermometer. Lubricants must be used for rectal insertion to avoid patient discomfort. Gloves are required under Standard Precautions when there is potential exposure to body fluids or excretions.

9. Ensure privacy. Place the patient in a side-lying position facing toward the examination room door. Drape appropriately.

This procedure may embarrass the patient. If the door is opened inadvertently, it will be less embarrassing if the patient is facing the door with less chance of exposure. The patient must be side-lying to expose the anus.

10. Expose only the buttock area. With the nondominant hand, lift the topmost buttock. Visualize the anus.

Never expose the patient unnecessarily. Never insert the thermometer without a clear view of the anus.

11. Touch the thermometer to the anus lightly. The anus will usually reflexively tighten against the intrusion. When the anus relaxes, insert the thermometer gently past the sphincter. Have the patient breathe deeply with the mouth opened.

Never force the thermometer; forcing may perforate the rectal canal. Breathing through the mouth will relax the patient.

12. Insert the thermometer about 1½ inches for an adult, 1 inch for a child, and ½ inch for an infant older than 2 months. *Note:* Infants younger than 2 months should have temperatures taken by the tympanic or axillary method to avoid damage to the rectal canal.

These depths make it less likely that the rectal canal will be perforated.

13. Release the upper buttock and drape the sheet back over the patient. Hold the thermometer in place for 3 minutes.

The patient must be covered for privacy. The thermometer will not stay in place if not held.

14. At the end of 3 minutes, remove the thermometer. Offer the patient a tissue for cleaning or assist as needed. Remove the sheath by turning it inside out as it is pulled from the thermometer. Wipe the thermometer from stem to bulb. Discard sheath in appropriate container.

The patient may be uncomfortable with extra lubricant around the anal area. Lubricant or the sheath will obscure the mercury column. Turning the sheath inside out will reduce the transmission of pathogens.

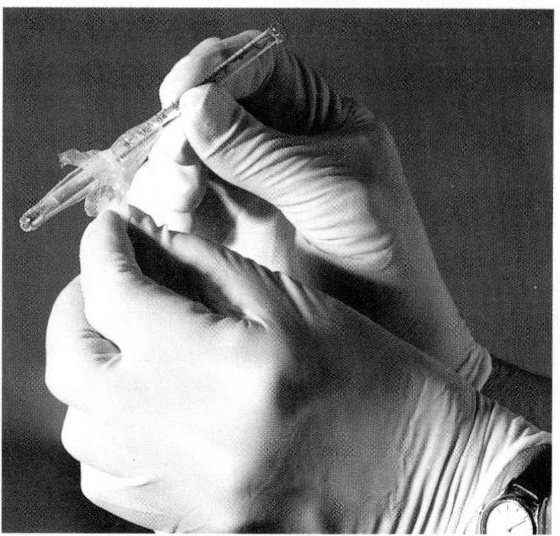

15. Note the reading. Remove and dispose of gloves. Wash your hands.

Hands are washed after removing gloves to prevent the spread of microorganisms.

continued

Procedure 3-4 Continued Measuring Rectal Temperature Using a Glass Mercury Thermometer

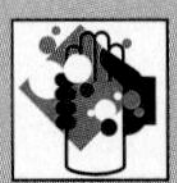
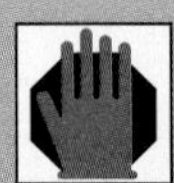

3

16. Thank the patient and provide appropriate instructions.

Courtesy encourages the patient to have a positive attitude about the physician's office.

17. Disinfect thermometer according to the facility's policy. Wash your hands.

This prevents the spread of microorganisms.

DOCUMENTATION GUIDELINES

- Date and time
- Patient complaints/concerns
- Temperature, indicate rectal (R)
- Other vitals as needed or required by office protocol
- Patient education/instructions
- Your signature

Charting Example

DATE	TIME 2½ y/o /c hx of exposure to
	chicken-pox. Mother concerned re: rash
	over trunk × 2 days. Child fussy and
	feverish × 3 days. T - 101.4 (R), P - 114
	(A), R - 30. Dr. Royal in to check child.
	Mother given pediatric temperature
	management brochure, expressed under-
	standing of instructions. Your Signature

Note: Infants older than 2 months and very small children may be held in the lap or over the knees for this procedure or may remain on the examining table with the parent close by. Hold the thermometer and the buttocks with the dominant hand while securing the child with the nondominant hand. If the child moves with the thermometer in place, the thermometer and the hand will move together with the buttocks and avoid perforating the rectal canal.

Procedure 3-5 Measuring Axillary Temperature Using a Glass Mercury Thermometer

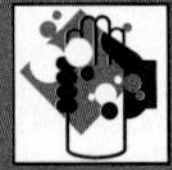

PURPOSE:

To evaluate the degree of heat produced and lost in patients for whom other methods of measurement are contraindicated

EQUIPMENT/SUPPLIES

- glass mercury thermometer (either oral or rectal, according to facility's policy)
- tissues or cotton balls
- sheaths if used

STEPS

1–7. Follow steps 1–7 as directed in Procedure 3-3.

8. Expose the axillary area. Do not expose more of the patient's chest or upper body than is necessary to ensure the proper placement of the thermometer.

The patient's privacy must be observed.

9. Dry the axilla with patting motions.

Friction will increase the surface temperature. The axilla should be dry to remove perspiration, which may cause the thermometer to slip.

continued

Procedure 3-5 Continued Measuring Axillary Temperature Using a Glass Mercury Thermometer

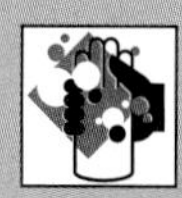

10. Place the bulb of the thermometer well into the axilla. Close the arm down over the axilla and cross the forearm over the chest. Drape the clothes or gown over the patient for privacy.

This position offers the best exposure to the mercury column and maintains a closed environment. The patient should never be exposed unnecessarily.

11. Leave the thermometer in place for 10 minutes. Stay with the patient.

Axillary temperatures take longer to register than oral or rectal. Staying with the patient ensures compliance.

12. Remove the thermometer after the prescribed time. Remove the sheath or clean from stem to bulb. Note the reading.

Clean the thermometer of any surface dirt or perspiration before reading. Clean from the cleanest area to the less clean.

13. Thank the patient and provide appropriate instructions.

Courtesy encourages the patient to have a positive attitude about the physician's office.

14. Disinfect the thermometer according to the facility's policy. Wash your hands.

This prevents the spread of microorganisms.

DOCUMENTATION GUIDELINES

- Date and time
- Patient complaints/concerns
- Temperature, indicate axillary (A)
- Other vitals as needed or required by office protocol
- Patient education/instructions
- Your signature

Charting Example

DATE	TIME
	S - Mother states 8 m/o congested × 3
	days. Tugging at ear × 1 day, fussy
	since last PM
	O - T - 100.6 (A), P - 124 (A), R - 32
	A - Febrile child
	P - Dr. Smythe in to check patient.
	—Your Signature

Note: This is an excellent method for assessing a child's temperature but is time consuming and requires that the child remain still. Have the parent hold the child with the arm holding the thermometer against the parent's body to keep the thermometer in place. The parent may read to the child during this time or may give the child a bottle if appropriate. This is the preferred method for assessing the temperature of patients younger than 2 months to avoid damage to the rectal canal.

Procedure 3-6 Measuring Temperature Using an Electronic Thermometer

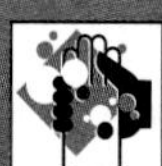
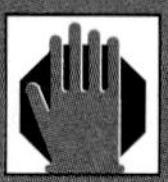

PURPOSE:

To evaluate the degree of heat produced and lost by the body as a basis for assessing the patient's health status

EQUIPMENT/SUPPLIES

- battery-powered unit with probes and covers
- gloves
- lubricant (for rectal temperature)

STEPS

1. Wash your hands.

Handwashing promotes infection control.

2. Assemble the equipment and supplies.

This ensures that everything you need is available.

3. Greet and identify the patient. Explain the procedure.

Identifying the patient prevents errors. Explaining the procedure helps ease anxiety and ensure compliance.

continued

3

Procedure 3-6 Continued Measuring Temperature Using an Electronic Thermometer

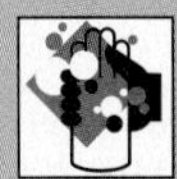
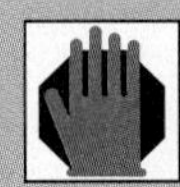

4. Choose the method most appropriate for the particular patient (eg, oral, rectal, axillary) and cover the probe to be used. Almost all units have one probe for oral and one for rectal. Covers are carried with the unit in a specially fitted box attached to the back of the unit. Put on gloves.

Comply with the facility's policy for the appropriate method for each patient. Standard Precautions must be observed when there is potential exposure to body fluids.

5. Place the thermometer as described for measuring an oral temperature (Procedure 3-3), rectal temperature (Procedure 3-4), or axillary temperature (Procedure 3-5).

6. If taking an oral temperature, help the patient hold the probe. If taking a rectal temperature, you must hold the probe.

The electronic probe is heavier than the glass thermometer and is harder for patients to hold in place. Taking a rectal temperature always requires that the assistant hold the thermometer in place.

7. Note that the electronic unit will emit a beep when the temperature shows no signs of rising beyond a certain point. This will usually be within 20–60 seconds.

8. Remove the probe. Note the reading; most will retain the reading until the probe is reinserted into the unit.

9. Discard the probe cover in a waste receptacle. If this was a rectal temperature, help the patient to clean away any remaining lubricant. Remove gloves. Wash your hands.

The probe cover will be contaminated and must be disposed of properly. Hands must be washed after removing gloves to avoid the spread of pathogens.

10. Thank the patient and provide appropriate instructions.

Courtesy encourages the patient to have a positive attitude about the physician's office.

11. Return the unit to the charging base.

The unit must be kept charged and ready for use.

DOCUMENTATION GUIDELINES

- Date and time
- Patient complaints/concerns
- Temperature, indicate axillary (A), oral (O), or rectal (R)
- Other vitals as needed or required by office protocol
- Patient education/instructions
- Your signature

Charting Example

DATE	TIME
	S: Pt c/o sore throat × 2 days, feels T
	may be elevated. Has Rxed/c OTC
	lozenges and ASA.
	O: T - 101.4 (A), P - 96, R - 24, BP - 122/74.
	Skin warm and flushed.
	A: Febrile pt
	P: Dr. Rogers in to see pt. Your Signature

Note: Electronic thermometers do not require the time limits set for glass thermometers. Most will provide a reading in well under 60 seconds.

Procedure 3-7 Measuring Temperature Using a Tympanic Thermometer

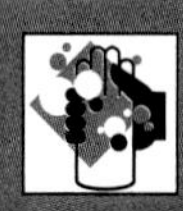

PURPOSE:

To evaluate the degree of heat produced and lost by the body as a basis for assessing the patient's health status

EQUIPMENT/SUPPLIES

- tympanic thermometer
- disposable probe covers

3

STEPS

1. Wash your hands.
   Handwashing promotes infection control.
2. Assemble the equipment and supplies.
   This ensures that everything you need is available.
3. Greet and identify the patient. Explain the procedure.
   Identifying the patient prevents errors. Explain the procedure to ease anxiety and ensure compliance.
4. Remove the tympanic thermometer from the base and put the disposable cover on the probe.
5. Insert the probe, sealing the opening of the ear canal. Press the button to take the temperature, which will be displayed on the digital screen in about 2 seconds.

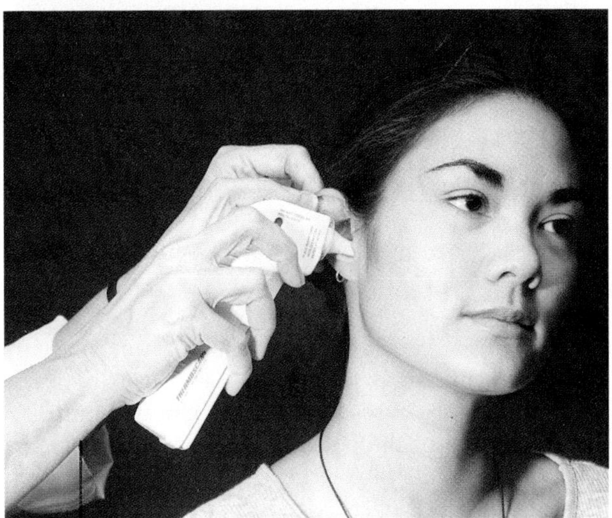

6. Remove the probe and note the reading. Discard the probe cover in a waste receptacle.
   The probe cover will be contaminated and must be disposed of properly.
7. Thank the patient and provide appropriate instructions.
   Courtesy encourages the patient to have a positive attitude about the physician's office.
8. Return the unit to the base.
   The unit must be kept charged and ready for use.

DOCUMENTATION GUIDELINES

- Date and time
- Patient complaints/concerns
- Temperature, indicate tympanic (T)
- Other vitals as needed or required by office protocol
- Patient education/instructions
- Your signature

Charting Example

DATE	TIME Mother reports 8 m/o BF list-
	less and feverish since last PM. Appetite
	poor × 2 days. Several loose stools
	but no watery stools. No vomiting. Skin
	flushed and moist. T - 101.3 (T),
	P - 114 (A), R - 30. Weight 20¾ lbs (last
	wt 19½ lbs 5 wks ago). Dr. Gay in to see
	patient. Mother given pt ed brochure for
	temp management and warning signs
	to report. Verbalized understanding of
	instructions. — Your Signature

Procedure 3-8 Disinfecting a Glass Thermometer

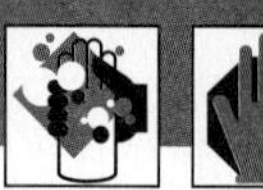

PURPOSE:

To eliminate surface pathogens and to avoid the spread of microorganisms between patients

EQUIPMENT/SUPPLIES

- thermometer to be disinfected
- soft tissue or cotton ball
- disinfectant soap
- soaking solution in basin or container

STEPS

1. Put on gloves.
   Gloves prevent the spread of infection.
2. Wipe the thermometer with a soft tissue or cotton ball from stem to bulb with a rotating friction.
   A soft material will remove more surface substances than a firmer material such as a paper towel. Friction will dislodge most substances. Wipe all surfaces from the cleanest area to the less clean.
3. Rub the thermometer briskly with cool or tepid soapy water.
   Water that is too warm causes mercury to rise too quickly and may damage the thermometer. Water that is too cool is not as effective as tepid water. Soap dissolves fats and oils that remain on the surface.
4. Rinse with cool water.
   The soap residue must be removed before placing in a soaking solution.
5. Dry well.
   Moisture left on the thermometer will dilute the soaking solution and render it ineffective.
6. Place in the disinfectant soaking solution of choice, such as 70% alcohol.
   Heat disinfection cannot be used with thermometers.
7. After the prescribed period of time for the soaking solution of choice, remove the thermometer, rinse and store in a covered instrument tray padded with gauze to prevent chipping.
   Chemicals left on the thermometer may irritate the patient's mucosa. Instructions will be provided with the solution stating the time for disinfection to occur; these times must be carefully observed.

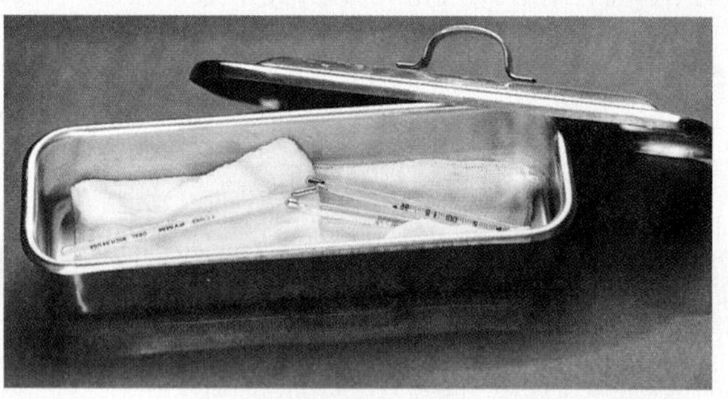

Note: Clean and disinfect the soaking basin and storage tray daily using hot soapy water. Many facilities suggest daily autoclaving as well.

PULSE (P)

As the heart beats, it forces blood into the arteries causing them to expand. As the heart relaxes, the arteries relax. Each heartbeat is counted at the point of expansion of the artery.

Although every artery in the body has a pulse, the pulse usually is measured only at a point where an artery may be pressed against a bone or other underlying firm surface. These are called pulse points.

There are several pulse points at which the heartbeat can be palpated (felt) or auscultated (heard). From head to foot, these are temporal, facial, carotid, apical, brachial, radial, femoral, popliteal, posterior tibialis, and dorsalis pedis. Figure 3-9 shows some of these pulse sites. The apical pulse usually cannot be palpated unless the patient has a circulatory abnormality, but it is easily auscultated and is considered the most accurate measurement. All of the others listed usually are palpated or may be auscultated with a Doppler unit.

Palpation of the pulse is performed by placing the index and middle finger, the middle finger and ring finger, or all three fingers, over a pulse point (Fig. 3-10). Auscultation usually requires a stethoscope to hear the pulse or a Doppler unit to broadcast the sound. For apical auscultation, the bell of the stethoscope is placed over the apex of the heart and the beats are counted for 1 minute.

Characteristics

Although you will know the terms that apply to the measurements of the pulse, it is not within the scope of practice for medical assistants to diagnose the read-

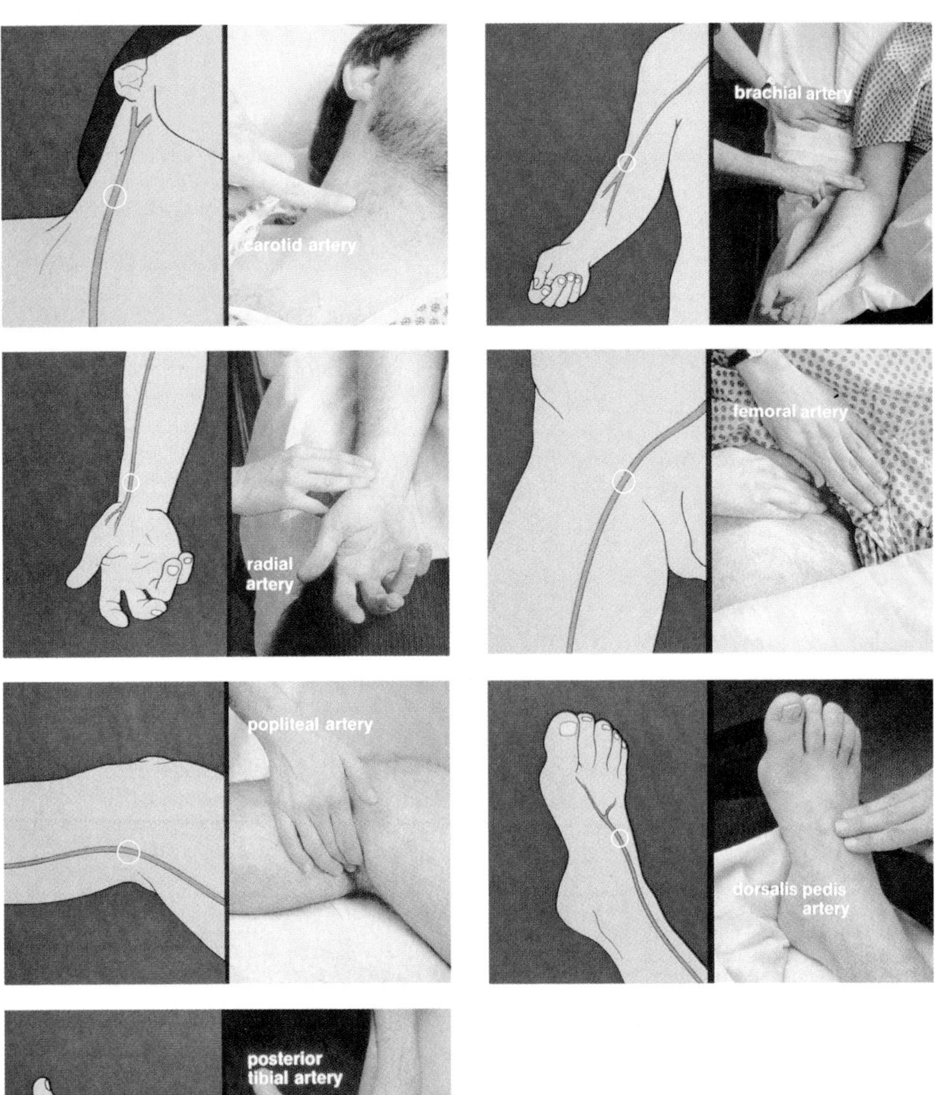

Figure 3-9 Sites for palpation of peripheral pulses (Lippincott Learning Systems).

ings. Observations will be made about the characteristics of the pulse. However, the rate should never be listed as bradycardia, a pulse of less than 60 beats per minute (bpm or beats/min), or tachycardia (an adult pulse of more than 100 bpm). Only the number should be listed with observations regarding the characteristics. The characteristics of the pulse to be assessed are rate, rhythm, and volume.

Rate is defined as the number of heartbeats occurring in 1 minute. You may observe that the rate is fast (rapid) or slow but should record only the number and let the physician diagnose beyond that point.

Rhythm is defined as the time interval between each heartbeat or the pattern of the beats. In the normal heartbeat, this pattern will be regular. A regular heartbeat will be recorded as such; an irregular beat will be recorded as irregular.

Volume is defined as the strength or force of the heartbeat and can be described as soft, bounding, weak, thready, feeble, strong, or full.

3

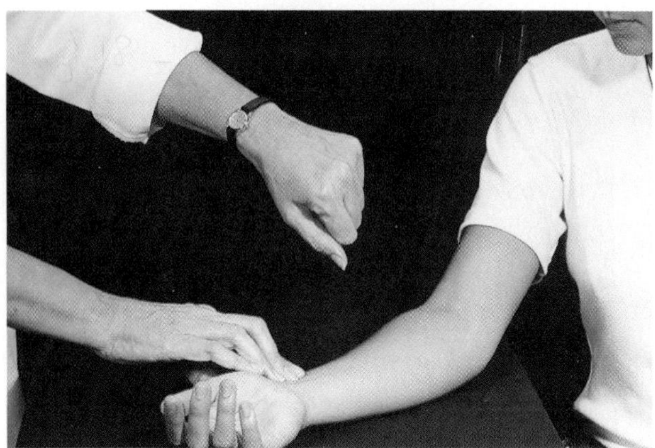

Figure 3-10 Measuring a radial pulse.

Averages and Ranges

In the healthy adult, the average pulse rate is 70 to 80 bpm. With other ages, there is a large variance of pulse rates as shown in Table 3-3.

Factors Affecting Pulse Rates

Many factors affect the force, speed, and rhythm of the heart. As noted in Table 3-3, young children and infants normally have a much faster heart rate than adults. It is not unusual for a conditioned athlete to present with a normal heart rate below 60 bpm. Older adults may very well exhibit an increased heart rate as the myocardium begins to compensate for decreased efficiency. Other factors that affect pulse rates are listed in Table 3-4.

The pulse is counted most often at the radial point for convenience and because most patients prefer this site (Procedure 3-9). If the radial pulse is irregular or hard to count or if cardiac disease is present, the apical pulse is the site of choice for pulse measurement (Procedure 3-10).

Note: Some peripheral pulses are counted using a Doppler ultrasound unit. The unit may be attached to earpieces such as found on stethoscopes so that only you can hear the pulse, or it may be set to broadcast the sound for counting purposes. These devices are battery powered. Follow these steps to use a Doppler unit:

1. Use a coupling or transmission gel on the probe to make an airtight seal and to promote ultrasound transmission.
2. With the machine "on," hold the probe at a 45-degree angle with light pressure to ensure contact but to avoid obliterating the pulse (Fig. 3-11). Arteries are usually loud with a pumping sound; veins have a lighter, whooshing sound.
3. If the vein sound interferes with the measurement, reposition the probe until the artery sound is dominant.
4. Assess the rate, rhythm, and volume and record.
5. Clean the patient's skin and the machine probe with warm water to remove the coupling gel.

Table 3-3 **Variations in Pulse Rates by Age**

Age	*Beats per Minute*
Birth to 1 y	110–170
1–10 y	90–110
10–16 y	80–95
16 y to midlife	70–80
Elderly adult	55–70

Table 3-4 **Factors Affecting Pulse Rates**

Factor	*Effect*
Time of day	The pulse is usually lower early in the morning than later in the day.
Gender	Women have a slightly higher pulse rate than men.
Body type and size	Tall, thin people usually have a lower pulse rate than shorter, stockier people.
Exercise	The heart rate increases with the need for increased cardiac output (amount of blood ejected from either ventricle per minute).
Stress or emotions	Anger, fear, excitement, and stress will raise the pulse; depression will lower it.
Fever	The increased need for cell metabolism in the presence of fever raises the cardiac output to supply oxygen and nutrients; the pulse may rise as much as 10 bpm per degree of fever.
Medications	Many medications raise or lower the pulse as a desired effect or an undesirable side effect.
Blood volume	Hemorrhage or loss of blood volume as in dehydration or loss of tissue fluid will increase the need for cellular metabolism and will increase the cardiac output to supply the need.

Checkpoint Question

4. *When measuring a patient's pulse, what characteristics are to be assessed? Briefly explain each.*

Procedure 3-9 Measuring the Radial Pulse

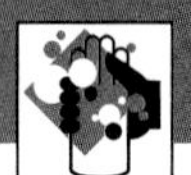

PURPOSE:

To detect the presence of possible pathologic cardiac disorders

EQUIPMENT/SUPPLIES

- watch with sweep second hand or other means of measuring seconds

3

STEPS

1. Wash your hands.
Handwashing promotes infection control.

2. Assemble the equipment.
This ensures that everything you need is available.

3. Greet and identify the patient. Explain the procedure.
Identifying the patient prevents errors. Explain the procedure to ease anxiety and ensure compliance.

4. Place the patient in a seated or supine position with the arm relaxed and supported.
If the arm is not supported and relaxed, or patient is uncomfortable, the pulse count may be affected.

5. With the index, middle, and ring fingers of the dominant hand, use the fingertips to press firmly enough to feel the pulse, but gently enough not to obliterate it.
The fingertips have greater sensitivity than other portions of the fingers. Using more than one finger increases the chance of finding the pulse. Avoid using the thumb; it has a slight pulse of its own and may be confused with the patient's. The thumb may be used on the opposite side of the patient's hand to steady the patient's hand and yours.

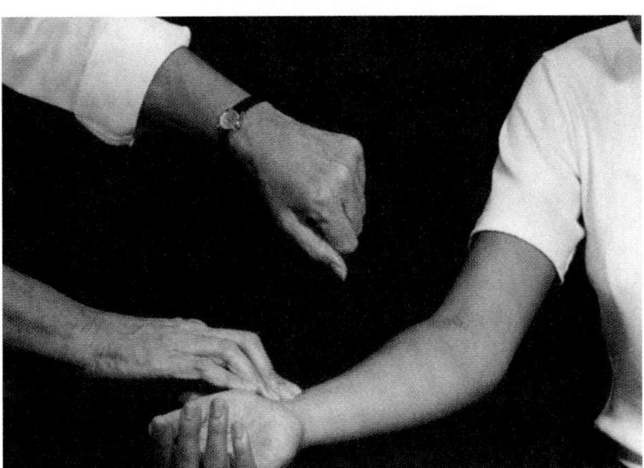

6. If the pulse is regular, count for 30 seconds and multiply by two. If this is a baseline pulse or if it is irregular, count for a full 60 seconds.
Counting an irregular pulse for less than 60 seconds will not give an accurate measurement. You may check at other sites if unsure of the assessment.

DOCUMENTATION GUIDELINES

- Date and time
- Patient complaints/concerns
- Heart rate at radius, rhythm, and volume
- Other observations appropriate to assessment of the cardiovascular system, such as skin color and skin temperature
- Other vital signs as needed or required by office protocol
- Your signature

Charting Example

DATE	TIME Pt c/o periods of racing heart-
	beats. Color pink, skin cool and dry, no
	apparent distress. P - 96 at radius, 96
	at apex, BP 114/82. Dr. Perkins notified.
	— Your Signature

Procedure 3-10 Measuring the Apical Pulse

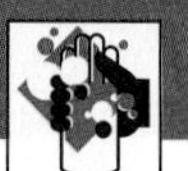

PURPOSE:

To detect the presence of possible pathologic cardiac disorders if measurement of the radial pulse is contraindicated or is not adequate

EQUIPMENT/SUPPLIES

- stethoscope
- watch with sweep second hand or other means of measuring seconds

3

STEPS

1. Wash your hands.

   Handwashing promotes infection control.

2. Assemble the equipment. Ensure that the stethoscope has clean earpieces.

   This ensures that everything you need is available. Dirty earpieces may spread disease.

3. Greet and identify the patient. Explain the procedure.

   Identifying the patient prevents errors. Explaining the procedure helps ease anxiety and ensure compliance.

4. Place the patient in a comfortable sitting or supine position. Remove the upper clothing or open sufficiently to allow access to the chest wall. Drape for privacy with a gown or sheet.

   If the patient is uncomfortable, the pulse rate may be affected. If clothing interferes with sound transmission or placement of the stethoscope, an inaccurate reading may result. Privacy for the patient must be ensured.

5. Locate the apex of the heart by palpating to the fifth intercostal space, between the fifth and sixth ribs. Move laterally to the left along the intercostal space to the nipple line or the midclavicular line.

   This will locate the cardiac apex where the sound is usually heard the loudest.

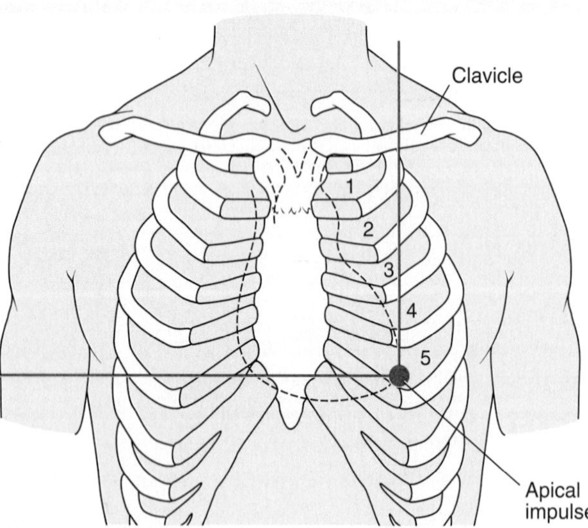

6. Clean the stethoscope diaphragm with alcohol and warm it in the palm of your hand.

   The stethoscope head should be cleaned between patients to avoid the spread of microorganisms. A cold stethoscope may cause the patient to be uncomfortable and may cause the heart rate to speed.

7. Insert the earpieces into the ear canals with the openings pointing slightly forward. A Doppler unit may also be used to broadcast the sound.

   The ear canal in adults angles slightly forward. Inserting the earpieces to follow the line of the canal will make it easier to hear. Broadcasting the sound will allow more than one worker to assess the pulse.

8. Position the stethoscope or Doppler unit until the sound is heard clearly. Listen for the S_1 and S_2 (sinus) sounds that will sound like "lubb, dubb." Together, they count as one beat.

   The "lubb" sound is made when the atrioventricular valves close; the "dubb" sound is made when the semilunar valves close.

9. Count for 1 full minute.

   If the heart rate must be counted by the apical pulse, it usually means that cardiovascular pathology is present and a full minute will be needed to assess the count properly.

continued

Procedure 3-10 Continued Measuring the Apical Pulse

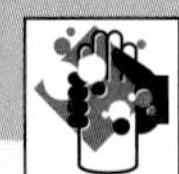

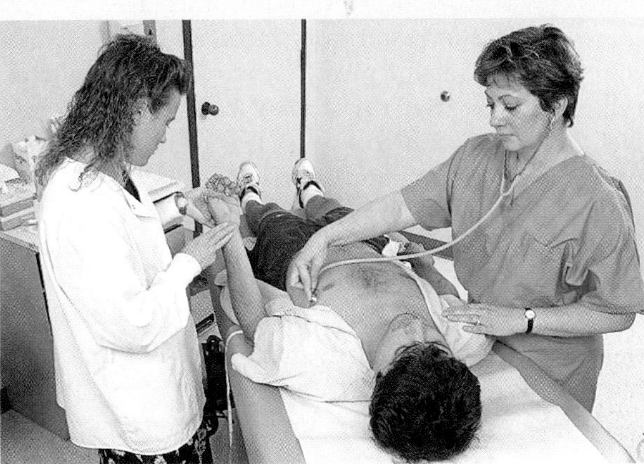

Two healthcare workers taking the apical and radial pulses to determine the pulse deficit (see Note 1).

DOCUMENTATION GUIDELINES

- Date and time
- Patient complaints/concerns
- Heart rate, rhythm, and volume
- Any observations appropriate for assessment of the cardiovascular system, such as skin color or skin temperature
- Other vital signs as needed or required by office protocol
- Patient education/instructions
- Your signature

Charting Example

DATE	TIME Recheck for medication evaluation.
	Unable to palpate radial pulse. Apical
	pulse 64, regular and full. BP - 104/62.
	Dr. Mendez notified. — Your Signature

Note 1: If cardiovascular disease is present, it may be necessary to compare the radial pulse with the apical pulse to evaluate the pulse deficit. This is the difference between the sounds heard at the apex and the pulse felt at the radius. If there is a difference, the apex will always be the higher number. Generally it works best to have two people take the opposite pulses simultaneously, one at the apex, the other at the radius. With the watch at a point that both may see the sweep second hand, the apical recorder will call "start," usually as the hand reaches 12, 3, 6, or 9, to make it easier to keep track. The assistant who called "start" will call "stop" at the appropriate time and the numbers will be compared and recorded. If two workers are not available, one worker may perform the procedure by counting first one pulse for 60 seconds, then counting the other. Pulses performed in this manner will be recorded as "Apical/Radial" or "A/R."

Note 2: If not otherwise noted in the patient's chart, most pulses are presumed to be radial.

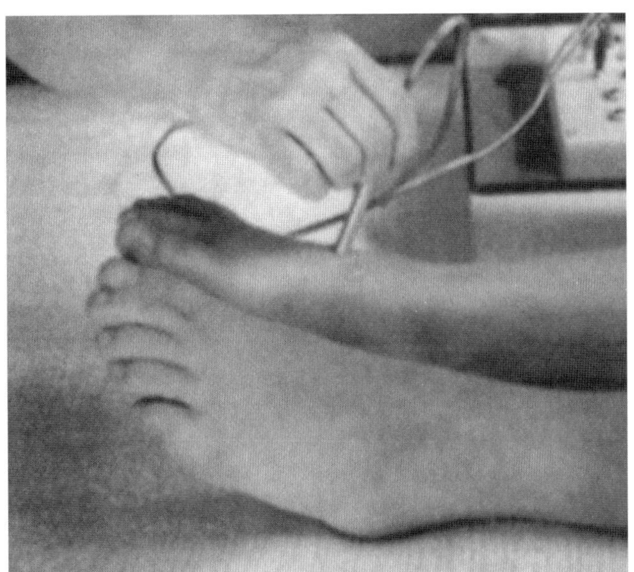

Figure 3-11 Auscultation of the pedal pulse using a Doppler unit.

RESPIRATION (R)

Respiration is defined as the exchange of gases between the atmosphere and blood of the body. External respiration involves the intake of air through the respiratory tract to the alveoli and bloodstream; internal respiration refers to the exchange of gases between the bloodstream and the tissue cells. The major gases exchanged are carbon dioxide (CO_2) and oxygen (O_2). Respiration is controlled by the respiratory center in the brain stem (primarily in the medulla oblongata), and by feedback from the chemosensors in the carotid that check for an increase in the CO_2 content of the blood.

As the body breathes, it brings into the lungs O_2 from the atmosphere by inspiration or inhalation. It forces out CO_2 and other wastes by expiration or exhalation. Inspiration and expiration are accomplished by the mechanical muscular action of the diaphragm and ribs. When you inhale, the diaphragm contracts and flattens as the rib cage lifts and expands, creating a negative pressure within the chest cavity that must be filled by the intake of air. When you exhale, the diaphragm relaxes and moves upward in a dome shape; the rib cage falls and compresses the pleura and the air is pressed out. Each respiration is counted as one full inspiration and one full expiration.

3

Observing the rise (inspiration) and fall (expiration) of the chest to count respirations is usually performed as a part of the pulse measurement to obtain an accurate reading. Patients can and usually do change the voluntary action of breathing if they are aware that they are being watched; therefore, it is generally considered best not to announce that you will now count the respirations. However, when appropriate, you may need to use a stethoscope to auscultate the respirations.

Characteristics

The characteristics of respiration are rate, rhythm, and depth. *Rate* is defined as the number of respirations occurring in 1 minute; the written descriptions medical assistants should use are normal, rapid, or slow. The physician may diagnose and record these as eupnea (easy, normal respirations), tachypnea (fast respirations), or bradypnea (slow respirations); this is not the responsibility of the medical assistant. (See Chapter 17, Assisting With Respiratory Patients, for more information about abnormal breathing patterns.)

When measuring respirations by auscultation and using a stethoscope, the count is performed for 1 minute and may be recorded as an odd number. When measuring respirations by observation in a patient without respiratory or cardiac symptoms, it is equally proper to count the respirations for 15 seconds and then multiply by four or for 30 seconds and multiply by two. This type of measurement is always recorded in even numbers.

Rhythm is defined as the period of time (spacing) between each respiration to determine a pattern. This interval or pattern will be equal in normal respirations and is written as regular. Any abnormal rhythm is described by what is detected and is written as irregular.

Depth is defined as the volume of air being inhaled and exhaled. When a person is at rest, the depth should be regular and consistent. There should be no noticeable sounds other than the regular exchange of air, and the written description should be either deep or shallow. If sounds are present, it is usually a sign of a disease process. Such sounds are referred to with specific descriptions, such as crackles, stridorous, stertorous, wheeze, and so on. (See Chapter 17, Assisting With Respiratory Patients, for more information about abnormal breath sounds.)

Averages and Ranges

In the healthy adult, the average respiratory rate is 14 to 20 breaths per minute. With other ages, there is a large variance of respiratory rates, as Table 3-5 shows. In fever states, as the pulse rises to satisfy the increased cellular needs, the respiratory rates will increase as well to bring in more oxygen. It is generally noted that each degree of temperature rise will increase the pulse by as many as 10 bpm; the respiratory rate will follow by increasing one respiration for each four to five bpm of the pulse.

A respiration rate that is significantly slower than the average is called bradypnea. A respiration rate that is much faster than the average is called tachypnea. Further descriptions that can be given are:

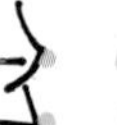

- Dyspnea—difficult or labored breathing
- Apnea—no respirations
- Hyperpnea—abnormally deep, gasping breaths
- Hyperventilation—a respiratory rate that greatly exceeds the oxygen demand
- Hypopnea—shallow respirations
- Orthopnea—inability to breathe or difficulty breathing in a supine or prone position; the patient usually has to sit upright to breathe.

The Cheyne-Stokes breathing pattern is a noticeable pattern that usually begins with slow shallow breathing, escalates to deep rapid breathing, then decreases to slow shallow breathing again. This pattern is followed by a period of apnea. The pattern continues until the apnea is permanent and death occurs. Cheyne-Stokes breathing sometimes precedes the "death rattle," which is caused by mucus accumulating in the throat as the cough reflex diminishes and the patient can no longer swallow this accumulation.

Procedure 3-11 lists the steps for counting respirations.

Checkpoint Question

5. *What happens within the chest cavity when the diaphragm contracts?*

Table 3-5 **Variations in Respiration Ranges by Age**

Age	*Respirations per Minute*
Infant	20 +
Child	18–20
Adult	14–20

Procedure 3-11 Counting Respirations

PURPOSE:

To detect the presence of possible respiratory pathology

STEPS

1. With patient already in position and sweep second hand in view, count a complete rise and fall of the chest as one respiration. *Note:* Some patients breathe at rest using the abdominal muscles more than the chest muscles. Observe carefully for the easiest area to assess for the most accurate reading.
   One complete cycle is counted as a respiration.
2. If the pattern is regular, count respirations for 30 seconds and multiply by two, or count for 15 seconds and multiply by four. If the pattern is irregular, count respirations for a full minute.
   A full 60 seconds will be necessary for accuracy if the rate is not regular.

DOCUMENTATION GUIDELINES

- Date and time
- Patient complaints/concerns
- Respiratory rate, rhythm, volume, and breath sounds
- Other observations appropriate to assessment of respiratory function, such as position assumed, effort required
- Other vital signs as needed or required by office protocol
- Patient complaints/concerns
- Patient education/instructions
- Your signature

Charting Example

DATE	TIME Pt c/o SOB, some pain on
	inspiration, difficulty breathing lying down.
	Color pale, skin warm and dry. T-99.4,
	P-60, R-26, BP 136/92. Dr. Morton in to
	check patient. — Your Signature

Respirations are usually counted just after measuring the radial pulse, with your hand still on the patient's wrist. If patients are aware that breaths are being counted, it is not unusual for them to alter the pattern.

BLOOD PRESSURE (BP)

Blood pressure is the pressure of the blood as it is forced against the arterial walls. The ventricles contract and eject the blood during a phase called **systole.** As the heart pauses briefly to rest and refill, the arterial pressure drops; this phase is called **diastole.**

Pressure is measured in both the contraction and relaxation phases. As the ventricles contract, the highest pressure level is recorded as systolic pressure. When the ventricles relax, the lowest pressure level is recorded as diastolic pressure.

Systolic and diastolic pressure are the two parts of the **cardiac cycle,** the period from the beginning of one heartbeat to the beginning of the next. The average adult blood pressure is 120/80 with a normal range between 100 and 140 systolic and 60 to 90 diastolic. Pressures of greater than 140/90 are considered hypertensive; pressures of less than 100/60 are considered hypotensive. A lower pressure may be normal for athletes with exceptionally well conditioned cardiovascular systems. A pressure that drops suddenly when the patient stands is referred to as **postural hypotension** or orthostatic hypotension. These patients will experience dizziness and may actually faint.

Diastolic and systolic pressures are measured by using a stethoscope, and an instrument called a sphygmomanometer (Procedure 3-12). There are two basic types of sphygmomanometers: the aneroid, which has a dial for the readings, and the mercury, which has a calibrated, mercury-filled glass tube for the readings (Fig. 3-12). The mercury is considered to be the more accurate. Each type measures blood pressure in millimeters of mercury, which is abbreviated "mmHg." Both are attached to a cuff by a rubber tube. A second rubber tube is attached to a pump with a screw valve used to blow up the rubber bladder held within the cuff. This arrangement of tubes and bladder presses the artery and records the pressure exerted by the blood as it flows through the vessel.

Electronic sphygmomanometers work well at home and either broadcast the sound or display a digi-

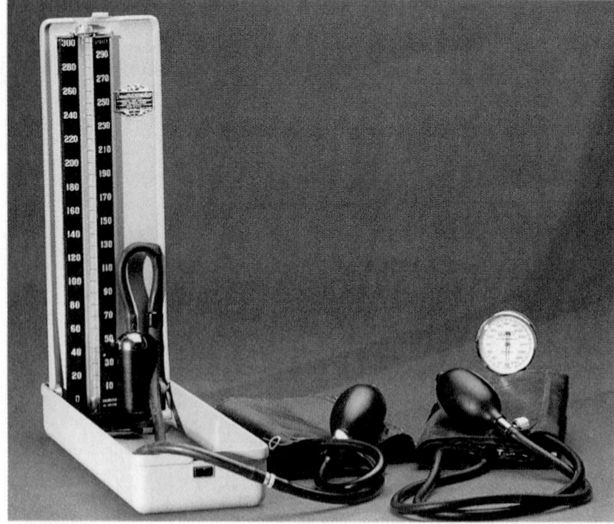

Figure 3-12 The mercury column sphygmomanometer and the aneroid sphygmomanometer.

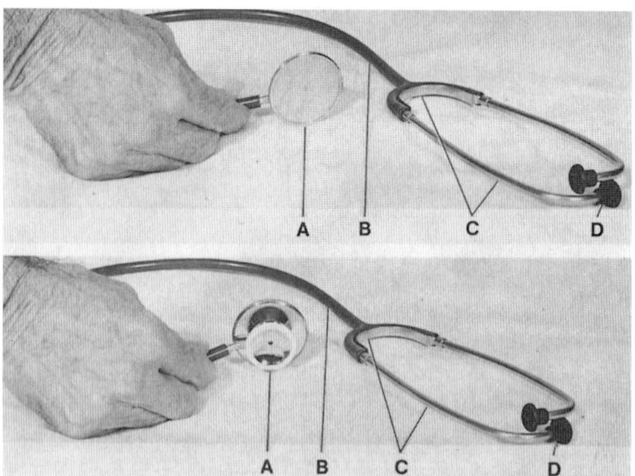

Figure 3-13 (A) The chest piece on this stethoscope contains both a diaphragm (*top*) and a bell (*bottom*). The diaphragm is used for listening to high-pitched sounds. The bell is better for detecting low-pitched sounds; it is used when obtaining the blood pressure. (B) The tubing may be rubber or plastic. Unnecessarily long tubing decreases good sound conduction. A length of about 50 cm (20 in) seems best. (C) The brace and biaural are the metal portions connecting the tubing and the chest piece. The biaural should clear the examiner's face. The brace prevents the tubing from kinking. (D) The eartips are rubber or plastic and should fit snugly but comfortably into the ears. They should be placed so that they are directed downward and forward. If the eartips are not properly positioned in the ear canal, sound quality will be poor, and when measuring blood pressure a falsely low systolic and falsely high diastolic pressure are likely to be obtained.

tal readout. Most offices currently prefer the more traditional and reliable aneroid or mercury equipment. As technology improves the electronic instruments, their use in the medical office will increase.

A stethoscope is needed for you to hear the pressure sounds with the standard methods of measurement (Fig. 3-13). Some offices may use a Doppler type of pressure measurement that will broadcast the sound of the systolic pressure without the use of a stethoscope.

A pressure of 120/80 indicates the force needed to raise a column of mercury to the 120 mark on the glass tube during systole and 80 during diastole. The pressure indicates the elasticity of the arteries, the strength of the heart muscle, and the quantity or viscosity (thickness) of the blood in the circulatory system.

The results of a blood pressure measurement are recorded as a fraction, with the systolic as the numerator and the diastolic as the denominator (eg, 120/80).

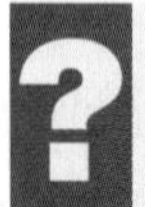

Checkpoint Question

6. *What is happening in the heart during systole and during diastole?*

Korotkoff Sounds and the Five Phases of Blood Pressure

Korotkoff sounds are those sounds heard through the stethoscope during the measurement of blood pressure. These sounds consist of two basic types: the first sound producing a "lubb" reflects the systolic period of the cardiac cycle and the second sound producing a softer "dubb" reflects the diastolic period of the cardiac cycle. Thus, one heartbeat consists of the "lubb-dubb" sound and reflects one cardiac cycle of contraction and relaxation. The Russian neurologist Nicolai Korotkoff classified these sounds into five phases as described in Table 3-6.

Pulse Pressure

Pulse pressure is the difference between systolic and diastolic readings. For example, the difference in the normal adult average blood pressure of 120/80 is 40. The range for pulse pressure normal values is 30 to 50 mmHg and a general rule is that the difference should be no more than one-third of the systolic reading.

Table 3-6 **Five Phases of Blood Pressure**

Phase	*Sounds*
I	Faint tapping sounds heard as cuff deflates (systolic)
II	Soft swishing sounds
III	Rhythmic, sharp, distinct tapping sounds
IV	Soft tapping sounds that become faint
V	No sounds (diastolic)

What If?

What if a patient has a dialysis shunt (a surgically made venous access port allowing the patient to be connected to a dialysis machine) in his left arm? Could you use that arm to take his blood pressure?

NO! By taking blood pressure in that arm, you could cause the shunt to be permanently damaged. The patient's chart should clearly indicate the shunt's location. Also, most dialysis patients are keenly aware of their conditions and will alert you to the location of their shunts. Additionally, you should not draw blood from the affected arm.

Auscultatory Gap

An auscultatory gap may be observed in patients who have a history of **hypertension** (elevated blood pressure) and occurs in phase II of the cardiac cycle. An auscultatory gap is the loss of sounds for as many as 30 mmHg or more during the fall of the needle or mercury. The beat is then heard again and continues to fade away. If this is not properly measured, the blood pressure may be tragically undermeasured. The recording of an auscultatory gap should be written as the first sound heard/the second sound heard (after the gap)/the last sound heard (eg, 210/130/120).

Factors Influencing Blood Pressure

Atherosclerosis and arteriosclerosis are two factors that greatly influence blood pressure. These diseases affect the size of the vessel lumen and the elasticity of the vessels. The general health of the patient is also a major factor and includes dietary habits, alcohol and tobacco use, the amount and type of exercise, previous heart conditions or myocardial infarctions, and family history for cardiac dysfunction or coronary heart disease.

Other factors affecting blood pressure include:

- *Age*—As the body ages, vessels begin to lose elasticity and will require more force for expansion. The buildup of atherosclerotic patches will also increase the force needed for blood flow.
- *Activity*—Exercise raises the pressure; depression will lower it. It is best to have the patient rest quietly in the examination room for a few moments before taking his or her pressure.
- *Stress*—The sympathetic nervous system raises the pressure in response to the flight-fright-fight syndrome.
- *Position*—Pressure is usually lower in the supine position. Crossing the legs may elevate the reading.
- *Medications*—Some medications will lower and others will raise the pressure.

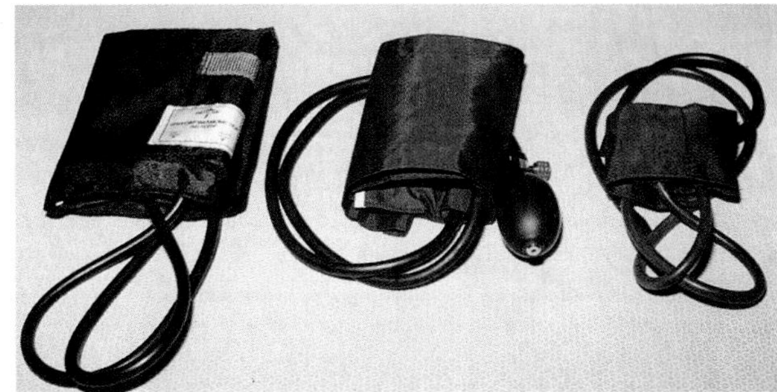

Figure 3-15 Three sizes of blood pressure cuffs (from left): a large cuff for an obese adult, a normal cuff, and a pediatric cuff.

Choosing the Correct Cuff Size

Choose the correct size of cuff before beginning to measure blood pressure. The blood pressure measure-

text continues on page 71

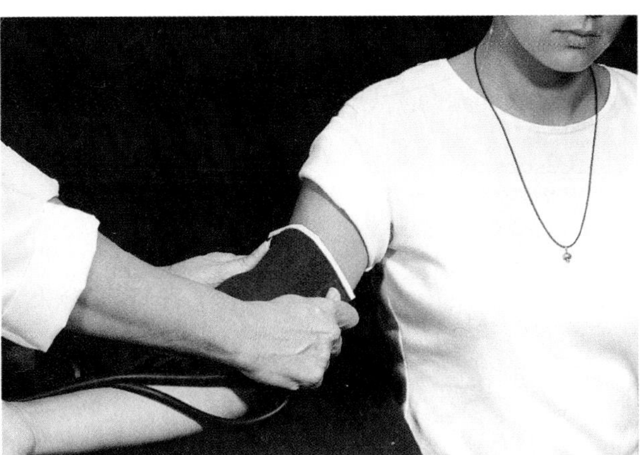

Figure 3-14 Choosing the right blood pressure cuff.

Box 3-2
Causes of Errors in Blood Pressure Readings

- Wrapping the cuff improperly
- Failing to keep the patient's arm at heart level
- Failing to support the patient's arm on a stable surface
- Recording auscultatory gap for diastolic pressure
- Failing to maintain the gauge at eye level
- Pulling the patient's sleeve up tightly above the cuff
- Listening through clothing
- Allowing the cuff to deflate too rapidly or too slowly
- Failing to wait 1–2 minutes before rechecking

Procedure 3-12 Measuring Blood Pressure

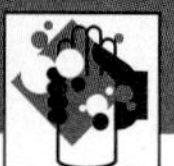

PURPOSE:

To provide an objective assessment of the patient's cardiovascular status and to detect possible cardiac pathology

EQUIPMENT/SUPPLIES

- sphygmomanometer
- stethoscope
- alcohol wipe

STEPS

1. Wash your hands.

Handwashing promotes infection control.

2. Assemble the equipment and supplies.

This ensures that everything you need is available.

3. Identify the patient and explain the procedure. Ask the patient about recent smoking, caffeine, exercise, or emotional upset.

Identifying the patient prevents errors. Explain the procedure to ease anxiety and ensure compliance. The listed factors affect pressure levels.

4. Position the patient. Have the patient's arm supported and slightly flexed with the palm upward. The upper arm should be level with the heart. The patient's legs should not be crossed, and the feet should be flat on the floor.

Patients are usually sitting unless the physician specifies a standing or lying pressure. (Always record the position if it is other than sitting.) Positioning the arm with the palm upward makes it easier to palpate the brachial artery. If the muscles are tensed to support the arm, the pressure will be affected. If the upper arm is higher than heart level, the pressure will be inaccurate. If the legs are crossed, the pressure may be higher than normal.

5. Expose the area. Remove the garment if the sleeve is too tight to raise above the area.

Tight clothing may act as a tourniquet and decrease the flow of blood. If clothing remains over the area, the sounds may be obscured.

6. Center the deflated cuff over the brachial artery on the medial aspect of the upper arm. To assess the center of the cuff, fold the bladder in half; place the midpoint just above the brachial artery. The lower edge of the cuff should be 1–2 inches above the antecubital area.

Pressure must be applied over the artery for the correct reading. If the cuff is too low on the arm, it may interfere with the stethoscope placement and increase the environmental noises to obscure the pressure sounds.

7. Wrap the cuff smoothly. It should fit snugly against the arm without being too tight. (Cuffs vary. Some fasten with Velcro, some fasten with hooks, and others with long cloth tails.)

The cuff must be wrapped smoothly and snugly to ensure an accurate reading.

8. If using a mercury manometer, keep it vertical and at eye level. An aneroid dial must register with the needle at zero before beginning.

If the meniscus of the mercury is read other than eye level, reading may be falsely high or low. If the aneroid needle doesn't register zero, it shouldn't be used until professionally calibrated.

9. Palpate the brachial pulse with the fingertips of the nondominant hand in the antecubital area.

It will be easier to hear the pulse sounds if the stethoscope is directly over the artery.

10. With the air pump in the dominant hand and valve between the thumb and forefinger, turn the screw clockwise (right to tighten). Do not tighten it to the point that it will be difficult to turn back.

The cuff will not fill with the valve open. If the valve is too tight, it will be difficult to release with one hand.

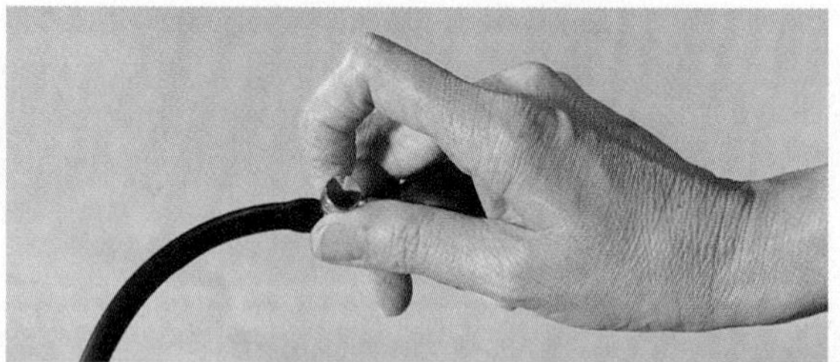

continued

Procedure 3-12 Continued Measuring Blood Pressure

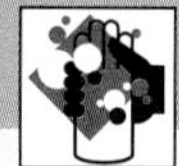

11. With the fingers of the nondominant hand still at the pulse, inflate the cuff and note the point at which the brachial pulse is no longer felt. This number will be slightly below the first Korotkoff sound heard on auscultation.
    Noting this point will give you a reference for assessing the pressure and a goal for reinflating the cuff.

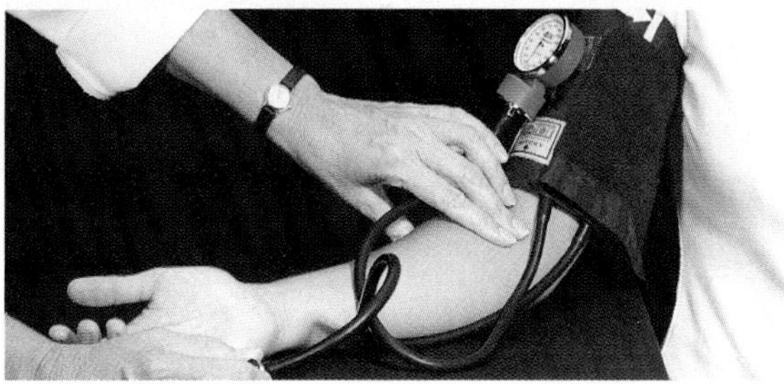

12. Deflate the cuff by turning the knob counterclockwise (left to loosen). Wait at least 30 seconds before reinflating the cuff.
    This interval allows the circulation to return to normal. The patient may raise or flex the arm and hand briefly to restore full circulation.
13. Clean the stethoscope chest piece with alcohol. Place the stethoscope earpieces in the ear canal with the openings pointing slightly forward. Stand or sit about 3 ft from the manometer, with the gauge at eye level. The stethoscope tubing should hang freely and should not rub against anything.
    A clean chest piece prevents cross-contamination. With earpieces pointing forward, the openings will follow the line of the ear canal. With the manometer at eye level, there is less chance of error. If the stethoscope rubs against objects, extraneous environmental noises may obscure the sound of the pulse.
14. Place the bell or diaphragm against the brachial artery but do not press hard. Hold with the nondominant hand.
    The bell magnifies low-pitched sounds better than the diaphragm. The diaphragm covers more area, which may assist with finding the pulse if the brachial has been hard to palpate. If not pressed firmly enough, the sounds may not be heard; if pressed too firmly, the pulse may be obliterated.

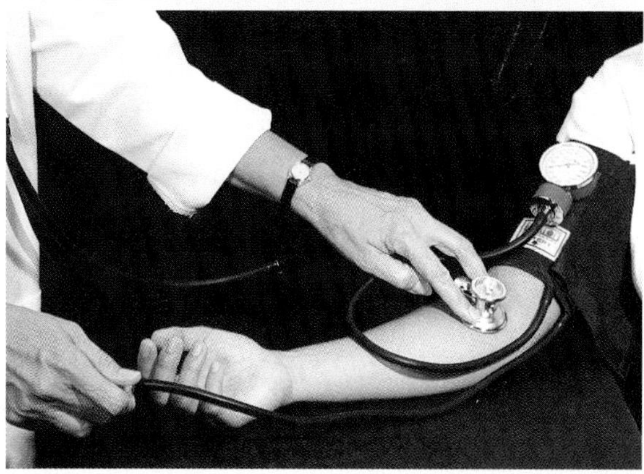

15. With the valve in the dominant hand, thumb and forefinger on the valve screw, turn the screw just tightly enough to inflate the cuff. Pump the valve to about 30 mmHg above the number felt on palpation.
    If the screw is tightened too much, it will be difficult to release. Inflating above the 30 mmHg point is uncomfortable for the patient and is unnecessary; inflating less than 30 mmHg may cause the highest systolic reading to be missed.
16. With the thumb and forefinger remaining on the screw, slowly release the air at about 2–4 mmHg per second.
    Releasing too fast will cause missed beats; too slow will interfere with circulation.
17. Listening carefully, note the point on the gauge at which the first clear tapping sound is heard. This is the first systolic sound or Korotkoff I.
18. Read at the top level of the meniscus (curved surface) of the mercury or at the number indicated by an arrow on the aneroid. Aneroid and mercury measurements are usually recorded as even numbers.
    Reading at an angle will give an inaccurate measurement.

continued

3

Procedure 3-12 Continued Measuring Blood Pressure

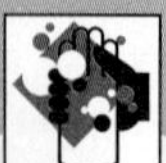

19. Maintaining control of the valve screw, continue to deflate at about 2–4 mmHg per second and identify each of the Korotkoff sounds.

Many physicians will require that all sounds be recorded rather than the traditional systolic/diastolic.

20. When the last sound is heard, note the reading and quickly deflate the cuff. *Note:* Never immediately reinflate the cuff if you are unsure of the reading. Totally deflate the cuff and wait at least 1 minute before repeating the procedure. Have the patient raise the arm and flex the fingers of that hand to restore circulation and relieve vasocongestion if the pressure must be reassessed.

This will be the diastolic or Korotkoff V sound.

21. Remove cuff and press the air from the bladder.

22. If this is the first recording or the first patient visit, the physician may want a reading in the opposite arm also or in a position other than sitting.

Pressures will vary from arm to arm or according to position.

23. Clean and store the equipment. Wash your hands.

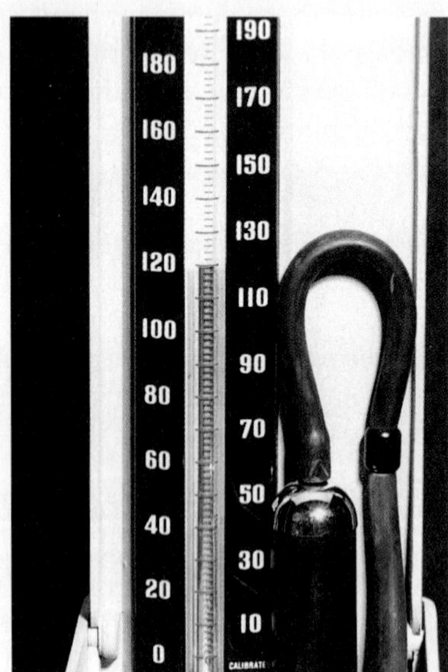

The meniscus reads 120 mmHg.

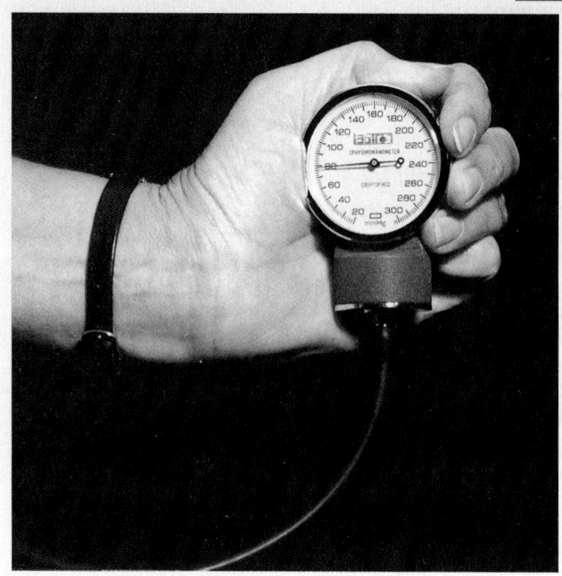

The gauge reads 80 mmHg.

DOCUMENTATION GUIDELINES

- Date and time
- Patient complaints/concerns
- Pressure reading and observations, such as patient position if other than sitting and arm used. Record the result with the systolic over the diastolic, and other sounds that might have been heard eg 160/110/80, if an auscultatory gap was heard.
- Other vitals as needed or required by office protocol
- Action taken, as needed
- Patient education/instructions
- Your signature

Charting Example

DATE	TIME Pt arrived c/o headache X 3 days,
	worse today. Has Rxed /c ASA.
	BP 180/120. Dr. Rodriquez notified
	immediately. — Your Signature

Note: The palpatory method may be used if the Korotkoff sounds cannot be heard. Using the properly placed cuff, pump 30 mmHg above the last felt pulse. Watching the mercury column or the aneroid needle as they drop, record the number at which the systolic pulse is felt at the radius. The diastolic cannot be assessed in this manner.

ment may be inaccurate by as much as ±30 mmHg if the cuff size is incorrect. The width of the cuff should be 40% to 50% of the circumference of the arm. To determine the correct size, hold the narrow edge of the cuff at the midpoint of the upper arm. Wrap the width, not the length, around the arm. The cuff width should reach not quite half way around the arm (Fig. 3-14). Varying widths of cuffs are available, from about 1 inch for infants to 8 inches for obese adults (Fig. 3-15). It is your responsibility to choose carefully the size most appropriate for the patient.

Errors in blood pressure readings may be caused not only by the wrong cuff size, but also by other factors. Box 3-2 lists additional causes of errors in blood pressure readings.

CHARTING VITAL SIGNS IN THE HOSPITAL SETTING

Medical assistants who are employed as unit clerks in the hospital setting usually will not perform vital sign assessments but will record on graphic sheets the readings brought to them by the nurses on the unit. The vital signs are recorded in the TPR form, with temperature first, pulse second, and respiration third (eg, 98.6–80–18) and *never* in any other order.

The medical assistant records the data on special graphic forms with areas for the temperature, pulse, respiration, blood pressure, height, and weight on admission and as needed through the hospital stay (Fig. 3-16). Most forms also include an area for bowel elimination and intake and output. There will be dates across the top with space for the day of the hospital stay, postoperative day, or postpartum day. The first day in the hospital will be listed as ADM (day of admission), the second day will be listed as Day 1. If surgery is performed or if this is a maternity patient, the first full day after noting PO (postoperative) or PP (postpartum) will be listed as Day 1 in the spaces below the listing for the hospital stay.

The graphic record gives an instant picture of the vital sign fluctuations during the hospital stay. The graph usually has heavy lines for full numbers or degrees and lighter lines for fractions of degrees of temperature, multiples of five for pulse (eg, 50, 55, 60, 65,

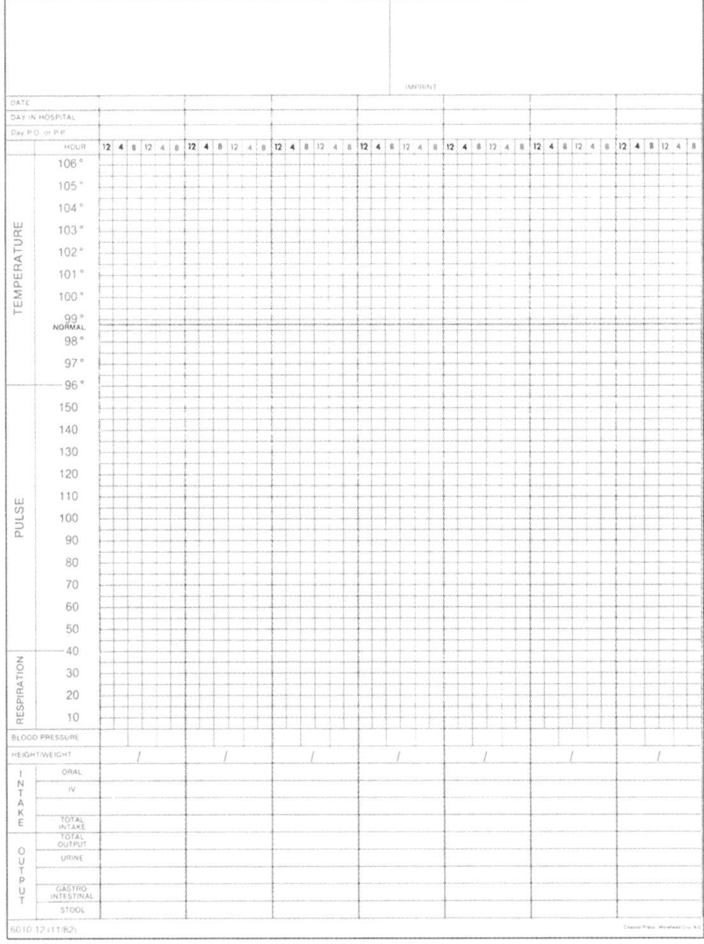
IMPRINT
DATE
DAY IN HOSPITAL
Day P.O. or P.P.
HOUR 12 4 8 12 4 8 | 12 4 8 12 4 8 | 12 4 8 12 4 8 | 12 4 8 12 4 8 | 12 4 8 12 4 8 | 12 4 8 12 4 8 | 12 4 8 12 4 8
TEMPERATURE 106° 105° 104° 103° 102° 101° 100° 99° NORMAL 98° 97° 96°
PULSE 150 140 130 120 110 100 90 80 70 60 50 40
RESPIRATION 30 20 10
BLOOD PRESSURE
HEIGHT/WEIGHT
INTAKE ORAL IV TOTAL INTAKE
OUTPUT TOTAL OUTPUT URINE GASTRO INTESTINAL STOOL
6010 12 (11/82)

Figure 3-16 A graphic sheet for recording vital signs.

70, 75), and whole number multiples of 10 for respirations. The forms will vary by the facility. The variety of information required and the structure for recording are infinite.

In all cases, the medical assistant will enter dots on the perpendicular hour line and the horizontal reading line. Line the dot under the time and across from the reading. A straight edge corner aligned with the reading and moved across the page to the time column will help avoid errors. Make a dot at this point and connect it to the dot for the previous reading. If the temperature is axillary or rectal, note an A or an R beside the dot; if the pulse is apical, note this also. The lines are small and errors are easy to make, even using a straight edge guide. If an error is made, mark X through the dot, initial the space and make the correction.

Some facilities use military time for graphic sheets and for charting. The day starts at 1 minute past midnight as 0001. One AM is recorded as 0100; 10 minutes past 2:00 AM is recorded as 0210. Noon is 1200 and midnight is 2400.

Many hospitals and clinics now use computers for recording the vital sign data. You will need to familiarize yourself with the system used by the facility in which you work.

Answers to Checkpoint Questions

1. *Rectal temperatures are usually 1° higher than oral temperatures because of the rectum's vascularity and tightly closed environment.*
2. *A child's body temperature is usually higher than an adult's because of the child's higher metabolism.*
3. *Temperature taken by the tympanic route measures the temperature of the blood in the tympanic membrane on its way to the hypothalamus. The ear canal is a closed environment with the probe in place, resulting in a rapid, noninvasive, and accurate reading.*
4. *Measuring a patient's pulse involves assessing the rate (number of heartbeats in 1 minute), rhythm (time between each heartbeat), and volume (strength of the heartbeat).*
5. *When the diaphragm contracts, a negative pressure results and must be filled with inhaled air.*
6. *During systole, the ventricles contract and force out the blood. During diastole, the ventricles relax and fill with blood.*

Critical Thinking Challenges

1. You are asked to teach a patient, Mr. Stone, how to take his blood pressure at home. Create a patient education brochure that explains the procedure in understandable terms and that includes normal blood pressure values. In addition, the physician wants Mr. Stone to record his blood pressure readings for 1 month. Design a sheet that Mr. Stone can easily use to record these readings.
2. Ms. Black has had a bad morning. She had car trouble on the way to the office. She could not find a parking place in the office lot. She was late for her appointment and had to be worked in. How would you expect this to affect her vital signs? Explain your response.
3. Mrs. Cooper is an elderly woman with very little muscle mass. She weighs 90 lb. Which type of sphygmomanometer cuff will she likely need? Why?

Suggestions for Further Reading

Earnest, V. V. (1993). *Clinical Skills in Nursing Practice,* 2nd ed. Philadelphia: Lippincott-Raven.

Kerschner, V. L. (1992). *Health Unit Coordinating, Principles and Practices.* Albany, NY: Delmar Publishers.

Kozier, B., & Erb, G. (1993). *Techniques of Clinical Nursing,* 4th ed. Redwood City, CA: Addison-Wesley.

Memmler, R. L., Cohen, B. J., & Wood, D. L. (1996). *Structure and Function of the Human Body,* 6th ed. Philadelphia: Lippincott-Raven.

Rosdahl, C. B. (1995). *Textbook of Basic Nursing,* 6th ed. Philadelphia: Lippincott-Raven.

Smeltzer, S. C., & Bare, B. G. (1996). *Brunner and Suddarth's Textbook of Medical-Surgical Nursing,* 8th ed. Philadelphia: Lippincott-Raven.

Taylor, C., Lillis, C., & LeMone, P. (1997). *Fundamentals of Nursing: The Art and Science of Nursing Care,* 3rd ed. Philadelphia: Lippincott-Raven.

Timby, B. K. (1996). *Fundamental Skills and Concepts in Patient Care,* 6th ed. Philadelphia: Lippincott-Raven.

4 Physical Examination

Chapter Outline

Components of the Physical Examination
Basic Instruments and Supplies
- Percussion Hammer
- Tuning Fork
- Nasal Speculum
- Otoscope
- Ophthalmoscope
- Audioscope or Audiometer
- Examination Light
- Gooseneck Lamp
- Tape Measure
- Gloves
- Stethoscope
- Tongue Depressor
- Penlight or Flashlight

Special Instruments and Supplies
- Headlight or Head Mirror
- Laryngeal Mirror
- Laryngoscope
- Vaginal Speculum
- Ayre Spatula and Histobrush
- Cotton-Tipped Applicators
- Fixative
- Slides, Slide Covers, and Laboratory Request Forms
- Lubricant
- Anoscope
- Proctoscope
- Sigmoidoscope

Examination Techniques
- Inspection
- Palpation
- Percussion
- Auscultation
- Mensuration
- Manipulation

Responsibilities of the Medical Assistant
- Room Preparation
- Patient Preparation
- Assisting the Physician
- Postexamination Duties

Physical Examination Format
- Head
- Neck
- Eyes
- Ears
- Nose and Sinuses
- Mouth and Throat
- Chest
- Reflexes
- Supine Chest
- Breasts
- Abdomen
- Genitalia and Rectum
- Legs
- Posture, Gait, Coordination, Balance, and Strength

General Health Guidelines and Checkups

Role Delineation

CLINICAL

Patient Care

- Prepare and maintain examination and treatment areas.
- Prepare patient for examinations, procedures, and treatments.
- Assist with examinations, procedures, and treatments.

Chapter Competencies

Learning Objectives

Upon successfully completing this chapter, you will be able to:

1. Spell and define the Key Terms.
2. Identify and state the function of the instruments and supplies used for the physical examination.
3. Describe six methods used to examine the patient.
4. List the basic sequence of the physical examination.
5. State the responsibilities of the medical assistant before the examination.
6. Summarize the assisting duties of the medical assistant during the physical examination.

Chapter Competencies *(continued)*

Performance Objectives

Upon successfully completing this chapter, you will be able to:

1. Assist the physician in all aspects of the physical examination (Procedure 4-1).

Key Terms

(See Glossary for definitions.)

applicators	**digital**	**manipulation**	**PERRLA**
asymmetry	**extraocular**	**mensuration**	**range of motion**
auscultation	**fixative**	**nasal septum**	**rectovaginal**
baseline	**gait**	**occult**	**sclera**
bimanual	**hernia**	**palpation**	**speculum**
bruit	**inguinal**	**Papanicolaou**	**symmetry**
cerumen	**inspection**	**percussion**	**transillumination**
diagnosis	**lubricant**	**peripheral**	**tympanic membrane**

The purpose of the complete physical examination is to assess the patient's general state of health by examining each body system. Early signs of disease may be detected during this procedure. New patients usually receive a complete physical examination, which gives the physician **baseline** information about the patient. Baseline information is valuable for future comparison; it can aid the physician in **diagnosis** (identifying a disease or condition). Routine examinations are then performed at regular intervals to maintain health and prevent disease. As a medical assistant, you will be responsible for assisting the physician in the performance of routine physical examinations.

COMPONENTS OF THE PHYSICAL EXAMINATION

The three components to the complete physical examination are medical history, actual physical examination, and laboratory and diagnostic tests.

The specific procedures for obtaining a medical history and performing routine diagnostic and laboratory tests are described elsewhere in this text. (See pertinent chapters in Unit 1: Performing Clinical Duties; Unit 2: Assisting With Diagnostic and Therapeutic Procedures; and Unit 5: Performing Laboratory Procedures.) The details of a complete physical examination follow. Once the data from the medical history, physical examination, and diagnostic tests are evaluated, a judgment about the patient's conditions is made, and a plan of care is devised.

BASIC INSTRUMENTS AND SUPPLIES

The basic instruments used for the general physical examination enable the physician to examine the body. These should be stored in a special tray or drawer and kept in a convenient location in each examination room. The exact equipment used will vary from office to office according to the preference of the physician. The use and the purpose of the most common instruments and supplies used for the physical examination are described below.

Percussion Hammer

The percussion hammer is used to test neurologic reflexes. Also called the reflex hammer, this instrument has a stainless steel handle with a hard rubber head. The head is used to test reflexes by striking the tendons of the ankle, knee, wrist, and elbow. The tip of the handle is used to

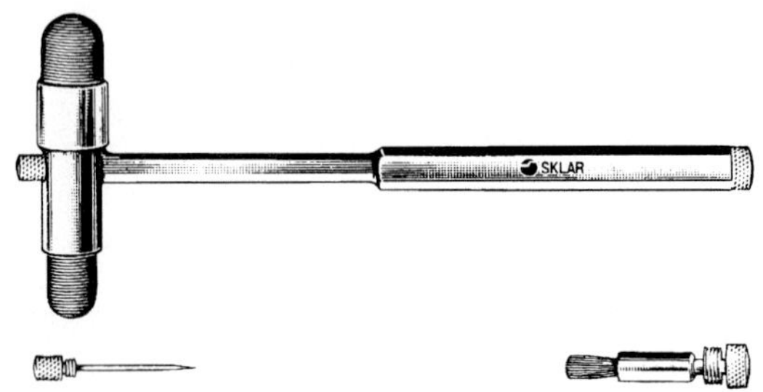

Figure 4-1 The Buck neurological hammer. Note the pin and brush that fit within the frame of the hammer and are used to assess sensory perception. (Sklar Instruments, West Chester, PA.)

stroke the sole of the foot. Some hammers are equipped with a brush and needle in their handles for testing sensory perception (Fig. 4-1).

Tuning Fork

The tuning fork is used to test hearing and vibratory sensations. It is a stainless steel instrument consisting of a handle and two prongs. The examiner strikes the prongs against his or her hand, which causes them to vibrate and produce a humming sound (Fig. 4-2).

Nasal Speculum

The nasal speculum is a stainless steel instrument that is inserted into the nose for visual inspection (examination) of the lining of the nose, nasal membranes, and septum. By squeezing the handles, the tips open to dilate the nostrils for visualization (Fig. 4-3). Nasal spec-

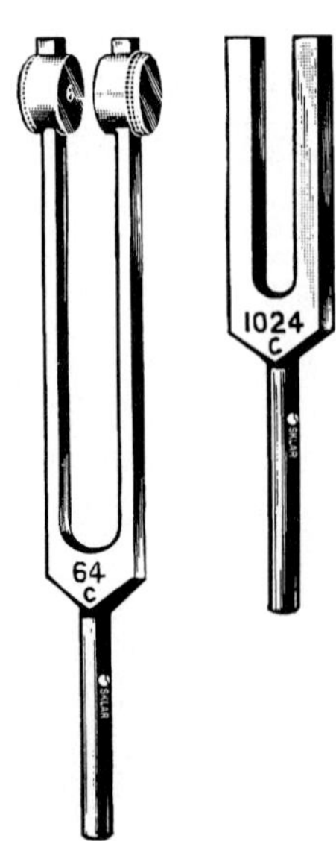

Figure 4-2 Tuning forks. (Sklar Instruments, West Chester, PA.)

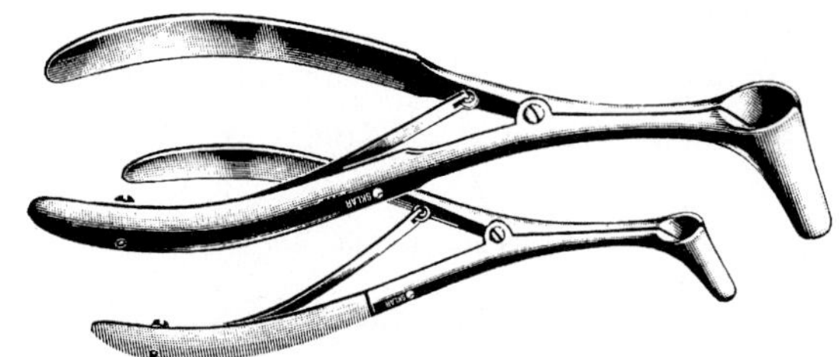

Figure 4-3 Nasal specula. (Sklar Instruments, West Chester, PA.)

ula are available in a disposable form also. In addition, an otoscope with a special attachment may be used.

Otoscope

The otoscope permits visualization of the ear canal and tympanic membrane—a thin membrane in the middle ear that transmits sound vibrations (also called the eardrum). The otoscope has a stainless steel handle containing batteries and a head with a light, a magnifying lens, and a cone-shaped hollow-tipped speculum that is placed into the ear canal. The interchangeable specula come in a variety of widths and are numbered according to size. They must be thoroughly cleaned with a disinfectant, such as alcohol, after each use. Most offices use disposable covers so the tip does not directly contact the patient. Disposable specula are also available. The nose may also be examined with the otoscope by attaching specialized nasal specula tips.

Ophthalmoscope

The ophthalmoscope is used to examine the interior structures of the eye. It has a stainless steel handle containing batteries and a head with a light, magnifying lenses, and an opening through which to view the eye.

The examination of the eye, ear, and nose can be accomplished by using a common handle or base unit and changing only the head (or tip) for each part of the examination.

The otoscope and the ophthalmoscope operate on batteries located in the handle. A unit with rechargeable batteries must be placed in a charger when not in use. Some offices are equipped with wall-mounted electrical units to which the scopes are attached. Batteries are not necessary with these units (Fig. 4-4).

Audioscope or Audiometer

The audioscope or audiometer is used to screen patients for hearing loss. It looks very much like an otoscope. The examiner places the tip into the patient's

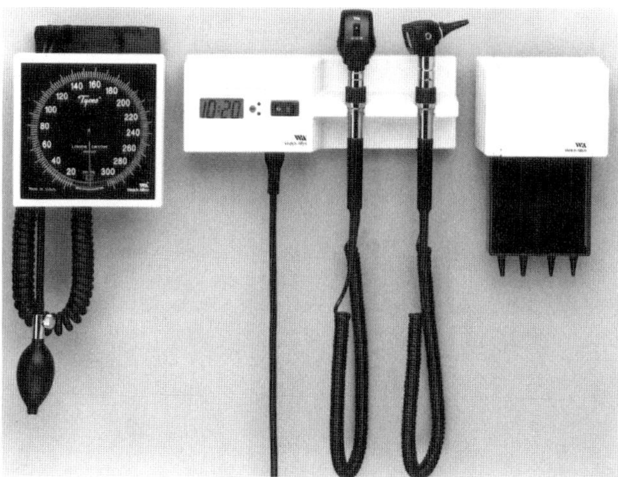

Figure 4-4 Wall-mounted examining instruments. From left: sphygmomanometer with cuff, ophthalmoscope, otoscope, and dispenser for disposable otoscope covers. (Welch Allyn, Skaneatels Falls, NY.)

ear, and the instrument produces a variety of tones. The patient is asked to respond as each tone is heard.

Examination Light

Some offices are equipped with an adjustable overhead examination light. As a medical assistant, you have the responsibility to see that light is directed toward the area of the patient's body that the doctor is examining.

Gooseneck Lamp

The gooseneck lamp is a flexible floorlamp on a movable stand. It is capable of movement in a variety of directions to provide good visibility. Again, you have the responsibility to see that light is directed toward the area of the patient's body that the doctor is examining.

Tape Measure

The tape measure is a flexible ruler that is measured in inches and feet or centimeters and meters. It is used to measure head circumference and height in the infant, height of the uterus (fundus) during pregnancy, and the size of body parts or abnormalities.

Gloves

Disposable examination gloves are used when the mouth, vagina, and rectum are examined to protect the patient and physician from microorganisms. Under Standard Precautions, gloves should be worn when touching blood, body fluids, secretions, excretions, mucous membranes, nonintact skin, and contaminated items.

Stethoscope

The stethoscope is used for listening to body sounds. At its end is a chestpiece with a diaphragm or bell that is placed on the patient's body. This is connected to two earpieces by flexible rubber or vinyl tubing. The examiner uses the stethoscope to auscultate the sounds of the heart, lungs, and intestines. It is also used for taking blood pressure readings.

Tongue Depressor

The tongue depressor (tongue blade) is a thin, flat, smooth piece of wood about 6 inches long used to hold down the tongue to inspect the mouth and throat. Illuminated tongue blade holders allow the tongue blade to be inserted into a lighted stainless steel holder at the end of a handle containing batteries.

Penlight or Flashlight

The penlight and flashlight are used to provide light during the examination. The penlight is the shape and size of a ballpoint pen. It is battery operated and has a clip on its side that is pressed to produce light. It is usually used for inspecting the eyes, nose, and throat. Other uses include shining a light through the sinuses and scrotum for the purposes of examination; this is called **transillumination.** The base previously described for the otoscope and ophthalmoscope can also be used for a transilluminating head that is attached in the same manner as the other two units. The common flashlight may also be used for the same purposes.

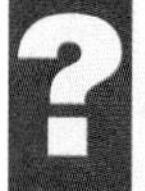

Checkpoint Question

1. *Which instruments are used to test hearing, and how do they work?*

SPECIAL INSTRUMENTS AND SUPPLIES

In addition to the basic instruments and supplies described previously, other specialized equipment may be used for the physical examination.

Headlight or Head Mirror

An ear, nose, and throat specialist (otorhinolaryngologist) may wear a headlight or head mirror for the examination. This consists of a light or mirror attached to a headband that fits over the head (Fig. 4-5). Because the examiner needs a light source to examine the ear, nose, and throat, this provides illumination for these areas either directly or reflected from the examining light.

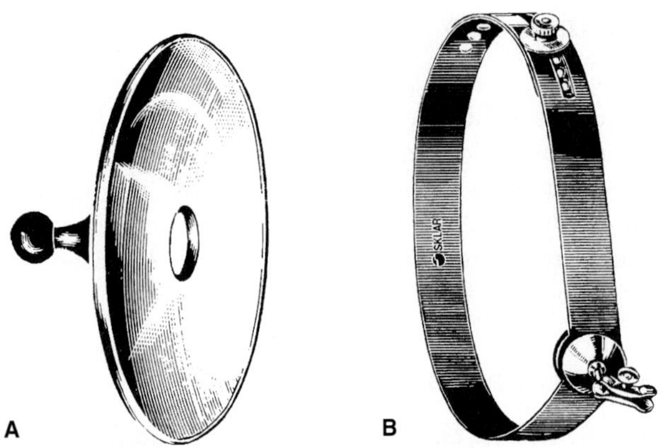

Figure 4-5 A head mirror (A) and head band (B). (Sklar Instruments, West Chester, PA.)

Laryngeal Mirror

The laryngeal mirror is a stainless steel instrument with a long, thin handle. Attached to its end is a small round mirror. It is used to examine the throat and larynx (Fig. 4-6).

Laryngoscope

The laryngoscope is an instrument with lights and mirror used to visualize the larynx.

Vaginal Speculum

The general physical examination for the female may include a pelvic examination and **Papanicolaou** (Pap) smear, a simple smear method of examining tissue cells for cancer (especially of the cervix). The vaginal **speculum** is a broad-billed bivalved instrument that is inserted into the vagina to expand the vaginal opening (Fig. 4-7). It permits the physician to visualize the cervix and vaginal walls and to obtain specimens. It is made of reusable stainless steel or disposable plastic.

Ayre Spatula and Histobrush

The Ayre spatula, or cervix scraper, is a thin, flat, smooth piece of wood about 6 inches long. One tip has an irregular shape that is placed in the cervical opening and rotated to collect the specimen for a Pap smear.

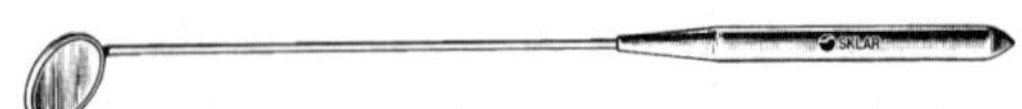

Figure 4-6 Laryngeal mirror. (Sklar Instruments, West Chester, PA.)

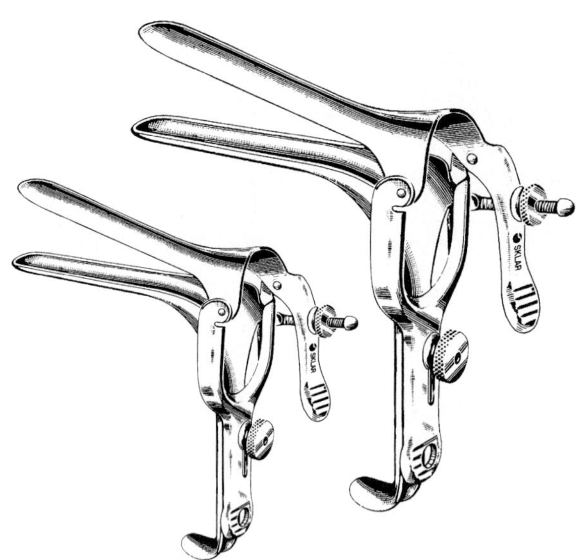

Figure 4-7 Two sizes of vaginal specula. (Sklar Instruments, West Chester, PA.)

The other end is rounded and is used to collect cells from the vaginal cul-de-sac.

The histobrush is about 6 inches long, made of nylon or plastic, and tipped with soft bristles in a spiral that can be rotated in the cervical os to remove cells for a Pap smear (Fig. 4-8). Both are often used to obtain an adequate sample of cells for microscopic inspection.

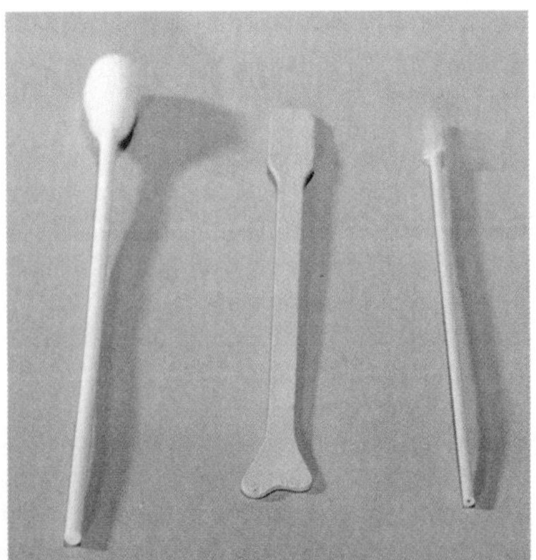

Figure 4-8 Cotton swab (*left*), Ayre spatula (*center*), and histobrush (*right*). Cotton swabs of this size are frequently used to remove excess vaginal secretions or to apply medications during the gynecologic examination.

Cotton-Tipped Applicators

Cotton-tipped **applicators** are bits of cotton or rayon attached to a slender wooden or plastic stick. They may be small for specimen collection or may be large for medication application or for removing excess secretions that may interfere with treatment or visualization (see Fig. 4-8).

Fixative

A **fixative** is a chemical spray made of 50% alcohol and 50% ether or 95% ethyl alcohol. It "fixes" the Pap smear specimen on the slide and preserves it for cytology testing.

Slides, Slide Covers, and Laboratory Request Forms

Glass microscope slides are used for specimens. Slides are placed into covers to preserve and protect them for transportation to the laboratory for analysis. Laboratory request forms are necessary to identify the patient and to provide patient data.

Lubricant

A **lubricant** is a gel used to reduce friction and provide for easy insertion. It may be used to facilitate speculum insertion or the **bimanual** (two hand) examination after the Pap smear is completed. It is also used for the rectal examination.

Anoscope

The anoscope is a stainless steel speculum that is inserted into the anus to inspect the rectal canal. Clear plastic disposable anoscopes are available and allow better visualization of the rectal mucosa. An obturator with a rounded tip extends beyond the anoscope to guide it into the rectum. After the instrument is inserted, the obturator is removed for visualization. Some anoscopes have a knob that rotates the inserted end without having to turn the handle (Fig. 4-9).

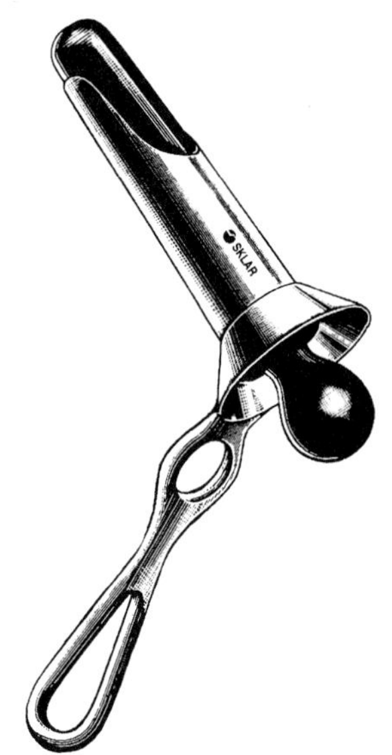

Figure 4-9 Anoscope. (Sklar Instruments, West Chester, PA.)

Proctoscope

The proctoscope is a speculum used to visualize the rectum and the distal portion of the colon. It consists of a straight tube with an obturator with a rounded tip that extends beyond the tube to direct or guide it along the canal. After the instrument is inserted, the obturator is removed and a fiberoptic light handle and magnifying lens are attached so that the physician can see through the tube. The tube is marked in centimeters so that any abnormalities noted may be located according to their depth in the canal. The proctoscope is longer than the anoscope and shorter than the sigmoidoscope.

Sigmoidoscope

The sigmoidoscope is an instrument used to inspect visually the rectum and sigmoid colon. It consists of a tube with an obturator, fiberoptic light handle, and magnifying lens. A suction machine, cotton-tipped applicators, glass microscope slides, slide covers, and laboratory request slips should be available when any rectal procedures are done. Tissue or stool specimens may be obtained.

In most offices, the larger, inflexible scopes have been replaced with flexible fiberoptic instruments that are smaller in diameter and are more comfortable for the patient. These newer instruments also allow for greater depth of examination and better visualization of the intestinal mucosa.

Checkpoint Question

2. *What are the different uses of the anoscope, proctoscope, and sigmoidoscope?*

EXAMINATION TECHNIQUES

The physician uses six basic techniques to gather information during the physical examination.

Inspection

Inspection means looking at areas of the body to observe physical features. The examiner inspects the patient's general appearance, movements, coloring, contours, **symmetry** (equality in size or shape) or **asymmetry** (inequality in size or shape), deformities, injuries, and skin condition. Inspection may be done with the naked eye, with instruments, or with a light source.

Palpation

Palpation involves touching the body with the fingers or hands. The examiner palpates the body to determine pulse rate; the size, shape, and location of organs; the presence of masses; and the existence of swelling, tenderness, or pain. Skin temperature, moisture, texture, and elasticity may also be assessed. Palpation may be performed with both hands (bimanual), the full length of the fingers (**digital**), one hand, the fingertips, or the palm of the hand. Palpation ranges from lightly touching the fingers over the skin to a deep probe to assess internal organs, such as the liver and spleen.

Percussion

Percussion is tapping or striking the body with the hand or an instrument to produce sounds. Direct percussion is performed by directly striking the body with a finger. Indirect percussion is done by placing a finger or fingers on the area and then striking with a finger of the other hand. In both methods, the examiner listens to the sounds and feels for vibrations produced to determine the position, size, and density of body organs and cavities. Percussion may be done with the fingers, knuckles, or side of the hand. A percussion hammer is used to test reflexes.

Auscultation

Auscultation involves listening to the sounds of the body. The examiner uses a stethoscope to hear heart sounds (such as the heartbeat and murmurs), lung sounds (such as respirations and signs of infection), blood vessel sounds (such as the movement of blood through the vessels), and abdominal sounds (such as the movement of gases and fluids). Direct auscultation may be done by placing the ear directly on the patient's body.

The above methods are usually performed in the order given for each area of the body as it is examined. For the abdominal examination, auscultation is performed before palpation and percussion because doing these first may alter the normal bowel sounds.

Mensuration

Mensuration refers to the measurement of height, weight, length, diameter, flexion, extension, hearing, vision, and pressure.

Manipulation

Manipulation is the passive movement of the joints of the body to determine extent of movement, or **range of motion**. The examiner moves the joints of the head, arms, hands, legs, and feet.

Checkpoint Question

3. *Why is auscultation of the abdomen performed before palpation?*

RESPONSIBILITIES OF THE MEDICAL ASSISTANT

Room Preparation

As a medical assistant, you are responsible for seeing that the room is prepared for the examination. The examination room should be clean, well lighted and ventilated, and at a comfortable temperature for the patient. The examining table should be covered with clean paper and all evidence of previous patients removed.

Patient Preparation

Once the examining room is ready, call the patient by name from the waiting room and escort him or her to the examining room. It is important that you develop rapport with your patients and practice good interpersonal skills. This will help to put patients at ease and will increase their confidence in you. Your goal is to create a positive, supportive, caring, and friendly atmosphere. Assess the patient's facial expression and level of anxiety by noting verbal and nonverbal behavior. Treat the patient as an individual and speak clearly with a confident tone of voice as you explain the procedure.

Take and record the patient's history and chief complaint if this is your responsibility. Take and record the vital signs and the results of the visual acuity and blood tests. Explain how to obtain a urine specimen and direct the patient to the restroom. Label the specimen and see that it arrives in the laboratory. Return the patient to the examining room and give instructions for disrobing and gowning. Some physicians have preferences for the gown opening in the front or the back. Leave the room while the patient undresses un-

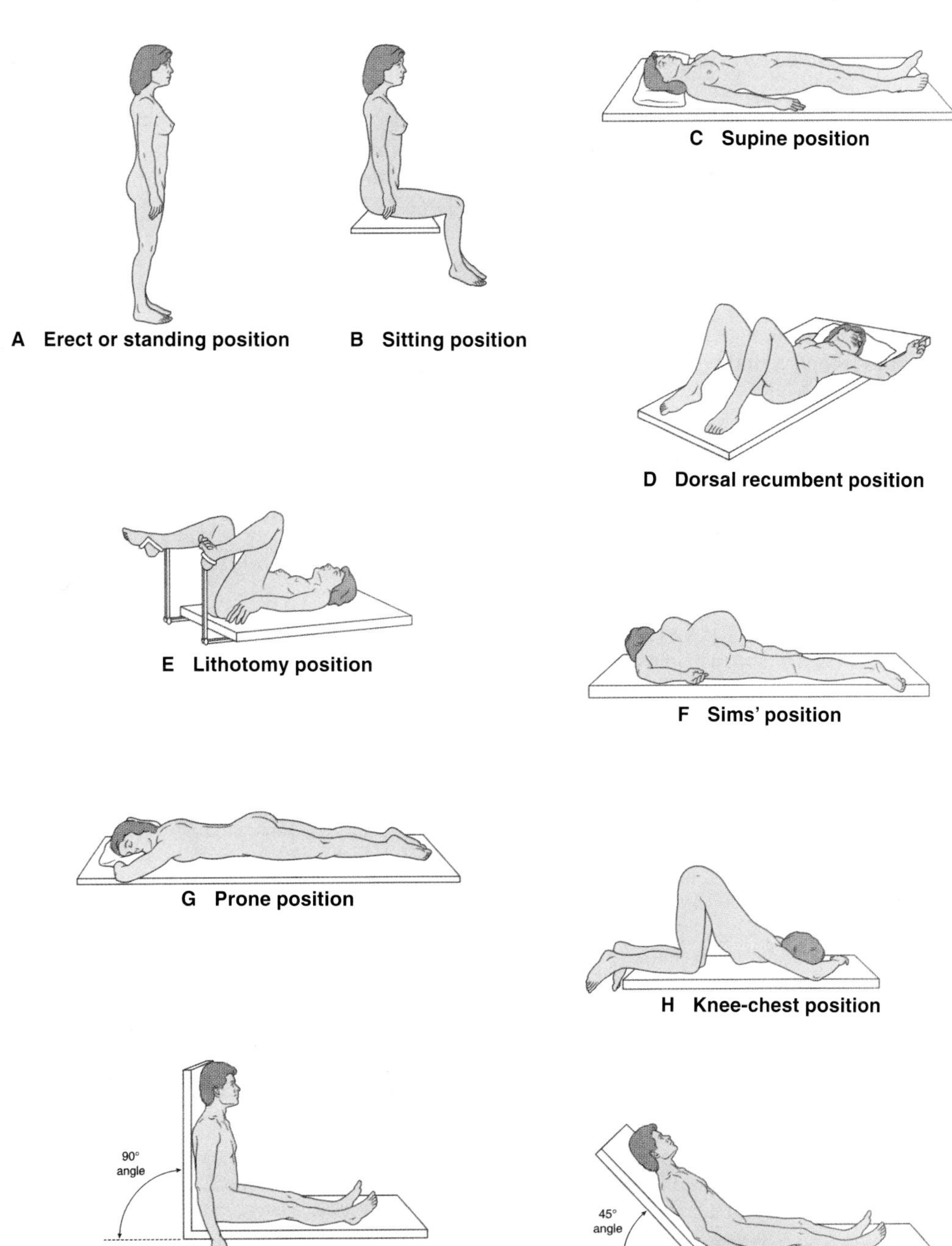

Figure 4-10 Patient examination positions. (A) Erect or standing position. The patient's body is erect and facing forward with the arms down at the sides. (B) Sitting position: The patient sits erect at the end of the examining table with the feet supported. (C) Supine position: The patient lies on the back with arms at the sides. A pillow is usually placed under the head for comfort. (D) Dorsal recumbent position. The patient is in the supine position with the legs separated, the knees bent, and the feet flat on the table. (E) Lithotomy position. This position is similar to the dorsal recumbent position except the patient's feet are placed in stirrups rather than flat on the table. The stirrups should be level with each other and about 1 foot from the edge of the table. The patient's feet should be moved into or out of the stirrups simultaneously to avoid back strain. (F) Sims' position. The patient lies on the left side with the left arm and shoulder behind the body, the right leg and arm sharply flexed on the table, and the left knee slightly flexed. (G) Prone position. The patient lies on the abdomen with the head supported and turned to one side. The arms may be placed under the head or by the sides, whichever is more comfortable. (H) Knee–chest position. The patient kneels on the table with the arms and chest on the table, hips in the air, and back straight. (I) Fowler's position. The patient is in a sitting position with the head of the table elevated 80°–90°. (J) Semi-Fowler's position. The patient is in a semi-sitting position with knees slightly bent and with the head of the table elevated 30°–45°.

4

less your assistance is needed. When the patient is ready, obtain an electrocardiogram if one is ordered. Then, have the patient sit on the edge of the examining table and cover the legs with a drape sheet. Place the chart outside the door of the examining room and notify the physician that the patient is ready.

Assisting the Physician

During the physical examination, for legal reasons you must remain in the room when a male physician examines a female patient. In every examination, your responsibility is to assist the physician by handing the instruments and supplies needed and directing the light appropriately.

4

You must also assist the patient in assuming appropriate positions (Fig. 4-10) as the doctor proceeds, making sure to adjust the drapes to expose only those body parts being examined. Patient support and reassurance are also vital assisting duties during the examination. Table 4-1 lists the various examination positions, the body parts usually examined in the positions, and the instruments needed by the physician.

Postexamination Duties

At the completion of the physical examination, you are expected to perform follow-up treatments and procedures if necessary. Direct the patient to dress. Leave the room unless your assistance is required. Return to the examining room and ask if the patient has any questions. Reinforce any instructions that have been given and provide patient education. Escort the patient to the front office, where any future

Table 4-1 **Examination Positions and Their Uses**

Patient Position	*Body Part(s) Examined*	*Instruments Needed*
Sitting	General appearance	
	Head, neck	Stethoscope, glass of water
	Eyes	Ophthalmoscope, penlight
	Ears	Otoscope, tuning fork
	Nose	Nasal speculum, penlight, substances to test sense of smell
	Sinuses	Penlight
	Mouth	Glove, gauze square, tongue blade, penlight
	Throat	Glove, tongue blade, laryngeal mirror, penlight
	Axilla, arms	
	Chest	Stethoscope
	Breasts	
	Upper back	Stethoscope
	Reflexes	Percussion hammer
Supine	Chest	Stethoscope
	Abdomen	Stethoscope
	Breasts	
Lithotomy, dorsal recumbent, or Sims'	Female genitalia and internal organs	Glove, vaginal speculum, Ayre spatula, histobrush, slides, fixative, slide covers, requisition form, lubricant
	Female rectum	Glove, lubricant, slides, slide covers, requisition form or occult blood test
Standing, dorsal recumbent, or Sims'	Male genitalia and hernia	Glove
	Male rectum	Glove, lubricant, slides, slide covers, requisition form
	Prostate	Glove, lubricant
	Legs	Percussion hammer
	Spine, posture, gait, coordination, balance, strength, flexibility	
Prone	Back, spine, legs	
Knee–chest (genupectoral)	Rectum	Glove, lubricant, sigmoidoscope (optional)
	Female genitalia	Glove, lubricant, vaginal speculum, Ayre spatula, histobrush, slides, fixative, slide covers, requisition form
	Prostate	Glove, lubricant
Fowler's (used for patients with breathing difficulties)	Head, neck, chest	Stethoscope

Patient Education

The Body's Warning Signals

Teach patients to recognize the following early warning signs of cancer:

C—change in bowel or bladder habits
A—a sore that does not heal
U—unusual bleeding or discharge
T—thickening, lump, or change in shape of the breasts or testes
I—indigestion or difficult swallowing
O—obvious change in a wart or mole; bleeding, enlargement, or itching
N—nagging cough or hoarseness

Frequent severe headaches and persistent abdominal pain are other signals that should not be ignored.

Instruct parents not to overlook the following signs in their children:

- Continual crying for no obvious reason
- Unexplained nausea and vomiting
- General failure to thrive
- Spontaneous bleeding or bleeding that does not stop in the normal amount of time
- Bumps, lumps, masses, or swelling anywhere on the body
- Frequent stumbling for no apparent reason

appointment may be scheduled and billing questions clarified.

Return to the examining room and clean all used instruments and equipment and dispose of used supplies. Clean the examining table and counter surfaces with disinfectant. (See Chap. 1, Asepsis and Infection Control.) Cover the examination table with clean paper, and prepare the room for the next patient. Check the patient's medical record to be sure that all data have been accurately documented.

Procedure 4-1 describes the steps for assisting the physician with the physical examination.

Checkpoint Question

4. *What are the four basic responsibilities of the medical assistant in the performance of the physical examination?*

PHYSICAL EXAMINATION FORMAT

The physical examination of the patient by the physician begins with the patient seated on the examining table with a drape sheet over the lap and covering the legs. The doctor usually progresses through the examination in orderly and methodical sequences. The patient's general appearance, behavior, speech, posture, nutritional status, hair distribution, and skin are observed throughout the examination.

Head

The patient's skull, scalp, hair, and face are inspected and palpated for size, shape, and symmetry. The examiner is looking for nodules, masses, or local trauma.

Neck

The patient may be asked to roll the head around in all directions to assess for range of motion and to check for any limitations of movement. The lymph nodes are located in the neck and are palpated. The trachea is inspected and palpated. The thyroid gland is inspected and palpated for size and symmetry.

The patient may be asked to swallow several times and small sips of water may be offered so the physician may palpate the thyroid gland. However, this is not always necessary because just the normal act of swallowing produces the same result. The carotid arteries are palpated and auscultated on both sides to check for any bruits (abnormal sounds) caused by possible blockage.

Eyes

The visual acuity test is usually performed by the medical assistant before the doctor's examination. (See Chap. 13, Procedures Associated With the Sensory System, for the procedure for visual acuity testing.) The physician inspects the **sclera,** the fibrous tissue covering the eye, for normal color (white in Caucasians and lightly yellow in African Americans). The pupils are inspected with a light to see if they are equal in size and round, and their reaction to light and accommodation are evaluated. Normal pupil reaction is indicated as **PERRLA** (pupils equal, round, reactive to light and accommodation). Eye movement is assessed by having the patient follow the examiner's fingers or the ophthalmoscope light. If this is normal, it is abbreviated EOM intact, for **extraocular** (outside the eye) movement intact. **Peripheral** vision (side vision) is also assessed to test the horizontal and vertical fields of vision.

Using the ophthalmoscope, the physician is able to examine the interior of the eye (Fig. 4-11). The condition of the retina can be assessed. Pathology of the intraocular vessels will also be evaluated.

Ears

The ears are inspected and palpated for size, symmetry, lesions, and nodules. The otoscope is used to examine

4

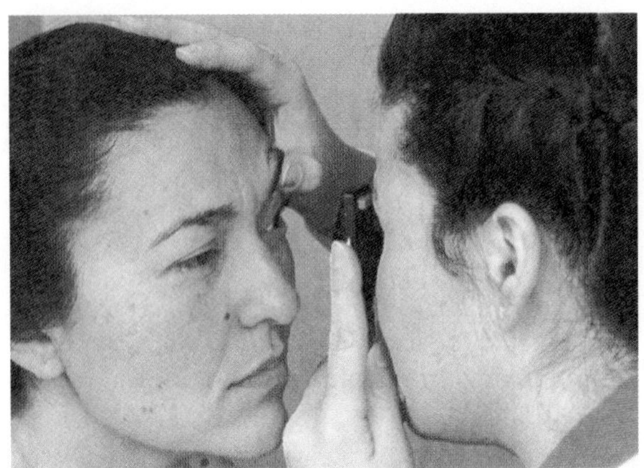

Figure 4-11 Ophthalmoscopic examination.

the interior of the ear canal (Fig. 4-12). The examiner is able to visualize the ear canal, noting the presence of **cerumen** (ear wax). The tympanic membrane can also be checked for coloration and scarring and to see if it is intact. Normally, the tympanic membrane is pearly gray and concave in appearance, but infection may cause discoloration and fluids from infection behind the eardrum may cause the membrane to bulge. Auditory acuity is tested with the tuning fork.

Nose and Sinuses

The external nose is inspected and palpated for abnormalities. The interior of the nose is examined using a nasal speculum and light. The position of the **nasal septum** is noted for deviation to the right or left. The nasal septum divides the nostrils. Each nostril is inspected for coloration of the mucosa, discharge, lesions, obstruction, polyps, swelling, or tenderness. The sense of smell may be assessed by having the patient close his or her eyes and identify a common substance, such as alcohol, lemon, strawberry, or peppermint.

The paranasal sinuses are inspected and palpated. The technique of transillumination may be used to visualize the sinuses by darkening the room and placing a penlight against the upper cheek or periorbital ridge and looking in the mouth for the degree of light penetration through the sinuses.

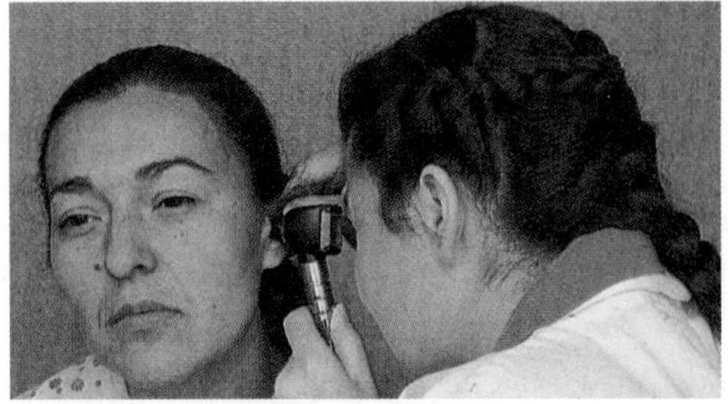

Figure 4-12 Visual otoscope examination.

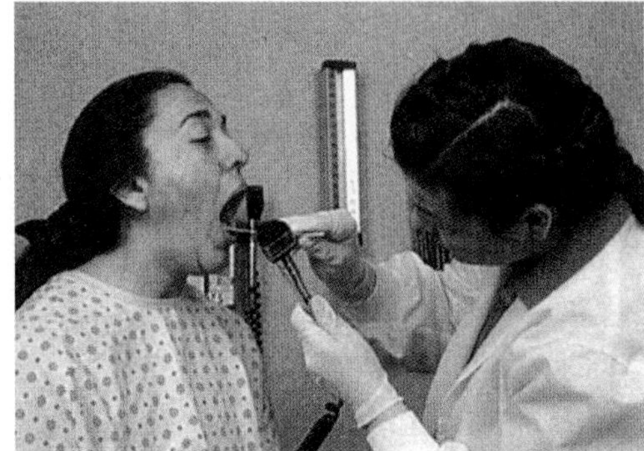

Figure 4-13 Examination of the oral cavity and throat.

Mouth and Throat

The physician inspects the mucous membranes, gums, tongue, teeth, tonsils, and throat using clean gloves, a light source, and a tongue blade (Fig. 4-13). A laryngeal mirror may be used to inspect the throat. The mucous membranes and tongue may be palpated using a gauze square. The examiner is also assessing general dental hygiene and salivary gland function and is looking for ulcerations, nodules and abnormalities in color.

Checkpoint Question

5. *What is the tympanic membrane, and how does the presence of infection affect it?*

Chest

The anterior chest is examined with the gown removed to the waist. The physician inspects the anterior chest and breasts, observing the general appearance, symmetry, respiratory rate and pattern, and obvious masses or swelling. Palpation is then performed and includes the axillary (underarm) lymph nodes and the area over the heart. Percussion of the underlying structures follows. Using a stethoscope, the examiner auscultates the lungs for abnormal sounds, and the patient may be asked to take deep breaths. The heart sounds and apical pulse are also assessed.

The posterior areas of the chest are inspected. Palpation includes assessment of the respiratory pattern and the muscles of the back and spine. This is followed by percussion of the back to assess lung fields. Then, using a stethoscope, the examiner listens to the lung sounds, and the patient is asked to take deep breaths.

Reflexes

Before having the patient lie back on the table, the physician usually will progress to the reflexes. The examiner uses the percussion or reflex hammer to strike the biceps, triceps, patellar, Achilles, and plantar tendons to evoke a response. The physician may prefer to test the plantar reflexes with the patient supine.

Supine Chest

After the reflexes have been assessed, the patient is assisted to the supine position with the anterior chest exposed and the drape sheet placed from the waist down. The heart may be reexamined in this position using inspection for visible external movements and an auscultation of the heart sounds. The patient may be asked to turn briefly onto his or her left side while the examiner listens to the heart sounds with the stethoscope.

Breasts

The breasts may be palpated in both the male and female. The supine position is preferred for palpation of the breasts because the breast tissue flattens out so that abnormalities, if present, are felt more easily.

Abdomen

To examine the abdomen, the drape sheet is lowered to the pubic area. A drape is placed across the chest, or the gown is replaced and raised to just beneath the breasts. The abdomen is inspected for contour, symmetry, and pulsations. Auscultation follows. The examiner uses the stethoscope to listen to the bowel sounds and abdominal blood vessels. Percussion determines the outlines of the abdominal organs. Palpation evaluates for enlargement, masses, pain, or tenderness (Fig. 4-14).

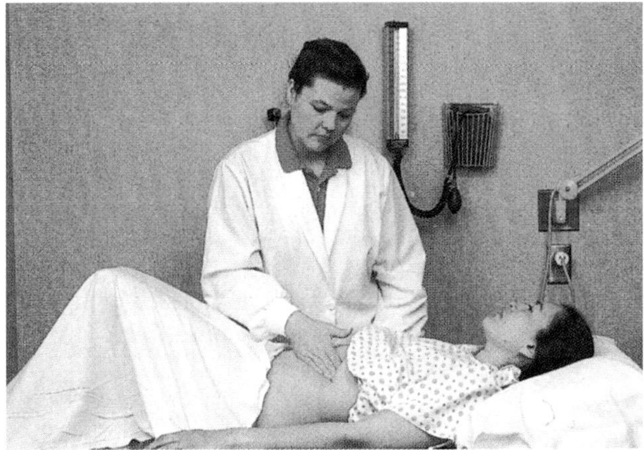

Figure 4-14 Abdominal palpation. Note that the patient's knees are raised to reduce tension in the abdominal muscles.

The groin area is palpated for enlargement of **inguinal** lymph nodes or the presence of a **hernia.** A hernia is the protrusion of an organ through the muscle wall of the cavity that normally surrounds it. The femoral blood vessels may also be palpated and auscultated.

Checkpoint Question

6. *Why is the patient asked to assume the supine position for palpation of the breasts?*

4

Genitalia and Rectum

The physician wears clean gloves to examine the external male genitalia and rectum. Inspection is done to note symmetry, lesions, swelling, masses, and hair distribution. The scrotal contents may be visualized using transillumination in a darkened room. In addition, the scrotum is palpated for testicular size, contour, and consistency. The patient is then asked to stand and bear down while the examiner places a gloved index finger upward along the side of the scrotum into the inguinal ring to assess for a hernia. The patient is then asked to bend over the examination table. The examiner inspects the anus for lesions or hemorrhoids and then places a lubricated and gloved index finger into the rectum to palpate the anal sphincter muscle tone and the prostate for size, consistency, or masses. An **occult** (hidden) blood test is obtained from stool on the gloved finger.

The female genitalia and rectum are examined with the patient in the lithotomy position and draped appropriately. The examiner wears a clean latex glove on the dominant hand. The gooseneck or overhead lamp is adjusted to direct light on the perineal area. The external genitalia are inspected for lesions, edema, cysts, discharge, and hair distribution. The vaginal speculum is inserted to inspect the condition of the cervix and vaginal mucosa. A Pap smear is obtained and possibly a sample of the secretions in the vagina. After the speculum is removed, a bimanual examination is done to palpate the internal reproductive organs for size, contour, and masses. Two fingers of the gloved hand are inserted into the vagina while the ungloved hand is placed on the lower abdomen to compress the internal organs. Sometimes a **rectovaginal** examination is necessary to palpate the posterior uterus and vaginal wall. The examiner places a gloved index finger in the vagina and the middle finger in the rectum at the same time.

The rectum is inspected and palpated for lesions, hemorrhoids, and sphincter tone. A stool specimen is obtained for occult blood.

4

Procedure 4-1 Assisting With the Physical Examination

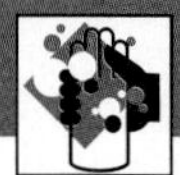
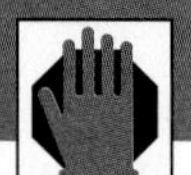
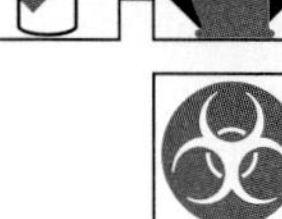

PURPOSE:

To reduce patient anxiety and increase patient cooperation
To assist the physician in evaluating the patient's health status with maximum efficiency and minimal interference

EQUIPMENT/SUPPLIES

- appropriate instruments may include stethoscope, ophthalmoscope, penlight, otoscope, tuning fork, nasal speculum, tongue blade, laryngeal mirror, percussion hammer, speculum
- glass of water (optional)
- substances for testing sense of smell (optional)
- gloves
- gauze squares
- lubricant
- vaginal spatula/histobrush
- slides, slide covers, and fixative
- requisition slips as appropriate
- tissues
- specimen container
- gown
- drape
- electrocardiograph

STEPS

1. Wash your hands.
   Handwashing promotes infection control.
2. Prepare the examining room.
   A clean room that is free from contamination prevents transfer of microorganisms.
3. Assemble the equipment.
   This ensures that all supplies are available.
4. Greet the patient by name and escort to the examining room.
   Identifying the patient by name acknowledges the patient as a person and prevents errors.
5. Explain the procedures.
   Explaining the procedure helps ease anxiety and ensure compliance.
6. Obtain and record the medical history and chief complaint if that is your responsibility.
   A medical history gives the physician important background information about the patient's health and symptoms.
7. Take and record the patient's temperature, pulse, respirations, blood pressure, height, weight, and visual acuity. Draw blood if necessary.
   The vital signs and diagnostic tests give the physician an overall picture of the patient's health.
8. Instruct the patient in obtaining a urine specimen and escort to the restroom.
   The urinalysis provides data on the patient's general health. An empty bladder facilitates the palpation of the abdomen.
9. See that the specimen is properly labeled and received in the laboratory.
   Proper labeling of specimens helps to prevent errors.
10. Escort the patient back to the examining room. Instruct patient to disrobe completely and put on a gown opening down the back or front as directed by the physician. Leave the room unless the patient needs assistance.
    The gown must open in the direction that provides accessibility for the examination. Patients often prefer to disrobe in private; elderly and disabled patients may need assistance in disrobing and gowning.
11. Perform an electrocardiogram if ordered.
    The electrocardiogram gives the physician information about the heart's conduction system.
12. Assist the patient into a sitting position on the edge of the examination table. Cover the lap and legs with a drape sheet.
    Greeting the physician in a sitting position is psychologically beneficial to the patient, and it is the position in which the physician begins the examination. A drape sheet provides privacy by covering body parts not being examined.
13. Place the patient's chart outside the examination room door, and notify the physician that the patient is ready.
    Good communication between office personnel helps to prevent delays.
14. Assist the physician during the examination by handing the instruments needed for examination of each body area and ensuring proper patient positioning.
    Anticipating the physician's needs promotes efficiency and saves time.
    a. Begin by handing the physician the instruments necessary for examining the:
       - head and neck—stethoscope and glass of water

continued

Procedure 4-1 Continued Assisting With the Physical Examination

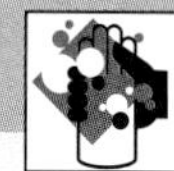 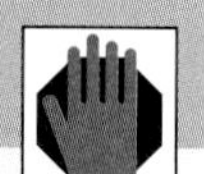 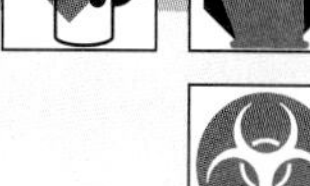

- eyes—ophthalmoscope, penlight
- ears—otoscope, tuning fork
- nose—nasal speculum, penlight, substances for testing sense of smell
- sinuses—penlight
- mouth—glove, gauze square, tongue blade, penlight. *Note:* Hand the tongue blade to the physician by holding it in the middle. When it is returned to you after use, grasp it in the middle again so that you do not touch the end that was in the patient's mouth
- throat—glove, tongue blade, laryngeal mirror, penlight. *Note:* Warm the laryngeal mirror by placing it in warm water before handing it to the physician.

Holding the tongue blade in the center allows the physician to grasp one end of it so that the clean end may be placed in the patient's mouth. Warming the laryngeal mirror prevents fogging.

b. Assist the patient in removing the gown to the waist so the physician can examine the chest and upper back. Hand the physician the stethoscope for sounds within the thorax.

Only those parts being examined are exposed; the rest of the body remains covered.

c. Assist the patient in putting on the gown, and remove the drape sheet from the legs so the physician may test the reflexes. Hand the physician the reflex hammer.

d. Assist the patient to a supine position, opening the gown at the top to expose the chest once again. Place the drape sheet from the waist down to the toes. Hand the physician the stethoscope to assess cardiac sounds.

e. Cover the patient's chest and lower the drape sheet to the pubic area to expose the abdomen. The physician will use the stethoscope to assess bowel sounds.

f. Assist with genital and rectal examinations. Hand the patient tissues following these examinations.

For females:

- Assist the patient into the lithotomy position and drape appropriately.
- For examination of the genitalia and internal reproductive organs, provide a glove, lubricant, speculum, spatula or brush, slides, fixative, slide covers, and requisition slip.
- For rectal examination, provide a glove, lubricant, slides, slide covers, and requisition slip.

For males:

- Assist the patient to a standing position. In this position, the physician can check for a hernia; by having the patient bend over the table, the physician can perform a rectal and prostate examination.
- For hernia examination, provide a glove.
- For rectal examination, provide a glove, lubricant, slides, slide covers, requisition slip.
- For prostate examination, provide a glove and lubricant.

Tissues may be used to wipe off excess lubricant used in the examination.

15. Help the patient to return to a sitting position at the edge of the examining table.

The physician often discusses the findings with the patient at this time and provides instruction.

16. Perform any follow-up procedures or treatments.

17. Leave the room while the patient dresses unless needed for assistance with clothing.

This provides privacy.

18. Return to the room to answer questions, reinforce instructions, and provide patient education.

Patient compliance depends on full understanding of the treatment plan. Patient education is the responsibility of all health care workers.

19. Escort the patient to the front office.

You can help clarify appointment scheduling or billing questions, if any.

20. Properly clean or dispose of all used equipment. Clean the room with disinfectant and prepare for the next patient.

All instruments, supplies, and equipment that come into direct contact with patients must be appropriately decontaminated or placed in disposal container.

21. Wash your hands.

continued

4

4

Procedure 4-1 Continued **Assisting With the Physical Examination**

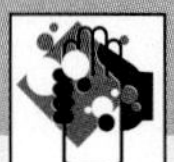
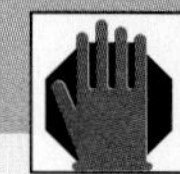
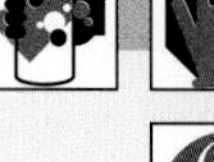

DOCUMENTATION GUIDELINES

- Date and time
- Patient complaints/concerns
- Anthropometric measurements and vital signs as required by office protocol
- Results of routine office laboratory procedures
- Special preparations or procedures for the examination
- Patient education/instructions
- Your signature

Charting Example

DATE	TIME Pt. presents for annual PE. No
	complaints. T-98.6, P-94, R-16,
	BP-109/66. U/A collected. Essentially
	negative. Dr. Williamson in to exam. pt.
	—Your signature

What If?
The physician will be performing a genital examination on a disabled female patient. What if she is unable to assume the lithotomy position?

Both the genital and rectal examinations may be performed in the dorsal recumbent or Sims' position for those patients (such as the elderly or those with disabilities) who cannot assume the more uncomfortable positions, such as the lithotomy position.

Legs

The legs are inspected and peripheral pulse sites are palpated in the supine position. The patient is then assisted to the standing position where the peripheral pulse sites may be palpated again and the legs observed for varicose veins and edema.

Posture, Gait, Coordination, Balance, and Strength

The spine may be inspected and palpated and general posture assessed in the standing position. In addition, the patient may be asked to walk and perform other movements so that **gait** and coordination may be observed. A balance test may be done by having the patient stand with feet together and eyes closed. Range of motion and muscle strength are assessed on both the arms and the legs.

Each physician has an established pattern for performing physical examinations. The sequence may vary, or certain aspects may be added or deleted based on the findings for each patient.

Checkpoint Question
7. *What is the purpose of the rectovaginal examination?*

GENERAL HEALTH GUIDELINES AND CHECKUPS

Physicians vary as to how often they recommend a complete physical examination for their patients. For patients aged 20 to 40, physical examinations are scheduled about every 1 to 3 years. Annual examinations are typical for patients over age 40, unless an existing medical condition requires more frequent visits.

For women, the first Pap smear is recommended between ages 18 and 20 or at the onset of sexual activity and then annually thereafter. A breast examination by a doctor is recommended every 3 years from ages 20 to 40 and annually after that. Breast self-examination should be performed monthly. A baseline mammogram is recommended between ages 35 and 40, every 2 years during the forties, and then annually after 50 years of age. These guidelines are being reassessed currently and mammograms soon may be performed more frequently. If the patient is at risk for breast cancer, the doctor may recommend mammograms earlier and more often.

All patients should have a baseline electrocardiogram at age 40 and follow-up only as necessary. A rectal examination and stool for occult blood are recommended annually beginning at age 40. At age 50 a flexible sigmoidoscopy examination is recommended and then every 3 to 5 years after that if the initial tests are negative.

Adult immunizations are recommended according to the following guidelines:

- Tetanus booster every 10 years or if the patient sustains a severe injury
- One injection of pneumonia vaccine (Pneumovax) between 60 and 65 years of age or earlier at the physician's discretion
- After age 65, annual flu shot (influenza A and B)
- Some doctors also recommend a series of three hepatitis B injections for their adult patients.

Patients should be instructed regarding signs and symptoms that may signal health problems and when to call the physician.

Answers to Checkpoint Questions

1. *The tuning fork and the audioscope are used to test hearing. To use the tuning fork, the examiner strikes its prongs against the hand, causing them to vibrate and produce a humming sound. To use the audioscope, the examiner places the tip into the patient's ear; as the instrument produces various tones, the patient responds when each tone is heard.*
2. *The anoscope is used to inspect the rectal canal. The proctoscope is used to visualize the rectum and anus. The sigmoidoscope is used to inspect visually the rectum and sigmoid colon.*
3. *Auscultation involves listening to body sounds. Palpation stimulates bowel sounds, so if it is performed before auscultation, it may alter the normal bowel sounds.*
4. *As a medical assistant, you are responsible for preparing the examination room, preparing the patient, assisting the physician during the examination, and cleaning the room and equipment afterward.*
5. *The tympanic membrane, also called the eardrum, is a thin membrane in the middle ear that transmits sound vibrations. Normally, it is pearly gray and concave in appearance. However, in the presence of infection, it may become discolored. Also, infected fluids behind the eardrum may cause the membrane to bulge.*
6. *When the patient is in the supine position, the breast tissue flattens out. This makes it easier for the physician to feel any abnormalities, if present.*
7. *The rectovaginal examination is done to palpate the posterior uterus and vaginal wall.*

Critical Thinking Challenges

1. During the physical examination, the physician asks the patient to walk across the room. What can be determined about the patient's health from observing the patient's way of walking?
2. After the physical examination, the patient asks you: "Why did the physician strike my chest and listen?" How would you explain this?
3. Why is it possible for the physician to assess vascular health by checking the eyes?

Suggestions for Further Reading

Bates, B., Buckley, L. S., & Hoekelman, R. A. (1995). *A Guide to Physical Examination and History Taking,* 6th ed. Philadelphia: Lippincott-Raven.

Rosdahl, C. B. (1995). *Textbook of Basic Nursing,* 6th ed. Philadelphia: Lippincott-Raven.

Smeltzer, S. C., & Bare, B. G. (1996). *Brunner and Suddarth's Textbook of Medical-Surgical Nursing,* 8th ed. Philadelphia: Lippincott-Raven.

Taylor, C., Lillis, C., & Lemone, P. (1997). *Fundamentals of Nursing,* 3rd ed. Philadelphia: Lippincott-Raven.

Timby, B. K., & Lewis, L. W. (1996). *Fundamental Skills and Concepts in Patient Care,* 6th ed. Philadelphia: Lippincott-Raven.

5 Instruments and Equipment

Chapter Outline

Instruments
- Forceps
- Scissors
- Scalpels and Blades
- Towel Clamps
- Probes and Directors
- Retractors

Instruments and Equipment Used by Specialists

Care and Handling of Instruments

Principles and Practices of Asepsis

Sanitation

Disinfection

Sterilization
- Sterilization Equipment
- Autoclave
- Sterilization Indicators
- Loading the Autoclave
- Operating the Autoclave

Boiling

Storage and Recordkeeping

Maintaining Surgical Supplies

Role Delineation

CLINICAL

Fundamental Principles

- Apply principles of aseptic technique and infection control.
- Comply with quality assurance practices.

Patient Care

- Prepare and maintain examination and treatment areas.

GENERAL

Operational Functions

- Evaluate and recommend equipment and supplies.

Chapter Competencies

Learning Objectives

Upon successfully completing this chapter, you will be able to:

1. Spell and define the Key Terms.
2. Identify an instrument by its characteristics.
3. Categorize instruments based on use.
4. State the difference between reusable and disposable instruments.
5. Define sanitation.
6. Distinguish between the need for disinfection and sterilization.
7. Name several methods used for sterilization.
8. Identify instruments specific to designated specialties.
9. Maintain adequate maintenance checkups and servicing of equipment.
10. Keep adequate supplies (light bulb, lens, and so on) on hand for equipment needs.
11. Identify the need for special storage of supplies (ie, disinfectants and sterilants), instruments, and equipment.
12. Maintain adequate documents and records of maintenance or sterilization for instruments and equipment.

Chapter Competencies *(continued)*

Performance Objectives

Upon successfully completing this chapter, you will be able to:

1. Sanitize equipment for disinfection or sterilization (Procedure 5-1).
2. Properly wrap equipment in preparation for sterilization in an autoclave (Procedure 5-2).
3. Operate an autoclave observing protocol for pressure, time, and temperature appropriate for the material to be sterilized (Procedure 5-3).

Key Terms

(See Glossary for definitions.)

autoclave
disinfectants
disinfection
ethylene oxide
forceps
germicide
hemostat
instruments
needle holder
obturator
ratchets
sanitation
sanitizing
scalpel
scissors
serrations
sterile field
sterilization

As a medical assistant, you will be responsible for assisting with medical procedures and minor surgical procedures in an office or clinical setting. To manage this responsibility effectively, you must:

- Become familiar with many types of instruments
- Understand the principles and practices of asepsis
- Have a working knowledge of disinfection and sterilization techniques
- Be able to use equipment designed for sterilization, treatment, and diagnostic purposes

You must also be competent in maintaining accurate records of the purchases and maintenance performed on office equipment, performing routine equipment maintenance, and maintaining inventory to ensure adequate supplies are available for diagnostic testing, medical and surgical treatment, and sterilization and disinfection procedures.

INSTRUMENTS

In an office or clinical setting, you must be able to identify medical or surgical **instruments** by their design and function. Medical instruments are used for treatment, assessment, and examination purposes. Surgical instruments are tools or devices designed to perform specific functions such as cutting, dissecting, grasping, holding, retracting, or suturing. Surgical instruments are designed to perform specific tasks based on their shape; they may be curved, straight, sharp, blunt, serrated, toothed, or smooth. Many are made of steel and are designed to be durable. Medical and surgical instruments are made to be either reused or disposed of, depending on the instrument's use and the manufacturer's recommendations.

You should be able to name or identify and know the proper use and care of the instruments used for clinic or office procedures. Most can be identified for use by carefully examining the instrument and its parts; instruments are so specifically designed that the configurations will usually give clues to their uses. The most widely used surgical instruments include several types of forceps, scissors, scalpels, and clamps.

Forceps

Forceps are surgical instruments used to grasp, handle, compress, pull, or join tissue, equipment, or supplies. There are several different types of forceps including, but not limited to, the following:

- **hemostat** *clamp*—a surgical instrument with slender jaws used for grasping blood vessels and establishing hemostasis
- *Kelly clamp*—a curved or straight forceps or hemostat; those with long handles are frequently used in gynecologic procedures
- *sterilizer forceps*—used to transfer sterilizer supplies, equipment, and other surgical instruments
- **needle holder**—used to hold and pass a suturing needle through tissue
- *spring or thumb forceps*—usually consist of a spring handle and a serrated or toothed point used for grasping tissue for dissecting or suturing; examples: tissue forceps and splinter forceps

Figure 5-1 shows various types of forceps.

All forceps are available in a multitude of sizes, with or without **serrations** or teeth, with curved or straight blades, with ring tips, blunt tips, or sharp tips. Many have **ratchets** in the handles to hold the tips tightly together. These are notched mechanisms that click into position to maintain tension. Some have spring handles that are compressed to grasp objects.

Most physicians will use a variety of forceps for procedures performed in the office. You must spend time studying the names and purposes of each to assist the physician when a specific instrument is requested.

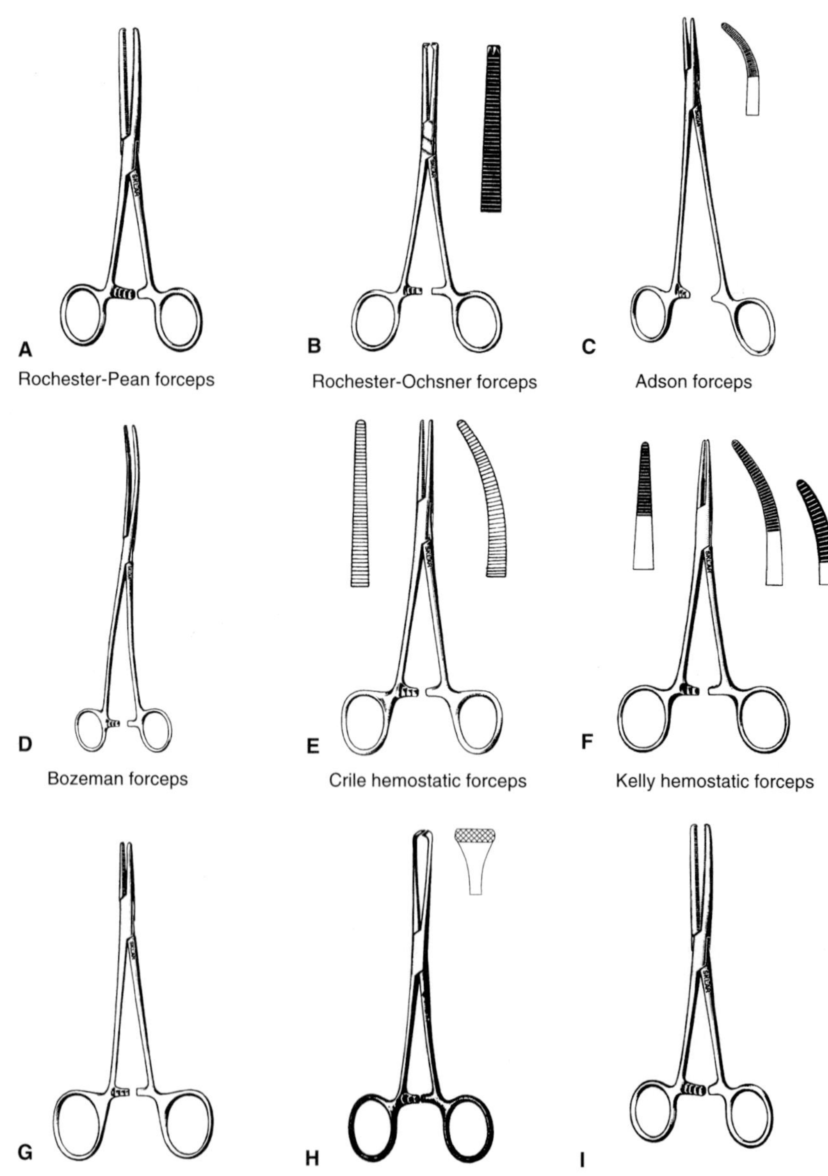

Figure 5-1 Types of forceps. (Sklar Instruments, West Chester, PA.)

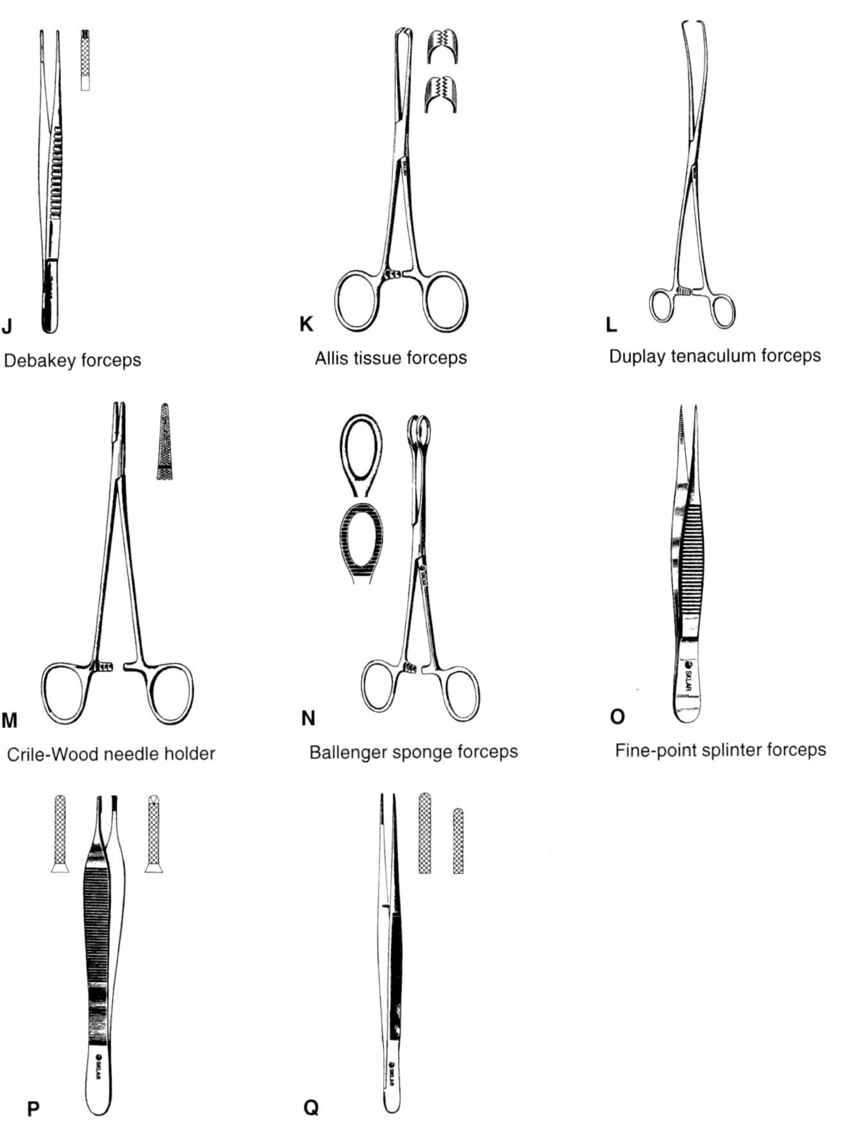

Figure 5-1 *(continued)*

Scissors

Scissors are sharp instruments composed of two opposing cutting blades, held together by a central pin on which the blades pivot. Scissors are used for dissecting superficial, deep, or delicate tissues and for cutting sutures and dressing. Scissors have blade points that are blunt or sharp or a combination of both, depending on the use of the instrument. The several types of scissors include:

- *straight scissors*—used during operations or procedures to cut deep or delicate tissue and for cutting sutures
- *curved scissors*—used for dissecting superficial and delicate tissues
- *suture scissors*—used to cut sutures; made with a straight top blade and a "curved-out" or hooked, blunt-shaped bottom blade to fit under, lift, and grasp sutures for snipping
- *bandage scissors*—have a flattened blunt tip on the bottom longer blade for fitting under bandages safely. These are usually angled to maneuver more easily under bandages. The most common type is the Lister bandage scissors.

Figure 5-2 shows various types of scissors.

Scalpels and Blades

A **scalpel** is a small surgical knife with a straight handle and a sharp blade edge. The scalpel handle can use interchangeable blades, based on the type of surgical procedure to be performed. Straight or pointed blades are used for incision and drainage purposes; curved

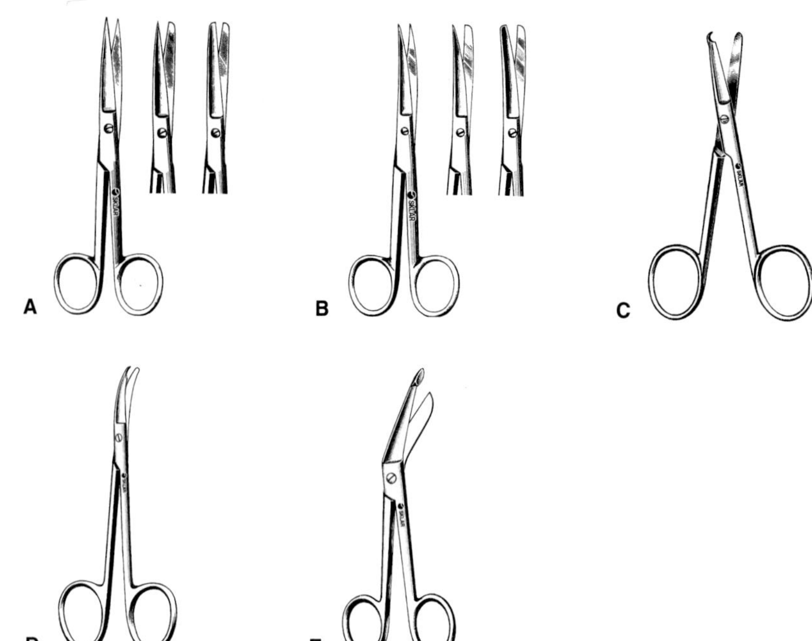

Figure 5-2 Types of scissors. (**A**) Straight-blade operating scissors, *left to right:* sharp/sharp (S/S), sharp/blunt (S/B), blunt/blunt (B/B). (**B**) Curved-blade operating scissors, *left to right:* sharp/sharp (S/S), sharp/blunt (S/B), blunt/blunt (B/B). (**C**) Spencer stitch scissors. (**D**) Suture scissors. (**E**) Lister bandage scissors. (Sklar Instruments, West Chester, PA.)

blades are used to excise tissue. If a reusable handle is used, the blade will always be disposable. Many offices use disposable handles and blades. Figure 5-3 shows various scalpels and blades.

Towel Clamps

Towel clamps are used to maintain the integrity of the **sterile field** by holding the sterile drapes in place, allowing exposure of the operative site (Fig. 5-4). A sterile field is a specific area that is considered free of microorganisms.

Probes and Directors

Before entering a cavity or site for a procedure, the physician may first probe the depths and direction of the operative area. The probe will show the angle and depth of the operative area, and the director will guide the knife or instrument once the procedure has begun (Fig. 5-5).

Retractors

Retractors hold open layers of tissue, exposing the areas underneath to view. They may be plain or toothed; the toothed retractor may be sharp or blunt. Retrac-

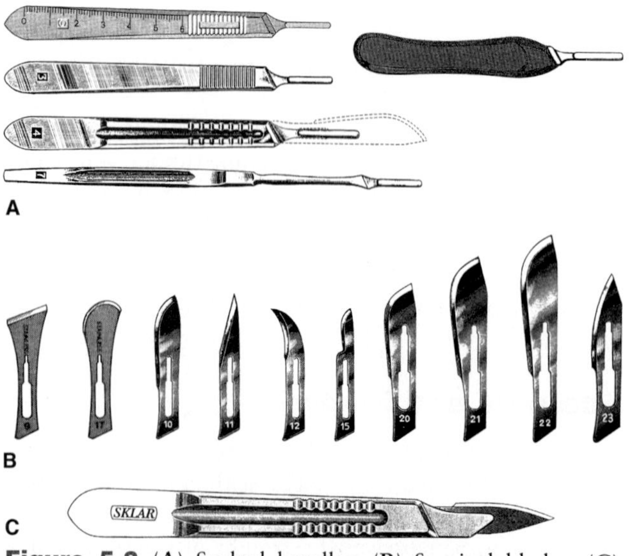

Figure 5-3 (**A**) Scalpel handles. (**B**) Surgical blades. (**C**) Sterile disposable scalpel-complete. (Sklar Instruments, West Chester, PA.)

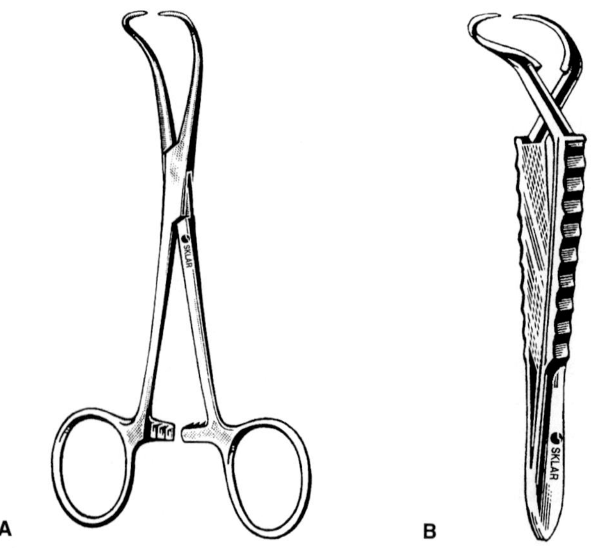

Figure 5-4 (**A**) Backhaus towel clamp. (**B**) Jones cross-action towel clamp. (Sklar Instruments, West Chester, PA.)

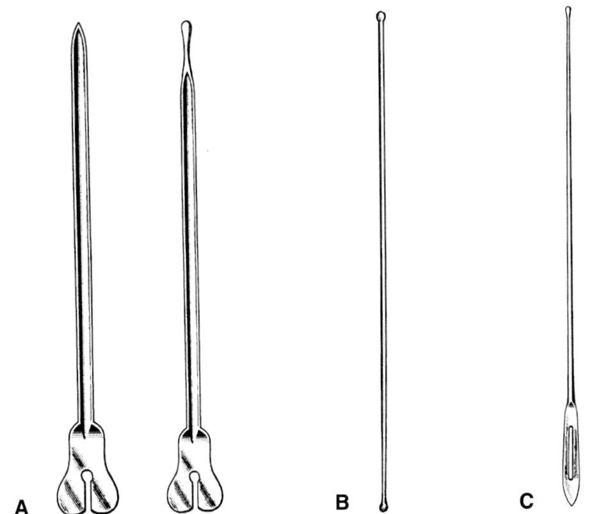

Figure 5-5 (A) Director and tongue tie. (B) Double-ended probe. (C) Probe with eye. (Sklar Instruments, West Chester, PA.)

tors may be designed either to be held by an assistant or screwed open to be self-retaining. Figure 5-6 shows several types of retractors.

Checkpoint Question

1. *Describe the uses for forceps, scissors, scalpels, and towel clamps.*

INSTRUMENTS AND EQUIPMENT USED BY SPECIALISTS

Physicians have preferences for certain types of instruments specific to their practices. An obstetrician usually will not have equipment normally used only by orthopedists, such as cast cutters and splints. Nor would the orthopedist have equipment usually used by an otologist, such as Buck's ear curet or otic lavage equipment.

As a medical assistant, you will not be required to identify a large assortment of instruments or equipment, but you must know the names, uses, and care of the equipment, instruments, and supplies used by the specific practice in which you work. Table 5-1 shows, by specialty, the most commonly used instruments and equipment.

Many of the instruments listed in Table 5-1 and in the section on instruments (above) may be reused. However, many are manufactured for "single-use only" and must be disposed of properly. Disposable instruments should not be reprocessed. Reusable items should be processed according to the designated use of the instrument or based on the manufacturer's recommendations.

In selecting the method of cleaning, disinfecting, or sterilizing, you must consider the uses for the instrument (medical asepsis versus surgical asepsis) and know any effects that certain chemicals may have on the equipment (ie, etching of glass or metal by solvents).

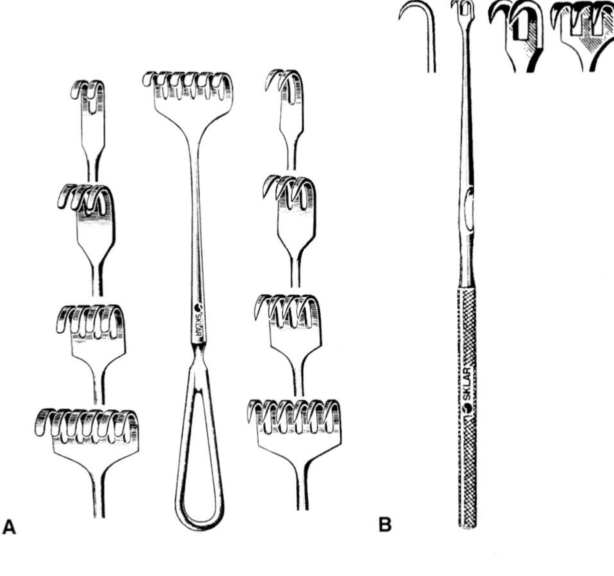

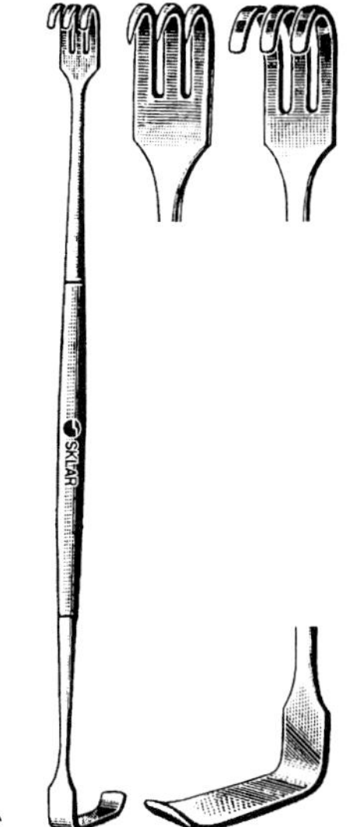

Figure 5-6 (A) Volkman retractor. (B) Lahey retractor. (C) Senn retractor. (Sklar Instruments, West Chester, PA.)

CARE AND HANDLING OF INSTRUMENTS

To ensure that surgical instruments always function properly, follow these guidelines:

1. Avoid dropping or tossing instruments into basins or sinks. Surgical instruments are delicate and may have sharp blades or pointed tips easily damaged by improper handling. Should an instrument be

text continues on page 99

Table 5-1 **Commonly Used Instruments and Equipment, by Specialty**

Instruments	*Use*
Obstetrics and Gynecology	
Speculum (pl. specula)	Opening the vagina for viewing the vaginal walls and cervical os and to perform procedures; are sized and may be reusable metal or disposable plastic
Fetal monitor	Assessing the health of the fetus
Ultrasound	Visualizing the fetus
Vaginal swabs	Applying or removing substances from the vagina or cervix
Tenaculum	Grasping and holding a part with hooklike tips and clasps tightly with ratchets
Uterine sounds	Assessing the depth of the uterus or location of the fundus; are graduated in inches or centimeters
Uterine dilators	Widening the cervical os; usually sized 3–18 mm
Curet	Scraping the endometrium; may be blunt or sharp
Dressing forceps	Sponging the area clean or applying treatments; may be ring forceps or Kelly forceps
Biopsy forceps or curet	Securing bits of tissue for microscopic study

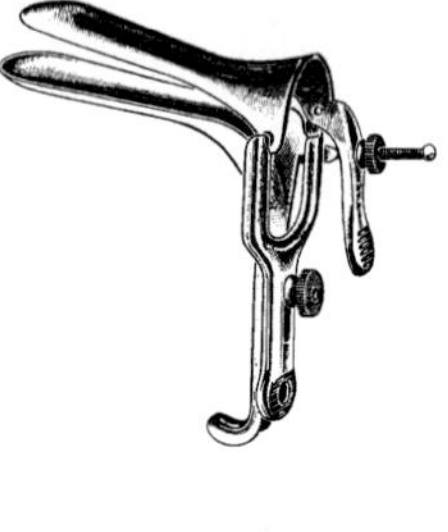

Graves vaginal speculum

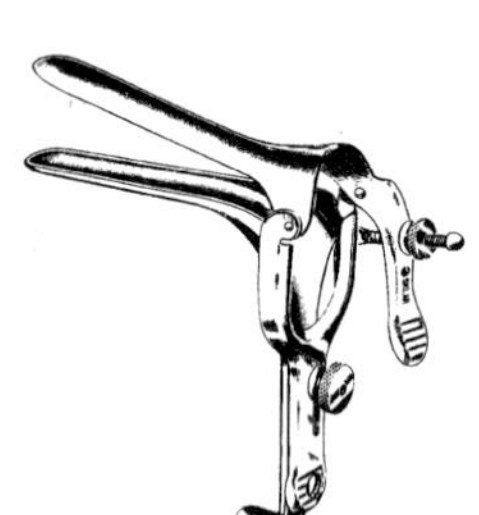

Pederson vaginal speculum

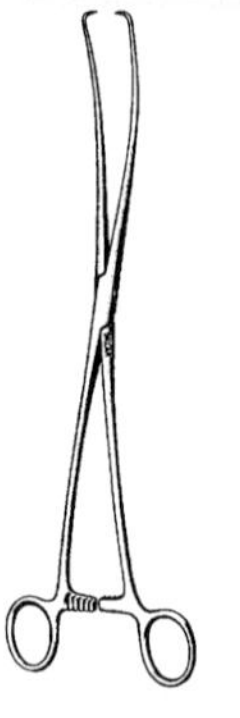

Duplay tenaculum forceps

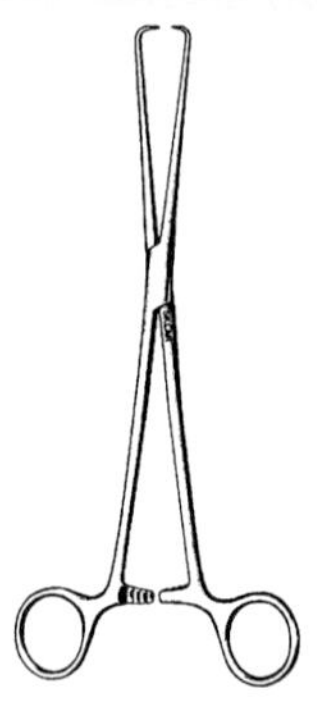

Schroeder tenaculum forceps

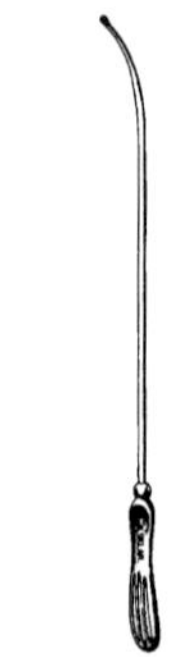

Sims uterine sound

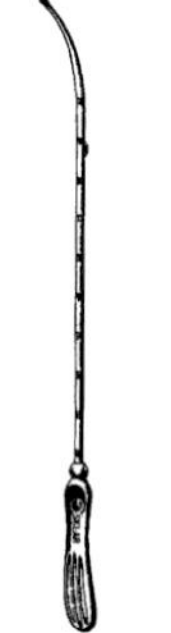

Simpson uterine sound-malleable

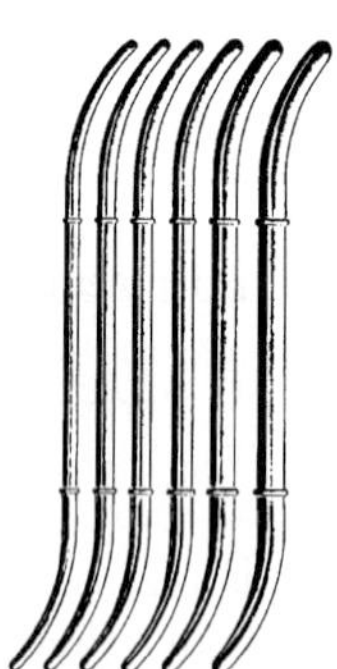

Hank uterine dilator

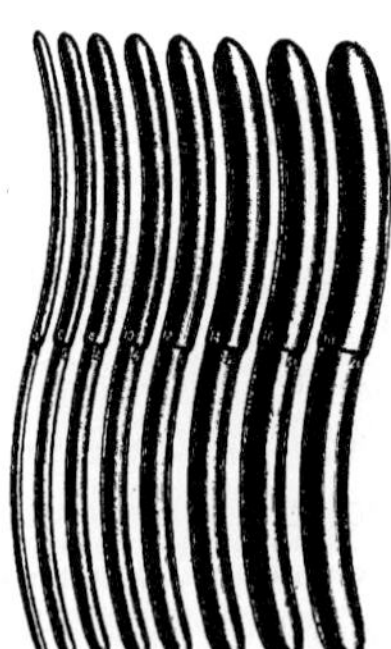

Hegar uterine dilator

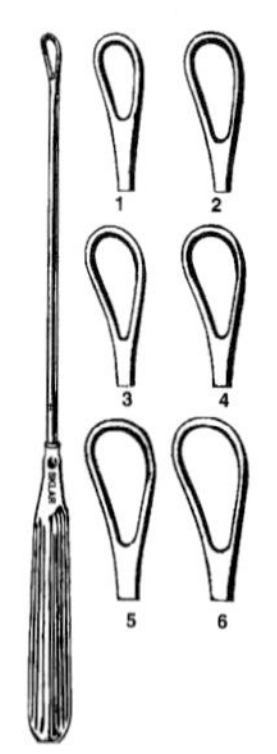

Thomas uterine curets

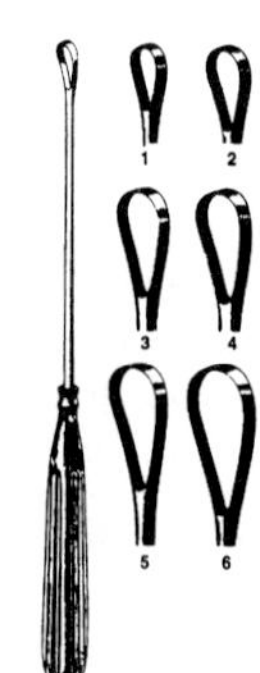

Sims uterine curets

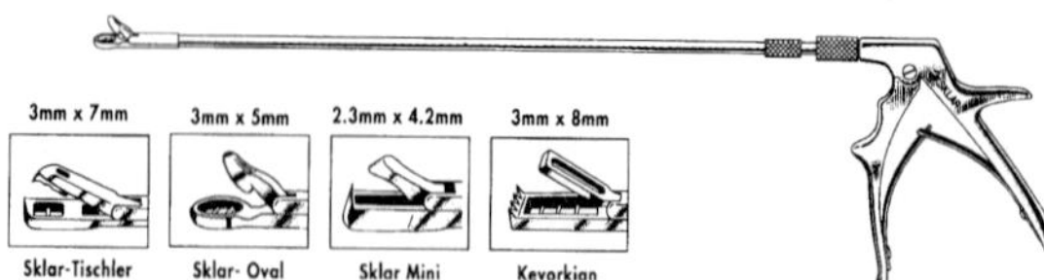

Universal style biopsy instruments

(continued)

Table 5-1 **Commonly Used Instruments and Equipment, by Specialty** *(Continued)*

Instruments	*Use*
Orthopedics	
Splints, braces, straps, supports, and immobilizers	Securing a part to prevent movement during healing
Cast saw or cutters and spreaders	Removing the cast at the completion of treatment
Dust collector or suction	Minimizing the debris of cast removal
Goniometer	Measuring range of motion and joint function
Rachiometer	Measuring spinal curvature

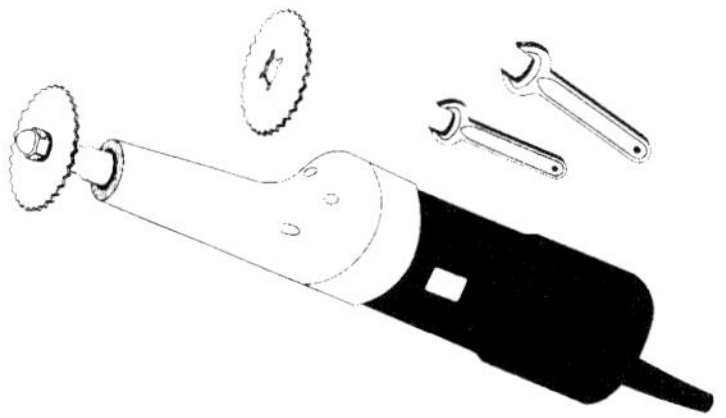
Oscillating plaster saw

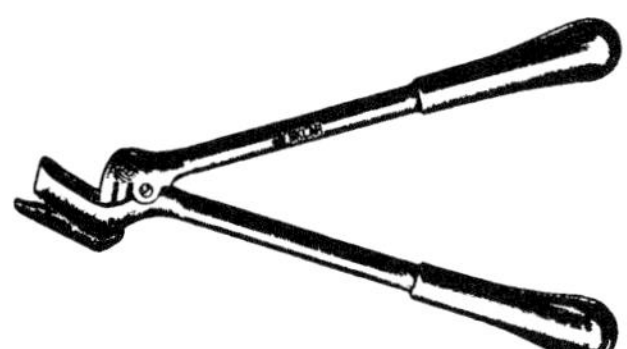
Stille plaster shears

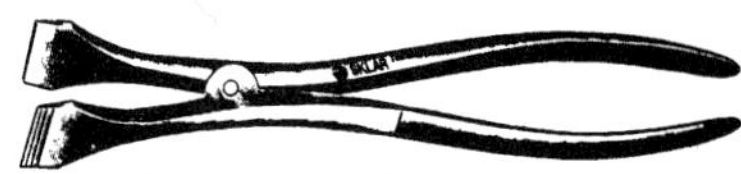
Hennig plaster spreader

Instruments	*Use*
Urology	
Cystoscope	Viewing the interior of the bladder
Catheter kits	Emptying the bladder for procedures or for securing a sterile specimen for diagnostic procedures; may be straight for one use, or may be Foley to remain in the bladder for a period of time
Prostate biopsy instruments	Removing bits of tissue for further microscopic study
Urethral sounds	Exploring the bladder depth and direction and for meatal dilation in cases of urethral stenosis; sized Fr 8–26
Microscopes, culture media, strip testing supplies	Diagnosing disorders

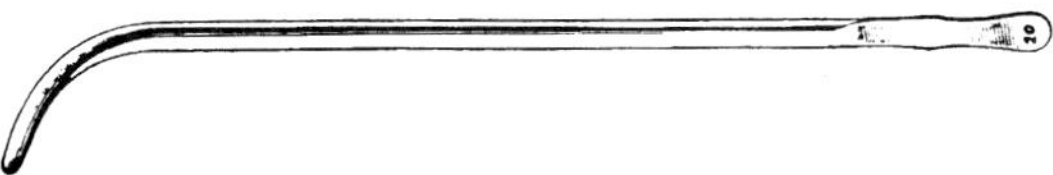
Otis/Dittel urethral sound

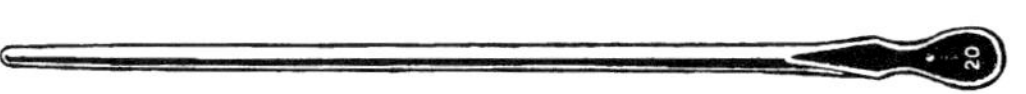
Dittel urethral sound

Instruments	*Use*
Proctology	
Anoscopes, sigmoidoscopes, proctoscopes	Visualizing the interior of the lower intestinal tract; are usually lighted and primarily flexible fiberoptic with a power source. Most will have an **obturator** for ease of insertion and patient comfort. Some will be equipped with suction devices.
Anal specula	Opening the anal walls for visualization
Biopsy instruments (punch or alligator)	Removing tissue (punch biopsy involves removing a small piece of tissue by making a small circular hole; alligator biopsies use an instrument with jaws that grasp and excise tissue)
Hemorrhoidal ligator	Applying a band to the base of the hemorrhoid to cause it to necrose and slough off

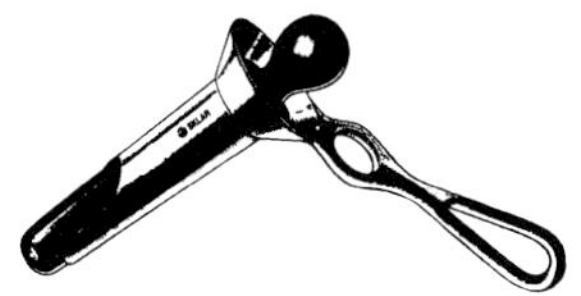
Ives rectal speculum (Fansler)

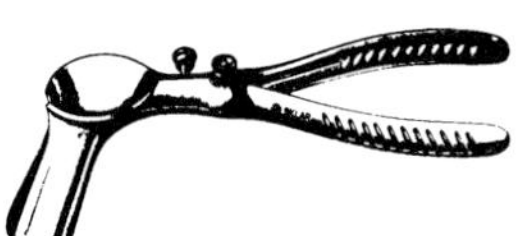
Pratt rectal speculum

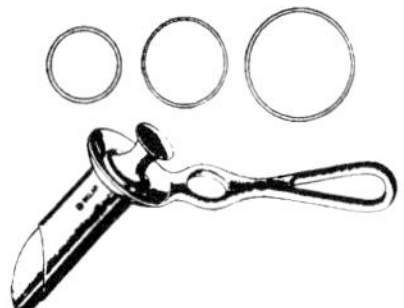
Hirschman anoscope

(continued)

Table 5-1 **Commonly Used Instruments and Equipment, by Specialty** *(Continued)*

Instruments	*Use*
Otology and Rhinology	
Audioscope/Audiometer	Viewing the tympanic membrane and screening for decibel level losses
Tympanometer	Detecting otitis media and other middle ear pathologies; equipped with a printer for hard copy to assess the status of tympanic membrane pressure
Nasal or ear forceps	Visualizing the site of concern
Curets	Removing cerumen or scraping the nasal passages
Syringes	Washing out the ear canal; may be either bulb or plunger type
Nasal speculae	Extending the nostrils to visualize the nasal passages

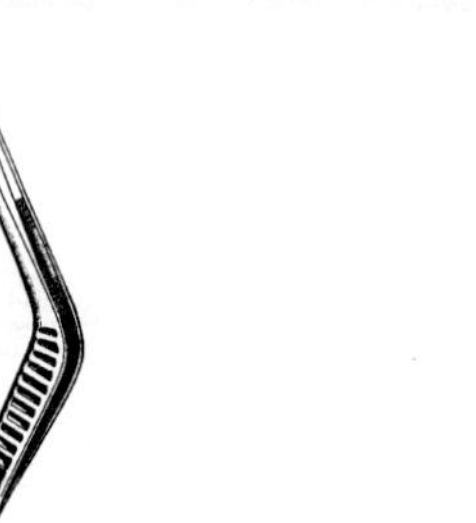

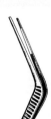

Wilde ear forceps

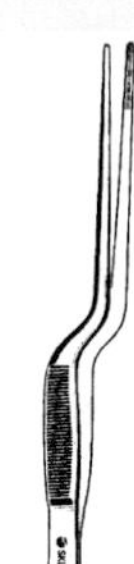

Lucae bayonet forceps

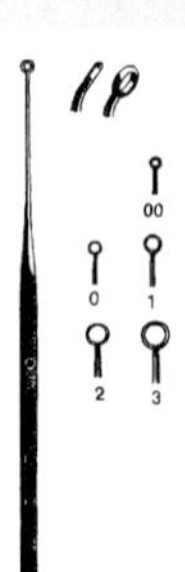

Buck ear curet

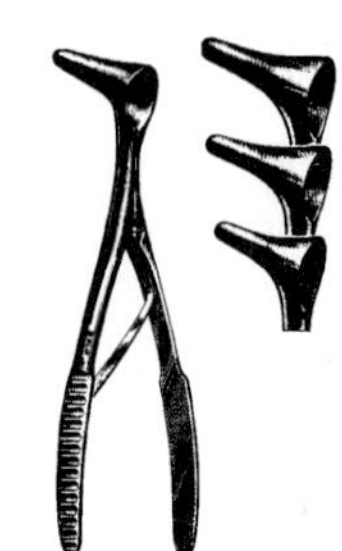

Vienna nasal speculum

Instruments	*Use*
Ophthalmology	
Iris and strabismus scissors	Performing surgery
Eye loop and lid retractor	Assisting with finding and removing foreign bodies
Tonometer	Measuring the intraocular pressure to diagnose glaucoma

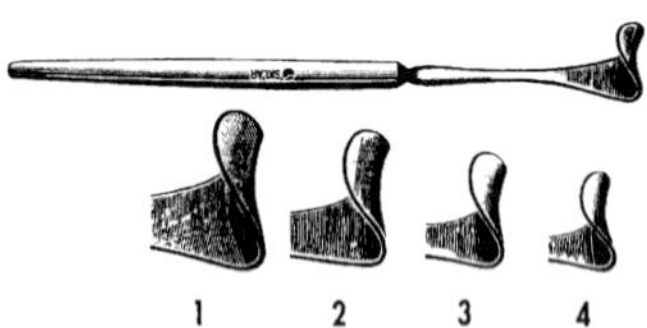

Desmarres lid retractor

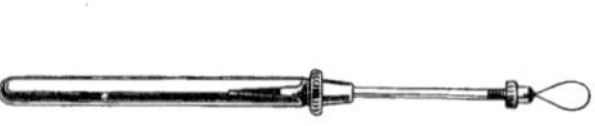

Bailey foreign body remover

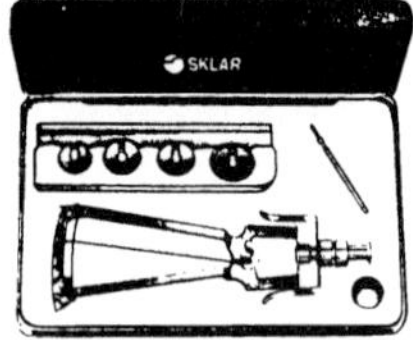

Schiotz tonometer

Instruments	*Use*
Dermatology	
Punch biopsy	Removing small circular sections of skin for microscopic studies; sized 2–8 mm, either disposable or reusable
Comedone extractors	Removing blackheads and opening pustules

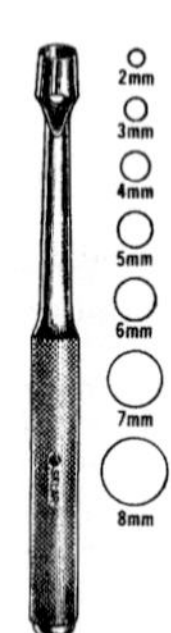

Keyes cutaneous punch

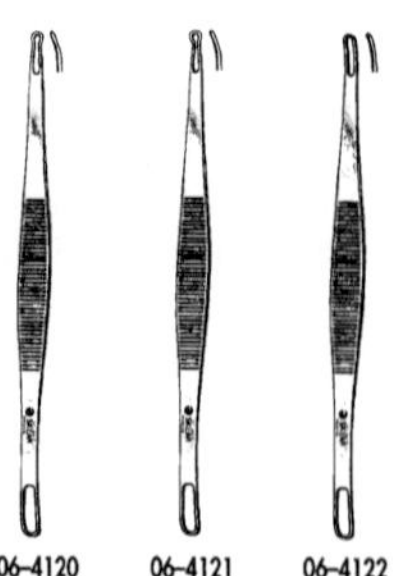

Schamberg comedone extractor

Instruments courtesy of Sklar Instruments, West Chester, PA.

dropped accidentally, it should be carefully inspected to identify damage. Damaged instruments usually can be repaired and should not be discarded unless repair is not feasible.

2. Avoid stacking instruments into a pile. They may become tangled and be damaged when separated.
3. Sharp instruments should always be stored separately to prevent dulling or damaging the sharp edges and to prevent accidental injury. Disposable scalpel blades should be removed from reusable handles and placed in puncture-proof sharps containers; if the handle is also disposable, the whole unit is discarded in the container. Syringes with needles attached and suture needles are placed in an approved sharps container and never placed in the trash or with other instruments for processing. Delicate instruments, such as those with lenses, delicate scissors, or tissue forceps, are kept separate so they may be processed appropriately.
4. Keep ratcheted instruments in an open position when not in use to avoid damage to the ratchet mechanism.
5. Rinse gross contamination from instruments as quickly as possible to prevent drying and hardening, which makes the cleaning process more difficult.
6. Check instruments before sterilization to ensure that they are in good working order; this allows you to identify instruments in need of repair.
   a. Blades or points should be free of bends and nicks.
   b. Tips should close evenly and tightly.
   c. Instruments with box locks should move freely but should not be too loose.
   d. Instruments with spring handles should have enough tension to grasp objects tightly.
   e. Scissors should close in a smooth, even manner with no nicks or snags. (Scissors may be checked by cutting through gauze or cotton to be sure there are no rough areas.)
   f. Screws should be flush with the instrument surface. They should be freely workable but not loose.
7. Use instruments only for the purpose for which they were designed. For instance, surgical scissors should never be used to cut paper or open packages because this may damage the cutting edges.
8. Sanitize instruments before they are sterilized so that sterilization procedures will work effectively.

Checkpoint Question

2. *Why should you avoid dropping surgical instruments, and what should you do if one drops accidentally?*

PRINCIPLES AND PRACTICES OF ASEPSIS

As a medical assistant, you are responsible for minimizing the onset and spread of infection based on the principles and practices of asepsis as it relates to instruments, equipment, and supplies. Asepsis is the absence of microorganisms, infection, or infectious material. Asepsis is classified as either medical asepsis or surgical asepsis.

Medical asepsis (clean technique) is the removal or destruction of disease organisms or infected material. Surgical asepsis (sterile technique) refers to practices designed to render and maintain objects and areas maximally free from microorganisms. (See Chap. 1, Asepsis and Infection Control, for a detailed discussion of medical and surgical asepsis and handwashing.)

You must be able to distinguish between the need for disinfection versus the need for sterilization. By becoming familiar with the manufacturer's recommendations for processing instruments and equipment based on the purposes for which the items will be used, you will be able to determine the level of asepsis appropriate in each instance. The method of sterilization to be used in any procedure depends on the nature of the material to be sterilized and the type of bacteria to be destroyed. It is recommended that procedures of sterilization be assigned to one or two workers in the facility. The occasional worker may not have the experience or knowledge to ensure that true sterilization will be accomplished.

SANITATION

Surgical instruments and equipment have to be cared for and cleaned according to the recommendation of the manufacturer and with their eventual uses in mind. All instruments and equipment must be sanitized, which means they will be cleaned with warm soapy water and mechanical action to remove all organic matter and other residue.

Sanitation is the science of maintaining a healthful, disease-free, and hazard-free environment. Sanitation results in the reduction of the microbial population on an inanimate object to a safe or relatively safe level. Cleaning or **sanitizing** must precede **disinfection** and **sterilization** procedures (Procedure 5-1). Disinfection destroys most pathogenic organisms; sterilization destroys all microorganisms.

DISINFECTION

Disinfection describes a process that eliminates many or all pathogenic microorganisms on inanimate objects, with the exception of bacterial spores. The

Procedure 5-1 Sanitizing Equipment for Sterilization or Disinfection

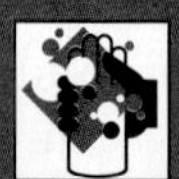
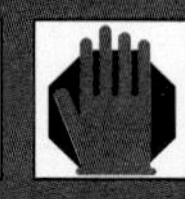
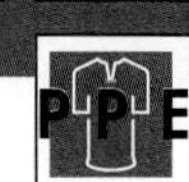

PURPOSE:

To render surfaces optimally free of pathogens

EQUIPMENT/SUPPLIES

- equipment to be sanitized
- gloves
- impervious gown
- eye protection (goggles, face shield)
- soaking solution
- brushes or gauze
- basin

STEPS

1. Put on gloves, gown, and eye protection.
   These devices protect against splattering and prevent contamination of your clothing.
2. Take apart pieces that require assembly. If cleaning is not possible immediately, disassemble the pieces and soak the sections to avoid having them stick together.
3. Check for the operation and integrity of the equipment. If the equipment is defective, it should be repaired or discarded.
4. Rinse with cool water.
   Hot water "cooks" proteins onto the equipment.
5. After the initial rinsing, force streams of soapy water through any tubular or grooved instruments to clean the inside and the outside.
6. After the cool rinse, use a hot soapy soak to dissolve fats or lubricants left on the surface. Use the soaking solution of choice for the facility.
7. Use friction with a soft brush or gauze to loosen transient microorganisms. Abrasive materials should not be used on delicate instruments and equipment. Brushes work well on grooves and joints. Open and close the jaws of scissors or forceps several times to ensure that all material has been removed.
8. Rinse well.
   Proper rinsing removes soap or detergent residues.
9. Dry well before autoclaving or soaking.
   Excess moisture will cause super wet steam and decrease the effectiveness of the autoclave process by delaying drying; it may also wick microorganisms into the damp packs. Moisture will dilute the soaking solution, if the instrument is disinfected in that manner.
10. Be aware that any items used in the sanitation process (such as basins and brushes) are considered grossly contaminated and must be properly sanitized or discarded.

process kills pathogenic organisms or renders them inert.

In the health care setting, disinfection is generally accomplished by the use of liquid chemicals or wet pasteurization (Table 5-2). **Disinfectants are chemicals that can be applied to instruments and equipment to destroy microorganisms.** Disinfection is affected by a number of factors, any of which may limit the effectiveness of the process. These include:

- Prior cleaning of the object
- The amount of organic material on the object
- The type and level of microbial contamination
- The concentration of the **germicide** (chemical that kills pathogens)
- The length of exposure to the germicide
- The shape or complexity of the object
- The temperature of the disinfection process

Categories of disinfection include:

- High level—destroys all microorganisms, with the exception of bacterial spores
- Intermediate—inactivates *Mycobacterium,* tuberculin bacilli, vegetative bacteria, most viruses, and some fungi, but does not necessarily kill bacterial spores
- Low level—can kill most bacteria, some viruses, and some fungi, but cannot be relied on to kill resistant microorganisms, such as tuberculin bacilli or bacterial spores

(See Chap. 1, Asepsis and Infection Control, for a more complete description of these categories.)

Disinfectants or germicides inactivate virtually all recognized pathogenic microorganisms but not necessarily all microbial forms, such as spores, on inanimate objects.

Table 5-2 **Disinfection Methods**

Method	*Uses and Precautions*
Alcohol (70% isopropyl alcohol or ethyl alcohol)	Used for noncritical items (countertops, thermometers, stethoscopes) Flammable Damages some rubber, plastic, and lensed equipment
Chlorine (sodium hypochlorite or bleach)	Dilute to 1:10 (1 part bleach to 10 parts water) Used for a broad spectrum of antimicrobial activity Inexpensive and fast acting Corrosive, inactivated by organic matter, relatively unstable
Formaldehyde	Disinfectant and sterilant Regulated by OSHA Presence must be marked on all containers and storage areas
Glutaraldehyde	Alkaline or acid based Effective against bacteria, viruses, fungi, and some spores OSHA regulated; requires adequate ventilation, covered pans, gloves, and masks Must display biohazard or chemical label
Hydrogen peroxide	Stable and effective when used on inanimate objects Attacks membrane lipids, DNA, and other essential cell components Can damage plastic, rubber, and some metals
Iodine or iodophores	Bacteriostatic agent used for skin surfaces Not to be used on instruments May cause staining
Phenols (tuberculocidal)	Used for environmental items and equipment Requires gloves and eye protection Can cause skin irritation and burns

DNA, deoxyribonucleic acid; OSHA, Occupational Safety and Health Administration

5

STERILIZATION

Disinfection practices are not sufficient to process instruments and equipment for sterile technique; objects requiring surgical asepsis must be sterilized. Sterilization is the complete elimination or destruction of all forms of microbial life, including spore forms. It is accomplished by either physical or chemical processes. Steam under pressure, dry heat, **ethylene oxide** (a gas), and liquid chemicals are principle sterilizing agents. Critical medical devices or patient care equipment that enter normally sterile tissue or the vascular system, or through which blood flows, should be sterilized before each use.

Two types of bacteria are major concerns in sterilization: spore formers and nonspore formers. Spores are extremely resistant to heat. They can be destroyed most effectively by steam under pressure in an **autoclave,** an appliance used to sterilize medical instruments. Nonspore formers vary widely in their reaction to heat, but most of them are destroyed by boiling water, chemical agents, or gases. The method of sterilization to be used in any procedure depends on the nature of the material to be sterilized and the type of bacteria to be destroyed.

The most frequently used sterilant in the clinic or office setting is the autoclave, which uses steam under pressure. Other types of sterilants include liquid chemicals (glutaraldehyde or formaldehyde) and gas solvents (ethylene oxide). The liquid chemical form is the second most frequently used sterilant for instruments with successful sterilization after 10 hours of total submersion in the chemical liquid agent. Ethylene gas is rarely used in clinics or offices because of the dangers associated with its use. The Occupational Safety and Health Administration (OSHA) has issued stringent guidelines for its use, and workers must be specially trained in safety measures.

Table 5-3 describes various methods of sterilization.

Table 5-3 **Sterilization Methods**

Method	*Concentration or Levels*
Heat	
Moist heat (steam under pressure)	250°F or 121°C for 30 min
Boiling	100°C or 212°F at least 30 min
Dry heat	171°C for 1 h 160°C for 2 h
Liquids	
Glutaraldehyde Formaldehyde	Follow manufacturer's recommendation or OSHA requirements and guidelines
Gas	
Ethylene oxide	450–500 mg/L 50°C

OSHA, Occupational Safety and Health Administration

What If?

What if, while pouring glutaraldehyde into a container, the chemical spills?

OSHA and state regulations have defined a specific law to protect you from hazardous materials. The law is termed "The Right to Know" and requires that all companies using hazardous materials have Material Safety Data Sheets (MSDS) available to their employees. MSDS forms are prepared by the chemical manufacturer and clearly state how to handle and dispose of the chemical. These forms also include a list of potential health hazards to workers and identify the safety equipment needed when using the chemical. Never handle any type of chemical spill without first reading the MSDS form.

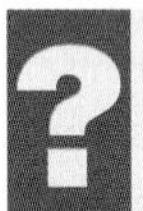

Checkpoint Question

3. *What are the differences between sanitation, disinfection, and sterilization?*

Sterilization Equipment

Several different types of sterilization equipment are necessary in the clinic or office setting. As a medical assistant, it is your responsibility to:

- Become familiar with the uses and operation of each piece of equipment
- Schedule periodic preventive maintenance or servicing of the equipment
- Maintain adequate supplies for general operational needs

Autoclave

The most frequently used piece of equipment for sterilizing instruments today is the autoclave (Fig. 5-7). The autoclave consists of two chambers, an outer unit where pressure builds and an inner chamber where the actual sterilization occurs. Water is added to a reservoir where it is converted to steam as the preset temperature is reached. The steam is forced into the inner chamber, increasing the pressure, which raises the temperature of the steam to a higher degree than that of boiling water (212°F or 100°C). (The pressure has no effect on sterilization; its purpose is to increase the temperature of the steam. The higher the pressure, the higher the temperature of the steam, which allows for more rapid destruction of most spores and viruses.)

An air vent exhaust at the bottom of the autoclave allows the air present in the chamber to be pushed out and replaced by the pressurized steam. When no more air is present, the chamber seals and the temperature gauge begins to rise. Newer automatic autoclaves can be set to vent, time, turn off, and exhaust at preset

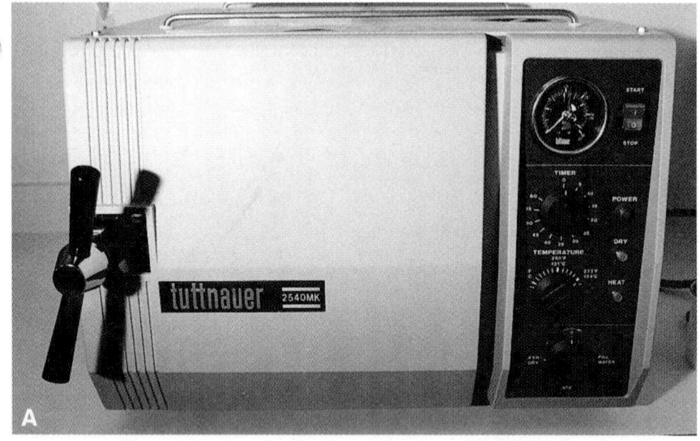

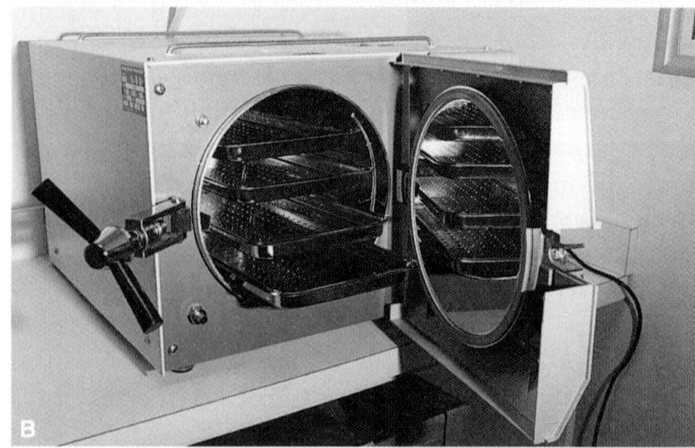

Figure 5-7 (**A**) An office-sized autoclave; note the clearly marked dials and gauges. (**B**) The interior of the autoclave.

times and levels. Older models may require that the steps be advanced manually. All manufacturers provide instructions for operating the machine and recommendations for times necessary to sterilize different types of loads. These instructions should be posted in a prominent place near the machine.

Remember: Sterilization is required for surgical instruments and equipment that will come in contact with internal body tissues or cavities that are considered sterile. The autoclave is commonly used to sterilize minor surgical instruments, surgical storage trays and containers, and some surgical equipment, such as cystoscopes (lighted instruments guided through the urethra to visualize the bladder) and proctoscopes (lighted instruments guided through the anus to visualize the lower colon). Autoclaving is not recommended for many types of scopes; follow the manufacturer's recommendations.

You must be knowledgeable not only about the use of, the need for, and the care of the autoclave, but you also must know how to operate the equipment

Box 5-1

Preparing Equipment and Supplies for Sterilization

After sanitizing and checking the equipment and supplies, dry them well and prepare them to be wrapped. The wrapping material must have certain properties. For example, it must:

- Be permeable to steam but not contaminants
- Resist tearing and puncturing during normal handling
- Allow easy opening to prevent contamination of the contents
- Maintain sterility of the item during storage

The wrap may be double layers of cotton muslin, special paper, or appropriately sized instrument pouches. The pouches are gaining wide acceptance because of their convenience. They are sized for a small, single instrument or for an entire tray or setup and all sizes in between. They are transparent on one side so that the contents can be checked before opening. The pouches offer many benefits: They provide good protection from contamination, are easy to use, take up little space, and when opened properly, form a sterile field from which to work. However, they are somewhat stiff to work with, and if a large sterile field must be set up, an additional barrier drape must be wrapped within the package to form the table drape.

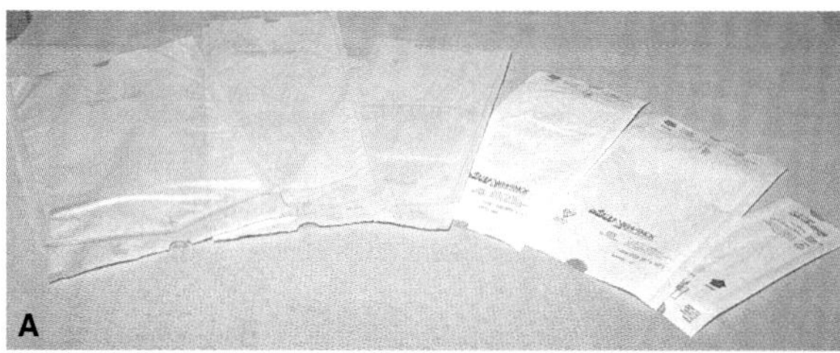

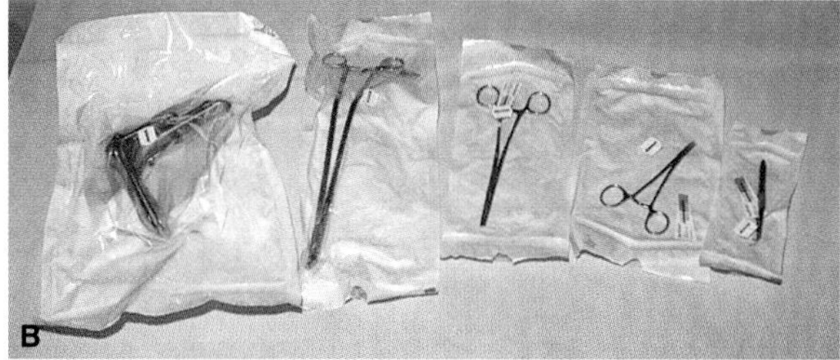

(**A**) Instrument pouches in a variety of sizes and (**B**) after autoclaving.

To facilitate the wrapping process, prepare note cards listing items to include in packages. Pull the appropriate card and assemble the equipment to ensure that each package is complete.

5

properly and how to prepare the items for sterilization (Box 5-1). No matter how well the equipment is operated, if the items are not properly prepared for the autoclaving process, the sterility of the items cannot be ensured (Procedure 5-2).

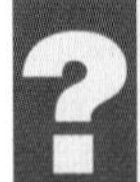

Checkpoint Question

4. *What is an autoclave and how does it work?*

Sterilization Indicators

Tapes applied to the outside of the packets will indicate that the items have been exposed to heat and pressure but will not ensure sterility of the contents (Box 5-2). Sterilization indicators placed in the packs will register that the proper pressure and temperature were present for the required time to allow steam to penetrate to the inner parts of the pack (Fig. 5-8). Improper wrapping, loading, or operation of the autoclave will prevent the indicator from registering properly.

5

Box 5-2
Autoclave Indicator Tape

Autoclave tape is designed to change color in the presence of heat and steam. In extreme instances, tapes may change appearance when stored too near heat sources. Most tapes have lines imprinted that will deepen in color after exposure to gas or autoclave sterilization. However, sterilization of the package contents is not ensured by a color change. Proper sterilization can only be assumed if accompanying sterilization indicators have registered that all elements of the sterilization process have been achieved.

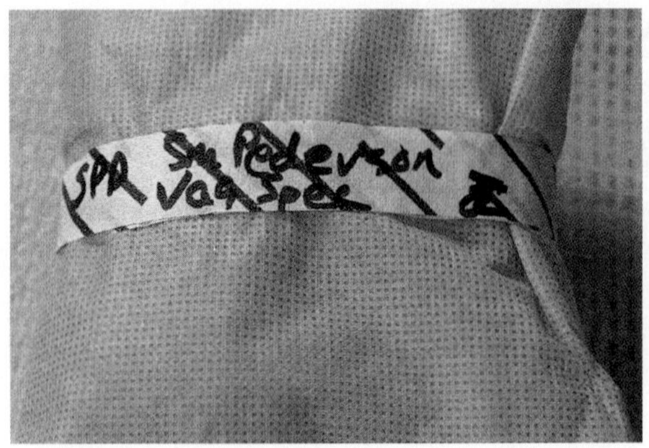

Color indicator strips change color, indicating sterilization has occurred.

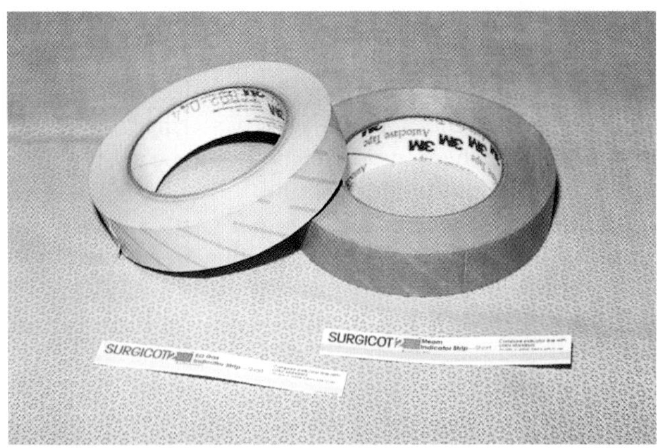

Figure 5-8 Sterilization indicators and tape. Gas indicator and tape (*left*) and steam indicator and tape (*right*).

Forms of indicators include those that change colors as higher temperatures are reached. If the required temperature is reached, it will register within the safe zone on the indicator. Specially designed tubes containing wax pellets are also used to indicate by the melted wax that the required temperature was reached.

Although most types of sterilization indicators work well, the best method of determining the effectiveness of sterilization is the culture test. Strips impregnated with heat-resistant spores are wrapped and placed in the center of the autoclave between the packages in a specific load. The strips are removed from their packets and placed in a broth culture to be incubated according to the instructions of the manufacturer. At the end of the incubation period, the culture is compared to a control to determine that all spores have been killed. If sterilization was incomplete, the entire load processed with the indicators must be reprocessed.

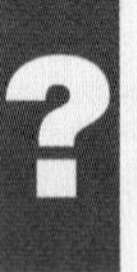

Checkpoint Question

5. *What is a sterilization indicator and what can prevent it from registering that sterilization has occurred?*

Loading the Autoclave

Load loosely to allow steam to circulate throughout the items. If too many items are packed in, steam will not penetrate to those items in the center.

Place containers on their sides with lids off. If containers are placed in the autoclave in an upright position, air, which is heavier than steam, will settle into the interior of the container and keep steam from circulating to the inner surfaces.

Place all packs vertically (on their sides) to allow for the maximum steam circulation and penetration. Like materials should be autoclaved together—soft with soft, metal with metal—as much as possible. Items should be packed on a perforated tray for steam circulation.

Figure 5-9 shows a properly loaded hospital autoclave.

Checkpoint Question

6. *How would you load an autoclave?*

Operating the Autoclave

All components of the autoclaving process—temperature, pressure, steam, and time—must be in place for the items to reach a state of sterility. Follow the instruction manual carefully. All machines use the same principles, but operation may vary. Become familiar with the function of the machine in your facility. Instructions may be covered in plastic or laminated and posted beside the machine for easy reference. Procedure 5-3 outlines the general steps for operating an autoclave.

Use distilled water only. Tap water contains chemicals that will coat the interior, clog the exhaust valves, and hinder operation. Fill the reservoir only to the fill

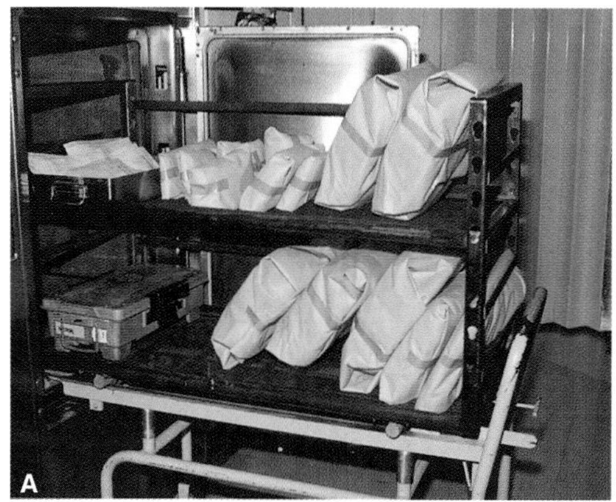

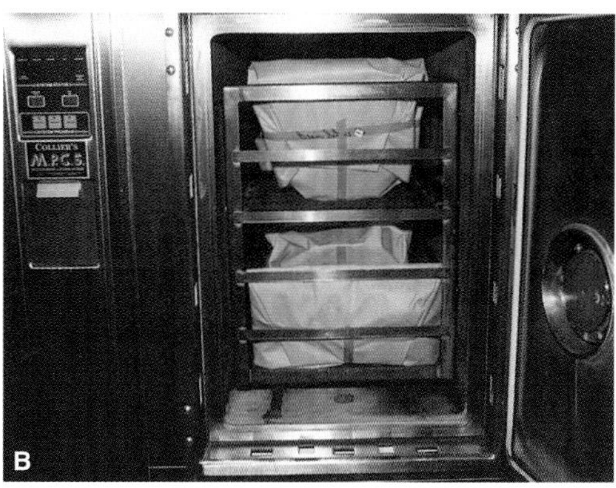

Figure 5-9 (**A**) A properly loaded hospital autoclave. Note the arrangement of the packs. Small packs are placed in a perforated tray to allow steam to circulate. (**B**) There is room on all sides for steam circulation.

5

Procedure 5-2 Wrapping Equipment and Supplies for Sterilization

PURPOSE:

To ensure the sterility of surgical instruments
To facilitate opening properly wrapped packages to maintain a sterile field

EQUIPMENT/SUPPLIES

- sanitized items
- list of items to be included in pack, as needed
- sterilization wrap preferred by the facility, appropriate size for items
- sterilization indicator
- heat-sensitive sealing tape

STEPS

1. Open all hinged instruments.

Packing hinged instruments in the open position ensures that steam penetrates all surfaces.

2. Place a barrier cloth on the bottom of trays to be used as a surgical field.

The barrier cloth absorbs condensation.

3. If multiple items are to be wrapped together, place the larger, heavier items on the bottom.

Placing the instruments in this manner protects them from damage.

4. If sharp pointed, hinged instruments are to be sterilized, place a cotton ball between the tips before wrapping.

The cotton ball prevents the tips from piercing the wrap.

continued

Procedure 5-2 Continued **Wrapping Equipment and Supplies for Sterilization**

5. Wrap the instruments as follows:

a. Place the items to be sterilized diagonally on the barrier wrap. Include a sterilization indicator. If possible or practical, place the items in an order that will facilitate the procedure for which they are prepared.

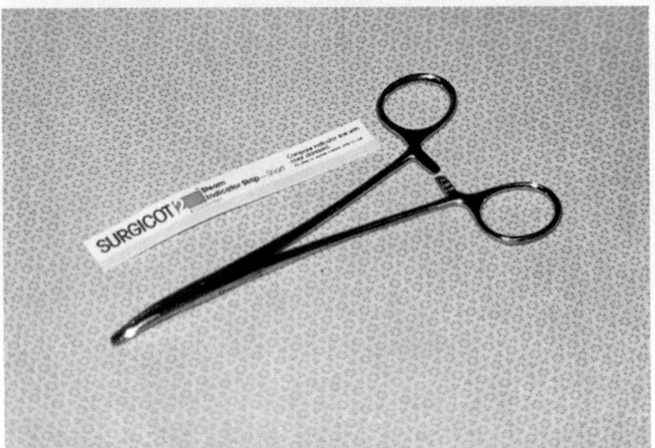

b. Fold the closest corner over with a tab folded back.

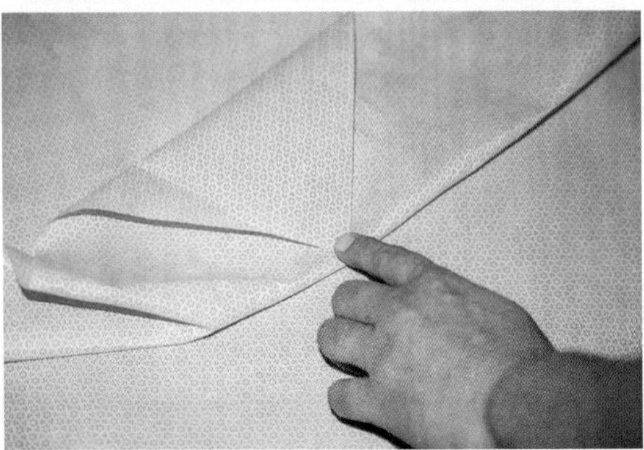

c. Fold in the left corner, then fold in the right corner, each with a folded tab.

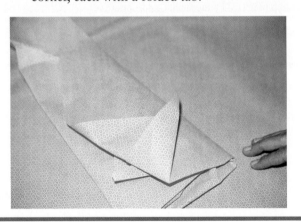

d. Fold the last corner over the pack or item and tuck the last corner under the preceding flaps. If the pack is to be double wrapped, follow the same procedure.

This ensures that items can be unwrapped or opened properly to prevent contamination.

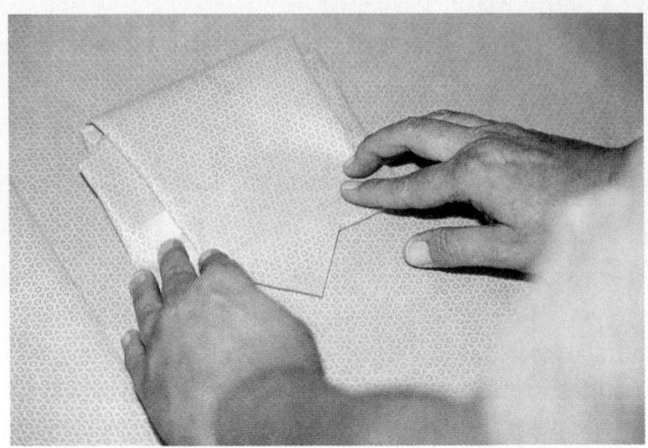

7. Seal the items with sterilization indicator tape. Indicate on the tape the contents of the pack, the date of processing, and your initials.

This provides a means of determining that items have been exposed to autoclave, the contents of the pack, and the person responsible for preparing the pack.

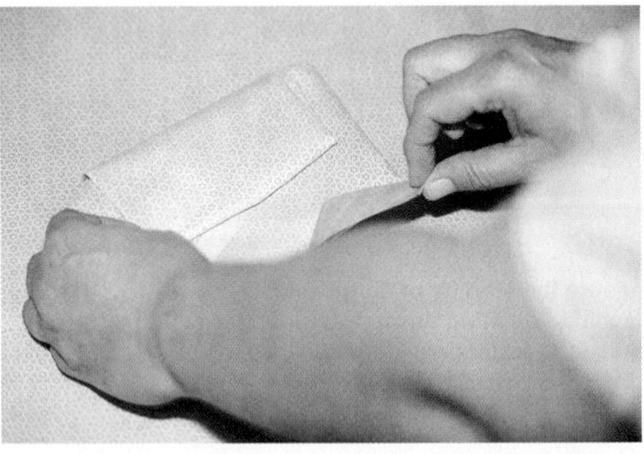

Note: *Wrap dressings for surgical setups in multiples of 5 or 10 to be counted at completion of the procedure. Be aware that site-prepared packs are considered sterile for 30 days.*

Procedure 5-3 Operating an Autoclave

PURPOSE:

To ensure that objects processed by this method are free of all microorganisms

EQUIPMENT/SUPPLIES

- sanitized, wrapped articles sealed with indicator tape (packs should each contain sterilization indicator)
- distilled water
- autoclave operating manual
- separately wrapped sterilization indicator

STEPS

1. Assemble the equipment. An indicator should be wrapped within each pack. An indicator may also be included and wrapped separately to check the efficiency of the process without disturbing the wrapped packages.
   Doing this ensures that all supplies are available. Including a wrapped indicator separately will allow you to check that the procedure was performed properly.
2. Check the water level and add more if needed, just to the fill line.
   Too little water causes too little steam, too much water causes saturated steam that will extend the drying time and may wick microorganisms into the damp packs.
3. Load the autoclave:
   a. Place trays and packs on their sides, from 1 to 3 inches from each other and from the sides of the autoclave.
      Steam circulation is not possible if items are tightly packed. Placing items vertically allows heavier air to be forced out rather than pooling in containers.
   b. Put containers on their sides with the lids ajar.
      Containers on their sides with lids ajar allow steam to circulate within.
   c. In mixed loads, place hard objects on the bottom shelf and softer packs on the top racks.
      Harder objects may form condensation that will drip onto softer items and cause them to be wet.
   d. Pack an indicator in the middle of the load.
4. Read the instructions that should be available near the machine. Almost all machines follow the same protocol:
   a. Close the door and secure it.
   b. Switch on the machine.
   c. When the temperature gauge reaches the temperature required for the contents of the load (usually 250°F or 121°C), set the timer. Many autoclaves can be preprogrammed for the required time.
   d. When the timer indicates that the cycle is over, vent the machine. (Most autoclaves do this automatically.)
   e. Most loads dry in 5–20 minutes. Hard items dry faster than soft items.
5. When the load has cooled, remove the items. Wear thermal gloves to prevent burns.
6. Check the separately wrapped indicator for proper sterilization.
   If the indicator registers that the load was properly processed, the items should be sterile; if the indicator has not registered, the load will need to be reprocessed.
7. Store the items appropriately in a clean, dry, dust-free area. Site-prepared packs are considered sterile for 30 days.
8. Clean the autoclave by manufacturer's suggestions, which usually involve scrubbing with a mild detergent and a soft brush. Attention to the exhaust valve will prevent lint from occluding the outlet. Rinse the machine thoroughly and allow it to dry.

line. Too much water will cause saturated steam and will not be as efficient; too little water will not produce the required amount of steam.

The temperature and pressure are usually 250°F at 15 lb pressure for 20 to 30 minutes. Follow the manufacturer's instructions for the load content. Solid or metal loads will take slightly less time than soft, bulky loads.

Be sure to vent when the timer sounds to allow the pressure to drop safely. Open the door slightly to allow the temperature to drop and the load to cool and dry. If the door is opened more than ¼ to ½ inch, colder air will rush in and cause condensation on the items. Newer autoclaves vent automatically.

Do not remove the items until they are dry. Bacteria from your hands will wick through the moist coverings and contaminate the items. Handle the packs with hand protectors to prevent burns.

Post a routine maintenance schedule near the machine. At recommended intervals, clean the lint trap, wash out the interior with a cloth or soft brush, and check the function of all components.

BOILING

Boiling kills many of the pathogens found in an office but will not kill spores and the hepatitis virus. Water will boil to a temperature of 212°F or 100°C and no higher. Rapidly boiling water is no hotter than slowly bubbling water; it is simply evaporating faster.

Items to be boiled are usually metal or firm rubber. Only items that will not be used to enter sterile surfaces are to be boiled; most specula fit this description. They must be thoroughly sanitized, and all parts must be under the boiling water. Set the timer when the water reaches a full boil. Time is usually set for at least 20 minutes. Efficiency is increased with the addition of a 2% solution of sodium carbonate.

Boiling is rarely used in medical offices today. It is not considered a safe method of sterilization. More efficient methods of eliminating microorganisms have replaced the office boiler.

STORAGE AND RECORDKEEPING

When using and maintaining sterilization and treatment equipment, the facility and staff are responsible for providing appropriate storage of these items, for keeping accurate records of warranties and maintenance agreements, and for keeping reordering information on hand.

Familiarize yourself with the manufacturer's recommendation for proper storage of instruments and equipment. Does this equipment need to be sterilized and stored wrapped in barrier protection? Can it be stored in a clean area with a dustcloth or dustcover, such as electrocardiograph machines and ultrasound equipment? Is this an article of supply that warrants the need for special storage? Should the item be labeled and displayed so that employees are aware of potential hazards?

Most facilities have specific storage or supply rooms for housing sterile and nonsterile instruments and equipment. This area should be kept clean and dust free; it is usually located close to the area of need. Clean and sterile supplies and equipment must be separated from soiled items and waste.

In addition to providing proper storage for instruments and equipment, medical assistants are also responsible for keeping accurate records of sterilized items and equipment. Information that must be recorded includes maintenance records and "load" or sterilization records. Load or sterilization records should include:

- Date and time of the cycle
- General description of the contents of the load
- Exposure time and temperature
- Name or initials of the operator
- Results of the sterilization indicator
- Expiration date of the load (usually 30 days)

The maintenance records will include service by the manufacturer's representative and daily maintenance or maintenance as recommended to keep the equipment in optimum working condition.

Checkpoint Question

7. *What six items should be included on a sterilization record?*

MAINTAINING SURGICAL SUPPLIES

As a medical assistant, you should keep an up-to-date master list of all supplies with all purchases and replacements. It is best to have one person responsible for maintaining the inventory, for keeping maintenance schedules, and for placing orders. If too many workers are involved, the care and handling of the facility equipment may either be overlooked or efforts may be duplicated.

Instruction manuals for all equipment should be kept on file and used when ordering supplies for replacement or maintenance. Equipment records for each item should include:

- Date of purchase
- Model number and serial number of the equipment
- Time period that service is recommended
- Date that service was requested
- Name of the individual requesting the service
- Reason for the service request
- Description of the service performed and any parts replaced
- Name of the person performing the service and the date the work was completed
- Signature and title of the person who acknowledged completion of the work

Warranties and guarantees should be kept with the equipment records. It is helpful also to have the name of the manufacturer's contact person attached to the records.

A tickler file should be kept to remind the staff of the need for manufacturer service maintenance and concurrent or periodic maintenance to be performed by the facility personnel.

Parts and supplies for items that are vital to the operation of the facility should always be kept on hand. The shelf life of the item, the storage space available, and the time required to order and receive an item should be considered in maintaining an inventory. If the piece of equipment cannot function without all of its components—and if some of those components have a short life span—replacements must be readily available. For example, an ophthalmoscope without a light is virtually useless.

Answers to Checkpoint Questions

1. *Forceps are used to grasp, handle, compress, pull, or join tissue, equipment, or supplies. Scissors are used for dissecting superficial, deep, or delicate tissues and for cutting sutures and dressings. Scalpels are small knives used for surgery. Towel clamps are used to maintain the integrity of the sterile field by holding sterile drapes in place, allowing exposure of the operative site.*
2. *Because surgical instruments are delicate, improper handling may easily damage sharp blades or pointed tips. If you do drop an instrument, check it carefully to identify any damage. Note that damaged instruments usually can be repaired.*
3. *Sanitation is the science of maintaining a healthful, disease-free, and hazard-free environment. Disinfection is a process that destroys pathogenic organisms. Sterilization is a process that destroys all microorganisms.*
4. *An autoclave is an appliance for sterilizing medical instruments using steam under pressure. It consists of two chambers, an outer unit where pressure builds and an inner chamber where the actual sterilization occurs. Water is added to a reservoir, where it is converted to steam. This steam is then forced into the inner chamber, thereby increasing the pressure, which in turn raises the temperature of the steam. The higher the steam temperature, the more rapid is destruction of microorganisms.*
5. *A sterilization indicator, which is placed inside a pack to be autoclaved, registers the effectiveness of the sterilization process. Improper wrapping of packages, loading, or operation of the autoclave can prevent the indicator from registering correctly.*
6. *Load the autoclave loosely; do not try to pack in too many items because the steam cannot penetrate to those in the center. Place containers on their sides with the lids off. Place all packs on their sides to allow for maximum steam circulation and penetration.*
7. *The six items to include on a sterilization record are date and time of the cycle, general description of the load contents, exposure time and temperature, name or initials of the operator, results of the sterilization indicator, and load expiration date.*

Critical Thinking Challenges

1. You are the senior medical assistant at Dr. Will's office. She instructs you to orient new employees on various aspects of the practice and requests that you develop an orientation booklet for all staff members. Design a booklet that contains the following information:
   - Basic explanations of the instruments commonly used in the practice
   - Procedures for sanitizing, disinfecting, and sterilizing the instruments
   - Operating instructions for the autoclave
2. Create a record that can be used to document sterilization.
3. Develop a system for maintaining the office's surgical supplies.

Suggestions for Further Reading

APIC. (1990). *APIC Guidelines for Selection and Use of Disinfectants and Sterilants.*

Caldwell, E., & Hegner, B. (1991). *The Nursing Assistant: A Nursing Process Approach,* 6th ed. Albany, NY: Delmar.

Donowitz, L. (1994). *Infection Control for the Health Care Worker.* Chicago: Mosby–Year Book.

Preventing Disease Transmission in Personal Service Worker Occupations. (1994). Rockville, MD: U.S. Department of Health and Human Services, Public Health Service.

6 Assisting With Minor Office Surgery

Chapter Outline

Preparing and Maintaining a Sterile Field
- Sterile Surgical Packs
- Ensuring Package Sterility
- Sterile Transfer Forceps
- Pouring a Sterile Solution
- Adding Sterile Items from Peel-Back Packages

Preparing the Patient for Minor Office Surgery
- Patient Instructions and Consent
- Positioning and Draping
- Preparing the Patient's Skin

Local Anesthetics

Scalpels and Blades
- Attaching a Scalpel Blade
- Discarding Sharps

Wound Closure
- Needles
- Sutures
- Assisting with Wound Closure
- Steri-strips
- Adhesive Closure

Assisting with Suture Removal

Assisting with Staple Removal

Sterile Dressings

Bandaging
- Types of Bandages
- Bandage Application Guidelines
- Montgomery Straps

Commonly Performed Office Surgical Procedures
- Excision of a Lesion
- Incision and Drainage (I & D)

Electrosurgery
- Safety Measures
- Care of Equipment

Laser Surgery

Specimen Collection During Office Surgery

Postsurgical Procedures
- Cleaning the Examination Table
- Cleaning the Operative Area

Role Delineation

CLINICAL

Fundamental Principles

- Apply principles of aseptic technique and infection control.

Diagnostic Orders

- Collect and process specimens.

Patient Care

- Prepare and maintain examination and treatment areas.
- Prepare patient for examinations, procedures, and treatments.
- Assist with examinations, procedures, and treatments.

GENERAL

Professionalism

- Project a professional manner and image.
- Work as a team member.

Communication Skills

- Treat all patients with compassion and empathy.
- Adapt communications to individual's ability to understand.

Legal Concepts

- Practice within the scope of education, training, and personal capabilities.
- Document accurately.
- Maintain and dispose of regulated substances in compliance with government guidelines.
- Comply with established risk management and safety procedures.

Instruction

- Instruct individuals according to their needs.
- Teach methods of health promotion and disease prevention.

Chapter Competencies

Learning Objectives

Upon successfully completing this chapter, you will be able to:

1. Spell and define the Key Terms.
2. List your responsibilities in the performance of minor office surgery.
3. List the guidelines and procedures for preparing and maintaining sterility of the field and the surgical equipment.
4. Explain the difference between dressings and bandages and give the purposes for both.
5. Describe the guidelines for the application of dressings and bandages.
6. State your responsibility in relation to informed consents and patient preparation.
7. Identify types and sizes of sutures and needles and give reasons for the selections of each.
8. Explain the purpose of local anesthetics and list three commonly used in the medical office.
9. Describe methods of skin closure performed in the medical office.
10. Describe the procedure for attaching a scalpel blade to a reusable handle.
11. State your responsibility during surgical specimen collection.
12. List the types of laser and electrosurgery in the medical office and explain procedures and precautions for each.
13. Practice environmental disinfection to prevent cross-contamination between patients and personnel.

Performance Objectives

Upon successfully completing this chapter, you will be able to:

1. Open sterile surgical packs (Procedure 6-1).
2. Use sterile transfer forceps (Procedure 6-2).
3. Add sterile solution to a sterile field (Procedure 6-3).
4. Open sterile packets.
5. Add the contents of peel-back packets to the sterile field.
6. Perform hair removal and skin preparation (Procedure 6-4).
7. Attach a surgical blade to a scalpel handle.
8. Remove sutures (Procedure 6-5).
9. Remove staples (Procedure 6-6).
10. Apply a sterile dressing (Procedure 6-7).
11. Change an existing sterile dressing (Procedure 6-8).
12. Wrap roller bandages using various techniques.
13. Apply tubular gauze bandage (Procedure 6-9).
14. Assist with excisional surgery (Procedure 6-10).
15. Assist with incision and drainage (Procedure 6-11).

Key Terms

(See Glossary for definitions.)

approximate
atraumatic
bandages
coagulate
dressings
electrocautery
electrodes
preservative
ratchets
swaged needle
traumatic

As a medical assistant, you will have many responsibilities when minor surgery is performed in the physician's office. These include:

1. Reinforcing the physician's instructions regarding preparation for surgery, including at-home skin preparation, fasting, bowel preparations, and so on.
2. Identifying the patient and the procedure before the physician arrives to gather the proper equipment and supplies.

3. Preparing the treatment room, instruments, supplies, and equipment.
4. Assisting the physician during the procedure.
5. Applying the **dressing** (wound covering).
6. Instructing the patient in postoperative wound care (eg, frequency of dressing changes, application of topical medication, observation of the wound for changes indicating healing or infection).
7. Assisting the patient as needed before, during, and after the procedure.
8. Assisting with postoperative instructions, prescriptions, medications; scheduling return visits.
9. Removing and caring for instruments, equipment, and supplies, including disposable items, "sharps," and contaminated and unused instruments.
10. Preparing the room for the next patient.

In addition, frequently you will be asked by the physician to witness the patient signing the informed consent document.

PREPARING AND MAINTAINING A STERILE FIELD

Minor office surgery involves procedures that penetrate the body's normally intact surface. Whenever there is an open wound, surgical asepsis must be maintained. (See Chap. 1, Asepsis and Infection Control.) Because hands can never be sterilized, sterile transfer forceps or sterile gloved hands must be used to handle sterile objects during a sterile procedure.

Follow the guidelines below during a sterile procedure:

1. Do not let sterile packages become damp or wet. Microorganisms can be drawn into the package by a wicking action. If a package sterilized in the medical office becomes moist, it must be repackaged in a clean, dry wrapper and resterilized. Damp, wet, or torn disposable packages must be discarded.
2. Always face a sterile field. If you must leave the area or work with your back to the sterile field, cover the field with a sterile drape using sterile technique.
3. Hold all sterile items above waist level. When sterile items are not in the field of vision, they may become contaminated without your knowledge.
4. Place sterile items in the middle of the sterile field. A 1-inch border around the field is considered contaminated.
5. Do not spill any liquids, even sterile liquids, onto the sterile field. Remember, the surface below the field is not sterile, and moisture will allow microorganisms to wick up to the surgical field.
6. Do not cough, sneeze, or talk over the sterile field. Microorganisms from the respiratory tract can contaminate the sterile field.
7. Never reach over the sterile field. Dust or lint from clothing can contaminate the sterile field.
8. Be aware that soiled supplies, such as gauze or instruments, should not be passed over or placed on the sterile field.
9. If you know or suspect that the sterile field has been contaminated, alert the physician. Sterility must be reestablished before the procedure can continue.

Sterile Surgical Packs

Many medical offices keep a box with index cards or a loose-leaf binder listing surgical procedures that are commonly performed in the office and the items needed for setup. Most medical offices prepackage sterile setups in a suitable wrapper and prepare them in the office by autoclave sterilization. (See Chap. 5, Instruments and Equipment, for autoclaving procedure.) These setups are labeled according to the type of procedure (eg, lesion removal, suture setup) and contain the general instruments for these procedures. Some basic supplies (eg, gauze sponges, cotton balls, and towels) may also be included before autoclaving.

Because of the time and effort involved in the strict quality control that must be maintained to ensure that items autoclaved on site are sterile after processing, many offices use commercially packaged, disposable surgical packs. Disposable surgical packs have become increasingly popular because they are convenient and come in an almost infinite variety of forms with a wide assortment of contents. They may contain one sterile article (such as a 4 × 4 sterile dressing) or a complete sterile surgical setup.

Many of the supplies will be packaged in peel-apart wrappers with two loose flaps to be pulled apart and the sterile item dropped carefully onto the operative field. The insides of the wrappers may be opened out and used as sterile fields. If the sides of the packages are pulled completely part, items left within the wrapper may be set out to the side of the procedural setup for use as needed. Some of the packages are enclosed in plastic and wrapped inside with barrier material that can be used as a sterile field.

Directions for opening are clearly marked on the outside of the pack and should be read and understood. If the surgical pack is opened improperly, the contents will be contaminated and cannot be used. Commercially prepared sterile packs are generally more expensive than medical practice site-prepared packs; therefore, take care to avoid waste. Large surgical packs contain items specific for various types of surgery; the contents of the pack will be noted on the label. Commercially prepared packs list the contents item by item; site-prepared packs usually only state the type of setup. Procedure 6-1 describes the steps for opening sterile surgical packs.

Ensuring Package Sterility

There should be a sterilization indicator inside each site-prepared surgical package to show that it has been properly sterilized. Tapes, strips, and packaging with indicator stripes or dots on the outside of the packs are not 100% accurate and do not guarantee sterility. These devices are designed to change color when exposed to high temperatures, as in an autoclave. Indicator strips, tapes, and packages should never be stored near the autoclave or in other unusually warm areas because the indicators may change colors as if the package had gone through a sterilization cycle.

In the autoclave, sterility is achieved only by the right combination of temperature, pressure, steam, and time. All four elements must be present at the proper levels in the autoclave cycle to ensure sterility. In addition, an improperly packed autoclave can impede steam penetration to the articles, which will prevent sterilization but will allow the package indicator to change colors. Therefore, sterilization indicators should be packaged within each site-prepared pack and must be checked before beginning the surgical procedure. (See autoclaving procedures in Chap. 5, Instruments and Equipment.) When opening a package of sterile objects, the procedure is the same whether the items are site-prepared reusables or commercially prepared disposables. For all sterile packs or supplies, keep in mind that:

1. The unsterile area is the outside surface of the outside wrapper.
2. The sterile area includes the inside surface of the outside wrapper, the inside wrapper (if included), and the contents of the package.
3. Items are considered contaminated and should be repackaged and resterilized:
   a. When moisture is present
   b. When they have been dropped from the sterile field
   c. If they are out of date (Site-prepared packages expire 30 days from preparation; commercial packs have a posted expiration date.)
   d. If the sterilization indicator has not turned color
   e. If the wrapper is torn or damaged
   f. When any area is known or thought to have been touched by an unsterile item

Checkpoint Question

1. *What are nine guidelines that must be followed to maintain a sterile field?*

Sterile Transfer Forceps

Sterile transfer forceps can be used to move sterile articles from one sterile area to another sterile area. The forceps' tips and the sterile articles being transferred must both remain sterile. The handles of the forceps are considered medically aseptic and are not considered sterile because these are touched by bare hands (Fig. 6-1).

Sterile transfer forceps are stored either in a dry sterile container, in a wrapped sterile package, or in a sterile solution in a closed container system, such as Bard Parker, which helps protect the forceps from contamination and slows evaporation of the soaking solution. In a closed dry container system, the forceps and container must be sanitized and autoclaved daily. In a closed sterile solution system, the forceps and the container are resterilized at least every day, or more often if needed, and fresh solution is added daily. Only one forceps should be stored per container because separate containers decrease the chance of contamination when removing forceps and avoid damage caused by tangling.

Proper use of sterile transfer forceps requires that certain guidelines be followed (Procedure 6-2).

Pouring a Sterile Solution

Whether site-prepared or commercially prepared, trays are not processed or stored with liquids in open containers. Solutions must be added as needed at the time of setup. Some procedures require sterile water or saline, others may require an antiseptic solution. These will be poured into containers already arranged into position by using transfer forceps (Procedure 6-3).

Adding Sterile Items from Peel-Back Packages

Procedure packages are frequently prepared with supplies (eg, cotton balls, gauze squares, and so forth) to eliminate the need to add more at the time of setup.

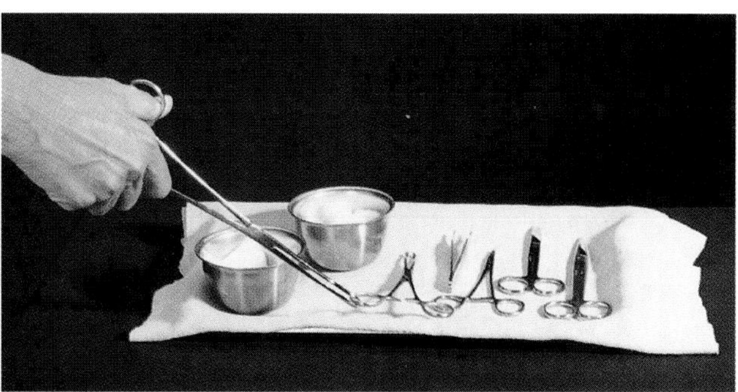

Figure 6-1 Sterile transfer forceps may be used to move items on the sterile field.

However, patient assessment at the time of surgery may suggest the need for additional items. These small supplies are usually provided commercially in peel-apart packages.

Peel-apart packages containing small or single items to be added to a surgical field have an upper edge with two flaps that are used to open the package in a manner that maintains the sterility of the contents. The package is properly opened by using both hands. With the thumbs just inside the tops of the edges, the flaps are separated using a slow, outward motion of the thumbs and flaps (Fig. 6-2). Keep in mind that the inside of the sealed package and the contents are sterile; they will become contaminated if they are touched by any unsterile object.

There are three ways in which the contents of peel-back packages can be added to the sterile field:

1. *By using sterile transfer forceps.* Peel the edges apart with a rolling motion as described above. With the two edges held down, the contents may be lifted up and away with forceps (Fig. 6-3).
2. *By using the sterile gloved hand.* This method requires two people, usually the medical assistant who will open the package and the physician who will remove the contents with sterile gloved hands. You must carefully hold the edges to avoid contaminating the physician's gloves (Fig. 6-4).
3. *By flipping the contents onto a sterile field.* To do this, you must step back from the sterile field to prevent the hands and the unsterile outer wrapper of the pack from crossing over the sterile field. The edges are pulled down and away from the package contents and the item is carefully tossed or flipped onto the field without crossing the sterile area.

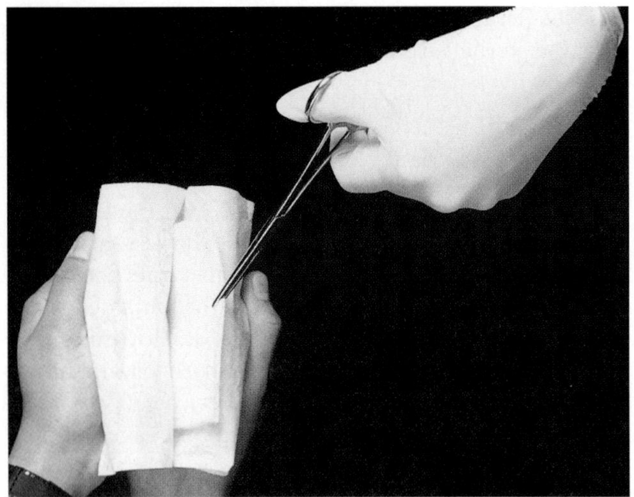

Figure 6-3 The physician may use forceps to remove small supplies.

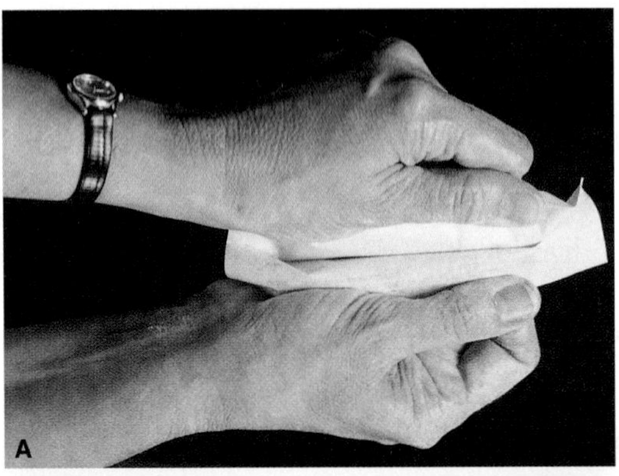

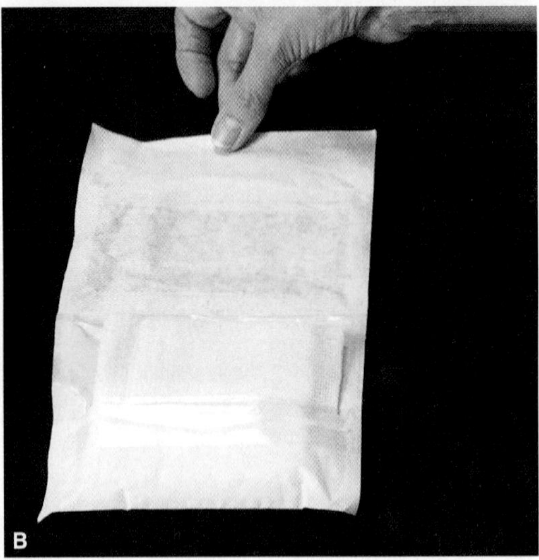

Figure 6-2 Sterile packets. (**A**) Open sterile packets by grasping the edges and rolling the thumbs outward. (**B**) Opening the packet properly forms a sterile field.

In most cases, items in presterilized peel-back envelopes cannot be resterilized and must be discarded when opened even if not used. Because such items are relatively expensive to purchase, they should not be

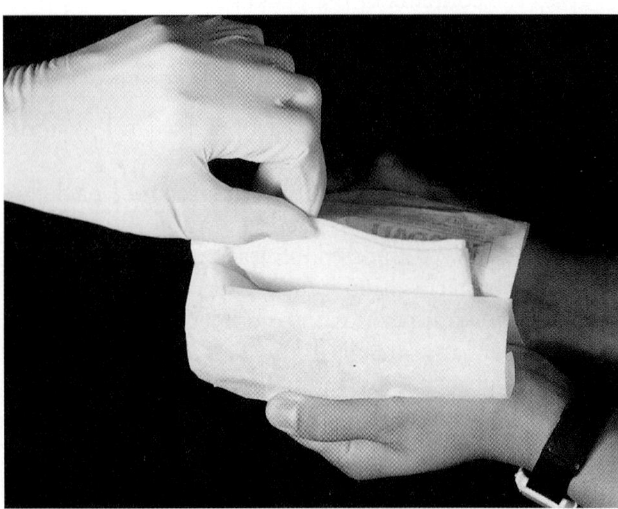

Figure 6-4 Sterile gloved hands may be used to remove small items.

6

Procedure 6-1 Opening Sterile Surgical Packs

PURPOSE:

To maintain sterility of instruments and supplies used for surgical procedures
To prevent contamination of body areas entered during surgical procedures

EQUIPMENT/SUPPLIES

- surgical pack
- surgical stand

STEPS

1. Check the surgical procedure to be performed. Remove the appropriate tray or item(s) from the storage area.
   a. Check the label for contents and expiration date.
      Packages that have passed the expiration date should not be used.
   b. Check for tears or areas of moisture.
      Areas that have tears or are moist will contaminate the contents of the package.

2. Place the package, with the label facing up, on a clean, dry, flat surface, such as a Mayo or surgical stand.
   Even though the field will be protected by a barrier undersurface, keep microorganisms at a minimum by using an area as free of pathogens as possible. The surgical stand makes it easy to move the field for the physician's convenience.

3. Without tearing the wrapper, carefully remove the sealing tape. If the package is commercially prepared, carefully remove the outer protective wrapper.
   Many disposable packages are wrapped in a barrier wrap that will become the sterile field when properly opened. They are then sealed in see-through plastic film. Packages prepared in the medical office will be sealed using tape designed to indicate that the package has been through the autoclave procedure.

4. Loosen the first flap of the folded wrapper. Open the first flap by pulling it up, out, and away; let it fall over the far side of the table.
   By doing this, you avoid having to reach across the field again.

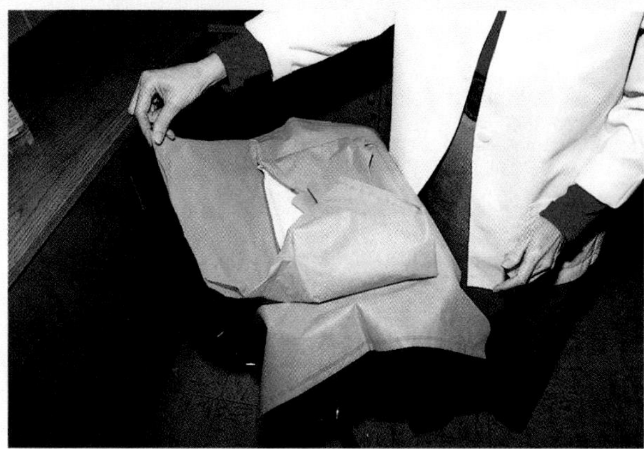

5. Open the side flaps in a similar manner using the left hand for the left flap; right hand for right flap. Touch only the unsterile outer surface; do not touch the sterile inner surface.
   This decreases movement over the sterile areas of the package.

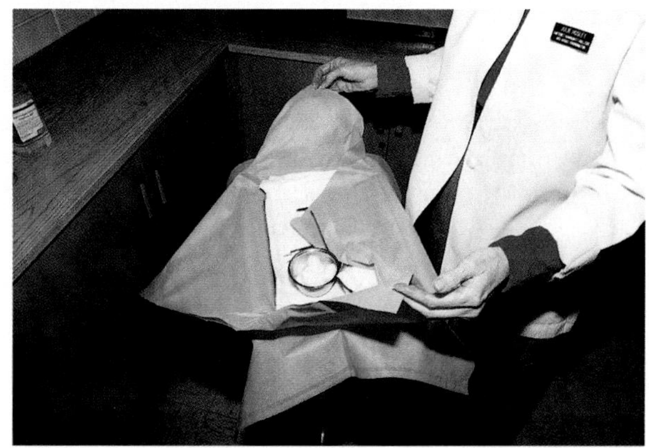

continued

opened unnecessarily. A supply of items that might be needed during the procedure should be conveniently close to the area and added only if needed.

text continues on page 118

Checkpoint Question

2. *What are three ways that contents of peel-back packages can be added to the sterile field?*

Procedure 6-1 Continued Opening Sterile Surgical Packs

6. Pull the remaining flap down and toward you by grasping the unsterile surface only. The unsterile surface of the wrapper is now against the surgical stand; the sterile inside surface of the wrapper forms the sterile field.

7. Repeat steps 4 through 6 for packages with a second or inside wrapper. This sterile inside wrapper also provides a sterile field on which to work. The field is now ready for additional supplies as needed or is ready for the procedure to begin.

Note: If it is necessary to leave the area after opening the field, cover the tray and its contents with a sterile drape. At the completion of the procedure, discard any commercially wrapped items that are not used for the sterile procedure for which they were opened.

Procedure 6-2 Using Sterile Transfer Forceps

PURPOSE:

To move items on the sterile field for the physician's convenience
To maintain sterility of items used for surgical procedures

EQUIPMENT/SUPPLIES

- forceps and container
- item(s) to be transferred

STEPS

1. Slowly lift the forceps straight up and out of the container without touching the inside above the level of the solution or the outside of the container.
   The area above the soaking solution and the rim are considered unsterile.
2. Hold the forceps with the tips down.
   This avoids having the solution run toward the unsterile handles and then back to the grasping blades and tips, thus contaminating them.
3. Keep the forceps above waist level.
   This prevents accidental and unnoticed contamination.
4. Pick up the article to be transferred and drop it onto the sterile field so that the forceps will not come in contact with the sterile field.
   The forceps may still be moist from the soaking solution, which may cause microorganisms to wick from the surface below the sterile field.

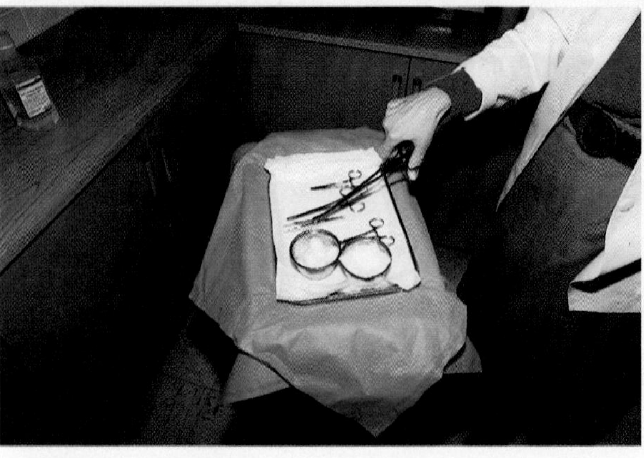

Note: Sterile transfer forceps that have been wrapped and autoclaved may be placed with tips on the sterile field with handles extending beyond the 1-inch contaminated perimeter. You may then grasp the handles that extend beyond the perimeter if you need to move objects around the field for the physician's convenience.

6

Procedure 6-3 Adding Sterile Solution to the Field

PURPOSE:

To make available sterile solutions required in the performance of sterile procedures

EQUIPMENT/SUPPLIES

- container of sterile solution
- sterile setup

STEPS

1. As with any drug or medication, identify the correct solution by carefully READING THE LABEL.
   The label should be checked three times to avoid errors: when taking the container from the shelf, before pouring the solution, and when returning the container to the shelf.
2. Check for an expiration date on the label; do not use the solution if it is out of date, if the label cannot be read, or if the solution appears abnormal. *Note:* Sterile water and saline bottles must be dated when opened and must be discarded if not used within 48 hours.
   Out-of-date solutions may have changed chemically and deteriorated and are no longer considered sterile.
3. If you are adding medications into the solution (eg, Xylocaine, a local anesthetic), show the medication label to the physician now.
   This allows for verification of the contents.
4. With sterile transfer forceps, move any solution receptacles close to the edge of the sterile field but well within the 1-inch border.
   This prevents reaching across the sterile field to pour the solution.
5. Remove the cap or stopper. Hold the cap with the fingertips, with the cap opening facing downward, to prevent accidental contamination of the inside. If it is necessary to put the cap down, place it with the opened end facing up. If you are pouring the entire contents of the container onto the sterile field, you may discard the cap. Retain the bottle to keep track of amount added to the field and for charting purposes later. You can then discard it.
   If the cap becomes contaminated and is returned to the bottle, the contents are considered contaminated. Placing the cap on a surface with the opening facing upward prevents contamination of the interior of the cap.

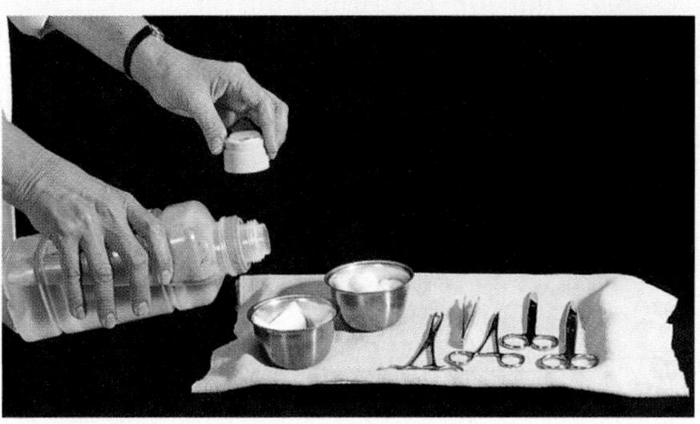

6. Grasp the container so that the label is facing the palm of the hand ("palm the label").
   If solution runs down the side of the bottle in this position, it will not obscure the label.
7. Pour a small amount of the solution into a separate container or waste receptacle.
   The lip of the bottle is considered contaminated; pouring off this small amount cleanses the bottle tip.
8. Carefully and slowly pour the desired amount of solution into the sterile container from not less than 4 inches and not more than 6 inches above the container. Do not allow the bottle of solution to touch the sterile container or tray because this will cause contamination.
   Pouring the solution slowly reduces the chance of splashing and over-filling. Solution poured too quickly or from an improper height may splash. Touching the container to objects on the sterile field contaminates the field. If the solution splashes onto the field, a wicking action will cause contamination from the surface below.
9. After pouring the desired amount of solution into the sterile container, recheck the label for contents and expiration date.
   This ensures accuracy.
10. Replace the cap carefully to avoid touching the bottle rim with any unsterile surface of the cap.
    Careful replacement of the cap ensures that the contents remain sterile.
11. Return the solution to its proper storage area and recheck the label again.
    This ensures accuracy.

6

PREPARING THE PATIENT FOR MINOR OFFICE SURGERY

Patient Instructions and Consent

Many of the minor surgical procedures (eg, suture insertion or removal, incision and drainage, sebaceous cystectomy) that are performed in the medical office require only a full explanation of the procedure and informed consent. The patient either agrees and the procedure is performed, or the patient refuses and the procedure is not done.

In today's litigious society, prudent physicians routinely obtain signed informed consent documents even for minor office procedures. Preprinted forms can be obtained or specially designed to contain all the information needed for informed consent and may be used for procedures requiring legal, witnessed signatures and for those requiring only that the patient review the procedure. Other forms can be rather general with blank spaces to add information relevant to the procedure to be performed. Both should provide spaces for the date and signatures of patient, physician, and witness(es) (Fig. 6-5).

Other data usually found in informed consent documents include procedure and purposes, expected results, alternative therapies, possible side effects, risks, and complications. The medical assistant is not responsible for obtaining informed consent from the patient but will probably be required to witness the signing of the document by the patient. It is the physician's legal responsibility to obtain informed consent from the patient. If a procedure is performed on a date after the consent is signed, you may be asked to verify the consent at that time, but should not obtain the initial informed consent from the patient.

The patient may ask how long the procedure will last, what preparations are needed, if fasting is necessary, and other questions. You may answer queries of this nature for the patient after verifying the information with the physician. It is always a good practice to give specific written instructions to the patient for any necessary fasting or bowel preparation so that a procedure can be done on schedule and with no preventable risk to the patient. The physician may prescribe medication or may dispense medications to be taken by the patient at home before the surgery.

You should notify the physician if the patient expresses confusion or misunderstanding about the instructions. Encourage the patient to call the office should questions arise later.

Positioning and Draping

Before positioning the patient for a minor surgical procedure, have the patient void; this helps avoid discomfort during the procedure. Offer to help the patient remove whatever clothing is necessary to expose the operative site. Expose only the area necessary for the procedure to ensure the patient's privacy. Be aware that the air-conditioned office may become uncomfortably cool for patients. Additional sheets or a blanket may be added for comfort.

Assist the patient to assume a comfortable position on the examining table that will allow exposure of and access to the operative site. Pillows may be used for comfort and support. Patients should not be expected to maintain uncomfortable positions, such as lithotomy or knee–chest, while waiting for the physician. They should be positioned only when the physician is ready to begin the procedure. (See Chap. 4, Physical Examination, for more information about positioning.) At the end of the procedure, assist the patient from the table, allowing as much time as needed. Often patients who did not need help removing clothing will require assistance dressing following minor surgery. Be aware of this and assist as necessary.

The type of procedure and the position in which the patient is placed for minor surgery will determine the type of drapes used to expose the operative site and cover the patient. Disposable paper drapes are most commonly used in the medical office. They come in many different sizes and shapes, each suited for specific uses. Paper drapes can be used alone, in combination, or with separate drape sheets and towels. Fenestrated (window) drapes have an opening to expose the operative site while covering adjacent areas. Fenestrated drapes may be small, such as those used for suture insertion or removal, or rather large, as in lithotomy drapes used to cover the legs and lower abdomen but expose the perineal area. Some sterile drapes are combined with adhesive-backed clear plastic, which adheres to the patient's skin and eliminates the need for towel clamps, such as Backhaus clamps or nonperforating towel clamps. (See Chap. 5, Instruments and Equipment, for illustrations of these clamps.)

When removing contaminated drapes from the patient following a procedure, put on protective gloves and carefully roll the items away from your body, keeping the contaminated areas innermost. This helps to surround the dirtier areas of the sheet with the cleaner area and helps prevent contaminated clothing. Because the sheets and towels will likely be contaminated with blood and/or bodily fluids, Standard Precautions must be followed. (See Chap. 1, Asepsis and Infection Control.)

Preparing the Patient's Skin

The goal of preoperative skin preparation is to remove as many microorganisms from the skin as possible to decrease the chance of wound contamination. Skin

SPECIAL CONSENT TO OPERATION OR OTHER PROCEDURE

PATIENT ______________________ PATIENT NUMBER ________

DATE ______________ TIME ______________

1. I HEREBY AUTHORIZE DOCTOR ______________ AND/OR SUCH ASSISTANTS AS MAY BE SELECTED BY HIM, TO PERFORM THE FOLLOWING PROCEDURE(S): ______________________

   ON ______________________
   (NAME OF PATIENT OR MYSELF)

2. THE PROCEDURE(S) LISTED ABOVE HAVE BEEN EXPLAINED TO ME BY DR. ________ AND I UNDERSTAND THE NATURE AND THE CONSEQUENCES OF THE PROCEDURE(S).

3. I RECOGNIZE THAT, DURING THE COURSE OF THE OPERATION, UNFORESEEN CONDITIONS MAY NECESSITATE ADDITIONAL OR DIFFERENT PROCEDURES THAN THOSE SET FORTH. I FURTHER AUTHORIZE AND REQUEST THAT THE ABOVE NAMED SURGEON, HIS ASSISTANTS, OR HIS DESIGNEES PERFORM SUCH PROCEDURES AS ARE IN HIS PROFESSIONAL JUDGMENT NECESSARY AND DESIRABLE, INCLUDING, BUT NOT LIMITED TO, PROCEDURES INVOLVING PATHOLOGY AND RADIOLOGY. THE AUTHORITY GRANTED UNDER THIS PARAGRAPH SHALL EXTEND TO REMEDYING CONDITIONS NOT KNOWN TO DR. ______________ AT THE TIME THE OPERATION IS COMMENCED.

4. I AM AWARE THAT THE PRACTICE OF MEDICINE AND SURGERY IS NOT AN EXACT SCIENCE AND I ACKNOWLEDGE THAT NO GUARANTEES HAVE BEEN MADE TO ME AS TO THE RESULTS OF THE OPERATION OR PROCEDURE.

5. TISSUE REMOVED DURING SURGERY SHALL BE SENT TO PATHOLOGY TO BE EXAMINED AND DISPOSED OF IN ACCORDANCE WITH THE RULES AND REGULATIONS OF THE MEDICAL STAFF OF THE SURGERY CENTER.

______________________ ______________________
Procedure has been discussed with patient. (Surgeon's Signature) SIGNATURE OF PATIENT

PATIENT IS UNABLE TO SIGN BECAUSE ❑ HE (SHE) IS A MINOR ______ YEARS OF AGE

❑ OTHER (SPECIFY) ______________

______________________ ______________________
WITNESS PERSON AUTHORIZED TO SIGN FOR PATIENT

______________________ ______________________
RELATIONSHIP OF ABOVE TO PATIENT

Figure 6-5 Sample consent form.

preparation may range from simply applying an antiseptic solution to the skin to removing gross contamination and hair from the operative area. Hair can be removed with depilatory creams but often requires shaving the skin (Procedure 6-4).

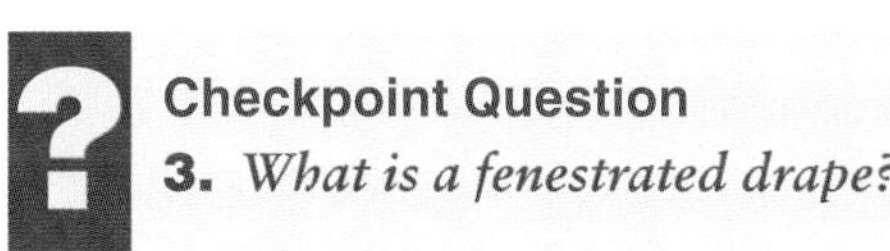

Checkpoint Question

3. *What is a fenestrated drape?*

LOCAL ANESTHETICS

When office surgery of any kind is performed, the site is first anesthetized (numbed) with a local anesthetic to minimize the pain and discomfort felt by the patient. Occasionally, when a wound contains imbedded debris that must be removed prior to repair, the local anesthetic will be injected before preparing the wound site to facilitate wound cleaning.

Procedure 6-4 Performing Hair Removal and Skin Preparation

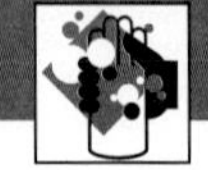
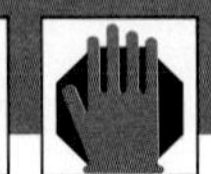

6

PURPOSE:

To render the surgical area maximally free of microorganisms
To aid in the prevention of postprocedure infection

EQUIPMENT/SUPPLIES

- nonsterile gloves
- shave cream or lotion
- new razor
- gauze or cotton balls and warm rinse water
- antiseptic
- sponge forceps

STEPS

1. Wash your hands.

2. Assemble the equipment.

A new razor must be used for each patient to avoid the transmission of pathogens and to ensure the closest possible shave.

3. Greet and identify the patient. Explain the procedure and answer any questions.

4. Put on gloves.

5. Prepare the patient's skin.

a. If the patient's skin is to be shaved:

(1) Apply shaving cream or soapy lather to the area to be shaved.

Shaving cream or soapy lather on the skin reduces friction and helps prevent scratching the skin.

(2) Pull the skin taut and shave by pulling the razor across the skin in the direction of hair growth.

Shaving in the direction in which the hair grows gives the closest shave while reducing the chance of nicking the skin.

(3) Repeat this procedure until all hair is removed from the operative area. Rinse and pat the shaved area thoroughly dry using a gauze square.

Rinsing removes soap residue and hair from the shaved area. Pat dry rather than rubbing to prevent abrasions. Using gauze squares for drying will pick up stray hairs that might remain after rinsing.

b. If the patient's skin is not to be shaved:

(1) Rinse away any soapy solution used for general cleaning.

(2) Dry the skin before applying antiseptic solution to avoid diluting the antiseptic.

6. Apply antiseptic solution of the physician's choice to the skin surrounding the operative area using sterile gauze sponges, sterile cotton balls, or antiseptic wipes.

a. With the gauze or cotton ball grasped in the sterile sponge forceps, wipe the skin in circular motions starting at the operative site and working outward.

b. Discard each sponge after making a complete sweep.

Discarding sponges after each stroke will prevent contamination of the wound by microorganisms brought back to the area from the surrounding skin.

c. If the area is large or circles are not appropriate, wipe the sponge straight outward from the operative site, then discard it.

d. Repeat the procedure until the entire area has been thoroughly cleaned. At no time should a wipe that has passed over the skin be returned to the already cleaned area or to the antiseptic solution.

7. With dry sterile gauze sponges grasped in the sponge forceps, pat the area thoroughly dry. In some instances, the area may be allowed to air dry.

If the area is moist, the sterile drapes may become wet also, causing wicking to contaminate the operative site.

8. Instruct the patient not to touch or cover the prepared area.

This avoids contaminating the operative site, which would require repeating the procedure.

9. Drape the prepared area for the procedure or cover it with sterile drapes if the procedure will be delayed for a short time. Longer delays may require reapplication of the antiseptic solution.

DOCUMENTATION GUIDELINES

- Date and time
- Area of skin preparation
- Any lesions, open areas, or rashes in the skin preparation area
- Patient education/ instructions
- Your signature

Charting Example

DATE	TIME Pt in for excision of mole rt
	shoulder. Skin shaved, prepped with
	Betadine solution. Area clear of lesions.
	Dr. Spencer in for surgical procedure.
	—Your signature

Note: Commercially packaged skin preparation kits are available with most of the listed items provided. Gloves must be worn for shaving to prevent contact with blood or body fluids if nicks or cuts occur. If the skin is not to be shaved, you will need only antiseptic solution, gauze or cotton balls, or antiseptic wipes.

Lidocaine (Xylocaine) and Xylocaine with epinephrine (0.5%–2%) are two of the many local anesthetics commonly used in the medical office. Others include lidocaine (Baylocaine), mepivacaine (Carbocaine), and bupivacaine (Marcaine). Epinephrine is added to local anesthetics to slow absorption by the body and lengthen its effectiveness and as a vasoconstrictor to help provide hemostasis. It is used when the physician anticipates a longer procedure.

There are two procedures used for the administration of local anesthesia. In one procedure, the assistant may draw the anesthetic for the physician, retaining the vial beside the syringe for the physician's approval. In this case, the anesthetic usually is given before the physician gloves for the procedure.

The second option is used if the physician gloves before the anesthetic is given. In this procedure, a sterile syringe will be included in the sterile field setup. When the physician is ready to administer the anesthetic, show the label, clean the stopper, and hold the vial while the physician draws the required amount into the syringe. There are many methods of holding the vial securely for the physician during this procedure. A team that works well together will develop a method that ensures that surgical asepsis is maintained.

SCALPELS AND BLADES

Disposable scalpel blades with permanently attached handles are frequently used in the medical office. Less commonly seen in offices today are reusable scalpel handles with disposable blades attached. Figure 5-3 shows various types of scalpel handles and blades. Because of the possibility of serious injury to the assistant, the process of attaching or removing the blade should be performed very carefully and according to procedure. The blade should never be attached or removed by hand.

Attaching a Scalpel Blade

Scalpel blades, which are small and extremely sharp, are difficult to grasp. To attach a blade to a scalpel handle, put on sterile gloves and follow these steps:

1. Grasp the *blunt* side of the blade (*not* the sharp side) in the jaws of a hemostat held in the dominant hand (Fig. 6-6).
2. With the hemostat and blade in the dominant hand and the scalpel handle in the nondominant hand, slide the opening in the blade into the grooves in the handle tip in one smooth, continuous motion.
3. Note a click sound, which can be heard when the blade is correctly seated.

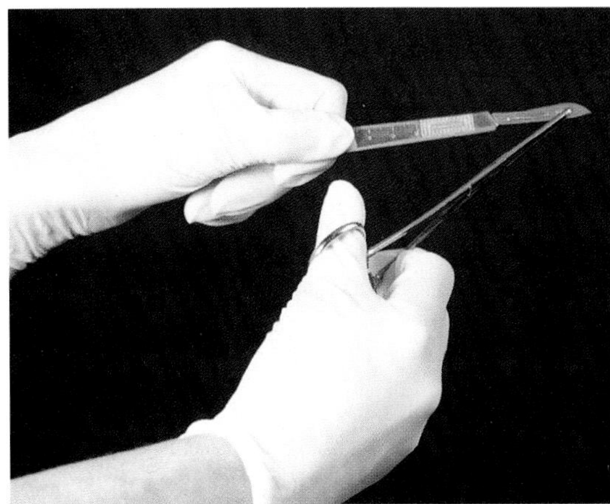

Figure 6-6 Place or remove a scalpel blade by grasping the blunt side with a hemostat.

4. If the blade does not click, or if it does not lie flat against the handle tip, remove the blade with the hemostat and repeat the procedure. (To remove the blade, reverse the procedure.). Never place or remove blades without a hemostat. Instruments are available to remove blades in the safest manner possible.

Blades range in size for various procedures; the physician determines the size needed for any incision. Most medical office surgical procedures require the use of small-sized blades.

Discarding Sharps

When "sharps" or any other used instruments are discarded from the surgical field, they should be placed in a basin rather than tossed into a sink or waste receptacle (Fig. 6-7). Contaminated instruments are not returned to the field but must be cared for with safety in

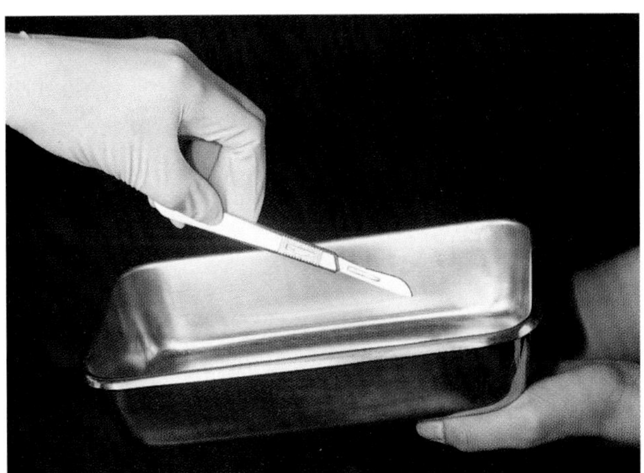

Figure 6-7 Instruments should be placed in a basin after use. They should never be tossed into a wash basin or returned to the field.

mind. For instance, when the physician has made the incision and no longer needs the scalpel, hold a basin to receive the soiled instrument. At the completion of the procedure, the instrument and other sharps from the field can be cared for or safely discarded into an appropriate sharps container.

WOUND CLOSURE

Many types of wounds require closure to ensure rapid healing with minimal scarring. This is accomplished by bringing the edges of the wounds as closely together as possible in their original position (**approximate**). Skin closure procedures are performed after cyst or tissue sample removal, in response to lacerating injuries, or anytime that skin surfaces require assistance in the healing process. Skin closures performed in the office usually include the insertion of sutures or staples or the use of Steri-strips. Supplies used to suture skin closure will include needles and sutures.

What If?

What if while you are separating a contaminated blade from a scalpel handle you accidentally cut your finger?

Remove your gloves and immediately wash your hands with an antiseptic solution. Then have the physician evaluate the wound. He or she may suggest that you perform a surgical scrub or irrigate the wound, or antibiotics may be ordered. The patient should be asked permission to obtain a blood sample to test for hepatitis and HIV. (State laws vary regarding the legality of health care workers demanding a blood sample for testing.) Many states require that health care workers be immunized against HBV at their employer's expense. Finally, be sure to notify your supervisor of any work-related injury so that it may be appropriately documented.

Needles

Needles used in minor office surgery are chosen for the type of surgery to be performed. Needles are classified by:

- Shape—curved or straight
- Point—tapered or cutting
- Eye—***atraumatic*** (*swaged*) or **traumatic** (with an eye)

Cutting needles are used on tough tissue such as skin. Round or tapered (noncutting) needles are used on tissues such as subcutaneous, peritoneum, or muscle.

Atraumatic, or **swaged needles** have suture material that has been mechanically attached to the needle by the manufacturer and do not require threading. They are called atraumatic because they cause less trauma as they pass through the tissues. Unlike atraumatic or swaged needles, threaded needles have an eye with a double thickness of suture that must be pulled through tissues. The double thickness of suture makes a larger, therefore more traumatic, opening in the tissues than a swaged suture. Swaged needles have the appropriate size suture material attached by the manufacturer.

Swaged needles are used far more often than any other type of needle in the medical office. It is considered rare to use any needle other than a curved, swaged needle in minor office surgery. Swaged needles are selected for a procedure according to the size and length of the suture material. The attached needle gauge is a corresponding size. Suture and needle selection is usually done by the physician; you should know your physician's preferences and anticipate needs whenever possible.

Sutures, needles, and suture/needle combinations are contained in peel-apart packages that are sterile on the inside so that they can be added to the sterile field (Fig. 6-8). This may be done by sterile transfer forceps, a sterile gloved hand, or by carefully flipping them onto the sterile field.

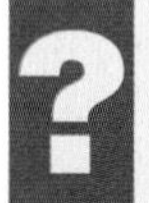

Checkpoint Question

4. *How do swaged needles differ from threaded ones?*

Sutures

Sutures are used to close wounds and incisions and to bring tissue layers into close approximation. Sutures come in various gauges (diameters) and lengths. Very large gauge (diameter) suture is given a number from 1 to 5; 5 is the largest. Sutures smaller than size 1 are expressed in zeros. Suture sizes, which become progressively smaller, range from 0 to 10, or smaller (ie, 1-0, 2-0, 3-0, and so forth). A very fine 10-0 suture, which is about the diameter of a human hair, is generally used for microsurgical procedures. When fine suture is needed, such as on the face and neck, 5-0 and 6-0 suture are commonly used. Very fine suture decreases obvious scarring and gives a better cosmetic result. Heavier suture is needed for areas that exert strain on the wound, such as limbs and hands.

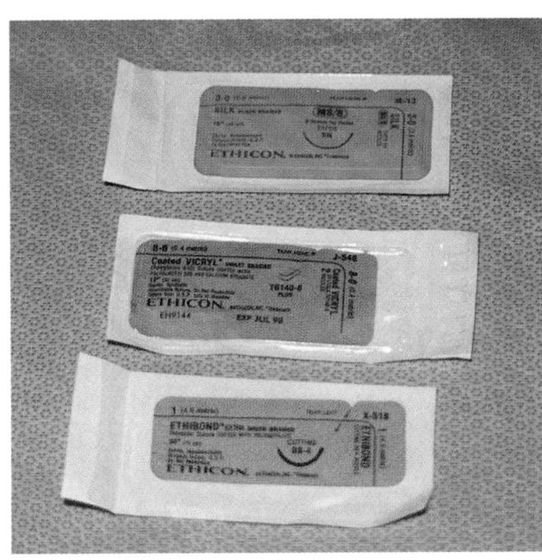

Figure 6-8 Suture material and suture needles are supplied in see-through packs, with the size of suture material and the type of needle listed on the packet. The inside of the packet is sterile.

Sutures also come in absorbable and nonabsorbable forms. Absorbable suture, or catgut (made from the intestines of sheep or cattle), is readily broken down by body processes and usually does not require a removal procedure. There are two forms of absorbable gut suture: chromic, which is chemically treated to delay absorption, and plain, which is not treated and is the most quickly absorbed of the two. Absorbable sutures are used most frequently in the hospital setting during surgery on deep tissues.

Nonabsorbable sutures come in the greatest variety of brands, sizes, lengths, and swaged needles; they are the most versatile. Nonabsorbable sutures either remain in the body permanently or are removed after healing has occurred. Nonabsorbable sutures are used on the skin, intestines, or bone; to ligate larger vessels; and to attach heart valves and various artificial and natural grafts. Nonabsorbable sutures are made from fibers (eg, silk, nylon, Dacron, cotton) and from stainless-steel wire.

Another form of nonabsorbable suture is the metal skin clip or staple; these may be made of stainless steel. There are very specialized types of metal clips made of sterling silver for use in neurosurgery and other procedures. When nonabsorbable sutures or staples are used to close skin wounds, they must be removed when the wound has healed.

Depending on the location of the skin wound, sutures will remain in place for varying lengths of time; the head and neck may require 3 to 5 days, whereas the arms and legs may require 7 to 10 days.

Sutures if not swaged to the needle are packaged individually in see-through peel-apart packages. These packages are labeled according to the type, size, and length of the enclosed suture material; whether it is absorbable or nonabsorbable; and the type of needle if this material is swaged. The insides of these packages are sterile until opened. Some are supplied in dual peel-apart packages so that the inside package can be reused if it has not been damaged or opened.

Assisting With Wound Closure

When a wound is sutured in the office, you will be required to set up a sterile field. The physician will inspect the wound and decide what type and size suture material to use. You may be required to assist the physician during the procedure.

Added to the sterile field may be items such as surgical drapes, hemostats, needle holders, tissue (thumb) forceps, scissors (dissecting or operating), suture material (probably swaged suture/needle combinations), gauze sponges, sterile gloves, and equipment to inject local anesthetic (syringe, needle, wipe, and anesthetic). If the physician requires assistance during the insertion of sutures, you will be required to scrub, glove, and pass instruments as needed during the procedure. (See Chap. 1, Asepsis and Infection Control.)

In almost all instances in the medical office, swaged needles will be used. If you are assisting, hand the needle to the physician in the functional position, clamped in the needle holder with the point upward. Click the **ratchets** (parts that lock together) twice for a secure hold. If the physician is right-handed, the suture material will extend to the right and the needle will point to the left. If the physician is left-handed, the reverse will be true.

Suture material must be cut during the procedure. This is usually done by the physician. If you are scrubbed to assist, the scissors will be passed in a functional position, which means that you will grasp the closed blades with the handles downward. The physician will indicate when scissors are needed and expects the handles to be placed firmly in the palm with the blades pointing upward (Fig. 6-9). Thumb and tissue forceps will be passed in the opposite manner, tips downward when gripped by the physician. In all instances, the physician's personal preference will guide the assistant.

Steri-strips

Steri-strips are adhesive skin closures used to approximate the edges of a small wound if sutures are not needed. Steri-strips are appropriate where there is little tension on the skin edges. The strips are placed transversely across the line of the wound to bring the wound edges in close approximation (Fig. 6-10). When removing Steri-strips, carefully lift the edges distal to the wound and pull gently toward the wound.

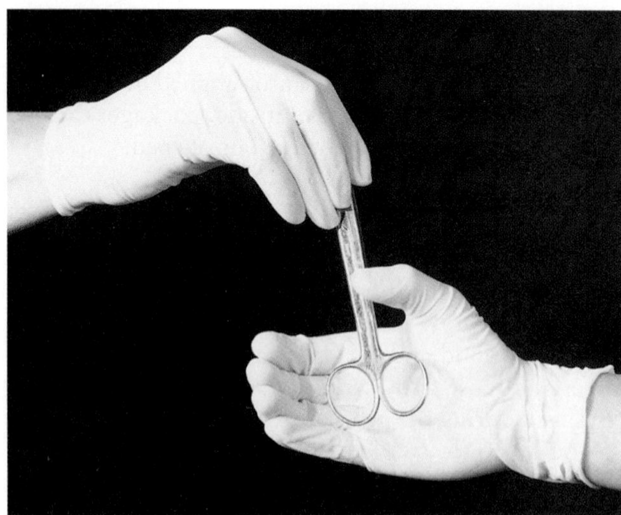

Figure 6-9 Instruments are passed in the functional position. Grasp blades or tips and pass the instrument to the physician, with the handle to the palm.

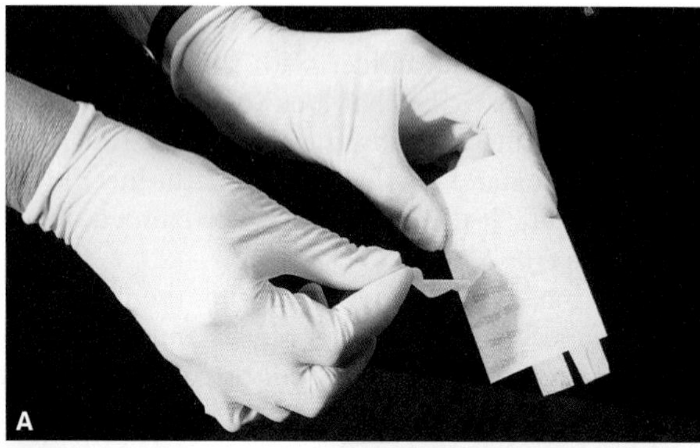

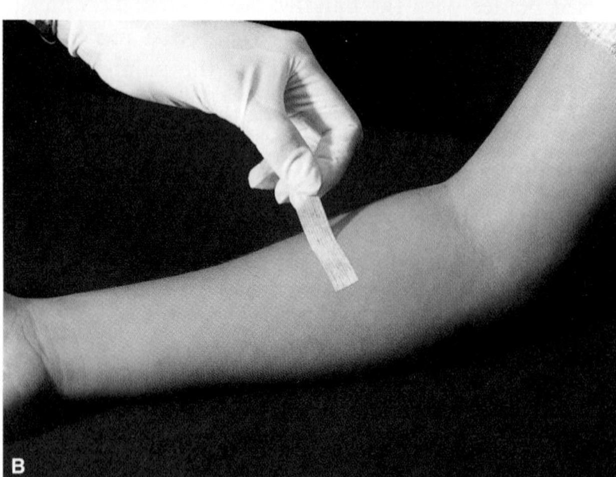

Figure 6-10 Steri-strips. (A) These light-weight lengths of porous tape are used for small wounds. (B) Steri-strips are placed transversely across a wound.

Never pull the strips away from the wound as tension on the wound site may disrupt the healing process.

Adhesive Closure

Surgical glue, or wound adhesive, has recently been introduced to replace sutures in certain types of wounds. Studies show that preclosure anesthetics are not needed, eliminating one of the most dreaded aspects of suture wound closure. After preliminary skin preparation and any necessary wound cleaning, the physician simply approximates the edges of the wound and spreads the site with the fast-drying glue, supplied in sterile single-use ampules. The glue is relatively waterproof, which helps keep the wound cleaner, reducing the risk of infection. It is flexible, which increases patient comfort. In most instances, the glue will slough off in about 10 to 14 days.

Your responsibility will be limited to preprocedure skin preparation and setting up the minimal supplies, such as providing the ampule of sterile glue and selecting the sterile gloves for the physician. Postprocedural instruction may also be your responsibility and may include directives to protect the wound from additional trauma and instructions about when to return for a wound recheck. There is no return visit needed for removal of the glue as required for suture removal.

Checkpoint Question

5. *How do you hand a right-handed physician a needle for suturing?*

ASSISTING WITH SUTURE REMOVAL

In many instances, you will be required to remove sutures from a wound. Patients should understand that there might be a "pulling" sensation during suture removal but there should not be pain. The area must first be cleaned with an antiseptic solution. Either gloved with sterile gloves or using a sterile transfer forceps, clean the area in a circular motion away from the wound or in straight wipes away from the suture line (Fig. 6-11). Discard the wipe after each sweep, and use a new one for the next sweep across the area. Either sterile disposable suture removal kits, which contain all of the equipment needed for suture removal (Fig. 6-12), or sterile reusable equipment may be used (Procedure 6-5).

text continues on page 128

Procedure 6-5 Removing Sutures

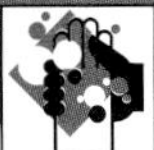
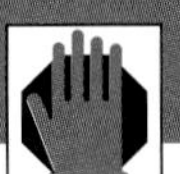
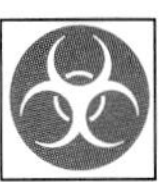

PURPOSE:

To restore the integrity of the operative site after the healing process

EQUIPMENT/SUPPLIES

- thumb forceps
- gauze
- antiseptic
- sterile gloves
- suture scissors
- Option: Sterile, disposable suture removal kits contain all needed supplies.

STEPS

1. Wash your hands.
2. Assemble the equipment.
3. Greet and identify the patient. Explain the procedure and answer any questions.
4. If dressings have not been removed previously, do so (see Procedure 6-8). Properly dispose of dressings. *Note:* At this point in the procedure, the physician may be called to assess the healing process. The wound may need to be assessed both before and after exudate is removed. Then clean the wound area as directed.
   The skin must be as free of pathogens as possible before the removal of the sutures to prevent contamination of the wound. If exudate is present, the stitches may not be easily visualized.
5. Open the suture removal packet using surgical asepsis or set up a field for on-site sterile equipment. Put on sterile gloves.
   Suture removal is a sterile procedure.
6. Note that the knots will be tied in such a way that one tail of the knot will be very close to the surface of the skin while the other will be closer to the area of suture that is looped over the incision.
7. Remove the sutures.
   a. Grasp the end of the knot that is closest to the skin surface and lift slightly and gently up from the skin.

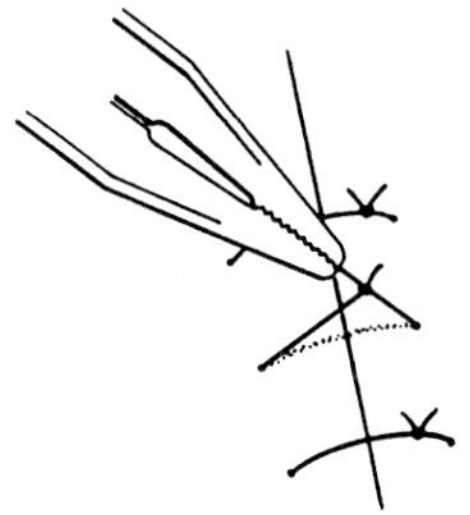

   b. Cut the suture below the knot as close to the skin as possible.

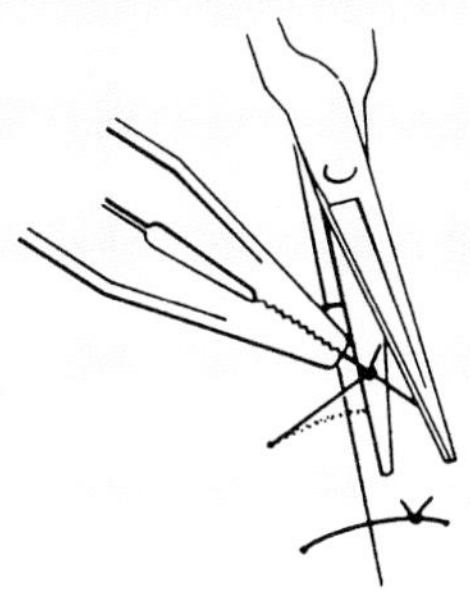

   Cutting below the knot and close to the skin frees the knot at an area that has not been exposed to the outside surface of the body. The only part of the suture that will pull through the tissues will be the suture that was under the skin surface.

   c. Use the thumb forceps to pull the suture out of the skin with a smooth, continuous motion at a slight angle in the direction of the wound.

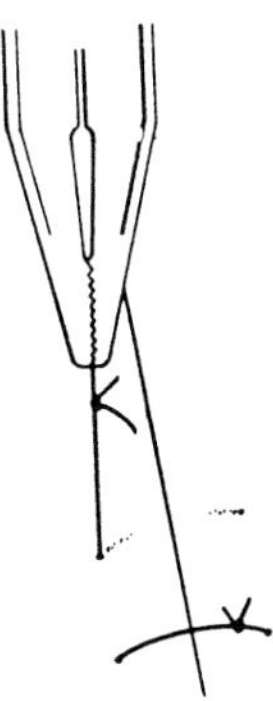

   This avoids tension on the healing tissue.

8. Place the suture on a gauze sponge. Repeat the procedure for each suture.
   This helps in counting the number removed; if six sutures previously inserted are now to be removed, there should be six sutures on the gauze sponge at the end of the procedure.

continued

Procedure 6-5 *Continued* Removing Sutures

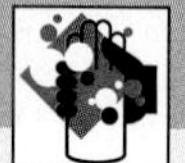
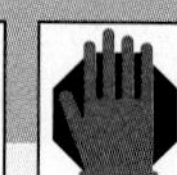

9. Clean the site with an antiseptic solution, and if the physician has indicated, cover with a sterile dressing.

    Some wounds need to be protected for a while longer; some wounds will have healed well enough to be left uncovered.

10. Properly care for or dispose of equipment and supplies. Clean the work area. Remove gloves and wash your hands.

DOCUMENTATION GUIDELINES

- Date and time
- Location of sutures
- Number of sutures removed
- Any difficulty with suture removal
- Any signs or symptoms of infection
- Patient complaints/concerns
- Patient education/instructions
- Your signature

Charting Example

DATE	TIME Pt arrived for suture removal. Six
	sutures removed from (L) elbow by order
	of Dr. Serratt. Wound appears to be
	healing, no drainage noted. Dr. Serratt in
	to check wound. Wound cleaned with
	antiseptic solution. Steri-strips and
	sterile dressings applied to wound. Pt
	instructed to continue prescribed
	ointment and RTC in 5 days for F/U.
	—Your signature

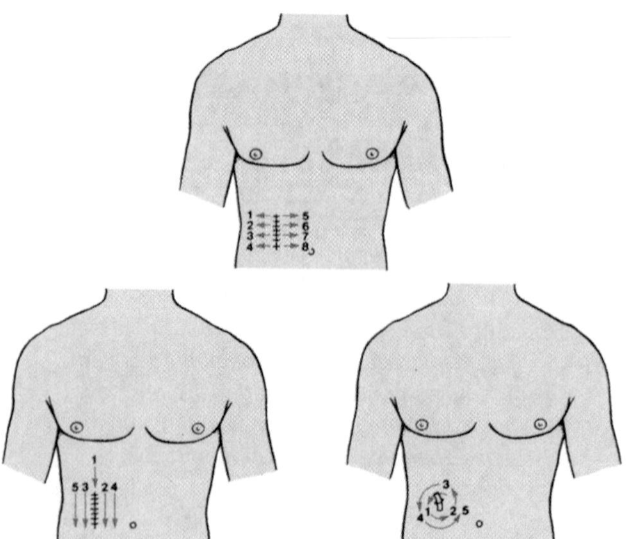

Figure 6-11 Clean the wound outward from the site following any of the numbered patterns shown here.

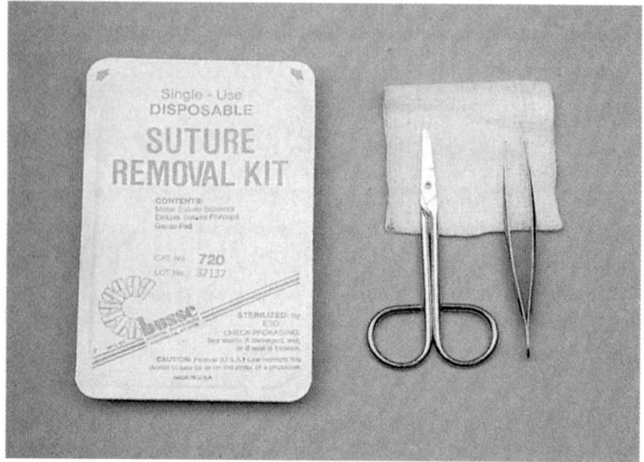

Figure 6-12 Suture removal kit.

Procedure 6-6 Removing Staples

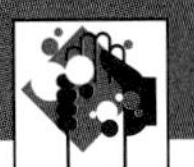
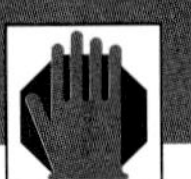
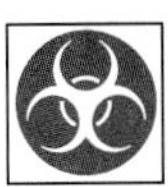

PURPOSE:

To restore the integrity of the operative site after the healing process

EQUIPMENT/SUPPLIES

- antiseptic solution or wipes
- gauze squares
- sponge forceps
- instrument for removing staples
- sterile gloves
- Option: Sterile, disposable staple removal kits contain all needed supplies.

STEPS

1. Wash your hands.
2. Assemble the equipment.
3. Greet and identify the patient. Explain the procedure and answer any questions.
4. If the dressing and bandages have not been removed, do so (Procedure 6-8). Dispose of dressings properly in a biohazard container. *Note:* At this point in the procedure, the physician may be called to assess the healing process. The wound may need to be assessed both before and after exudate is removed.
   The dressings will be contaminated and must be handled using Standard Precautions.
5. Clean the incision with antiseptic solution using the previously described method for wound care. Pat dry using dry sterile gauze sponges.
   The incision must be cleaned before removing the staples to avoid possible infection. If exudate is present, the staples may not be easily visualized.
6. Put on sterile gloves.
   Staple removal is a sterile procedure.
7. Gently slide the end of the staple remover under each staple to be removed. Press the handles together to lift the ends of the staple out of the skin and remove the staple.
   The remover is designed to open the staple so that the ends will lift free and minimize patient discomfort.

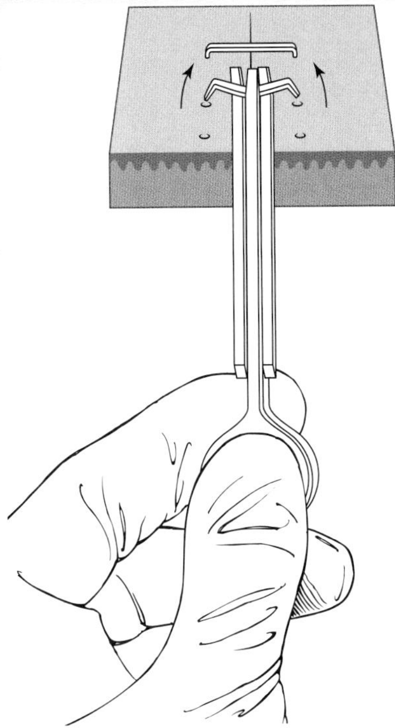

8. Place each staple on a gauze square as it is removed.
   This helps in counting the staples. If three staples were inserted, then three staples should now be removed.
9. When all of the staples are removed, gently clean the incision as instructed for all procedures. Pat dry. Dress the site if required by the physician.
   The area should be cleaned and dried before applying new dressings to avoid wicking microorganisms. The healing process may be far enough along to allow the wound to remain uncovered.

continued

Procedure 6-6 Continued Removing Staples

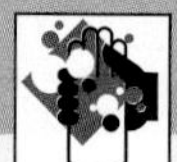

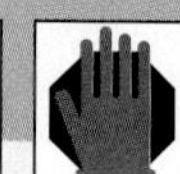

10. Properly care for or dispose of all equipment and supplies. Clean the work area. Remove gloves and wash your hands.

Standard Precautions must be followed.

DOCUMENTATION GUIDELINES

- Date and time
- Location of staples
- Number of staples removed
- Any difficulty with staple removal
- Any signs or symptoms of infection
- Patient complaints/concerns
- Patient education/instructions
- Your signature

Charting Example

DATE	TIME
	S: "I get my staples out today."
	O: Incision on abdomen in right lower
	quadrant. Four staples in place. No
	drainage or redness noted.
	A: Staple removal needed.
	P: 1. Four staples removed without problem.
	2. Antiseptic solution applied.
	3. D/c instructions given by surgeon.
	—Your signature

ASSISTING WITH STAPLE REMOVAL

Following hospital surgery, many incisions will be closed with metal staples rather than fiber sutures. Patients frequently leave the hospital before the staples can be removed safely and need to return to the physician's office for their removal. Frequently it will be your responsibility to remove the staples. Most offices use staple removal kits similar to the kits supplied for suture removal. These include a special instrument for removing the staples rather than thumb forceps and suture scissors included in the suture removal kits. Some offices will assemble equipment on site (Procedure 6-6).

STERILE DRESSINGS

Sterile **dressings** are items such as 4 × 4 absorbent gauze sponges, nonadhering dressings, and so on that have been processed for use on open wounds (Fig. 6-13). Sterile dressings are generally prepackaged in small quantities but may come in bulk containers. They are manufactured in different sizes and shapes, each for a specific use. Dressings should be handled using sterile technique to maintain their sterility. Procedure 6-7 describes the steps for applying a sterile dressing.

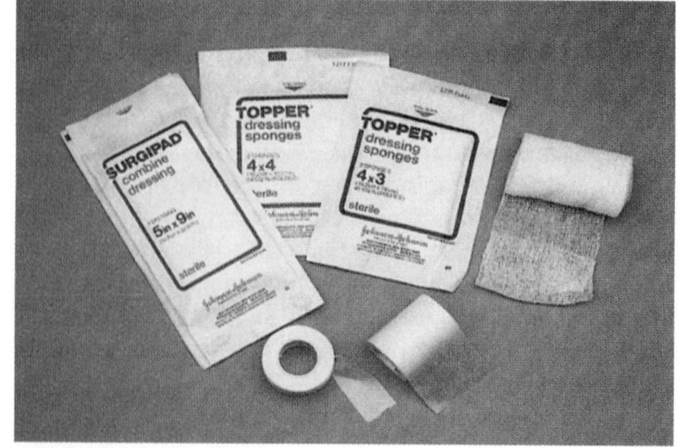

Figure 6-13 Various types of gauze dressings and tape. (Photo © Ken Kasper.)

Procedure 6-7 Applying a Sterile Dressing

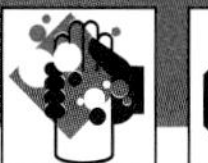
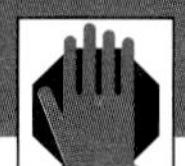
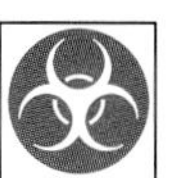

PURPOSE:

To avoid infection and promote healing by providing a sterile wound environment
To protect the wound from trauma

EQUIPMENT/SUPPLIES

- sterile gloves
- dressings
- scissors
- appropriate bandages and tapes
- any medication to be applied to the dressing
- Option: Disposable dressing change kits contain all needed supplies.

STEPS

1. Wash your hands.
2. Assemble equipment.
3. Greet and identify the patient. Ask about any tape allergies before deciding on the type of tape to use.

   Patients must be identified to avoid errors in treatment. Some patients are sensitive to the adhesive on tapes and may develop skin irritation. Many types of hypoallergenic tapes are available to avoid this problem.
4. With the size of the dressing and bandage in mind, cut or tear lengths of tape to secure the bandage. Set the tape aside in a convenient location.

   Having tape prepared saves time and may prevent the dressing from slipping if tape must be torn after the dressing is applied.
5. Explain the procedure and instruct the patient to remain still during the procedure and to avoid coughing, sneezing, or talking until the procedure is complete.

   Unexpected movements by the patient may result in contamination of the sterile supplies and the wound. Talking, coughing, and sneezing release droplets of moisture containing microorganisms from the respiratory tract which may contaminate the sterile field and the wound.
6. Open the dressing pack to create a sterile field. Observe the principles of surgical asepsis. Many packets are designed to be opened by the peel-apart method.

   Observing sterile technique is necessary to ensure the sterility of the dressing after it has been opened. Packages of dressings are sterile on the inside surfaces; if opened in a manner that allows the inside of the package to remain sterile, the inner surface may be used as a sterile field on which the dressing may remain until it is needed.
7. a. If sterile gloves are to be used for the procedure, open the appropriate size package of sterile gloves. Using sterile technique, put on the gloves. (See procedure for applying sterile gloves in Chapter 1, Asepsis and Infection Control.)

   It is necessary to wear sterile gloves during a sterile procedure to prevent contamination of the dressings or wound site.

   b. If using a sterile transfer forceps to apply the dressing (the "no-touch" method), use sterile technique to arrange the dressing on the wound site, and do not touch the dressing or the site with the hands.

   Using proper technique avoids contamination of the dressings or the wound.
8. Using the already opened sterile dressings and principles of sterile technique, apply to the wound the number of dressings needed to cover and protect the wound properly. Be sure to place sterile dressings carefully on the wound; do not drag them over the skin into position.

   If the dressing is dragged over the skin and into position, the dressing will be contaminated by microorganisms from the surrounding skin and may cause infection.
9. Apply the bandage so that it completely covers the sterile dressing and conforms to the patient's contours. The bandage should extend at least 1 inch beyond the border of the dressing.

   The opportunity for wound contamination is greatly reduced when the bandage is placed so that it completely covers the wound dressing from outside contaminants.
10. Apply the previously cut lengths of tape over the bandage in a manner that secures both bandage and dressing. Apply tape sufficiently to secure the bandage, but avoid overuse of tape. When the wound is completely covered, you may remove your gloves, or you may prefer to keep them on during the taping. Discard them in the proper receptacle.

    Tape is used only to keep the dressings and bandages in place. Tape should not completely obscure the bandage, but should allow for the observation of any bleeding or drainage. Too much tape can cause perspiration to dampen

continued

6

Procedure 6-7 Continued **Applying a Sterile Dressing**

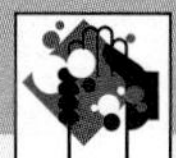 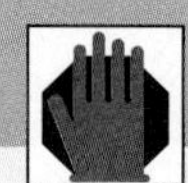 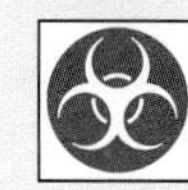

the dressing and compromise sterility. Tape should not obstruct blood circulation. More tape used to secure dressings and bandages means more must be removed, which may cause discomfort to the patient.

11. When the patient is required to change dressings at home, provide appropriate instructions. Dressings and bandages should be kept clean and dry and changed when wet or soiled. Otherwise, dressings should be changed as frequently as instructed by the physician. *Note:* The physician will describe to the patient the signs of infection, such as redness, swelling, pain, or undue warmth at the site; what to do regarding excess bleeding or drainage; and how to manage any drains that might be present.

Microorganisms may be transported to the wound by capillary action when the dressing becomes wet or soiled. To decrease the chance of contamination and infection, dressings should be changed as they become wet or soiled in addition to the prescribed schedule.

12. Assist the patient from the examination table.

Patients may become dizzy or unsteady upon sitting up. To prevent falls, it is important to stay with the patient in case this occurs.

13. Properly care for or dispose of equipment and supplies. Disposable articles contaminated with blood or wound drainage require special disposal protocol. Clean the work area. (See Chapter 1, Asepsis and Infection Control.)

14. Return reusable supplies (unopened sterile gloves or dressings, bandages, tape) to their appropriate storage areas; all others should be discarded correctly.

Unopened, reusable supplies should be returned to the appropriate storage areas for reuse. Discarding uncontaminated reusables is wasteful.

DOCUMENTATION GUIDELINES

- Date and time
- Location and type of dressing
- Any signs or symptoms of infection
- Presence and type of drainage
- Patient complaints/concerns
- Patient education/instructions
- Your signature

Charting Example

DATE	TIME Six sutures inserted by Dr. Cater
	following excision of sebaceous cyst (R)
	shoulder. Minimal sanguineous drainage.
	Sterile dressings applied to site. Pt's
	spouse observed the application and
	verbalized understanding of procedures
	as outlined in pt ed brochure.
	—Your signature

Note: For the purposes of this procedure, it will be presumed that the skin and the lesion have been cleaned in the manner preferred by the physician. If medication is to be applied to the wound, it should be applied first to the dressing and then the dressing applied to the wound. This avoids touching the wound, which might cause discomfort to the patient.

A sterile dressing is considered contaminated, or unsterile, when it is damp or wet, its wrapper is damaged, it is outdated, or it is removed improperly from its wrapper or container. Sterile dressings are used directly over a wound to:

1. Cover and protect from contamination
2. Absorb drainage such as blood, serum, pus
3. Exert pressure (eg, direct pressure on an open wound to slow bleeding)
4. Hide disfigurement during the healing process
5. Hold medications against the wound to facilitate healing

A sterile dressing may be accompanied by various bandages (sling, cravat, roller, tubular gauze) to hold the dressing in place, protect the injured part, or restrict movement.

When you remove a sterile dressing or change an existing one (Procedure 6-8), carefully observe for any drainage or exudate, and note this in the patient's chart (Box 6-1). Notify the physician when the wound is uncovered so that it can be examined and a decision made regarding appropriate healing. Box 6-2 discusses the types and phases of wound healing.

text continues on page 134

Procedure 6-8 Changing an Existing Sterile Dressing

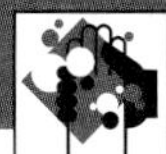
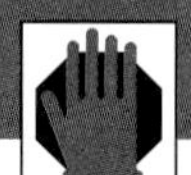
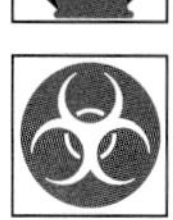

PURPOSE:

To avoid infection and promote healing by providing sterile wound environment
To protect the wound from trauma

EQUIPMENT/SUPPLIES

- sterile dressings and sterile gloves (for applying the new dressing)
- unsterile gloves (for removing the old dressing and bandage)
- skin antiseptic solution with sterile gauze squares or sterile cotton balls or premedicated antiseptic wipes
- sterile basin (to receive the solution and gauze or cotton)
- tape, torn to appropriate lengths and set aside as in Procedure 6-7
- approved biohazard containers for contaminated waste
- Option: Disposable dressing change kits contain all needed supplies.

STEPS

1. Wash your hands.
2. Assemble the equipment.
3. Greet and identify the patient. Explain the procedure and answer any questions.
4. Prepare a sterile field. If using a sterile container and solution, open the package containing the basin using sterile technique and use the inside of the wrapper as the sterile field for the basin. Peel apart the wrappers for the gauze or cotton balls and flip them into the basin or use sterile transfer forceps to place them in the basin.
   This avoids wound contamination.
5. Prepare antiseptic solution by first pouring off a small amount of the solution into a waste receptacle; then pour the solution from the stock bottle into the sterile container on the sterile field.
   The first bit of solution to cross the mouth of the container should be poured away to remove any pathogens that may be in that area.
6. Instruct the patient not to talk, cough, sneeze, laugh, or move during the procedure.
   Respiratory droplets may contaminate the sterile field. Movement may cause the field to be accidentally contaminated.
7. Wearing clean gloves, carefully remove the tape from the bandage by pulling it toward the direction of the wound. Large bandages that encircle a limb may first be cut with bandage scissors on the side of the limb away from the wound. Remove the old bandage and dressing. *Note:* If the dressing is difficult to remove because of dried wound exudate or blood, soak it with sterile water or saline for a few minutes to loosen it. Gently pull the edges of the dressing toward the center. Never pull on a dressing that does not come off easily; the healing process will be disrupted. If this procedure does not loosen the dressing or causes undue discomfort to the patient, notify the physician immediately.
   Gloves must be worn during any procedure involving contact with blood or body fluid. Tape pulled away from the direction of the wound may pull the healing edges of the wound apart.
8. Discard the soiled dressing in a biohazard container. Do not pass it over the sterile field.
   The dressing will be soiled with blood and body fluid and must be considered potentially hazardous. Dressings passed over the sterile field will shed microorganisms and contaminate the area.
9. Inspect and observe the wound for degree of healing, amount and type of drainage, appearance of wound edges, and so on.
   Inspections and observations are made now because following proper wound cleaning, most wound exudate will be removed. Make a mental note for charting when the procedure is complete.
10. Observing medical asepsis, remove and discard gloves. *Note:* At this point, the physician should inspect the wound before exudate or drainage is removed. Decisions must be made regarding the healing process. If a culture is ordered, it must be taken before the wound is cleaned to ensure the most reliable test results.
    Proper removal of gloves helps prevent contamination.

continued

Procedure 6-8 Continued **Changing an Existing Sterile Dressing**

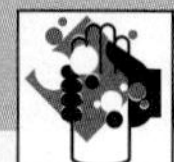
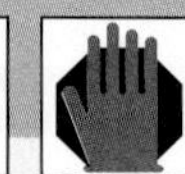
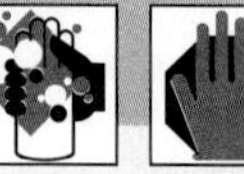

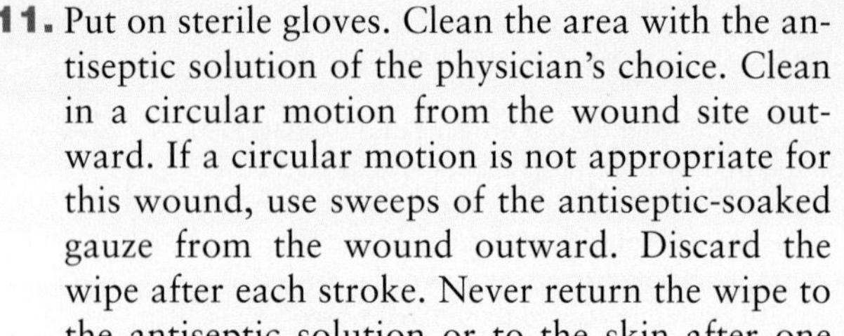

11. Put on sterile gloves. Clean the area with the antiseptic solution of the physician's choice. Clean in a circular motion from the wound site outward. If a circular motion is not appropriate for this wound, use sweeps of the antiseptic-soaked gauze from the wound outward. Discard the wipe after each stroke. Never return the wipe to the antiseptic solution or to the skin after one sweep across the area.

The area must be cleaned before fresh dressings are applied. Returning the wipe to the wound area or the solution brings microorganisms from the surrounding skin to the open lesion.

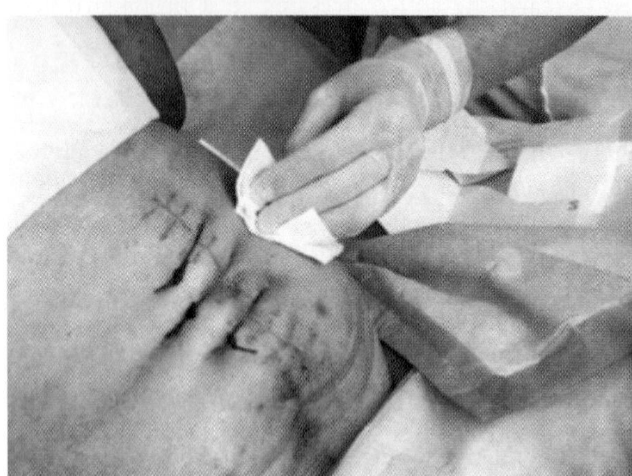

12. Replace the dressing using the procedure for sterile dressing application (Procedure 6-7).

DOCUMENTATION GUIDELINES

- Date and time
- Location and type of dressing
- Any signs or symptoms of infection
- Presence and type of drainage
- Patient complaints/concerns
- Patient education/instructions
- Your signature

Charting Example

DATE	TIME Pt arrived in office for sterile
	dressing change. Ulcerated wound noted
	on (R) heel. Yellow drainage noted.
	Dr. Carson notified. Culture taken as
	ordered. Wound cleaned with Betadine
	solution. Sterile dressing applied. Pt
	instructed to keep limb elevated and keep
	wound dry. RV in a.m. for dressing change.
	—Your signature

Box 6-1
Wound Drainage

When observing wound drainage, be sure to note:

Color
- Serous (clear)
- Sanguineous (blood-tinged)
- Serosanguineous (pinkish or clear and red mixed)
- Purulent (white, green, or yellow-tinged drainage; usually has an unpleasant odor characteristic of infection)

Amount
- Copious (large amount)
- Medium (moderate amount)
- Scant (small amount)

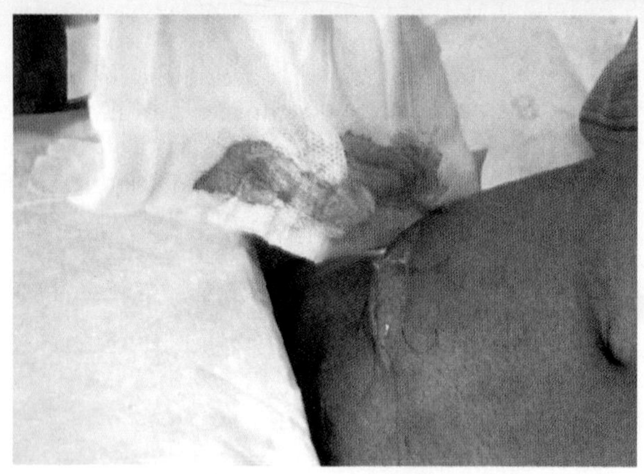

Box 6-2
The Healing Process

Types of Wound Healing

- *Healing by Primary Intention:* This simplest form of healing results from wounds that are closely approximated, allowing the entrance of little or no bacteria to complicate the process. The edges of the wound lie closely together, new cells form quickly to bind the site, and capillaries expand themselves across the tissue break to restore circulation to the tissues. There is usually little scarring.
- *Healing by Secondary Intention:* Granulation of tissue is present, and the edges of the wound join indirectly. Because the area is not closely approximated, additional new cells are required to fill spaces in the lesion. Capillaries may not be able to reach across the gap to restore full circulation. Nerves may not rejoin, which results in diminished nerve stimulus through the area. A large scab forms to protect the area while healing goes on below it. Scarring is more severe than with primary intention healing.
- *Healing by Tertiary Intention:* The wound initially is left open to fill in with granular tissue, then sutured at a later time. There is considerable scar formation.

Phases of Wound Healing

- *Phase I (inflammatory, lag, or exudative phase):* This phase usually lasts from 1 to 4 days. The body attempts to heal itself by increasing the circulation to the part and by beginning to reroute or repair the supplying vessels. The increased circulation brings with it more white blood cells to mount a defense

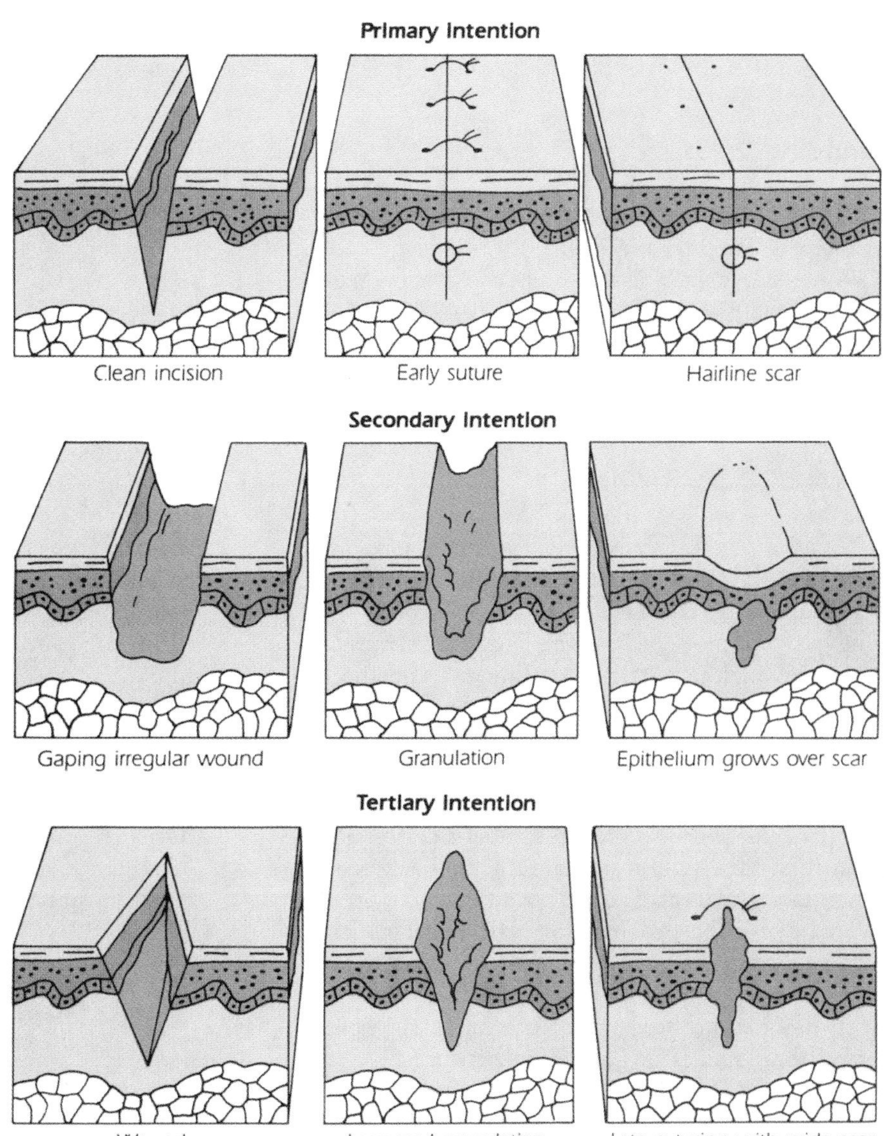

Types of wound healing.

continued

6

Box 6-2
The Healing Process *(Continued)*

against pathogens. Serum and red blood cells brought by the additional blood form a gluelike fibrin to plug the wound. As the fibrin dries, it pulls the edges of the wound closer together and forms a scab. Signs that this phase is working are edema from the tissue fluid, warmth from the extra blood, redness from the vasodilation, and pain from the pressure on the nerve endings caused by the edema.

- *Phase II (proliferative, healing, or granulation phase):* This phase may last from several days to several weeks. The vessels continue to repair themselves and may reroute if damage is severe. The scab from phase I continues to dry and to pull the edges as closely together as possible.
- *Phase III (remodeling, maturation, or scarring phase):* This phase may take from weeks to years, depending on the severity of the wound. Fibroblasts build scar tissue to guard the area.

Checkpoint Question

6. *When are sterile dressings used?*

BANDAGING

Bandages are strips of woven materials. Typically absorbent, they are used for many purposes, including:

1. Applying pressure to control bleeding
2. Holding a dressing in place
3. Protecting dressings and wounds from contamination
4. Immobilizing an injured part of the body
5. Supporting an injured part of the body

Types of Bandages

- *Roller bandages* are soft woven materials wound on themselves to form a roll. Roller bandages are available in various lengths and widths from 1 inch to 6 or more inches. The bandage size selected depends on the part being bandaged and the desired thickness of the completed bandage. Most bandages are made of a porous, lightweight material and are either sterile or clean (unsterile). Most gauze bandages conform easily to angular surfaces of the body. Loosely woven standard cotton roller gauze, which is not stretchy and has edges that fray easily, is rarely used in offices today.

  To avoid the problems of plain roller gauze, a crepelike, stretchy gauze is made to adjust to various body contours and resists unrolling much better than plain roller gauze. Kling and Conform are two brand names that are frequently used.
- *Elastic bandages,* such as the Ace brand, are special bandage rolls that have elastic woven throughout the fabric; they are generally brownish-tan. Unlike other types of roller gauze, elastic bandages can be washed and reused many times. Because of the elastic fibers, you must use great care when applying the bandage to prevent compromising circulation and still give support to the injured part. Apply elastic bandages so that there is no wrinkling of the concentric layers. Never stretch or pull on the elastic bandage during application to avoid applying it too tightly. Always watch for signs of impaired circulation and ask the patient for comments as the bandage is being applied.

  Bandages should fit snugly but not too tightly. Adjust the bandage accordingly if it seems too loose or when the patient expresses discomfort if it is too tight. Some elastic bandages are available with an adhesive backing, which helps keep the layers in place and provides a secure, snug, and comfortable fit.
- *Tubular gauze bandages* are used to enclose rounded body parts. The bandage resembles a hollow tube and is woven to give it an extremely stretchy quality. It is used to enclose fingers, toes, arms, and legs and even the head and trunk. Tubular gauze bandages are available in various widths from ⅝ inch to 7 inches to fit any part of the body.

  Tubular gauze is applied using a metal or plastic tubular framelike applicator. The applicator is available in various sizes and should be slightly larger than the body part to be covered. This enables the gauze to slide easily over the body part. Applicators are marked according to a size number that corresponds to the boxes of different size tubular gauze. Procedure 6-9 discusses the specific steps for applying a tubular gauze bandage.

Bandage Application Guidelines

When properly applied, bandages should feel comfortably snug and should be fastened securely enough to remain in place until removed. Bandages can be fastened with safety pins, adhesive tape, or clips, such as those supplied with elastic bandages. A patient's confidence in your professional ability is greatly enhanced

6

Box 6-3
Six Techniques for Wrapping a Roller Bandage

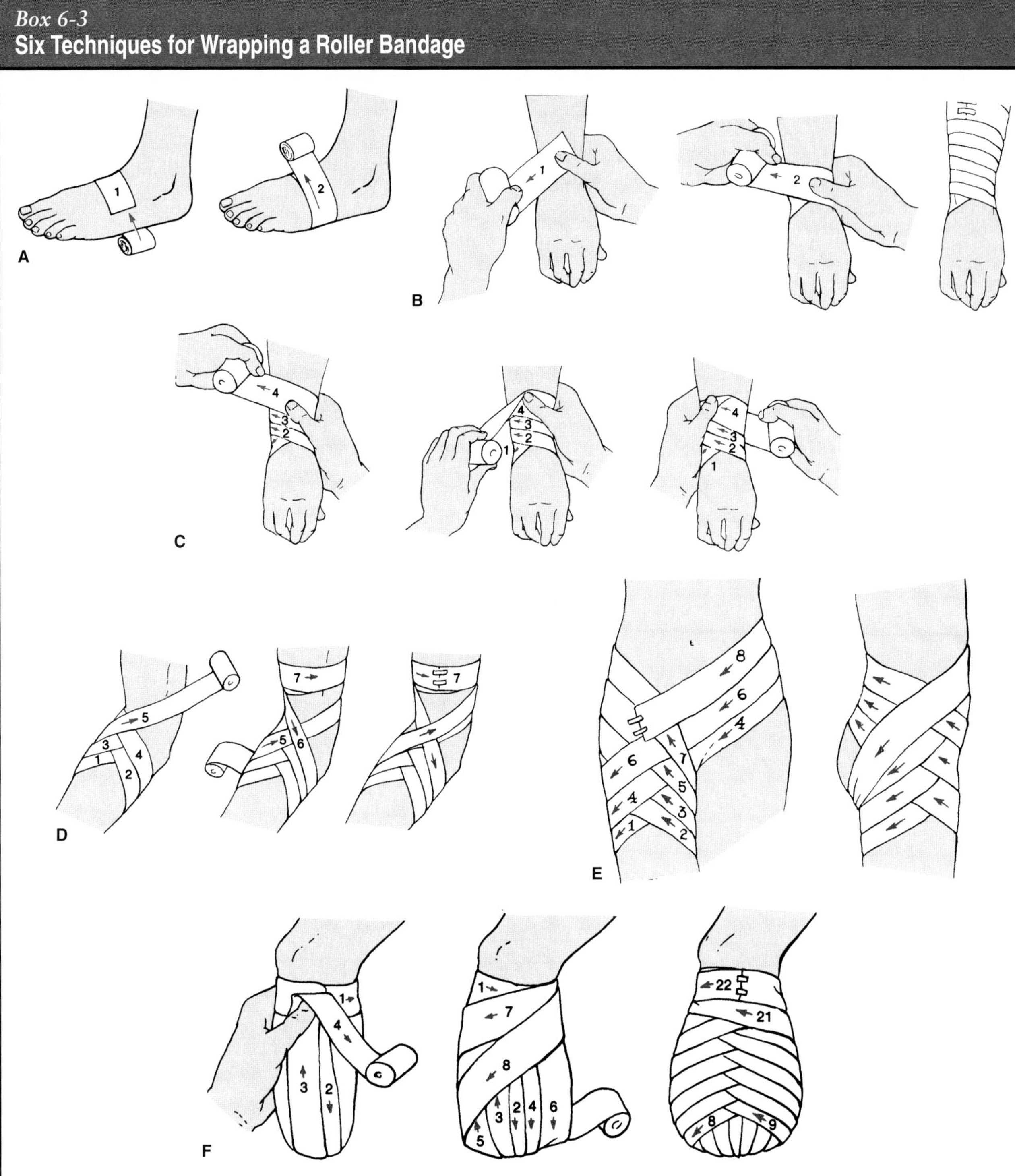

(*A*) A *circular turn* is used to anchor and secure a bandage when it is started and ended. It simply involves holding the free end of the rolled material in one hand and wrapping it about the area, bringing it back to the starting point. (*B*) A *spiral turn* partly overlaps a previous turn. The overlapping varies from one-half to three-fourths of the width of the bandage. Spiral turns are used when wrapping a cylindrical part of the body like the arms and legs. (C) A *spiral reverse turn* is a modification of a spiral turn. The roll is reversed halfway through the turn. This works well on tapered body parts. (*D*) A *figure-of-eight turn* is best used when an area spanning a joint, like the elbow or knee, requires bandaging. It is made by making oblique turns that alternately ascend and descend, simulating the number "8." (*E*) A *spica turn* is a variation of the figure-of-eight turn. It differs in that the wrap includes a portion of the trunk or chest. (*F*) The *recurrent turn* is made by passing the roll back and forth over the tip of a body part. Once several recurrent turns have been made, the bandage is anchored by completing the application with another basic turn like the figure-of-eight. A recurrent turn is especially beneficial when wrapping the stump of an amputated limb.

when a bandage is applied comfortably, neatly, and securely. Patients become understandably upset when bandages fall off through normal use. Below are general guidelines for applying bandages.

1. Observe the principles of medical asepsis to prevent the transfer of pathogens. Surgical asepsis is not necessary; the bandage may be used on the outside to cover a sterile dressing or may be used alone in cases where there is no open wound.
2. Keep the area to be bandaged and the bandage itself dry and clean because moisture may wick bacteria onto the area of concern. A moist bandage, which also encourages the growth of pathogens, will be uncomfortable for the patient.
3. Never place bandages directly over a wound. Sterile dressings are applied first and then are covered with a bandage for protection. The bandage should extend approximately 1 to 2 inches beyond the edge of the dressing.

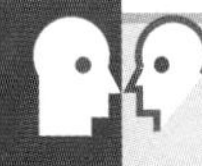

Patient Education

At-Home Wound Care

Patients with dressings and bandages that must be changed between office visits will need instructions to ensure that healing is not compromised and to avoid the spread of pathogens. When patients understand the purpose for instructions and health care directives, they are more likely to comply and to make decisions that lead to better self-care.

- Demonstrate to the patient or caregiver proper handwashing techniques to avoid the spread of pathogens either to or from the patient.
- If special supplies must be purchased, help the patient find financial aid, if necessary, and provide him or her with a list of sources for medical supplies.
- If the procedure appears to be too complicated at this time for the patient or caregiver to master, speak with the physician regarding your concerns, and suggest a home health service until the procedure can be simplified.
- Show the patient or caregiver ways to make wound care and dressing changes more comfortable for the patient and safer for those around him or her. Urge the use of impervious bags for dressings, gloves for dressing changes, and clean or aseptic technique as the situation requires. Demonstrate the entire procedure, and check frequently for questions and comprehension.
- Educate the patient or caregiver to signs that should be reported, such as increased drainage, odor, and so forth.

4. Never allow skin surfaces of two body parts to touch each other because wound healing may cause opposing surfaces to adhere and result in scar tissue formation. For example, burned fingers are each dressed separately, but may be bandaged together.
5. Pad joints and any bony prominence to help prevent skin irritation caused by the bandage rubbing against the skin over a bony area.
6. Bandage the affected part in the normal position: joints should be slightly flexed to avoid muscle strain, discomfort, or pain. Otherwise, muscle spasms may occur if the limb is made to assume an unnatural position.
7. Apply bandages beginning at the distal part and extending to the proximal part of the body. Bandage turns that extend distal to proximal aid in the return of venous blood to the heart and help make the bandage more secure.
8. Always communicate with the patient. If the patient complains that the bandage is too tight or too loose, adjust the bandage. The bandage should fit snugly, but if it is too tight, it may impair circulation. If it is too loose, it may fall off.
9. When bandaging hands and feet, leave the fingers and toes exposed whenever possible to make it easier to check for circulatory impairment. If there is coldness, pallor, or cyanosis of the nail beds or pain, swelling, numbness, or tingling of the toes or fingers, remove the bandage immediately and reapply it correctly.

Box 6-3 illustrates various techniques for wrapping bandages.

Montgomery Straps

Surgical patients who are discharged from the hospital with draining wounds that require frequent dressing changes will probably be dressed with Montgomery straps. This type of bandage consists of opposing pairs of straps, or tapes, with gauze ties that cross over thick layers of absorbent dressings (Fig. 6-14). When the dressings are soiled, the ties are loosened, the soiled dressings removed, and new dressings applied. The adhesive tapes, or straps, are not removed unless grossly soiled. Montgomery straps have many advantages over conventional dressings and bandages for the heavily draining wound, including ease of dressing change and maintenance of skin integrity at the operative site.

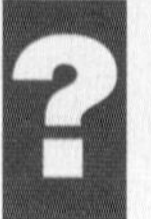

Checkpoint Question

7. *When applying a bandage, at which end of the extremity must you begin? Why?*

Procedure 6-9 Applying a Tubular Gauze Bandage

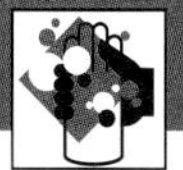
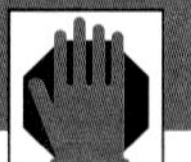

PURPOSE:

To reinforce and secure dressings applied to wounds
To protect the wound from trauma

EQUIPMENT/SUPPLIES

- tubular gauze
- applicator
- tape
- scissors

STEPS

1. Wash your hands.
2. Assemble the equipment.
3. Greet and identify the patient. Explain the procedure and answer any questions.
   Tubular gauze may be applied after a sterile dressing change, in which case, this step will have been completed.
4. Choose the appropriate size tubular gauze applicator and gauze width. Manufacturers of tubular gauze supply charts with suggestions for the most appropriate size to use for various body parts.
   The applicator and gauze should slip easily over the body part. Choose an applicator slightly larger than the part to be covered. The gauze designed to fit the chosen applicator will provide a secure fit.
5. Select and cut or tear adhesive tape in lengths to secure the gauze ends.
   Tape ensures that the gauze will not slip off. Having it at hand before beginning the procedure saves time and effort.
6. Place the gauze bandage on the applicator in the following manner:
   a. Be sure the applicator is upright (open end up) and placed on a flat surface.
   b. Pull a sufficient length of gauze from the stock box; do not cut it at this time.
   c. Open the end of the length of gauze and slide it over the upper end of the applicator. Continue pushing until all of the gauze needed for this procedure is on the applicator.
   d. Cut the gauze when the required amount of gauze has been transferred to the applicator.
7. Place the applicator over the distal end of the affected part (finger, toe, leg) and begin to apply the gauze. Hold it in place as you move to step 8.
   The application should begin distally and work proximally.
8. Slide the applicator containing the gauze up to the proximal end of the affected part. Holding the gauze at the proximal end of the affected part, pull the applicator and gauze toward the distal end.
   This keeps the bandage from slipping. If the bandage is not held in place at the early stages of application, it may not completely cover the part.

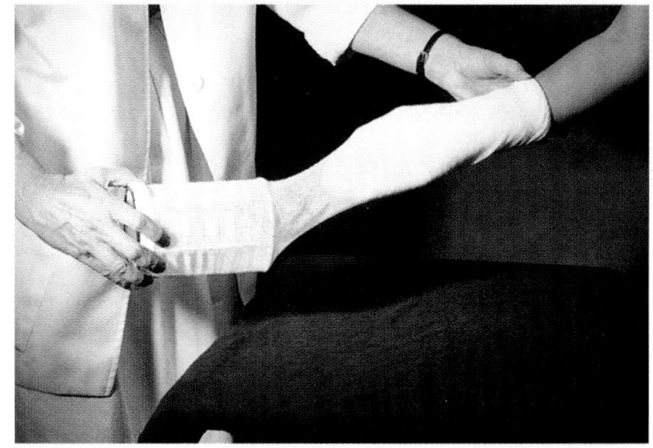

continued

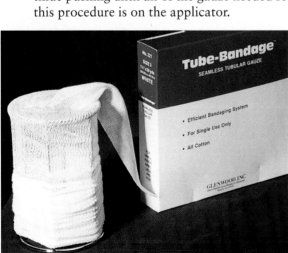

Procedure 6-9 Continued Applying a Tubular Gauze Bandage

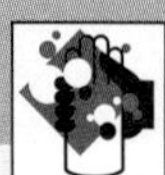
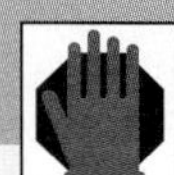

9. Continue to hold the gauze in place. Pull the applicator 1 to 2 inches past the end of the affected part if the part is to be completely covered. In many instances, the gauze will not be required to extend beyond a limb and may cover only the area around the wound.

   The bandage will be secured at the distal end if the part is to be completely covered. If the distal portion of the limb is not to be covered, the bandage must extend at least 1 inch beyond the wound site and dressing to ensure adequate coverage.

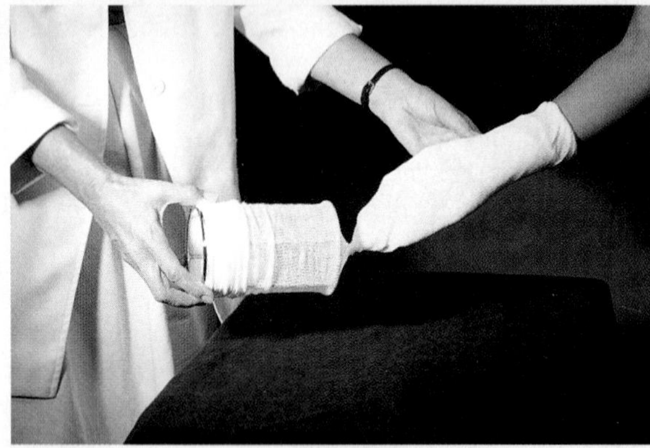

10. Turn the applicator one full turn to anchor the bandage.

    The bandage will be securely held in place by the twist.

11. Move the applicator toward the proximal part as before.

    This allows for a double layer of bandage for protection.

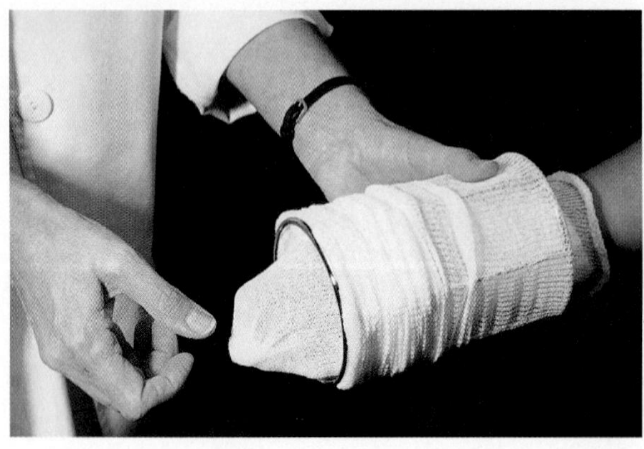

12. Move the applicator forward about 1 inch beyond the original starting point. Anchor the bandage again by turning it as before.

    Anchoring provides a secure fit.

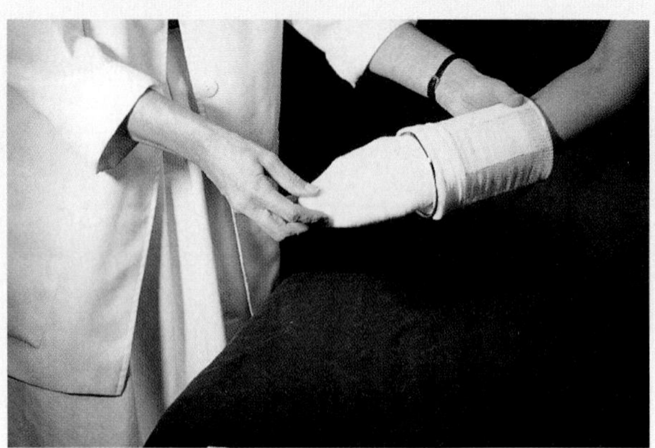

13. Repeat the procedure until the desired coverage is obtained. The final layer should end at the proximal part of the affected area. Any extra length of gauze not needed can be cut from the applicator. Remove the applicator.

    The part should be adequately covered to protect the wound.

14. Secure the bandage in place with adhesive tape or cut the gauze into two tails and tie them at the base of the tear. Tie the two tails around the closest proximal joint. Use adhesive tape sparingly to secure the end if not using a tie.

    The bandage must be securely fastened to keep it in place until it must be changed.

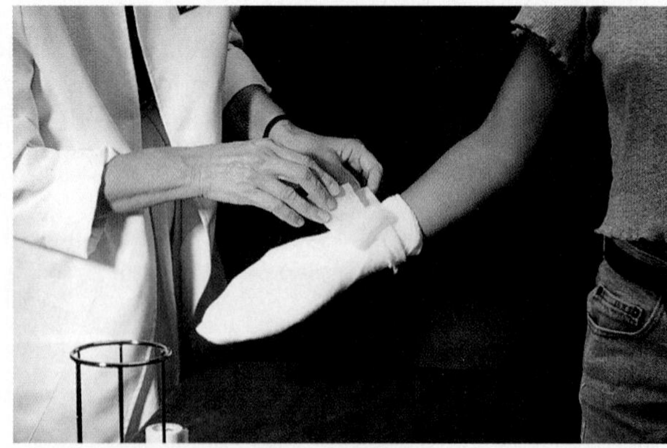

15. Properly care for or dispose of equipment and supplies. Clean the work area. Wash your hands.

continued

Procedure 6-9 Continued **Applying a Tubular Gauze Bandage**

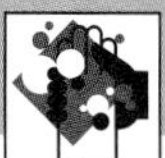
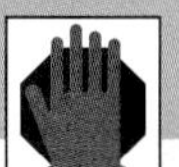

DOCUMENTATION GUIDELINES

- Date and time
- Location and type of dressing
- Any signs or symptoms of infection
- Presence and type of dressing
- Patient complaints/concerns
- Patient education/instructions
- Your signature

Charting Example

DATE	TIME Pt arrived /c laceration to (R)
	palm by kitchen knife. Wound cleaned with
	antiseptic solution. Tetanus booster
	current. Dr. Preston sutured /c #1-0 silk.
	Sterile dressings applied, tubular gauze
	to cover. Pt to keep wound dry and
	elevated. RTC in 3 days for recheck.
	—Your signature

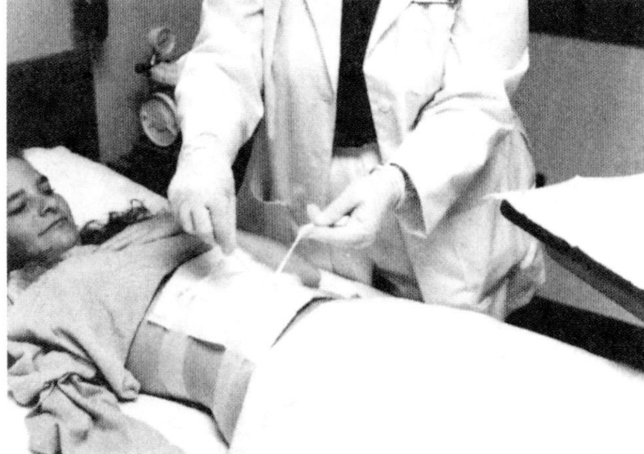

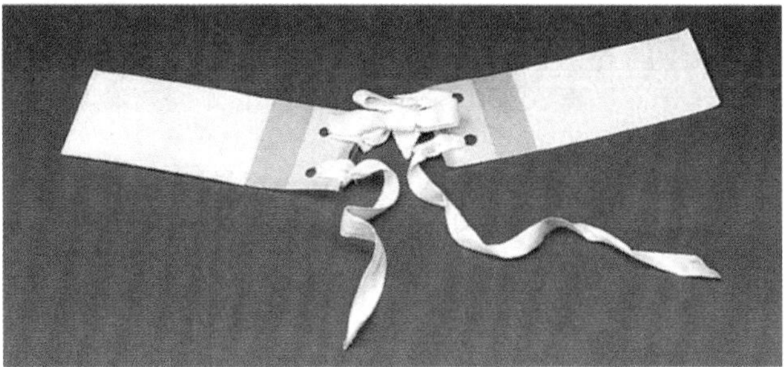

Figure 6-14 Montgomery straps or ties are used to prevent skin breakdown from frequent tape removal when dressings need to be changed often.

COMMONLY PERFORMED OFFICE SURGICAL PROCEDURES

Two of the most frequently performed minor surgeries in the general medical office are the excision of skin lesions (moles, lentigines, keratoses, and skin tags) and the incision and drainage of abscesses. Incisions may be closed with sutures or may be left to heal without interference, depending on the size and position of the wound. Surgical setups may be purchased prepackaged with many of the supplies needed for minor excisional procedures. Supplies listed with the procedures are site-prepared and include sutures. Standard Precautions must be followed when assisting with these procedures.

Excision of a Lesion

Physicians may excise lesions with electrocautery (see below) or with standard surgical equipment (Procedure 6-10). If the lesion does not require analysis, it can be desiccated or fulgurated (see below). Many lesions are referred to pathology for diagnosis after excision.

6

Procedure 6-10 Assisting with Excisional Surgery

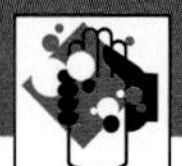
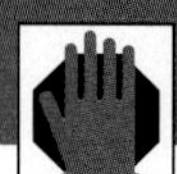
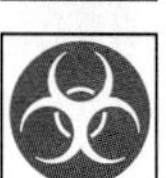

PURPOSE:

To assist the physician in procedures requiring surgical asepsis
To reduce patient anxiety and to increase patient cooperation and comfort
To maintain sterility of equipment and supplies

EQUIPMENT/SUPPLIES

At the side
- sterile gloves
- local anesthetic
- antiseptic wipes
- adhesive tape
- bandages
- specimen container with completed laboratory request

On the field
- basin for solutions
- gauze sponges and cotton balls

On the field (continued)
- antiseptic solution
- sterile drape
- dissecting scissors or iris scissors
- scalpel blade and handle of physician's choice
- mosquito forceps
- tissue forceps
- needle holder
- suture and needle of physician's choice

STEPS

1. Wash your hands.
2. Assemble the equipment.
3. Greet and identify the patient. Explain the procedure and answer any questions.
4. Step up a sterile field on a surgical stand with the at-the-side equipment close at hand. Cover the field with a sterile drape if necessary until the physician arrives.
5. Position the patient appropriately.
   The position required depends on the location of the lesion.
6. Put on sterile gloves or use transfer forceps for the aseptic process.
   Sterile gloves or the "no touch" technique protects from contamination.
7. Cleanse the site with sterile antiseptic solution in the manner described for skin preparation (Procedure 6-4). *Note:* The physician may do this before gloving. Some physicians prefer that the site be cleaned and made ready by an assistant; others prefer doing it themselves after gloving and using the supplies on the field. In all instances, the physician's preference takes precedence over any outlined procedure.
   The antiseptic discourages the entrance of microorganisms into the wound.
8. The physician will perform the procedure; you may be asked to assist during the procedure. This usually involves adding supplies as needed, watching closely for opportunities to assist the physician and comforting the patient, or putting on sterile gloves and passing instruments to the physician from the field. *Note:* If the lesion is to be referred to pathology for analysis, you will be required to assist with the specimen container during the procedure.
9. At the end of the procedure, dress the wound using the procedure for applying a sterile dressing (see Procedure 6-7).
   The wound must be covered to protect the incision from contamination during the healing process.
10. Assist the patient from the table and offer to help with clothing as needed.
    Depending on the site of the lesion, it may be difficult for the patient to replace clothing.
11. Clean the examining room in preparation for the next patient. Discard all disposables in appropriate biohazard containers. Return unused reusable items to their proper place. Wash your hands.

DOCUMENTATION GUIDELINES

- Date and time
- Location of procedure
- Type of specimen and routing procedure
- Type of dressing
- Patient complaints/concerns
- Patient education/instructions
- Your signature

Charting Example

DATE	TIME Pt scheduled for removal nevus (R)
	periorbital ridge. Excised by Dr. Myers /s
	difficulty. 2 sutures #6-0 silk. Nevus
	routed to Path lab. Sterile dressing
	applied to wound site. Pt instructed to
	keep wound clean and dry and RTC in 2
	days. —Your signature

Procedure 6-11 Assisting with Incision and Drainage (I & D)

PURPOSE:

To assist the physician with procedures requiring surgical asepsis
To reduce patient anxiety and to increase patient cooperation and comfort
To maintain sterility of equipment and supplies

EQUIPMENT/SUPPLIES

At the side
- sterile gloves
- local anesthetic
- antiseptic wipes
- adhesive tape
- additional sterile dressings
- packing gauze
- bandages

(If the wound is to be cultured, a culture tube will also be included at the side.)

On the field
- basin
- sterile cotton balls or gauze
- antiseptic solution
- sterile drape
- syringes and needles for local anesthetic (unless the physician prefers that the site be numbed before gloving)
- commercial I & D set or scalpel, dissecting scissors or operating scissors, hemostats, tissue forceps, 4 × 4 gauze sponges, probe (optional)

STEPS

1–4. Follow steps 1–4 of Procedure 6-10: Assisting With Excisional Surgery.

5. Position the patient appropriately.
The position required depends on the location of the abscess.

6–8. Follow steps 6–8 of Procedure 6-10: Assisting With Excisional Surgery.

9. At the end of the procedure, dress the wound using the procedure for applying a sterile dressing (see Procedure 6-7).
The wound must be covered to avoid further contamination and to absorb drainage. The exudate is a hazardous body fluid requiring Standard Precautions.

10. Assist the patient from the table and offer to help with clothing as needed.
Depending on the site of the abscess, it may be difficult for the patient to replace clothing.

DOCUMENTATION GUIDELINES

- Date and time
- Location of procedure
- Type of specimen (eg, wound culture) and routing procedure
- Patient's temperature or other vital signs, if indicated by the infectious process or patient complaints
- Any complications with procedure
- Patient education/instructions
- Your signature

Charting Example

DATE	TIME Pt arrived in office with an abscess
	on (L) hand, third digit. Finger was
	prepped by the physician. Abscess was
	I&D. Pt tolerated procedure well. Tubular
	gauze dressing applied. Pt instructed to
	return for wound check in 3 days. Written
	instructions given to pt. Pt verbalized
	understanding of all instructions.
	—Your signature

Incision and Drainage (I&D)

An abscess is a localized collection of pus in a cavity surrounded by inflamed tissue. It is the body's response to an infectious process when pathogens have entered through a break in the skin. Abscesses may be referred to as boils, furuncles (one lesion), or carbuncles (several lesions grouped closely together) and are very painful. The site must be incised and the infected material drained before healing can take place (Procedure 6-11).

ELECTROSURGERY

Electosurgery uses high-frequency, alternating electric current to destroy or cut and remove tissue. It also is used to **coagulate** small bleeding vessels. Electrosurgery is considered an alternative to traditional office surgery and is rapidly gaining favor for many procedures. An advantage of electrical surgery is the cautery effect produced by the electricity that seals

6

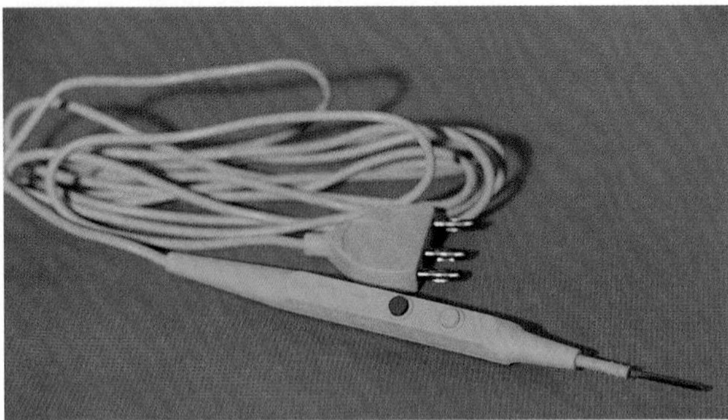

Figure 6-15 A disposable electrosurgical unit. The blade is designed to either cut or cauterize.

small bleeding vessels and coagulates nearby cells to reduce bleeding and loss of cell fluid. Electrosurgical units use disposable **electrodes** (medium for conducting electrical current) tips of different sizes and shapes to deliver the desired amount of electric current to the tissues (Fig. 6-15).

The following procedures are considered to be electrosurgery:

- *Fulguration* destroys tissue using controlled electric sparks. As the physician holds the electrode tip 1 to 2 mm away from the site, a series of sparks destroys the superficial cells at the site.
- *Electrodesiccation* dries and separates tissue using an electric current. In this procedure, the electrode is placed directly on the site.
- ***Electrocautery*** causes quick coagulation of small blood vessels with the heat created by the electric current. Electrocautery is commonly referred to as electrocoagulation.
- *Electrosection* is used for incision or excision of tissue. There is minimal bleeding with this type of procedure, but more damage can occur to surrounding tissues.

Physicians frequently use electrosurgery to remove moles, cysts, warts, and certain types of skin and cervical cancers. Electrosurgical equipment includes various electrode tips, such as blades, needles, loops, and balls, each having specific uses.

During electrosurgery, your responsibilities are to ensure the safety and comfort of the patient and to pass the electrode to the physician as needed. As with all instruments, the electrode must be passed in its functional position. The electrode is handed with the tip in a downward position.

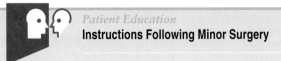

Patient Education

Instructions Following Minor Surgery

After minor surgery, instruct patients to report the following conditions:

- Excessive bleeding (additional teaching should include how to stop bleeding, eg, direct pressure, elevation)
- Redness, red streaks, or excessive swelling in the area
- Temperature elevation

Also explain that dressings must be kept clean and dry. If the dressing is to be changed, include instructions for dressing changes. Finally, make sure the patient understands the date, time, and place of suture or staple removal.

Safety Measures

Because electric current is delivered to the tip by the electrosurgical machine, great care should be exercised to prevent injuries. Although the device is always activated by the physician, it is possible to cause injury to the patient, physician, or medical assistant if the device is handled carelessly. Care must be taken to ground the patient before electrosurgery. Metal conducts electricity and can cause serious burns. When assisting with electrosurgery, follow these safety measures:

- Ensure that all working parts are in good repair. The electrical current is carefully regulated; if the machine is defective, serious injury to the patient might occur.
- Ensure that all metal is removed from the patient. The patient must be asked if metal implants are present or if a cardiac pacemaker is in place. Metal implants may become very hot, and pacemakers may malfunction during the procedure.
- Ensure that the patient is grounded with a pad supplied by the manufacturer. This should be attached at a site recommended by the manufacturer (some recommend placing the pad far from the operative site; others suggest placing it near the site). Improper placement can result in injury.
- Place the grounding pad firmly and completely against the patient's skin. A conducting gel must be applied to the pad and to the physician's skin, or an adhesive-backed pad can be used to facilitate conduction through the grounding pad. Areas of skin against the pad that are not well connected will result in "hot spots" and may burn the patient.

Care of Equipment

Although tips in use today are usually disposable, reusable tips are still used in some offices. Reusable tips are processed in the autoclave. They may be polished with steel wool if they become dull. Disposable tips should be discarded after use. Electrosurgical machines should be inspected periodically to ensure they are in good working order. The operating manual will suggest periods of maintenance to be performed by office staff and routine inspections by technicians trained to avoid potential malfunctions. Surfaces should be kept clean and dry; machines should be kept covered when not in use.

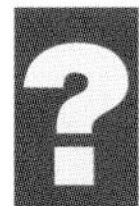

Checkpoint Question

8. *Which type of electrosurgery is used for incision or excision of tissue?*

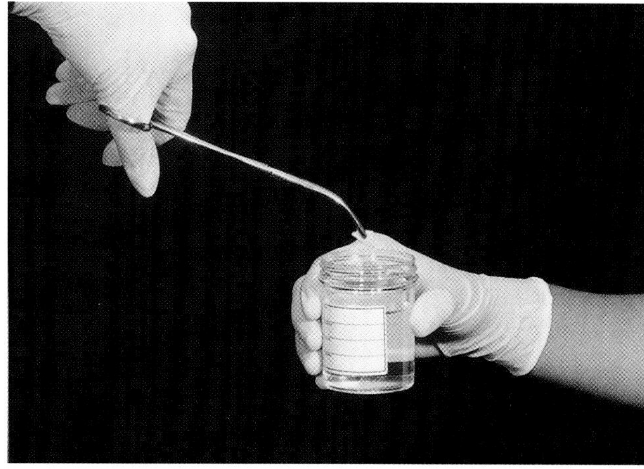

Figure 6-16 Tissue samples are placed in preservative by the physician.

LASER SURGERY

Lasers are devices that focus high-intensity light in a narrow beam to create extreme heat and energy. In medicine, lasers can be used to cut tissue and coagulate small bleeding vessels. There are many types of lasers, each with fairly specific applications in medicine. The more common types of lasers encountered in the medical office include:

- Argon laser—used for coagulation
- Carbon dioxide (CO_2) laser—used for cutting tissue
- Nd:YAG—used for coagulation and to separate warts and moles from surrounding tissues

Light from the laser usually is not visible. Colored filters are used to illuminate the laser's target, enabling the physician to direct the light to the affected area.

As with other electronic devices used in the medical offices, attention to care and handling of the laser will ensure that it is in good working order when it is needed. It is important to read and follow the manufacturer's recommended maintenance procedures described in the instruction manual that accompanies the equipment.

Everyone who is in the room while the procedure is in progress is required to wear goggles for eye protection. It is generally recommended that health care workers complete a training program before assisting with laser procedures to ensure that safety precautions are followed.

SPECIMEN COLLECTION DURING OFFICE SURGERY

Many minor office surgical procedures yield specimens that must be referred to a laboratory to be examined by a pathologist. Specimens include samples of tissue, wound exudate, foreign bodies, and so on.

The medical assistant usually chooses the proper container with the appropriate **preservative** (substance that delays decomposition) for the type of procedure being performed. The open container must be held steady to avoid touching the sides of the container as the physician drops the specimen into the preservative (Fig. 6-16).

The medical assistant is usually responsible for labeling the pathology request form with the correct patient and specimen data. Laboratory request forms usually require information such as patient name, age, sex, identification number or Social Security number, date, type of specimen to be examined, type of laboratory examination requested, where the specimen was obtained (ie, L cheek, R leg), and the physician's name or laboratory contract number. Specimens must be transported to the pathology laboratory as quickly as possible.

POSTSURGICAL PROCEDURES

In preparation for the next patient, discard all used equipment properly or transport it to the equipment room for sanitizing before sterilization. Clean the room as part of the procedure. Always put on gloves for environmental cleaning.

Follow "low-level disinfection" procedures as part of routine housekeeping between each patient use of the examining rooms to reduce the opportunity for cross-contamination between patients. (See Chap. 1, Asepsis and Infection Control, for more information about levels of infection control.) Inspect examining rooms prior to each use to ensure that the area has been properly cleaned after the previous patient.

6

Cleaning the Examination Table

Remove papers and sheets in a rolling movement so outside surfaces cover the interior of the bundle. Avoid having table covers and sheets come into contact with your clothing. Discard the sheets and covers appropriately. Wipe down the surfaces of the table with an approved disinfectant solution and allow to dry. Replace the covers and sheets for the next patient.

Cleaning the Operative Area

Wipe down the surgical stand, sink, counter, examining table, and other surfaces used during the procedure with an approved disinfectant solution and allow to dry before re-use. When environmental disinfection procedures are completed, examine the room with a critical eye to be sure that it is neat, clean, and ready for the next patient.

Answers to Checkpoint Questions

1. *To maintain a sterile field, you must keep sterile packages dry, face the sterile field, keep sterile items above waist level, keep items in the middle of the field, avoid spills, do not cough or sneeze near the field, never reach over the field, do not pass contaminated items over the field, and alert the physician if the field becomes contaminated.*
2. *Contents from a peel-back package can be added to a sterile field by sterile forceps, by a sterile gloved hand, and by flipping.*
3. *A fenestrated drape has an opening to expose the treatment site while covering adjacent areas.*
4. *Swaged (atraumatic) needles have the appropriate size suture material attached by the manufacturer. Threaded needles have an eye with a double thickness of suture that must be pulled through tissues.*
5. *To hand a right-handed physician a needle for suturing, place the needle in the needle holder, click the ratchets twice, and hand the needle holder with the suture material to the right and the needle to the left.*
6. *Sterile dressings are used to cover and protect a wound, absorb drainage, exert pressure, hide disfigurement, and hold medications against the skin.*
7. *Apply bandages beginning at the distal part and extending to the proximal part of the body. Bandage turns that extend distal to proximal aid in the return of venous blood to the heart and help make the bandage more secure.*
8. *Electrosection is the type of electrosurgery used for incision or excision of tissue.*

Critical Thinking Challenges

1. Dr. Brown has just informed Mrs. Levine that she should return tomorrow for office surgery. While you are alone with the patient, Mrs. Levine begins to cry and expresses great concern about the procedure. What should you do in this situation?
2. Review the anatomy of a hair follicle. Why are skin nicks more likely if the hair is shaved in the opposite direction as its natural growth?
3. Why would wounds in the head and face heal faster than those in the arms and legs?
4. Review the properties of epinephrine. Which of its actions would slow the absorption of medications in the tissues?
5. Why is it preferable for infected wounds to heal with delayed surface closure?

Suggestions for Further Reading

Kozier, B., & Erb, G. (1993). *Techniques in Clinical Nursing,* 4th ed. Redwood City, CA: Addison-Wesley.

Scherer, J. C., & Timby, B. K. (1995). *Introductory Medical-Surgical Nursing,* 6th ed. Philadelphia: J.B. Lippincott.

Smeltzer, S., & Bare, B. (1996). *Brunner and Suddarth's Textbook of Medical-Surgical Nursing,* 8th ed. Philadelphia: Lippincott-Raven.

Smith-Temple, J., & Johnson, J. Y. (1994). *Nurse's Guide to Clinical Procedures,* 2nd ed. Philadelphia: J.B. Lippincott.

Timby, B. K. (1996). *Fundamental Skills and Concepts in Patient Care,* 6th ed. Philadelphia: Lippincott-Raven.

7 Pharmacology

Chapter Outline

Role Delineation

GENERAL

Professionalism

- Adhere to ethical principles.

Communication Skills

- Treat all patients with compassion and empathy.

Legal Concepts

- Practice within the scope of education, training, and personal capabilities.
- Document accurately.
- Maintain and dispose of regulated substances in compliance with government guidelines.

Instruction

- Locate community resources and disseminate information.

Operational Functions

- Maintain supply inventory.
- Evaluate and recommend equipment and supplies.

Chapter Competencies

Learning Objectives

Upon successfully completing this chapter, you will be able to:

1. Spell and define the Key Terms.
2. Identify chemical, trade, and generic drug names.
3. Name the regulations that historically have affected the manufacture, sale, and prescribing of medications.
4. List and explain the branches of the government that regulate both standard and controlled drugs.
5. List and identify the categories of controlled substances and give an example of each.
6. Describe the sources of drugs and give examples.
7. Explain how drugs are categorized by action and effect.
8. List factors that affect drug action.

Chapter Competencies *(continued)*

9. Explain pharmacokinesis and describe the steps.
10. Describe how drugs may interact for an increased or decreased effect.
11. Explain and define terms related to drug effects.
12. List sources for information on pharmacology.

Key Terms

(See Glossary for definitions.)

antagonism
chemical name
drug
generic name
pharmacodynamics
pharmacokinesis
pharmacology
potentiation
synergism
trade name

Pharmacology is the term given the study of drugs: their actions, dosages, and side effects. A **drug** is a chemical substance that, when administered, affects body function(s). Pharmaceutical companies are required to list the chemical compound, actions, dosages, adverse effects, indications, and contraindications of the medications they manufacture so that those who work with these drugs and those for whom these drugs are prescribed are informed of all aspects of the drugs' properties. Medications are available in many forms and are administered in various ways to produce therapeutic effects. As a medical assistant, you are responsible for knowing about the drugs used by your physician.

MEDICATION NAMES

Most medications have a **chemical name** or an organic name, a **generic name**, and a **trade name** (Box 7-1). The chemical name, the first name given to any medication, identifies the chemical components of the drug. If the medication is primarily organic, such as digitalis, this name may be listed in addition to or in place of a chemical name. The generic name is assigned to the medication when it is manufactured during research and development. When the drug is available for commercial distribution by the original manufacturer, a brand name or trade name is given. The trade name is registered by the U.S. Patent Office and has the official mark of this office after its name. For 17 years, the manufacturer has the exclusive rights to produce the drug. After that time, other companies may combine the same chemicals and produce their own equivalent (generic) of the drug. Each company marketing the generic form of the trade name drug then assigns its own trade name to its generic equivalent. Trade names are always capitalized; generic names begin with lower case letters.

Drugs can be classified according to their actions and effects on the body. Table 7-1 provides examples of commonly prescribed drugs and their classifications.

Checkpoint Question

1. *What is the difference between a drug's chemical name and trade name?*

7

Box 7-1
Drug Names

Chemical name	7-chloro-1, 3-dihydro-1-methyl-5-phenyl-2H-1, 4-benzodiaxepin-2-one
Trade name	Valium
Generic name	diazepam

LEGAL REGULATIONS

Consumers in the United States are protected by federal regulations regarding drugs. The Pure Food and Drug Act was passed in 1906 and amended in 1938. The amended law, called the Federal Food, Drug, and Cosmetic Act, required that the safety of a drug must be proven before it is distributed to the public. An amendment, called the Durham-Humphrey Amendment, was passed in 1952. This addition banned many drugs from being dispensed without a prescription. The Kefauver-Harris Amendment of 1962 required testing of prescription and nonprescription medications for effectiveness before their release for sale.

Food and Drug Administration

The Food and Drug Administration (FDA) was established to review drug applications and petitions for food additives; to inspect facilities where drugs, cosmetics, and foods are made; and to remove unsafe drugs from the market. The FDA also ensures that the ingredients listed on food, drugs, and cosmetics are correct as labeled.

Drug Enforcement Agency

In 1970, the Controlled Substances Act was passed to regulate the manufacture and distribution of drugs whose use may result in dependency or abuse. This act also requires that anyone who manufactures, prescribes, administers, or dispenses such controlled substances must register annually with the United States Attorney General under the Bureau of Narcotics and Dangerous Drugs (BNDD).

The Drug Enforcement Agency (DEA) is a branch of the Justice Department designated to exercise strong regulatory control over all drugs listed by the BNDD. This authority extends to prescribing, refilling, and storing controlled substances in the medical office. The DEA is concerned with controlled substances only; medications not subject to abuse are not regulated by this agency. The DEA is also responsible for revising the list of drugs included in the Schedule of Controlled Substances (Table 7-2). Officials at regional DEA offices are available to answer any questions regarding the drugs under its control. As a medical assistant, you should make sure that the physician's office is on the DEA's periodic mailing list to keep abreast of changes.

Registration

When the physician registers with the U.S. Attorney General under the BNDD, a registration number (DEA number) is issued. Physicians are registered for a period of 3 years after application and acceptance. Near the end of the 3 years, the DEA will mail a renewal registration form to the physician. As a medical assistant, you may be responsible for maintaining professional records and licensure, including this form. If the form does not arrive before the physician's registration expires, you must notify the DEA. The DEA does not take responsibility if the physician's registration expires. Instructions for completing the initial registration or a renewal are printed on the form. If medications are administered and dispensed by the same physician at different offices, a separate form must be completed for each site. The registration retires with the physician; it does not stay with the medical office.

Inventory

Controlled substances in Schedule II are received from suppliers using a Federal Triplicate Order Form DEA 222. Schedules III through V do not require triplicate forms, but invoices for receipt of these substances must be maintained for 2 years.

As controlled substances are received, they are listed on a special inventory form in the office. Their receipt should be signed by two employees. Every time a controlled substance leaves the medical office inventory, it must be recorded; include the drug name, patient, dose, date, ordering physician, and the employee who handled the procedure. At regular intervals decided at the site, two employees should reconcile the inventory list with the medications on hand and sign that both are correct. These inventory forms must be kept for 2 years.

If controlled substances are administered and dispensed, records must be maintained separate from the patients' charts and must be readily available for inspection by the authorities of the DEA. If only an occasional controlled substance is administered and none are dispensed, the procedure must be recorded on the patient's chart and be available for DEA review. If controlled substances are prescribed and not administered

7

Table 7-1 **Classifications of Drugs**

Therapeutic Classification	*Effect or Action/Uses*	*Common Examples*
Adrenergic blocking agents/antiadrenergics	Affect the beta receptors of adrenergic nerves that control the vascular system; used to treat hypertension, cardiac arrhythmias, glaucoma	Metoprolol tartrate (Lopressor), propranolol hydrochloride (Inderal), timolol (Timoptic)
Adrenergics	Mimic the activity of the sympathetic nervous system; used to treat hypotensive episodes, bronchial asthma, cardiac arrest, heart block, ventricular arrhythmias, and allergic reactions	Epinephrine (Adrenaline), phenylephrine hydrochloride (Neo-Synephrine), ephedrine sulfate
Analgesics	Used to relieve pain; available in nonnarcotic and narcotic varieties (see also antipyretic and anti-inflammatory agents)	Aspirin, acetaminophen (Tylenol), codeine
Anesthetics	Various actions and effects according to type of anesthesia indicated. Local anesthesia provides a pain-free state in a specific area or region; general anesthesia is administered to the patient with the aim of loss of consciousness.	Procaine hydrochloride (Novocain), thiopental sodium (Pentothal), halothane (Fluothane)
Antacids	Neutralize or reduce the acidity of the stomach by combining with hydrochloric acid and producing salt and water	Magnesia (Milk of Magnesia), calcium carbonate (Tums)
Antihelminthics	Actions vary; prime purpose of antihelminthic drugs is to kill parasitic worms	Piperazine citrate, mebendazole (Vermox)
Antianginal agents	Promote vasodilation, which relieves the symptoms of angina	Nitroglycerin, diltiazem hydrochloride (Cardizem)
Antianxiety agents	Act on subcortical areas of the brain; exact mechanism of action not fully understood; used in the short-term treatment of symptoms of anxiety	Alprazolam (Xanax), chlordiazepoxide (Librium), diazepam (Valium), clorazepate dipotassium (Tranxene)
Antiarrhythmics	Various actions and effects; used to treat disturbances or irregularities of the heart rate, rhythm or both	Disopyramide (Norpace), procainamide hydrochloride (Pronestyl), esmolol (Brevibloc), bretylium tosylate (Bretylol), verapamil hydrochloride (Calan)
Antibiotics	Destroy, interrupt, or interfere with the growth of microorganisms; used to treat bacterial infections	Penicillin, ampicillin, cefaclor, tetracycline, sulfadiazine
Anticoagulants and thrombolytics	Anticoagulants used to prevent the formation of blood clots; thrombolytics used to dissolve blood clots	Heparin sodium, streptokinase (Streptase), coumadin (Warfarin)
Anticonvulsants	Reduce the excitability of the nerve cells of the brain; used to treat convulsive disorders, epilepsy	Phenobarbital, phenytoin (Dilantin), carbamazepine (Tegretol)
Antidepressants	Generally increase stimulation of the central nervous system; used in the management of various types of depression	Amitriptyline hydrochloride (Elavil), fluoxetine hydrochloride (Prozac), phenelzine (Nardil), sertraline (Zoloft)
Antidiarrheals	Decrease intestinal peristalsis	Loperamide hydrochloride (Imodium A-D)
Antiemetic agents	Used to treat or prevent nausea or vomiting; some are also useful as antivertigo agents (used to treat or prevent motion sickness)	Dimenhydrinate (Dramamine), promethazine hydrochloride (Phenergan)
Antifungals	Destroy, slow, or retard the growth of fungi; used to treat fungal infections	Ketoconazole (Nizoral), miconazole nitrate (Monistat 3 or 7), fluconazole (Diflucan)
Antihistamines	Used to counteract the effects of histamine on body organs and structures; used to treat allergies and allergic reactions. Some provide relief from nausea and vomiting; some have sedative effects.	Chlorpheniramine maleate (Chlor-Trimeton), diphenhydramine hydrochloride (Benadryl), loratadine (Claritin)
Antihypertensives	Lower blood pressure by increasing the size of arterial blood vessels; used in the treatment of high blood pressure	Diltiazem (Cardizem), prazosin (Minipress), propranolol hydrochloride (Inderal)
Anti-inflammatory agents	Reduce irritation and swelling of tissues	Aspirin, acetaminophen (Tylenol), ibuprofen (Advil), naproxen (Naprosyn)
Antineoplastic agents	Slow the rate of tumor growth and delay metastasis; used to treat malignant diseases (cancer)	Cyclophosphamide (Cytoxan), mitoxantrone hydrochloride (Novantrone)
Antiparkinsonism agents	Used to treat the symptoms associated with parkinsonism	Benztropine mesylate (Cogentin), levodopa (Larodopa)

(continued)

7

Table 7-1 **Classifications of Drugs** *(Continued)*

Therapeutic Classification	*Effect or Action/Uses*	*Common Examples*
Antipsychotics (neuroleptics)	Exact mechanism not understood; used to treat various acute and chronic psychoses	Chlorpromazine hydrochloride (Thorazine), haloperidol (Haldol)
Antipyretics	Decrease body temperature	Aspirin, acetaminophen (Tylenol)
Antitussives, mucolytics, and expectorants	Antitussives relieve coughing, mucolytics loosen respiratory secretions, and expectorants aid in removing thick mucus from the respiratory passages; medications may have one or more combinations of the three; used to relieve the discomfort of upper respiratory infections	Codeine sulfate, diphenhydramine hydrochloride (Benylin Cough), guaifenesin (Entex)
Antivirals	Appear to inhibit viral replication; only effective against a small number of specific viral infections	Acyclovir (Zovirax), zidovudine (AZT)
Bronchodilators	Dilate the bronchi and allow more air to enter the lungs; used in the treatment of acute and chronic asthma, chronic bronchitis, and emphysema	Albuterol sulfate (Ventolin), metaproterenol sulfate (Alupent), theophylline
Cardiotonics	Increase the force of contraction of the myocardium of the heart; used in the treatment of congestive heart failure, atrial fibrillation, atrial flutter, and paroxysmal atrial tachycardia	Digoxin (Lanoxin), milrinone lactate (Primacor)
Cholinergic blocking agents/anticholinergics	Affect the autonomic nervous system; used to treat peptic ulcers, ureteral and biliary colic, and preoperatively to reduce secretions of the upper respiratory tract	Atropine sulfate, scopolamine hydrobromide, propantheline bromide (Pro-Banthine)
Cholinergics	Mimic the activity of the parasympathetic nervous system; used to treat glaucoma and myasthenia gravis	Neostigmine (Prostigmin), pilocarpine hydrochloride
Decongestants	Reduce swelling of the nasal passages to enhance drainage of the sinuses; used to treat nasal congestion	Oxymetazoline hydrochloride (Dristan), pseudoephedrine hydrochloride (Sudafed)
Diuretics	Increase the excretion of urine by the kidneys; used to release excess fluid in body tissues	Furosemide (Lasix), hydrochlorothiazide (Diuril)
Emetics	Promote vomiting by acting on the chemoreceptor trigger zone of the medulla	Ipecac syrup
Histamine H_2 antagonists	Inhibit the action of histamine at the histamine H_2 receptor cells of the stomach, thereby reducing the secretion of gastric acid	Cimetidine (Tagamet), ranitidine (Zantac), famotidine (Pepcid)
Hormones (female)	Used to prevent symptoms of menopause, female castration, ovarian failure, and amenorrhea; combinations of estradiol, norethindrone, and other hormones used for contraception	Estradiol (Estraderm), medroxyprogesterone acetate (Provera)
Hormones (male)	Androgen therapy treats testosterone deficiency. Anabolic steroids are chemically related to androgens and promote the tissue-building process.	Fluoxymesterone (Halotestin), nandrolone decanoate (Deca-Durabolin)
Immunologic agents (vaccines)	Stimulate the immune response to create protection against a specific disease or to supply ready-made antibodies that provide passive immunity	Pneumococcal vaccine, influenza virus vaccine, diphtheria and tetanus toxoids
Insulin and oral hypoglycemics	Injectable insulin is used to control type I diabetes mellitus; type II diabetes mellitus controlled with oral hypoglycemics	Intermediate-acting insulin (NPH Insulin), long-acting insulin (Ultralente U), mixed insulin (Novolin 70/30), glipizide (Glucotrol), metaformin (Glucophage)
Sedatives and hypnotics	Sedatives relax and calm, hypnotics induce sleep; available in barbiturate and nonbarbiturate varieties	Butabarbital; sodium, phenobarbital, chloral hydrate, temazepam (Restoril)
Stimulants	Increase the activity of the central nervous system; used to increase respiration and to treat narcolepsy, attention deficit disorder, and exogenous obesity	Methylphenidate hydrochloride (Ritalin), amphetamine sulfate, methamphetamine hydrochloride (Desoxyn)
Thyroid and antithyroid agents	Used to increase or decrease the amount of thyroid hormones manufactured and secreted into the body; used to treat hypothyroidism or hyperthyroidism	Levothyroxine sodium (T_4), levothyroxine sodium (Synthroid), propylthiouracil (PTU)

Adapted from Scherer, J. C., & Roach, S. S. (1996). *Introductory Clinical Pharmacology,* 5th ed. Philadelphia: Lippincott-Raven.

Table 7-2 **Controlled Substances**

Schedule	*Description*	*Examples*
I	These drugs have the highest potential for abuse and have no currently accepted medical use in the United States. There are no accepted safety standards for use of these drugs or substances even under medical supervision, although some are used experimentally in carefully controlled research projects.	Opium, marijuana, lysergic acid diethylamide (LSD), peyote, mescaline
II	These drugs have a high potential for abuse. They have a current accepted medicinal use in the United States, but with severe restrictions. Abuse of these drugs can lead to dependence, either psychological or physiologic. Schedule II drugs require a written prescription and cannot be refilled or called into the pharmacy by the medical office. Only in extreme emergencies may the physician call in the prescription. A handwritten prescription must be presented to the pharmacist within 72 h.	Morphine, codeine, secobarbital (Seconal), cocaine, amphetamines, hydromorphone (Dilaudid), methylphenidate (Ritalin)
III	These drugs have a limited potential for psychological or physiologic dependence. The prescription may be called in to the pharmacist by the physician and refilled up to five times in a 6-month period.	Paregoric, Tylenol with Codeine, Fiorinal
IV	These drugs have a lower potential for abuse than those in Schedules II and III. They can be called into the pharmacist by a medical office employee and may be filled up to five times in a 6-month period.	Chlordiazepoxide (Librium), diazepam (Valium), propoxyphene (Darvon), phenobarbital
V	These drugs have a lower potential for abuse than those in Schedules I, II, III, and IV.	Diphenoxylate (Lomotil), brompheniramine (Dimetane Expectorant DC), guaifenesin (Robitussin-DAC)

*Five schedules, or categories, of controlled substances were established by the Bureau of Narcotics and Dangerous Drugs. Medications in the five schedules may be revised periodically after review.

or dispensed, some states require only that the information be recorded on the patient's chart; others require that a separate file be kept of prescription copies of controlled substances.

The DEA number should not be preprinted on the prescription. Cautious physicians write it in rather than risk patients having easy access to it.

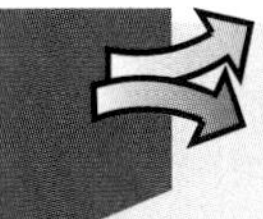

Ethical Tips

Controlled Substances

If you suspect that a physician or health care professional is illegally diverting controlled substances, you have an ethical and, in some states, a legal responsibility to report this suspicion. Gather and document evidence and reasons to suspect diversion of substances. You should have a clear and compelling case to present to the proper authorities. If a physician is involved, report this evidence to the Drug Enforcement Agency (DEA) and the American Medical Association (AMA). The state medical society should also be notified. If the suspected health care worker is not a physician, report it to the appropriate supervisor or superior. Most states have programs to assist the health care professional in obtaining appropriate help. In most instances, you may remain anonymous.

Most physicians avoid keeping controlled substances in their offices because of the risk of theft. Controlled substances kept in the medical office must be locked in a safe or in a secure, locked box bolted to a shelf in a locked cabinet. The number of people with access to the keys or to the cabinet should be limited. Many offices keep the DEA prescription pad, the state triplicate forms, and the inventory forms in the cabinet also.

If drugs are lost or stolen, the local law enforcement agency must be notified immediately. If drugs are expired and must be destroyed, two employees must witness the destruction of the medication and sign and date the form for destroyed substances. An option for the disposal of controlled substances requires that the regional DEA office send a representative to your office to retrieve and dispose of the drugs.

Checkpoint Question

2. *What information needs to be documented when a controlled substance is administered?*

PRESCRIPTIONS

Medications may be administered (given in the office), dispensed (a supply given for later use), or prescribed (a written order to be filled by a pharmacist). An established protocol and traditional form must be followed when filling out the prescription:

Date. Prescriptions must be filled within 6 months of the date listed.

Patient's name and address

Superscription. The emblem Rx means "take."

Inscription. Includes the name of the medicine, the desired form (eg, liquid, tablet), and the strength (eg, 250 mg, 500 mg).

Subscription. Notes amount to dispense (eg, 60 tabs, 120 mL).

Signature. Notes instructions for taking (eg, with meals, tid, qid).

Refills. Notes number of times prescription can be refilled, generally no more than five times within 6 months, but this will vary.

Physician's signature. Physicians are responsible for prescriptions written in their offices and should check and sign any that will be given to patients. The medical assistant may prepare the prescription for the physician, but it is in the best interest of all concerned for the physician to sign it.

Generic. Some physicians will allow generic substitutes for certain medications but not for others.

All medications prescribed in the medical office must be documented in full on the patient's chart. Prescriptions that are called or faxed to the pharmacist must also be documented. The chart is a legal document and may be called into court in the event of legal action. If the medication order is not recorded, it will be presumed that the medication was never ordered. Figure 7-1 shows a sample prescription form.

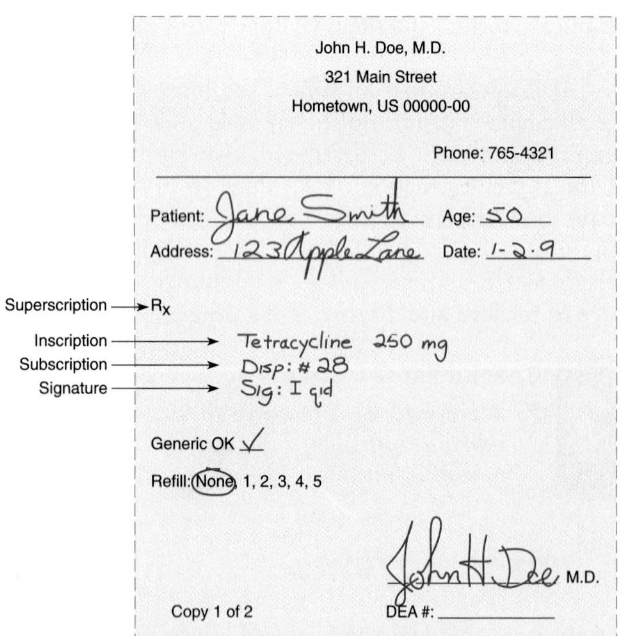
John H. Doe, M.D.
321 Main Street
Hometown, US 00000-00

Phone: 765-4321

Patient: Jane Smith Age: 50
Address: 123 Apple Lane Date: 1-2-9

Superscription → Rx
Inscription → Tetracycline 250 mg
Subscription → Disp: # 28
Signature → Sig: I qid

Generic OK ✓

Refill: (None) 1, 2, 3, 4, 5

John H. Doe M.D.

Copy 1 of 2 DEA #:

Figure 7-1 Sample prescription form.

Checkpoint Question

3. *What does the inscription on the prescription indicate, and how does this differ from the subscription?*

SOURCES OF DRUGS

Drugs are available from numerous natural sources, such as plants, minerals, and animals. They may also be synthetic (prepared in the laboratory by artificial means). Table 7-3 lists a number of commonly prescribed drugs and their sources.

PHARMACODYNAMICS

Drugs are commonly categorized by their action and effect on body function. **Pharmacodynamics** is the term used to describe the study of how drugs act within the body. All drugs cause cellular change (drug action) and a degree of physiologic change (drug effect).

An action of a drug administered for a local effect is limited to the area where it is administered. Drugs that exert local effects may be ointments, such as zinc oxide. A drug administered for a systemic effect is absorbed into the blood and then carried to the organ or tissue on which it will act. A systemic effect can be produced by administering drugs orally, sublingually, rectally, parenterally, transdermally, or by inhalation. (See Chap. 8, Preparing and Administering Medications, for more information.)

In addition, certain topical drugs will produce a systemic effect; these include drugs applied to the mucous membranes in the vagina, rectum, eyes, or nose. Because mucous membranes are bathed in watery solutions and are very vascular, they are more receptive to drugs than skin.

A number of factors can influence a drug's action in the body. These are described in Box 7-2.

PHARMACOKINETICS

Drugs undergo numerous changes within the body from the time of transport from the site of administration until they are inactivated and excreted. **Pharmacokinesis** is the term given the study of the action

7

Table 7-3 **Common Drugs and Their Sources**

Source	Drug	Use
Plants		
Cinchona bark	Quinidine	Antiarrhythmic
Purple foxglove	Digitalis	Cardiotonic
Opium poppy	Paregoric	Antidiarrheal
	Morphine	Analgesic
	Codeine	Antitussive, analgesic
Minerals		
Magnesium	Milk of magnesia	Antacid, laxative
Silver	Silver nitrate	Placed in eyes of newborns to kill *Neisseria gonorrhoeae* Chemical cautery of lesions
Gold	Solganal	Arthritis treatment
Animal Proteins		
Porcine or bovine pancreas	Insulin	Antidiabetic hormone
Porcine or bovine stomach acids	Pepsin	Digestive hormone
Animal thyroid glands	Thyroid, USP	Hypothyroidism
Synthetics		
	Demerol	Analgesic
	Lomotil	Antidiarrheal
	Gantrisin	Sulfonamide
Semisynthetic		
Escherichia coli bacteria and altered DNA molecules	Humulin	Antidiabetic hormone

Box 7-2
Factors Influencing Drug Action

Age Elderly people have slower metabolic processes. Age-related kidney and liver dysfunctions also extend the breakdown and excretion times in these patients, so it is necessary to monitor the cumulative effects of drugs in the elderly. Children may have a more immediate response to drugs and therefore must be assessed frequently.

Weight Many drug dosages are calculated and administered according to the patient's weight. As a general rule, the larger the patient, the greater the dose; however, individual sensitivity to the effects of drugs will be taken into consideration.

Sex Women may react differently to certain drugs than men because of the ratio of fat/body mass or fluctuating hormone levels.

Existing Pathology If the body is compromised by a disease process, absorption, distribution, metabolism, and excretion may be altered.

Tolerance Some medications given over a long period may cause the body to become resistant to their effects, requiring larger doses to achieve the desired response.

Other Medications Certain medications will increase and others will decrease the effects of interacting medications. Older patients on multiple medications with contributory disease processes and delayed metabolism are at significant risk for altered drug action.

Note: Medical assistants should *always* administer medications under the direct order of the physician. Under *no* circumstances should a medical assistant adjust a dosage unless specifically instructed to do so by the physician.

of drugs within the body, from administration to excretion. Pharmacokinetic processes are described below.

Absorption

Absorption gets the drug into the bloodstream. Absorption usually occurs in the mucosa of the stomach, small intestine, mouth, rectum, the dermal layers of the skin, the subcutaneous tissue, or blood vessels in the muscles. If a drug is not administered correctly, it might be destroyed before it reaches its site of action. An example would be administering with a meal a medication that should only be given on an empty stomach.

Distribution

Distribution moves the drug from the bloodstream into the tissues and fluids of the body.

Metabolism

Metabolism is the physical and chemical alterations that the drug undergoes within the body. During the process of metabolism, the liver breaks down the drug and alters it to more water-soluble by-products so it can be excreted by the kidneys. In the presence of hepatic disease, the liver may not be able to break down the drug properly for excretion by the kidneys. In this case, the patient may experience toxic effects caused by an accumulation of the drug in the liver or bloodstream. In some instances, drugs may bypass the metabolic processes. Some drugs reach the kidneys relatively unchanged; these drugs can be detected in the urine.

Excretion

Excretion eliminates the waste products of drug metabolism from the body. Most drugs are excreted by the kidneys. Unless the drug is excreted before a repeat dose is given, a cumulative effect can occur, possibly resulting in toxic levels of medications in the body.

Digoxin, a cardiotonic, has the potential for causing a toxic cumulative effect. If digoxin accumulates, the patient's heart rate may slow to a dangerously low level. For this reason, patients taking digoxin must be monitored. Digoxin levels in the blood are checked periodically to avoid toxicity. In some instances, the accumulation of the drug in the body may be the desired effect, to build a therapeutic blood level not possible without the cumulative effect.

If the kidneys are compromised by disease, medication may not be properly eliminated, adding to the danger of a cumulative effect and possible toxicity.

What If?

Mrs. Jones calls your office and asks that her prescription for digoxin be refilled. As you are talking with her, you pull her chart to record the call. What if, while reviewing her chart, you notice that she has not had digoxin levels determined as scheduled? How would you handle this situation?

Because digoxin may cause a toxic cumulative effect, it is important that patients taking this drug have their digoxin levels monitored regularly. Explain to Mrs. Jones that you will check with the physician regarding her request and that you will call her back. You should note your conversation in Mrs. Jones' chart, then place the chart on the physician's desk or discuss it personally at a convenient time. When the physician has made a decision, call Mrs. Jones with instructions for the drug's renewal and her course of action.

Checkpoint Question

4. *What are the four pharmacokinetic processes? Explain each.*

DRUG INTERACTIONS

When two or more drugs are taken simultaneously, one drug may increase, decrease, or cancel the effects of the other. The following discussion explains common drug interactions and the terms used to describe these interactions. Table 7-4 lists other important drug-related terms you should know.

Synergism refers to two drugs working together. One drug helps the action of the other for an effect that neither produces alone. For example, small doses of promethazine (Phenergan), a nonnarcotic sedative, and meperidine (Demerol), a synthetic narcotic analgesic, are more effective for pain relief than the same dose or an increased dose of Demerol alone.

Potentiation describes the effect in which one drug prolongs or multiplies the effect of another drug. For example, probenecid (Benemid), an antigout medication is given with penicillin (an antibiotic) to delay its excretion and to build up a high level of penicillin in the blood.

Table 7-4 **Drug-Related Terms to Know**

Term	*Meaning*
Therapeutic classification	States the purpose for the drug's use (eg, cardiotonic, anti-infective, antiarrthymic).
Teratogenic category	Relates the level of risk to fetal or maternal health. These rank from Category A through D, with increasing danger at each level. Category X indicates that the particular drug should never be given during pregnancy.
Indications	Gives disorders for which the particular drug would be prescribed.
Contraindications	Indicates conditions or instances for which the particular drug should not be used.
Adverse reactions	Refers to undesirable side effects of the particular drug.
Hypersensitivity	Refers to an excessive reaction to a particular drug; also known as a drug allergy. The body must build this response; the first exposures may or may not indicate that a problem is developing.
Idiosyncratic reaction	Refers to an abnormal or unexpected reaction to a drug peculiar to the individual patient; not technically an allergy.

Antagonism refers to an effect in which one drug decreases the effect of another. For example, naloxone (Narcan), a narcotic antagonist, is used to treat some narcotic overdosages.

All of these examples of drug interactions are considered to be desirable interactions. However, on some occasions drug interactions produce undesirable effects. For example, sedatives and barbiturates given together can cause central nervous system depression (synergism). Cimetidine (Tagamet), a gastric antisecretory drug, given with the antidepressant imipramine (Tofranil) will increase the levels of Tofranil in the blood (potentiation). Antacids taken with the antibiotic tetracycline prevent the absorption of tetracycline (antagonism).

Checkpoint Question

5. *How does synergism differ from antagonism?*

MEDICATION ALLERGIES

When gathering a patient's medical history (see Chap. 2, Medical History and Patient Interview), you must always ask about allergies of any sort, particularly allergies to medications. Existing drug allergies must be noted prominently on the front of the patient's chart. Stickers are available with spaces to write the name(s) of the medication(s). These may also be posted on each page of the patient's order sheets.

If the patient is receiving allergy medications, or any medication that has a high incidence of allergic reactions (eg, penicillin), the patient must wait for 20 to 30 minutes and be rechecked before leaving the office. Leave the medication and the chart in the medication station until the patient has been checked and cleared to leave. The reaction, positive or negative, must be fully documented on the chart, including the lot number of the medication from the container. If a positive reaction is noted, it should be checked by the physician before the patient is allowed to leave the office.

Allergic reactions commonly noted include:

- Redness and swelling at the injection site
- Itching, either at the site or generalized
- Dyspnea
- Nausea
- Dizziness

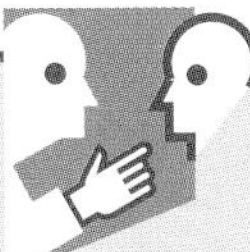

Advice and Tips

Understanding Drug Dependence

Drug dependence, sometimes referred to as addiction, can be either physical or psychological. After the medication is stopped, a patient who is physically dependent will experience mild to severe physiologic symptoms that gradually decrease in intensity.

Patients who are psychologically dependent have acquired a need for the feeling brought on by the drug. After the drug is stopped, there will be no physiologic withdrawal; however, patients may experience depression for a time.

To help control these symptoms, physicians will sometimes substitute a placebo for the drug. Placebos are inactive substances that resemble the actual medication but contain no drugs. Sugar tablets or saline solution (for injections) are commonly used as placebos.

SOURCES OF INFORMATION IN PHARMACOLOGY

The *Physician's Desk Reference* (PDR) is widely used as a reference for drugs in current use. The book is written to be used by physicians, but it is readily available in offices, libraries, and bookstores. It is clearly written to identify the drug's chemical name, brand

7

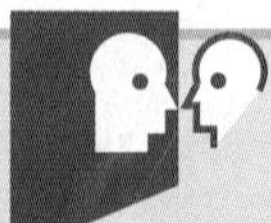

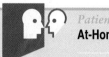

Patient Education

At-Home Medication Administration

Patients are responsible for their own care once they have left your office. To continue the treatment begun by the physician, patients need to understand the importance of proper medication administration.

Help them in this manner:

- Remind patients to bring a list of all medications to each visit. This includes over-the-counter (OTC) preparations, such as vitamins and minerals, cold relief preparations, laxatives, and indigestion aids. Any of these preparations may interfere with the therapeutic effect of prescribed medications. Some patients may choose to bring all of their medications with them to each visit for evaluation.
- Alert patients to the need to report any symptoms or suspected side effects they experience and let the physician decide if it is medication related.
- Make patients feel welcome to ask questions about their medications. Patients who are made aware of the purpose and action of the medication will be more likely to follow health care directives.
- Caution patients to check all prescriptions as they are filled. If the medication does not look like it has before, urge patients to question the pharmacist or contact the physician's office. Errors do happen.
- Help patients set up individualized dosage schedules. Many memory aids are available for sorting a day's or week's worth of medications in compartmentalized boxes to remind patients to take each of their medications on time.
- Caution patients about taking medications at night. Educate patients to turn on lights, and read medication labels, wear glasses, if needed, and drink a full glass of water. Remind patients to sit with both of their feet on the floor to avoid choking.
- Unless otherwise indicated, tell patients to take all medications from each prescription.
- Encourage questions!

name, and generic name. It also lists the properties, indications, contraindications, dosages, and so on.

The *United States Pharmacopeia Dispensing Information* (USPDI) consists of two paperback volumes providing drug information for the health care provider. It defines drugs in respect to sources, chemistry, physical properties, tests for identity, method of assay, storage, and dosage. It also provides directions for compounding and general use. The USPDI, however, does not contain photographs of the medications, and, unlike the PDR, which is sometimes distributed to physicians at no charge, must be purchased.

The *American Hospital Formulary Service* (AHFS) is distributed to practicing physicians and contains concise information arranged according to drug classifications.

Compendium of Drug Therapy is published annually and is distributed to practicing physicians. It includes photographs of the drugs and phone numbers of major pharmaceutical companies and poison control centers. It also includes copies of some package inserts.

Answers to Checkpoint Questions

1. *A drug's chemical name identifies the chemical components of the drug; the trade name is the name under which the manufacturer distributes the drug commercially.*
2. *When a controlled substance is administered, you must document the drug name, patient, dose, date, ordering physician, and the employee who performed the procedure.*
3. *The inscription indicates the medication name, desired form, and strength. The subscription indicates the amount of medication to dispense.*
4. *The four pharmacokinetic processes are absorption, distribution, metabolism, and excretion. Absorption is the process by which the drug gets into the bloodstream. Distribution moves the drug from the bloodstream into body tissues and fluids. During metabolism, the drug undergoes chemical and physical changes within the body. The waste products of drug metabolism are eliminated during excretion.*
5. *Synergism refers to a drug interaction in which one drug helps another drug's action. Antagonism is a drug interaction in which one drug decreases another drug's effects.*

Critical Thinking Challenges

1. How would you educate patients regarding prescribed medications? What type of information do they need to know? Is there anything that they do not need to know?
2. Using PDR, look up a medication that you have taken. (Your school's library will have a PDR.) What is the medication's chemical name? Explain what you learned about this medication that you did not already know. Is it a good idea for PDRs to be sold in bookstores for patients to buy? Justify your response.

Suggestions for Further Reading

Craven, R. F., & Hirnle, C. J. (1996). *Fundamentals of Nursing: Health and Human Function,* 2nd ed. Philadelphia: Lippincott-Raven.

Dawe, R. (1993). *Math and Dosage Calculations for Health Occupations.* New York: Glencoe.

Kozier, B., & Erb, G. (1993). *Techniques of Clinical Nursing,* 4th ed. Redwood City, CA: Addison-Wesley.

Lane, K. (1992). *Medications: A Guide for the Health Professions.* Philadelphia: F.A. Davis.

Scherer, J. C., & Roach, S. S. (1995). *Introductory Clinical Pharmacology,* 5th ed. Philadelphia: J.B. Lippincott.

Smeltzer, S. C., & Bare, B. G. (1996). *Brunner and Suddarth's Textbook of Medical-Surgical Nursing,* 8th ed. Philadelphia: Lippincott-Raven.

Taylor, C., Lillis, C., & LeMone, P. (1997). *Fundamentals of Nursing: The Art and Science of Nursing Care,* 3rd ed. Philadelphia: J.B. Lippincott.

Timby, B. (1996). *Fundamental Skills and Concepts in Patient Care,* 6th ed. Philadelphia: Lippincott-Raven.

8

Preparing and Administering Medications

Chapter Outline

Role Delineation

CLINICAL

Fundamental Principles

- Apply principles of aseptic technique and infection control.

Patient Care

- Prepare patients for examinations, procedures, and treatments.
- Prepare and administer medications and immunizations.
- Maintain medication and immunization records.

GENERAL

Communication Skills

- Treat all patients with compassion and empathy.

Legal Concepts

- Practice within the scope of education, training, and personal capabilities.
- Document accurately.

Instruction

- Instruct individuals according to their needs.

Chapter Competencies

Learning Objectives

Upon successfully completing this chapter, you will be able to:

1. Spell and define the Key Terms.
2. List safety guidelines for medication administration.

Chapter Competencies *(continued)*

3. List and explain the "seven rights" of medication administration.
4. Explain the procedure for a charting error or a medication error.
5. Explain the differences between the oral and parenteral routes of medication administration and note why one method may be preferable to another in a specific situation.
6. Give examples of solid and liquid oral forms of medication.
7. List the parts of a syringe and name those parts that are to be kept sterile.
8. List the types of injections and their angles.
9. Describe the needle lengths, gauges, and preferred site for each type of injection.
10. Describe how to calculate dosages using the metric and apothecary systems of measurement and how to convert measurements within and between systems.
11. Describe the various methods for calculating pediatric dosages.

Performance Objectives

Upon successfully completing this chapter, you will be able to:

1. Administer oral medications (Procedure 8-1).
2. Administer sublingual or buccal medications (Procedure 8-2).
3. Administer rectal medications.
4. Administer vaginal medications.
5. Apply transdermal medications (Procedure 8-3).
6. Apply topical medications (Procedure 8-4).
7. Prepare an injection (Procedure 8-5).
8. Administer an intradermal injection (Procedure 8-6).
9. Administer and read a tine or Mantoux test (Procedure 8-7).
10. Administer a subcutaneous injection (Procedure 8-8).
11. Administer an intramuscular injection (Procedure 8-9).
12. Administer an intramuscular injection using the Z-track method (Procedure 8-10).

Key Terms

(See Glossary for definitions.)

ampules
diluent
gauge
Mantoux
meniscus
nebulizer
vials

As a medical assistant, you may be responsible for administering medications under the supervision of the physician. It is important that you acquire a knowledge of medications, their uses and abuses, range of dosages, methods of administration, symptoms of overdosage, adverse effects, and untoward effects that may occur. Because medication administration is an exact science and can be harmful to the patient when errors are made, you must perform this procedure with strict attention to safety.

COMMON ABBREVIATIONS

You must be thoroughly familiar with the terminology, abbreviations, symbols, and signs used in prescribing and administering medications and in documenting such procedures. The abbreviations listed in Table 8-1 are among those most commonly used and should be memorized.

Table 8-1 **Abbreviations**

Abbreviation	*Meaning*	*Abbreviation*	*Meaning*	*Abbreviation*	*Meaning*
aa	of each	IV	intravenous	qh	every hour
ac	before meals	kg	kilogram	q2h	every 2 hours
ad lib	as desired	L, l	liter	q3h	every 3 hours
AM, am	morning	lb	pound	qid	four times a day
amp	ampule	m, min	minim	qod	every other day
amt	amount	mcg, μg	microgram	qs	quantity sufficient
aq	aqueous	mEq	milliequivalent	qt	quart
bid	twice a day	ml, mL	milliliter	R	right, rectal
/c	with	n	normal	Rx	take, prescribe
cap	capsule	NaCl	sodium chloride	/s	without
cc	cubic centimeter	NKA	no known allergies	SC, subcu, subq, S/Q	subcutaneously
DC, disc, d/c	discontinue	noc	night	sig	label
disp	dispense	NPO	nothing by mouth	SL	sublingual
dl, dL	deciliter	NS	normal saline	sol	solution
dr	dram	OD	right eye	SOS	once if necessary
DW	distilled water	OS	left eye	sp	spirits
elix	elixir	OU	both eyes	ss	one-half
et	and	os	mouth	stat, STAT	immediately
ext	extract	oz	ounce	supp	suppository
fl, fld	fluid	p	after	syr	syrup
g, GM	gram	pc	after meals	tab	tablet
gr	grain	PM, pm	afternoon or evening	T, tbsp	tablespoon
gt(t)	drop(s)	po, PO	by mouth	t, tsp	teaspoon
h, hr	hour	prn, PRN	whenever necessary	tid	three times a day
hs, HS	hours of sleep	pt	pint	tinc	tincture
Id	intradermal	q	every	ung	ointment
IM	intramuscular	qd	every day		

SAFETY GUIDELINES

To ensure safety when administering medications, follow these guidelines:

1. Know the policies of your office regarding the administration of medications.
2. Give only the medication(s) that the physician has ordered in writing. Do not accept verbal orders.
3. Check with the physician if you have any doubt about a medication or an order.
4. Avoid conversations or other distractions while drawing up and administering medication. It is important to remain attentive during this task.
5. Work in a quiet, well lighted area.
6. Check the label when taking the medication from the shelf, pouring it, and replacing it on the shelf. This is known as the "three checks" for safe medication administration (Box 8-1).
7. Place the order and the medication side by side to compare for accuracy.
8. Check strengths of the medication (eg, 250 mg versus 500 mg) and the routes (eg, ophthalmic, otic, topical).
9. Read labels carefully. Do not scan labels or orders.
10. Check the patient's chart for allergies to components of the medication.
11. Check the medication's expiration date.
12. Be alert for color changes, precipitation, odor, or any indication that the medication's properties have changed.
13. Measure exactly; there should be no bubbles.
14. Have sharps containers as close to the area of use as possible.
15. Put on gloves for all procedures that might result in contact with blood or body fluids.
16. Stay with the patient while oral medication is being taken. Watch for any reaction, and record the patient's response.
17. Never return a medication to the container.
18. Never recap, bend, or break a used needle.
19. Never give a medication poured or drawn up by someone else.
20. Never leave the medication cabinet unlocked when not in use.
21. Never give the keys for the medication cabinet to an unauthorized person. Limit access to the medication cabinet by limiting access to the cabinet keys.

Box 8-1
Reading Medication Labels

Many medications are supplied in unit dose packs, one single dose per single package. These are the most commonly prescribed dosages and usually do not require calculation once you have identified the proper drug, route, and dosage. Other medications are supplied in stock bottles with multiple doses to be dispensed as ordered.

If the drug preparation is a trade preparation, the medication label lists both a trade name (eg, Lanoxin) and a generic name (eg, digoxin). If the drug form is generic, usually only one name is listed. This is common among older drugs. Remember that trade names are capitalized and generic names are in lower case letters. Be sure to check the label against the physician's order before administering any medication.

The medication dosage strength and the unit of measure (eg, 300 mg) can be found beneath the drug name (or names) on the label. Some older medications may list both metric and apothecary measures. For instance, aspirin may list 300 to 325 mg (gr v); phenobarbital may list 15 mg (gr 1/4).

If the medication is a trade combination with two or more generic or trade preparations, these also are listed on the label. For instance, Percocet is a combination of the generic drugs oxycodone and acetaminophen, both of which are listed in smaller letters under the trade name Percocet. Combinations usually contain varying doses of their components and are ordered as numbers of tablets or capsules, not as units of measure. For instance, the order may state, "Give tabs ii," rather than a number of milligrams.

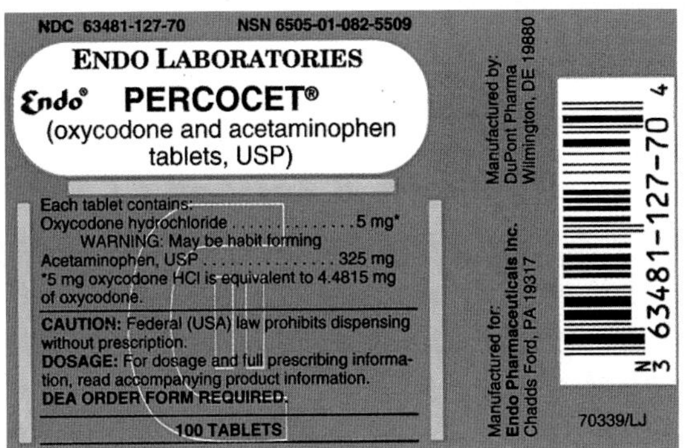

Courtesy Endo Pharmaceuticals, Chadds Ford, PA. Used with permission.

If the combination is available in varying strengths, these also are listed on the label (eg, Sinemet CR [a combination of carbidopa and levodopa] 25–100, 50–200), reflecting increasing doses of the drug components.

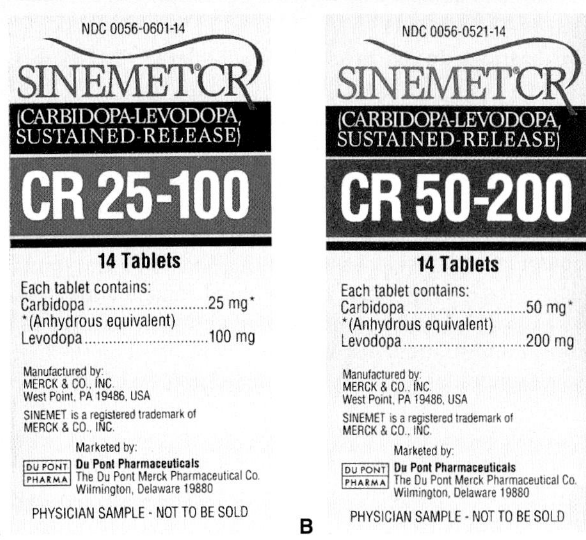

Courtesy DuPont Pharmaceuticals Company, Wilmington, DE. Used with permission.

The medication label also lists the administration route (if other than oral), the expiration date, the manufacturer's name, and a control or lot number. The control or lot number is used to trace or identify medications in case of recalls or other concerns. If the drug container holds more than one dose, the quantity also is included (eg, 100 tablets, 50 capsules).

Depending on space, some labels contain warnings and/or precautions (eg, Federal law prohibits dispensing without a license.), storage requirements (eg, Store at room temperature.), handling (eg, Shake well before using.), or the usual dose.

Oral Solution Labels

For liquid oral preparations, the weight or the amount of medication is dissolved and contained in a certain volume of carrier or solution. For instance, one tablet of medication may contain 500 mg, but its liquid counterpart may be dissolved as 500 mg per 10 mL (500 mg/10 mL). The label shows the name of the trade and/or generic medication and those items included on the solid preparation label—manufacturer, expiration date, lot number, and the total contents (eg, 30 mL, 100 mL). The dose strength is listed as dosage per volume (eg, 200 mg per 5 mL, 50 mg per 10 mL, written 200 mg/5 mL, 50 mg/10 mL). These dosages are dispensed into calibrated medicine cups or oral syringes, commercial medicine spoons may be used in the home. Oral liquid preparations also may be given as drops with an attached and appropriately calibrated dropper. Because drop size varies, droppers not designed for a specific medication may dispense an improper quantity.

continued

Box 8-1
Reading Medication Labels *(Continued)*

Parenteral Labels

Medications to be given intramuscularly (IM), subcutaneously (SC), intradermally (ID), and intravenously (IV; not usually drawn by the medical assistant and never given by a medical assistant) usually are supplied in much smaller containers than oral preparations, making the information displayed on the label appear crowded and requiring very fine print in some cases. The label information is the same—trade and/or generic name, manufacturer, lot number, expiration date, total volume—plus the preferred route for the medication (eg, IM, ID). If the medication must be reconstituted before administration, instructions may be listed on the label if space allows, or they may be included in the package insert.

Solution Reconstitution

Chemicals in dry form usually last longer than those in liquid form. If the medication must be reconstituted before administration, the label may give the information regarding the amount and type of liquid (eg, 5 mL sterile saline), the length of time the preparation will last after mixing, and the storage directions. For example, the label may state: Add 9.5 mL of sterile water for injection for 10 mL per vial. The total vial may contain 1 g (1000 mg) of medication; now each milliliter contains 100 mg of medication. The volume of the drug in the vial before reconstitution accounts for the additional 0.5 mL.

The vial may be reconstituted to varying degrees of dosage strength by altering the amount of diluent (the liquid added to the vial). For instance, it may be recommended that the vial above may also be mixed with 4.5 mL of sterile water for a total volume of 5 mL. Now each milliliter contains 200 mg of the medication. The assistant mixing the medication must write on the label the medication strength after reconstitution, the solution used as a diluent, the time and date it was mixed, and his or her initials.

Reading a medication label should never be done automatically. Skimming over a familiar label without carefully checking all of the items listed above may result in a serious error and injury to your patient. READ THE WHOLE LABEL CAREFULLY!

Checkpoint Question

1. *When are the "three checks" for safe medication administration performed?*

SEVEN RIGHTS FOR CORRECT MEDICATION ADMINISTRATION

Medication errors should not occur during careful preparation or administration. By adhering to the policy of observing the "seven rights" during medication administration, you will eliminate the potential for many errors (Box 8-2). The "seven rights" include the following:

1. **Right patient.** Ask the patient to state his or her name. Some patients will answer to any name.
2. **Right time and frequency of administration.** Most medications are given immediately (stat) in the medical office.
3. **Right dose.** Check dosages. Many medications come in various strengths. Should it be 250 mg or 500 mg?
4. **Right route of administration.** Some medications may be formulated for various routes. Check the medication. Is it otic, ophthalmic, topical?
5. **Right drug.** Many medication names are very much alike; for instance, Orinase and Ornade may be confused if care is not taken.
6. **Right technique.** Check how the medication is to be given. With food? With juice? Intramuscularly? Subcutaneously?
7. **Right documentation.** The medical record is a legal document. If the procedure is not documented, it is presumed that it was not performed.

All medications given in the office must be documented immediately with the medication name, dosage,

Box 8-2
Medication Errors

Even if you are extremely careful, you may make an error when administering a medication. It is imperative that you report the error to the physician and that intervention measures start immediately. The error and all corrective actions must be documented thoroughly on the patient's chart. An incident report must be completed for the error and filed in the patient's chart as verification that all possible precautions were taken for the patient.

Errors made in charting medications must be corrected using a standard procedure. If you discover a charting error, mark it through with one line. Then mark the correction above the error and sign it.

P.O. J. Smith, M.A.
Tetracycline 250 mg ~~I.M.~~ given stat as ordered.
———————————— J. Smith, M.A.

route, site (if injected), and signature of the medical assistant. The patient's response may be charted as well when appropriate.

SYSTEMS OF MEASUREMENT FOR MEDICATION ADMINISTRATION

The two systems most frequently used to measure medications for drug dosage are the metric and apothecary systems. Although often used by patients, household measurements are not accurate and should be avoided in the administration of medication (Box 8-3).

You may find it necessary to convert from the apothecary to the metric system or to convert measurements within one of the systems. Although many medications are supplied in various dosages and in unit packs of the dosages most often ordered, occasionally you may be required to calculate a dosage by using mathematical equations. It will be necessary to master the elements of the systems of measurement before calculations can be attempted.

The Metric System

The metric system is used throughout the world. Because the system is based on multiples of 10, decimals are often used but never fractions. In the metric system, the base unit of LENGTH is the METER (m). The base unit of WEIGHT is the GRAM (g or gm, either capitalized or lower case). LITER (L or l) is used to measure volume. Prefixes show a fraction of the base. Prefixes often used are:

- micro (0.000001)
- milli (0.001)
- centi (0.01)
- deci (0.1)
- kilo (1000)

For example, using the base unit of a GRAM, fractional measurements would be:

- microgram (mcg, μg)—one millionth of a gram
- milligram (mg)—one thousandth of a gram
- kilogram (kg)—1000 grams

(Decagram and centigram are not used in medication administration.)

Using the base unit of a METER (m = 39.37 inches), fractional measurements would be:

- millimeter (mm)—one thousandth of a meter (about 0.04 inches)
- centimeter (cm)—one hundredth of a meter (about 0.4 inches)

(Other measures are not used in medical practice.)

Using the base unit of a LITER (l or L = approximately 1.06 quarts), fractional measurements would be:

- milliliter (ml, mL)—one thousandth of a liter (about 0.03 ounces)

(Other liquid measures are rarely used in medical practice.)

Note: One cubic centimeter takes up the same space as one milliliter. The measures are used interchangeably at times. An order may read 5 mL or 5 cc, and the measure would be the same.

The Apothecary System

The apothecary system is used less frequently now than in the past and is gradually being replaced by the metric system. In the apothecary system, liquid measurements include DROP(S) (gt[t]), MINIM (min, m), FLUID DRAM (fl dr), FLUID OUNCE (fl oz), PINT (pt), QUART (qt), and GALLON (gal) (Fig. 8-1). Mea-

Box 8-3
Household Measurements

Household measurements include cups, medicine droppers, teaspoons, and tablespoons. Some of the approximate equivalents to household measurements are:

1 teaspoon = 1 fluid dram = 5 mL
1 tablespoon = ½ fluid ounce = 4 fluid drams = 15 mL
2 tablespoons = 1 fluid ounce = 30 mL

Caution patients who will be using household measurements to avoid using table flatware and regular cups. Standard measuring spoons and cups are more accurate.

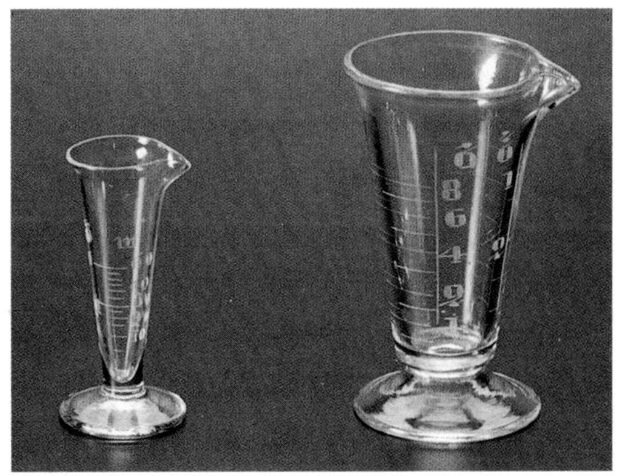

Figure 8-1 Apothecary measures. Minim glass (*left*) and dram/ounce glass.

Table 8-2 **Most Commonly Used Approximate Equivalents***

Metric	*Apothecary*	*Household*
0.06 g	gr i	
0.06 mL	min i	1 drop
1.0 g	gr xv	
1.0 mL	min xv	⅕ tsp
5 mL	(1 dr) ʒ i	1 tsp
15 mL	(½ oz) ℥ ss	1 Tbs
30 mL	(1 oz) ℥ i	2 Tbs
500 mL	(16 oz) ℥ 16	1 pt
1000 mL	(32 oz) ℥ 32	1 qt

*There are many discrepancies among these approximate equivalents. For example, 30 mL is the accepted equivalent for 1 oz (29.57 mL is the exact equivalent); however, multiplying 5 mL per dram by 8 (ʒ viii per ounce) results in an equivalent of 40 mL for 1 oz rather than the accepted equivalent of 30 mL = 1 oz.

Such discrepancies are inevitable when two systems are used whose equivalents are not exact. The discrepancies are within a 10% margin of error, which usually is acceptable in pharmacology.

From Taylor, C., Lillis, C., & Le Mone, P. (1993). *Fundamentals of Nursing: The Art and Science of Nursing Care,* 2nd ed., p. 1347. Philadelphia: J.B. Lippincott.

surements for solid weights include GRAIN (gr), DRAM (dr), OUNCE (oz), and POUND (lb). Roman numerals may be used for smaller numbers, such as gr v or gtt ii. Fractions may be used when necessary.

Table 8-2 lists commonly used equivalents in the metric, apothecary, and household systems of measurement.

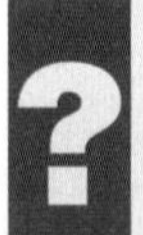

Checkpoint Question

2. *What are three systems of measurement for medication administration? Which one should be avoided and why?*

CONVERTING MEASUREMENTS

Metric to Metric

In the metric system, it is sometimes necessary to convert measurements to the same unit of measure. For example, the physician may order 0.5 g of medication, and the medication label reads 500 mg. To convert within the metric system, use the following rules:

- To change grams to milligrams, multiply grams by 1000 or move the decimal three places to the right.

  (Example: 0.5 g × 1000 = 500 mg)

- To change milligrams to grams, divide the milligrams by 1000 or move the decimal three places to the left.

  (Example: 500 mg ÷ 1000 = 0.5 g)

- To change milligrams to micrograms, multiply the milligrams by 1000 or move the decimal three places to the right.

  (Example: 5 mg × 1000 = 5000 μg)

- To change micrograms to milligrams, divide the micrograms by 1000 or move the decimal three places to the left.

  (Example: 500 μg ÷ 1000 = 0.5 mg)

- To change liters to milliliters, multiply the liters by 1000 or move the decimal three places to the right.

  (Example: 0.01 L × 1000 = 10 mL)

- To change milliliters to liters, divide the milliliters by 1000 or move the decimal three places to the left.

  (Example: 100 mL ÷ 1000 = 0.1 L)

There is no conversion necessary when changing milliliters to cubic centimeters; they are approximately the same.

Apothecary to Metric/Metric to Apothecary

To convert from one system to another system, such as from the apothecary to the metric system, use the following rules:

- To change grains to grams, divide the grains by 15.

  (Example: gr 30 ÷ 15 = 2 g)

- To change grains to milligrams, multiply the grains by 60. Use this rule when there is less than one grain.

  (Example: gr 1/4 × 60 = 15 mg)

- To change ounces to cubic centimeters (or mL), multiply the ounces by 30.

  (Example: 4 oz × 30 = 120 cc)

- To change cubic centimeters (or mL) to fluid ounces, divide the cc (or mL) by 30.

  (Example: 150 cc ÷ 30 = 5)

- To change kilograms to pounds, multiply the kilograms by 2.2.

  (Example: 50 kg × 2.2 = 110.0 lb)

- To change pounds to kilograms, divide the pounds by 2.2.

  (Example: 44 lbs ÷ 2.2 = 20 kg)

- To change drams to milliliters (or cc), multiply the drams by 4.

  (Example: 3 drams × 4 = 12 mL)

- To change drams to cubic centimeters (or mL), multiply drams by 4.

  (Example: 2 drams × 4 = 8 cc)

- To change cubic centimeters to minims, multiply the cc by 15 or 16.

  (Example: 0.5 cc × 16 = 8 m)

- To change minims to cubic centimeters, divide the minims by 15 or 16.

  (Example: 30 m ÷ 15 = 2 cc)

Table 8-3 lists approximate equivalents in the metric and apothecary systems.

Table 8-3 **Commonly Used Metric Units and Their Approximate Apothecary Equivalents**

Metric	*Metric*	*Apothecary*
1 g	1000 mg	gr xv
0.6 g	600 mg	gr x
0.5 g	500 mg	gr viiss
0.3 g	300 mg	gr v
0.2 g	200 mg	gr iii
0.1 g	100 mg	gr iss
0.06 g	60 mg	gr i
0.05 g	50 mg	gr ¾
0.03 g	30 mg	gr ½ or gr ss
0.02 g	20 mg	gr ⅓
0.015 g	15 mg	gr ¼
0.016 g	16 mg	gr ¼
0.010 g	10 mg	gr ⅙
0.008 g	8 mg	gr ⅛
0.006 g	6 mg	gr 1/10
0.005 g	5 mg	gr 1/12
0.003 g	3 mg	gr 1/20
0.002 g	2 mg	gr 1/30
0.001 g	1 mg	gr 1/60
	0.6 mg	gr 1/100
	0.5 mg	gr 1/120
	0.4 mg	gr 1/150
	0.3 mg	gr 1/200

From Taylor, C., Lillis, C., & Le Mone, P. (1993). *Fundamentals of Nursing: The Art and Science of Nursing Care,* 2nd ed., p. 1347. Philadelphia: J.B. Lippincott.

CALCULATING ADULT DOSAGES

Administration of medication is an exacting science; errors in calculation could prove fatal to the patient. There are two methods by which dosages are most frequently calculated: the ratio method and the formula method. It is important to note that measurements must be in the same system, either apothecary or metric, and in the same unit of measurement before a calculation can be made. When using the metric system, be careful to keep the decimal point in the correct position for calculation, and be sure to convert fractions to decimals (eg, ½ should be converted to 0.5).

Ratio and Proportion

Proportion shows the relationship between two equal ratios. The first and fourth terms of a proportion are called the extremes. The second and third terms are called the means. In a proportion, the product of the means equals the product of the extremes. Ratio and proportion are sometimes used in dosage calculations. When the ratio and proportion method is used to calculate dosages, the problem is set up as:

Dose on Hand : Known Quantity =
Dose Desired : Unknown Quantity

EXAMPLE 1. The physician orders 250 mg erythromycin. On hand is 100 mg/mL. State the equation:

100 mg : 1 mL = 250 mg : X

Multiply the extremes = 100X.

Multiply the means = 250 mg.

250 = 100X

To arrive at X, divide 250 by 100.

250 ÷ 100 = 2.5

In this example, you would administer 2.5 mL of erythromycin at 100 mg/mL.

EXAMPLE 2. The physician orders phenobarbital 25 mg. On hand are 12.5-mg tablets. State the equation:

12.5 mg : 1 tab = 25 mg : X

Multiply the extremes = 12.5X.

Multiply the means = 25 mg.

25 = 12.5X

To arrive at X, divide 25 by 12.5.

25 ÷ 12.5 = 2

In this example, you would administer 2 tablets of phenobarbital.

The Formula Method

The formula method is written as:

$$\frac{\text{Desired}}{\text{On Hand}} \times \text{Quantity}$$

EXAMPLE 1. The physician orders ampicillin 0.5 g. On hand is ampicillin 250 mg/capsule. How much ampicillin should be administered? Remember, both dosages must be in the same unit of measure. Change grams to milligrams following the rules for conversion within the metric system (eg, multiply the grams by 1000 or move the decimal three places to the right). To change 0.5 g to milligrams, multiply 0.5 by 1000. The answer is 500 mg.

$$\frac{500 \text{ mg (Desired)}}{250 \text{ mg (On Hand)}} \times 1 \text{ (Quantity)} = 2 \times 1 = 2$$

In this example, you would administer 2 capsules.

EXAMPLE 2.

Desired: 0.35 g
On Hand: 700 mg/mL
How many mL?

Remember, measurements must be in equivalent units, so 0.35 g must be changed to milligrams (eg, multiply the grams by 1000 or move the decimal three places to the right. In this case, 0.35 g become 350 mg.)

$$\frac{350 \text{ mg}}{700 \text{ mg}} \times 1 \text{ mL} = \frac{1}{2} \text{ mL} = 0.5 \text{ mL}$$

Checkpoint Question

3. *Before calculating dosages, what must be done with the measurements?*

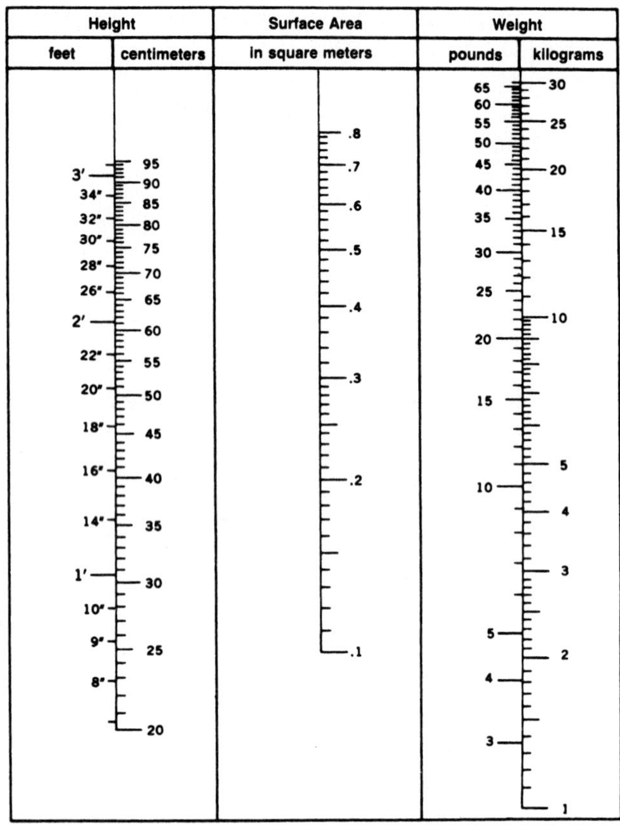

Figure 8-2 Nomogram for estimating surface area of infants and young children. To determine the surface area of the patient, draw a straight line between the point representing the height on the left vertical scale and the point representing the weight on the right vertical scale. The point at which this line intersects the middle vertical scale represents the patient's surface area in square meters. (Used with permission of Ross Products Division, Abbott Laboratories, Columbus OH 43216 from Nomogram. © 1999 Ross Products Division, Abbott Laboratories.)

CALCULATING PEDIATRIC DOSAGES

Several formulas are used for pediatric dosage calculation. The method considered to be the most accurate involves calculating dosage by body surface area (BSA) and requires a scale known as a nomogram. The following formulas are used in calculating dosage for infants and children.

The Nomogram

Pediatric dosages using the BSA are easily and accurately calculated on a nomogram such as the one illustrated in Figure 8-2. This method is considered to be one of the most accurate and can be used for children up to 12 years of age. Some medications are designed to be calculated by this method for adults who are below normal percentiles for body weight. The nomogram chart estimates the BSA according to height and weight. BSA is expressed in square meters.

The chart has three columns. A straight line is drawn from the patient's height in inches or centimeters (column one) to the patient's weight in kilograms or pounds (column three). The straight line will then intersect on the BSA column (column two). This column gives the estimated BSA of the child. After obtaining the BSA average, the following formula is used:

$$\frac{\text{BSA in m}^2 \times \text{Adult Dose}}{1.7} = \text{Child's Dose}$$

EXAMPLE 1. The child weighs 65 lb, or 30 kg, and his height is 50 inches, or 128 cm. Therefore, his BSA is 1.02. If the adult dose is 250 mg, then:

$$\frac{1.02 \times 250}{1.7} = 150 \text{ mg}$$

After obtaining the child's dose, use ratio and proportion or the short formula and compute the amount of medication to be administered from the amount on hand.

Young's Rule

Using Young's rule, the age of the child, divided by the age of the child plus 12, multiplied by the average adult dose equals the child's dose.

$$\text{Pediatric Dose} = \frac{\text{Child's age in years}}{\text{Child's age in years} + 12} \times \text{Adult Dose}$$

Young's rule is not used when the child is over the age of 12 years or under 12 months. If a child over 12 years is small enough to need a smaller dose, Clark's rule may be used.

Clark's Rule

This calculation is more accurate than Young's rule and allows for variations in body size and weight for different ages. Using Clark's rule, the weight of the child divided by 150 (presumed weight of average adult) multiplied by the average adult dose equals the child's dose.

$$\text{Pediatric Dose} = \frac{\text{Child's weight in pounds}}{150 \text{ pounds}} \times \text{Adult Dose}$$

For calculating dosages for infants less than 2 years of age, Fried's rule may be used.

Fried's Rule

This calculation is used only occasionally for children under 2 years of age and bases the dosage on age in months. In this case, the 150 used in calculations is the age in months of a 12½-year-old child and presumes that a child of that age would be eligible for an adult dose. Using Fried's rule, the child's age in months divided by 150 multiplied by the average adult dose equals the child's dose.

$$\text{Pediatric Dose} = \frac{\text{Child's age in months}}{150 \text{ months}} \times \text{Adult Dose}$$

Note: Young's, Clark's, and Fried's rules are used less frequently than the BSA method of calculation and may soon be phased out of use.

Dosage Per Kilogram

Many medications that require careful calibration and that are based on weight are prepared with directions for administering a dosage per kilogram of body weight. Instructions for calculation will be included in the package insert. For instance, the insert may state: *Adults and children over 25 kg (55 lb), give 300 mg q 12 h per day in divided doses. Children less than 25 kg, give 25 mg/kg per day in divided doses q 12 h.*

EXAMPLE 1. The child to whom this medication is to be given weighs 20 lb. This weight must be converted into kilograms. Remember that 1 kg is 2.2 lb; therefore, the child weighs 9 kg.

State the equation as follows: 25 mg/9 kg/d divided by 2 (medication is given twice in 24 hours).

$$25 \text{ mg} \times 9 = 225 \text{ mg/d} \div 2 = 112.5 \text{ q } 12 \text{ h}$$

(In many cases it will be necessary to "round off" the dosage.)

Remember that some recommended doses are calculated for a day's total dose, then must be divided into recommended dose divisions, such as qid or bid. For example, the recommended dose for a 24-hour period may be 300 mg, but should be given in q 8 h increments of 100 mg each. A serious overdose might result if this final calculation step is not taken.

8

What If?

What if a child arrives at the medical office in cardiac arrest? How does the physician have time to calculate the child's body weight?

In such a situation, the physician does not have the time to perform the calculations and instead may rely on printed graphs that list precalculated emergency drug doses. Also, some hospital emergency departments use computer software that will automatically calculate and print a list of all pediatric emergency medications and their doses.

MEDICATION ROUTES

Medication can be administered in many ways. The route of administration is chosen after considering many factors. Sometimes the route is chosen because of cost, safety, or degree of speed by which the drug will be absorbed into the system. Certain drugs may be administered by only one route. Some drugs may be toxic if given by a certain route, some may be effective only if given by a specific route, and sometimes absorption will only occur through one particular route.

ORAL ADMINISTRATION

Of all the medication routes, the oral route is the easiest and most preferred by patients; however, oral medication is usually slow to take effect and cannot be

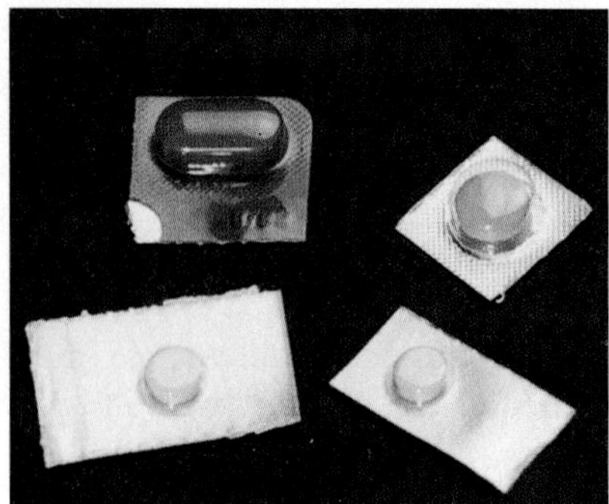

Figure 8-3 Unit dose packages.

used for unconscious patients, those with nausea and vomiting, or those who are NPO (nothing by mouth).

Drugs given orally may be administered as tablets, capsules, pills, or liquids (Procedure 8-1). They are usually absorbed through the walls in the gastrointestinal tract.

Many drugs are available in unit-dose packages that contain the amount of the drug for a single dose and in the proper form for administration (Fig. 8-3). Unit-dose packages are labeled with the trade name, generic name, precautions, instructions for storage, and an expiration date. Liquid medications may be measured in a graduate, minim glass, medicine glass, or plastic cup.

Table 8-4 lists common solid and liquid forms of oral medications.

Table 8-4 **Forms of Oral Medications**

Form	*Description*
Solids	
Buffered	Agents are added to decrease or counteract the medication's acidity to prevent gastric irritation.
Caplet	Medication is compressed into the shape of a capsule. It may be coated for ease in swallowing, but it does not have a gelatin covering.
Capsule	Powdered or granulated medication is enclosed in a gelatin capsule designed to dissolve in gastric enzymes or high in the small intestines.
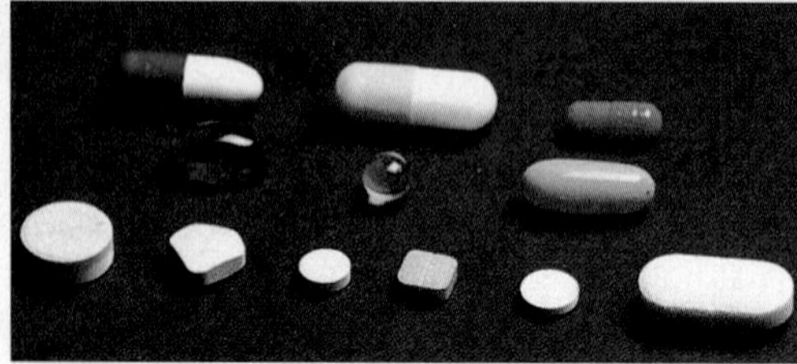	Oral medications. Tablets (*front*), gelcaps (*middle*), and capsules.
Enteric-coated tablet	A compressed dry form of a medication coated to withstand the gastric acidity and dissolve in the intestines. These may be medications that would be destroyed by the gastric enzymes or might be damaging to the gastric mucosa. Never crush or break enteric-coated tablets.
Gelcap	An oil-based medication is enclosed in a soft gelatin capsule.
Lozenge	A firm, compressed form of medication, usually for a local effect in the mouth or throat. Caution patients to let lozenges dissolve slowly and avoid drinking any fluids for a period of time after using the lozenge.
Powder	A finely ground form of medication; may be difficult for many patients to swallow.
Spansule or time-release capsule	Gelatin capsules are filled with forms of the medication that will dissolve over a period of time rather than all at once. Never open spansules unless this is recommended or allowed by the manufacturer.
Tablet	Medication is formed into many shapes and colors for easy identification. Tablets usually dissolve high in the gastrointestinal tract. These may be broken into halves only if they have been scored for that purpose (see photo).
Liquids	
Elixir	Medication is dissolved in alcohol, and flavoring is added. These are less sweet than syrups and are usually preferred by adults. They should not be used for alcoholics or diabetics.
Emulsion	Medication is combined with water and oil. Emulsions must be thoroughly shaken to disperse the medication evenly.
Extract	This is a very concentrated form of medication made by evaporating volatile plant oils. Extracts may be administered as drops and are usually given in a liquid to disguise their strong taste.
Gel	Medication is suspended in a thin gelatin or paste base.
Suspension	Particles are dissolved in a liquid that must be shaken well before administering.
Syrup	This very sweet form of medication is used frequently for children's medications and is usually flavored in addition to having a high sugar content.

Procedure 8-1 Administering Oral Medications

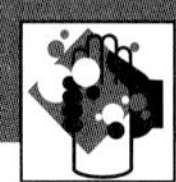

PURPOSE:

To provide medication by the route most appropriate for optimum medication metabolism with minimal discomfort

EQUIPMENT/SUPPLIES

- medication
- medication tray
- disposable calibrated cup
- physician's instructions
- glass of water

STEPS

1. Wash your hands.

2. Assemble the equipment and supplies.

3. Select the medication. Compare the label to the physician's instructions. Check the expiration date. Check the label three times: when taking it from the shelf, while pouring, and when returning to the shelf.

Carefully dispensing medications helps prevent errors. Outdated medication should not be administered to a patient.

4. Calculate the correct dosage to be given, if necessary.

5. Remove the cap from the container, touching only the outside of the lid.

The inside of the lid will become contaminated if touched.

6. Remove the correct dose of medication from the container.

a. *For solid medications:*

(1) Pour the capsule or tablet into the bottle cap to prevent contamination of the cap and the medication. *CAUTION:* If the dosage requires that a scored tablet be broken, use a gauze square for breaking. Never break the tablet by using bare hands. Never crush enteric-coated tablets, and never open time-release capsules.

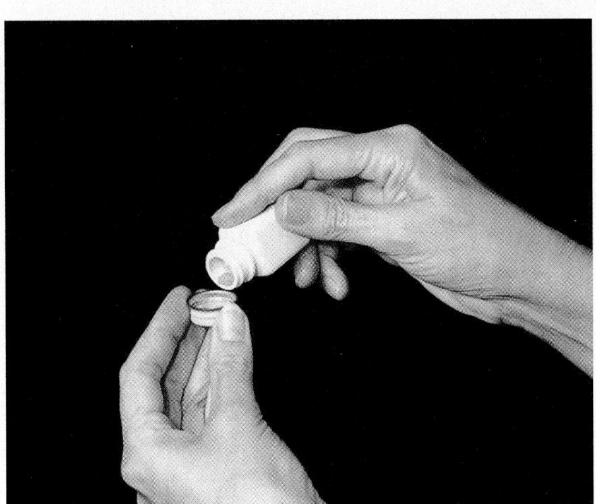

(2) Transfer the medication to a disposable cup without touching the inside of the cup or the medication.

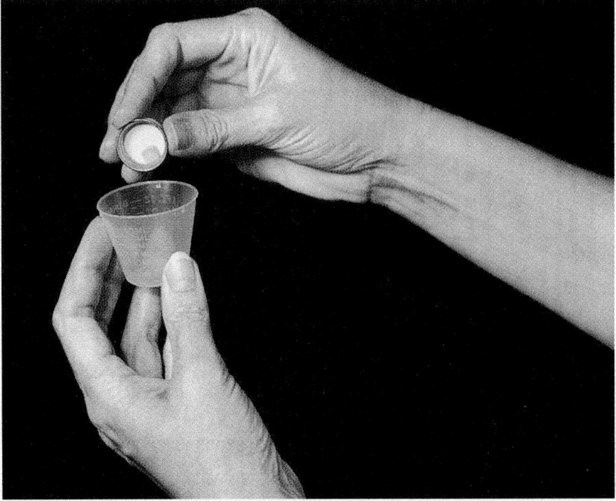

b. *For liquid medications:*

(1) Open the bottle lid and place it on a flat surface with the open end facing up to prevent contamination of the inside of the cap.

(2) Palm the label to prevent liquids from dripping onto the label and obscuring the writing.

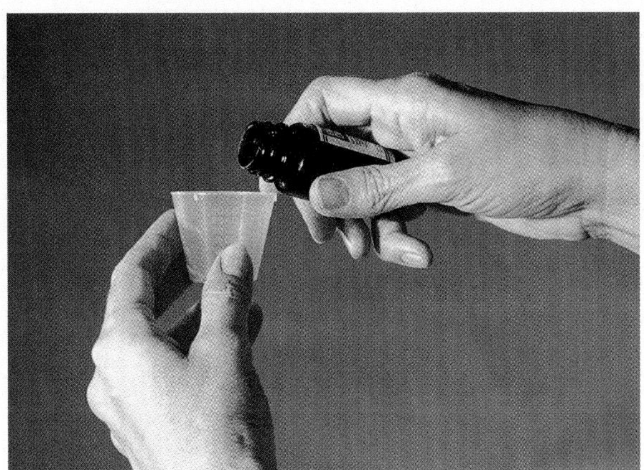

(3) With the opposite hand, place the thumbnail at the correct calibration on the cup. Holding the cup at eye level, pour the medication.

continued

8

Procedure 8-1 Continued Administering Oral Medications

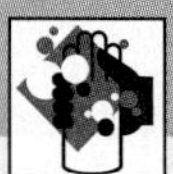

(4) Read the level at the lowest level of the **meniscus,** the curved surface of the medication in the container. The lowest level of the meniscus gives the proper amount of medication.

7. Greet and identify the patient. Explain the procedure. Ask the patient about medication allergies that might not be noted on the chart.
Allergies may exist that have not been noted.

8. Give the medication to the patient.

9. Give the patient a glass of water for swallowing the medication unless contraindicated.
Water helps the patient swallow the medication. However, water is contraindicated when giving medications intended for local effect (such as cough syrup or lozenges) or when giving buccal or sublingual medications, which are absorbed locally for a systemic effect and must not be swallowed (see Procedure 8-2).

10. Remain with the patient to be sure that all of the medication is swallowed. Observe any unusual reactions, and report them to the physician. Record any unusual reactions on the patient's chart.
You cannot assume that the patient swallowed the medication unless you observe it. Unusual reactions may signal a developing hypersensitivity to the medication.

11. Wash your hands.

DOCUMENTATION GUIDELINES

- Date and time
- Medication name
- Dose
- Route
- Reactions to medication as indicated
- Patient education/instructions
- Your signature

Charting Example

DATE	TIME Ampicillin 125 mg PO given stat to
	pt NKA. Pt reminded to complete course
	of prescription and RTC in 10 days.
	—Your signature

Sublingual Route

Medication given sublingually is placed under the patient's tongue; it must not be swallowed. The medication is dissolved by the saliva in the mouth and is absorbed directly into the bloodstream through the mucosa covering the sublingual vessels. The number of medications administered sublingually is limited. Caution the patient not to eat or drink until the medication has totally dissolved.

Buccal Route

Medication given by the buccal route is placed in the pouch between the cheek and gum at the side of the mouth for absorption through the vascular oral mucosa. Few medications are manufactured for this route. The patient must not drink fluids until the medication is completely absorbed.

Procedure 8-2 describes the steps to follow for administration of sublingual or buccal medications.

Checkpoint Question

4. *What are the disadvantages of the oral route for medication administration?*

MUCOSAL ADMINISTRATION

Many medications administered to the mucous membranes are designed for a local effect. Examples include local fungicides in vaginal suppositories or local irritants to cause defecation in rectal suppositories. However, because of the vascularity of the mucous membranes, certain systemic drugs can be administered by the rectal route as well.

Rectal Route

Rectal medications can be in the form of suppositories or liquids (administered as a retention enema). They can provide a local effect, or they may be absorbed through the rectal mucosa for a systemic effect. Rectal medications may be used for patients who are NPO or who have nausea and vomiting, but they are never used for patients who have diarrhea.

Most rectal suppositories use a cocoa butter or glycerin base that melts at body temperature (Fig. 8-4*A*). These should be inserted about 2 inches into the rectum, above the internal rectal sphincter to avoid the urge to evacuate (see Fig. 8-4*B*). If insertion is difficult, lubricating gel may be applied, but never petrolatum

Procedure 8-2 Administering Sublingual or Buccal Medications

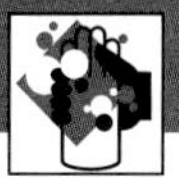

PURPOSE:

To provide medication by the route most appropriate for optimum medication metabolism with minimal discomfort

To provide a route that bypasses the gastrointestinal tract and its enzymes to reach the circulatory system

EQUIPMENT/SUPPLIES

- medication
- medication tray
- disposable cup
- physician's instructions

8

STEPS

1–7. Follow steps 1–7 as described in Procedure 8-1, Administering Oral Medications.

8. Administer the medication.

a. *For sublingual medications:* Have the patient place the medication under the tongue.

b. *For buccal medications:* Have the patient place the medication between the cheek and gum.

9. Remain with the patient to be sure that the medication is *not* swallowed and is allowed to dissolve completely. Do not allow the patient to ingest any food or water until the medication is completely absorbed.

You cannot assume that the medication was taken properly unless you observe it. Unusual reactions may signal a developing hypersensitivity to the medication.

10. Observe any unusual reactions, and report them to the physician. Record any unusual reactions on the patient's chart.

11. Wash your hands.

DOCUMENTATION GUIDELINES

- Date and time
- Medication name
- Dose
- Route
- Reactions to the medication as indicated
- Patient education/instructions
- Your signature

Charting Example

DATE	TIME Pt c/o chest pain. BP-148/84,.
	P-86. NTG 1/150 SL × 3. Pain subsided.
	Dr. Fleming in to ck. pt. Referred stat to
	General Hospital Cardiology Clinic.
	—Your signature

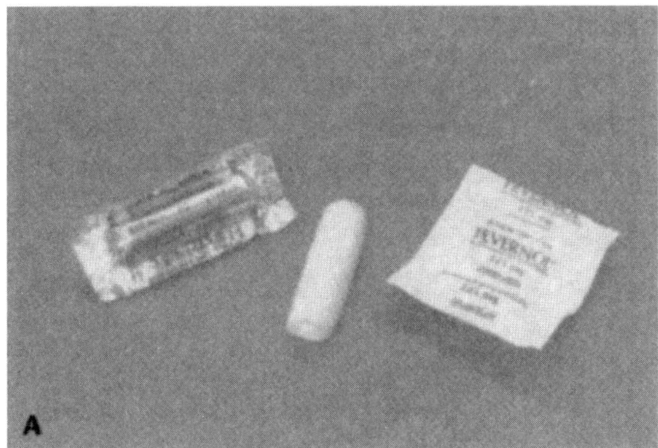

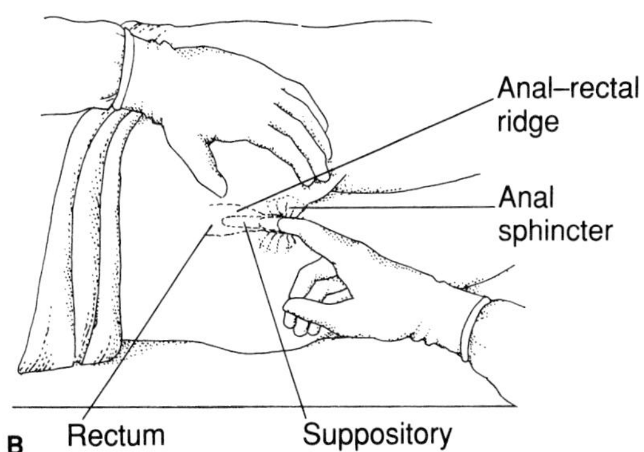

Figure 8-4 (A) These are examples of suppositories. They are made in a variety of sizes and shapes. (B) Rectal suppositories should be introduced into the anus well beyond the internal sphincter.

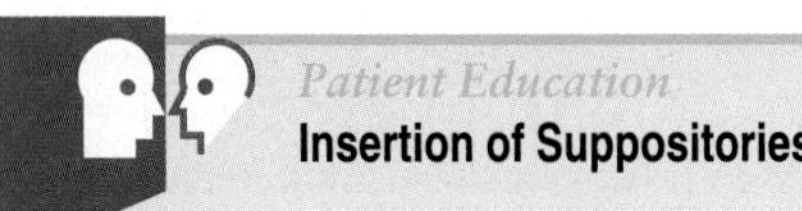

Patient Education

Insertion of Suppositories

Some patients are not proficient with the insertion of suppositories and may require specific instructions or simple drawings. Medication errors have occurred because patients did not know the difference between their various orifices. Take a few moments to ensure that the patient understands the route of application, methods to make application easier (lubricating gel or warm water to moisten), and that the foil wrapper is to be removed and is not part of the treatment.

Remember: If you are helping the patient to insert either rectal or vaginal suppositories, or if you are administering solutions by either route, you must follow Standard Precautions and wear gloves.

(petrolatum interferes with absorption and is damaging to the mucosa). Never force the insertion of a suppository because this could be dangerous to the patient. At the very least, it would cause unnecessary discomfort.

Both enemas and suppositories should be retained by the patient for about 20 to 30 minutes before elimination.

Vaginal Route

Vaginal medications may be creams, tablets, cocoa butter-based suppositories, or solutions for douches. Examples include hormonal creams and antibiotic or antifungal preparations. Very few medications other than those for local effects are prescribed for the vaginal route. All are more effective if inserted the full length of the vagina, preferably into the posterior fornix (Fig. 8-5).

The patient should remain lying for a period of time after insertion; therefore, instructions may suggest that the medication be inserted at bedtime. For the patient's comfort, she may need a light pad to absorb drainage.

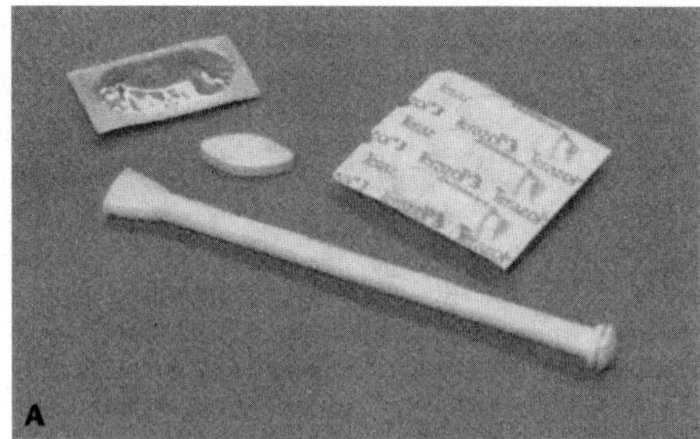

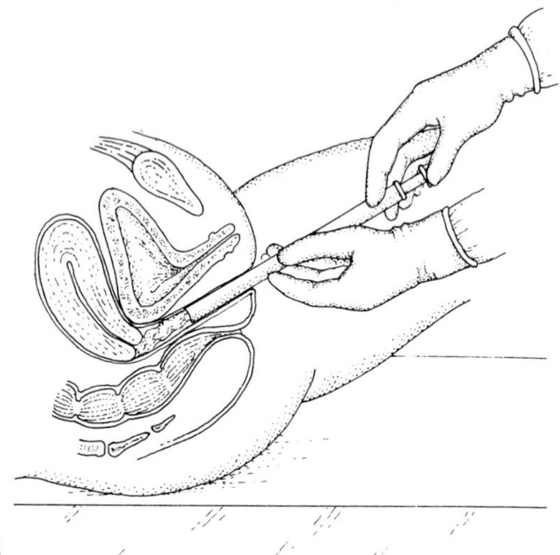

Figure 8-5 Insertion of vaginal medication. (**A**) Vaginal suppository and applicator. (**B**) Insertion of vaginal cream using applicator.

DERMAL ADMINISTRATION

Dermal medications are applied to the skin. They include topical creams, lotions, and ointments and transdermal medications. Topical medications produce localized effects, such as coating or soothing. Transdermal medications produce systemic effects.

Transdermal Medications

Medication administered transdermally is delivered to the body by absorption through the skin. Delivery is slow and maintains a steady, stable level of medication. Dermal patches are placed on the skin, usually on the chest or back, upper arm, or behind the ear (for prevention of motion sickness). Antiangina medications placed anywhere on the chest wall are effective by this route.

Procedure 8-3 describes the steps to follow when applying transdermal medication. Procedure 8-4 describes the steps to follow when applying topical medication.

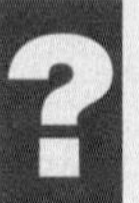

Checkpoint Question

5. *How do the effects of topical and transdermal medications differ?*

Procedure 8-3 Applying Transdermal Medications

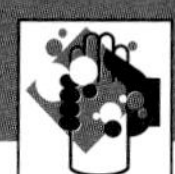
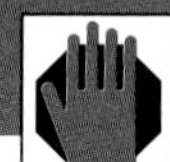

PURPOSE:

To administer over a period of time a medication that requires a sustained action

EQUIPMENT/SUPPLIES

- medication
- medication tray
- physician's order

8

STEPS

1. Wash your hands.
2. Assemble the equipment and supplies.
3. Greet and identify the patient. Explain the procedure. Ask the patient about medication allergies that might not be noted on the chart.
   Allergies may exist that have not been noted.
4. Select the site for administration, and perform any necessary skin preparation. The sites are usually the upper arm, the chest or back surface, or behind the ear; these should be rotated. Ensure that the skin is dry, clean, and free of any irritation. Do not shave areas with excessive hair; trim the hair closely with scissors.
   Shaving may abrade the skin and cause the medication to be absorbed too rapidly.
5. You may glove at this point. If there is a patch already in place, remove it carefully. If you choose not to glove, do not touch the inside of the patch to avoid absorbing any remaining medication. Discard the used patch in the trash container. Inspect the site for irritation.
   Touching the medication may cause it to be absorbed into your skin, causing undesirable reactions.
6. Open the medication package by pulling the two sides apart. Do not touch the area of medication.
7. Apply the medicated patch to the patient's skin following the manufacturer's directions. Press the adhesive edges down firmly all around, starting at the center and pressing outward. If the edges do not stick, fasten with paper tape.
   Starting at the center eliminates air spaces that may prevent contact with the skin.
8. Wash your hands.

DOCUMENTATION GUIDELINES

- Date and time
- Medication name
- Dose
- Location of patch
- Reactions to the medication as indicated
- Patient education/instructions
- Your signature

✓Charting Example

DATE	TIME Transdermal NTG patch applied to
	L anterior chest. Pt instructed in
	application of patches and received pt ed
	brochure. Verbalized understanding.
	—Your signature

PARENTERAL ADMINISTRATION

If a patient is NPO, if the drug cannot be absorbed through the gastrointestinal system, or if a more rapid or controlled response is needed, the parenteral route is used. Parenteral administration refers not only to injections, but to all the ways in which drugs are administered other than by swallowing for absorption in the gastrointestinal tract.

The intramuscular route is often used for this type of administration because the muscles are highly vascular, and absorption is fairly rapid (see "Types of Injections and Injection Sites," p. 180). Administration by injection is the most efficient method of drug administration, but it can also be the most hazardous. The effects may be quite rapid, the medication cannot be retrieved, and, because the skin is broken, it is possible for infections to develop. You must use aseptic technique whenever administering medications by the injection route (Box 8-4).

If an injection is placed incorrectly, nerve damage could occur, or the penetration of blood vessels could cause formation of a hematoma. Incorrect placement of the needle during an intramuscular injection could cause the medication to be delivered intravenously.

8

Procedure 8-4 Applying Topical Medications

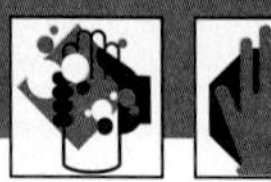

PURPOSE:

To provide medication by the route most appropriate for optimum medication metabolism and minimal patient discomfort
To reduce itching, lubricate or soften the skin, induce vasodilation or vasoconstriction
To prevent or treat infection, reduce inflammation, or administer sustained transdermal medication

EQUIPMENT/SUPPLIES

- medication
- medication tray
- physician's order
- washing solution (optional)
- tongue blade
- large cotton-tipped swab
- gloves
- dressing, bandage, tape (optional)

STEPS

1. Wash your hands.
2. Assemble the equipment and supplies. Check the medication label three times.
3. Greet and identify the patient. Explain the procedure. Ask the patient about medication allergies that might not be noted on the chart.
   Allergies may exist that have not been noted.
4. Assess the area to record observations regarding the condition of the skin.
   Observations must be made before applying medication.
5. Put on gloves, in most instances.
   Wearing gloves prevents contact with lesions or absorption of the medication through your skin if you inadvertently touch the medication.
6. If the area is soiled, clean the skin according to the steps for skin preparation outlined in Procedure 6-4: Performing Skin Preparation and Hair Removal in Chapter 6, Assisting with Minor Office Surgery.
   Medication must be applied to clean skin.
7. If old medication remains in the area from a previous treatment, remove it by the same procedure.
   New medication should not be applied over old medication.
8. If the lesion requires a dressing and bandage, apply the medication to the dressing using a tongue blade.
   Medication is applied to the dressing, not to the wound, to avoid patient discomfort.
9. If the medication is to be applied directly to the area, lightly spread it with a tongue blade or a large cotton-tipped swab working from the center of the area outward.
   Work from the area of concern outward.
10. Use clean technique or medical asepsis if there are no open lesions. Use no touch technique or surgical asepsis if the skin is broken.
    This avoids the spread of pathogens.
11. Bandage if necessary.
    This protects the area.
12. Clean the treatment room, and dispose of equipment and supplies appropriately. Wash your hands.

DOCUMENTATION GUIDELINES

- Date and time
- Medication name
- Dose
- Location of application
- Reactions to the medication as indicated
- Patient education/instructions
- Your signature

Charting Example

DATE	TIME Delacort to lesions on R forearm
	as directed. Pt education re: procedure.
	Verbalized understanding of instructions
	and pt ed brochure.—Your signature

Box 8-4
Injections: Maintaining Sterility

The following parts of the hypodermic setup must be kept sterile:

- Syringe tip
- Inside of barrel
- Shaft of plunger
- Needle

EQUIPMENT NEEDED FOR GIVING INJECTIONS

Medications used for injections are supplied in **ampules, vials,** and cartridges (Fig. 8-6).

Ampules

Ampules are small, glass containers that must be broken at the neck to aspirate the solution into the syringe. When the ampule is opened, all medication from it must be either used or discarded. It must not be saved for later use because once the ampule is broken, sterility cannot be maintained.

Vials

Vials are glass or plastic containers sealed at the top by a rubber stopper. They may be single-dose or multiple-dose containers. The contents of vials may be in solution or in powder or crystal form, which requires reconstitution with a specific amount and type of **diluent** (diluting agent), usually sterile water or saline. Certain drugs such as phenytoin (Dilantin) require a special diluent supplied by the manufacturer.

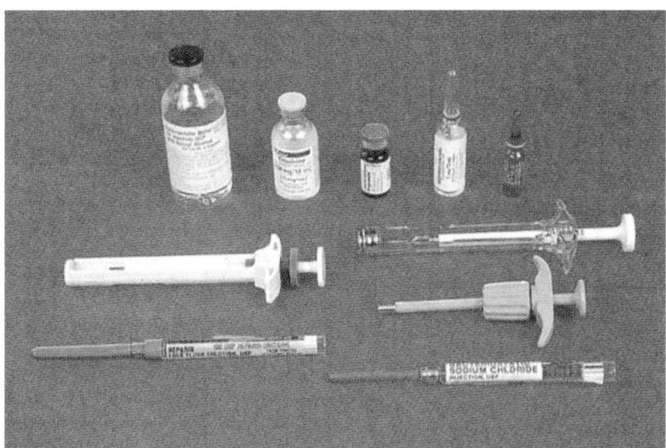

Figure 8-6 Ampules, vials, prefilled cartridges, and holders.

When a powdered drug is reconstituted, the following must be written on the label:

1. Date of the reconstitution
2. Initials of the person who reconstituted the drug
3. Diluent used

To reconstitute a dry form of medication, withdraw from the vial the amount of air that will be replaced by the diluent. Inject the required amount of diluent into the air space in the vial and not into the medication to avoid bubbles or foam. Withdraw the needle, and gently roll the bottle between the palms to dissolve the medication. Shaking the bottle may cause bubbles.

8

Vials may be intended for multiple doses or for a unit dose. Vials intended for multiple dose use may be up to 50 mL and may be used repeatedly by entering through the rubber stopper to remove a portion of the solution. Unit-dose vials usually contain 1 to 2 mL, and all of the solution is removed for a single injection. Some single-dose vials are designed to include the dry form of the medication and the solution required for its reconstitution in separate compartments. Instructions for combining the two in these specially designed vials will be included by the manufacturer. These are usually to be reconstituted just before being administered.

Cartridges

Prefilled syringes contain a premeasured amount of a medication in a disposable cartridge with a needle attached. The prefilled cartridge and needle are placed in a holder for administration (Fig. 8-7). Examples of units are the Tubex and the Carpuject.

Needles and Syringes

A variety of needles and syringes are used for injections. The 3-mL or cubic centimeter (cc) hypodermic syringe is the most common type used for injections. Syringes designed to hold 10 mL or more are usually used in the medical office for irrigation. All syringes consist of a plunger, body or barrel, flange, and tip (Fig. 8-8). The other types of syringes used for parenteral administration are tuberculin and insulin. Reusable glass syringes may be used for surgical procedures, but disposable plastic syringes will be used for injections.

Needle lengths vary from ⅜ to 1 inch or 1½ inch, for standard injections. **Gauge** refers to the diameter of the needle lumen. Needle gauge varies from 18 (large) to 30 (small); the higher the number, the smaller the gauge.

Most companies prepackage hypodermic syringes in color-coded envelopes with the needle attached (Fig.

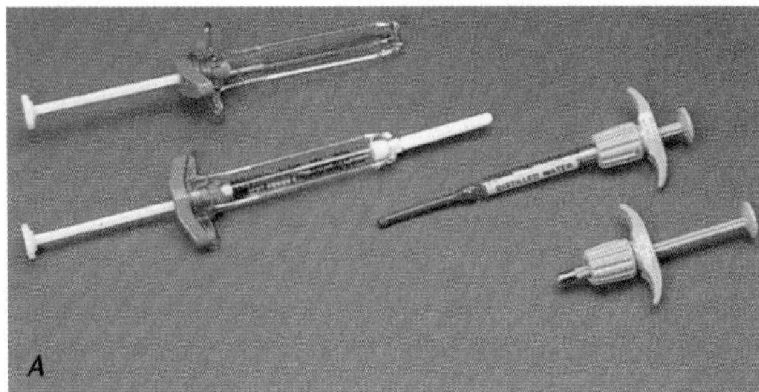

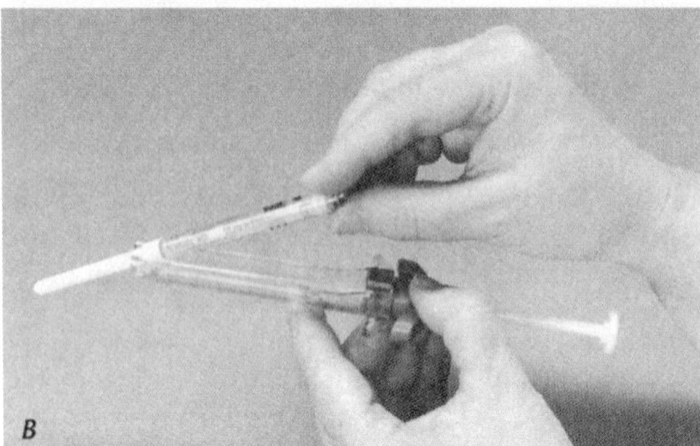

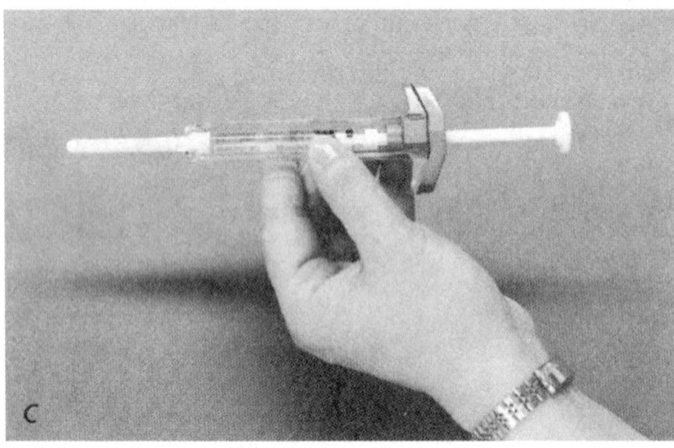

Figure 8-7 Prefilled syringes. (**A**) Prefilled medication cartridges and injector devices. (**B**) Inserting the cartridge into the injector device. (**C**) Ready for injection.

8-9). Separate needles and syringes may be purchased as needed. This type of syringe may be used for either subcutaneous or intramuscular injections.

It is necessary to choose the package with a needle length and gauge appropriate for the route of the injection to be given. For example, an intramuscular injection requires a needle length of at least 1 inch, depending on the size of the patient and the fat/muscle ratio. The needle will vary from 20 to 25 gauge, depending on the medication to be administered. Thick medications, such as penicillin, are difficult to draw into a syringe using a small-gauge needle and will be supplied in a prefilled cartridge with the appropriate-sized needle. Subcutaneous injections are generally given using a short, small-gauge needle: 25 gauge ⅝ inch or 23 gauge ½ inch.

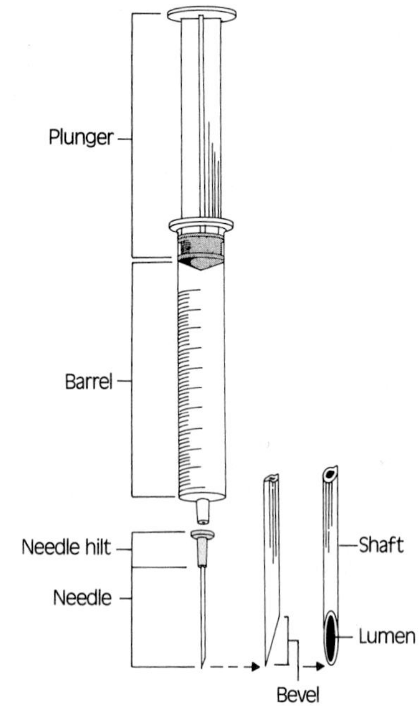

Figure 8-8 Parts of a syringe and needle.

All hypodermic syringes are marked with 10 calibrations per milliliter or cubic centimeter on one side of the syringe. Each small line represents 0.1 (one-tenth) mL or cc. The other side of the syringe may be marked in minims (Fig. 8-10).

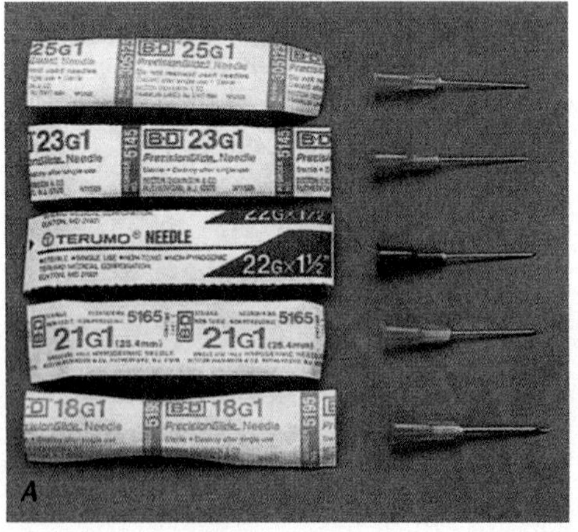

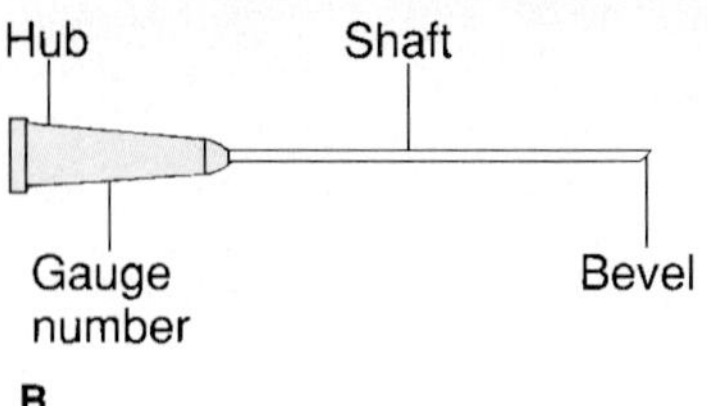

Figure 8-9 Needles. (**A**) Different gauges and lengths. (**B**) Parts of a needle.

Procedure 8-5 Preparing an Injection

PURPOSE:

To withdraw a precise amount of medication without introducing contamination to the medication

EQUIPMENT/SUPPLIES

- medication
- medication tray
- antiseptic wipes
- appropriate-sized needle and syringe
- physician's instructions

8

STEPS

1. Wash your hands.
2. Assemble the equipment and supplies. Be careful to choose the needle and syringe according to the route of administration, type of medication, and patient's size.
3. Select the proper medication. Check the expiration date, and check the medication three times: when taking it from the shelf, while drawing it up, and when returning it to the shelf.
   Never administer a medication that is out of date. Checking the medication ensures accuracy.
4. If necessary, calculate the correct dosage to be given.
5. Open the sterile syringe/needle package. Assemble if necessary.
   Needles and syringes often come preassembled in a package, or they may be purchased separately and assembled as needed.
6. Check to make sure the needle is firmly attached to the syringe by grasping the needle at the hub and turning it clockwise onto the syringe held in the other hand. Remove the needle guard.
   A needle not firmly attached may become detached during the procedure.

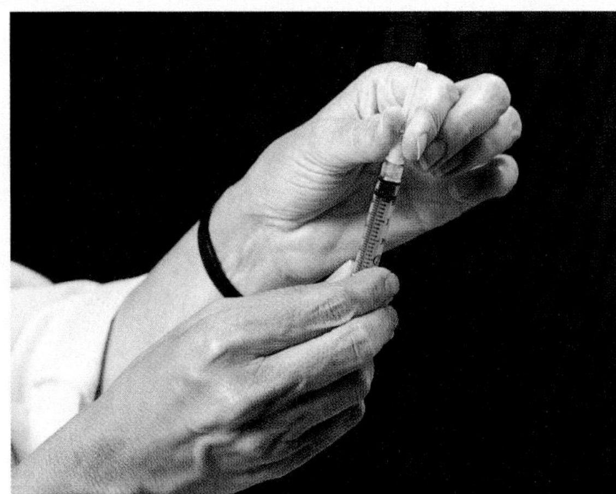

7. Withdraw the correct amount of medication from the ampule or vial.
   a. *From an ampule:*
      (1) With the fingertips of one hand, tap the stem of the ampule lightly to remove any medication in or above the narrow neck.
      (2) Place a piece of gauze around the ampule neck to protect your fingers from broken glass. Grasp the gauze and ampule firmly with the fingers. Snap the stem off the ampule with a quick downward movement of the gauze. Be sure to aim the break away from your face. Set the ampule top aside to discard.

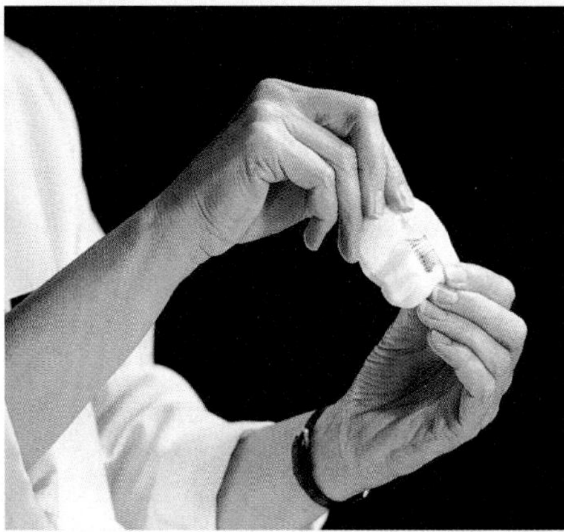

      (3) Insert the needle lumen below the level of the medication. Withdraw the medication by pulling back on the plunger of the syringe without letting the needle touch the unsterile broken edge of the ampule to avoid contaminating the needle. Withdraw the desired amount of medication; set the ampule aside to dispose of properly.
      (4) If there are air bubbles in the syringe, hold it vertically with the needle uppermost, and tap the barrel gently with the fingertips until the air bubbles rise to the top. Draw back on the plunger to admit a small amount of air, then gently push the plunger forward to eject all of the air in the syringe. Do not eject any of the medication if only the required dosage has been drawn up. *Note:* Special needle adapters are available with filters to guard against the possibility of aspirating minute glass particles into the medication to be administered. Discard the adapter needle after drawing up the medication, and attach the appropriate sized needle for the situation to the syringe for the administration of the medication.

continued

Procedure 8-5 Continued **Preparing an Injection**

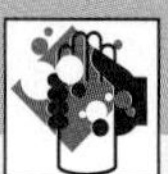

b. *From a vial:*

(1) Cleanse the rubber stopper of the vial with the antiseptic wipe to avoid introducing microorganisms into the medication.

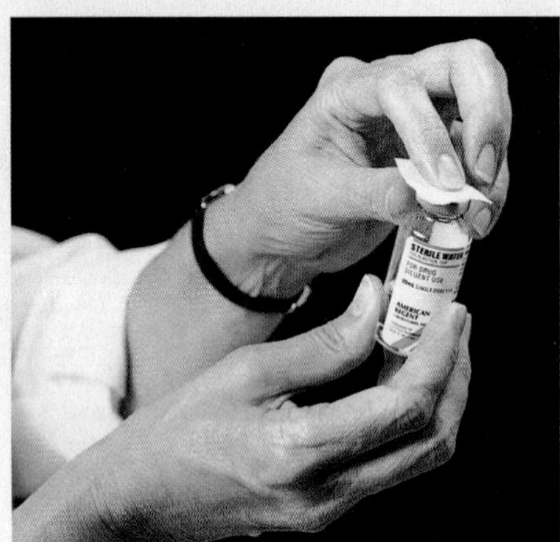

(2) Pull back on the plunger to aspirate an amount of air equal to the amount of medication to be removed from the vial.

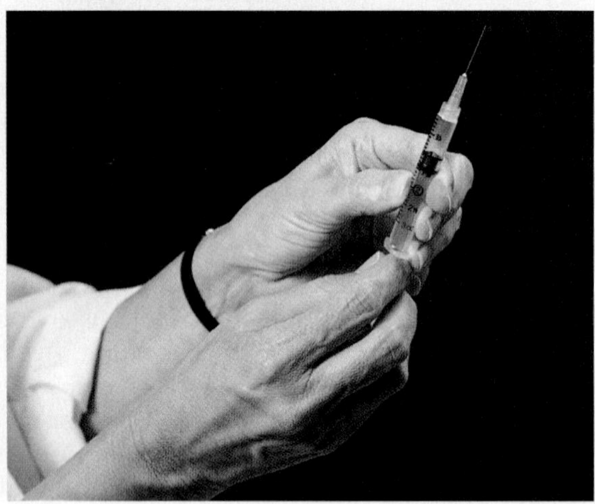

(3) Insert the needle through the cleansed center of the stopper and above the level of the medication to prevent foam or bubbles from forming in the medication. Inject the air from the syringe into the vial to avoid forming a vacuum in the vial, which would make withdrawal of the medication difficult.

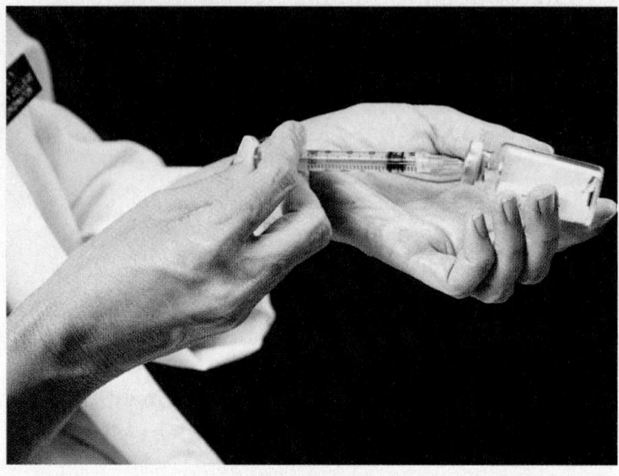

(4) Invert the vial, holding the syringe at eye level. Aspirate the desired amount of medication into the syringe.

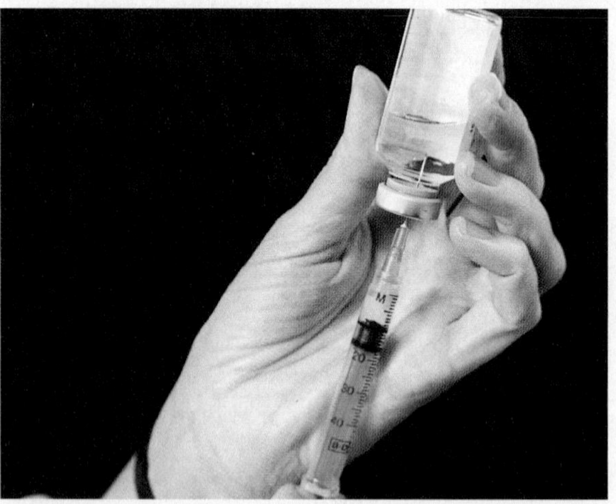

continued

Procedure 8-5 *Continued* Preparing an Injection

(5) Remove any air bubbles in the medication within the syringe by gently tapping with the finger tips on the barrel of the syringe held vertically. Remove any air remaining in the syringe by slowly pushing the plunger. Doing this allows the air to flow back into the vial to maintain the equalized pressure.

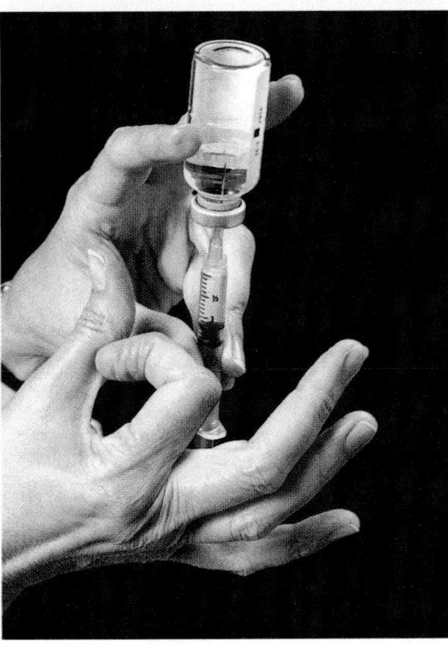

8. Carefully recap the needle.

Needles are never recapped after administering the medication. The purpose of recapping a newly filled unused syringe is to protect the sterility of the needle.

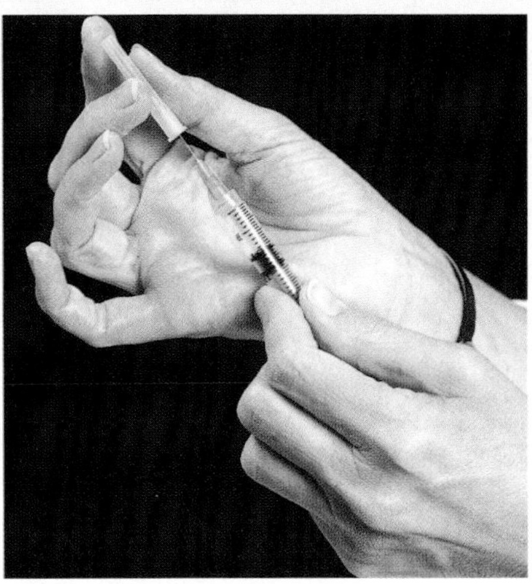

9. Place the syringe with the medication on the medication tray with the physician's instructions. Place an antiseptic wipe on the tray for administering the medication. You are now ready to proceed with administering the specific type of injection ordered by the physician (see Procedures 8-6 to 8-10).

8

The tuberculin (TB) syringe is narrow and has a total capacity of 1 mL or cc. There are 100 calibration lines marking the capacity. Each line represents 0.01 mL. Every tenth line is longer than the others to indicate 0.1 mL. TB syringes are used for newborn and pediatric doses, for intradermal skin tests, and any time that minute amounts of medication are to be given.

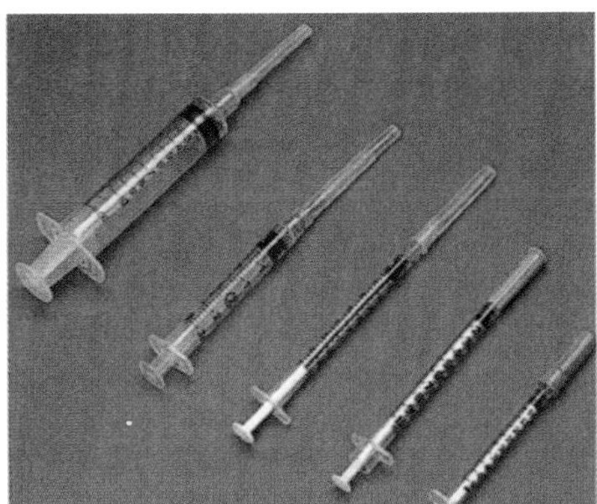

Figure 8-10 Syringes (*from top to bottom*): 10 mL, 3 mL, tuberculin, insulin, and low-dose insulin.

The insulin syringe is used strictly for administering insulin to diabetic patients. It has a total capacity of 1 mL. The 1-mL volume is marked as 100 units (U) to represent the strength of 100 U insulin/mL when full. Each group of 10 U is divided by five small lines. Each line represents 2 U. A smaller insulin syringe with a capacity of 0.5 mL can be used when less than 50 U insulin is ordered. The smaller insulin syringe has 50 small calibration lines, each representing 1 U insulin (Fig. 8-11).

Most of the insulin used today is U-100, which means that there are 100 U insulin in each mL (cc). It is important to remember that the insulin syringe must be marked U-100 to match the insulin used.

Procedure 8-5 describes the steps required for preparing an injection.

Checkpoint Question

6. *What are ampules and vials and how do they differ?*

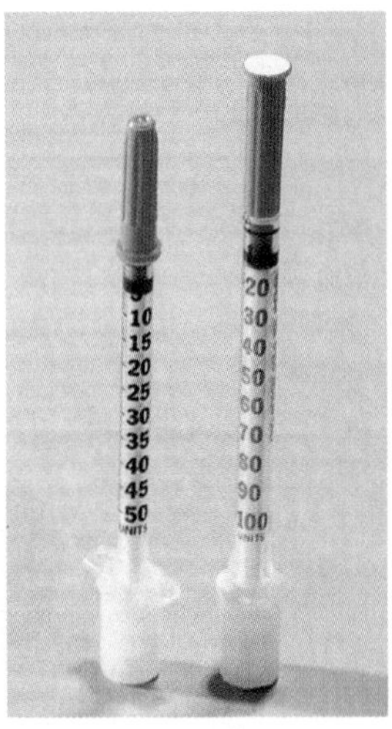

Figure 8-11 Insulin syringes. 50 U (*left*) and 100 U (*right*).

TYPES OF INJECTIONS AND INJECTION SITES

Intradermal Injections

Intradermal injections are inserted at a 10- to 15-degree angle, almost parallel to the skin surface (Fig. 8-12). When administered correctly, the needle will be slightly visible under the skin, and a small bubble (wheal or bleb) will be raised in the skin surface when the solution is injected. Recommended sites include the anterior forearm and across the back. Intradermal injections are used exclusively to administer skin tests, such as the tine or **Mantoux** tuberculin skin test or allergy tests.

The tine test is used for routine screening and is not considered as diagnostic as the Mantoux test. Both use purified protein derivative (PPD) from a live tuberculin bacillus culture to test for the presence of tuberculin antibodies. A positive tine test is usually followed by a Mantoux test. A positive Mantoux reaction with induration greater than 10 mm will indicate the possibility of active or dormant tuberculosis or exposure to the disease. Further testing by sputum culture and x-rays is required for a definitive diagnosis.

Procedure 8-6 describes the steps for giving an intradermal injection. Procedure 8-7 describes how to administer the tine or Mantoux test.

Subcutaneous Injections

Subcutaneous injections are given into the fatty layer of tissue below the skin by positioning the needle and syringe at a 45-degree angle to the skin (see Fig. 8-12). The subcutaneous route is chosen for drugs that should not be absorbed as rapidly as through the intramuscular or intravenous routes.

Common sites include the upper arm, thigh, back, and abdomen. Procedure 8-8 describes the steps for administering a subcutaneous injection.

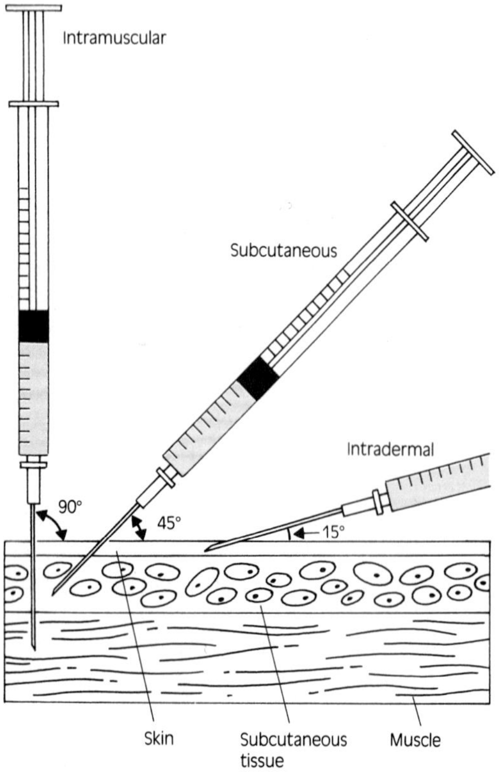

Figure 8-12 Comparison of the angles of insertion for intramuscular, subcutaneous, and intradermal injections.

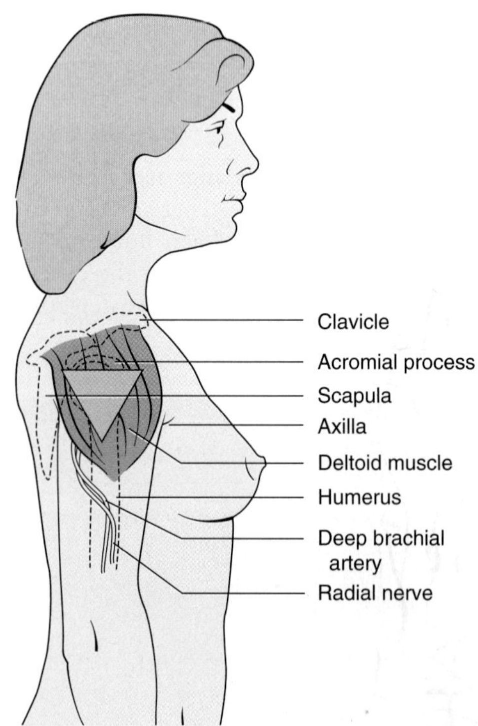

Figure 8-13 The deltoid muscle site for intramuscular injections is located by palpating the lower edge of the acromial process. At the midpoint, in line with the axilla on the lateral aspect of the upper arm, a triangle is formed.

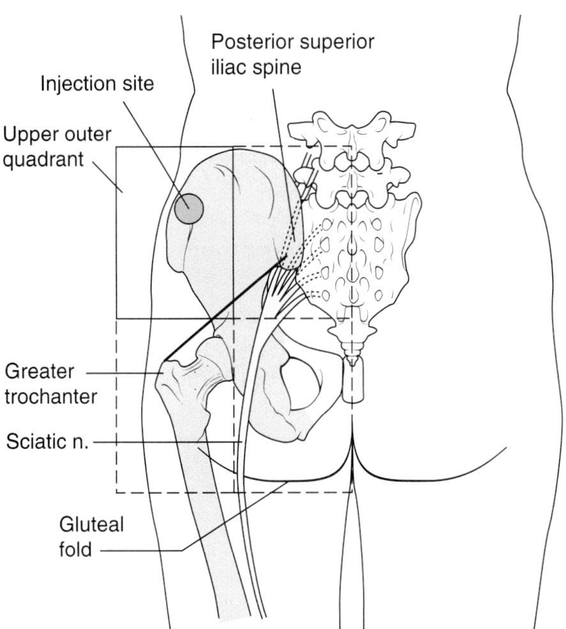

Figure 8-14 The dorsogluteal site for administering an intramuscular injection is lateral and slightly superior to the midpoint of a line drawn from the trochanter to the posterior superior iliac spine. Correct identification of this site minimizes the possibility of accidentally damaging the sciatic nerve.

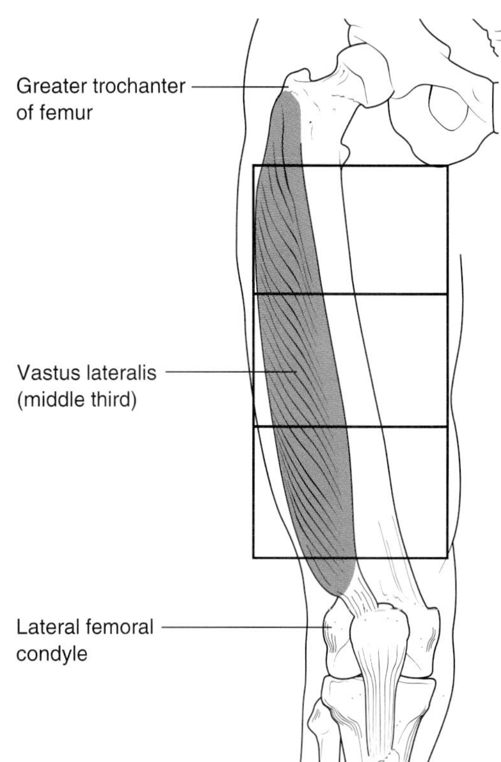

Figure 8-16 The vastus lateralis site for intramuscular injections is identified by dividing the thigh into thirds horizontally and vertically. The injection is given in the outer middle third.

Intramuscular Injections

Intramuscular (IM) injections are given into a muscle by positioning the needle and syringe at a 90-degree angle to the skin (see Fig. 8-12). Absorption of IM medications is fairly rapid because of the vascularity of

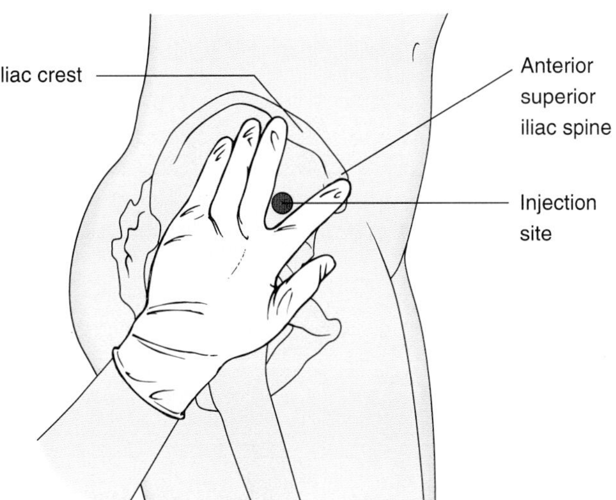

Figure 8-15 The ventrogluteal site is located by placing the palm on the greater trochanter and the index finger toward the anterior superior iliac spine. The middle finger is then spread posteriorly away from the index finger as far as possible. A "V" or triangle is formed by this maneuver. The injection is made in the middle of the triangle.

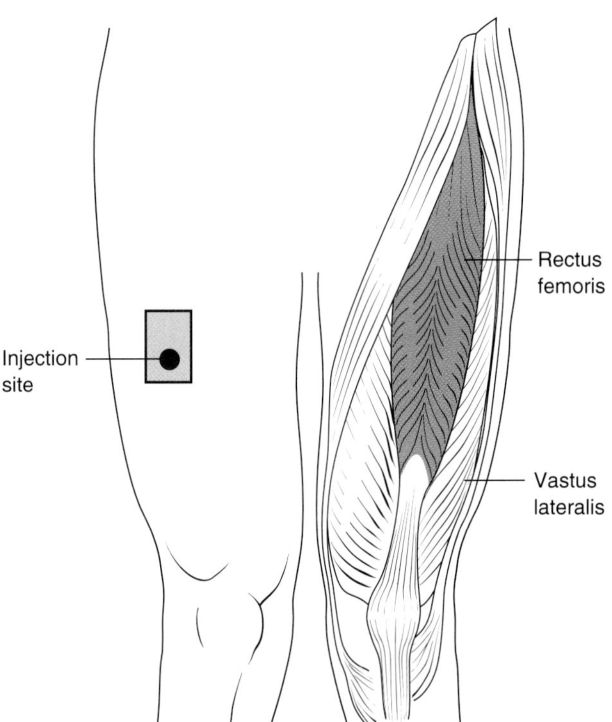

Figure 8-17 The rectus femoris site for intramuscular injections is used only when other sites are contraindicated.

muscle tissues. If absorption needs to be slower, the medication will be supplied mixed with an oil base rather than saline or water to prolong the absorption time.

Recommended sites include the deltoid (Fig. 8-13), dorsogluteal (Fig. 8-14), ventrogluteal (Fig. 8-15), and vastus lateralis (Fig. 8-16). The rectus femoris (Fig. 8-17) can also be used for giving IM injections but only when using the other sites is contraindicated. (It is recommended that no more than 1 mL be administered in the deltoid site.)

Procedure 8-9 describes the steps for administering an IM injection.

Z-Track Method of Intramuscular Injection

This method is used for IM administration of medications that may irritate or damage the tissues if allowed to leak back along the line of injection (Procedure 8-10). The Z-track method prevents leakage by sealing off the layers of skin along the route of the needle (Fig. 8-18).

If the medication is extremely caustic, directions may include changing the needle after drawing up the solution. The additional precaution of drawing up to

text continues on page 191

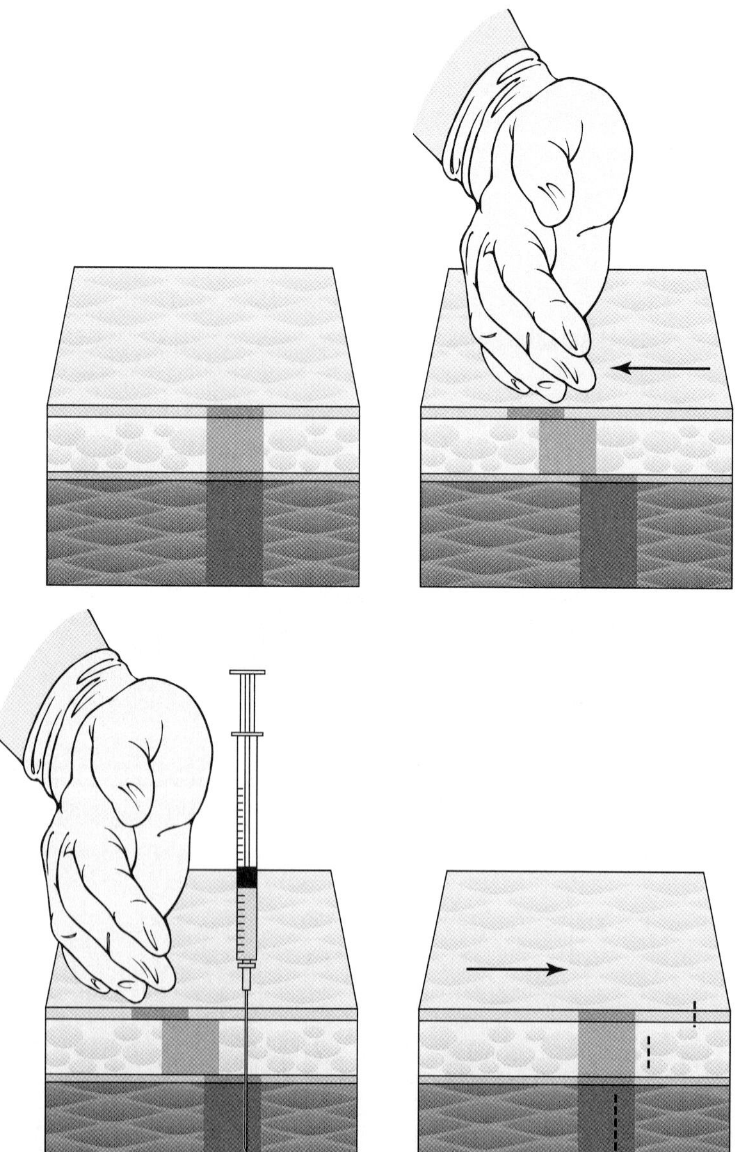

Figure 8-18 The Z-track technique is used to administer medications that are irritating to subcutaneous tissue. The skin is pulled to one side, the needle is inserted, and the solution is injected after careful aspiration. When the needle is withdrawn and the displaced tissue is allowed to return to its normal position, the solution is prevented from escaping from the muscle tissue.

Procedure 8-6 Administering an Intradermal Injection

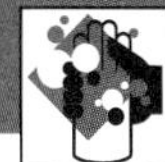
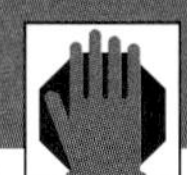
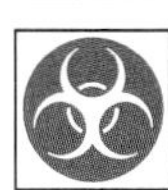

PURPOSE:

To administer medications to identify allergies and sensitivities

EQUIPMENT/SUPPLIES

- medication
- medication tray
- antiseptic wipe
- appropriate-sized needle and syringe (generally a ⅜-inch 26–28-gauge needle on a tuberculin syringe to administer 0.1–0.2 mL)
- physician's instructions
- gloves

8

STEPS

1. Prepare the injection according to the steps in Procedure 8-5.
2. Greet and identify the patient. Explain the procedure. Ask the patient about medication allergies that might not be noted on the chart.
   Allergies may exist that have not been noted.
3. Select the appropriate site for the injection. Recommended sites are the anterior forearm and the middle of the back. Make sure the entire site is exposed for safety and accuracy.
4. Prepare the site by cleansing with an antiseptic wipe. Use a circular motion starting at the injection site and working outward. Do not touch the site after cleaning. If the site is grossly contaminated, wash it first with soap and water, then clean with an antiseptic wipe.
   The site must be prepared by first removing microorganisms from the area. Wiping in a circular motion will carry the microorganisms away from the site. Touching the site after cleaning it will cause contamination.
5. Put on gloves.
6. Remove the needle guard. Using your nondominant hand, pull the patient's skin taut.
   Stretching the skin allows the needle to enter the skin with less resistance and secures the patient against movement.
7. With the bevel of the needle facing up, insert the needle at a 10- to 15-degree angle into the upper layer of the skin. When correctly placed for an intradermal injection, the needle will be slightly visible below the surface of the skin. It is not necessary to aspirate when performing an intradermal injection.
   The needle should be inserted almost parallel to the skin to ensure that penetration occurs within the dermal layer. The bevel of the needle facing up will allow the wheal to be formed. If the bevel faces downward, no wheal will be formed and the medication may be absorbed into the tissues.

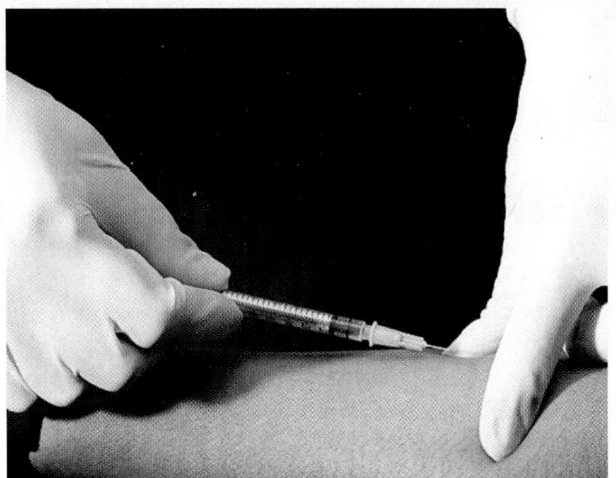

8. Release the skin held in the nondominant hand and secure the needle hub with the thumb and forefinger. Inject the medication slowly by depressing the plunger. A wheal will form as the medication enters the dermal layer of the skin. Hold the syringe steady for proper administration.
   Moving the needle once it has penetrated the skin will cause the patient to experience discomfort.

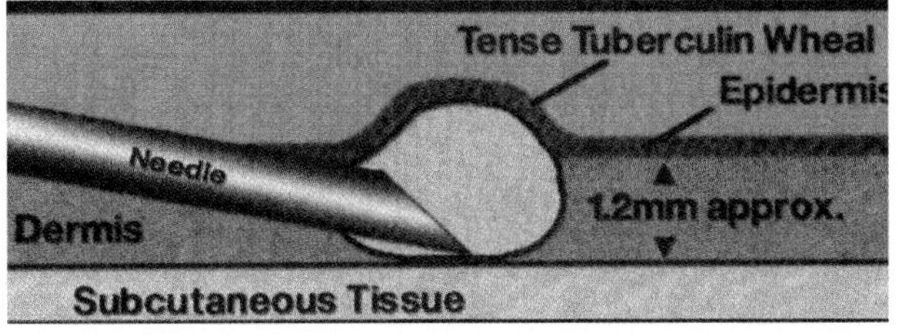

9. Remove the needle from the skin at the same angle at which it was inserted. Gently hold an antiseptic wipe over the site as the needle is withdrawn. Do not press or massage the site.
   Withdrawing the needle quickly and gently at the angle of insertion reduces the chance of discomfort. Pressure on the wheal may cause the medication to be pressed into the tissues or out of the line of injection.

continued

Procedure 8-6 Continued **Administering an Intradermal Injection**

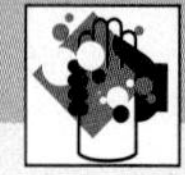
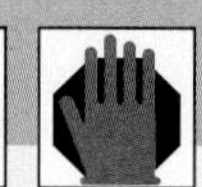

10. Dispose of the syringe and the needle in the approved container. Do not recap the needle. The sharps container should be placed where you have easy access to it after administration of an injection.
    Discarding without recapping helps reduce the risk of an accidental needle stick.
11. Caution the patient not to massage the site.
    Medication is not to be distributed into the tissues.
12. Remove gloves and wash your hands.
13. Remain with the patient following the administration of an intradermal injection to observe for any unusual reactions. *Note:* If the patient experiences any unusual reactions, notify the physician immediately.
14. Depending on the type of skin test administered, the length of time required for the body tissues to react, and the policies of the medical office, perform one of the following:
    a. Read the test results. Inspect and palpate the site for the presence and amount of induration.
    b. Tell the patient when to return (date and time) to the office to have the results read.
    c. Instruct the patient to read the results at home. Make sure the patient understands the instructions. Have the patient repeat the instructions if necessary.

DOCUMENTATION GUIDELINES

- Date and time
- Medication name
- Dose
- Location of injection
- Reactions to medication as needed
- Patient education and instructions for returning or reading results
- Your signature

Charting Example

DATE	TIME Allergy testing administered × 14
	across scapular area. Dr. Gray assessed
	reaction. Pt tolerated procedure well. To
	RTC in 3 days to begin immune therapy for
	allergies. —Your signature

Procedure 8-7 **Administering a Tine or Mantoux Test**

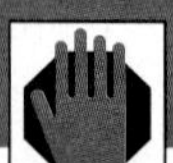

PURPOSE:

To test for sensitivity to the tuberculin bacillus

EQUIPMENT/SUPPLIES

- tine applicator or tuberculin syringe with ⅜–½-inch, 26–27-gauge needle with 0.1 mL purified protein derivative
- millimeter ruler
- acetone wipe or alcohol wipe
- gloves

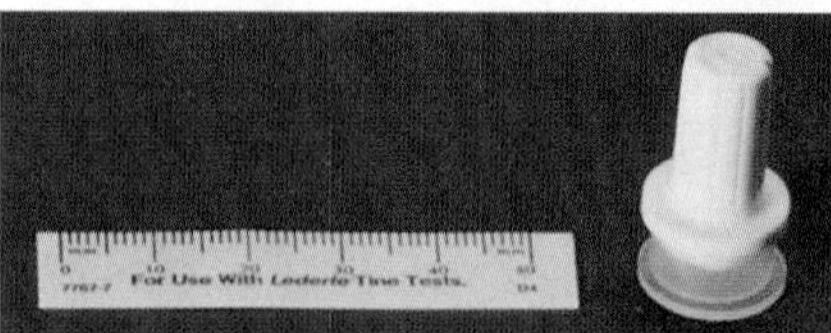

Tine applicator and millimeter ruler.

STEPS

1. Wash your hands.
2. For the tine test, obtain the tine applicator. For the Mantoux test, prepare the injection according to the steps in Procedure 8-5.
3. Greet and identify the patient. Explain the procedure.
4. Assess the area of the forearm about 4 inches below the antecubital area.
    Do this to ensure that the traditional site is appropriate and free of lesions.

continued

Procedure 8-7 Continued Administering a Tine or Mantoux Test

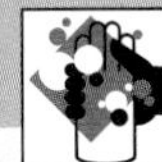
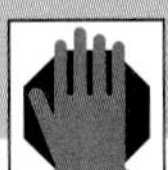

5. Clean the area with outward, circular strokes with the acetone wipe. Allow to dry.
   Cleaning from the area of injection outward carries the microorganisms away from the site. Allowing the area to dry prevents inoculation with the antiseptic. Acetone dries quickly, but alcohol may be used if allowed to dry completely.
6. Put on gloves.
7. Grasp the forearm with the nondominant hand to stretch the skin, secure the site, and make it easier to pierce the skin.
   a. *For the Mantoux test:*
      Follow steps 7–9 of Procedure 8-6, Administering an Intradermal Injection.
      The PPD must be inserted into the intradermal layer of the skin.
   b. *For the Tine test:*
      Uncap the tester and press it into the skin.
      The sharp tines of the tester must pierce the surface of the skin to introduce the PPD into the intradermal layer.
      Hold for 1–2 seconds, release the tension on the skin, and remove the tester.

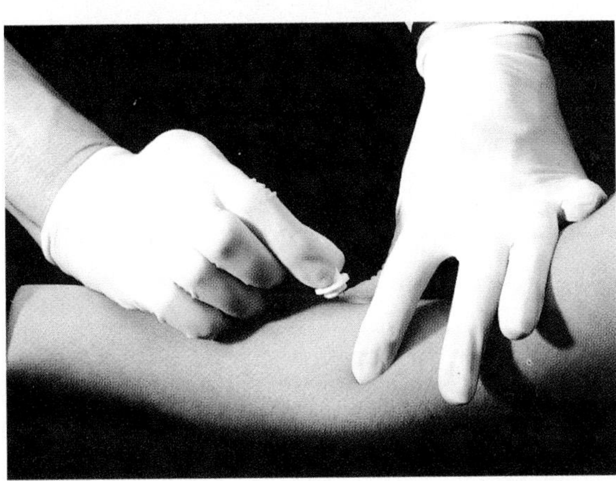

8. Do not massage the site in either method. Cover the site gently and briefly with an alcohol wipe but do not press or wipe.
   The testing material may be pressed into the lower layers or along the lines of injection.
9. Properly care for or dispose of equipment and supplies. Remove gloves and wash your hands.
10. Advise the patient regarding returning for evaluation of the test or give instructions regarding the evaluation card to be completed in 48–72 hours and returned by mail. *Note:* If the patient is to return for evaluation of the test, read the results in a good light with the arm slightly flexed. Palpate from the outside area to the center of induration and measure using a millimeter ruler. Disregard erythema and measure only the area of induration. Record the results.
   Results must be documented.

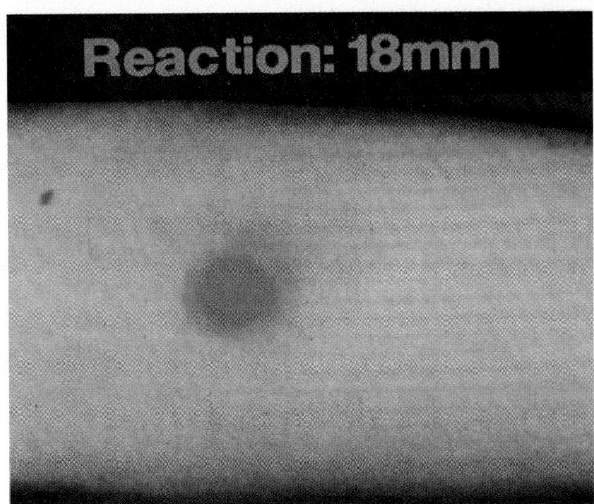

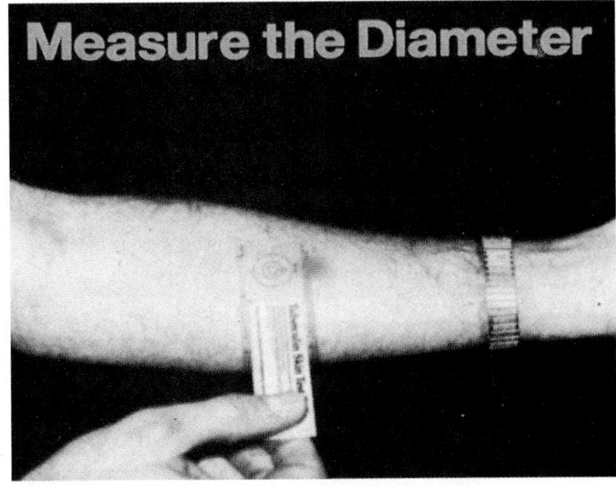

DOCUMENTATION GUIDELINES

- Date and time
- Medication name
- Dose
- Location of injection
- Reactions to the medication as needed
- Patient education and instructions for returning or reading results
- Your signature

Charting Example

DATE	TIME Mantoux test with PPD 0.1 mL Id
	in L anterior forearm. Pt instructed to
	return in 2 days for assessment of site,
	verbalized understanding of instructions.
	—Your signature

8

Procedure 8-8 Administering a Subcutaneous Injection

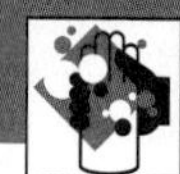

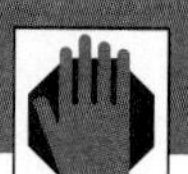

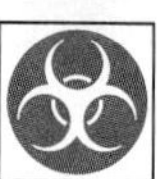

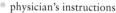

PURPOSE:

To provide medication by the route most appropriate for optimum medication metabolism with minimal patient discomfort

To provide a slower response than expected from an intramuscular injection of medication

EQUIPMENT/SUPPLIES

- medication
- medication tray
- antiseptic wipe
- appropriate-sized needle and syringe (generally a ½–⅝-inch, 24–28-gauge needle on a regular 2–3-mL syringe or tuberculin syringe)
- physician's instructions
- gloves

STEPS

1. Prepare the injection according to the steps in Procedure 8-5.
2. Greet and identify the patient. Explain the procedure. Ask the patient about medication allergies that might not be noted on the chart.
   Allergies may exist that have not been noted.
3. Select the appropriate site for the injection. The upper arm, thigh, back, and abdomen are common sites for subcutaneous injections. Make sure the entire site is exposed for accuracy and safety.
   Constricting clothing may cause an error in site identification.
4. Put on gloves.
5. Prepare the site by cleansing with an antiseptic wipe. Use a circular motion starting at the injection site and working outward. Do not touch the site after cleaning. If the site is grossly contaminated, wash it first with soap and water, then clean with an antiseptic wipe.
   The site must be prepared by first removing microorganisms from the area. Wiping in a circular motion will carry microorganisms away from the site. Touching the site after cleaning it will cause contamination.

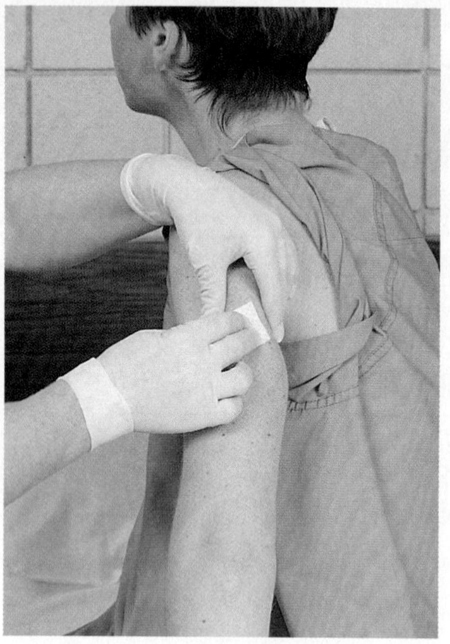

6. Remove the needle guard. Using the nondominant hand, hold the skin surrounding the injection site in a cushion fashion.
   Holding the skin up and away from the underlying muscle will ensure entrance into the subcutaneous tissues. Proper technique will help ensure that the subcutaneous tissue, not the muscle, is entered.

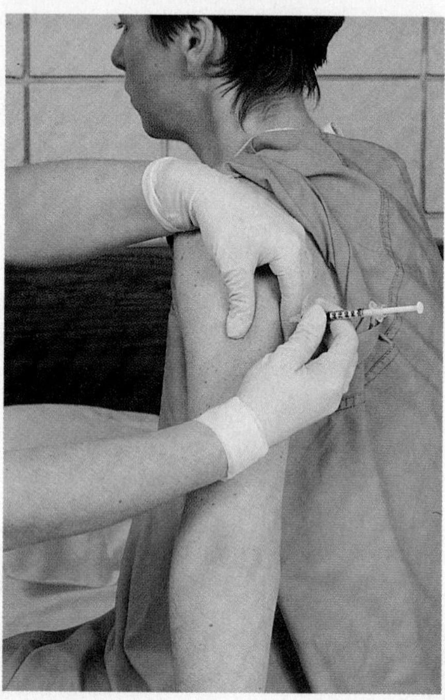

continued

Procedure 8-8 Continued Administering a Subcutaneous Injection

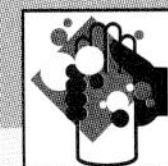
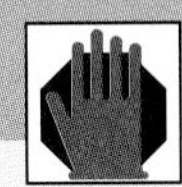

7. With a firm motion, insert the needle into the tissue at a 45-degree angle to the skin. Hold the barrel between the thumb and index finger of the dominant hand, and insert the needle up to the hub into the tissue.

   A quick, firm motion is less painful to the patient. Full insertion ensures that the medication is inserted into the proper tissue.

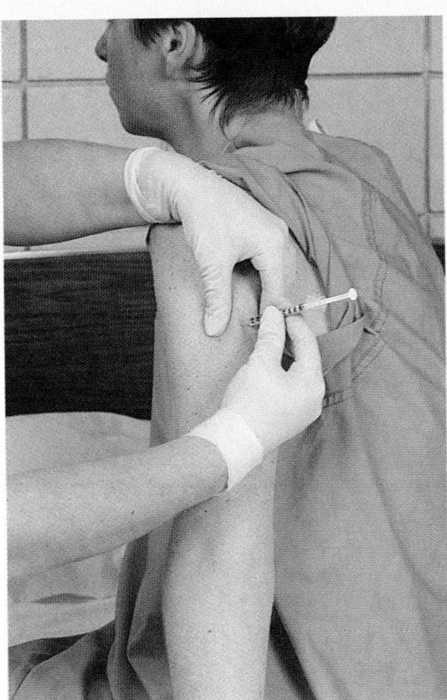

8. Remove your nondominant hand from the skin.

   Removing your hand will prevent medication from being injected into compressed tissue, which causes pressure against nerve fibers and increases discomfort to the patient.

9. With the thumb and forefinger of the nondominant hand on the hub of the needle to hold the syringe steady, pull back on the plunger slightly. If blood appears in the syringe, a vessel has been entered. If this occurs, prepare a new injection and repeat steps 4–9.

   Moving the syringe will cause discomfort to the patient. If medication intended for subcutaneous administration is administered into a vessel, the medication can be absorbed too quickly, producing undesirable results.

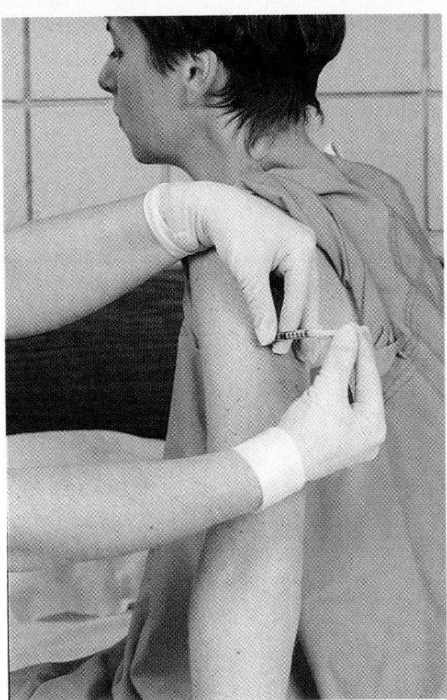

10. Inject the medication slowly and steadily by depressing the plunger.

    If the medication is injected rapidly, pressure is created which will cause patient discomfort and may cause tissue damage.

continued

Procedure 8-8 Continued Administering a Subcutaneous Injection

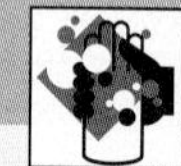
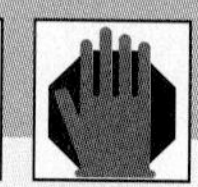

11. Place an antiseptic wipe over the injection site, and remove the needle at the same angle at which it was injected.

Withdrawing the needle quickly and at the same angle reduces patient discomfort. The antiseptic wipe helps prevent tissue movement when the needle is withdrawn.

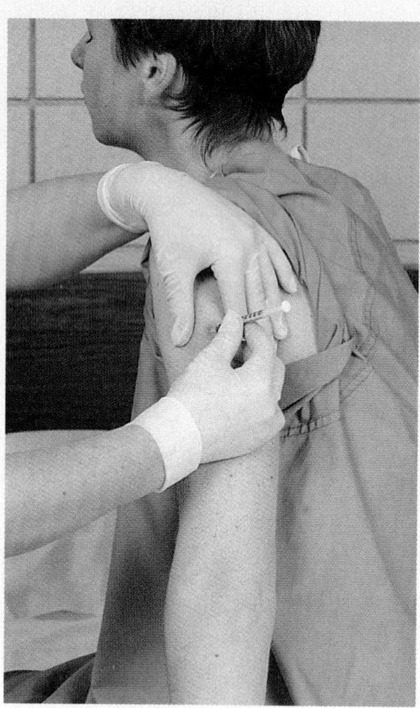

12. Properly dispose of the syringe and needle into an approved sharps container. Do not recap the needle. The sharps container should be placed where you have easy access to it after giving the injection.

Discarding without recapping helps reduce the risk of an accidental needle stick.

13. Gently massage the injection site with the antiseptic wipe. Apply pressure to the site and cover with an adhesive bandage if needed. Heparin, sometimes given subcutaneously, is not massaged because it may cause excessive bleeding into the site.

Massaging helps distribute the medication into the tissues so that it can be more completely absorbed.

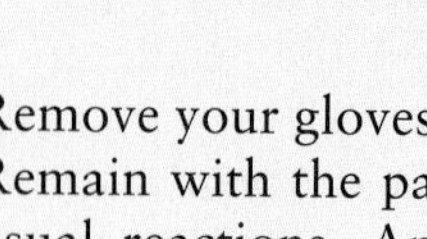

14. Remove your gloves and wash your hands.

15. Remain with the patient to observe for any unusual reactions. An injection given for allergy desensitization requires that the patient remain in the office for at least 30 minutes to be observed for a reaction. Assist the patient from the examination table if necessary. *Note:* If the patient experiences any unusual reactions, notify the physician immediately.

Patients may become faint after an injection or may have an adverse reaction to the medication. Reactions to allergy injections may build over time and may cause anaphylaxis.

DOCUMENTATION GUIDELINES

- Date and time
- Medication name
- Dose
- Location of injection
- Reactions to the medication as needed
- Patient education/instructions
- Your signature

Charting Example

DATE	TIME 0.5 mL of Vial A allergy medication
	administered subq L upper arm. Pt
	displayed no erythema or other
	symptoms at 30 minutes. Pt d/c to
	return for continuing series in 2 days.
	—Your signature

Procedure 8-9 Administering an Intramuscular Injection

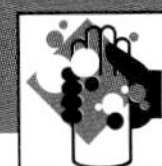
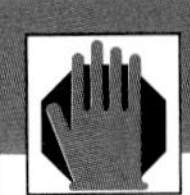

PURPOSE:

To provide medication by the route most appropriate for optimum medication metabolism with minimal discomfort
To provide a more rapid response than most other medication administration methods

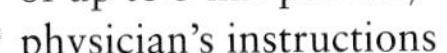

EQUIPMENT/SUPPLIES

- medication
- medication tray
- antiseptic wipe
- appropriate-sized needle and syringe (generally a 1–2 inch, 20–23-gauge regular 2–5-mL syringes for the injection of up to 3 mL per site)
- physician's instructions
- gloves

8

STEPS

1. Prepare the injection according to the steps in Procedure 8-5.
2. Greet and identify the patient. Explain the procedure. Ask the patient about medication allergies that might not be noted on the chart.
   Allergies may exist that have not been noted.
3. Select the appropriate site for the injection (see Figs. 8-14 through 8-18) and the appropriate syringe.
   Major nerves and blood vessels may lie near the sites for intramuscular injections. Skill and accuracy are crucial to avoid injury to the patient.

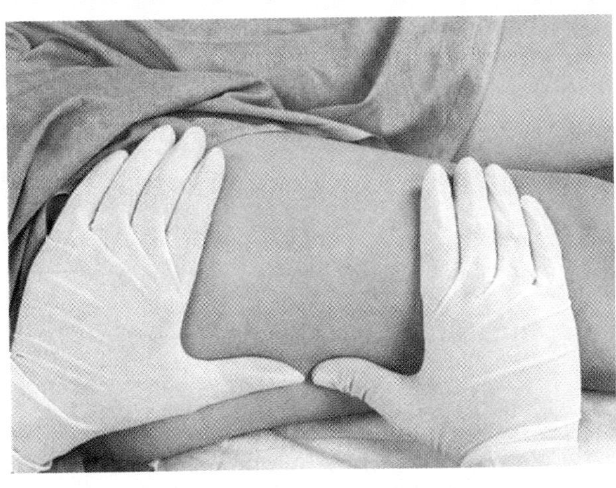

4. Prepare the site by cleansing with an antiseptic wipe. Use a circular motion starting at the injection site and working outward. Do not touch the site after cleaning. If the site is grossly contaminated, wash it first with soap and water, then clean with an antiseptic wipe.
   The site must be prepared by first removing microorganisms from the area. Wiping in a circular motion will carry the microorganisms away from the site. Touching the site after cleaning it will cause contamination.
5. Put on gloves.
6. Remove the needle guard. Pull the skin taut over the injection site using the thumb and index fingers of the nondominant hand. *Note:* Patients with meager muscle mass may require that you grasp the muscle and "bunch" it to ensure that the medication is inserted as deeply into the area as possible.
   Pulling the skin taut allows for easier insertion of the needle and helps ensure that the needle enters muscle tissue. "Bunching" the muscle affords a deeper mass in a very thin patient.
7. Hold the syringe like a dart. Using a quick, firm motion, insert the needle at a 90-degree angle to the skin.
   A quick, firm motion causes the patient less discomfort. A 90-degree angle ensures that the medication is injected into muscle tissue.
8. With the thumb and forefinger of the nondominant hand, hold the syringe steady, pull back slightly on the plunger with the dominant hand. If blood appears in the syringe, you must prepare a new injection and repeat steps 4–8.
   Moving the syringe will cause discomfort to the patient. If the medication intended for an intramuscular injection is injected into a vessel, it will be absorbed too quickly, producing undesirable results.
9. Slowly inject the medication by steadily depressing the plunger of the syringe.
   If the medication is injected too rapidly, it will cause discomfort and may cause tissue damage.
10. Place an antiseptic wipe over the injection site. Remove the needle quickly and at the same angle at which it was inserted.
    Withdrawing the needle quickly and at the same angle reduces patient discomfort. The antiseptic wipe helps prevent tissue movement when the needle is withdrawn.
11. Properly dispose of the needle and syringe in an approved sharps container. Do not recap the needle. The sharps container should be placed where you have easy access to it after the injection has been administered.
    Discarding the needle without recapping helps reduce the risk of an accidental needle stick.

continued

Procedure 8-9 Continued **Administering an Intramuscular Injection**

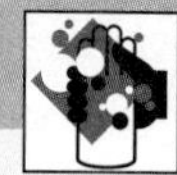
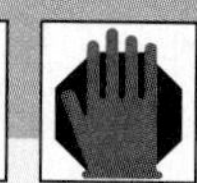

12. Gently massage the injection site with an antiseptic wipe. Apply pressure to the site and cover with an adhesive bandage if needed.

Massaging helps distribute the medication into the tissues for better absorption.

13. Remove gloves and wash your hands.

14. Remain with the patient to observe for any unusual reactions. Assist the patient off the examination table if necessary. *Note:* If the patient experiences any unusual reaction, notify the physician immediately.

Medications given intramuscularly may react quickly. The patient must be observed for reaction to the drug effects. Some patients become faint after injections.

DOCUMENTATION GUIDELINES

- Date and time
- Medication name
- Dose
- Location of injection
- Reactions to the medication as needed
- Patient complaints/concerns
- Patient education/instructions
- Your signature

✓Charting Example

DATE	TIME Penicillin 200,000u administered
	IM in L dorsogluteal area by order of
	Dr. Fleming. No redness or swelling at site
	at 30 minute assessment. Pt d/c to
	return for reck in 12 days. —Your signature

Procedure 8-10 **Administrating an Intramuscular Injection Using the Z-Track Method**

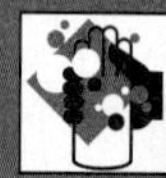
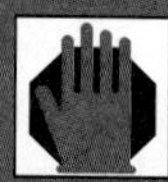

PURPOSE:

To provide medication by the route most appropriate for optimum medication metabolism with minimal discomfort

To provide a more rapid response than most other medication administration methods

EQUIPMENT/SUPPLIES

- medication
- medication tray
- antiseptic wipe
- appropriate-sized needle and syringe
- physician's instructions
- gloves

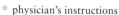

STEPS

1–5. Follow steps 1–5 as described in Procedure 8-9, Administering an Intramuscular Injection. *Note:* The ventrogluteal, vastus lateralis, and dorsogluteal sites work well for the Z-track method; the deltoid does not.

6. Remove the needle guard. Rather than pulling the skin taut or grasping the tissue as you would for an intramuscular injection, pull the top layer of skin to the side and hold it with the nondominant hand.

By displacing the top layer of skin, the puncture route will be sealed when the layers of tissue slide back to their proper alignment.

7. Insert the needle to the hub at a 90-degree angle in a quick, dartlike motion.

8. With the side of the nondominant hand holding the displaced skin, grasp the hub of the needle with the thumb and forefinger and aspirate by withdrawing the plunger slightly with the dominant hand. If no blood appears, push the plunger in slowly and steadily. Count to 10 before withdrawing the needle.

This allows time for the tissues to begin absorption of the medication.

9. Cover the area with an antiseptic wipe. Withdraw the needle and release the skin. Most Z-track medications must not be massaged to avoid forcing the medication into upper tissues. Check the manufacturer's guidelines.

10. Properly dispose of the needle and syringe in an approved sharps container. Do not recap the

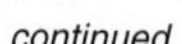
continued

Procedure 8-10 Continued Administrating an Intramuscular Injection Using the Z-Track Method

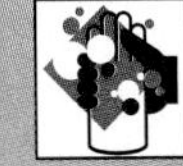
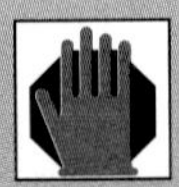

needle. The sharps container should be placed where you have easy access to it after the injection has been administered.

Discarding without recapping helps reduce the risk of an accidental needle stick.

11. Remove gloves and wash your hands.
12. Remain with the patient to observe for any unusual reactions. Assist the patient off of the examination table if necessary. *Note:* If the patient experiences any unusual reaction, notify the physician immediately.

    Medications given intramuscularly may react quickly. The patient must be observed for reaction to the drug effects. Some patients become faint after injections.

DOCUMENTATION GUIDELINES

- Date and time
- Medication name
- Dose
- Location of injection
- Reactions to the medication as needed
- Patient complaints/concerns
- Patient education/instructions
- Your signature

Charting Example

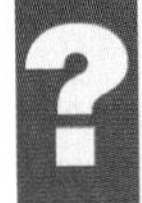

DATE	TIME Imferon 150 mg by Z-track in R
	dorsogluteal area by order of Dr. Lupton.
	No local reaction or staining noted.
	—Your signature

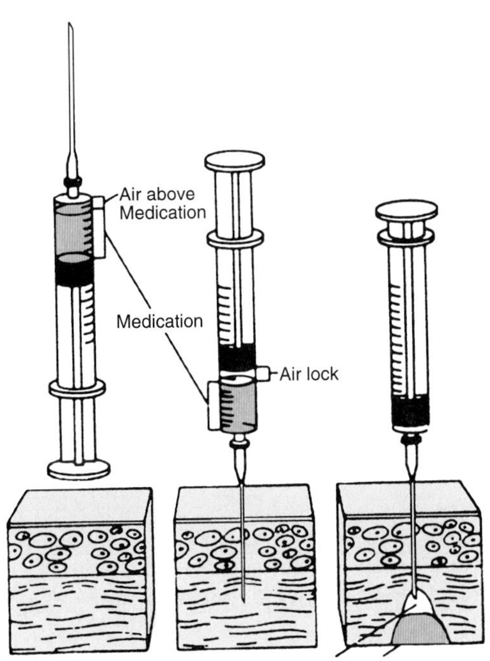

Figure 8-19 An air bubble added to the syringe after the medication has been accurately measured helps to expel solution that is trapped in the shaft of the needle when the injection is given. It also helps to trap the injected solution in the intramuscular tissue.

0.5 cc air into the syringe may be required. When the medication is injected at a 90-degree angle, the additional air will rise to the top of the syringe and be injected after the medication. This will clear the needle and the path of the injection (Fig. 8-19).

The ventrogluteal, vastus lateralis, and dorsogluteal sites work well for the Z-track method; the deltoid does not.

Checkpoint Question

7. *Name the types of injections. List possible sites for each type of injection.*

OTHER MEDICATION ROUTES

Inhalation

Inhalation involves administration of medications, water vapors, or gases by inspiration of the substance(s) into the lungs. Medication is absorbed quickly through the alveolar walls into the capillaries. Existing pathology may make absorption difficult to predict. Patients with chronic pulmonary conditions may self-administer

8

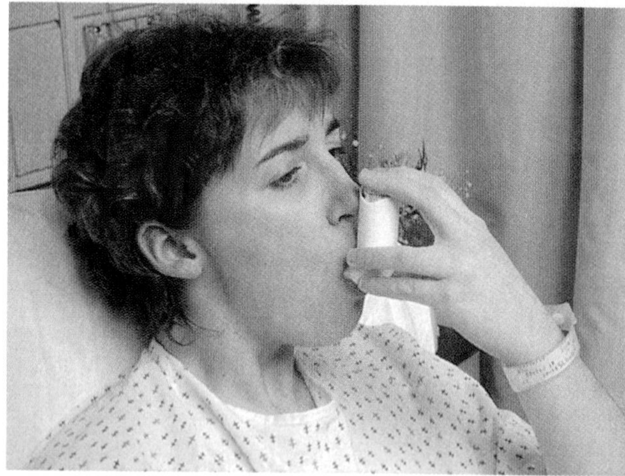

Figure 8-20 Nebulizer. A bottle of medication is attached to a mouthpiece. After the patient exhales, the mouthpiece is gripped with the lips, and while the patient takes a deep inhalation slowly, the bottle is firmly pushed down on the mouthpiece to release one dose of medication. (Photo © Ken Kasper.)

the medication with a hand-held **nebulizer,** which is an apparatus for producing a fine spray of medicated mist (Fig. 8-20).

Intravenous

With this route, a sterile solution of a drug is injected into the body by venipuncture; larger amounts of medication in solution may be administered intravenously than by most other methods. Intravenous medication has the quickest action because it enters the bloodstream immediately. Only drugs intended for intravenous administration should be given by this route.

Intravenous medications are NEVER administered by medical assistants; physicians, nurses, or paramedics may administer intravenous medications.

Intra-arterial

Medications given using this route are administered into an artery and will have immediate effects. This method will never be used by medical assistants.

Intrathecal

Medication administered intrathecally is injected into the space within the spinal meninges. This route is usually confined to methods of anesthesia or analgesia.

Intra-articular

Medication given by this route is administered into a joint space. This route is used exclusively for treatment of joint pain.

Intraosseus

Infusions of medications, fluids, or blood are made by the physician directly into the marrow (usually the tibia in children) in emergency situations when intravenous access is not an option.

Answers to Checkpoint Questions

1. *The three checks are performed when the medication is taken from the shelf, when it is poured, and when it is put back on the shelf.*
2. *The three systems used to measure medications are the metric, apothecary, and household systems. Household measurements, which are often used by patients, should be avoided because they are inaccurate.*
3. *To calculate dosages accurately, you must ensure that the measurements are in the same system (either metric or apothecary) and in the same unit of measurement.*
4. *Oral medication typically takes effect slowly. Also, the oral route cannot be used for patients who are unconscious, for those with nausea and vomiting, and for those who are NPO.*
5. *Topical medications produce local effects; transdermal medications have systemic effects.*
6. *Ampules and vials are medication containers. An ampule is a glass container with a narrow neck; it must be broken to obtain the medication, which is in solution form. A vial is a glass or plastic container sealed with a rubber stopper; it contains medication in either solution or in dry form (eg, powder or crystals).*
7. *Types of injections include intradermal, subcutaneous, and intramuscular. Sites for intradermal injections include the anterior forearm and the back. Sites for subcutaneous injections include the upper arm, thigh, back, and abdomen. Sites for intramuscular injections include the deltoid, ventrogluteal, and vastus lateralis; the rectus femoris is used only when the other sites are contraindicated.*

Critical Thinking Challenges

1. Create a conversion chart that you can carry with you to help with converting between the metric and apothecary systems.
2. Design a patient education brochure that will teach patients about taking oral medications.
3. You are giving an intramuscular injection. After inserting the needle, you aspirate by pulling back slightly on the plunger. As you do this, blood appears in the syringe. What has happened? What should you do?

Suggestions for Further Reading

Boyer, M. J. (1994). *Math for Nurses: A Pocket Guide to Dosage Calculation and Drug Administration,* 3rd ed. Philadelphia: J.B. Lippincott.

Craven, R. F., & Hirnle, C. J. (1996). *Fundamentals of Nursing: Health and Human Function,* 2nd ed. Philadelphia: Lippincott-Raven.

Dawe, R. (1993). *Math and Dosage Calculations for Health Occupations.* New York: Glencoe.

Henke, G. (1995). *Med-Math: Dosage Calculation, Preparation and Administration,* 2nd ed. Philadelphia: J.B. Lippincott.

Kozier, B., & Erb, G. (1993). *Techniques of Clinical Nursing,* 3rd ed. Redwood City, CA: Addison-Wesley.

Lane, K. (1992). *Medications: A Guide for the Health Professions.* Philadelphia: F.A. Davis.

Scherer, J. C., & Roach, S. S. (1995). *Introductory Clinical Pharmacology,* 5th ed. Philadelphia: J.B. Lippincott.

Smeltzer, S. C., & Bare, B. G. (1996). *Brunner and Suddarth's Textbook of Medical-Surgical Nursing,* 8th ed. Philadelphia: Lippincott-Raven.

Taylor, C., Lillis, C., & LeMone, P. (1997). *Fundamentals of Nursing: The Art and Science of Nursing Care,* 3rd ed. Philadelphia: Lippincott-Raven.

Timby, B. (1996). *Fundamental Skills and Concepts in Patient Care,* 6th ed. Philadelphia: Lippincott-Raven.

Unit 2

Assisting With Diagnostic and Therapeutic Procedures

9

Introduction to Anatomy and Physiology

Chapter Outline

Organization of the Body
- Chemicals
- Cells
- Tissues
- Organs
- Body Systems

General Plan of the Body
- Anatomic Position
- Body Planes
- Locations and Positions
- Body Cavities
- Areas and Regions

Homeostasis

Chapter Competencies

Learning Objectives

Upon successfully completing this chapter, you will be able to:

1. Spell and define the Key Terms.
2. Describe in ascending order the organization of the body, beginning at the atomic level and advancing to the systemic level.
3. Describe a cell and its components.
4. List the nine abdominal regions and name the organs included in each.
5. List the body cavities and their contents.
6. Describe the systems, the organs involved in each system, and the function of each system.
7. Define the anatomic position.
8. Explain the meaning of the terms homeostasis and positive and negative feedback.

Key Terms

(See Glossary for definitions.)

abdominal regions
anatomic position
anatomy
cell
element
homeostasis
negative feedback
organ
physiology
planes
positive feedback
quadrants
system
tissues

To function effectively in the medical field, you will need an understanding of the human body and how it works. To achieve this goal, you must study the body's normal structures and functions. Anatomy refers to the study of the body's structure; **physiology** is the study of the body's functions. Knowledge of the body in its normal state will enable you to evaluate and understand abnormal conditions observed and described in the medical practice.

ORGANIZATION OF THE BODY

Beginning at the most basic atomic structure, the body progresses through levels of organization that interact to maintain the functions necessary for life (Fig. 9-1).

Chemicals

The atom is the smallest component of an **element** that contains the physical properties of that element. An element is a substance made up of only one type of atom. For example, iron is an element. It may be broken down into individual iron atoms, but no other type of atom will be contained in the element. Everything in the world is made up of atoms in a multitude of arrangements.

An atom consists of a *nucleus* with positively charged *protons* and usually an equal number of neutral particles called *neutrons*. These are orbited by negatively charged *electrons* (Fig. 9-2). Positives and negatives attract each other, each possessing a property that the other needs. This attraction keeps the protons and electrons in constant motion and holds them close in an arrangement that resembles a galaxy with a sun (the nucleus) and orbiting planets (the electrons).

Each of the more than 100 elements currently identified (eg, iron, calcium, phosphorus, and so on) has a specific number of protons, neutrons, and electrons. The numbers are always consistent for each atom to be identified as a particular element. Each atom is given a number based on the number of protons in the nucleus. No other atom will have this number of protons. For instance, all hydrogen atoms have one proton and one electron, all carbon atoms have six of each, and all oxygen atoms have eight of each.

Each atomic element is also designated by a symbol (Table 9-1). The symbol may be an abbreviation of the element's name, such as O for oxygen or H for hydrogen. Or it may be an abbreviation of the element's Latin name, such as Fe for iron (from the Latin ferrum) or K for potassium (from the Latin kalium).

The arrangement of the atoms within their structure is consistent, with electrons always orbiting the nucleus in a certain pattern. The first orbit around the nucleus will hold only two electrons and the concentric orbits beyond will hold up to eight. If the outer orbit has fewer than eight electrons, the atom will look for another with fewer than eight to complete the outer orbit. If the atoms attracted to each other completely share the outer eight, they will form a very stable union. For example, sodium has an arrangement of 2-8-1 and chloride has 2-8-7, which means that chloride needs one electron to complete its outer orbit and sodium needs seven. When these two elements meet, they bond and become the very stable molecule known as sodium chloride or salt. A molecule is the combination of two or more atoms usually into something other than the original element.

To maintain life functions, atoms and molecules arrange and rearrange themselves constantly within the cells and the body fluids. The exchange of oxygen for carbon dioxide would not be possible nor would the transmission of nerve impulses or the release of body wastes without this effort to balance the normal composition of the internal environment. These minute elements are the basis of all physiologic functions within the body.

Cells

After the simplest structural level of the atom, combining then to the molecule, the body is organized in an orderly manner of ever-increasing complexity.

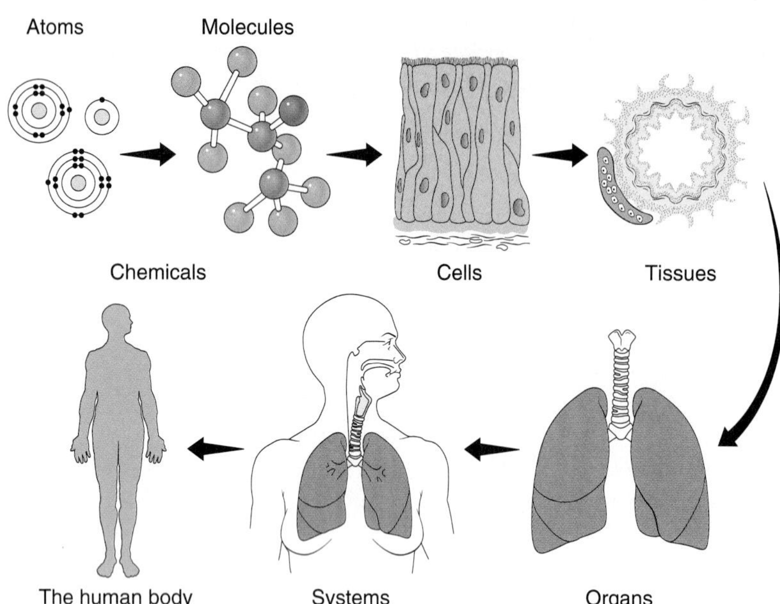

Figure 9-1 The body's level of structural organization.

9

The cell—the fundamental unit of all living tissue—is a complex arrangement of chemicals designed to carry out specific activities. Body cells range in size from the relatively large ovum, about the size of a period on this page (or 1000 μm), to the infinitely tiny red blood cells, which are only about 7.5 μm. Cell shapes range from the basic round shape normally associated with cells to the long nerve cells and multinucleated muscle cells.

Regardless of the shape, size, or function, each cell has three main parts: the cell membrane, the cytoplasm, and the nucleus.

Cell membranes are composed of phospholipids (phosphorus and fatty substances) and are selectively permeable. Selective permeability means that the cell membranes allow necessary substances to move in and wastes to move out, but the cytoplasm and the cell components are kept inside. Within the cell membrane is the cytoplasm, which contains the organelles (small organs) that move about and carry out the cell's functions (Fig. 9-3). If the cell is responsible for the manufacture of an enzyme or a hormone, the organelles are designed to create just that substance and no other. If the cell is responsible for the transmission of nerve impulses, its cellular components are designed for this purpose (Table 9-2).

The messages carried from one generation of cell to another are encoded in the deoxyribonucleic acid (DNA) contained within the nucleus and relayed to the

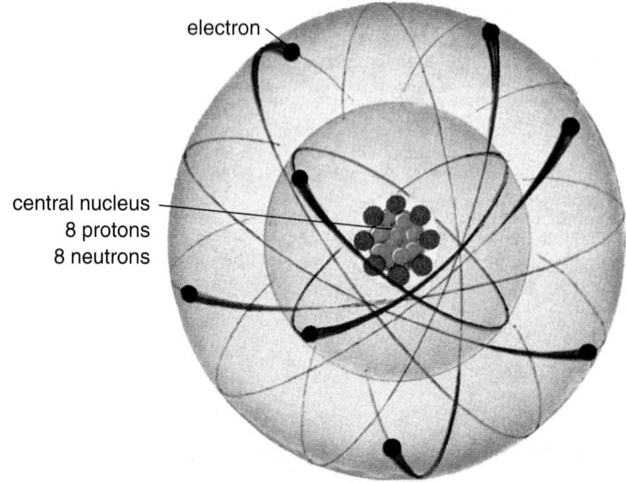

Figure 9-2 Representation of an oxygen atom. Eight protons and eight neutrons are tightly bound in the central nucleus, around which the eight electrons revolve.

Table 9-1 **Common Biochemical Elements**

Name	*Symbol*	*Atomic Number*
Hydrogen	H	1
Carbon	C	6
Nitrogen	N	7
Oxygen	O	8
Sodium	Na	11
Phosphorus	P	15
Sulfur	S	16
Chlorine	Cl	17
Potassium	K	19
Iron	Fe	26

These elements are essential to life. Our body functions depend on the interaction of their properties.

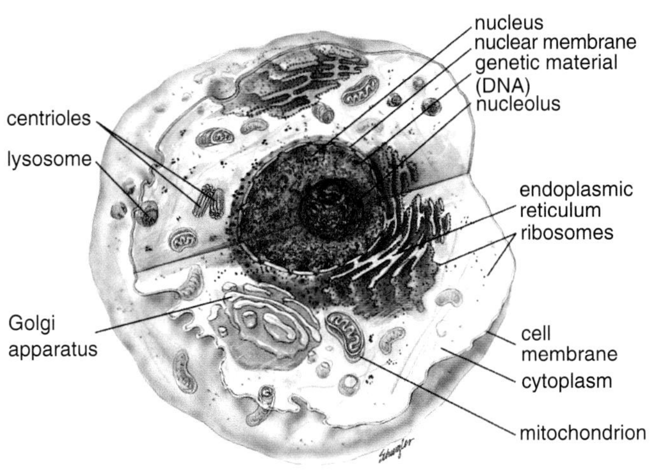

Figure 9-3 Diagram of a typical animal cell showing the main organelles.

organelles by the ribonucleic acid (RNA), which moves freely as a messenger from the nucleus to the cell parts. At each division, or reproduction cycle, of the cell (called *mitosis*), the information relating to that cell's functions will be carried by the DNA as it divides into two daughter cells. Functions of the cell include:

- Respiration
- Digestion of nutrients
- Elimination
- Energy production
- Reproduction

These functions, on a microscopic scale, are the same as those performed by the body.

Checkpoint Question

1. *What are the three main parts of the cell and their functions?*

Tissues

Body **tissues** are made up of a collection of similar cells and their supporting structures acting together to perform a particular function (Table 9-3). Tissues differ from each other by their cell shape and size, by the type and amount of supporting material between the cells, and by their specific functions. The four basic types of tissue are epithelial, connective, muscular, and nervous (Fig. 9-4).

9

Organs

An **organ** is more complex than a tissue and is formed by various tissues and cells working together to perform a specific function. For example, the heart is an organ made of special cardiac conduction cells formed into muscular tissue that work in a coordinated effort to pump blood throughout the body. Another example is the ovary, which is a collection of specialized cells capable of reproducing the species and contained within tissue designed to nurture and mature the cells as needed for ovulation.

Some organs are found in pairs, such as the kidneys and the lungs. Each one of the paired organs can function independently, if necessary, after injury or surgical removal of the organ. The liver, pancreas,

Table 9-2 **Cell Structures**

Name	*Description*	*Function*
Cell membrane	Outer layer of the cell; composed mainly of lipids and proteins	Limits the cell; regulates what enters and leaves the cell
Cytoplasm	Colloidal suspension that fills the cell	Holds the cell contents
Nucleus	Large, dark-staining body near the center of the cell; composed of DNA and proteins	Contains the chromosomes with the genes (the hereditary material that directs all cell activities)
Nucleolus	Small body in the nucleus; composed of RNA, DNA, and protein	Needed for protein manufacture
Endoplasmic reticulum (ER)	Network of membranes in the cytoplasm	Used for storage and transport; holds ribosomes
Ribosomes	Small bodies in the cytoplasm or attached to the ER; composed of RNA and protein	Manufacture proteins
Mitochondria	Large organelles with folded membranes inside	Convert energy from nutrients into adenosine triphosphate (source of stored energy)
Golgi apparatus	Layers of membranes	Put together special substances, such as mucus
Lysosomes	Small sacs of digestive enzymes	Digest substances within the cell
Centrioles	Rod-shaped bodies (usually 2) near the nucleus	Help separate the chromosomes in cell division
Cilia	Short, hairlike projections from the cell	Create movement around the cell
Flagellum	Long, whiplike extension from the cell	Moves the cell

Table 9-3 **Tissue Types and Functions**

Type	*Functions*	*Examples*
Epithelial	Covers body surfaces Lines cavities Forms glands	Skin surfaces, respiratory and gastrointestinal tracts, genitourinary system
Connective	Holds other tissues together Forms and supports all parts of the body Protects body parts	Fibrous, reticular, fatty (or adipose), bone, cartilage, blood
Muscular	Maintains posture Generates bone movement Helps produce heat to regulate body temperature	Skeletal, cardiac, smooth, involuntary muscles
Nervous	Conducts nerve impulses and messages to and from the brain Regulates body functions	Central and peripheral nervous systems

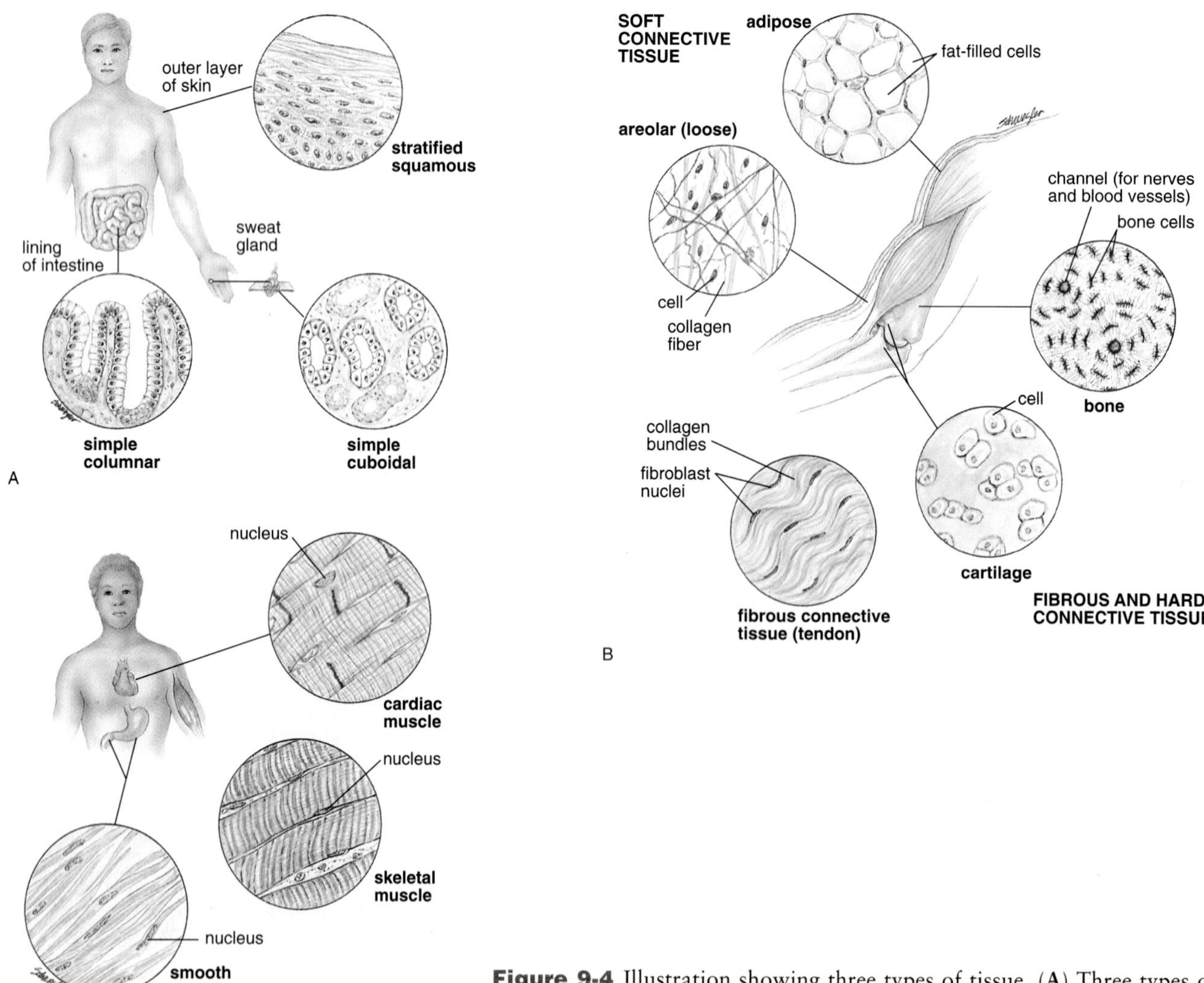

Figure 9-4 Illustration showing three types of tissue. (**A**) Three types of epithelium. (**B**) Connective tissue. (**C**) Muscle tissue.

spleen, and brain are so specialized that they can maintain near-normal functioning with over 30% of the organ damaged or excised.

Body Systems

A body **system** is composed of a group of organs that work together to perform a specific function for the body. For example, the nervous system includes the brain, the spinal cord, and the nerves. These organs function as a system to coordinate body activity through nerve stimulation. The circulatory system includes the heart, blood vessels, and blood, all working together to transport nutrients to areas of need and pick up wastes for transport to points of elimination (Table 9-4).

Checkpoint Question

2. *What makes up tissues and organs?*

GENERAL PLAN OF THE BODY

As a medical assistant, you must be able to locate accurately the various organs and structures to describe specifically the details of your observations and assessments. References must be consistent across the profession to avoid confusion in describing location, direction, position, and so on. The following discussion outlines the acceptable standards of references set by the allied health professions.

Anatomic Position

Anatomic position refers to a standing position with the body erect, facing forward, feet pointed forward and slightly apart, arms down at the sides with the palms facing forward and the thumbs outward. Anatomic position will always be the reference for direction, distance, or movement. Remember also that the patient will be facing you, so that the patient's right will be on your left.

9

Body Planes

Planes are imaginary lines drawn through the body and used to facilitate the study of individual organs or of the body as a whole. There are three planes at right angles to each other. These are:

1. *Transverse.* A line drawn from side to side horizontal to the floor divides the body into inferior and superior portions.
2. *Sagittal.* A line drawn through the body from the head to the feet divides the body into right and left. A mid-sagittal line divides the body exactly into halves.
3. *Frontal.* A line drawn from the head to the feet divides the body into front and back, or anterior and posterior (also referred to as ventral and dorsal).

Table 9-4 **Body Systems and Functions**

System	*Organs*	*Functions*
Circulatory	Heart, blood, and blood vessels	Carries oxygen and nutrients to the cells and removes waste
Endocrine	Pituitary, pineal body, thyroid, parathyroid, thymus, adrenal, ovaries, testes, islets of Langerhans (in pancreas)	Produces hormones that regulate body processes
Gastrointestinal	Salivary glands, teeth, tongue, pharynx, esophagus, stomach, intestines, liver, gallbladder, pancreas	Digests, transports, and absorbs nutrients Eliminates solid wastes
Integumentary	Skin, hair, nails, sweat and oil glands	Protects against infection Helps regulate body temperature Eliminates some waste
Musculoskeletal	Muscles, bones, joints, ligaments, tendons	Protects and supports the body Makes movement possible Produces some blood cells
Nervous	Brain, spinal cord, nerves	Coordinates body activity through nerve stimulation
Respiratory	Nose, pharynx, larynx, trachea, bronchi, lungs	Brings oxygen into the body and eliminates carbon dioxide
Reproductive	Male: testes, urethra, prostate gland, penis, and related structures Female: breasts, ovaries, uterus, vagina, and related structures	Regulates reproduction, sexual activity, and sexual identity
Urinary	Kidneys, ureters, urinary bladder, urethra	Eliminates liquid wastes

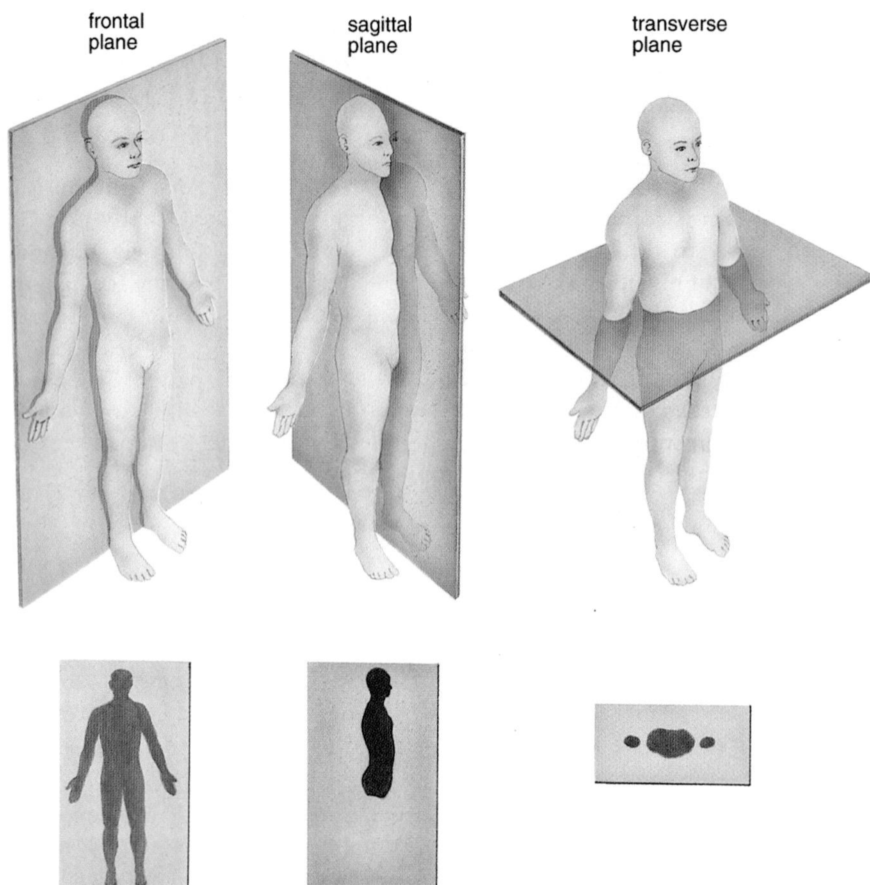

Figure 9-5 Planes of division.

Body planes locate areas on the body from left to right, from back to front, and from top to bottom (Fig. 9-5).

Locations and Positions

References to locations and positions on the body are made from the anatomic position (see above). With a transverse plane, the body is divided into superior and inferior sections. The heart is superior to the stomach, for example. The frontal plane divides the body into anterior (front) and posterior (back), or ventral (front) and dorsal (back). The chest is anterior, for example, and the spine is posterior. Positions and locations may also be described using the following terms:

- *Medial* (close to the midline of the body). The heart is medial to the lungs.
- *Lateral* (away from the midline, to the side of the body). The arms are lateral to the chest.
- *Superficial* (close to the surface). The epidermis is the most superficial layer of skin.
- *Deep* (far from the surface). The abdominal lymph nodes are deep within the peritoneum.
- *Proximal* (close to the point of origin). The elbow is proximal to the wrist.
- *Distal* (further from the point of origin). The ankle is distal to the knee.

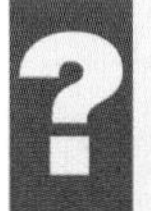

Checkpoint Question

3. *How many body planes are there? Name and describe each one.*

Body Cavities

The body has two major cavities, the ventral cavity and the dorsal cavity, that contain a compact arrangement of internal organs (Fig. 9-6). The dorsal cavity is further divided into the cranial cavity, which contains the brain, and the vertebral cavity, containing the spinal cord. The ventral cavity is the larger of the two and is further divided into more specific areas:

- The *thoracic cavity* contains the heart, lungs, esophagus, trachea, and large blood vessels.
- The *abdominal cavity* contains the stomach, most of the intestines, the liver, the gallbladder, the pancreas, and the spleen. The abdominal cavity is further divided into a retroperitoneal (behind the peritoneum) cavity, which contains the kidneys and ureters.

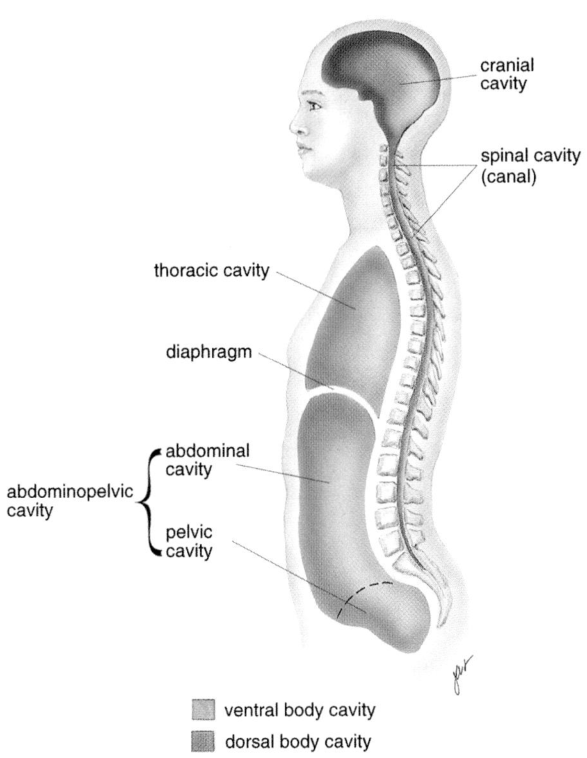

Figure 9-6 Side view of the body cavities.

Box 9-1
Body Areas and Regions

Abdominal	between thoracic and pelvic
Axillary	armpit
Brachial	upper arm
Buccal	between the cheek and gum
Cardiac	in the region of the heart
Cervical	neck
Cranial	head
Femoral	thigh
Gastric	stomach (not abdomen)
Hepatic	liver
Iliac	hip
Inguinal	groin
Lumbar	lower back
Mammary	breast
Occipital	back of the head
Pectoral	anterior chest
Pelvic	below the abdominal area
Perineal	floor of the pelvis
Plantar	sole of the foot
Popliteal	behind the knee
Pulmonary	lungs
Sacral	base of the spine
Temporal	side of the head
Thoracic	chest cavity

- The *pelvic cavity* lies below the abdominal cavity and contains the bladder, the rectum, and the internal reproductive system.

The thoracic and abdominal cavities are divided by the diaphragm—a thin, very muscular layer that assists with respiratory movements. All of the abdominal organs are maintained in place by the omenta, layers of peritoneum that stretch from the upper posterior wall of the abdominal cavity and loop around the organs to keep them in place.

Areas and Regions

Locations and positions may be described by the region involved. For instance, a patient complaining of neck pain has pain in the cervical region. Pain in the groin may be described as inguinal pain. Some of the more common areas and regions are listed in Box 9-1.

Because the abdominal cavity is so large an area, it is divided into nine areas—called the **abdominal regions**—to provide more accurate means of identifying underlying organs and structure locations. The three central regions include the:

- Epigastric region, located just below the breastbone
- Umbilical region, the area around the umbilicus (navel)
- Hypogastric region, the lowest of the midline regions

At each side are the right and left hypochondriac regions, just below the ribs, also known as the subcostal regions; the right and left lumbar regions; and the iliac, or inguinal regions. With this information, it is possible to be precise in identifying the exact location of a patient's abdominal complaints (Fig. 9-7).

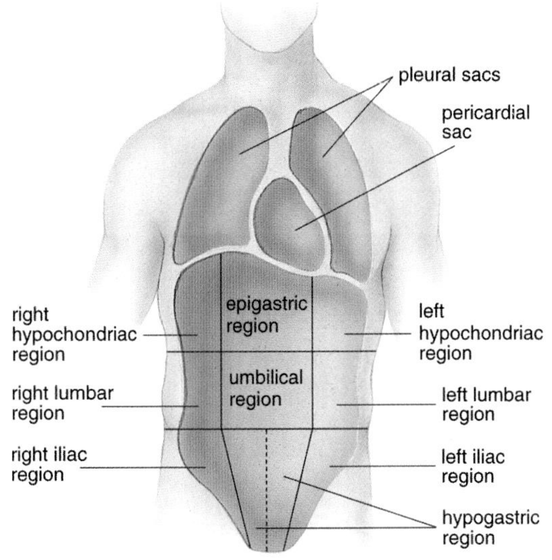

Figure 9-7 Nine abdominal regions.

What If?

A patient presents complaining of a "stomachache." What if, when asked to point where it hurts, the patient says "right down here" and points to the mid-abdominal area?

Be aware that many people confuse the term "stomach" with the term "abdomen" when describing the location of a complaint. Using the anatomic position and the regions, you can correctly interpret the position of incorrectly described symptoms.

The abdomen also may be divided into **quadrants,** or four parts. These are the right and the left upper quadrants and the right and left lower quadrants. These areas are also important in reporting findings and preparing documentation.

Checkpoint Question

4. *Why is the abdominal cavity divided into nine regions?*

HOMEOSTASIS

Homeostasis is the means by which the body maintains a relatively consistent internal environment necessary for survival. Some of the functions maintained by homeostasis can tolerate a fairly wide range. For example, the body will do fairly well with a blood glucose level between 60 and 100 mg/dL, but it cannot tolerate a blood pH (acid–base balance) lower than 7.35 or higher than 7.45. If either of those values ventures away from a normal range, the body mechanisms will begin to work to bring them back into acceptable ranges. Homeostasis manages the constant fluctuations of the body functions by keeping the internal environment within relatively narrow boundaries.

Feedback refers to the information that comes to the body's sensors from the internal or external environment. Feedback either stimulates or depresses the mechanisms that maintain homeostasis.

Positive feedback is an increase in a body function in response to a stimulus. Positive feedback reinforces, rather than opposes, the change that is occurring. Clot formation in response to an injury is an example of positive feedback.

Negative feedback works against a change and is a stabilizing mechanism. An example of negative feedback shows how the system is used to maintain homeostasis of blood carbon dioxide (CO_2) concentration. As CO_2 levels increase, the respiratory rate increases to permit CO_2 to exit the body in increased amounts through expired air. Without this homeostatic mechanism, the body's CO_2 content rapidly rises to toxic levels and may result in death. Consider also a change in body temperature. If the temperature sensors perceive the environment as too cool, shivering will generate warmth; if it is perceived as too warm, vasodilation will rush blood to the periphery for cooling to reduce the core temperature.

The healthy person's homeostasis can maintain a balance between the negative and positive feedback. This homeostatic balance is necessary for continued health and an ongoing steady internal environment.

Answers to Checkpoint Questions

1. *The three main parts of the cell are the cell membrane, cytoplasm, and nucleus. The cell membrane regulates what enters and leaves the cell through selective permeability. The cytoplasm holds the organelles that are responsible for the cell's function. The nucleus contains the chromosomes.*

2. *Tissues are made up of a group of similar cells working together. Organs are formed by different tissues working together to perform a specific function.*

3. *There are three body planes. The transverse plane is a line drawn from side to side horizontal to the floor that divides the body into inferior and superior positions. The sagittal plane is a line drawn through the body from the head to the feet to divide the body into right and left. The frontal plane is a line drawn from the head to the feet to divide the body into front and back, or anterior (ventral) and posterior (dorsal).*

4. *The abdominal cavity is divided into nine regions because it is so large and to provide a more accurate means of identifying and locating organs and structures.*

Critical Thinking Challenges

1. You have been asked to give a brief presentation to a group of students on the organization of the body. Develop a presentation that describes the body's organization in an ascending order. At what level would you start? At what level would you end?
2. While transcribing dictation from the physician, you note the following statements:
   - A bullet was surgically removed from the thoracic cavity. It was lodged in the superior aspect of the esophagus.
   - An incision was made medially in the right hypochondriac region.
   - The 3-cm laceration was sutured. It was located medial and proximal to the left knee.

Draw a stick figure to illustrate the correct location of each ailment described.

3. Compare and contrast the forms of regulatory feedback. Include several examples of each.

Suggestions for Further Reading

Carpenito, L. (1997). *Nursing Diagnosis,* 7th ed. Philadelphia: Lippincott-Raven.

Memmler, R. L., Cohen, B. J., & Wood, D. L. (1996). *The Human Body in Health and Disease,* 8th ed. Philadelphia: Lippincott-Raven.

Memmler, R. L., Cohen, B. J., & Wood, D. L. (1996). *Structure and Function of the Human Body,* 6th ed. Philadelphia: Lippincott-Raven.

Smeltzer, S., & Bare, B. (1996). *Brunner and Suddarth's Textbook of Medical-Surgical Nursing,* 8th ed. Philadelphia: Lippincott-Raven.

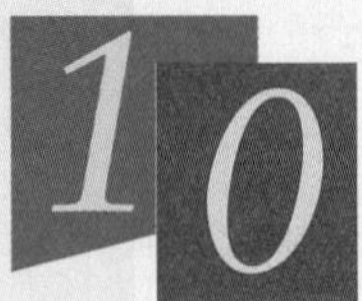

Assisting With Diagnostic and Therapeutic Procedures Associated With the Integumentary System

Chapter Outline

Role Delineation

CLINICAL

Fundamental Principles

- Apply principles of aseptic technique and infection control.

Diagnostic Orders

- Collect and process specimens.

Patient Care

- Prepare and maintain examination and treatment areas.
- Prepare patient for examination, procedures, and treatments.
- Assist with examinations, procedures, and treatments.

GENERAL

Professionalism

- Project a professional manner and image.

Communication Skills

- Treat all patients with compassion and empathy.

Legal Concepts

- Practice within the scope of education, training, and personal capabilities.
- Document accurately.

Instruction

- Instruct individuals according to their needs.
- Teach methods of health promotion and disease prevention.

Chapter Competencies

Learning Objectives

Upon successfully completing this chapter, you will be able to:

1. Spell and define the Key Terms.
2. List the major components of the integumentary system.
3. Describe the functions of the integument.
4. Recognize common skin disorders.
5. Describe common diagnostic procedures.
6. List precautions to observe during the application of warm or cold treatment.
7. Prepare the patient for examination of the integument.
8. Assist the physician with examination of the integument.
9. Understand how to instruct the patient on proper procedures for self-administering warm or cold applications at home.

Performance Objectives

Upon successfully completing this chapter, you will be able to:

1. Apply cold packs (Procedure 10-1).
2. Apply warm or cold compresses (Procedure 10-2).
3. Use a hot water bottle or commercial hot pack (Procedure 10-3).
4. Assist with therapeutic soaks (Procedure 10-4).
5. Obtain a wound culture.

Key Terms

(See Glossary for definitions.)

alopecia
abscess
adipose
allergens
arrector pili
benign
blisters
boil
bullae
collagen
comedos
cysts
dermatitis
dermatophytosis
dermis
elastin
epidermis
erythema
exudate
fascia
fissures
keratin
macules
malignant
melanin
melanocytes
neoplasm
nodule
papillomas
papillomavirus
papules
pediculosis
pruritus
pustules
scale
sebaceous glands
seborrhea
sebum
Staphylococcus
stratum corneum
stratum germinativum
Streptococcus
subcutaneous
sudoriferous gland
urticaria
verruca
vesicles
wheals
Wood's light

The skin, or integument, is the largest organ of the body. It has many functions and plays a vital role in maintaining homeostasis. This chapter covers the structure and function of the integument and its accessories, common skin disorders, and the role of the medical assistant in the examination and treatment of diseases of the integumentary system.

FUNCTION OF THE INTEGUMENTARY SYSTEM

One of the most important functions of the integumentary system is to protect the underlying tissues and organs of the body from the external environment. Unbroken skin provides a protective barrier that prevents the entrance of microorganisms and is the body's first line of defense against infection. In addition, the skin protects the body from mechanical injury, damaging substances, and the ultraviolet rays of the sun.

The integument assists in the regulation of body temperature. Increased sweat production in a warm environment lowers body temperature as sweat evaporates. Blood vessels in the skin dilate (vasodilation), bringing interior heat close to the body's surface to cool the body. In a cold environment, the blood vessels constrict (vasoconstriction) to conserve heat and shunt blood to the internal organs. In this way, the body's temperature tends to be maintained within a normal range.

The skin contains separate receptors for each of the cutaneous sensations, such as heat, cold, pain, touch, and pressure. It contains glands that secrete substances to prevent drying of the skin, hair, and ear canal. It is a storage site for fat, glucose, water, and certain salts. It excretes water, some salts, and waste products through the sweat glands. It converts cholesterol to vitamin D when exposed to ultraviolet rays. It cushions the body, and its waterproof surface prevents or regulates the loss or entry of fluids.

The integumentary system consists of the skin and its accessory organs, which include the hair, nails, sweat and oil glands, and the cutaneous nerve supply. The entire system defends against disease and helps to control temperature and regulate homeostasis.

> **Checkpoint Question**
>
> **1.** *How does the integument help to control body temperature?*

STRUCTURE OF THE INTEGUMENTARY SYSTEM

The skin is arranged in three basic layers: the **epidermis** (outer layer), the **dermis** (middle layer), and the **subcutaneous** tissue, which is beneath the skin. Each layer contains structures that perform specific functions for defense or homeostasis (Fig. 10-1).

Epidermis

The epidermis is the outer covering of the skin. It is composed of epithelial tissue and contains no blood vessels. The epidermis is relatively thin except in areas subjected to pressure, such as the palms of the hands and soles of the feet. Because of friction here, the rate of new cell production is greater than in other surfaces, and thick ridges called a callus may be formed.

The epidermis has two important layers. The outermost layer is called the **stratum corneum,** sometimes called the horny layer. Below this is the **stratum germinativum,** the area responsible for providing and nourishing new cell growth.

Stratum Corneum

The cells of the stratum corneum are composed of **keratin,** a nonliving waterproof substance that prevents loss of body fluid. These cells are constantly lost or worn off by friction or exposure to the environment, such as by bathing or from clothing.

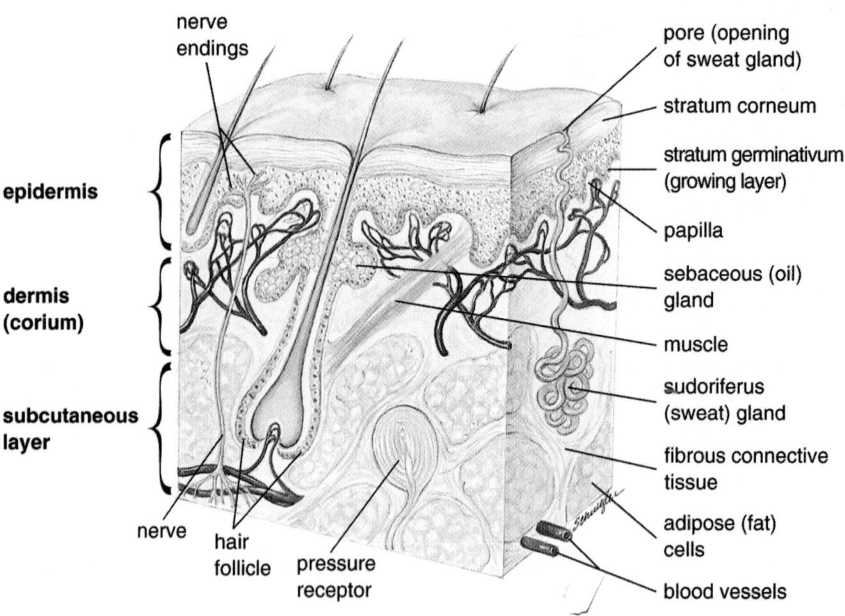

Figure 10-1 Cross section of the skin.

Stratum Germinativum

The stratum germinativum is the layer which, when intact and unbroken, provides protection against invading microorganisms. The acidity of the cells in this layer assists in destroying many of the microorganisms that come into contact with it, thus providing another avenue of protection. The cells of the stratum germinativum are constantly producing new skin cells by mitosis to replace those lost from the body surface.

Melanocytes are located in this layer. These cells produce **melanin,** a skin pigment. The activity of melanocytes is one of the inherited genetic characteristics. The amount of melanin produced determines the darkness of our skin. Light-skinned people produce less melanin; dark-skinned people produce more. Exposure to the ultraviolet rays of the sun increases melanin production and temporarily results in darker skin. Dark skin provides good protection for the stratum germinativum and underlying structures from damage by ultraviolet rays.

Dermis

The dermis is the middle layer of the skin. It is fibrous connective tissue made up of protein substances called **collagen** and **elastin.** Collagen provides strength, and elastin provides elasticity.

Papillary Layer

The papillary layer, which separates the epidermis and dermis, is richly supplied with capillaries. This blood supplies oxygen and nutrients to the stratum germinativum in the epidermis and to the structures in the dermis.

Arterioles located in the dermis, assisted by the nervous system (see Chap. 15, Assisting With Procedures Associated With the Cardiovascular System), aid in maintaining body temperature with their ability to constrict or dilate in response to the environment.

Sensory Receptors

Receptors for touch, pressure, heat, cold, and pain are located in the dermis. Each sensation has a specific receptor to detect information about the external environment. The number of receptors present in an area determines the sensitivity of the area.

Hair Follicles

Hair is found everywhere on the body except the soles, the palms, the lips, and the nipples. The base of each hair follicle is called the hair root and is located in the dermis. Capillaries provide oxygen and nutrients for new cell production. The hair shaft projects from the skin surface at an angle. It is made up of hard, nonliving, keratinized cells.

Attached to each follicle is the **arrector pili** or pilomotor muscle that contracts when the environment is cool, causing "goose bumps" as the skin tightens around the hair and the hair shaft is pulled erect. Oil glands open into hair follicles, helping to maintain moisture in the hair.

Hairs in the eyelashes and eyebrows help keep perspiration and dust out of the eyes. Nasal hair filters dust from the air that we breathe. Hair on the scalp provides insulation against heat lost through the vascular surfaces of the head.

Nail Follicles

Specialized follicles at the ends of the fingers and toes produce nails. New cells are formed in the matrix, called the nail bed, which is composed of living tissue. The nail beds produce keratinizing cells that push to the surface and adhere to one another. As they are pushed to the surface, the cells die so that the nails are composed of hard, keratinized dead cells. 10

Nails protect the ends of our fingers and toes from injury. When the nails are injured or lost, new nails will continue to be formed as long as the nail bed remains intact.

Sebaceous Glands

The **sebaceous glands,** or oil glands, open directly on the skin surface or into a hair follicle. Sebaceous glands secrete **sebum,** a thick, oily substance that acts as "waterproofing" for the skin. It lubricates the skin, keeping it soft to prevent drying and cracking. Muscle movement and the movement of the skin across under-

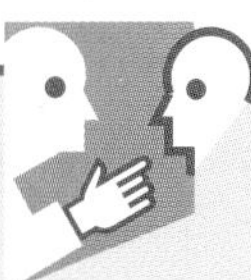

Advice and Tips

Dealing With Adolescents

Adolescents are acutely aware of their body appearance and any imperfections that they may have. The presence of acne can be a major concern for a teenager. Here are some tips for dealing with adolescents:

- Be understanding of their need for acceptance from their peers.
- Avoid condescending language. For example, never say, "It is *only* a pimple." To the teenager, this is a significant problem.
- Help the adolescent feel involved in making health care decisions. It will help to discuss health care issues in terms appropriate to their level of understanding.
- Give discharge instructions to both the adolescent and the caregiver, but focus the conversation to the young patient to ensure a feeling of participation.

lying tissues push sebum up from the glands to the skin surface.

Adolescents often have hyperactive sebaceous glands, which contribute to acne. Older adults have dry and fragile skin, resulting from hypoactivity of these glands.

Sudoriferous Glands

The **sudoriferous glands** are also known as sweat glands. They have a coiled base in the dermis, which extends as a tiny tube to form a pore in the skin through which sweat is excreted from the body. In the axillae and the groin, sudoriferous glands open into a hair follicle, rather than into a pore. Sweat, or perspiration, is made up mostly of water, some salts, and waste products. Through the sweat glands, the integumentary system helps the urinary system to maintain water balance and eliminate wastes.

Sudoriferous glands are located all over the body but are especially numerous in the axillae, on the palms and soles, and on the forehead. They are controlled by the nervous system. They may be activated by heat, pain, fear, and fever. Evaporation of perspiration from the body surface is an effective means of cooling the body.

One other function of the dermis is the conversion of a type of cholesterol to vitamin D when the body is exposed to ultraviolet rays. Vitamin D is necessary for the absorption of calcium and phosphorus from the small intestine.

Subcutaneous Tissue

The subcutaneous tissue, also called the superficial fascia (fibrous membrane tissue), connects the dermis to the underlying muscles.

The subcutaneous tissue contains collagen, elastin, blood vessels, and white blood cells that migrate throughout the tissues to search for and destroy pathogens. **Adipose** tissue is also located here. Adipose tissue stores fat as a potential energy source, cushions bony prominences, and helps to conserve body heat. The amount of adipose tissue varies from person to person and in thickness from one area of the body to another.

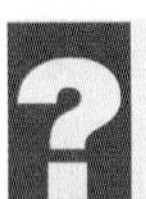

Checkpoint Question

2. *What are the three layers of the skin? Briefly describe each.*

COMMON INTEGUMENTARY DISORDERS

A number of integumentary disorders are manifested by lesions, or abnormalities in skin tissue (Fig. 10-3). These lesions may be primary or secondary (resulting from primary lesions).

Bacterial Skin Infections

Impetigo

Impetigo is a contagious bacterial infection of the skin that is usually seen in young children. It may be caused by ***Staphylococcus*** or ***Streptococcus*** organisms, types of bacteria commonly implicated in skin diseases. The lesions produced are usually seen on the face, neck, and exposed areas of the body (Fig. 10-2). They appear on the superficial layers of the skin as:

- **macules**—small, flat skin discolorations (see Fig. 10-3*A*)
- **vesicles**—small fluid-filled sacs (see Fig. 10-3*D*)
- **bullae**—large fluid-filled sacs (see Fig. 10-3*E*)
- **pustules**—pus-filled sacs (see Fig. 10-3*F*)

Patches of exudative impetigo vesicles produce honey-colored crusts (see Fig. 10-3*K*). These vesicles leave red areas when the crusts are removed.

Treatment involves washing the area two to three times a day and applying a topical antibiotic. Oral antibiotics may be prescribed for severe cases. Scratching must be discouraged. Towels, washcloths, and bed linens should be kept separate and must be washed daily to prevent spread of the disease. Individuals at risk for developing impetigo are those in poor health, those with conditions such as anemia or malnutrition, and those with poor hygiene.

Folliculitis

Folliculitis is a superficial infection of a hair follicle (see Fig. 10-3*N*). It is characterized by itching, burning, and pustule formation. Treatment is aimed at promoting drainage and healing. Saline soaks or compresses are ordered for 15 minutes twice a day. A topical anti-infective followed by application of a dressing is also recommended three times a day.

If folliculitis is left untreated, it may lead to **abscess** formation. An abscess is formed when a small sac of pus accumulates at the site of inflammation. The causative agent of these infections is often *Staphylococcus aureus*.

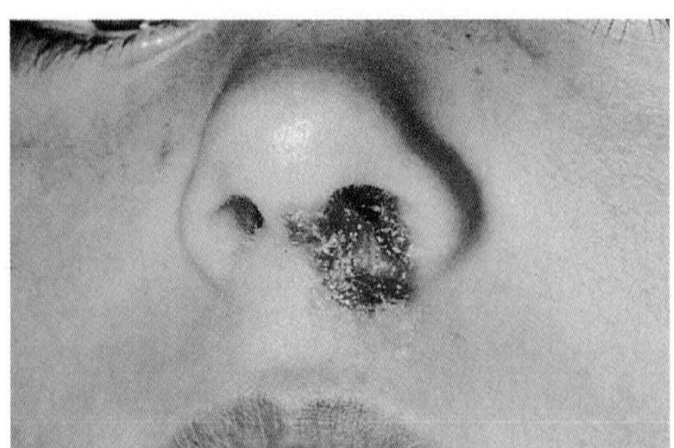

Figure 10-2 Impetigo of the nostril.

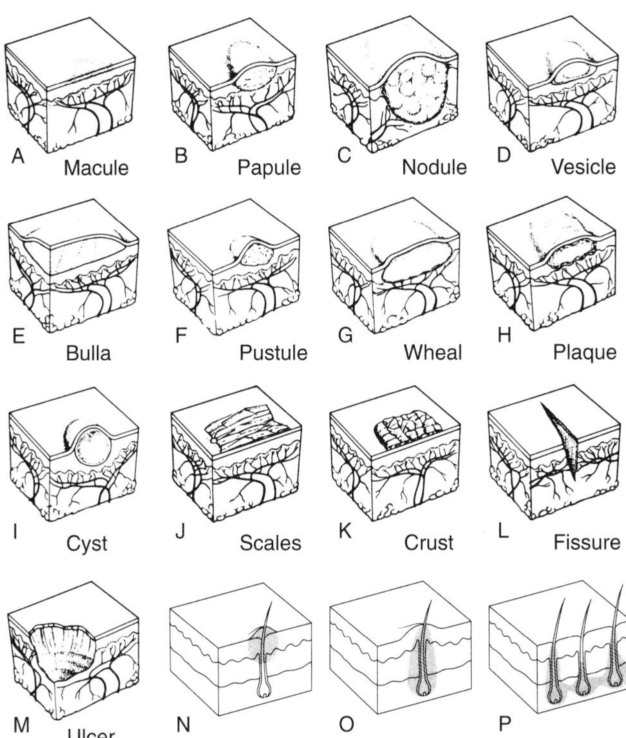

Figure 10-3 Skin lesions. *Primary lesions* (A) Macule. Flat, circumscribed discoloration. (B) Papule. Solid, elevated palpable lesion smaller than 1 cm; colors vary. (C) Nodule. Raised, solid lesion larger than 1 cm. (D) Vesicle. Small elevation filled with clear fluid. (E) Bulla. Large vesicle or blister; larger than 1 cm. (F) Pustule. Lesion containing pus. (G) Wheal. Transient elevation of the skin caused by edema of the dermis and surrounding capillary dilation. (H) Plaque. Solid, elevated lesion on skin or mucosa; larger than 1 cm. (I) Cyst. Tumor that contains semisolid or liquid material. *Secondary lesions* (J) Scales. Heaped up, horny layer of dead epidermis. (K) Crusts. Covering formed from serum, blood, or pus drying on the skin. (L) Fissures. Cracks in the skin. (M) Ulcer. Lesion formed by local destruction of the epidermis and part of the underlying dermis. *Other lesions* (N) Superficial folliculitis. Localized infection of hair follicle. (O) Furuncle. Acute inflammation deep within hair follicle. (P) Carbuncle. Infection involving subcutaneous tissues around several hair follicles.

Furuncle

A furuncle, or **boil**, is a deep-seated infection of a hair follicle (see Fig. 10-3O). Friction and pressure at the site may contribute to its formation. A hard, painful **nodule** (mass) forms (see Fig. 10-3C), enlarges for several days, then erupts with pus oozing from one site. Treatment of a furuncle includes application of moist heat to assist in "ripening" it or bringing it to a head. Often an incision and drainage (I & D) procedure is performed.

Carbuncle

A carbuncle consists of an interconnected group of hair follicles or several furuncles joined together in a mass (see Fig. 10-3*P*). The subcutaneous tissue in the surrounding area is also involved. These are hard, round, extremely painful swellings that take from several days to a week to enlarge. They eventually soften and erupt, discharging pus from several sites. When the skin sloughs away, a scarred cavity remains. The patient usually has an accompanying fever.

Treatment involves use of a systemic antibiotic, applications of moist heat, and incision and drainage once the lesion has matured. A topical anti-infective and loose bandages are applied. The site may require a wick to remain in the cavity for several days to facilitate healing by secondary intention.

Cellulitis

Cellulitis is a spreading infection of the connective tissue. It is caused by an infection of an existing wound. The skin becomes hot, red, and edematous. A systemic anti-infective usually provides rapid and successful treatment.

10

Checkpoint Question

3. *Which three bacterial skin infections develop in the hair follicles? Briefly describe each.*

Viral Skin Infections

Herpes Simplex

Herpes simplex infections are also called cold sores or fever **blisters**. (A blister is a collection of fluid in or beneath the epidermis.) The lesions, which appear on the lips, mouth, face, and nose, are small vesicles grouped together on a red base. They eventually erupt, leaving a painful ulcer, then a crust. They cause burning and stinging and may be precipitated by other infections, menstruation, fatigue, trauma, stress, or exposure to the sun.

Fever blisters are caused by herpes simplex virus I. They are recurrent, and no effective treatment eliminates or controls the disease. Acyclovir and other antivirals have shown promise in reducing the frequency and severity of the disease, but do not offer a cure. Treatment is aimed at relieving discomfort with topical ointments with varying degrees of effectiveness.

Herpes Zoster

It is commonly believed that herpes zoster, or shingles, is caused by the same virus that causes chickenpox. After exposure to chickenpox, the virus may lie dormant in the body for years until reactivated. It spreads down the length of a nerve to the skin, causing redness, swelling, and pain. After about 48 hours, a band of lesions develops, which begin as **papules,** small, red, solid elevations on the skin (see Fig. 10-3*B*). These progress to vesicles and pustules, then dry crusts. The lesions last for several weeks. Scarring and alterations in pigmentation are common. Pain often remains after the lesions have disappeared, in some cases as long as several months.

Shingles commonly appear on the face, back, and chest. Lesions are frequently unilateral. The disorder usually occurs in adults. The virus remains dormant in the nervous system of anyone who has had the disease and may recur in times of physical or emotional stress.

Treatment includes narcotic analgesics for the discomfort or nerve blocks for severe pain. Locally, calamine lotion may be used. The area must be protected from air and the irritation of clothing. Acyclovir is sometimes used to alleviate the severity of the disease and is most effective if started early in the course of the outbreak.

Verruca

A **verruca** is a wart. Warts are squamous cell **papillomas** (benign skin tumors) that appear as rough, raised lesions with a pitted surface. Warts occur singly or in groups and may be found anywhere on the skin or mucous membranes. They commonly appear on the fingers or hands. Warts vary in size, shape, and appearance and are thought to be caused by **papillomaviruses.**

Treatment of warts includes removal with keratolytic agents, liquid nitrogen, podophyllum resin, laser therapy, or surgery. They also may disappear spontaneously.

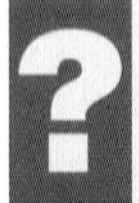

Checkpoint Question

4. *Which viral skin infection is linked to a common childhood disorder? Explain.*

Fungal Skin Infections

The most common fungal infections of the skin (**dermatophytosis**) are caused by a group of fungi molds called dermatophytes. There are several, and treatment is similar. The group of fungal diseases called tinea is collectively known to the lay public as ringworm.

Tinea Capitis

Tinea capitis affects the scalp. It is contagious and appears most frequently in children. It is characterized by round, gray, **scale** patches (dried skin flakes) and areas of **alopecia** (baldness). There are usually no symptoms, with the exception of light itching.

Tinea Corporis

Tinea corporis, or tinea circinata, is exhibited on nonhairy portions of the body (Fig. 10-4). It is characterized by itchy, red rings that are clear in the center with a scalelike border (see Fig. 10-3*J*). It is frequently found on the face and arms.

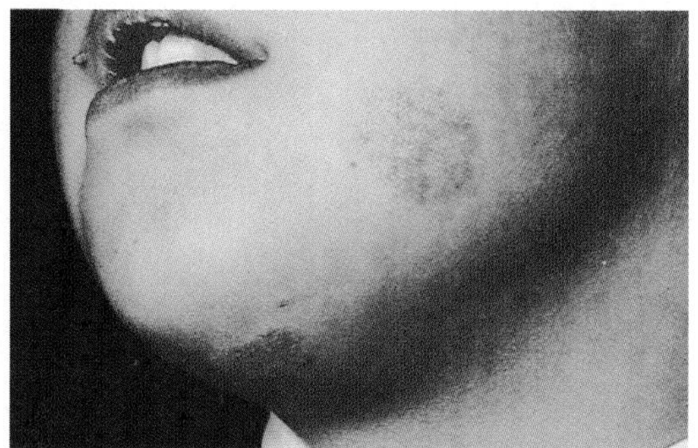

Figure 10-4 Tinea corporis (ringworm) of the face.

Tinea Cruris

Tinea cruris is known in lay terms as "jock itch." The lesions, which cause marked itching, are red macules with clear centers and scalelike borders. They are found on the skin in the groin area and the gluteal folds.

Tinea Pedis

Tinea pedis, or athlete's foot, is characterized by itching, burning, and stinging between the toes and on the soles. The lesions may appear as red, weepy vesicles; as chronic dry scales; or as **fissures** (cracklike lesions) between the toes (see Fig. 10-3*L*).

Tinea Unguium

Tinea unguium, also known as onychomycosis, causes thickening, discoloration, and crumbling of the nails, most often the toenails. It is difficult to cure and will take months of local antifungal preparations and systemic oral preparations for severe cases.

Tinea Versicolor

Tinea versicolor, also known as pityriasis versicolor, is not caused by dermatophytes. It is not known exactly what sort of fungus is the causative agent. The disease exhibits as a multicolor rash generally over the upper trunk. It is more common in young people in warm weather and is chronic. It varies from macular to raised, round or oval, from darkly pigmented to depigmented, and is slightly scalelike. There are usually no symptoms. Diagnosis of tinea versicolor is by **Wood's light,** an ultraviolet light that, when used in a darkened room, shows abnormalities in the skin as fluorescent colors. Treatment is with selenium sulfide daily for 7 days, antifungal creams or lotions, and oral antifungals for severe cases.

All of the tineas are treated with topical antifungal powders, creams, or shampoos and oral antifungals. Inflamed lesions may be treated with wet compresses or soaks. General measures for treating fungal infections and preventing transfer is to keep the area clean and dry because fungi thrive in moist conditions. Clothing should be loose fitting and laundered daily. Socks and underclothing should be changed frequently. Clothing should not be shared with others. Shower shoes should be worn in public showers and pools.

Checkpoint Question

5. *What is the difference between tinea capitis and tinea pedis?*

Parasitic Skin Infestations

Scabies

Scabies is a contagious skin disorder caused by the itch mite, *Sarcoptes scabiei*. It is spread by direct contact. The itching caused by the mite is worse at night when the female burrows under the epidermis to lay her eggs. The lesions are small red vesicles or pustules that occur between the fingers, at the inner wrist, elbows, axillae, waist, and groin.

Treatment for scabies is aimed at disinfestation. For adults, 1% lindane cream or lotion is applied from the neck down at bedtime. One application of Elimite cream is effective and is the drug of choice for children. All bedding and clothing for the whole family should be laundered daily until the infestation is clear.

Pediculosis

Pediculosis is an infestation of the skin with lice. Lice may be found in three body areas: the scalp (head lice), the body (body lice), or the pubic hairs ("crabs"). Wherever they are found, itching is intense, and the skin often becomes secondarily infected from scratching. Lice feed on human blood and lay eggs (nits) on body hairs or in clothing fibers. Nits may be seen on hair shafts close to the skin or in seams of clothing.

Pediculosis is commonly seen among populations with overcrowding and poor hygiene. The disorder is transmitted through physical contact with an infested person, by sitting on an infested toilet seat, or by sharing a comb, brush, clothing, or bedding that is infested. γ-Benzene hexachloride creams, lotions, or shampoos are used for all types of pediculosis. All clothing and linen must be dry cleaned or washed in hot water and ironed. Sealing items in plastic bags for 30 days or heating to 140°F will eliminate lice on items that cannot be laundered.

Inflammatory Reactions

Eczema

Eczema is an inflammatory skin disorder generally involving only the epidermal layer. It is more common in children than adults. It is characterized by itching, which may be prolonged. The lesions vary at different stages but generally begin as red patches, proceed to weepy vesicles, and end up as dry scale crusts. They appear on the face, neck, bends of knees and elbows, and the upper trunk. They usually run a chronic course of exacerbations.

The causes of eczema are many and varied, depending on the individual. Causes include:

- Food allergies to fish, eggs, and milk products
- Medication or chemical allergies
- Sensitivity to irritating soaps, household cleaning products, deodorants, and perfumes
- Inhalants, such as pollen, dust, or animal dander
- Poor circulation to a part
- Ultraviolet rays

Treatment involves removing the cause and promoting healing of the lesions. The causative agent should be avoided if it is known. The patient should maintain good hydration and keep the skin well moistened with emollients. A humid environment is recommended. Only one warm, not hot, bath should be taken daily with a nondrying soap. The skin should be patted dry and a topical emollient should be applied immediately. Scratchy clothing should be avoided.

Exudative lesions are treated with soaks, baths, or wet dressings for 10 to 30 minutes three or four times daily. Domeboro, Aveeno, or bicarbonate are good for these purposes. Topical corticosteroid lotions, creams, or ointments are usually applied twice a day. Bandages should be used at night to protect against scratching. Antihistamines may be necessary for severe **pruritus** (itching). For scales, a steroid ointment is recommended. Systemic corticosteroids, such as prednisone, are recommended only in severe cases.

Seborrheic Dermatitis

Seborrheic **dermatitis** (skin inflammation) is also known as **seborrhea**, which is an overproduction of sebum. It is a chronic dermatitis resulting in greasy yellow scales primarily on the scalp, where it is referred to as seborrheic dandruff. Underlying redness and pruritus may be present. The eyelids, face, chest, back, umbilicus, and body folds may also be affected. It is felt that seborrhea is caused by a genetic predisposition and a combination of hormones, nutrition, infection, or stress. It is treated with shampoos and topical corticosteroid lotions.

Urticaria

Urticaria, or hives, is characterized by acute inflammatory reaction of the dermis. It begins with itching, followed by **erythema** (redness) and swelling. The **wheals** (see Fig. 10-3G) that develop have a pale center with a red edge. They resemble a mosquito bite, and each lasts only a few hours. They appear in clusters anywhere on the body. Hives are self-limiting, lasting from a few days to a few weeks.

The most common causes are:

- Foods, such as shellfish, strawberries, tomatoes, citrus fruits, eggs, and chocolate
- Inhalants, such as feathers or animal dander
- Chemicals, cosmetics, and medications
- Sunlight
- Insect bites or stings
- Heat, cold, or pressure on the skin
- Infection
- Stress

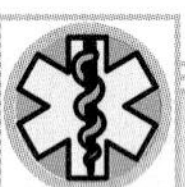

Action STAT!

Scenario: Cristina Tabernackle, 5 years old, is brought into the clinic by her mother. Ms. Tabernackle states that Cristina has a red rash over her body and is complaining of being itchy. You notice that Cristina's lips appear swollen also. Immediately you suspect the rash is urticaria (known to the lay public as hives). What should you do next?

1. As you assess Cristina's vital signs, question Ms. Tabernackle regarding the possible cause, when the rash began, and any other signs that she may feel are significant. (She states that Cristina started amoxicillin yesterday for otitis media, the rash began several hours ago, and that Cristina was restless for much of the night.)
2. Notify the physician immediately.
3. Assist the physician as necessary. This may include providing emergency supplies or administering medications, such as epinephrine or Benadryl.
4. Watch Cristina for signs of respiratory distress, such as cyanosis or dyspnea, and recheck her vital signs as needed.
5. When the physician confirms the allergic reaction, explain to Ms. Tabernackle that Cristina appears to be allergic to amoxicillin and that she will be given a different antibiotic. Be sure that Cristina's chart is clearly marked with the allergy according to office policy.
6. Document the incident and all patient/caregiver education in the patient's chart. Verify that Ms. Tabernackle understands the information provided.

It is important to note that allergic reactions presenting with urticaria may progress to anaphylaxis and can be life threatening. In certain situations, patients may need to be instructed in methods of self-administration of antihistamines or other means of reversing allergic reactions.

Treatment involves reducing the inflammation. The cause should be avoided if known. Antihistamines are usually given to reduce itching and swelling. A short course of prednisone is sometimes ordered. Starch or Aveeno baths twice a day may make the patient more comfortable. Epinephrine is given if symptoms of urticaria develop rapidly and are associated with dyspnea.

Acne Vulgaris

Acne vulgaris is an inflammatory disease of the sebaceous glands. Its cause is not known. It commonly occurs during adolescence and is characterized by pimples, **comedos** (blackheads), **cysts** (fluid sacs beneath the skin) (see Fig. 10-3*I*), and scarring. The lesions usually occur on the face, neck, upper chest, back, and shoulders. Overactive sebaceous glands cause excessive sebum to become trapped in the follicle, producing a dark substance that results in a blackhead. Leukocytes accumulate, and pus production results.

Treatment for acne includes a regimen of Retin-A, benzoyl peroxide, and tetracycline. Sunlamp treatments are sometimes used to dry the lesions. Accutane may be prescribed for severe acne that does not respond to ordinary treatments.

Psoriasis

Psoriasis is a chronic inflammatory skin disorder characterized by bright red plaques (see Fig. 10-3*H*) covered with dry, silvery scales. The cause is unknown. Psoriasis is usually found on the scalp, elbows, knees, base of the spine, palms, soles, and around the nails. There are usually no vesicles, and itching varies from mild to severe. It cannot be completely cured, and recurrences are likely. Exacerbations are common during cold weather, stress, or pregnancy. It is usually a chronic disorder and is difficult to treat.

Treatment includes tar preparations and topical steroid creams or ointments. Exposure to ultraviolet B light three times a week is also used.

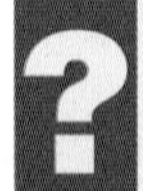

Checkpoint Question

6. *What is urticaria, and which layer of the skin does it affect?*

Disorders of Wound Healing

Cicatrix

A cicatrix is scar tissue that forms erratically and causes distortion of the wound. It usually occurs late in wound healing. It is an especially frequent occurrence after extensive burns. It may cause deformity and immobility of joints because it is less elastic than normal tissue.

Keloids

Keloids, an overproduction of scar tissue, occur as a complication of wound healing. The scar tissue forms as a result of excessive collagen accumulation. A raised nodule is formed that does not resolve with time. The cause is unknown. It occurs most frequently in young women, especially during pregnancy, and in African Americans. The most common sites are the neck and shoulders. Injections of cortisone are sometimes effective in treating keloids.

Disorders Caused by Pressure

Callus and Corn

A callus, sometimes called a callosity, is a raised painless thickening of the epidermis. It is caused by pressure or friction on the hands and feet. A corn is a hard, raised thickening of the stratum corneum on the toes. It results from chronic friction and pressure, especially from poorly fitting shoes. The pressure compresses the dermis, making it thin and tender and causing pain and inflammation. Soft corns can form between the toes.

The treatment for calluses and corns should begin with relieving pressure. Shoes should be made of soft leather and should fit properly. Liners may be inserted in shoes to relieve pressure. Bandages and corn pads are also available to correct the problem. Sometimes surgical intervention or chemical peeling with a keratolytic agent are recommended.

Decubitus Ulcers

Decubitus ulcers are also called bedsores or pressure sores. Decubiti are ulcers of the skin caused by prolonged pressure to an area of the body, usually over a bony prominence (see Fig. 10-3*M*). The pressure impairs blood supply and nutrition to the area. The most common sites are over the sacrum and hips, but they may also be seen on the back of the head, ears, elbows, heels, and ankles. They are most often seen in aged, debilitated, and immobilized patients. Bedridden patients are at risk for developing decubiti unless they are turned frequently to relieve pressure and the bed linen is kept clean and dry. Special mattresses, pads, and pillows are useful in prevention.

Decubitus ulcers are graded, or staged, according to the degree of involvement (Table 10-1). Treatment consists of topical antibiotic powders and adhesive absorbent bandages and dressings. Deep infections may require systemic antibiotics and possible surgical débridement.

Intertrigo

Intertrigo is a disorder of skin breakdown that occurs in the body folds of obese people. The combination of heat, moisture, and friction of the skin against itself in

Table 10-1 **Staging or Grading Scale for Decubitus Ulcers**

Stage	*Description*
I	Red skin that does not return to normal when massaged or when pressure is relieved.
II	Skin is blistered, peeling, or cracked superficially. 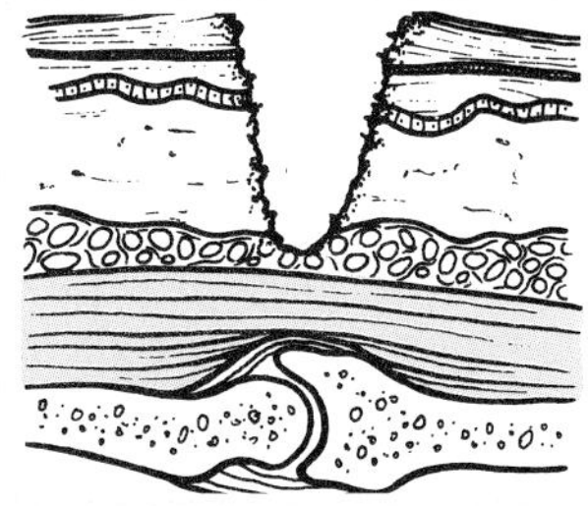
III	Skin is broken with loss of full thickness; subcutaneous tissue may be damaged; serous or bloody drainage may be present. 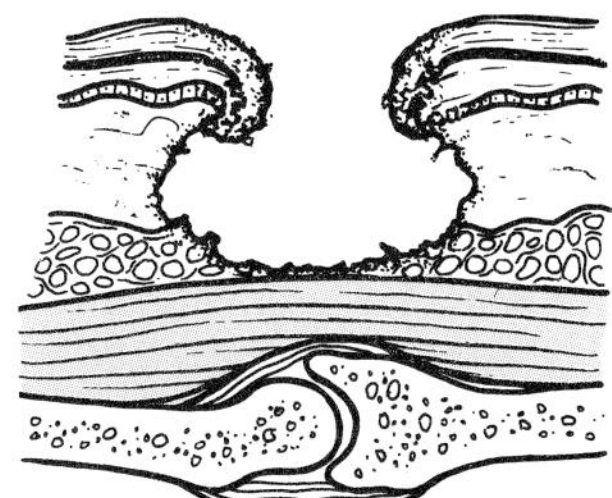
IV	Deep, crater-like ulcer with destruction of subcutaneous tissue; fascia, connective tissue, bone, or muscle are exposed and may be damaged. 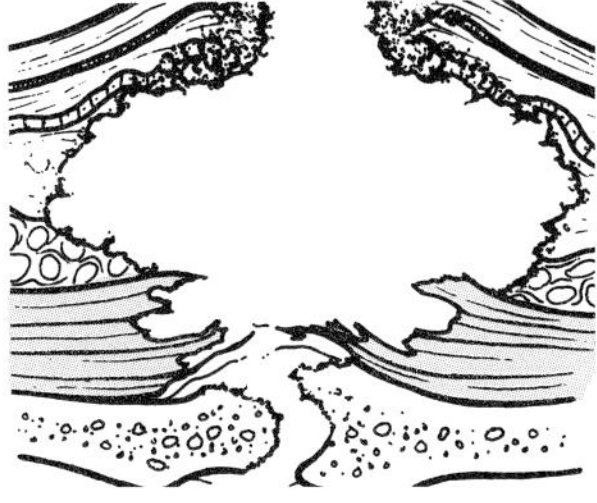

What If?

What if your elderly patient comes into the office with multiple decubitus ulcers? What should you do?

The geriatric population is always at risk for developing skin ulcerations; however, the physician must assess the situation to determine if the patient is receiving adequate care at home to prevent such breakdowns. Patients who arrive in a medical office with multiple ulcers in different stages of healing may be in situations of abuse or neglect. Elder abuse is less often identified, but some experts believe it is as common as child abuse. If you suspect elder abuse, contact your local Department of Social Services. An investigation will be initiated that may substantiate the abuse (requiring referral to law enforcement) or that may identify ways to alleviate the situation (caregiver education, respite care) without removing the patient from the home. In some states, not reporting elder abuse is against the law. The physician can be fined, or other penalties can be imposed.

these areas causes the skin to break down. Humid climates and poor hygiene are likely to aggravate the condition. Erythema and fissures of the skin result. The patient experiences itching, stinging, and burning.

Treatment for intertrigo involves proper hygiene and an attempt to keep the area clean and dry. Talcum powder is often recommended. Antibacterial or antifungal lotion or powder is necessary if secondary infection is present.

Alopecia

Alopecia refers to baldness. It may occur from physical trauma, systemic diseases (eg, lupus erythematosus, lymphomas, or hypothyroidism), bacteria or fungal infections, chemotherapy, excessive radiation, or genetic predisposition, as in male pattern baldness.

Baldness caused by scarring and male pattern baldness are permanent and cannot be reversed. For other causes of baldness, treatment of the underlying disorder often results in new hair growth.

Disorders of Pigmentation

Albinism

Albinism is a genetically determined condition in which there is a partial or total absence of the pigment, or melanin, in the skin, hair, and eyes. The skin is pale, the hair is white, and irises appear pink. The skin will not tan and is prone to sunburn. Eye problems are frequent because no pigment is present to protect the underlying structures from the ultraviolet rays of the sun. Albinism has no treatment.

Vitiligo

Vitiligo is a progressive, chronic destruction of melanocytes. It is thought to be an autoimmune disorder in patients with an inherited predisposition. The depigmented areas occur as white patches that sometimes have a hyperpigmented border. It usually occurs in exposed areas of the skin.

There is currently no effective method for treating vitiligo. Patients are advised to protect the areas from the sun because they are prone to sunburn in the absence of melanin. Waterproof cosmetics may be used to cover the areas.

Leukoderma

Leukoderma is the localized loss of skin pigment that results from damage caused by skin trauma. It is more common in African Americans. Frequent causes of leukoderma include contact with caustic chemicals or the healing of burns or infection.

Nevus

A nevus, also known as a birthmark or mole, is a congenital pigmented skin blemish. It is usually circumscribed and may involve the epidermis, connective tissue, nerves, or blood vessels. Nevi are usually **benign** (not cancerous) but may become **malignant** (cancerous). Patients should be cautioned to watch for changes in the color, size, and texture of any nevus. Bleeding and itching should also be reported (Box 10-1).

Checkpoint Question

7. *What are four disorders of pigmentation? Briefly describe.*

Skin Cancers

Basal Cell Carcinoma

Basal cell carcinoma is a slow-growing cancer that appears most frequently on exposed areas of the body, usually the face, but may also be found on the shoulders and chest, where sebaceous follicles are abundant. The lesions have a waxy appearance with a depressed center and a rolled edge where blood vessels may be apparent. Metastasis almost never occurs, but if left untreated, the lesions will grow locally and may ulcerate and damage surrounding tissues (Fig. 10-5).

Basal cell carcinoma is the most common malignant tumor of the skin of Caucasians. It commonly occurs in blond, fair-skinned men over age 40. Prolonged exposure to ultraviolet light or x-rays is thought to be

Box 10-1
Mole Inspection

On the lookout for malignant melanoma
Its incidence has doubled since 1980, and currently melanoma accounts for over 6000 deaths a year. Melanomas are usually pigmented, elevated skin lesions and frequently develop in a new or existing mole. The key to treatment of this potentially deadly cancer is early detection of changes in size, color, shape, elevation, texture, or consistency of any pigmented area—old or new—in any spot or bump (see illustrations below). By becoming familiar with what is normal for you, you'll be more apt to notice what is abnormal.

The eventual outcome of melanoma is governed by how deeply it has invaded the skin, which also determines how aggressively the cancer will be treated. That early detection can work to cut the mortality rate is clearly evident in the 90%-plus cure rate of malignant melanoma in Queensland, Australia, where an enormous incidence of the cancer led to excellent public education and screening campaigns. The cure rate in the United States is about 20%.

Mole patrol
Mole inspection becomes simpler if you keep in mind the American Cancer Society's ABCD rule for distinguishing a normal mole or other skin blemish from an abnormal one.

Normal *Abnormal*

Asymmetry. One-half of the mole does not match the other.

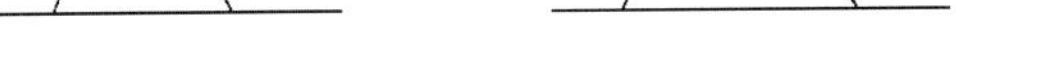

Border. The edges are irregular—ragged, notched, or blurred.

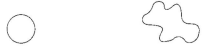

Color. The color is not uniform but may be differing shades of tan, brown, or black, sometimes with patches of red, white, or blue.

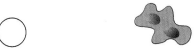

Diameter. The mole is larger than the size of a pencil eraser—about 6 mm or a quarter of an inch—or is increasing in size.

a predisposing factor for the development of basal cell carcinoma.

The most common treatment for basal cell carcinoma is surgical removal. Radiation therapy and cryosurgery are alternative treatments.

Squamous Cell Carcinoma

Squamous cell carcinoma is slightly less common than basal cell carcinoma. It may occur in any squamous epithelial area of the body, such as the lungs, cervix, or anus, but is more frequently found on the skin (Fig. 10-6). Squamous cell carcinoma is a slow-growing malignant **neoplasm** (tumor). The lesions are firm, red, horny or prickly, and painless and range widely in size. Those on exposed areas are thought to result from exposure to the sun. Those on areas not normally exposed, such as mucous membranes, are thought to be the result of frequent irritation. Treatment is the same as that used for basal cell carcinoma. Although basal cell carcinoma is not generally metastatic, squamous cell carcinoma, in contrast, can spread readily through underlying and surrounding tissues, depending on the

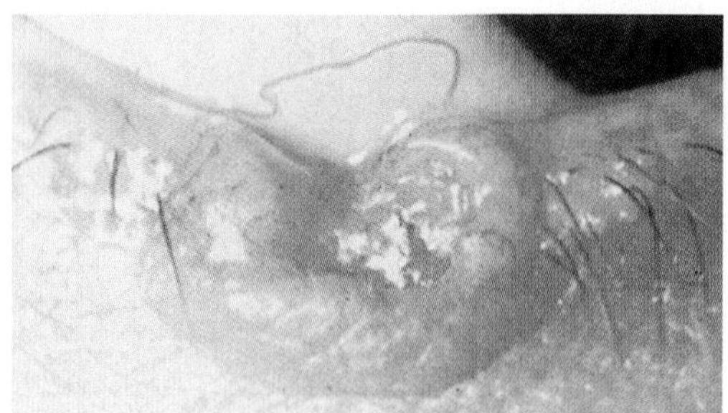

Figure 10-5 Basal cell carcinoma.

degree of cellular differentiation and depth of invasion.

Malignant Melanoma

Malignant melanoma is a cancer of the skin that forms from melanocytes. Lesions vary from macules to nodules and often have an irregular border and a variety of colors (Fig. 10-7). Mixtures of white, blue, purple, and red are the most common. The tumor grows both in radius and in depth into the dermis. In about 30% to 35% of cases, it grows in a pre-existing nevus.

Malignant melanoma, which is thought to be caused by excessive exposure to sunlight, is the leading cause of death due to skin disease. It is the ninth most common cancer. The incidence is 1 in 105 individuals in the United States. The peak age for malignant melanoma is between 50 and 70 years. Those at highest risk for developing the disease have blond or red hair, fair skin, blue eyes, a tendency to sunburn, and spend a lot of time outdoors (Box 10-2).

Treatment for malignant melanoma is surgical removal after a biopsy, possibly including lymph removal. Prognosis depends on the depth of the tumor. Tumors over 1.5 mm often metastasize to the lymph nodes, liver, lungs, and brain (see Box 10-1).

Checkpoint Question

8. *Which is more likely to metastasize—basal cell or squamous cell carcinoma?*

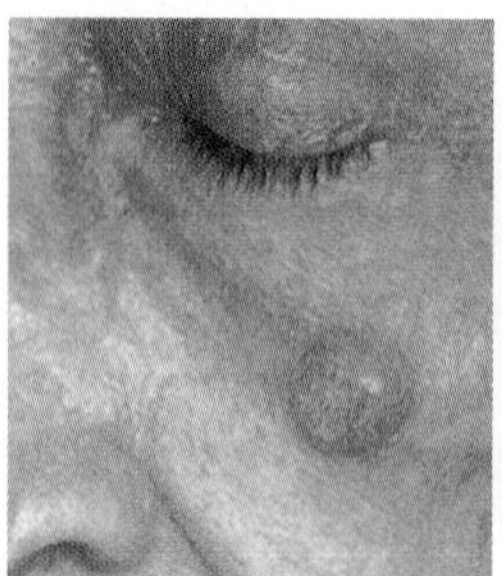

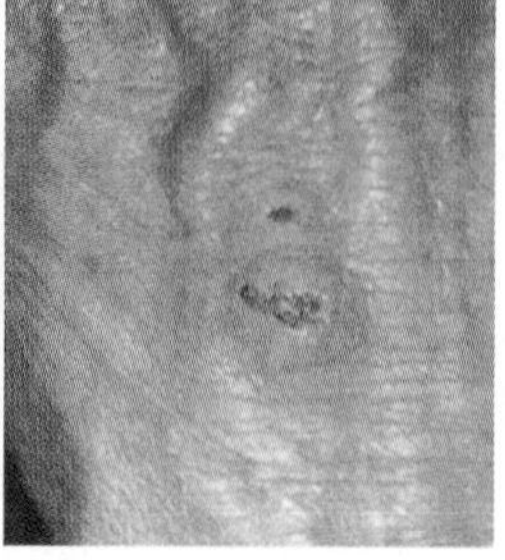

Figure 10-6 Squamous cell carcinoma.

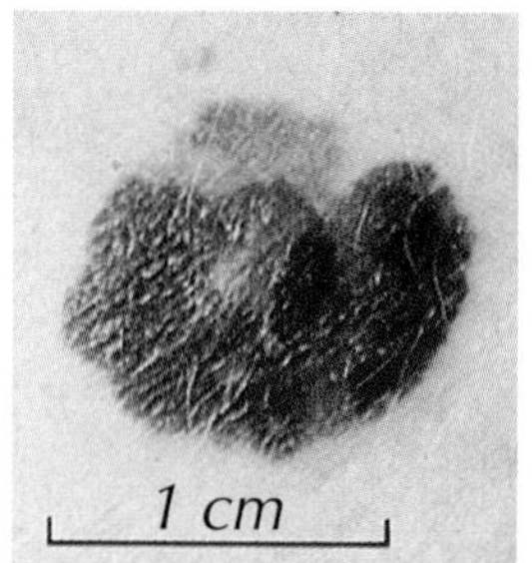

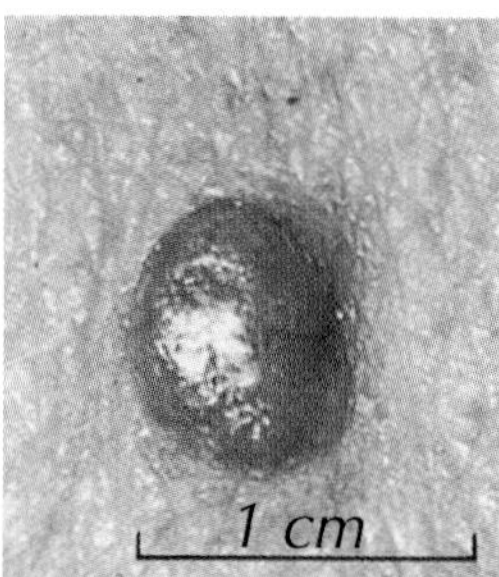

Figure 10-7 Malignant melanoma. (*Left*) Superficial melanoma. (*Right*) Nodular melanoma.

COMMON DIAGNOSTIC PROCEDURES AND THE MEDICAL ASSISTANT'S ROLE

Examination of the skin is performed mostly by inspection. This may be aided by palpation and the use of a diascope, a clear glass plate that allows the examiner to observe skin changes when pressure is applied.

Many skin lesions can be diagnosed by the history and the characteristic size, shape, and distribution on the skin. However, laboratory studies may be necessary to confirm a diagnosis. The medical assistant will be required to assemble equipment as directed by the physician, witness informed consent, and properly direct the specimens to appropriate laboratories. Standard Precautions must be observed when handling such specimens.

As the medical assistant, you will be responsible for preparing the room and the patient for the exami-

Box 10-2

Effects of Sunlight on the Skin

Exposure to the sun's ultraviolet rays is the major cause of skin cancers. In addition, ultraviolet rays cause sunburn and premature aging of the skin.

The incidence of skin cancers has risen dramatically in the last 20 years. This is thought to be due to the lack of sunscreen use and the increased tendency of people to spend more leisure time in the sun and sunbathing.

Primary prevention consists of limiting exposure to ultraviolet light by wearing proper clothing and using sunscreens. Exposure to the sun is not recommended during the five peak hours of the day, from 10:00 AM to 3:00 PM. A sunscreen with at least a 15 SPF (sun protective factor) is considered good protection in blocking ultraviolet rays. Most sunscreens contain PABA (*p*-aminobenzoic acid), which causes allergy in many people. However, a number of PABA-free sunscreens are available.

The use of sunlamps and tanning beds should be avoided.

nation. Gowning and draping should be appropriate to the patient's symptoms and body part to be examined.

During the examination, you will aid the physician by ensuring that the lighting is directed properly, handing necessary instruments and equipment, assisting in obtaining wound cultures, maintaining asepsis, and applying topical medications and dressings. Skin lesions must be protected from further infection by using medical asepsis or surgical asepsis as indicated. Again, Standard Precautions must be observed.

You will aid the patient in position changes and try to make the patient as comfortable as possible. To protect the patient's privacy, only body parts being examined are to be exposed.

After the examination, instruct the patient about home care, remove all soiled and contaminated supplies, and clean the room in the usual manner.

Wound Cultures

A wound culture consists of obtaining a specimen of wound **exudate** (drainage), which is then examined under a microscope to diagnose bacterial or fungal infection. To obtain a wound culture, follow these steps:

1. Wash your hands and put on gloves.
2. If a dressing is present, remove it, and dispose of it appropriately. Assess the wound for signs of infection by observing the color, odor, and amount of exudate.
3. Obtain a sample by either swabbing or aspirating the exudate. *For swabbing:* Obtain a sterile culture tube and remove the swab. Insert the swab into the exudate, being sure to saturate the swab (Fig. 10-8). Place the swab in the culture tube, and crush the ampule of transport medium (Fig. 10-9). Label the culture tube appropriately, and send it to the laboratory. *For aspirating:* Use a 1- to 5-mL syringe with needle removed to aspirate a sample of exudate, which is then placed in the culture tube for transport to the laboratory.

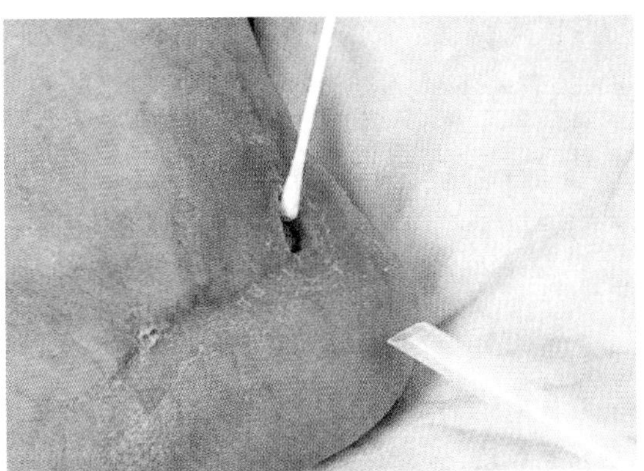

Figure 10-8 Insert culture swab into wound to obtain sample.

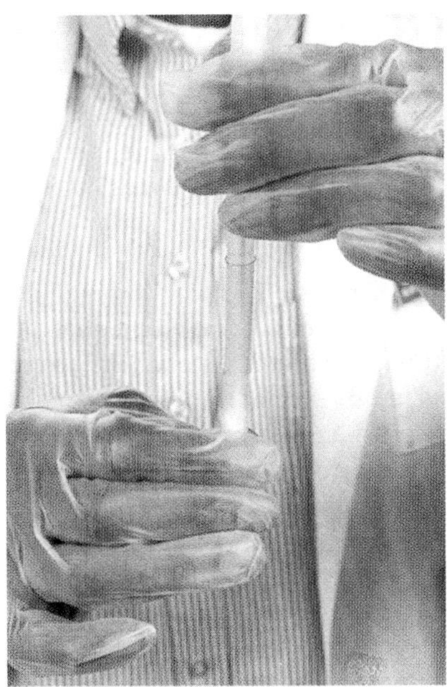

Figure 10-9 Crush ampule of medium.

4. Clean the wound and apply a sterile dressing according to the steps in Procedure 6-7: Applying a Sterile Dressing, in Chapter 6, Assisting With Minor Office Surgery.
5. Remove the gloves and wash your hands.

Skin Biopsy

The purpose of a skin biopsy is to remove a small piece of tissue from a lesion so that it may be examined under a microscope to differentiate between benign and malignant growths. A local anesthetic and sterile asepsis are used.

There are three types of skin biopsies: excision, punch, or shave biopsy. In an excision biopsy, the entire lesion is removed for study. When a punch biopsy is done, a small section is removed from the center of the lesion. A shave biopsy cuts the lesion off just above the skin line.

Your responsibility will be to assist the physician with equipment and supplies, observe surgical asepsis during the procedure, dress the wound, and route the specimen. Refer to Chapter 6, Assisting With Minor Office Surgery, for the procedure for assisting with excisional surgery.

Wood's Light Analysis

Wood's light is a black (ultraviolet) light. When it is directed 4 to 5 inches from the patient's skin in a darkened room, abnormalities in the skin and hair appear as fluorescent colors. It is used to detect fungal and bacterial infections, scabies, or alterations in pigment.

10

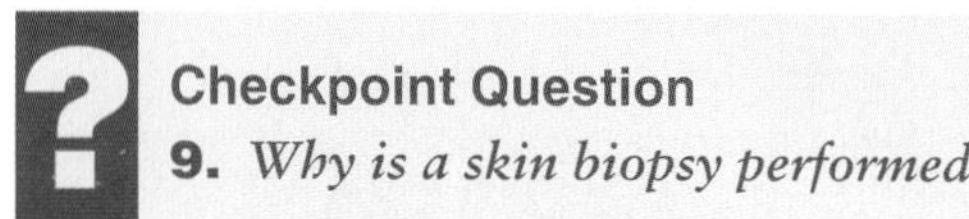

Checkpoint Question

9. *Why is a skin biopsy performed?*

Allergy Skin Testing

Scratch Test

Scratch or puncture tests are usually done on the outer surface of the upper arm or back to detect allergies. The skin surface is labeled or numbered in rows 1½ to 2 inches apart. A short scratch is then made with a needle or lancet and a drop of various **allergens** (substances that produce allergic reactions) is placed on each scratch or puncture. Fifty or more tests may be done at a time, and a certain pattern is followed so that the site of each allergen is identified. The test sites are examined after 15 to 20 minutes. A positive test for allergy to a substance is indicated by the development of a wheal at a site. Patients should not leave the office for at least 30 minutes after allergy testing so they can be observed for delayed allergic reactions (Box 10-3).

Intradermal Tests

Intradermal tests are done by injecting 0.01 to 0.02 mL of specific allergen extract intradermally on the anterior forearm. (See Chapter 8, Preparing and Administering Medications, for the procedure for intradermal injections.) Ten to 15 tests may be done on each arm. These are thought to be a more accurate method of testing for allergies than the scratch or puncture method.

Patch Tests

Patch tests, skin tests to identify allergens, are often done to determine the cause of contact dermatitis. A small amount of suspected allergen is placed on the anterior forearm, covered with cellophane, and taped down. Twenty to 30 tests may be done at a time. Results are read after 24 to 48 hours.

Box 10-3

Allergy Testing Safety Precautions

Allergy testing is usually performed by a trained technician in a controlled setting. The possibility of anaphylaxis is remote but must be considered. A well equipped and current emergency cart or tray must be on site and as close to the testing sites as possible. A basic setup includes:

- Injectable epinephrine with syringes and needles
- Various sizes of airways and intubation devices
- Oxygen and masks or ambubags
- Tourniquet

Additionally, some sites may require tracheotomy equipment, defibrillators, electrocardiography machines, and intravenous equipment.

Tuberculin Skin Testing

Tuberculin skin tests (Mantoux and tine tests) are used to screen for previous infection by the tuberculin bacillus, *Mycobacterium tuberculosis.*

- The Mantoux test consists of an injection of a minute amount of purified protein derivative (PPD) of the tuberculin bacillus given intradermally in the anterior forearm.
- The tine test is performed with a device that holds four tines, or prongs, impregnated with old tuberculin (OT) or PPD. This is pressed briefly into the anterior forearm. (Refer to Chap. 8, Preparing and Administering Medications, for the procedure for administering the Mantoux and tine tests.)

Tuberculin skin tests are read within 48 to 72 hours. A test is considered positive if redness and induration are present. The diameter of the indurated area should be measured in millimeters, usually with a guide provided by the manufacturer of the testing material. A positive test is usually indication for a follow-up chest x-ray and sputum studies.

WARM AND COLD APPLICATIONS

Because of the time involved in properly performing warm or cold soaks or compresses, these procedures are not often performed in the office setting. It frequently will be the medical assistant's responsibility to instruct patients who will be administering the treatments at home. Patients should understand the purpose for the procedure, the full performance of the procedure, the expected results, and precautions or danger signs.

Treatments may be warm or cold, moist or dry. Table 10-2 discusses types of heat and cold treatments and the purposes for each.

Precautions

The body quickly adapts to temperatures; for example, water in a pool feels cool at first, but the body soon becomes accustomed to the temperature. The water is no warmer, the body has simply adapted. By this reasoning, patients can be made to understand that it is not necessary to increase the temperature of treatments when they can no longer feel the initial benefits.

The body responds to extremes of temperature for extended periods of time by exerting an opposite ef-

Table 10-2 **Heat and Cold Treatments: Types and Purposes**

Dry Heat	*Moist Heat*	*Purposes*	*Dry Cold*	*Moist Cold*	*Purposes*
Heat Treatments			*Cold Treatments*		
Hot water bottle, heating pad, thermal pad, disposable heat pack, heat lamp	Compresses, warm packs, soaks, sitz bath	Relieve muscle spasm or tension Relieve pain Hasten healing by increasing blood flow to a part Provide local or systemic warming	Ice bag, ice collar, disposable cold pack	Compresses, cold soaks	Limit initial edema by decreasing capillary permeability (*Caution:* Cold retards relief of existing edema by decreasing blood flow to the part.) Decrease bleeding or hemorrhage Decrease inflammation formation Relieve pain by numbing the nerve pathways Provide local or systemic cooling

10

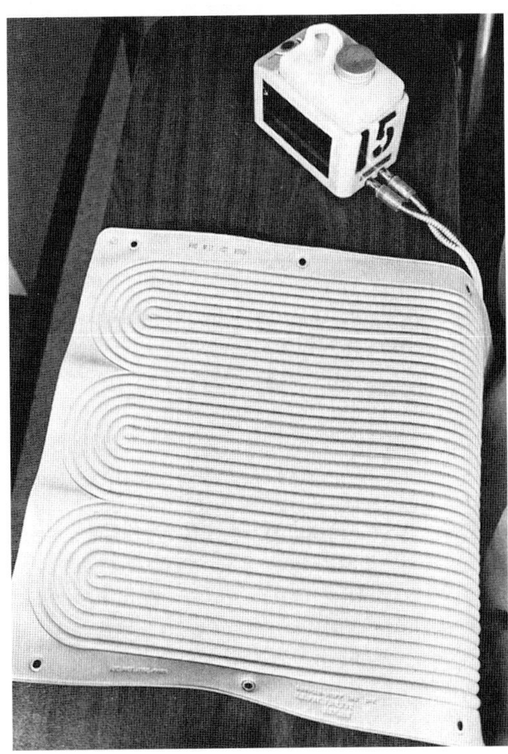

The Aquathermia (Aqua-K) pad is an electrical device that can be set to maintain water at a constant temperature and circulate it through the coils of the plastic pad. The pad can be used to provide dry heat, or it can be placed over a moist dressing to provide moist heat.

Table 10-3 **Proper Use of Heat and Cold: When *not* to Use Heat or Cold—and Why**

Do *not* use heat:	• Within 24 h after an injury because it may increase bleeding • For noninflammatory edema because increased capillary permeability will allow additional tissue fluid to build up • In cases of acute inflammation because increased blood supply will increase the inflammatory process • In the presence of malignancies because cell metabolism will be enhanced • Over the pregnant uterus because incidences of genetic mutation have been linked to heat applied to the gravid uterus • On areas of erythema or vesicles because it will compound the existing problem • Over metallic implants because it will cause discomfort
Do *not* use cold:	• On open wounds because decreased blood supply will delay healing • In the presence of already impaired circulation because it will further impair circulation

10

fect, called the rebound phenomenon. For example, beyond 30 minutes, heat applied to an area will cause vasoconstriction rather than vasodilation. Therefore, applications left on for longer periods of time than recommended will have an opposite effect than the one intended by the physician.

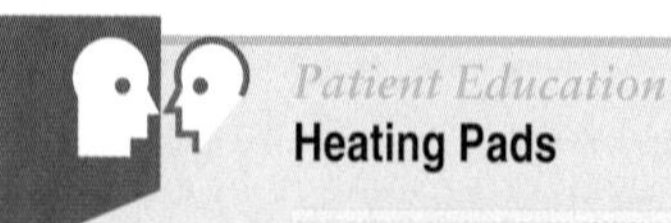

Patient Education

Heating Pads

Heating pads are not used in the office setting but may be recommended for home use. The patient must be aware of the potential for injury if strict guidelines are not followed. Share the safety tips below with your patient.

1. Be aware that most heating pads are equipped with a cover to ensure comfort and safety. If one is not provided, wrap the pad in a soft cover.
2. Do not fold or bend the pad; wires may break or short if not kept in alignment.
3. Do not pin the pad; pins may cause malfunction if they come in contact with wiring.
4. Never place pads under the body; heat may build up as it is reflected from the surface below and cause burns.
5. Set the temperature to be comfortably warm at first touch; do not turn the temperature up again as the body adjusts. (Explain to the patient in terms that can be understood the concept of adaptation to heat or cold and the dangers of ignoring warnings and guidelines.)
6. Alert the patient to the recommended time frame for heat treatments and the need for circulation to return to normal at intervals.

Heat applied to a large part of the body will decrease blood pressure due to peripheral vasodilation. Conversely, cold applied to large areas may cause the blood pressure to increase due to the shunting effect of vasoconstriction.

Some areas are more sensitive to heat than others. For example, areas of thin skin with few nerve receptors will not feel heat as quickly as the palms but because of the fragile skin in this area will be more likely to burn. The very young with immature nervous systems and the elderly with impaired nervous systems are more likely to suffer burns. Individuals with impaired mental states, such as the confusional states, are more prone to burns. Pre-existing pathology with compromised skin may also present a risk of burns.

Table 10-3 provides additional guidelines for proper use of heat and cold.

Temperature levels will vary by the length of application, method of application, the patient's general condition, and the condition of the skin. Temperature should be kept generally within the following guidelines:

- Warm—from tepid, 95/98°F, to a very warm 115°F (about 35°C to about 46°C)
- Cold—from neutral, 93/95°F, to a very cold 50°F (about 34°C to about 10°C)

Procedures 10-1, 10-2, and 10-3 describe the steps for applying cold, applying warm or cold compresses, and using a hot water bottle or commercial hot pack. For all of the procedures, observe Standard Precautions as necessary.

Soaks and Sitz Baths

Treatments may require that parts of the body be immersed in warm water or solutions for periods of time

text continues on page 228

Procedure 10-1 Applying Cold Treatments

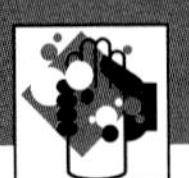

PURPOSE:

To decrease vasodilation or inflammation
To prevent edema after an injury
To reduce pain or bleeding

EQUIPMENT/SUPPLIES

- ice bag or ice collar or disposable cold pack
- cover
- ice chips or small cubes
- gauze or tape

STEPS

1. Wash your hands.
2. Assemble the equipment and supplies, checking the bag or collar for leaks. If using a commercial cold pack, read the manufacturer's directions.
   Check for leaks to avoid wetting and chilling the patient. Small bits of ice help the container conform to the patient's contours better than large pieces. The cover will add to the patient's comfort.
3. Fill the container about two-thirds full. Press it flat on a surface to expell excess air from within. Seal the container.
   If the container is too full of ice or air, it will not conform to the patient's contours.
4. Cover the bag.
   The cover will absorb condensation and be more comfortable for the patient.
5. Greet and identify the patient. Explain the procedure.
6. If using a commercial pack, activate it now.
7. Assess the area.
   The area must be assessed for documentation purposes and to ensure that the treatment can be successfully completed.
8. Ensure the patient's comfort.
   If the patient is comfortable when the treatment begins, compliance is more likely.
9. Secure the appliance with gauze or tape.
   It should be securely against the patient's skin for the greatest benefit. Pins may puncture the appliance.

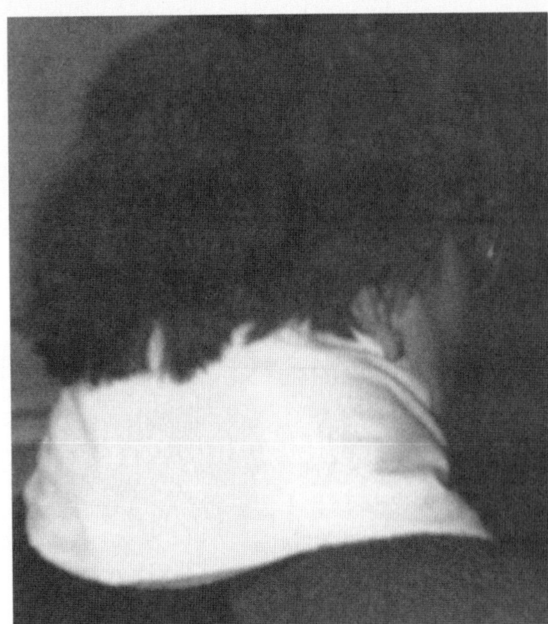

10. Apply for no longer than 30 minutes.
    Longer than the prescribed time may cause rebound, which will result in an adverse effect.
11. Assess the area for mottling, pallor, redness, or pain.
    Adverse effects should be reported to the physician immediately.
12. If the treatment is to be reapplied, wait 1 hour.
    Circulation must be allowed to return to normal in the area for proper nutrition and oxygen supply and removal of wastes.
13. Properly care for or dispose of equipment and supplies. Wash your hands.

continued

10

Procedure 10-1 Continued Applying Cold Treatments

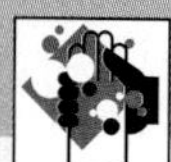

DOCUMENTATION GUIDELINES

- Date and time
- Location of treatment
- Time of treatment
- Observations of treatment site
- Complications or patient complaints/concerns
- Patient education/instructions
- Your signature

Charting Example

DATE	TIME Cold pack applied to left lower leg
	at 1400. Pack removed at 1430. No mot-
	tling, pallor, or redness noted. Pt states
	pain is less. Pt d/c to home by physician.
	—Your signature

10

Note: Ice bags are used for larger areas; ice collars are used for smaller areas. Disposable cold packs are convenient and safe for most uses.

Procedure 10-2 Applying a Warm or Cold Compress

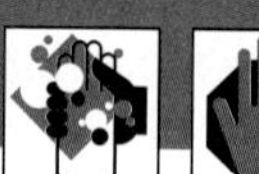

PURPOSE:

Warm: To hasten suppuration
To relieve muscle pain or spasms

Cold: To decrease vasodilation
To prevent edema after an injury
To relieve pain and slow bleeding

EQUIPMENT/SUPPLIES

- appropriate solution, warmed or cooled to recommended temperature
- absorbent material of the physician's choice
- waterproof barriers and insulators
- thermometer
- hot water bottle or cold pack
- clean or sterile basin
- sterile gloves or sterile transfer forceps, if appropriate

STEPS

1. Wash your hands. *Note*: If an open wound is present, observe surgical asepsis as outlined in Chap. 6, Assisting With Minor Office Surgery.

2. Assemble the equipment and supplies. Pour the solution into the basin. Check the temperature of the solution.

The solution must fall within the guidelines to avoid injury to the patient.

3. Greet and identify the patient. Explain the procedure.

4. Ensure patient comfort and privacy.

The patient is more likely to remain still for the procedure if comfort is ensured. Privacy must always be provided.

5. Protect the undersurface and clothing with waterproof barriers.

Wet bedding and clothing are uncomfortable for the patient and may cause chilling.

6. Put on gloves. Press or wring out excess moisture from the absorbent material. If using sterile procedure, this may be done with sterile gloves or with two sterile transfer forceps.

Compresses should be moist but not dripping to avoid wetting the patient.

continued

Procedure 10-2 Continued Applying a Warm or Cold Compress

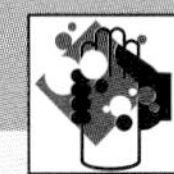
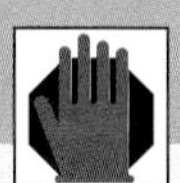

7. Touch the compress to the area lightly, and observe the patient's reaction or ask for a response.
Applying too rapidly to a compromised skin surface may cause pain or discomfort.

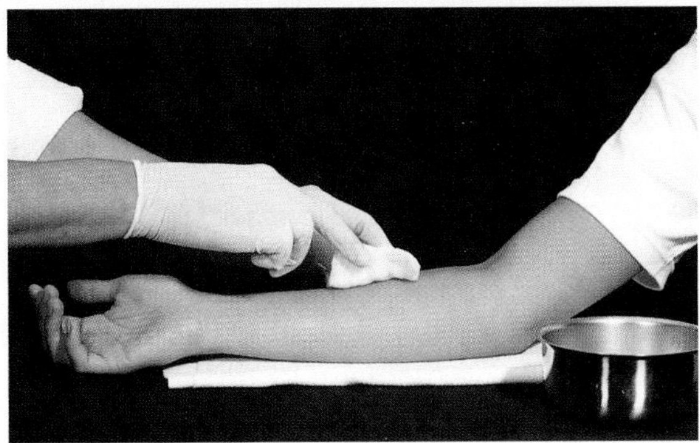

8. Check the surface of the skin.
If response to the solution is immediate, the temperature may be inappropriate.

9. Gently arrange the compress over the area and conform the material to the patient's contours. Insulate the compress with waterproof barriers.
Unless the material is against the skin, temperature will not be transferred to the area of concern. Insulating the area will retard temperature loss and will avoid wetting the patient.

10. Check frequently for moisture and temperature. Hot water bottles or ice packs may be used to maintain the temperature.
The temperature needs to stay fairly constant. If the material dries out, benefits will be lost.

11. Discontinue after 30 minutes. Wait 1 hour before reapplying.
Treatment longer than 30 minutes may result in rebound. The circulation should be allowed to return to normal for periods of time to avoid tissue damage.

12. Discard disposable materials, and appropriately disinfect reusable equipment. Wash your hands.

DOCUMENTATION GUIDELINES

- Date and time
- Solution used
- Temperature of solution
- Location of treatment
- Time period of treatment
- Observations of the treatment site
- Complications or patient complaints/concerns
- Patient education/instructions
- Your signature

Charting Example

DATE	TIME Warm saline compresses at 110°F
	(45°C) applied to lesion on R forearm at
	930. Compresses removed at 1000. Pt
	tolerated procedure well, skin warm and
	pink, lesion still intact. Pt instructed
	re: home compresses; verbalized under-
	standing of procedure and pt ed brochure.
	D/c to home by Dr. Cone. —Your signature

Note: Review Chapter 1, Asepsis and Infection Control, for gloving procedures or use of transfer forceps if an open lesion is present and if sterile technique is required for this procedure.

Note: Warm compresses will speed the suppuration process to increase healing. Cold compresses will slow bleeding and decrease inflammation.

10

Procedure 10-3 Using a Hot Water Bottle or Commercial Hot Pack

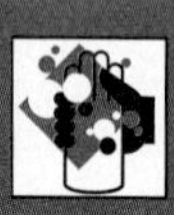

PURPOSE:

To warm a body part
To increase vasodilation and circulation to a part
To decrease pain and promote comfort

EQUIPMENT/SUPPLIES

- hot water bottle or commercial hot pack
- cover
- thermometer

STEPS

1. Wash your hands.
2. Assemble equipment, being sure to check the hot water bottle for leaks.
   Checking for leaks avoids wetting the patient.
3. Fill bottle about two-thirds full with water at appropriate temperature. Check temperature with thermometer.
   If the bottle is too full, it will not conform to the patient's contours. If water is too warm, it may cause tissue damage; if it is too cool, maximum benefits will not be achieved.
4. Place the bottle on a flat surface with the opening up and "burp" it by pressing out the excess air.
   Excess air will prevent the bottle from conforming to the patient's contours.

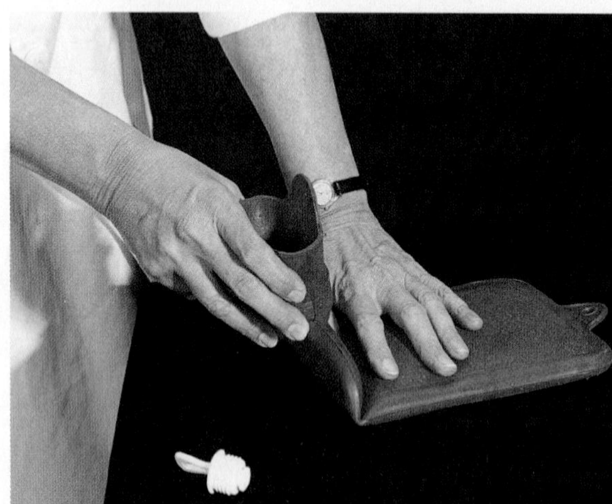

5. If using a commercial hot pack, follow the manufacturer's directions for activating it.
6. Wrap and secure the pack or bottle before placing on the patient's skin.
   Covering the bag will increase the patient's comfort and help to prevent burns.

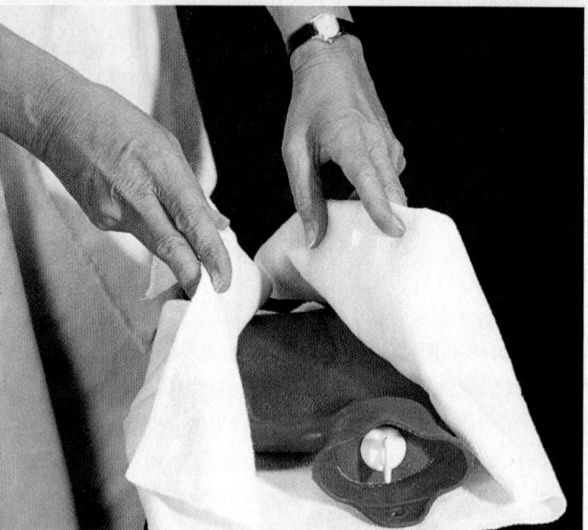

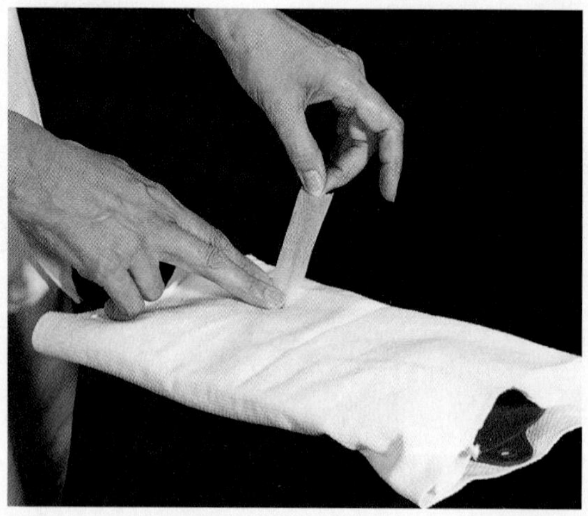

7. Greet and identify the patient. Explain the procedure.
8. If continuous heat has been ordered, follow the physician's instructions; otherwise, remove after 30 minutes. Assess the area every 10 minutes.
   General orders recommend removing sources of heat or cold after 30 minutes to avoid rebound and to allow circulation to return to normal.

continued

Procedure 10-3 Continued Using a Hot Water Bottle or Commercial Hot Pack

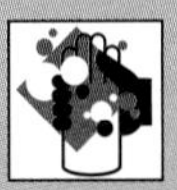

9. Report pallor (an indication of rebound), excessive redness (indicates temperature may be too high for this lesion), swelling (indicates that capillary permeability may contribute to tissue damage).

   Treatment may have to be re-evaluated for this patient.

10. Caution the patient that the body will adapt to the temperature and that it is not necessary to continually increase the temperature to achieve maximum benefits.

   This protects the patient from injury.

DOCUMENTATION GUIDELINES

- Date and time
- Location of treatment (if performed in the office)
- Time period of treatment
- Observations of the treatment site
- Complications or patient complaints/concerns
- Patient education/instructions
- Your signature

Charting Example

DATE	TIME Pt educated in proper application
	of hot water bottle. Written instructions
	given to pt. Pt verbalized understanding
	of all instructions. —Your signature

Procedure 10-4 Assisting With Therapeutic Soaks

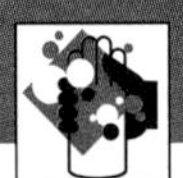

PURPOSE:

To relieve pain or muscle spasms
To increase vasodilation or circulation to a part

EQUIPMENT/SUPPLIES

- container large enough to contain the part to be soaked comfortably
- solution
- towels (for padding surfaces and drying the part)
- thermometer

STEPS

1. Wash your hands.
2. Assemble the equipment and supplies.

   If the container is uncomfortably small, proper application will be difficult and may cause muscle spasms. Surfaces should be padded for comfort.

3. Fill the container with the solution, and check the temperature with the thermometer. (The proper temperature is usually at no more than 110°F [about 45°C] because of the large surface involved and the possibility of blood pressure changes with vasodilation or vasoconstriction.)

   Burns or other tissue damage must be avoided.

4. Greet and identify the patient. Explain the procedure.
5. Slowly lower the part into the container and check for the patient's reaction. Arrange the part comfortably and in easy alignment. (The basin should be large enough to immerse the entire limb.) Check for pressure areas and pad the edges. The bottom may also be padded for comfort.

   Immersing too quickly can be shocking to the patient. If the patient is not comfortable, muscle spasms or strain may result.

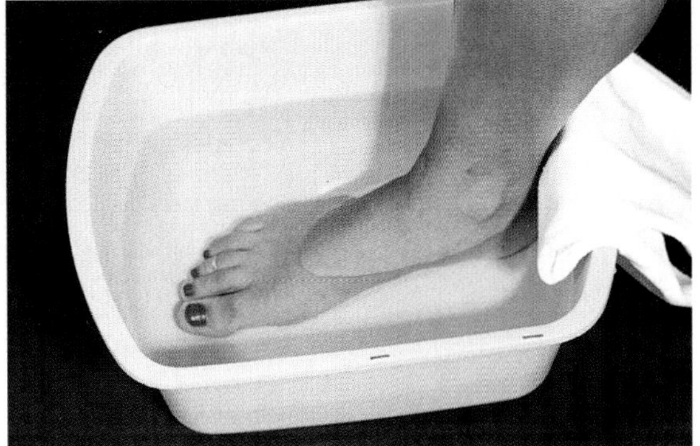

continued

Procedure 10-4 Continued Assisting With Therapeutic Soaks

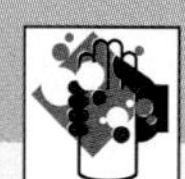

6. Soak for the prescribed period of time.
   Soaking too long may result in tissue damage or the rebound effect.
7. Check every 5–10 minutes for the proper temperature. If additional water or solution must be added to maintain the temperature, remove a quantity of the solution. With your hand acting as a shield between the patient and the stream of solution, add the required amount and swirl it quickly through the container.
   The proper temperature must be maintained for maximum benefit. Avoid pouring the solution or water against the patient.

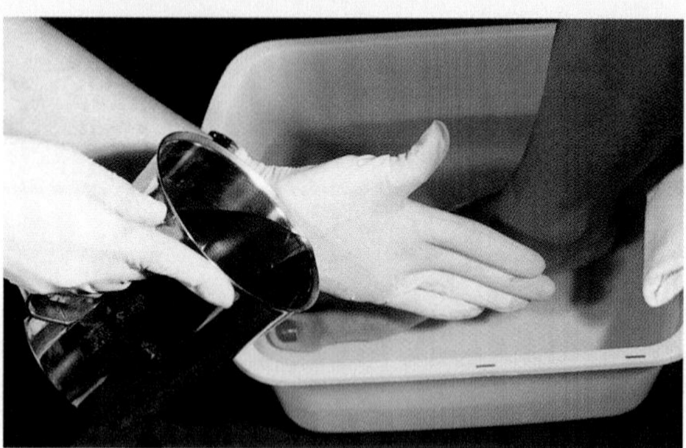

8. Soak for the prescribed time, usually 15–20 minutes.
   Soaking for longer may result in rebound or in tissue damage.
9. Carefully dry the part.
   The area may be sensitive to brisk rubbing after the treatment but must be dried to prevent chilling the patient or causing discomfort by remaining wet.
10. Assess the area.
11. Properly care for or dispose of equipment and supplies. Wash your hands.

DOCUMENTATION GUIDELINES

- Date and time
- Location of treatment
- Time period of treatment
- Type of solution
- Observations of the treatment site
- Complications or patient complaints/concerns
- Patient education/instructions
- Your signature

Charting Example

DATE	TIME Left foot was soaked for
	20 minutes in warm water. Pt tolerated
	procedure well. Skin warm and pink. Pt
	states muscle and joint pain slightly
	relieved. Pt verbalized understanding of
	procedural instructions and pt ed
	brochure. Pt d/c to home by Dr. Suratt.
	—Your signature

(Procedure 10-4). Disposable sitz bath containers are available at all medical supply stores for soaking the perineal area. They are equipped with detailed instructions from the manufacturer. If an extremity is to be soaked at home, the patient can use a Styrofoam chest to soak limbs. The chests are waterproof and are fairly large and deep and easy to clean. A towel draped over the opening will help to maintain the temperature of the treatment.

Checkpoint Question

10. *How does the body respond to prolonged exposure to temperature extremes?*

Answers to Checkpoint Questions

1. *The integument helps control body temperature through vasodilation and vasoconstriction. When the body is hot, blood vessels in the skin dilate, bringing interior heat close to the body's surface. When the body is cold, the vessels constrict to conserve heat.*
2. *The three basic layers of the skin are the epidermis (outer layer), the dermis (middle layer), and the subcutaneous tissue (connects the dermis to underlying muscles).*
3. *Folliculitis, furuncle, and carbuncle are bacterial skin infections that develop in the hair follicles. Folliculitis*

is a localized infection of a hair follicle. A furuncle is an infection deep within the hair follicle. A carbuncle is an infection involving subcutaneous tissue around several hair follicles.

4. *Herpes zoster, also known as shingles, is believed to be caused by the same virus that causes chickenpox. This virus can lie dormant for years after initial exposure. When reactivated, the virus spreads down a nerve to the skin, resulting in redness, swelling, pain, and eventual development of lesions.*

5. *Tinea capitis is a fungal skin infection that affects the scalp; tinea pedis is a fungal infection that affects the feet (it is also known as athlete's foot).*

6. *Urticaria (also known as hives) is an acute inflammatory reaction of the dermis; it is characterized by itching and the development of wheals.*

7. *Four pigmentation disorders are albinism (partial or total absence of pigment in the skin, hair, and eyes), vitiligo (chronic destruction of melanocytes), leukoderma (localized loss of pigment), and nevus (pigmented skin blemish).*

8. *Squamous cell carcinoma will spread through underlying and surrounding tissues.*

9. *A skin biopsy is used to examine a lesion for benign and malignant cells.*

10. *After prolonged exposure to temperature extremes, the body exerts the opposite effect. For example, heat applications lasting longer than 30 minutes will cause vasoconstriction rather than vasodilation. This is called the rebound phenomenon.*

Critical Thinking Challenges

1. Sunlight or ultraviolet rays are needed to convert vitamin D necessary for calcium and phosphorus absorption. Why would it be important that children be exposed to sunlight regularly during their growing years?
2. Why would molds and fungi thrive in a public shower or pool? Consider the factors needed for microorganisms to thrive.
3. Why would hot water be contraindicated in cases of eczema?

Suggestions for Further Reading

Craven, R. F., & Hirnle, C. J. (1996). *Fundamentals of Nursing: Health and Human Function,* 2nd ed. Philadelphia: Lippincott-Raven.

Professional Guide to Diseases, 4th ed. (1992). Springhouse, PA: Springhouse Corporation.

Schroeder, S. A., et al. (1992). *Current Medical Diagnosis and Treatment.* East Norwalk, CT: Appleton & Lange.

Smeltzer, S. C., & Bare, B. G. (1996). *Brunner and Suddarth's Textbook of Medical-Surgical Nursing,* 8th ed. Philadelphia: Lippincott-Raven.

Taylor, C., Lillis, C., & LeMone, P. (1997). *Fundamentals of Nursing: The Art and Science of Nursing Care,* 3rd ed. Philadelphia: Lippincott-Raven.

Timby, B. (1996). *Fundamental Skills and Concepts in Patient Care,* 6th ed. Philadelphia: Lippincott-Raven.

Walter, J. B. (1992). *An Introduction to the Principles of Disease,* 3rd ed. Philadelphia: W.B. Saunders.

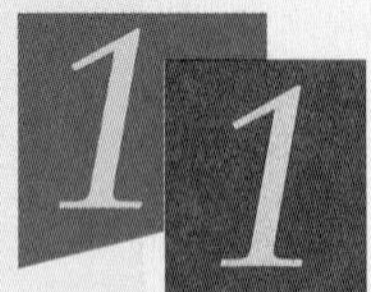

Assisting With Diagnostic and Therapeutic Procedures Associated With the Musculoskeletal System

Chapter Outline

Role Delineation

CLINICAL

Patient Care

- Prepare patient for examinations, procedures, and treatments.
- Assist with examinations, procedures, and treatments.

GENERAL

Professionalism

- Project a professional manner and image.

Communication Skills

- Treat all patients with compassion and empathy.

Legal Concepts

- Practice within the scope of education, training, and personal capabilities.

Instruction

- Instruct individuals according to their needs.

Chapter Competencies

Learning Objectives

Upon successfully completing this chapter, you will be able to:

1. Spell and define the Key Terms.
2. Describe the structure and function of the skeletal and muscular systems.
3. Identify the axial and appendicular skeletons.
4. List and describe the five types of bones.
5. Describe the curves of the spinal column using the appropriate terminology.
6. Explain the role of the intervertebral disks.
7. Name the three types of joints and give examples of each.
8. Name and locate the major muscles of the body.
9. List and describe types of fractures.
10. List and describe disorders of the musculoskeletal system.
11. Identify and explain diagnostic procedures of the musculoskeletal system.
12. List and describe types of ambulatory aids.

Performance Objectives

Upon successfully completing this chapter, you will be able to:

1. Prepare a patient for casting.
2. Assist the physician with cast application (Procedure 11-1).
3. Apply a triangular arm sling (Procedure 11-2).
4. Measure a patient for axillary crutches (Procedure 11-3).
5. Instruct a patient in the use of various crutch gaits (Procedure 11-4).
6. Transfer a patient to and from a wheelchair (Procedure 11-5).

Key Terms

(See Glossary for definitions.)

amphiarthroses
ankylosing spondylitis
antagonist
appendicular skeleton
arthrograms
arthroplasty
axial skeleton
bursae
callus
cancellous
contracture
contusions
diarthroses
electromyography
embolus
epiphyseal end plate
fixator
goniometer
insertion
intrinsic
iontophoresis
kyphosis
ligaments
lordosis
myofibrils
olecranon fossa
olecranon process
origin
Paget's disease
phonophoresis
prime mover
prosthesis
reduction
scoliosis
sesamoid
striated
synarthroses
synergist
tendons
tonus

Muscles allow movement of the body parts through contraction and relaxation. Bones provide the framework on which muscles and their supporting structures are attached. Because both systems depend on each other to function, they are often referred to as a single system—the musculoskeletal system. The integrity of the entire system is required for normal body movement.

STRUCTURE AND FUNCTION OF THE MUSCULOSKELETAL SYSTEM

The Skeletal System

The adult human has 206 named bones. These bones are grouped into two distinct structures known as the **axial skeleton** and the **appendicular skeleton** (Fig. 11-1). The axial skeleton—consisting of the 80 bones of the head, thorax, and trunk—is a fairly rigid structure that

11

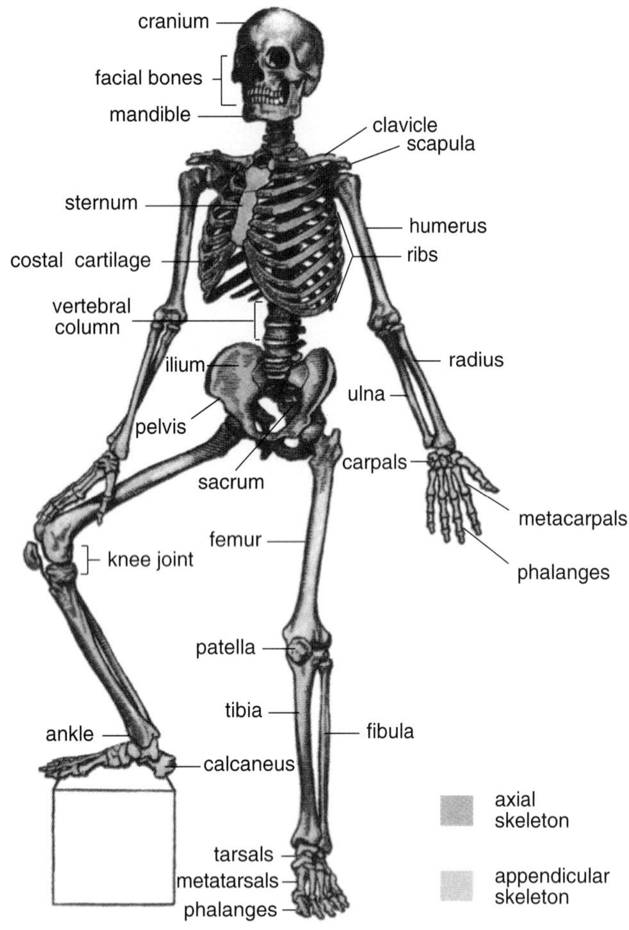

Figure 11-1 The skeleton.

supports and connects the two halves of the body. It includes the skull, the vertebral column, the thorax, and the hyoid bone. There are no long or short bones in the axial skeleton (see "Types of Bones," below).

The appendicular skeleton consists of the remaining 126 bones and provides a freely movable frame for the arms and legs. It includes the shoulder and pelvic girdles and all the bones of the arms, wrists, hands, thighs, legs, and feet. There are no irregular bones in the appendicular skeleton (see "Types of Bones," below). Fractures are more common in the appendicular skeleton; however, they are more serious in the axial skeleton (see "Common Musculoskeletal Disorders," below).

Types of Bones

The skeletal system consists of five types of bones: long, short, flat, **sesamoid,** and irregular.

Long bones are the largest bones in the body and make up most of the appendicular skeleton. Their length is greater than their width. These bones are tubular shaped with bulbous ends. The humerus and femur are long bones.

Short bones, unlike long bones, are generally more equal in height, length, and width. They usually articulate (join or attach) with more than one bone. The wrist and ankle bones are short bones.

Flat bones are thin bones with broad surfaces. Despite their name, these bones are more curved than flat. The scapula and ilium are flat bones.

Sesamoid bones are small bones that develop within **tendons** (tough, flexible fibers that bind muscle to bone), protecting them from undue wear and tear. They also change a tendon's angle of attachment to increase the leverage of the muscle force. The patella is a sesamoid bone.

Irregular bones are of mixed shapes and varieties that do not fit into the other categories. Vertebrae are classified as irregular bones.

Bone Structure

Bone is the hardest of all living tissue. Because bones are made up of different types of tissue, they are considered organs. Bone is composed of one-third organic (living) material, which provides elasticity and allows for partial deformation to help distribute forces, and two-thirds inorganic (nonliving) material, which provides strength and hardness.

Bone strength and integrity are maintained by a complex system that rebuilds osteocytes (bone cells) as they age and weaken. Osteoclasts are specialized cells that break down nonfunctional osteocytes and recycle the reusable components to rebuild new osteoblasts, the embryonic cells that will become mature osteocytes. Healthy bones are constantly removing old bone cells and building new ones.

Bone is either compact or **cancellous.** Compact bone is hard and dense and makes up the outer shell. Cancellous bone, which is porous and spongy, makes up the inside portion—a lattice-work space filled with marrow. Yellow marrow consists of fat cells and connective tissue. Red marrow fosters the production of blood cells.

Blood cell production occurs primarily in the epiphysis. The epiphysis is located at each end of a long bone; it is wider than the shaft (Fig. 11-2). Bones grow by producing new bone at the **epiphyseal end plate.** In children, this plate is easily seen on x-ray. It is not seen in adults, however, indicating that growth has stopped. If injury occurs at the epiphyseal end plate during the growth years, the bone may no longer grow, causing one limb to be shorter than the other.

The diaphysis is the shaft of the long bone. It is composed mainly of compact bone, making it very hard and strong. Its hollow center, called the medullary canal, lightens the weight of the bone. It contains yellow marrow and the blood vessels that supply the bone with nutrients. The metaphysis is the flared end of the

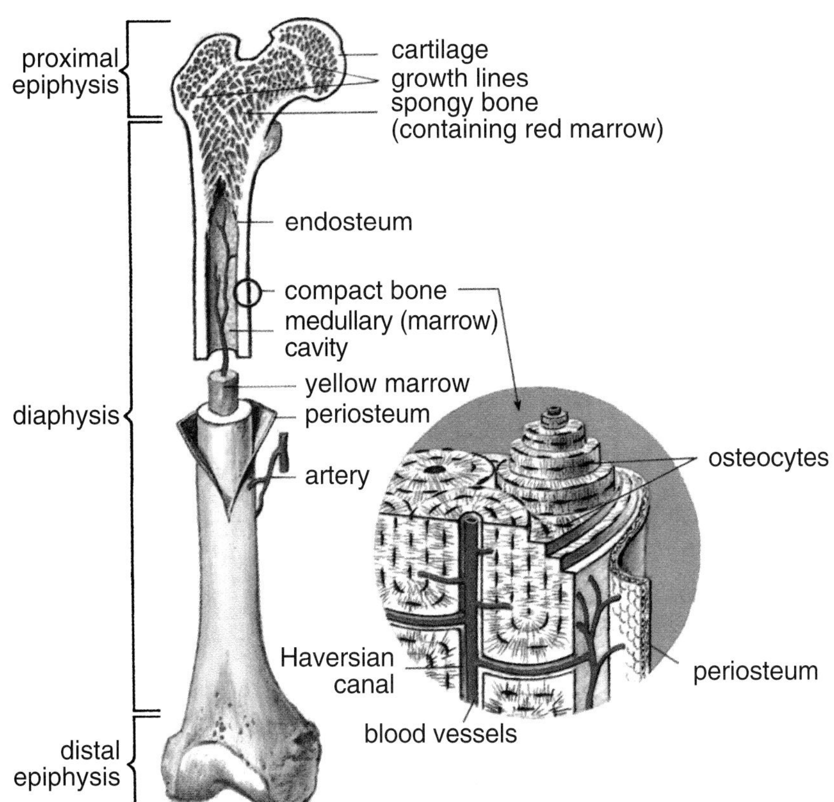

Figure 11-2 The structure of a long bone; the composition of compact bone.

diaphysis. It is mostly cancellous bone and supports the epiphysis.

Bones are covered by a tough fibrous layer called the periosteum. It is the life support system for the bone, providing the cells that form new bone after a fracture. It is well supplied with sensory nerves, which is the reason damage to a bone is so painful. Bones have a great capacity for healing themselves, more so than most other body structures.

Bones have many projections and depressions that serve various purposes. Table 11-1 describes the main bony landmarks and features.

Table 11-1 **Bony Landmarks and Features**

Bones are marked with various projections and depressions that serve a multitude of purposes. The main landmarks and features are listed below.

Landmark	*Features*
Condyle	A rounded projection on a bone that anchors ligaments and articulates with adjoining bones (eg, the olecranon condyle that fits into the olecranon fossa at the elbow to allow the forearm to straighten)
Crest	A ridge or long projection on a bone (eg, the iliac crest)
Epicondyle	A projection on a bone above the condyle (eg, the medial and lateral epicondyles at the elbow)
Facet	A smooth surface for articulation (eg, the facets of the vertebrae)
Foramen	An opening into a bone (or any body structure) as a passageway (eg, the foramen magnum at the base of the skull for the passage of the spinal cord)
Fossa	A hollow or depression in a bone, usually for the articulation of another bone (eg, the olecranon fossa that receives the olecranon process of the ulna to allow the forearm to straighten)
Head	The topmost part of a structure, the proximal end of a bone (eg, the head of the femur)
Neck	A constricted section, usually just below the head of a body part or a bone (eg, the neck of the femur)
Process	A projection or natural outgrowth of bone (eg, the acromion process)
Sinus	A hollow space within a bone; may serve to make the bone lighter (eg, the paranasal sinuses)
Spine	A sharp, bony process (eg, the sharp dorsal projection on a vertebra)
Suture	Union between nonmovable articulations (eg, the cranial sutures)
Tubercle	A small elevation on bone, usually for the attachment of muscles (eg, the greater tubercle of the humerus)
Tuberosity	Another name for a tubercle (eg, tibial tuberosity)

11

Bone Function

Bones support the body and act in response to the contraction of skeletal muscles, making movement possible.

Their overall functions include:

- Providing a supportive framework for the body
- Providing leverage for muscles
- Protecting vital organs
- Allowing for calcium metabolism and storage
- Facilitating blood cell production

All bones have particular functions. For example, the skull protects the brain and is a framework for the face. The ribs and sternum support the chest wall and protect the contents of the thorax. The scapula (shoulder blade) is joined to the humerus, the longest bone in the arm, which is attached at the elbow to the radius and the ulna (bones of the forearm). The wrist has eight carpal bones that attach to phalanges (bones of the fingers). All of these bones are necessary for the many movements involving the hands and arms.

The ilium and the ischium are the major bones of the pelvis. The femur (thigh bone) is the longest, strongest, and heaviest bone in the body. It attaches to the tibia, the longer bone of the lower leg. The patella (kneecap) covers this joint and protects it. The fibula articulates with the tibia and, at its distal end, forms the lateral ankle bone. The foot has seven tarsal bones, five metatarsal bones, and the toes, which are called the phalanges (like the fingers). All of these bones work together to keep us upright and give us mobility.

Checkpoint Question

1. *List five functions of the skeletal system.*

> *Box 11-1*
> **Types of Cartilage**
>
> - *Hyaline cartilage* is articular cartilage, covering the ends of opposing bones. It has no blood supply and gets its nutrients from the synovial fluid. It cannot heal itself when damaged.
> - *Fibrocartilage* functions as a shock absorber and fills the gap between two bones. In the knee, it is called the meniscus; in the shoulder, it is the labrum.
> - *Elastic cartilage* allows for specific limited movements. In the symphysis pubis, it stretches to allow for birth, and in the larynx, its motion is important for speech.

Joints

Joints hold the bones together. They are formed by connective tissue and cartilage, dense fibrous connective tissue that is capable of great tension and pressure (Box 11-1). In some joints, the bones are held together so tightly that little movement occurs. In joints in which the bones are held loosely, more movement is possible.

Types of Joints

Joints are grouped into three main types, according to the amount of movement they allow.

Synarthroses are immovable joints. They are formed by the direct union of bone to bone by dense fibrous tissue. Examples are the skull joints.

Amphiarthroses, slightly movable joints, are formed when two bones are joined directly by fibrocartilage or hyaline cartilage. Examples are the symphysis pubis and sacroiliac joint. Synarthrotic and amphiarthrotic joints function primarily to provide stability.

Diarthroses, or synovial joints, allow the bones to move freely in relation to one another because no structures directly connect the two bony surfaces (Table 11-2). The bones are connected indirectly to each other by **ligaments** that form a joint. Synovial joints make up the majority of the joints of the body. Examples include the shoulder, elbow, and knee.

The cavity of a synovial joint is filled by synovial fluid, which lubricates the joint, absorbs shock, reduces friction between the bones, and allows free, painless movement. It also nourishes the cartilage. The joint is surrounded by a capsule consisting of strong fibrous tissue that holds the joint together. The articular surface is smooth and covered with cartilage. The bones are held together and supported by ligaments; these are flexible but not elastic. The flexibility allows movement, and the absence of elasticity provides protection for the joint.

Bursae are small, padlike sacs that surround some joints. They are filled with a clear synovial fluid. Bursae are found in areas of excessive friction, such as under tendons and over bony prominences. Their primary purposes are to reduce friction between moving parts and to help prevent damage.

Joint Movement

The body is constantly moving and changing position. Movement in a joint occurs in a plane around an axis. The body has three planes—sagittal, frontal, and transverse—in which activity occurs. (See Chapter 9, Introduction to Anatomy and Physiology, for a discussion of body planes.) Various joint motions are described below and illustrated in Fig. 11-3.

In the sagittal plane:

- Flexion—bending one bone on another, causing a decrease in the angle of the joint (eg, bending the elbow or the knee)

Table 11-2 **Types of Joints**

Type	*Description*	*Movement*	*Examples*
Fibrous			
(immovable)	No synovial cavity Bones held together by fibrous tissue	No motion, or "give" only	Bones of skull fitted together with teethlike projections (sutures), roots of teeth in sockets of the maxillae and mandible
Cartilaginous			
(slightly movable)	No synovial cavity Bones held together by cartilage	Slight degree of flexibility	Intervertebral joints, costal cartilage, attachments of first 10 ribs to sternum, symphysis pubis
Synovial			
(freely movable)	Synovial cavity and articular cartilage present	Freely movable	Types of synovial joints listed below
Gliding	One bone slides over another Surrounding structures restrict the motion	Gliding motion without any angular or circular movements	Joints between carpal bones, tarsal bones, the sternum and clavicle, and the scapula and clavicle
Hinge	Spool-shaped process fits into concave socket	Motion like a door on a hinge; permits flexion and extension	Finger, elbow, and knee
Pivot	Arch-shaped process fits around peglike process	Motion like turning a doorknob; permits rotation	Joint between the first and second cervical vertebrae allows rotation of the head from side to side; joint between the head of the radius notch of the ulna allows for supination and pronation of the palms
Condyloid	Oval-shaped condyle of one bone fits into an elliptical cavity of another bone	Allows motion in two planes at right angles, permits flexion, extension in one plane, abduction, adduction in another plane	Radiocarpal joint of wrist
Saddle	Articular surface of one bone is saddle shaped and the articular surface of the other bone is shaped like a rider sitting in the saddle	Movements are side to side and back and forth; permits flexion, extension, abduction, adduction	Carpometacarpal joint of thumb, ankle
Ball-and-socket	Ball-like surface of one bone fitted into a cuplike depression of another bone	Rotating motions; permits widest range of motion; flexion, extension, abduction, adduction, rotation, circumduction	Shoulder and hip joints

From Jones, S. A., Weigel, A., White, R. D., McSwain, N. E., & Breiter, M. (1992). *Advanced Emergency Care for Paramedic Practice,* p. 364. Philadelphia: J.B. Lippincott.

11

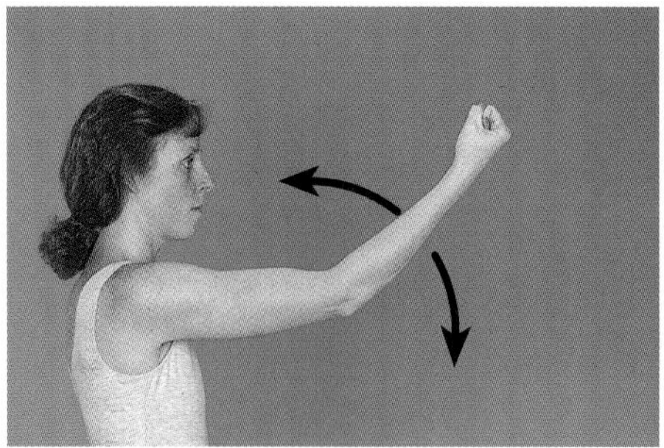

flexion/extension

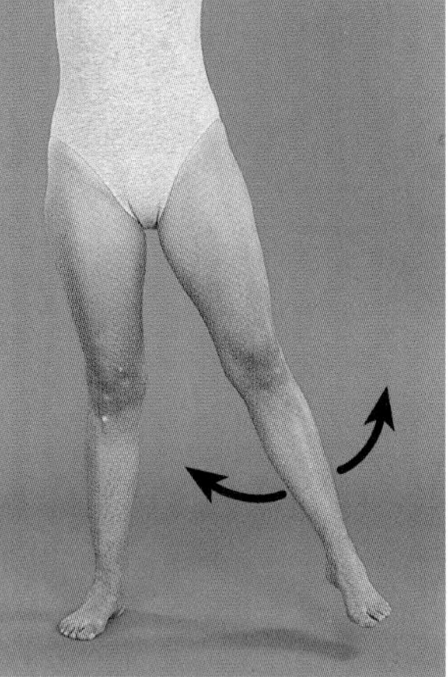

abduction/adduction

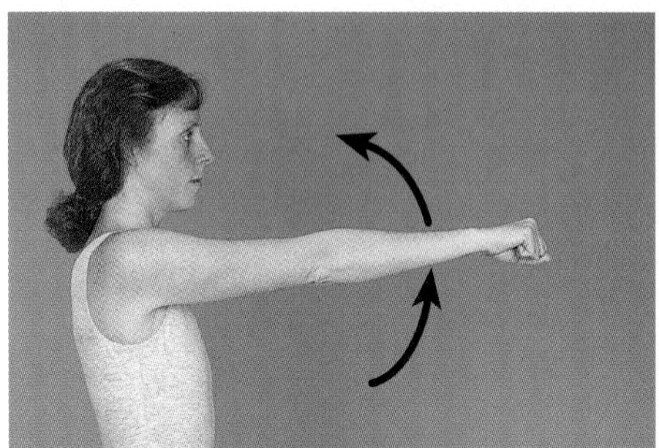

circumduction

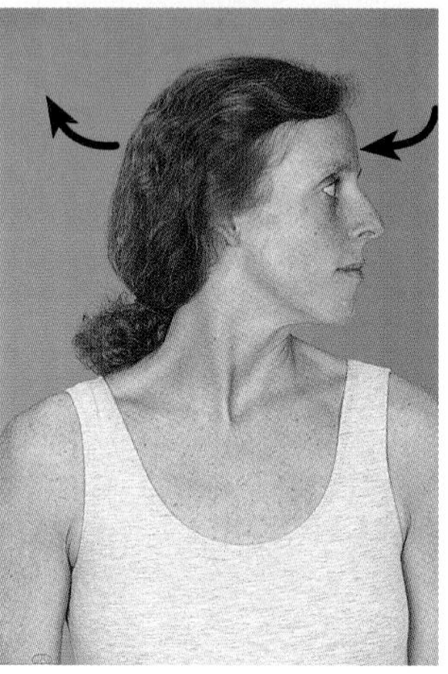

rotation

Figure 11-3 Normal range of motion of selected joints.

- Extension—straightening the joint, causing an increase in the joint angle. Extension usually returns the part of the body to the anatomic position.
- Hyperextension—straightening the body part beyond the anatomic position (eg, bending backward or raising the leg behind oneself)

In the frontal plane:

- Abduction—movement away from the midline of the body
- Adduction—movement toward the midline of the body

In the transverse plane:

- Rotation—movement around a fixed point. Internal or medial rotation occurs when the ball in a ball-and-socket joint moves into the joint (eg, reaching into one's back pocket). External or lateral rotation occurs when the ball moves back and away from the joint (eg, patting the back of the head). Internal and external rotation occur only in the shoulder and hip joint.

Circumduction combines all the movements, causing the distal end of the extremity to make a wide circle while the proximal end makes a small circle (eg, arm movements in swimming).

Some movements are specific to certain joints. For example, supination of the forearm occurs when the palms are turned up toward the face. Conversely, pronation occurs when the palms are turned down and away. Inversion occurs, for instance, when the foot is turned inward at the ankle so that the bottom of the big toe can be seen. Eversion is movement in the opposite direction. Dorsiflexion usually involves the foot or hand and describes a movement that shortens the angle at the back of the hand or top of the foot so that they point upward. The opposite is plantar flexion, which shortens the angle between the palm and the wrist, or pulls the foot downward to point the toes.

Range of Motion

Normal range of motion is the amount of motion possible in a joint within the limits of its anatomic structure. Many conditions can affect joint range, such as degenerative changes, injury, inflammation, disease, fractures, tumors, dislocations, nerve damage, deformities, and congenital anomalies (birth defects). When joint motion is limited, the joint is hypomobile. If

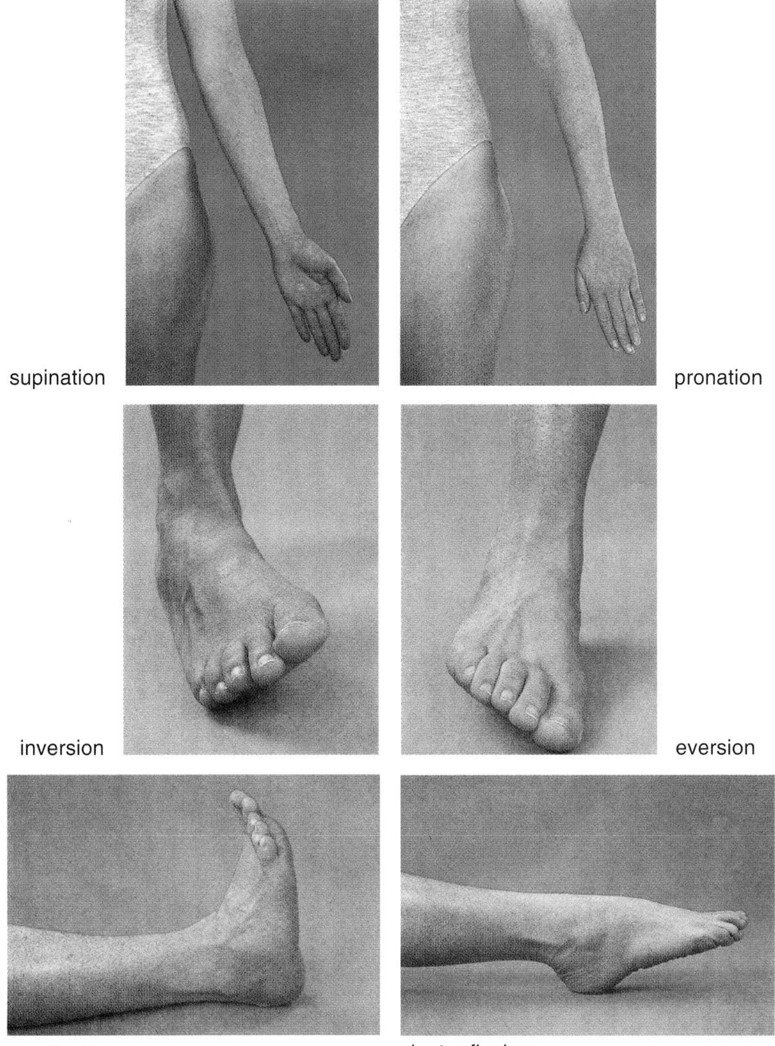

Figure 11-3 *(continued)*

movement is loose or greater than normal, the joint is hypermobile and is usually unstable.

The more complex the joint, the more likely it is to be affected by injury, degenerative processes, and disease. Anything that alters or disturbs the function of a specific part of a joint can eventually affect every part of the joint itself and its surrounding structures.

Checkpoint Question

2. *Name the three types of joints. Briefly describe each.*

Cranial Structures

The skull is considered to be two structures: the facial bones and the cranium.

The facial bones form the framework to give the face its shape. The *mandible,* the only movable bone in the skull, hinges at the temporomandibular joint (TMJ), forms the lower jaw, and holds our lower teeth (Fig. 11-4). The *maxillae* are two fused bones in the upper jaw that hold the upper teeth and form the anterior hard palate. The two *palatine* bones form the posterior hard palate. If the maxillae and palatine bones fail to fuse in the fetus, a cleft palate or hare lip will result, depending on the severity of the defect. The maxillae contain the maxillary sinuses. The *nasal* bones form the bridge of the nose and the *vomer* supports the lower nasal septum. The *zygomatic* bones are referred to as the cheekbones. On the lateral walls of the nasal cavity are the *conchae* (also part of the ethmoid bone in the cranium). When covered with mucous membrane, these structures are called the turbinates and are part of the respiratory system. Part of the medial eye socket is formed by the *lacrimal* bone that contains a channel for the tear duct to drain into the nasal cavity. The *hyoid* bone is considered part of the skull but joins with no other bone and is supported by the posterior attachment of the tongue.

The bones of the cranium form the floor of the brain pan and the protective outer structure of the

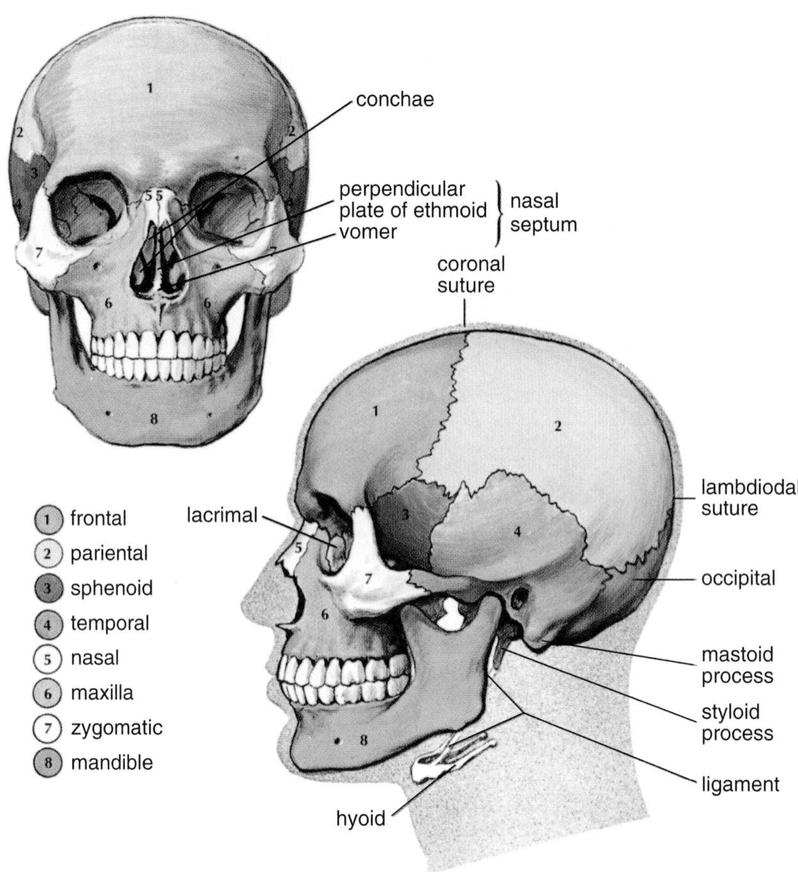

Figure 11-4 The skull, from the front and from the left.

skull. The forehead is formed by the *frontal* bone and contains the frontal sinuses. The *parietal* bones extend across the top and down the sides of the cranium. The *temporal* bones meet the parietal bones at the sides of the cranium and continue to enclose part of the base of the brain. Each contains a mastoid sinus and the structures of the ear (see Chap. 13, Assisting With Diagnostic and Therapeutic Procedures Associated With the Sensory System). The *ethmoid* bone encloses the medial eye socket, part of the nasal cavity, and, with the *sphenoid* bone, forms part of the base of cranium. The *occipital* bone is at the back of the skull and extends anteriorly to include part of the base. It also contains the foramen magnum, the opening through which the spinal cord and its structures exit the skull.

Major Skeletal Structures and Their Movements

The following discussion provides a description of the various joint structures and the specific kinds of movements permitted by each.

Vertebral Column (Spine)

The vertebral column (Fig. 11-5) is made up of 33 vertebrae and numerous joints. The vertebrae house and protect the spinal cord. They are separated from each other by 23 intervertebral disks, which make up 25% of the length of the spinal column. The vertebrae and their disks absorb and transmit the shock of running, walking, and jumping and keep the spine flexible for a high degree of mobility.

The four natural curves in the spine allow for great flexibility and significantly more strength (10 times) and resilience than that of a straight rod. These include:

- Cervical curve (projects anteriorly) C_1–C_7
- Thoracic curve (projects posteriorly) T_1–T_{12}
- Lumbar curve (projects anteriorly) L_1–L_5
- Sacral curve (projects posteriorly) S_1–S_5

One of the most important spinal joints involved for mobility is the facet joint. It is the point of posterior articulation between the vertebrae above and below. Each vertebra moves through four facet joints. The alignment of the facet joint determines the amount of rotation and other movements possible in the spine. Because of the shape of the facet joints, most of the flexion and extension occurs in the lumbar spine; most of the rotation and lateral side bending occurs in the thoracic spine.

Two vertebrae in the cervical spine differ from the others in shape and function. They are the first cervical (atlas) and second cervical (axis) vertebrae. The head

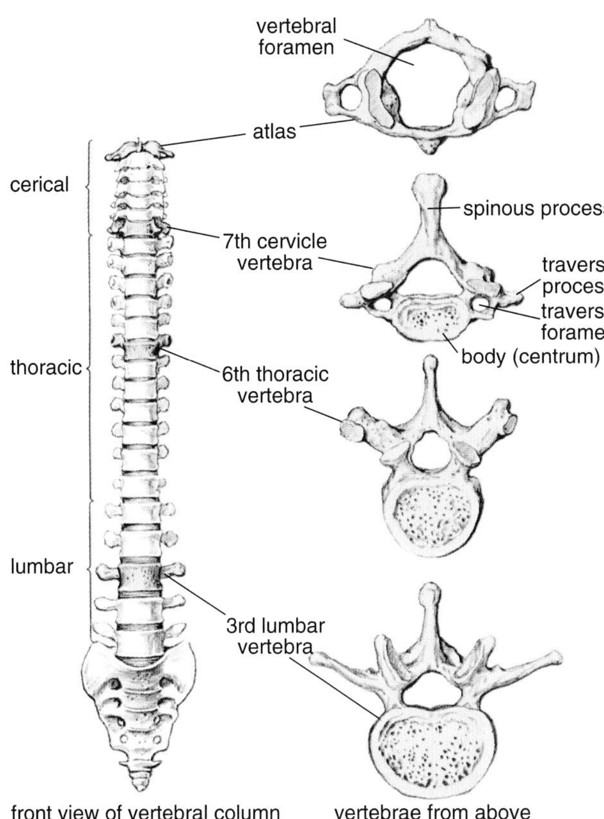

Figure 11-5 Front view of the vertebral column; vertebrae from above.

rests on the ring-shaped atlas, which has no body or spinous process. The axis forms the pivot on which the atlas rotates. Both support the weight of the head and allow for rotation.

Back strains are a leading cause of work-related injury among health care professionals because of the lifting, moving, and twisting often required while caring for patients. Box 11-2 offers some tips for avoiding back strain.

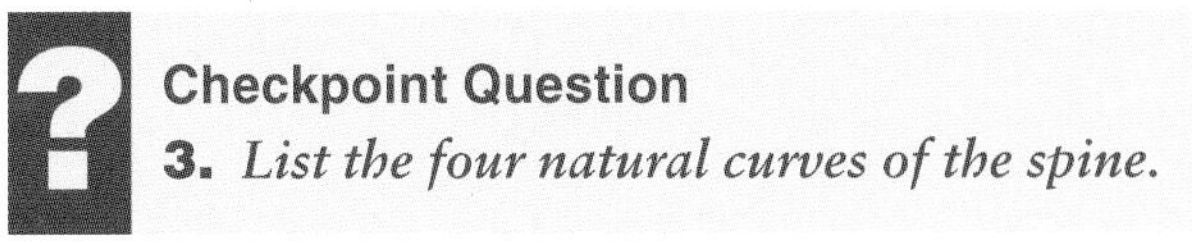

Checkpoint Question

3. *List the four natural curves of the spine.*

Shoulder

The shoulder, a ball-and-socket joint, is the most mobile joint in the body, allowing movement in three planes around three axes. It is made up of the head of the humerus articulating with the glenoid fossa (hollow or depression) of the scapula. Its articulating surface is surrounded by a joint capsule that is formed by an outer fibrous membrane and an inner synovial membrane. The joint capsule, the rotator cuff muscles, and surrounding support structures provide stability to the joint. (The rotator cuff is formed by the tendons of insertion of four muscles that hold the joint surfaces together during joint motion.)

The shoulder joint is capable of many movements, including horizontal abduction, horizontal adduction, and circumduction. Because it is so mobile, it is also one of the most unstable and easily injured joints in the body.

Box 11-2
Avoiding Back Strain

You can prevent back strain by using good body mechanics.

- When lifting a heavy object, keep the object close to your body. Never lift an object with extended arms.
- Never lift and twist at the same time. Lift the object, then reposition your feet by pivoting or taking two steps to turn.
- Learn the proper methods for transferring patients in and out of wheelchairs, stretchers, and examining tables.
- Bend your knees, not your back, when lifting.
- Ask for assistance from coworkers when you must lift or move obese patients or heavy objects.
- Maintain proper posture at all times; slouching causes muscle strain.
- Learn to use mechanical lifting devices, such as the Hoyer lift.

If you do sustain an injury at work, inform your supervisor immediately, and document what happened. Complete an incident report in accordance with the facility's policy.

Elbow

The elbow, a hinge joint, is made up of the articulation of the humerus, with the radius (lateral) and the ulna (medial). Flexion and extension are the only movements that occur in the elbow. The elbow is prevented from more than a few degrees of hyperextension by the fit of the **olecranon process** of the ulna into the **olecranon fossa** of the humerus. The radius and the ulna articulate at both the proximal and distal ends. These pivot joints allow pronation and supination of the forearm as the radius pivots around the ulna.

Wrist

The complex structure of the wrist allows for flexion, extension, and circumduction. The midcarpal joints allow gliding motions and aid wrist movement. The wrist is supported by ligaments and a joint capsule.

Hand

The hand performs the most intricate and specialized movements of the musculoskeletal system. Because the hand is the most significant point of function for the arm, all other joints of the upper extremity function mainly to place the hand in the many diverse positions necessary for it to accomplish its intended activities.

The thumb, the first digit, accounts for 50% of hand function. Its actions occur in different planes than do other joints. The thumb's carpal–metacarpal joint is a saddle-shaped joint that allows flexion, extension, abduction, adduction, opposition, and reposition. The fingers, the second through fifth digits, have four joints each. The carpal–metacarpal joints provide stability for the fingers. The metacarpal–phalangeal joints (knuckles) allow for flexion, extension, abduction, and adduction. The proximal interphalangeal joints and the distal interphalangeal joints can only flex and extend.

The thumb is shorter than the fingers because it has only three joints; however, this allows for greater function with opposition (touching the thumb to the little finger). It also allows the hand to grasp.

The muscles that control the precision movements and fine motor activities of the hand are known as **intrinsic** muscles because they have both of their attachments, origin and insertion, in the hand.

Hip

The hip, a ball-and-socket joint, is important for weight bearing and walking. Like the shoulder, it allows for flexion, extension, abduction, adduction, rotation, and circumduction. Unlike the shoulder, however, it is stable but not nearly as flexible.

The acetabulum is the socket of the hip joint. It receives the ball of the femur and is surrounded by a cylindrical joint capsule. The joint is strong and stable because the acetabulum is deep enough to hold most of the femoral head and is surrounded by three strong ligaments, the most important of which is the iliofemoral ligament. This ligament splits into two parts and is commonly known as the "Y" ligament. A person can maintain the upright position without using any muscles by thrusting the hips forward and resting on the Y ligaments. In this way, it is possible for an individual with paraplegia (paralysis of both lower extremities) to maintain the standing position using long leg braces.

The remaining structures of the pelvis include the *ilium,* the upper flared portion; the *ischium,* the posterior base of the pelvis; the *pubis,* the anterior portion fused with cartilage; and the *sacrum,* which is considered part of the vertebral column.

Knee

The largest joint in the body, the hinged knee joint allows for flexion and extension. It also has a rotational component that is caused by a small amount of rotation of the femur on the tibia and vice versa. "Locking" the knee into extension allows one to stand for long periods without using the muscles.

The patella is an integral part of the knee joint. It lies inside the quadriceps tendon and primarily protects the joint and increases the mechanism by which the quadriceps muscles facilitate lower leg movement.

The surface directly behind the knee is known as the popliteal space through which the arteries and nerves pass. The major muscles of support for the knee are the quadriceps (knee extension), hamstrings (knee flexion), and gastrocnemius muscles (calf muscle). The latter combines with the soleus muscle to form a common tendon known as the Achilles' tendon, which attaches on the heel bone (calcaneus). These serve to point the toes downward and help to propel the body forward while walking.

The knee joint is often injured because it is supported entirely by muscles and ligaments and has no bony stability. It also is one of the most stressed joints because it lies between the two longest bones in the body.

Ankle and Foot

The only true weight-bearing bone of the ankle is the tibia. It is the larger of the two bones of the lower leg and is medial to the fibula. The ends of the bones are called the medial and lateral malleoli (ankle bones). The muscles in the foot and ankle allow for dorsiflexion and plantar flexion, inversion, and eversion.

Weakness of these muscles, especially the tibialis anterior muscle, results in foot drop or a "flat, slap-footed" gait in which the person is unable to heel strike while walking and cannot clear the floor with the toes when swinging the leg forward while walking.

Because of its mobility and the weight it must bear, the ankle is the most frequently injured joint in the body.

Checkpoint Question

4. *What kind of joint is the knee? What are its two primary movements?*

The Muscular System

Types of Muscle Tissue

Muscle tissue makes up 40% to 50% of body weight. Muscles attached to bone are usually under conscious control and are called voluntary muscles. These muscles are composed of **myofibrils,** tiny threadlike structures with dark and light bands called striations. There are three types of muscle tissue, each with its own purpose and characteristics.

STRIATED OR SKELETAL MUSCLE. Most of the body's muscles are striated skeletal muscles (Fig. 11-6). The striations are the light and dark muscle fibers called myosin (thick fibers) and actin (thin fibers) that

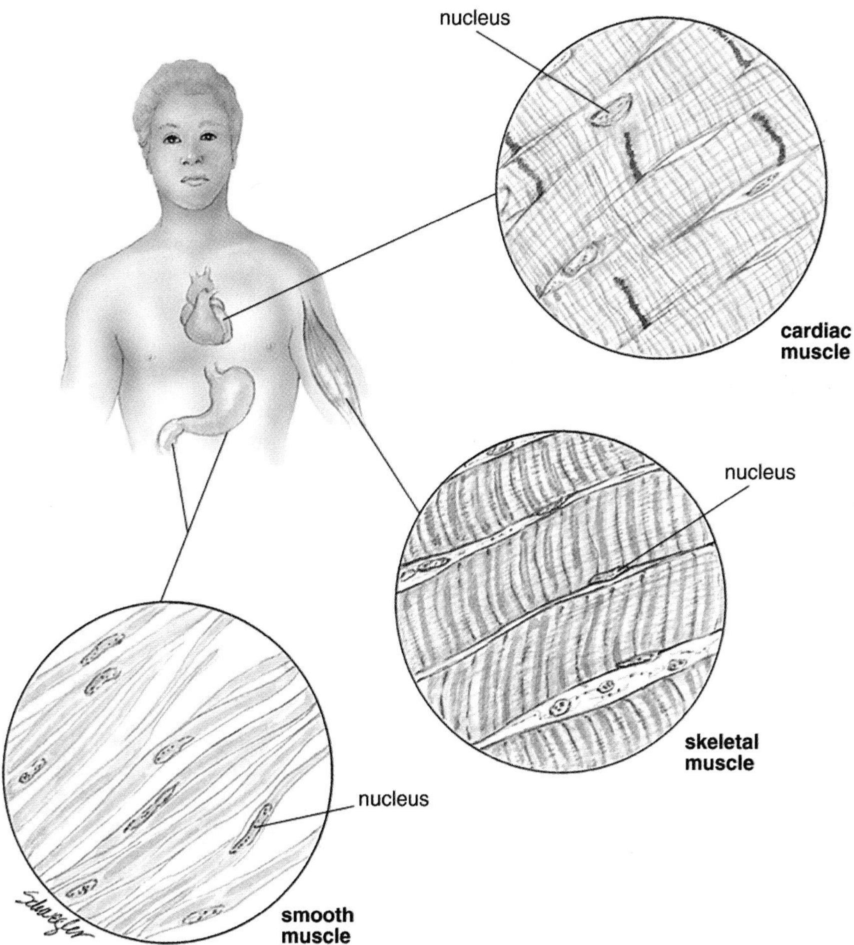

Figure 11-6 Muscle tissue.

slide back and forth across each other with contraction and relaxation.

Skeletal muscles are under voluntary control, are attached to bones, and facilitate movement. The muscles of the arms and legs are examples of skeletal muscles. The fibers of skeletal muscles can be aligned parallel with the line of pull, thus producing greater mobility, or they may be aligned at oblique angles for greater strength.

Very rarely does a skeletal muscle act alone. It may act as a **prime mover** at a joint, or it may work in cooperation with other muscles to perform a movement (**synergist**). It may fix or stabilize a joint (**fixator**) rather than cause it to move, or it may prevent movement by opposite muscles acting on a joint (**antagonist**).

SMOOTH MUSCLE. Smooth muscles are found in the wall of the hollow organs and viscera. They are present in the blood vessels and the large lymphatic vessels. Smooth muscle is controlled by the autonomic nervous system. (See Chap. 12, Assisting With Diagnostic and Therapeutic Procedures Associated With the Neurologic System.) Smooth muscles act in breathing, dilating pupils, contracting the uterus during childbirth, and moving food through the intestines. They are characterized by slow, rhythmic contractions.

CARDIAC MUSCLE. Cardiac muscle also is controlled by the autonomic nervous system. In the heart, these nerves regulate the activity of the specialized heart muscle, ensuring that the normal cardiac pacemaker and conductor cells keep the heart beating over 100,000 times daily. Cardiac muscle fibers make up the walls of the heart and usually do not regenerate or repair.

Muscle Structure

Muscles are attached to bones by tendons, which aid the body's mobility and stability. If the body had no muscles, the skeleton would collapse when placed in the erect position. When muscles are unable to function due to injury or disease, a person is unable to stand or walk independently. Figure 11-7 provides an anterior and posterior view of the muscles of the body.

Tendons begin within the muscles as part of the connective tissue surrounding individual muscle fibers. They extend and join to become the tough, flexible fibers that bind the whole muscle mass to its accompanying bone. Tendons can be cylindrical or flattened.

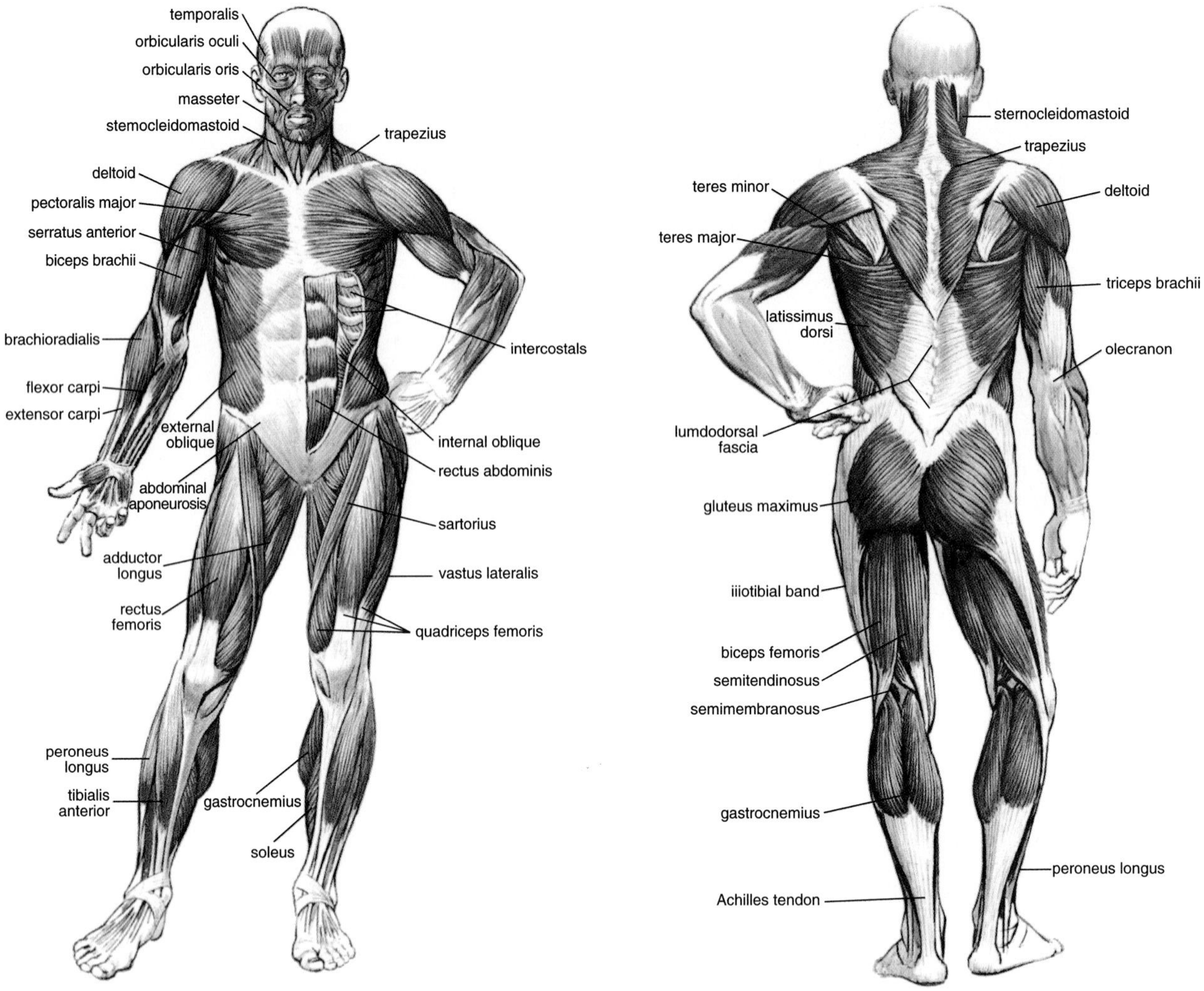

Figure 11-7 Muscles of the body. (**A**) Anterior (front) view. (**B**) Posterior (back) view.

Some tendons are encased in heavy fibrous sheaths for protection if they are subject to friction or pressure, such as when they pass between muscles, between bones, or through tunnels between bones. A broad tendinous sheet that attaches some muscles to bone is called an aponeurosis. The abdominal muscles, which arise from both sides of the body and attach to the midline where there are no bones, are attached to an aponeurosis called the linea alba (white line). The umbilicus lies within the linea alba.

Checkpoint Question

5. *What structure connects muscle to bone? What structure connects bone to bone?*

Muscle Function

Muscle tissue has four unique important properties:

- Irritability—the ability to respond to stimulus
- Contractibility—the ability to shorten
- Extensibility—the ability to lengthen or stretch on the application of force
- Elasticity—the ability to return to its normal length when the shortening or stretching force is removed

Muscles function by contracting and relaxing. Their function depends on their bony attachments, arising from one bone and inserting on another, usually crossing one or more joints. The end of the muscle that stays relatively fixed is said to be the **origin** of the muscle. The more movable end is the **insertion** of the muscle.

Muscles are capable of shortening to flex their bony attachments or may be stretched to extend these attachments. The force built up within a muscle is referred to as tension, which is required for a muscle to contract. The general steady, partial contraction of skeletal muscles, called **tonus,** helps us to remain upright and is maintained by an intact neurologic system. If the stimulus is disrupted, as in paralysis, the tension in the unaffected muscles will pull the body toward the unaffected side.

Muscles are complex and more adaptable than joints. A joint can be replaced, but no replacement

11

Table 11-3 **Review of Muscles**

Name	*Location*	*Function*
Muscles of the Head and Neck		
Orbicularis oculi	Encircles eyelid	Closes eye
Levator palpebrae superioris	Back of orbit to upper eyelid	Opens eye
Orbicularis oris	Encircles mouth	Closes lips
Buccinator	Flesh part of cheek	Flattens cheek; helps in eating, whistling, and blowing wind instruments
Temporal	Above and near ear	Closes jaw
Masseter	At angle of jaw	Closes jaw
Sternocleidomastoid	Along side of neck, to mastoid process	Flexes head, rotates head toward opposite side from muscle
Muscles of the Upper Extremities		
Trapezius	Back of neck and upper back, to clavicle and scapula	Raises shoulder and pulls it back, extends head
Latissimus dorsi	Middle and lower back, to humerus	Extends and adducts arm behind back
Pectoralis major	Upper, anterior chest, to humerus	Flexes and adducts arm across chest; pulls shoulder forward and downward
Serratus anterior	Below axilla on side of chest to scapula	Moves scapula forward; aids in raising arm
Deltoid	Covers shoulder joint, to lateral humerus	Abducts arm
Biceps brachii	Anterior arm, to radius	Flexes forearm and supinates hand
Triceps brachii	Posterior arm, to ulna	Extends forearm
Flexor and extensor carpi groups	Anterior and posterior forearm, to hand	Flex and extend hand
Flexor and extensor digitorum groups	Anterior and posterior forearm, to fingers	Flex and extend fingers
Muscles of the Trunk		
Diaphragm	Dome-shaped partition between thoracic and abdominal cavities	Dome descends to enlarge thoracic cavity from top to bottom
Intercostals	Between ribs	Elevate ribs and enlarge thoracic cavity
External and internal oblique; transversus and rectus abdominis	Anterolateral abdominal wall	Compress abdominal cavity and expel substances from body; flex spinal column
Levator ani	Pelvic floor	Aids defecation
Sacrospinalis	Deep in back, vertical mass	Extends vertebral column to produce erect posture
Muscles of the Lower Extremities		
Gluteus maximus	Superficial buttock, to femur	Extends thigh
Gluteus medius	Deep buttock, to femur	Abducts thigh
Iliopsoas	Crosses front of hip joint, to femur	Flexes thigh
Adductor group	Medial thigh, to femur	Adducts thigh
Sartorius	Winds down thigh, ilium to tibia	Flexes thigh and leg (to sit cross-legged)
Quadriceps femoris	Anterior thigh, to tibia	Extends leg
Hamstring group	Posterior thigh, to tibia and fibula	Flexes leg
Gastrocnemius	Calf of leg, to calcaneus	Extends foot (as in tiptoeing)
Tibialis anterior	Anterior and lateral shin, to foot	Dorsiflexes foot (as in walking on heels); inverts foot (sole inward)
Peroneus longus	Lateral leg, to foot	Everts foot (sole outward)
Flexor and extensor digitorum groups	Posterior and anterior leg, to toes	Flex and extend toes

From Memmler, R. L., Cohen, B. J., & Wood, D. L. (1996). *The Human Body in Health and Disease,* 8th ed., p. 125. Philadelphia: Lippincott-Raven.

for muscles has been found. The characteristics of a muscle can change in response to the demands placed on it. For example, weight lifting results in increased muscle size, whereas endurance training increases the capacity of the muscles to perform for long periods of time.

Lack of use over a short period of time (as little as 3 weeks) can cause muscles to atrophy (waste away). Muscles are resilient in that they can be stretched, tightened, molded, strengthened, and enlarged.

Table 11-3 lists the muscles and their locations and functions.

COMMON MUSCULOSKELETAL DISORDERS

Orthopedists and physical therapists specialize in treating musculoskeletal disorders and often are asked to provide appropriate treatment and rehabilitation procedures when a condition warrants specialized care. The most common disorders of the musculoskeletal system are sprains, dislocations, fractures, joint disruption, and degeneration. The musculoskeletal system reacts to injury or disease with pain (Box 11-3), swelling, inflammation, deformity, or limitation of range and function.

Sprains

Injury to a joint capsule and its supporting ligaments is called a sprain. (In contrast, injury to a muscle and its supporting tendons is called a strain.) Damage to muscle, ligament, or tendon fibers may result in joint instability. If the ligament is completely torn, it is unable to stabilize the joint efficiently. Common symptoms are inflammation and pain.

Applying ice at the time of injury helps reduce swelling and pain. For mild sprains, treatment includes exercise to prevent joint stiffness and muscle atrophy. Therapeutic devices and compression wraps reduce swelling. Moderate sprains must be treated with care to prevent further injury because the ligaments have been weakened. Healing takes 6 to 8 weeks. Severe sprains often require surgery and take much longer to recover.

In the spine, facet joint sprain can cause pain not only at the point of difficulty, but also radiating into an extremity (radicular pain) due to impingement on the nerve root that passes close to the joint.

In the knee, injury to the anterior ligament greatly compromises the joint's stability. The knee becomes unstable, swollen, and painful, and has limited motion. Complete tears require surgery and extensive rehabilitation. This kind of injury most commonly is caused by strong, forced hyperextension of the knee. The menisci, crescent-shaped fibrocartilage located on the proximal tibia, serve primarily as shock absorbers for the knee joint. Because they have no blood supply, they cannot repair themselves and usually require arthroscopic surgery (surgery through punctures into the joint to insert a scope rather than through an incision) to remove the torn parts.

Injury to the Achilles' tendon is extremely painful and limits the ability to walk. A complete tear usually requires surgery followed by immobilization.

Dislocations

Dislocation of a joint, called a luxation, occurs when the end of the bone is displaced from its articular surface. It can be caused by trauma or disease, or it may be congenital (eg, congenital hip dislocation in infants). Common sites for dislocations include the shoulders, elbows, fingers, hips, or ankles.

A subluxation is a partial dislocation in which the bone is pulled out of the socket, but all joint structures maintain their proper relationships. It can be the result of weakness, decreased muscle tone, gravity, or

Box 11-3

Relieving Musculoskeletal Pain

To relieve pain in acute, soft-tissue strains, sprains, and inflammations, rest or immobilization or both may be needed. Because painful movement may cause further damage to the injured tissue, restriction of movement may also be required. This can be accomplished by bed rest and by the use of casts, braces, slings, splints, collars, elastic wraps, or corsets. If weight bearing is painful or inadvisable due to fractures or musculoskeletal pathology, ambulatory aids (eg, canes, walkers, or crutches) may be used. (See "Ambulatory Aids and the Medical Assistant's Role" for more information.)

The use of hot moist packs, heating pads, or warm baths can help increase circulation, relax spasms, or ease sore muscles. Ice packs help prevent swelling, decrease inflammation, and reduce **contusions,** which may occur when there is a direct blow on a muscle.

With contusions, the capillaries (small blood vessels) rupture and bleed into the tissue. Swelling and inflammation may result. Reduction of the bleeding is crucial and is accomplished by applying cold packs and a pressure bandage. Immobilization to prevent further injury is also important. Within a few days, pain-free exercises and heat applications should be introduced to begin the healing process.

Generally, movement should begin as soon as possible after a soft-tissue injury to maintain a healthy joint and resilient muscles. Gentle active or passive movement in the pain-free range, mild joint mobilization, traction, and exercise are effective in maintaining normal range, function, and strength.

Table 11-4 **Types of Fractures**

Type	*Description*
Simple or closed	A break in the bone that does not protrude through the skin. It is usually treated with a closed reduction.
Compound or open	A break in the bone in which the broken end protrudes through the skin; infection is a major concern. Surgery is often required to reduce a compound fracture.
Spiral	A fracture that occurs with torsion or twisting type injures. It appears to be "S" shaped on x-ray.
Impacted	A fracture in which one bone segment is driven into another.
Greenstick	A common injury in children involving a partial or incomplete break in which only one side of a bone is broken like a "green stick."
Transverse	A fracture that is at right angles to the axis of the bone. It is generally caused by an excessive bending force or a direct hit on the bone.
Oblique	A fracture that is slanted across the axis of the bone.
Comminuted	A fracture occurring when a bone is fragmented, usually by a great deal of direct force. A comminuted fracture is difficult to reduce because of the many pieces of bone that must be held in proper alignment. Because it is more complicated to treat a fracture if the articular surface is involved, surgical intervention is usually required. Severe soft-tissue damage frequently accompanies this type of fracture because the force necessary to cause the fracture is so great that it causes a small explosion within the soft tissue.
Compression	Results from damage to the bone by the application of a strong force against both ends, such as a fall. Vertebrae are susceptible to compression fractures, especially in the elderly.
Depressed	A fracture of flat bones (usually the skull), causing the fragment to be driven below the surface of the bone.
Avulsion	A fracture caused by a strong force applied to the bone by the sharp, twisting-pulling motion of the attached ligaments or tendons.
Pathologic	These types of fractures are usually the result of a disease process, such as osteoporosis (brittle bone), **Paget's disease** (a chronic skeletal disease in the elderly with bowing of the long bones), bone cysts, tumors, or cancer.

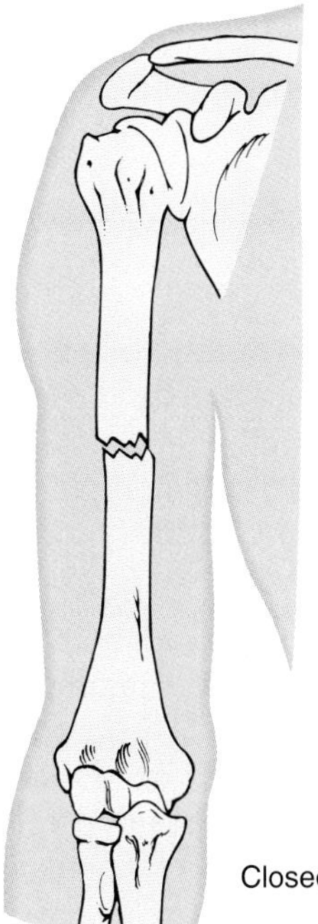

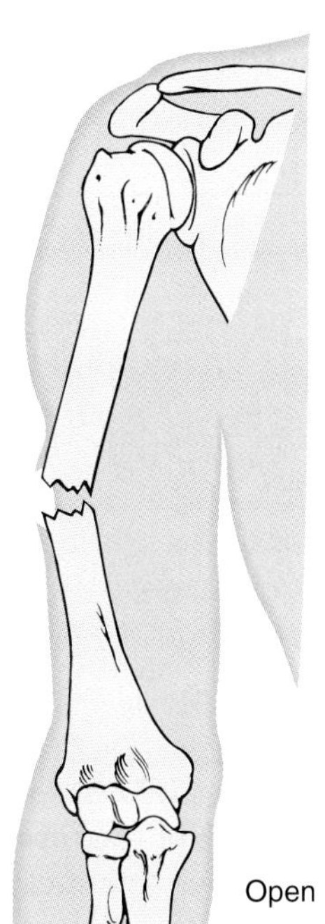

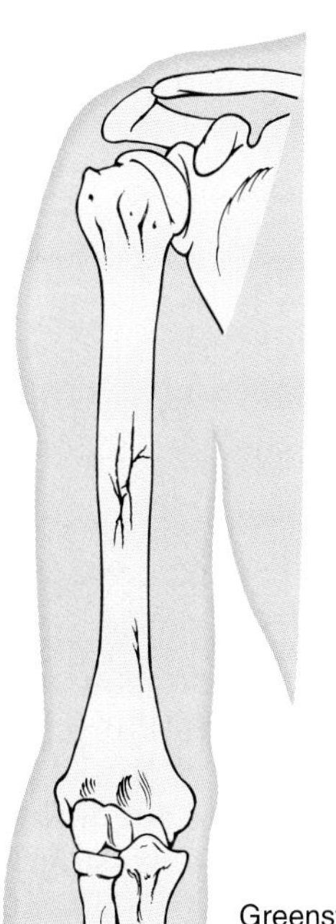

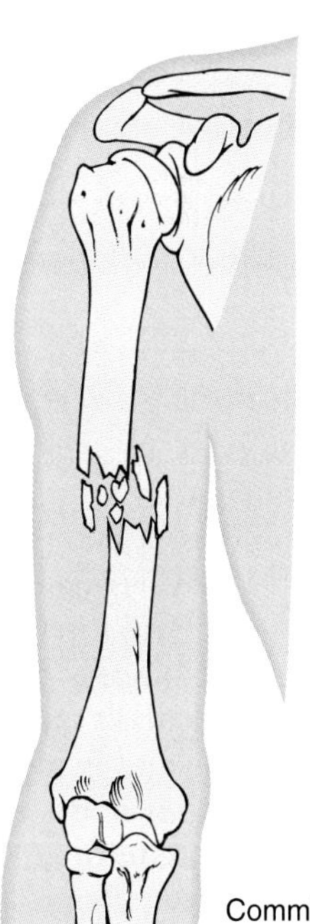

A

Types of fractures.

(continued)

Table 11-4 **Types of Fractures** *(Continued)*

Depressed fracture

Compression fracture

Avulsion fracture

Oblique fracture

Impacted fracture

Spiral fracture

Transverse fracture

B

neurologic deficit. The muscles bear most of the responsibility for preventing subluxation. Subluxations are often seen in the weakened shoulder joints of stroke patients.

In children, a common subluxation site is the elbow. The injury, termed "nurse-maid's elbow," results from a sudden and forceful longitudinal pull on an extended arm. It often is caused by a parent or caregiver pulling on the child's outstretched arm. The injury usually is painless and is identified by lack of arm movement. Reductions of the elbow usually are not difficult and do not require pain medications or surgery. Parental teaching should be done in a nonjudgmental manner. Parents often feel guilty for this injury and should be consoled accordingly.

Common symptoms of dislocations include pain, pressure, limited movement, and deformity. Numbness and loss of pulse to the part can also occur. Treatment may include reduction and immobilization of the joint. The patient may be taught exercises to strengthen supporting muscles to avoid recurrences.

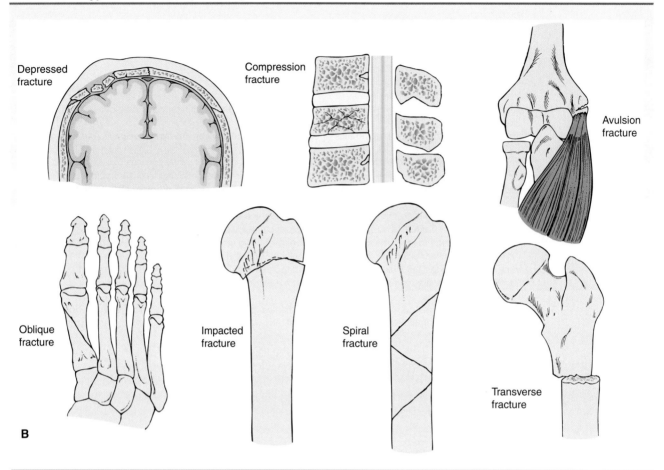

Checkpoint Question

6. *How does a luxation differ from a subluxation?*

Fractures

A fracture is a break or a disruption in a bone. Causes include falls or other trauma, disease, tumors, and unusual stress. There are many types of fractures, each presenting with its own set of problems (Table 11-4). However, all fractures have one symptom in common: pain. Other manifestations include swelling, hemorrhage, lack of movement or unusual movement, contusions, and deformity of the body part involved.

Treatment involves **reduction** (correction) by placing the broken ends into proper alignment. Casting, splinting, wrapping, and taping are means of obtaining a closed reduction. If it is not possible to obtain proper alignment by a closed reduction, surgery is required and the procedure is called an open reduction. Fractures in the shoulder joint are serious injuries because the immobilization necessary for healing causes adhesions in the capsule, resulting in a severe loss of motion and function.

Casts

Fractures must be immobilized to facilitate healing in the proper alignment. In many instances, both proximal and distal joints are included in the cast to further ensure that movement is restricted. Box 11-4 describes various types of casts. The casting material used can be either plaster or fiberglass.

The traditional *plaster* bandages are impregnated with calcium sulfate crystals and are supplied as rolls of material in widths (eg, 2–6 inches) appropriate to a variety of sites. When water is added to the dry rolls of bandage, a chemical reaction generates heat that may be uncomfortable to the patient for a short time, usually less than 30 minutes, but is necessary to produce a rigid dressing when dry. The bandage will mold smoothly to the casting site as it is applied.

The cast will be rather soft until it is fully dry, which can take as long as 72 hours. Patients must be cautioned not to exert pressure on the drying cast to avoid pressure sores from indentations. The cast must be kept dry at all times.

Because of its lighter weight, water resistance, and durability, *fiberglass* is the material of choice for casting uncomplicated fractures or as a progression from the more stable plaster cast for an unstable fracture. The polyurethane additives harden in minutes, eliminating the extended drying time. After the cast has set, the material will not soften when wet but if it does become wet, it must be dried to prevent skin lesions. The fabric has a more open weave than plaster, which helps maintain skin integrity.

ASSISTING WITH CAST APPLICATION. Position the patient comfortably before the procedure begins. Drape to expose only the part to be casted to avoid unnecessary exposure and protect other skin areas from the casting material. The part should be clean and dry; lesions, if present, should be attended and dressed appropriately before casting. (See Chap. 6, Assisting With Minor Office Surgery, for the procedure for dressing a wound.)

Box 11-4
Types of Casts

- *Short arm cast* extends from below the elbow to mid-palm.
- *Long arm cast* extends from the axilla to the mid-palm; the elbow is usually at a 90-degree angle.
- *Short leg cast* extends from below the knee to the toes; the foot is in a natural position.
- *Long leg cast* extends from the upper thigh to the toes; the knee is slightly flexed and the foot is in a natural position.
- *Walking cast* may be either a short leg cast or a long leg cast; the cast is extra strong to bear weight and may include a walking heel.
- *Body cast* encircles the trunk, usually from the axilla to the hip.
- *Spica cast* encircles part of the trunk and one or two extremities.

Note: Body and spica casts are not usually seen in the medical office because transporting these patients as outpatients is very difficult.

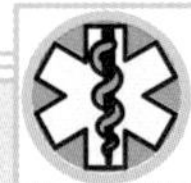

Action STAT!

Patient Fall

Scenario: Mr. Brown has a return appointment in your office today. Just before his scheduled arrival, Mrs. Brown runs into the office shouting, "My husband fell in the parking lot. Help!" You run outside and find Mr. Brown on the ground screaming in pain and holding his left arm. What should you do?

1. Instruct Mrs. Brown to go back into the office and to tell your coworkers what has happened and that you need help in the parking lot.
2. Reassure Mr. Brown, and try to keep him calm as you assess the situation and survey his injuries.
3. Do not move Mr. Brown until you complete a head to toe assessment. Check for possible injuries to his neck, back, pelvis, legs, or other body parts. If you suspect injuries to the neck, back, or hips, do not move him—have someone call for an ambulance.
4. Examine Mr. Brown's left arm closely. Look for deformities, color changes (cyanosis), open areas. Check for a radial pulse; assess sensation and hand mobility. Carefully immobilize the arm—gauze or a cravat sling are good choices—and recheck the pulse and circulation after immobilization.
5. Ask Mr. Brown what caused his fall. You need to determine if it resulted from external factors (snow, ice, uneven surfaces) or physical reasons (dizziness, chest pain).
6. Evaluate the options available. If the physician is not on site, call for an ambulance, and have the patient transferred to an emergency center. If the physician is present, he or she will decide how to handle this situation.
7. Complete an incident report, including all information regarding the accident.

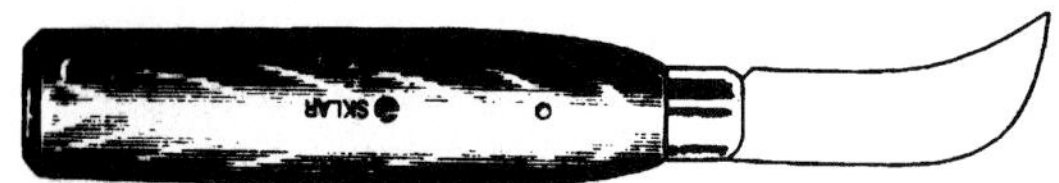

Figure 11-8 Plaster or cast knife. (Sklar Instruments, West Chester, PA.)

The limb is covered first with soft knitted tubular material with extra fabric above and below the projected casting length to allow for a padded fold at each end. The soft roller padding is applied in fairly thick layers over the knitted material with extra layers over bony prominences. The physician wraps the limb from distal to proximal with the soaked casting material. You may be responsible for soaking the material in cool or tepid water until bubbles no longer form around the rolls. Wear utility gloves to protect your hands from the material. Press—do not wring—the rolls until they are wet through but not dripping. Hand them to the physician as needed. When the site is adequately covered, the physician trims rough edges with a plaster knife (Fig. 11-8) and folds the knitted fabric back to form cuffs at each end. The skin is cleansed of casting material to avoid discomfort and skin breakdown. Procedure 11-1 details the steps required for assisting with cast application.

Because the unsupported weight of a short or long arm cast may put undue stress and strain on the shoulder muscles, slings are ordered to relieve and redistribute the weight. Slings also are used in situations that do not require a cast but do require that the arm be immobilized to facilitate healing. Procedure 11-2 describes the steps for applying a sling.

CAST REMOVAL. Cuts are made in the cast through its length on opposite sides, dividing it into halves. An electric oscillating circular saw known as a cast cutter is used. Assure the patient that this will not cut the skin. Protect your eyes from flying particles, and caution the patient also. The cast is split apart with a cast spreader. The padding is cut with utility scissors. Warn the patient that the skin will be pale and dry, and the muscle will be wasted from disuse. The skin will be sensitive to touch and temperature. Creams and lotions help alleviate the dryness, and physical therapy helps restore muscle tone. (See Chap. 5, Instruments and Equipment, for illustrations of an oscillating saw, plaster shears, and a plaster spreader.)

Checkpoint Question

7. *Explain the difference between an open and closed reduction.*

Healing of Fractures

The most important criterion for successful healing of a fracture is an adequate blood supply. The blood secretes an important gluelike substance known as **callus,** which is deposited around the break. Callus holds the ends of the bones together; with time, the callus turns to bone. Cells mold the callus and smooth the fracture site to close to its original size. Immobilization of the fracture site allows the molding and reshaping process to occur successfully.

If the blood supply is inadequate, delayed union or nonunion may occur. If damage is sufficient (eg, soft tissue, vascular, or neurologic) or if severe trauma, disease, tumor, or complications are involved, amputation may be necessary. Amputation is a drastic measure that is performed only when all other avenues are exhausted. A **prosthesis** enables the amputee to resume functional activities, such as walking, grasping, or holding.

A potentially life-threatening complication of a fracture of the long bones is a fat **embolus,** which results from the release of fat droplets from the yellow

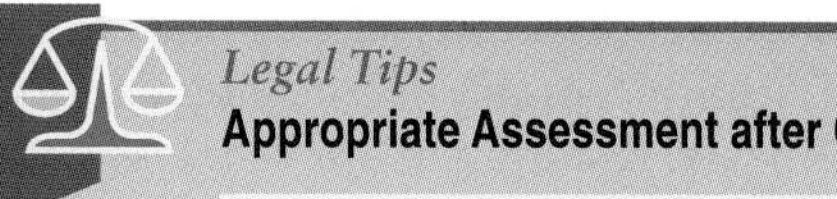

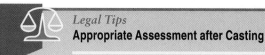

Legal Tips

Appropriate Assessment after Casting

Casts that are applied improperly can lead to nerve and vascular damage, resulting in permanent loss of function to the extremity. (In extreme situations, a surgical amputation may be required.) To ensure proper patient care and to avoid potential lawsuits, it is essential that distal extremity circulation be assessed and documented before and after reductions and casting.

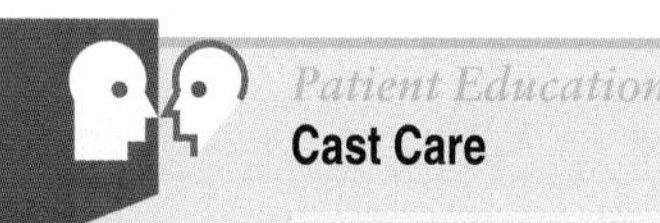

Patient Education

Cast Care

Instruct patients with casts to:

- Be aware of the initial warmth of the drying cast; this will diminish in 20 to 30 minutes.
- Keep the cast dry, if plaster.
- Avoid indentations by allowing the cast to dry completely before handling or propping on hard surfaces.
- Note that the extremities (ie, fingers and toes) are left uncovered to check for color, swelling, numbness, and temperature; report any impairment to the physician immediately.
- Report odors, staining, or prolonged warmth.
- Prevent swelling by elevating the limb for at least 24 hours after casting and as often as possible after that time.
- Never insert any object under the cast to scratch. Breaks in the skin may become infected and require that the cast be removed prematurely.

marrow of these bones. If the embolus becomes lodged in the coronary or pulmonary vessels or in a large vessel in the brain, it can totally block the vessel, causing an infarction and resulting in death. The elderly require longer periods for healing. Prosthetic joint replacements may be necessary if bone restructuring will not be adequate (Box 11-5).

What If?
What if your patient has a cervical fracture?

Fractures to the cervical spine can be life threatening or seriously disabling. There are seven cervical vertebrae. Fractures to cervical one (C-1), the most superior vertebra, tend to be fatal unless immediately and aggressively treated by emergency services personnel before transport to a trauma center. Fractures to cervical two (C-2) and three (C-3) often result in permanent or long-term respiratory dependency. Vertebrae fractures of cervical four through seven will result in various levels of paralysis and motor impairment. If you suspect a patient has a cervical fracture or other vertebral fractures, immobilize the patient and call for emergency personnel. Never move the patient unless the patient is in immediate danger. The ambulance technicians will properly immobilize the patient for transport to a hospital where radiographic tests will determine the extent of the injury.

Abnormal Spinal Curvatures

Exaggerated or abnormal curvatures of the spine affect the posture and the alignment of the shoulders and hips (Box 11-6). An abnormally deep lumbar curvature is referred to as **lordosis** or swayback. Abnormal thoracic curvature, particularly the upper portion, is called **kyphosis** or hunchback. A side-to-side or lateral curve is called **scoliosis;** this is relatively common during adolescence (Fig. 11-9).

Treatment involves the use of devices (eg, braces) to assist with the straightening of the curve to a more normal position. Transcutaneous muscle stimulation devices cause the muscles on one side to contract and draw the spine into its proper position.

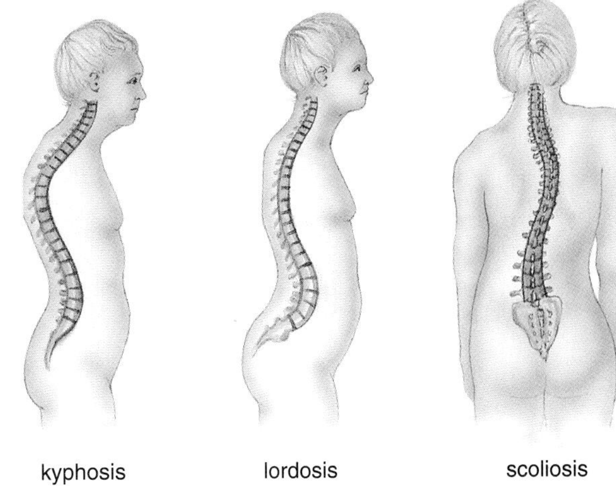

Figure 11-9 Abnormalities of the spinal curves.

Herniated Intervertebral Disk

The lumbar spine is one of the most frequently injured parts of the body because it absorbs the full weight of the upper body and the weight of anything that is carried. Because most of the movement in the lumbar spine occurs at the L-4 to L-5 and L-5 to S-1 segments, most herniated disks are seen at these levels, but injury can also occur anywhere in the spine.

A herniated disk occurs when the soft center of the disk (nucleus) ruptures through its tough outer layer to protrude into the spinal canal, sometimes pressing on the spinal cord. It is usually caused by severe trauma, degenerative changes, or strenuous strains. Common symptoms include severe back pain, numbness in the extremities, spasms, weakness, and limitation of movement. Flexion causes pain to radiate into the extremities; extension is restricted and causes pain at the spinal segment. The straight leg raise test will be positive for pain at 45 degrees to 60 degrees. A flattened lumbar curve and a lateral shift are not uncommon. On x-ray, the disk space may be narrowed.

Bone strength throughout the body is diminished during periods of confinement or inactivity; therefore, total bed rest is no longer the treatment of choice for the majority of musculoskeletal disorders, including herniated disks. Activity is limited by pain. Patients are instructed to perform simple ankle pumps and encouraged to take short walks from room to room. Therapy, traction, massage, and mild extension exercises help to relieve muscle guarding, which causes a compression force on the disk. Most disk herniations and bulges can be treated successfully without surgery. Severe, unremitting pain; numbness; and progressive weakness of an extremity are indications for surgery.

Checkpoint Question

8. *Name the three abnormal curvatures of the spine. Briefly describe each.*

Rotator Cuff Injury

Injury to the rotator cuff muscles in the shoulder can cause severe pain, weakness, and loss of function. Sur-

11

Box 11-5

Bone Healing in the Elderly

A fracture of the femur in the elderly raises special concerns. Bone-repairing osteoblasts are less able to use calcium to restructure bone tissue at any site in the elderly, but the neck of the femur, the most common fracture site, is especially vulnerable to delayed or imperfect healing due to poor blood supply. Fractures through this area, involving the femoral head or neck or just inferior to the greater trochanter, may require hip **arthroplasty** or total hip replacement.

Hip joint replacement prostheses are usually metal or polyethylene molded to conform to the joints they are designed to replace. Total hip replacement, usually used for degenerative joint disease or rheumatoid arthritis, replaces the head and neck of the femur and the acetabular surface. Knee replacement replaces both the head of the tibia and the distal epiphysis of the femur.

Early repair and return to mobility prevents contractures and atrophy of the supporting muscles. Postoperative ambulation prevents many of the complications associated with prolonged confinement in the elderly, such as pathologic fractures, static pneumonia, and renal calculi.

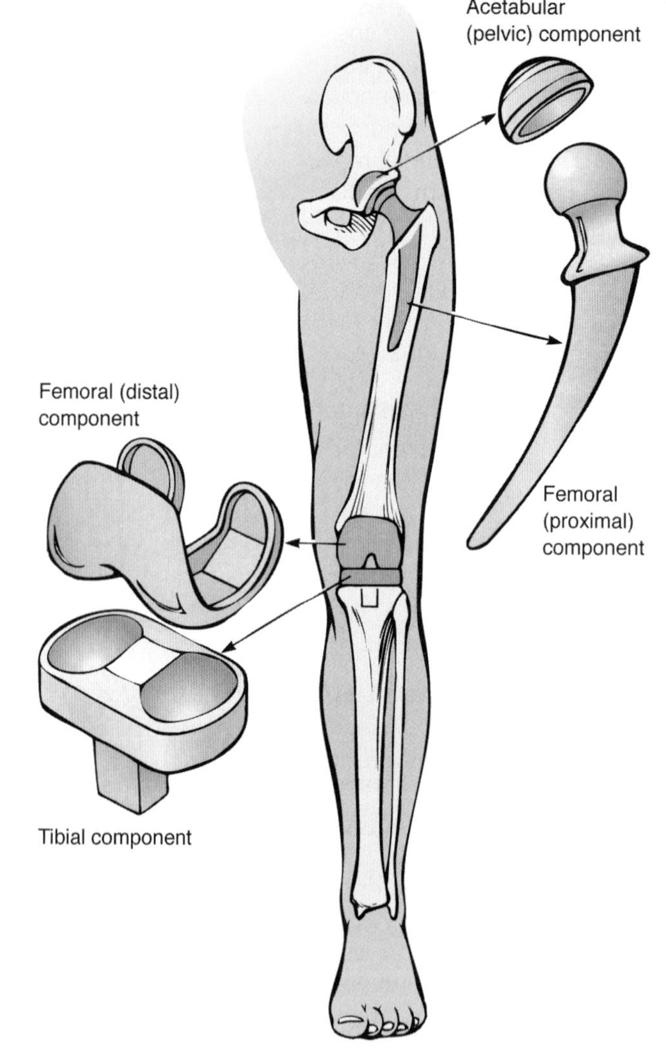

Hip and knee replacement.

gical intervention is often necessary because the tendons do not heal on their own. An extended period of postoperative rehabilitation is usually needed to increase range and strength and to regain the use of the shoulder. Professional athletes, particularly baseball pitchers, are prone to rotator cuff injuries.

Adhesive Capsulitis (Frozen Shoulder)

This condition affects the entire shoulder joint and its capsule. It involves a **contracture** (binding by shortening) of the joint structures, which usually results from

Box 11-6
Posture and Back Pain

Poor posture can lead to back pain, and pain and injury can lead to poor posture. Also, as people age, natural changes occur in the body that may affect posture. For example, the disks become less resilient and give in to forces such as gravity and body weight. Muscles are less flexible, and degenerative changes occur in the spine. In addition, more sedentary lifestyle causes weakness and shortening in some muscles and overstretching in others. The most common posture faults are the forward head posture and rounded shoulders.

In patients with poor posture, the bones are not aligned properly, and the muscles, joints, and ligaments become strained and stressed. Weak, tight, and inflexible muscles cannot support the back's natural curves. Years of poor posture can affect the position and function of the vital organs.

Maintaining good posture—or correcting poor posture—can help reduce a bulging disk or relieve the biomechanical stress caused by poor skeletal alignment, thus greatly aiding musculoskeletal system functioning.

a fracture or disease process that prevents movement. Anything that causes pain or restricts motion (eg, tendinitis, bursitis, nerve damage, strokes, sprains, or strains) can lead to a frozen shoulder.

Contractures develop when the joint is immobilized causing the fibers to stick to each other, thereby limiting the movement in the joint. Adhesions and additional collagen are produced in response to injury, thus resulting in a painful, tight, and constricted capsule.

The shoulder movements most restricted are abduction and external rotation. Because full active range of motion is not possible, weakness and atrophy are often present. Prolonged immobility can lead to joint degeneration. Women commonly find it difficult to fix their hair; men complain of the inability to reach their wallets in their back pockets.

Treatment consists of administration of anti-inflammatory medications, heat or cold applications, ultrasound, mobilization (gentle gliding of the joint surfaces) or manipulation, and stretching exercises. The recovery process is slow and typically painful. Contractures in the joints are often preventable with proper management and by moving the joint through a full range of motion each day.

Bursitis

The subdeltoid bursa lies between the deltoid muscle (the muscle that covers the cap of the shoulder) and the joint capsule. The subdeltoid bursa is the most common site for bursitis, an inflammation of the bursa. Other frequent sites are the olecranon process, the trochanter, the heel, and the prepatellar bursae. The most common symptom is pain during range-of-motion movement.

Treatment for bursitis usually consists of administration of anti-inflammatory medication, rest, heat or cold applications, ultrasound to promote healing, range-of-motion exercises, and activities within the pain-free range.

Tendinitis

Tendinitis is inflammation of the tendons. This disorder and others involving inflammation of contractile tissue or their attachments (eg, myositis [muscles] and tenosynovitis [sheaths covering the tendon]) usually occur after strains, sprains, overuse, or overstretching of the tissue. Pain does not occur with passive movement. Active movement is painful, and resistance to movement is intensely painful because the tissue must contract during active and resisted movement. Localized tenderness usually is present.

Treatment consists of rest, heat or cold applications, ultrasound, **iontophoresis** (electrical transfer of ions), massage, and transverse friction massage (deep massage across the fibers of the tendons).

Lateral Epicondylitis (Tennis Elbow)

Lateral epicondylitis, often called tennis elbow, is a common elbow injury involving a sprain or strain of the tendons of origin of the wrist and finger extensor muscles. Symptoms include extreme pain with extension of the wrist (such as when trying to lift a cup or glass) and exquisite pain on palpation over the extensor tendons at the elbow joint. Resistance to wrist extension and supination are the diagnostic tests for tennis elbow because both movements greatly increase the pain.

Treatment consists of ice applications, **phonophoresis** (ultrasound with cortisone) or iontophoresis, avoiding movements that cause the pain, use of a forearm strap just distal to the elbow joint to take the pressure off the tendon, transverse friction massage, and gentle passive exercise to maintain mobility. In prolonged, extreme cases, surgery may be indicated.

Carpal Tunnel Syndrome

A repetitive motion injury, carpal tunnel syndrome occurs when the carpal bones and transverse carpal ligaments compress the median nerve at the wrist. It is very

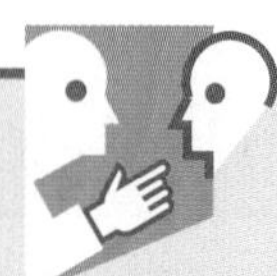

Advice and Tips

Living With Carpal Tunnel Syndrome

Question patients who are diagnosed with carpal tunnel syndrome about their work environments. This syndrome is common among typists, computer operators, assembly line workers, or other individuals whose professions demand frequent grasping, twisting, and flexion of the wrist. Many job sites can be re-engineered to be worker friendly. For example, caution a patient who is a typist to maintain good body alignment at all times in a properly proportioned and well-constructed chair. Note that palm supports for computer keyboards decrease the degree of wrist flexion. Advise the patient to take breaks and, if possible, to alternate computer work with other tasks. A physical therapist may offer range-of-motion exercises that the patient can do throughout the day to alleviate wrist tension and may also suggest changes in the working environment. Always consult the physician before making patient referrals.

commonly observed in those who flex their wrists repeatedly or who hold their hands in an unnatural position for long periods. Symptoms include numbness in the thumb and the index and middle fingers, pain, and weakness. Often, pain awakens the patient at night.

Diagnostic tests for carpel tunnel syndrome include Phalan's test, in which holding the wrist in flexion reproduces the symptoms; Tinel's test, in which the wrist is held in hyperextension and the transverse carpal ligament is thumped, thereby causing tingling into the hand and fingers; and nerve conduction velocity tests. Treatment can be conservative (eg, administration of anti-inflammatory medications and immobilization) or can require surgical release of the transverse carpal ligament.

Dupuytren's Contracture

Dupuytren's contracture results in flexion deformities of the fingers, most often the ring and little fingers, caused by contractures of the palmar fascia due to the overgrowth of fibrous tissue. Function is lost because the fingers cannot be straightened. Dupuytren's contracture is easily diagnosed by sight and palpation. Surgery is often required to release the contractures. Stretching the tight structures in the early stages may help to slow the progression.

Chondromalacia Patella

Chondromalacia patella is a degenerative disorder affecting the cartilage underlying the kneecap. It usually occurs in young women or in athletes who perform running, jumping, and bicycling activities. A common complaint is pain when walking down stairs or getting out of a chair. Rest, therapy, bracing or taping, and exercises can help to relieve the symptoms.

Plantar Fasciitis

This disorder, the most frequent cause of pain in the bottom of the foot, often is associated with heel spurs on the calcaneus. Deep palpation over the plantar (sole) surface of the heel bone will elicit pain. Treatment of choice is a foot orthosis (splint or heel pad) to support the arch and distribute the weight evenly. Heat, massage, and ultrasound are often effective. Surgery is rarely done because of the high incidence of recurrence.

Foot Deformities

Bunions, corns, and calluses form on the toes at pressure points or over points of excessive, prolonged friction. They usually are caused by poorly fitting shoes. Treatments of choice include well fitting shoes, pads, and topical medications. Hallux valgus, a great toe deformity, results in painful lateral deviation of the toe. It can be caused by excessive pressure on the foot, most often from shoes that are too narrow. In the early stages, hallux valgus can be corrected with straightening devices and properly fitting shoes. Surgery may be required for severe bone deformities.

Gout

Gout, a metabolic disease involving an overproduction of uric acid, usually affects the joint of the great toe. Gout presents as a painful, hot, inflamed joint; symptoms progressively worsen unless treated. Periods of remission and exacerbation may occur. The condition may become chronic and can lead to multijoint involvement with chronic pain, degeneration, and deformity. Symptoms are relieved by avoidance of purine-rich foods and alcohol-related products. Medication to prevent uric acid formation or foster its excretion from the body also may be prescribed.

Osteoarthritis

Osteoarthritis, or degenerative joint disease (DJD), is caused by wear and tear on the weight-bearing joints in which the articular cartilage degenerates and the ends of the bones enlarge. This overgrowth of bone intrudes into the joint cavity, causing pain and restricted movement. If the articular cartilage is inflamed, it is called osteochrondritis.

Treatment includes administration of anti-inflammatory medications, intra-articular corticosteroid injections, and use of ambulatory aids (eg, crutches, cane, walker) to decrease joint stress.

Rheumatoid Arthritis

Rheumatoid arthritis is a systemic autoimmune disease that attacks the synovium of the joint. Ultimately, it leads to inflammation, pain, stiffness, and crippling deformities. It usually begins on the non–weight-bearing joints but eventually affects most of the joints of the appendicular skeleton.

Rheumatoid arthritis of the spine is also called **ankylosing spondylitis,** and is characterized by extreme forward flexion of the spine and tightness in the hip flexors. Rheumatoid arthritis in children is known as Still's disease.

Checkpoint Question

9. *How does osteoarthritis differ from rheumatoid arthritis?*

Procedure 11-1 Assisting With Cast Application

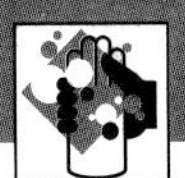

PURPOSE:

To assist in the realignment of a fracture or the immobilization of an area during healing

EQUIPMENT/SUPPLIES

- tubular soft stockinette fabric, sized to fit the limb
- roller padding/sheet wadding
- casting material, sized to fit the limb
- bucket of cool or tepid water
- plaster cast knife
- utility gloves for physician and assistant

STEPS

1. Wash your hands.
2. Assemble the equipment.
3. Greet and identify the patient. Explain the procedure and answer any questions.
4. Assess the need for size and lengths of fabric stocking, cotton padding, and casting material.
   Initial assessment of the patient's needs ensures that the material is appropriate for the patient.
5. At the physician's instructions, glove with the heavy utility gloves and begin to soak the casting material in the water. Remove the material when no more bubbles rise from the roll. Do not wring the roll; press the excess water from the roll, and pull free one corner of the first layer of the roll.
   Soaking in this manner adequately wets the material without overwetting; turning back a corner provides the physician with a starting edge.
6. Pass the cast knife to the physician at the completion of the procedure to trim away rough edges of the material.
   Rough edges may cause skin irritation.
7. Educate the patient regarding cast care for the type of cast applied. Ask for and answer any questions.
   Patient education prevents avoidable problems with cast care.
8. Help the patient reclothe if clothing has been removed for the procedure.
   Clothing may be difficult to replace after casting.
9. Care for and properly dispose of equipment and supplies. Wash your hands.

DOCUMENTATION GUIDELINES

- Date and time
- Location of cast
- Assessment of circulation to part
- Patient complaints/concerns
- Patient education/instructions
- Your signature

Charting Example

DATE	TIME Short leg cast with walking heel
	applied by Dr. Menendez. Pedal pulse
	strong before cast application; healing of
	fracture progressing since last cast
	application. Pt voiced no complaints. Toes
	have full range of motion with good
	sensory perception after casting; skin
	warm and pink. Pt reminded to report
	signs as outlined in pt ed brochure.
	Verbalized understanding of all
	instructions. —Your signature

11

Procedure 11-2 Applying a Triangular Arm Sling

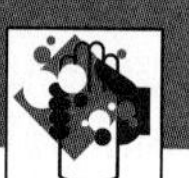

PURPOSE:

To assist in weight support and immobilization of an injured limb

EQUIPMENT/SUPPLIES

- sling as ordered by the physician
- pins

STEPS

1. Wash your hands.
2. Assemble the equipment.
3. Greet and identify the patient. Explain the procedure and ask for questions.
4. Position the affected limb with the hand at slightly less than a 90-degree angle so that the fingers are higher than the elbow.
   A slightly upward angle helps reduce swelling.
5. Place the triangle with the uppermost corner at the shoulder on the unaffected side (extend the corner across the nape), the middle angle at the elbow of the affected side, and the final lowermost corner pointing toward the foot on the unaffected side.
   This procedure allows for proper positioning.
6. Bring the lowermost corner up to meet the upper corner at the side of the neck, never at the back of the neck.
   This will avoid pressure from the knot against the neck.
7. Tie or pin the sling. Secure the elbow by fitting any extra fabric neatly around the limb and pinning it.
   Pinning helps to secure the sling.

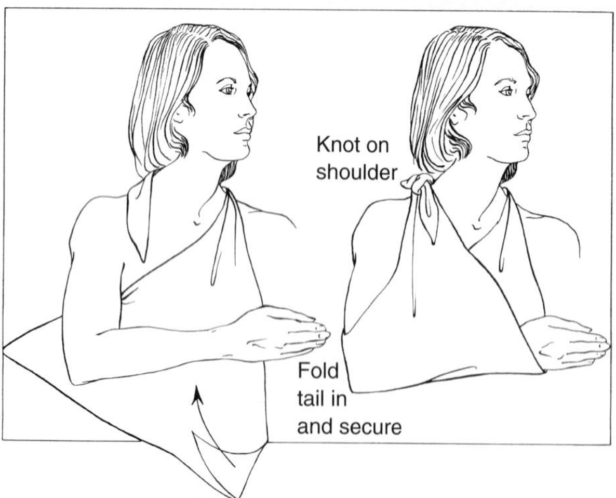

8. Check the patient's comfort level and distal extremity circulation.
   Assessing patient comfort and circulation helps ensure compliance and promotes patient safety.
9. Wash your hands.

DOCUMENTATION GUIDELINES

- Date and time
- Location of cast or injury
- Sling application
- Patient complaints/concerns
- Patient education/instructions
- Your signature

Charting Example

DATE	TIME Pt returned for cast change (L)
	arm. Healing progressing well. Fingers
	warm, pink with good mobility. Arm sling
	applied. Pt instructed on maintaining
	proper arm position. —Your signature

Note: Fitted canvas slings with Velcro or buckles are also available and are becoming the appliances of choice.

Treatment involves rest, hot and cold applications, physical therapy, and administration of anti-inflammatory medications.

Muscular Dystrophy

The congenital disorders collectively known as muscular dystrophy are characterized by varying degrees of progressive wasting of skeletal muscles. There is no neurologic involvement. The wasted, weakened muscles tend to be hypertrophic (an abnormal increase in size). The most common type, Duchenne's, is apparent in early childhood and usually is fatal by young adulthood. Mixed forms of muscular dystrophy occur in the middle adult years and may be fatal. Several forms, such as fascioscapulohumeral and limb girdle dystrophy, progress slowly from a childhood onset and result in varying degrees of disability. Duchenne's, fascioscapulohumeral, and limb girdle dystrophies are genetically transmitted; the cause of the mixed form is not known.

Diagnosis is based on family and patient history. Electromyography and muscle biopsy are used to rule out neurologic involvement. The characteristic signs are frequently the most obvious diagnostic indicators of the disease. There is no known cure for any form of muscular dystrophy.

Osteoporosis

If the rate of bone resorption by osteoclastic activity is greater than bone formation by osteoblasts, bones became lacy and porous rather than dense and solid. Porous bones deficient in calcium and phosphorus are brittle and vulnerable to fractures. The cause may be dietary with general deficiencies in calcium, vitamin D, or phosphorus, or may be a primary progressive inability to metabolize calcium brought on by estrogen deficiency in elderly women, a sedentary lifestyle, alcoholism, liver disorders, or rheumatoid arthritis.

There are few signs other than a gradual loss of stature with progressive kyphosis; the most severe sign is spontaneous, nontraumatic fractures. Diagnosis includes bone scans, densitometry (measuring the density of the bones), thyroid and parathyroid studies, and serum calcium and phosphorus determinations.

Treatment involves preventing fractures by increasing appropriate levels of exercise. Estrogen is usually prescribed for postmenopausal women if therapy can begin within 3 to 5 years of menopause. Calcium and vitamin D supplements are beneficial to arrest the progression but will not cure the underlying degenerative factors.

Bone Tumors

Bone tissue is rarely the primary site for malignancies but is frequently a secondary site for metastasis. Primary osteosarcomata occur most often in young men, although they may occur less frequently at any age in either sex. Osteogenic sarcomata originate in the bony tissue; nonosseous tumors seed to the bones from other primary sites. Ewing's sarcoma, originating in the marrow and invading the shaft of the long bones, is a common form of nonosteogenic sarcoma.

There is no known cause, but theories suggest that rapid development of bone tissue during growth spurts is a predisposing factor. Bone pain is the most common early sign. The pain is more intense at night, is usually dull and centered at the site, and is not relieved by resting the body part. Depending on the site, the mass may be palpable through the skin and muscles.

Biopsy is the definitive diagnostic route after bone scans suggest the need. Treatment is excision of the tumor, including a large margin of surrounding bone structure and nearby lymph nodes. Chemotherapy and radiation are usually indicated also.

COMMON DIAGNOSTIC PROCEDURES AND THE MEDICAL ASSISTANT'S ROLE

Physical Examination

The physician's evaluation of the musculoskeletal system usually includes an assessment of the patient's structure and function, movement, and pain. An important part of the evaluation involves the patient history, which includes the patient's description of the events and circumstances that led to the decision to seek medical help.

The physician observes the patient's overall physical state by noting how the patient walks, sits, stands, and moves. Concentrating on the area of concern, the physician then evaluates the problem by visual inspection, palpation, and diagnostic tests or reports. Pain and limited or compromised functions are warning signals. Strength also affects function and is a part of any musculoskeletal evaluation. Other important considerations are skin color, temperature, tone, and tenderness; abnormal findings might indicate underlying pathology.

Diagnostic Studies

The most frequently used tools for detecting disorders of the musculoskeletal system are radiology and diagnostic imaging, which are used for diagnosing fractures, dislocations, and degeneration or diseases of the

11

bones and joints. Other radiographic studies include **arthrograms,** which show joint pathology, and myelograms, which help detect intervertebral disk conditions. A bone scan analyzes bone growth, density, tumors, or other pathology.

Computed tomography scans and magnetic resonance imaging reveal soft-tissue pathology, such as tumors, metastatic lesions, strokes, and ruptured or bulging disks.

Electromyography and nerve conduction velocity tests measure the health and fitness of the nerves as they relate to conduction of nerve impulses and muscle function.

Bone densitometry measures the bone mineral density using small amounts of radiation, less than a chest x-ray. There is no preparation required of patients, though they may need to remove clothing with metal buckles or buttons and any jewelry that might interfere with assessment of the image. The readings are compared to a reference population based on age, weight, sex, and ethnic background to determine the bone status and fracture risk (Fig. 11-10).

Goniometry is the measurement of the amount of movement available in a joint by a protractor-like device called a **goniometer.** As the patient progresses through range of motion exercises, the angle of joint movement is measured to the point of pain and to the limitation of movement.

A bone or muscle biopsy is also a valuable diagnostic tool. It allows intense examination of the tissue under a microscope to determine cell damage, neoplasms (tumor or growth), or other types of diseases.

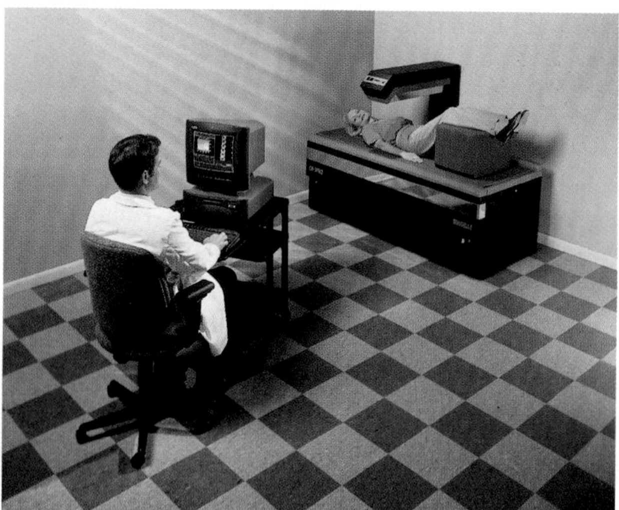

Figure 11-10 Bone densitometry measures bone mineral density. (By permission of the Lunar Corporation, Madison, WI.)

Checkpoint Question

10. *Name 11 procedures that can be used to diagnose musculoskeletal disorders?*

AMBULATORY AIDS AND THE MEDICAL ASSISTANT'S ROLE

Patients may lose their ability to move normally due to accidents and injuries, disease processes (eg, cerebrovascular accidents), neurologic or muscular defects, or degeneration. Patients who require assistance to maintain mobility may use crutches, canes, or walkers. Medical assistants often are responsible for teaching patients how to use these kinds of ambulatory aids safely (Box 11-7).

Crutches

Crutches may be either wooden or tubular aluminum. The most common form is the axillary crutch, which extends from the patient's axillae to the floor, with hand rests to distribute the weight to the palms. The Lofstrand or Canadian crutch is usually aluminum and reaches just to the forearms, with a metal cuff to maintain its position on the arms and a covered hand grip to distribute the weight (Fig. 11-11). The Lofstrand allows the patient to release and use his or her hands

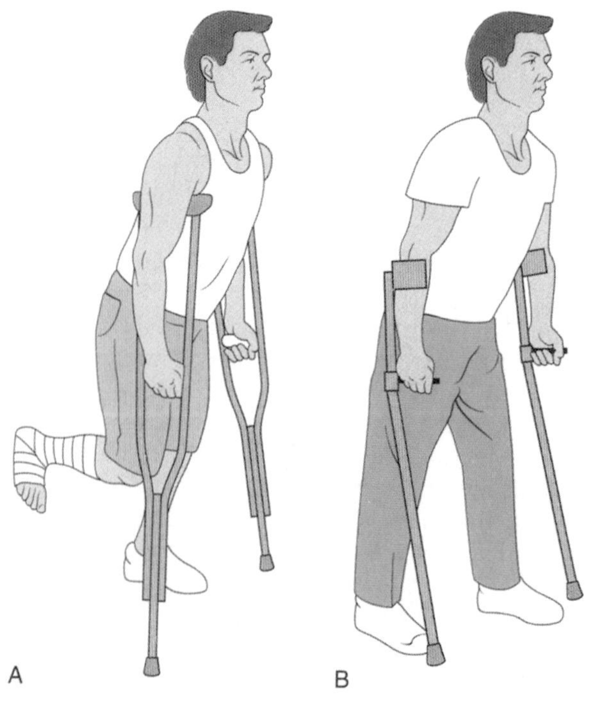

Figure 11-11 Types of crutches. (**A**) Axillary crutches. (**B**) Lofstrand, Canadian or forearm crutches.

Box 11-7
Safety Tips for Using Ambulatory Aids

- Check the rubber tips frequently, and replace worn tips immediately. (Most ambulatory aids require rubber tips, although some walkers are equipped with rollers.)
- Check screws and bolts frequently; tighten as needed.
- Remove scatter rugs and small pieces of furniture that may cause falls.

without losing the crutches. These work well for patients who will require crutch use for a long period of time or who have poor coordination.

Procedures 11-3 and 11-4 describe how to measure a patient for axillary crutches and how to teach a patient various crutch gaits. The Patient Education box offers tips for ascending and descending stairs with crutches and for sitting down safely.

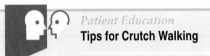

Patient Education
Tips for Crutch Walking

TO GO UP STAIRS:

- Stand close to the bottom step.
- With weight on the hands, step up to the first step with the unaffected leg.
- Bring the affected side and the crutches up to the step at the same time.
- Resume balance before proceeding to the next step.
- *Remember:* The good side goes up first!

TO DESCEND STAIRS:

- Stand close to the edge of the top step.
- Bend from the hips and knees to adjust to the height of the lower step. *Do not* lean forward (leaning forward may cause a fall).
- Carefully lower the crutches and the affected limb to the next step.
- Next, lower the unaffected leg to the lower step and resume balance. If a handrail is available, hold both crutches in one hand and follow the steps above.
- *Remember:* The affected foot goes down first!

TO SIT:

- Back up to the chair until you feel the edge on the backs of the legs.
- Move both crutches to the hand on the affected side and reach back for the chair with the hand on the unaffected side.
- Lower yourself slowly into the chair.

Canes

Canes are used when the patient needs extra support and stability but requires only a small measure of assistance with weight bearing. The standard cane may be used when the patient needs very slight assistance. The tripod (three legs) or quad cane (four legs) is useful when the patient needs greater stability (Fig. 11-12). The tripod and quad canes can stand alone if the patient needs free hands and can find other support. They tend to be bulkier and heavier, but because they offer greater stability and safety, they are good choices for patients who need greater support than the standard cane.

To measure for the proper cane length, have the patient stand erect. The cane should be level with the patient's greater trochanter, and the patient's elbow should be bent at a 30-degree angle.

To walk with a cane, the patient should:

1. Position the cane on the unaffected side, about 4 to 6 inches to the side and about 2 inches ahead of the foot.
2. Advance the cane and the affected leg together.
3. Bring the unaffected leg forward to a position just ahead of the cane.
4. Repeat the steps.

text continues on page 263

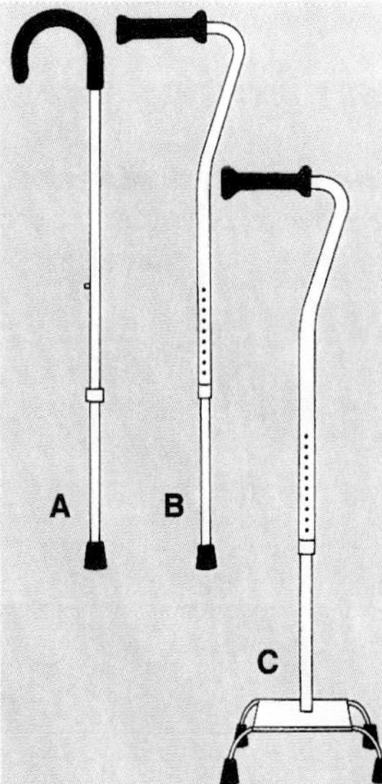

Figure 11-12 Three types of canes. (**A**) Single-ended canes with half-circle handles are recommended for patients requiring minimal support. (**B**) Single-ended canes with straight handles are recommended for patients with hand weakness. (**C**) Three- or four-prong canes are recommended for patients with poor balance.

11

Procedure 11-3 Measuring a Patient for Axillary Crutches

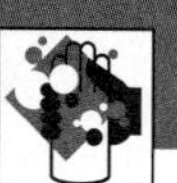

PURPOSE:

To ensure patient safety while using ambulatory aids

EQUIPMENT/SUPPLIES

- crutches with safety tips
- pads for the axilla and hand rests, as needed
- tools to tighten bolts

STEPS

1. Wash your hands.
2. Assemble the equipment.
3. Greet and identify the patient. Explain the procedure.
4. Ensure that the patient is wearing low-heeled shoes with safety soles.

   Low-heeled shoes with good soles will help prevent falls and ensure proper height measurement. While using crutches, patients should wear shoes with the same heel height to avoid an improper crutch fit.
5. Have the patient stand erect. Support the patient as needed.

   Providing support ensures patient safety.
6. Have the patient hold the crutches naturally with the tips about 2 inches in front of and 4–6 inches to the side of the feet. This is called the tripod position, and all crutch gaits start from this position (see Procedure 11-4: Teaching a Patient Crutch Gaits).
7. Using the tools as needed, adjust the crutches to the patient's height:
   a. Remove the wing nut and bolt, and move the extensions.

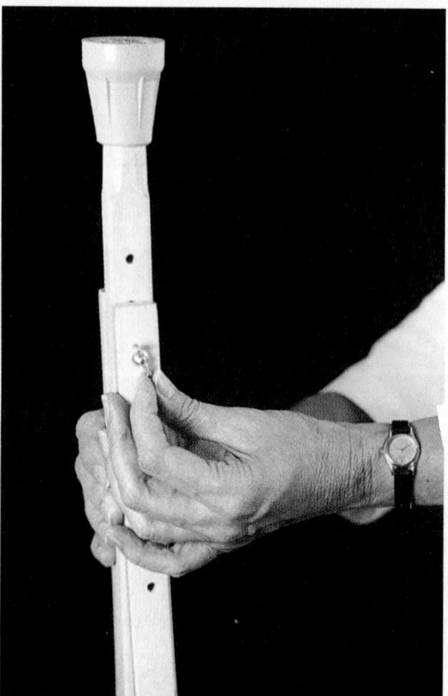

   b. Ensure that the axillary bar is about 2 fingerbreadths below the patient's axilla.
   c. Tighten the bolts for safety when the proper height is reached.

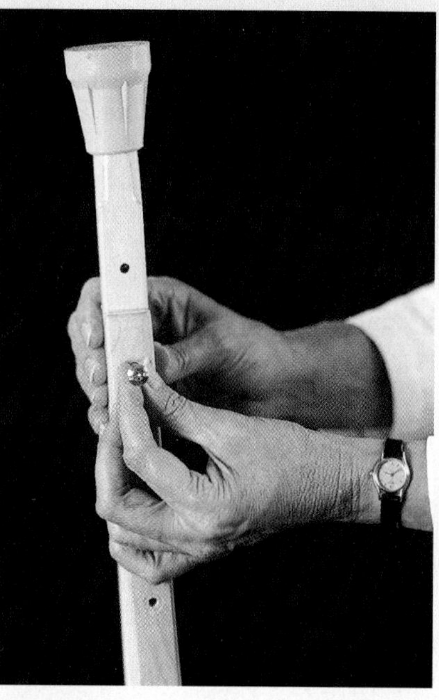

8. Adjust the handgrips.
   a. Raise or lower the bar along the shaft of the crutch.

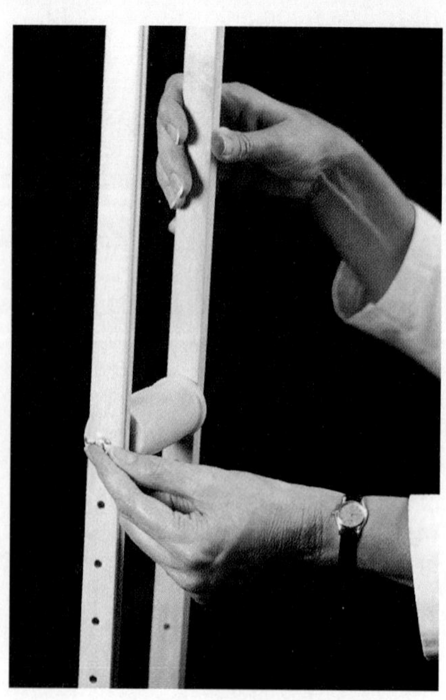

continued

Procedure 11-3 *Continued* Measuring a Patient for Axillary Crutches

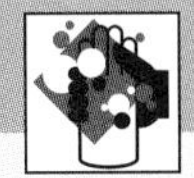

11

b. Check the adjustment. Crutches are properly adjusted when the patient's elbow is at a 30-degree angle when the bar is gripped and two fingers can be inserted at the axilla.

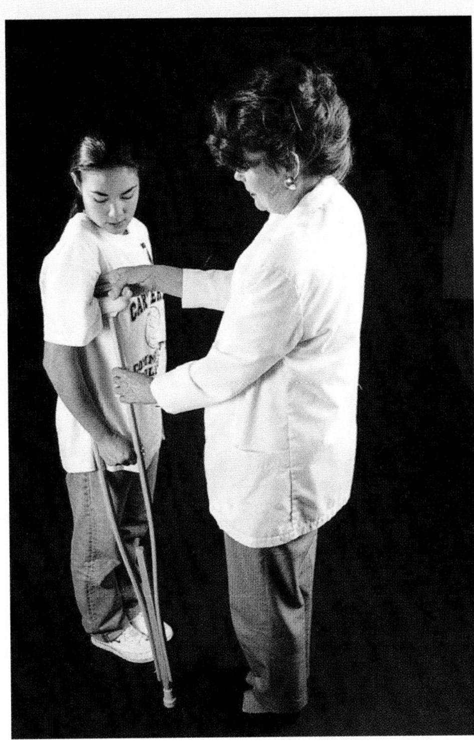

c. Tighten the bolts for safety.

9. If needed, pad axillary bars and handgrips with soft material to prevent friction.

10. Properly care for or dispose of equipment and supplies. Wash your hands.

Note: See Procedure 11-4, Teaching a Patient Crutch Gaits, for documentation guidelines and charting example.

Procedure 11-4 Teaching a Patient Crutch Gaits

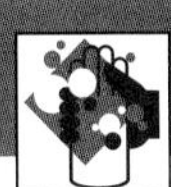

PURPOSE:

To increase the patient's independence with minimal patient energy expenditure while achieving the greatest degree of safety

The gait chosen will depend on the patient's weight-bearing ability, coordination, and general state of health. All gaits start with the tripod position (see Procedure 11-3: Measuring a Patient for Axillary Crutches).

STEPS

1. Wash your hands.

2. Have the patient stand up from a chair. To do this, the patient holds both crutches on the affected side, then slides to the edge of the chair. The patient pushes down on the chair arm on the unaffected side, then pushes to stand. Weight should be rested on the crutches until balance is restored.

3. Ensure that the crutches are in the tripod position.

To ensure safety and proper balance, crutches should be in this position before proceeding with any gait.

4. Have the patient begin the appropriate gait.

a. *Three-point gait:*

This gait is the most commonly used gait for crutch training. This gait is used when only one

continued

Procedure 11-4 Continued Teaching a Patient Crutch Gaits

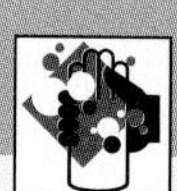

leg can be used for weight bearing or when only partial weight bearing is allowed on the affected leg. Amputees, those with injury to one leg, or patients who have had limb surgery will use this gait. This gait requires coordination and upper body strength.
   (1) The affected leg can be held clear of the floor or used in concert with the crutches. Both crutches are moved forward with the unaffected leg bearing the weight.
   (2) With the weight supported by the crutches, the unaffected weight-bearing leg is brought past the level of the crutches. The affected leg may be lightly touched down with no weight or may be supported.
   (3) The steps are repeated.

b. *Two-point gait:*
   This gait requires partial weight bearing and good coordination. Two points will be raised, and two points will be on the floor in this gait.
   (1) The right crutch and left foot are moved forward.
   (2) As these points rest, the right foot and left crutch are moved forward.
   (3) The steps are repeated.

c. *Four-point gait:*
   This gait is the slowest and safest of the gaits. At least three points are on the ground at all times. The patient must be capable of partial weight bearing. Patients with degenerative diseases, spasticity, and poor coordination will use this gait.
   (1) The right crutch moves forward.
   (2) The left foot is moved to a position just ahead of the left crutch.
   (3) The left crutch is moved forward.
   (4) The right foot moves to a position just ahead of the right crutch.
   (5) The steps are repeated.

d. *Swing-through gait:*
   (1) Both crutches are moved forward.
   (2) With the weight on the hands, the body swings through to a position ahead of the crutches.
   (3) The crutches are moved ahead.
   (4) The steps are repeated.

e. *Swing-to gait:* This gait may be used until the patient is ready for the swing-through gait.
   (1) Both crutches are moved forward.
   (2) With the weight on the hands, the body swings to the level of the crutches.
   (3) The crutches are moved ahead.
   (4) The steps are repeated.

5. Wash your hands.

DOCUMENTATION GUIDELINES

- Date and time
- Type of gait taught
- Measurement of crutches to fit patient
- Patient complaints/concerns
- Patient education/instructions
- Your signature

Charting Example

DATE	TIME Pt fractured (L) distal tibia.
	Fracture reduced and casted by
	Dr. Miranda. Postreduction—left toes
	warm to touch and pink in color. Able to
	wiggle toes. Pt fitted for axillary crutches
	—2 finger breadths below the axilla.
	Handgrips adjusted keeping elbows flexed
	at 30-degree angle. Two-point gait
	demonstrated. Pt returned demonstra-
	tion without problem. Written instruc-
	tions given to pt on crutch walking.
	Verbalized understanding of all
	instructions. —Your signature

continued

Procedure 11-4 Continued Teaching a Patient Crutch Gaits

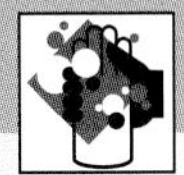

11

4 POINT GAIT • Partial weight bearing both feet • Maximal support provided • Requires constant shift of weight	2 POINT GAIT • Partial weight bearing both feet • Provides less support than 4 point gait • Faster than a 4 point gait	3 POINT GAIT • Non weight-bearing • Requires good balance • Requires arm strength • Faster gait • Can use with walker	SWING TO • Weight bearing both feet • Provides stability • Requires arm strength • Can use with walker	SWING THROUGH • Weight bearing • Requires arm strength • Requires coordination/ balance • Most advanced gait
4. Advance right foot	4. Advance right foot and left crutch	4. Advance right foot	4. Lift both feet/ swing forward / land feet next to crutches	4. Lift both feet / swing forward / land feet in front of crutches
3. Advance left crutch	3. Advance left foot and right crutch	3. Advance left foot and both crutches	3. Advance both crutches	3. Advance both crutches
2. Advance left foot	2. Advance right foot and left crutch	2. Advance right foot	2. Lift both feet / swing forward / land feet next to crutches	2. Lift both feet / swing forward / land feet in front of crutches
1. Advance right crutch	1. Advance left foot and right crutch	1. Advance left foot and both crutches	1. Advance both crutches	1. Advance both crutches
Beginning stance	Beginning stance	Beginning stance	Beginning stance	Beginning stance

11

Procedure 11-5 Transferring to and From a Wheelchair

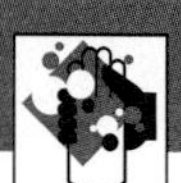

PURPOSE:

To increase patient independence and mobility
To promote safety and prevent injury

EQUIPMENT/SUPPLIES

- wheelchair
- transfer belt (optional, but preferred)
- sliding board (optional)

STEPS

1. Wash your hands.
2. Explain to both the patient and caregiver how you will facilitate the transfer and how they both may help.
   The transfer will be safer if all involved understand the procedure.
3. Organize the setting to ensure the shortest transfer distance possible and ease of maneuvering. If the wheelchair is placed facing the direction the patient either is facing or will need to face, there will be no need to turn the patient.
   Transferring the patient for the shortest distance possible decreases the risk of injury.
4. Align the wheelchair as close as possible to the point of transfer at either a 45-degree angle or parallel to the patient, preferably on the patient's strongest side. Lock the wheels, and raise the foot rests.
   Locking the wheels prevents rolling. If the chair is on the patient's strongest side, he or she will be better able to help with the move.
5. Assist the patient into position as needed.
   a. From a vehicle: Standing at the patient's side, slide one arm under his or her thighs, and brace the patient's shoulders with your other arm. In one smooth movement, turn the patient in the seat until his or her feet are toward the ground.
   b. From the table: With one arm under the patient's shoulders, assist him or her to sit. Help the patient to slide to the end of the table until his or her feet are on the table step. You may require assistance if the patient cannot step down.
   Note: To assist the patient into the vehicle or onto the table, reverse the procedure.
6. Help the patient put on a transfer belt. Secure it snugly.
   A transfer belt gives you a better grasp for the patient and reduces the risk of injury.
7. Grasp the transfer belt at the back by reaching around the patient's body, or reach under the patient's arms and place your hands on his or her chest wall, not his axilla.
   Using the transfer belt or lifting by the patient's chest wall helps support the upper body without causing discomfort to the axilla.
8. Have the patient grasp your shoulders, or have him reach with one hand for the far chair arm for partial support while grasping your shoulder with the other.
   This position allows the patient to assist with leverage.
9. Brace your feet apart with your right foot slightly forward. The patient's foot placement should mirror yours.
   The foot position is important to provide a wide base for support.
10. Keep your spine straight. Flex your knees and hips, and brace your knees against the patient's knees. Grasp the transfer belt or tighten your grip on the patient.
    This position provides stability and prevents twisting the spine.
11. Rock the patient back and forth to an agreed upon count of three. At the signal, encourage the patient to straighten his or her knees and hips. If possible, have the patient push off with the back foot.
    The rocking motion provides momentum to make lifting easier.
12. As you straighten, rock your weight onto your back foot, and pivot the patient with his or her back to the destination. Keep your knees against the patient's knees. Support the patient in this position for a moment until balance is restored.
    The patient is now in a stable position for transfer.
13. Have the patient step back to the chair (table or other seat), and grasp the arms of the chair or other surface while you continue to provide stability with your knees against the patient's.
    The patient will feel more secure if he or she can feel his or her destination. Maintaining contact with the patient's knees provides for greater safety.

continued

Procedure 11-5 Continued Transferring to and From a Wheelchair

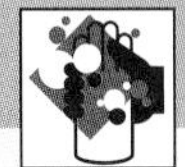

14. Shift your weight to your forward foot as the patient lowers to the sitting position.

As you shift your weight, you will provide momentum for sitting.

15. Have the patient sit well back into the seat. If in the wheelchair, lower the foot rests and help the patient position his or her feet. If you are to push the patient, make sure the patient's hands are in his or her lap.

The patient will be less likely to fall from the chair in this position. Feet and hands must be within the chair to avoid injury.

DOCUMENTATION GUIDELINES

- Date and time
- Patient complaints/concerns
- Procedures performed, as appropriate
- Patient education/instructions
- Your signature

Charting Example

DATE	TIME Pt arrived via WC for wound
	dressing L tibial ulcer. Wound appears
	pink, no undue redness. Minimal clear
	drainage. Pt has no complaints of dis-
	comfort. Dr. Sutton in to check wound.
	Sterile dressings applied. Pt to RTC in
	3 days for recheck. —Your signature

Walkers

Walkers are comfortable aids for the elderly or others with weakness or poor coordination. They consist of a lightweight aluminum frame in an open square. Because walkers are somewhat bulky, maneuvering in close quarters can be difficult. The walker frame should be level with the patient's hip, and the patient's elbow should be bent at about a 30-degree angle (Fig. 11-13).

To use a walker, the patient should:

1. Stand erect and move the walker ahead about 6 inches.
2. Using an easy walking gait with hands on the walker grips, step into the walker.
3. Move the walker ahead again.
4. Repeat the steps.

Checkpoint Question

11. *On which side of the body is the cane positioned?*

Wheelchairs

Though most patients arriving at the medical office are ambulatory, some may require wheelchair assistance. Chronic wheelchair-dependent patients and their caregivers usually have adapted to the situation and are likely to be adept at transfer and ensuring safety and comfort. In contrast, acute patients, who require the wheelchair for only a short time, usually are not quite as proficient and need more help from you. Compounding the problem is the need to transfer from vehicles not designed to be wheelchair accessible. In the examining room, examination tables are not designed to lower to the wheelchair level, then raise to a standard examination height. All of these factors make proper body mechanics and safety guidelines extremely important.

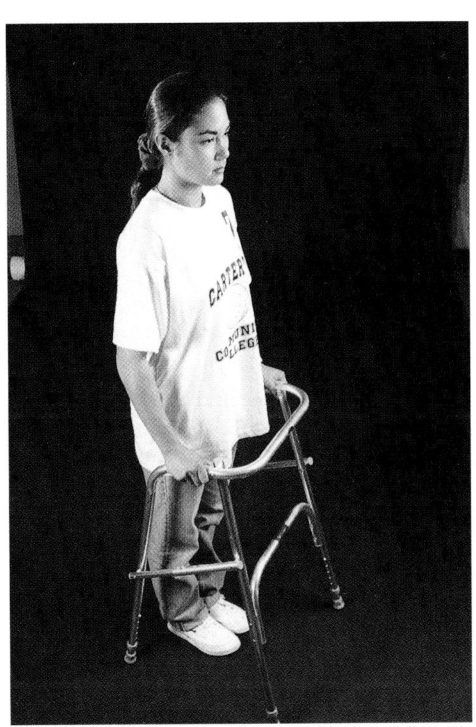

Figure 11-13 A properly adjusted walker.

11

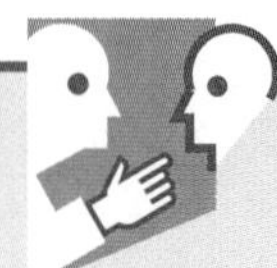

Advice and Tips
Wheelchair Rental

A patient who needs a wheelchair only for a short time can rent the equipment. Provide the names of local sources of rental medical equipment. If funds are a concern, resources are available to help patients who qualify for aid. For example, agencies such as the American Cancer Society, the American Heart Association, the American Lung Association, and hospice organizations assist with rental equipment or have equipment to lend to patients.

Assess the situation before you begin the transfer. How much can the patient and caregiver help? Does the patient understand what is expected of him or her? Is the scene set for the shortest, safest transfer possible? All offices are now wheelchair accessible, but you should check before you begin the transfer to ensure that the paths to and through the building are unobstructed. Decide before you enter the examining room how the transfer will work best to avoid having to maneuver the chair any more than necessary in the confined space. The transfer to and from the table may be more difficult than the transfer to and from the vehicle because of the table height. If the patient must be transferred to the table (some procedures may be completed with the patient in the chair) and is unable to assist, enlist aid and decide before you begin how each person—worker, patient, caregiver—can help facilitate the move. Never try to move or lift more than you realistically feel you can manage. Procedure 11-5 describes how to transfer a patient to and from a wheelchair.

To make the move easier, a sliding board assists with movement if the transfer is from two relatively comparable heights. Many wheelchair arms are designed to lower for this maneuver. The board is secured beneath the patient's buttocks on the chair seat. The patient grasps the opposite chair arm and, with your assistance, slips into the chair. The procedure is easily reversed. When the transfer is complete, be sure to secure the arm into the locked position before you begin to wheel the patient. Box 11-8 provides additional safety guidelines for wheelchair use.

Box 11-8
Safety Guidelines for Wheelchair Use

- Never pull on a weak or paralyzed limb. Muscle support at the joints usually is weak in these limbs, and the pull may result in a dislocation.
- If possible, move the patient's stronger side first; the stronger side can pull the weaker side.
- Always lock the wheels and raise the foot plates before beginning the transfer.
- Never begin to transport (roll) the patient without lowering the foot plates. Check to be sure that the patient's feet are supported by the foot plates and that his or her hands are within the confines of the chair.
- Pull the patient's hips far back into the chair seat, and secure the patient if he or she is confused or likely to fall.
- Back into and out of elevators. Approach corners with caution.
- Back the wheelchair down an incline, and push it up an incline. Always place yourself between the patient and the bottom of the incline to avoid having the patient pitch forward.

Answers to Checkpoint Questions

1. *The skeletal system provides a supportive framework for the body, provides leverage for the muscles, protects vital organs, allows for calcium metabolism and storage, and facilitates blood cell production.*
2. *Types of joints are synarthroses (immovable), amphiarthroses (slightly movable), and diarthrosis (freely movable).*
3. *The four natural curves of the spine are the cervical, thoracic, lumbar, and sacral curves.*
4. *The knee is a hinge joint. Its two primary movements are flexion and extension.*
5. *Tendons connect muscle to bone. Ligaments connect bone to bone.*
6. *Luxation is a complete dislocation; subluxation is a partial dislocation.*
7. *An open reduction involves surgery; a closed reduction does not.*
8. *Abnormal spinal curvatures include scoliosis (lateral curve), kyphosis (hunchback), and lordosis (swayback).*
9. *Osteoarthritis is a degenerative joint disease caused by wear and tear on the weight-bearing joints in which the articular cartilage degenerates and the ends of the bones enlarge. Rheumatoid arthritis is a systemic autoimmune disease that attacks the synovium of the joint, ultimately leading to inflammation, pain, stiffness, and crippling deformities. It usually begins in the non–weight-bearing joints, but eventually affects most of the joints of the appendicular skeleton.*
10. *Eleven procedures that can be used to diagnose musculoskeletal disorders are physical examination, computed tomography scans, magnetic resonance imaging, electromyography, nerve conduction velocity, goniometry, arthrograms, myelograms, bone scans, x-rays, and bone densitometry.*
11. *The cane is positioned on the unaffected side of the body.*

Critical Thinking Challenges

1. Create a patient education brochure for using ambulatory aids. Include a brief description of the purpose of each aid along with the procedure steps.
2. The youth baseball league playoffs are coming to your town and you are asked to participate in the first aid station. What kinds of orthopedic injuries would you expect to see and why? Develop a list of the first aid supplies that you would want to have available, and explain the reasons for your selections. What other health care professionals would you want to have at the first aid station with you?

Suggestions for Further Reading

Cohen, B. J. (1994). *Medical Terminology: An Illustrated Guide,* 2nd ed. Philadelphia: J.B. Lippincott.

Colburn, G. L., & Lause, D. B. (1993). *Musculoskeletal Anatomy: A Text and Guide for Dissection for Students in the Allied Health Sciences.* New York: Parthenon.

Iglarsh, A., Kendall, F., Lewis, C., & Sharman S. (1994). *The Secret of Good Posture.* Alexandria, VA: American Physical Therapy Association.

Kendall, F. P., McCreary, E., & Provance, P. (1993). *Muscle Testing and Function,* 4th ed. Baltimore: Williams & Wilkins.

Lippert, L. (1994). *Clinical Kinesiology for Physical Therapist Assistants,* 2nd ed. Philadelphia: F.A. Davis.

Memmler, R. L., Cohen, B. J., & Wood, D. L. (1996). *The Human Body in Health and Disease,* 8th ed. Philadelphia: Lippincott-Raven.

Scully, R., & Baynes, M. (1989). *Physical Therapy.* Philadelphia: J.B. Lippincott.

Wolf, R. (1991). *The Rehabilitation Specialists' Handbook.* Philadelphia: F.A. Davis.

12

Assisting With Diagnostic and Therapeutic Procedures Associated With the Neurologic System

Chapter Outline

Role Delineation

CLINICAL

Fundamental Principles

- Apply principles of aseptic technique and infection control.

Diagnostic Orders

- Collect and process specimens.

Patient Care

- Prepare patients for examinations, procedures, and treatments.
- Assist with examinations, procedures, and treatments.

GENERAL

Professionalism

- Project a professional manner and image.
- Work as a team member.
- Prioritize and perform multiple tasks.

Communication Skills

- Treat all patients with compassion and empathy.
- Adapt communications to individual's ability to understand.

Legal Concepts

- Practice within the scope of education, training, and personal capabilities.
- Document accurately.

Instruction

- Instruct individuals according to their needs.
- Teach methods of health promotion and disease prevention.

Chapter Competencies

Learning Objectives

Upon successfully completing this chapter, you will be able to:

1. Spell and define the Key Terms.
2. Differentiate between the functions of the central, peripheral, and autonomic nervous systems.
3. Explain the reflex arc.
4. Identify the three main components of the brain and list their individual functions.
5. Compare the functions of the parasympathetic and sympathetic systems.
6. Identify infectious diseases that involve the nervous system.
7. Identify physical and emotional effects of degenerative nervous system disorders.
8. Describe the medical assistant's role in caring for a patient having a seizure.
9. List potential complications of a spinal cord injury.
10. Name common diagnostic procedures for nervous system disorders and briefly explain each.

Performance Objective

Upon successfully completing this chapter, you will be able to:

1. Assist with performance of a lumbar puncture (Procedure 12-1).

Key Terms

(See Glossary for definitions.)

afferent
alpha-fetoprotein
amniocentesis
arachnoid
autonomic
axon
basal ganglia
cerebellum
cerebrum
concussions
convulsions
cranium
dendrite
diencephalon
dura mater
dysphagia
dysphasia
efferent
electroencephalogram (EEG)
gyri
hypothalamus
insula
medulla oblongata
meninges
meningocele
midbrain
migraine
myelogram
myelomeningocele
neurons
neurotransmitters
parasympathetic
pia mater
pons
Queckenstedt test
Romberg test
seizures
spina bifida occulta
sulci
sympathetic
synapses
thalamus

The nervous system is the chief communication and command center for all parts of the body. Its responsibilities range from controlling vital homeostatic functions to processing memory and logical thought.

The nervous system has two divisions: the central nervous system (CNS) and the peripheral nervous system (PNS). The CNS is composed of the brain and spinal cord and is the body's command center. Messages are relayed to and from the CNS by the cranial and spinal nerves that make up the PNS. A division of the PNS, the **autonomic** nervous system, functions automatically without conscious awareness. Respiratory and circulatory rates, blood pressure, and digestive processes are controlled by the autonomic nervous system (Fig. 12-1).

STRUCTURE AND FUNCTION OF THE NERVOUS SYSTEM

Structure of a Neuron

The fundamental functioning units of the nervous system are special cells called **neurons**, designed to carry electrical nerve impulses. A neuron is composed of three main parts: **dendrite**, **axon**, and cell body (Fig. 12-2).

1. The dendrite conducts impulses *toward* the cell body. Dendrites range from less than an inch to over a foot in length. A neuron may have one or more dendrites.
2. The cell body consists of the nucleus, the brain of the cell, and the cytoplasm, which contains the organelles of the cell. (See Ch. 9, Introduction to Anatomy and Physiology)

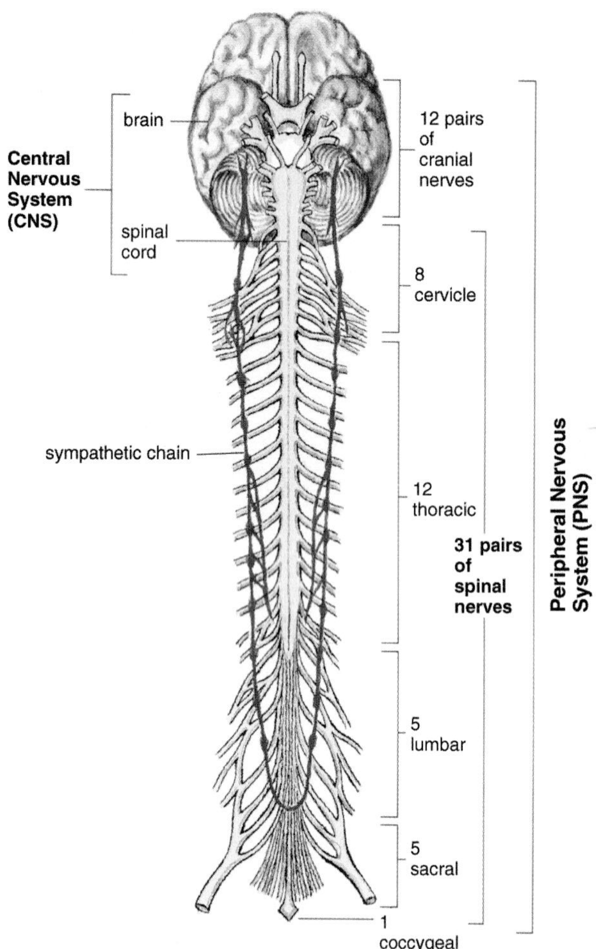

Figure 12-1 Anatomic division of the nervous system.

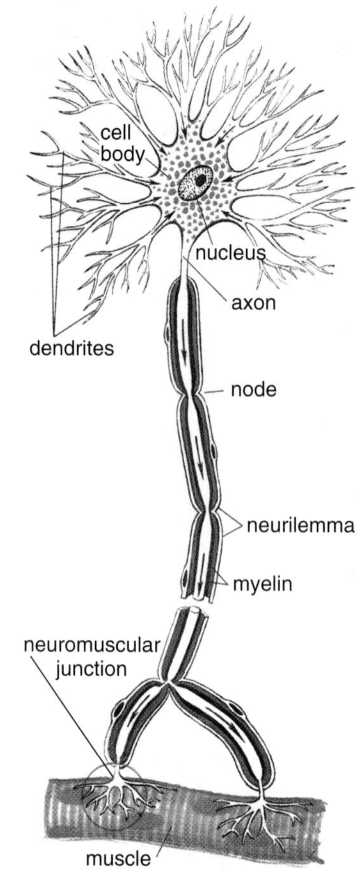

Figure 12-2 Diagram of a motor neuron. The break in the axon denotes length. The arrows show the direction of the nerve impulse.

3. The axon transmits impulses *away* from the cell body. A neuron has only one axon that may then branch into collateral axons. Some axons are covered with a cellular material called the myelin sheath, a fatty insulator formed by Schwann cells that wraps around the axon at intervals and increases the rate of impulse conduction. Myelinated cells are referred to as white cells because the fatty sheath gives them a white appearance. Neurons without the myelin sheath conduct impulses more slowly than the myelinated cells. They are called gray cells because, in the absence of the myelin sheath, they appear gray.

Neurons located outside the CNS are combined in pathways to form what is commonly called a nerve. Nerves are classified according to their functions:

- Sensory (**afferent**) nerves conduct impulses to the brain.
- Motor (**efferent**) nerves conduct impulses away from the brain.
- Mixed nerves are capable of both motor and sensory functions.

Nervous System Communication

Because communication within the internal environment is essential for life, the nervous system must be able to communicate with itself and with the rest of the body systems. It does so in two ways—through **synapses** (the junction of two neurons) and reflexes.

Neurons transmitting impulses do not actually touch the receiving neuron. They are divided by a small space, called a synapse, between the axon of one neuron and the dendrites and cell body of the next neuron. Communication between neurons occurs when a message is released by the axon of one neuron and then "jumps" across the synapse to the dendrite of another. Chemicals called **neurotransmitters** transmit messages across the synapse in the form of an electrical charge. Neurotransmitting substances include epinephrine (adrenaline), norepinephrine (noradrenaline), acetylcholine, and dopamine. Neurotransmitters rely on the presence of electrolytes, specifically sodium, potassium, and chlorine, to conduct the electrical impulse through the cell body to the point of synapse.

Internal communication also occurs through the reflex arc. A reflex is the body's involuntary response to a given stimulus. Reflex arcs are tested during routine office visits in what is commonly called reflex testing. The most common example is the tapping of the knee with a reflex hammer. Listed below is the sequence of events in this instance.

1. The skin of the knee and the nerve below it are stimulated by a tap with a percussion hammer just below the patella. (The knee is usually flexed and dangling.)
2. The sensory neuron transmits the impulse along the dendrite to the cell body of the neuron.
3. The sensory axon carries the impulse to the spinal cord.
4. The message is received within the spinal cord by the central (associative or connecting) neuron, and transmission begins to the motor neuron dendrite. A nerve pathway ascending the spinal column sends the information to the brain for grading and interpretation while the reflex impulses flash through the peripheral motor neuron responsible for the muscles in the knee area.
5. The message is received and processed by the cell body of the motor neuron and passed on to its axon.
6. The motor neuron axon stimulates the muscles in the knee to contract, causing movement to occur before the brain has had time to interpret the message sent by the ascending spinal nerves that the blow or knee tap has occurred.

Although the reflex arc sounds highly technical, it occurs without our conscious awareness, and the results are evident in milliseconds (Fig. 12-3).

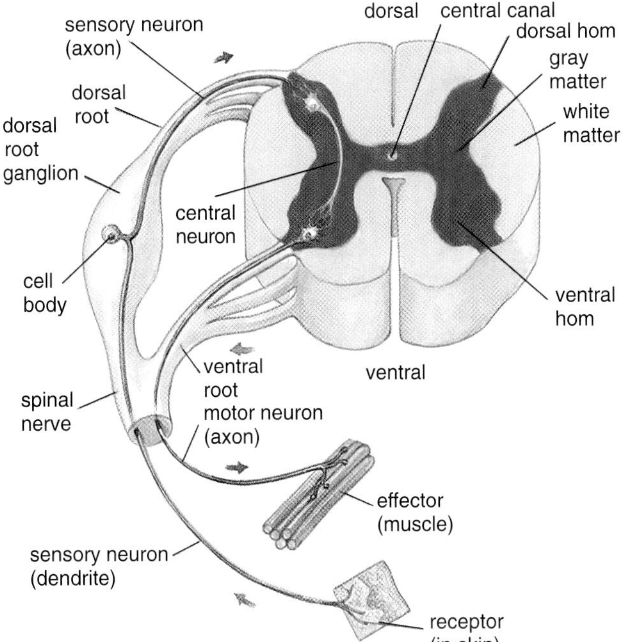

Figure 12-3 Reflex arc showing the pathway of impulses and cross-section of the spinal cord.

Checkpoint Question

1. *How does communication between two neurons occur?*

CENTRAL NERVOUS SYSTEM

The CNS consists of the brain and the spinal cord. The brain is situated in the skull and is protected by the strength of the **cranium.** The spinal cord begins at the base of the brain and travels through the vertebral column until about the second lumbar vertebra, referred to as L-2.

The Brain

Protective Coverings

The brain is covered by three layers of connective tissue called the **meninges**, which completely enclose the brain and spinal cord.

1. The outermost layer, the **dura mater,** is composed of fibrous tissue and is the thickest and toughest protective layer.
2. The middle layer, the **arachnoid,** is loosely attached to the dura mater by fine fibers that allow movement of cerebrospinal fluid (CSF) in the spaces between the membranes. This layer cushions and protects the brain and spinal cord from external injury.
3. The innermost layer, the **pia mater,** is closest to the brain. It is a very thin membrane of connective tissue that weaves in and out of the grooves in the brain, carrying most of the brain's blood supply.

Cerebrospinal Fluid

The brain is cushioned by CSF, which is formed in spaces deep within the brain called ventricles. CSF is filtered from the bloodstream and contains water and nutrients to nourish the tissues of the brain and spinal cord. It is clear and colorless, unless a disease process is present. CSF circulates from the ventricles out to the meninges, through the spinal cord, and back to the brain spaces. It is then reabsorbed into the bloodstream to be replenished by newly filtered fluid. CSF levels remain fairly constant; an elevation indicates the presence of a disease process or trauma (Fig. 12-4).

Major Divisions of the Brain

The brain has three main divisions or components: the cerebrum, brain stem, and cerebellum.

CEREBRUM. The **cerebrum** is the largest part of the brain. It is composed of the right and left hemispheres, the corpus callosum, and the **diencephalon,** which lies

12

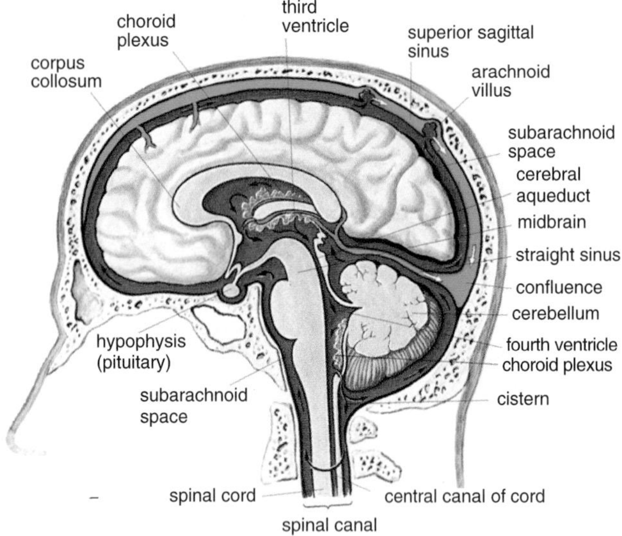

Figure 12-4 Flow of cerebrospinal fluid (CSF) from choroid plexuses back to the blood in dural sinuses is shown by the black arrows; flow of blood is shown by the white arrows.

beneath the hemispheres. It is important to note that the right hemisphere of the brain controls the left side of the body, and vice versa. The hemispheres are covered with an outer layer of nerve tissue called the cerebral cortex, also referred to as the gray matter. The cerebral cortex appears gray because the neurons in this area are not myelinated. This gray matter forms valleys that are called **sulci** and ridges that are called **gyri.** Under the gray matter is white matter, consisting of myelinated axons covered with fatty Schwann cells and dendrites that connect the areas of the cerebrum to one another and to other parts of the brain (Fig. 12-5).

Located deep in the white matter of each hemisphere is a band of gray matter called the **basal ganglia.** The basal ganglia neurons secrete a fluid called dopamine, one of the neurotransmitters essential for controlling body movement and facial expressions.

The cerebral cortex has many functions. As the brain's "memory bank," it sorts and stores knowledge for recall. It facilitates thought processes, judgment, word association, and the highest reasoning powers.

The cerebral cortex is divided into four areas or lobes. Each lobe is bilateral and is divided centrally by the longitudinal fissure. Each is associated with certain functions and is named according to the cranial bone under which it lies.

1. The *frontal lobe* lies below the frontal bone in the cranium and is the largest lobe. One of its main functions is generating impulses for voluntary movement. Other functions include intellectual reasoning, abstract thinking, and speech control.
2. The *parietal lobe* is found below the parietal skull bones. Its main function is sensory interpretation. It receives impulses from the nerves in the skin for touch, pain, and temperature and from the lingual papillae for taste. This lobe also interprets shapes, distances, and sizes.
3. The *temporal lobe* is located beneath the temporal bone. Its main function is sound interpretation within its auditory area. Also within this lobe is the olfactory area, which analyzes the stimuli perceived by the olfactory nerve bulbs in the nose.
4. The *occipital lobe* is located at the base of the cerebrum. Its main function is interpreting visual stimuli received from the optic nerve (Fig. 12-6).

Recent research has revealed the existence of an additional lobe, called the **insula,** which is thought to be responsible for visceral, or body organ, functions.

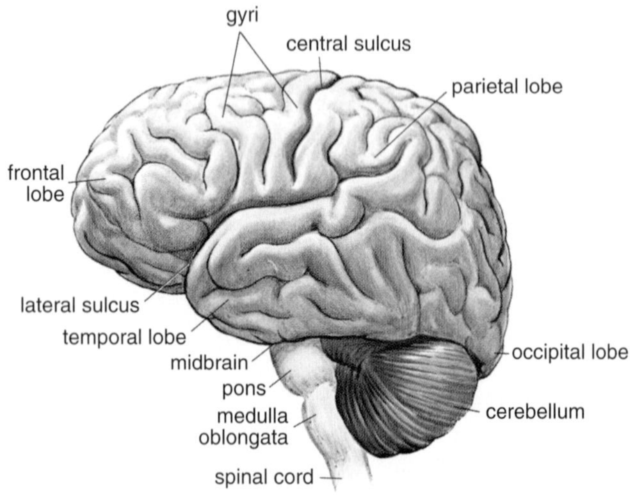

Figure 12-5 External surface of the brain showing the main parts and some of the lobes and sulci of the cerebrum.

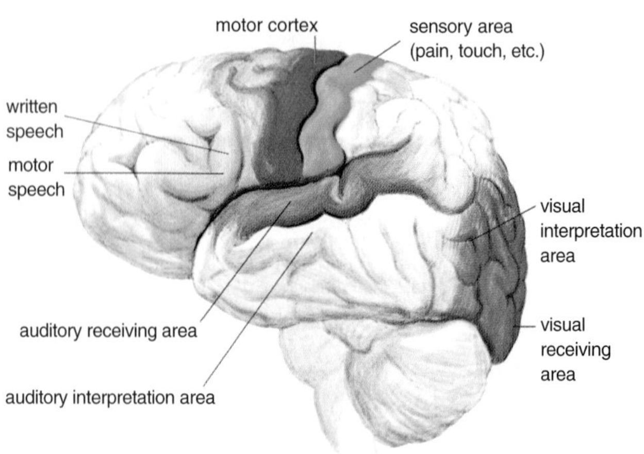

Figure 12-6 Functional areas of the cerebral cortex.

Under the gray matter of the cerebral cortex is the white matter. In it lies a band of nerve fibers called the corpus callosum, responsible for connecting the two hemispheres and transmitting information back and forth between them.

Between the two hemispheres lies the diencephalon. It is made of two parts called the **thalamus** and the **hypothalamus.** Most sensory impulses arrive by way of the thalamus. The thalamus sorts the impulses and sends them to the correct areas of the cerebral cortex for interpretation. Located below the thalamus is the hypothalamus, which is responsible for regulating body temperature, appetite, sleep patterns, and assisting with autonomic responses. It also helps regulate various body functions, including heart rate and blood pressure. In addition, the hypothalamus (in close cooperation with the pituitary) helps regulate several hormones, including secretion of the antidiuretic hormone that maintains the body's fluid balance.

Checkpoint Question

2. *Name the four lobes of the cerebral cortex and list their functions.*

BRAIN STEM. The brain stem, although apparently one continuous organ, is composed of three overlapping areas of function. They are the **midbrain, pons,** and **medulla oblongata.**

The midbrain serves primarily as a relay center for messages that control certain eye and ear reflexes. This part of the midbrain is composed of gray matter. The rest of the midbrain, made up of white matter, transmits impulses from the cerebrum to the other parts of the brain stem, cerebellum, or spinal cord.

The pons is a key communication center, relaying messages between the cerebellum and the entire nervous system. The pons also helps control some of the involuntary muscles used for breathing. In addition, the pons has control over the reticular formation cycle (also referred to as the reticular activating network), which initiates and maintains alertness and awareness. This mechanism wakes us when a threatening sound is perceived, even in deep sleep.

The medulla oblongata—perhaps the most important part of the brain in terms of life maintenance—contains three vital centers that regulate breathing, heart rate, and blood pressure. The respiratory center regulates the muscles used for breathing. The cardiac center regulates heart rate and the force of contractions of the heart muscle. The vasomotor center regulates blood pressure by controlling the smooth muscles of the blood vessels, causing either vasoconstriction or vasodilation.

CEREBELLUM. The **cerebellum** is composed of both gray and white matter. It has three basic involuntary functions:

1. *Maintaining equilibrium.* Equilibrium is required for standing, sitting, walking, and all body position changes. The cerebellum coordinates equilibrium by receiving the impulses from the semicircular canals in the inner ear and from various proprioception receptors in the body.
2. *Regulating muscle tone.* The cerebellum ensures that all muscles are ready for impulse reaction. If muscle response is compromised, the state of *tonus* (the condition that maintains the upright position with a state of partial muscle contraction) will collapse, causing paralysis.
3. *Ensuring muscle coordination.* The cerebellum is responsible for the quality of movement of the voluntary muscles.

The cerebellum gives the body its grace and coordination, translating impulses from the cerebrum into muscle movement. Essentially, the cerebrum tells the muscles what to do, and the cerebellum tells them how to do it.

Spinal Cord

The spinal cord is located in the vertebral column. It consists of both gray and white matter for transmitting impulses to and from the brain. The gray matter forms two columns called the ventral and the dorsal horns (see Fig. 12-3). This formation gives the gray matter an "H" appearance. The nerve cell bodies are located here. The white matter fills the rest of the cord and houses the nerve tracts and fibers.

The spinal cord has three distinct functions: sensory, motor, and reflex control. The sensory function carries messages to the brain by way of ascending nerve pathways. The motor function carries messages away from the brain or spinal cord by way of descending nerve pathways. The reflex function requires a stimulus, transmission of the stimulus, and a response. This is possible through connections with a sensory neuron, a connecting or associative neuron, and a motor neuron.

➤ PERIPHERAL NERVOUS SYSTEM

Both the brain and the spinal cord have nerves that transmit impulses. These nerves, called the cranial and spinal nerves, make up the PNS.

Cranial Nerves

Cranial nerves (Fig. 12-7) function as either sensory, motor, or mixed nerves. Sensory cranial nerves are re-

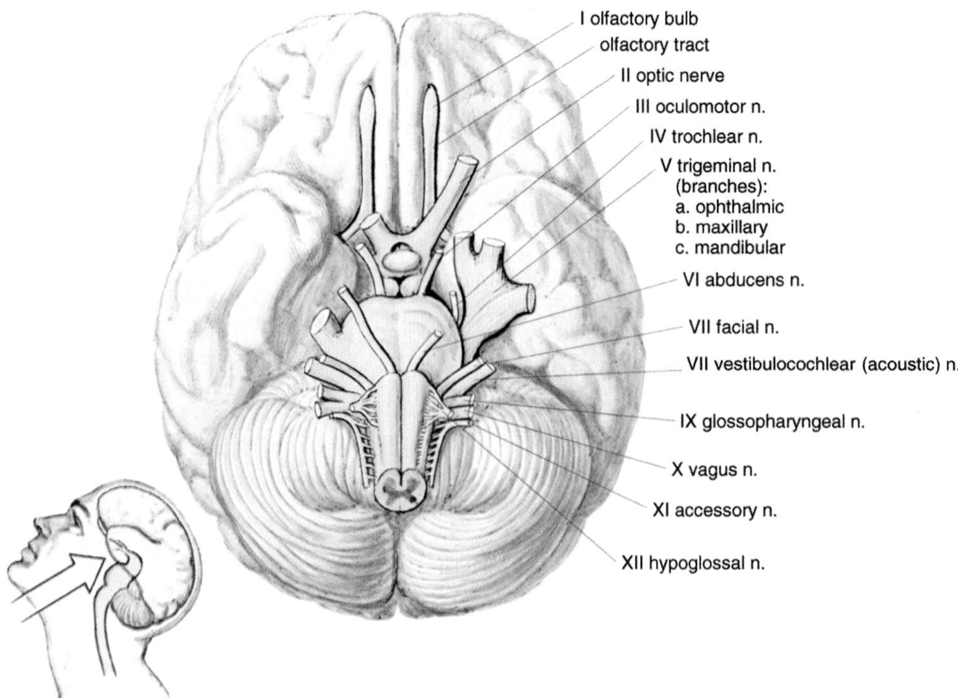

Figure 12-7 Base of the brain showing cranial nerves.

sponsible for functions such as smell, taste, hearing, touch, pain, and vision. The motor cranial nerves are related to both involuntary and voluntary muscle movements and to gland functions. The cranial nerves have specific names and are numbered using Roman numerals. Sensory cranial nerves are I, II, VIII; motor nerves are III, IV, VI, XI, XII; and the mixed are V, VII, IX and X (Table 12-1).

Checkpoint Question

3. *List the specific function of each cranial nerve.*

Table 12-1 **Cranial Nerves**

Nerve (Number)	*Type*	*Functions*	*Methods for Examining Nerve*
Olfactory (I)	Sensory	Sense of smell	Test each nostril for smell reception and interpretation.
Optic (II)	Sensory	Sense of vision	Test vision for acuity and visual fields.
Oculomotor (III)	Motor	Pupil constriction Raise eyelids	Test pupillary reaction to light and ability to open and close eyelids.
Trochlear (IV)	Motor	Downward inward eye movement	Test for downward and inward movement of the eye.
Trigeminal (V)	Motor	Jaw movements—chewing and mastication	Ask client to open and clench jaws while palpating the jaw muscles.
	Sensory	Sensation on the face and neck	Test face and neck for pain sensations, light touch, temperature.
Abducens (VI)	Motor	Lateral movement of the eyes	Test ocular movement in all directions.
Facial (VII)	Motor	Muscles of the face	Ask the client to raise eyebrows, smile, show teeth, puff out cheeks.
	Sensory	Sense of taste on the anterior two-thirds of the tongue	Test for the taste sensation with various agents.
Acoustic (VIII)	Sensory	Sense of hearing	Test hearing ability.
Glossopharyngeal (IX)	Motor	Pharyngeal movement and swallowing	Ask the client to say "ah," and have client yawn to observe upward movement of the soft palate; elicit gag response; note ability to swallow.
	Sensory	Sense of taste on the posterior one third of the tongue	Test for taste with various agents.
Vagus (X)	Motor	Swallowing and speaking	Ask the client to swallow and speak; note hoarseness.
Accessory (XI)	Motor	Movement of shoulder muscles	Ask the client to shrug shoulders against your resistance.
Hypoglossal (XII)	Motor	Movement of the tongue; strength of the tongue	Ask the client to protrude tongue; ask client to push tongue against cheek.

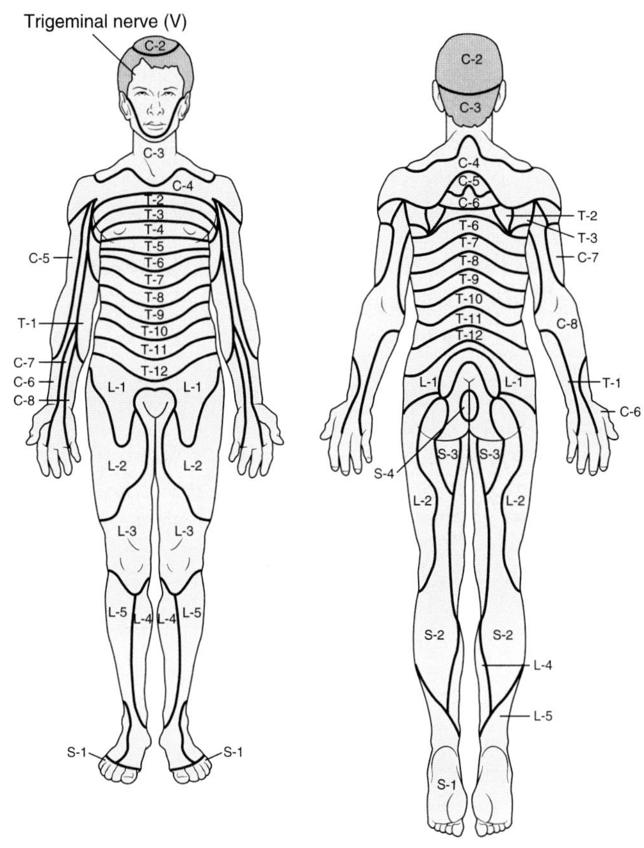

Figure 12-8 Spinal dermatomes.

Spinal Nerves

The spinal cord has 31 pairs of spinal nerves. Each nerve is attached to the spinal cord by a dorsal and a ventral root. The dorsal root carries the sensory impulses; the ventral root carries the motor impulses. Therefore, all spinal nerves are mixed nerves. The nerves are numbered by their exit between the vertebrae. The area served by each spinal nerve is referred to as a dermatome (Fig. 12-8).

12

AUTONOMIC NERVOUS SYSTEM

The autonomic nervous system is a specialized part of the PNS and works without conscious control. It regulates the action of the heart, certain glands, and the smooth muscle hollow organs. It is divided into two systems: **sympathetic** and **parasympathetic.** These systems work either to stimulate certain body functions or to reduce activity (Fig. 12-9).

Sympathetic System

The sympathetic system dominates in times of intense physical or mental stress, automatically producing cer-

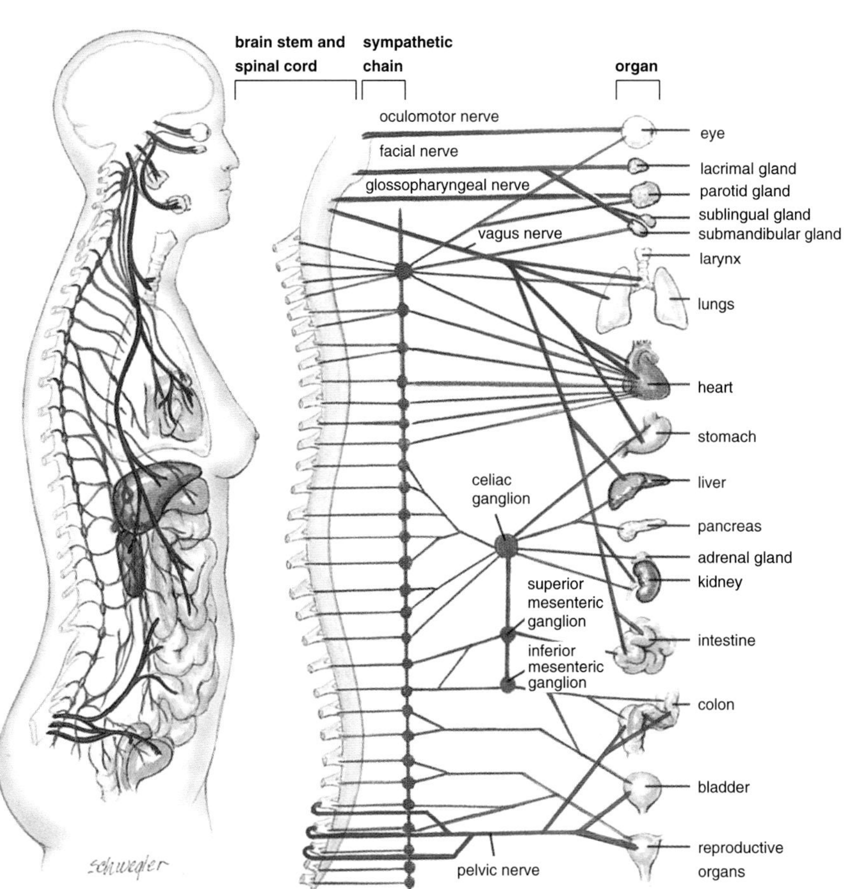

Figure 12-9 Autonomic nervous system (only one side is shown). The sympathetic system is shown in green; the parasympathetic system is shown in blue.

12

tain stimuli to the vital organs (ie, the "fright, flight, or fight response"). For example, the following responses help to ensure survival:

1. The adrenal glands are stimulated to produce epinephrine, or adrenaline, a hormone required for the response to stress.
2. Because the brain and muscles need more oxygen to respond to the emergency, the heart rate increases, and the force of each contraction becomes stronger. (This is due to the effect of epinephrine on the cardiovascular system.)
3. The bronchioles dilate in response to the epinephrine, and the respiratory rate increases to allow more oxygen into the lungs.
4. Blood pressure increases to speed blood to areas that must respond to the stressor.
5. Metabolism increases for extra glucose to supply energy for the crisis.
6. The pupils dilate, allowing more visual information to be gathered.
7. The gastrointestinal muscles and kidneys slow to conserve energy and shunt blood where it is most needed.
8. Sweat glands are stimulated to produce perspiration.
9. The blood vessels in the skin constrict to shunt blood away from the skin and to the vital organs.
10. The arrector pili muscles contract, pulling hair follicles upright and causing "goose bumps."

Parasympathetic System

In contrast to the sympathetic system, the parasympathetic system is involved with nonemergency automatic functions. Under normal circumstances or after the stress of a crisis, the following mechanisms take over:

1. The heart slows and the bronchioles constrict with the decreased physiologic need.
2. Saliva production increases and becomes thinner, allowing easier food digestion and nutrient absorption.
3. Blood flow increases to the stomach to aid digestion and nutrient absorption.
4. Kidneys resume urine production and excretion.

Table 12-2 compares body responses to a sympathetic and parasympathetic stimulus.

The sympathetic nerves are connected by a chain that makes it possible for a stimulus perceived by one receptor to connect instantly with all other functions of the system. This is a valuable survival reflex that in some instances allows us to begin our response to danger before our brains have fully processed the information needed for a reaction.

Unfortunately, our bodies are not always able to distinguish between some of our stressors and will initiate a sympathetic response to stressors such as an examination (physical or academic), a frustrating family or social situation, physical illness, and a multitude of minor stressors. Long-term overload of the sympathetic nervous system results in general exhaustion and a decreased immune response.

COMMON NERVOUS SYSTEM DISORDERS

The complexity of the nervous system makes it subject to many disorders. These disorders, which range from

Table 12-2 **Autonomic Nervous System—Body Response to Sympathetic and Parasympathetic Stimulus**

	Sympathetic Stimulus	*Parasympathetic Stimulus*
	Response	*Response*
Blood vessels to:		
Skeletal muscles	Dilation	Constriction
Skin	Constriction	No effect
Respiratory	Dilation	Constriction
Digestive tract	Constriction	Dilation
Pupils	Dilation	Constriction
Heart	Increased rate	Decreased rate
Bronchi (lungs)	Dilation	Constriction
Sweat glands	Stimulation	No effect
Kidneys	Decreased output	No effect
Liver	Glucose release	No effect
Adrenal medulla	Stimulation	No effect

minor inconveniences to lethal diseases, can be organized into the following groups: infectious, degenerative, convulsive (seizures), developmental, traumatic, neoplastic, and headaches.

Infectious Disorders

Meningitis

This disorder is characterized by inflammation of the meninges covering the spinal cord and the brain. It can result from either a bacterial or a viral infection. Viral meningitis is usually not life threatening and is short lived, but bacterial meningitis is often severe and may be fatal. The infectious process is usually precipitated by upper respiratory, sinus, or ear infections. Because these infections occur frequently in children, they are the most likely age group to develop meningitis. Meningitis also can result from head trauma in which an open area allows the organisms to enter the nervous system.

The patient with meningitis presents with a variety of symptoms, including nausea, vomiting, fever, headaches, and a stiff neck. The patient may complain of photophobia (intolerance to lights). A rash with small, reddish purple dots may appear. As patients become sicker, they may slip into a coma, and **seizures** (involuntary contractions of voluntary muscles) may occur.

To diagnose meningitis, the physician usually orders a complete blood count (see Chap. 30, Hematology). If the white blood cell count is high, a lumbar puncture (see below) is performed, and CSF is analyzed to determine the infectious organism. The treatment of meningitis is based on the organism. For viral meningitis, fluids and bed rest are encouraged. Bacterial meningitis is treated with antibiotics and requires hospitalization.

To identify other potential carriers, a thorough patient history is taken. The local health department must be notified of the diagnosis; some states require that an infectious disease form be completed. Depending on the type of meningitis, others who have had contact with the patient may be treated prophylactically.

Checkpoint Question

4. *How does the treatment of viral meningitis differ from that of bacterial meningitis?*

Encephalitis

Encephalitis is an inflammation of the brain. Frequently, it results from a viral infection that follows varicella (chickenpox), measles, or mumps. A strain of the virus is transmitted by mosquitoes. This type primarily is seen on the eastern and gulf coasts. Symptoms for all forms include drowsiness, headaches, and fever. Seizures and coma may occur in the later stages. Diagnosis is made through a lumbar puncture (see below) and analysis of CSF.

Treatment requires hospitalization for intravenous fluid therapy and supportive care. The prognosis is usually good if the diagnosis is made early and treatment begins quickly.

As with meningitis, the local health department should be notified to identify those who may have been exposed.

Poliomyelitis

Commonly called polio, this highly resistant virus affects the brain and spinal cord. It can live outside the body for several months, making it almost impossible to eliminate once it has appeared in a community. It is transmitted by direct contact and usually enters by the mouth. In the United States, its incidence has been greatly reduced as a result of aggressive immunization programs. However, because not all children have received the proper schedule of immunizations, and because some adults have not been immunized at all, concern about the disease still exists.

In the acute phase, the patient complains of a stiff neck, fever, headaches, and a sore throat. Nausea, vomiting, and diarrhea may also be noted. As the disease progresses, paralysis may develop. Muscle atrophy occurs, leading to eventual deformities. If the respiratory muscles are affected, the patient is unable to breathe without artificial assistance.

A new dimension to the disease, postpoliomyelitis muscular atrophy (PPMA) syndrome, has been documented in some individuals who had polio as children. These patients often present with symptoms similar to those that signaled the onset of the original disease. They usually complain of muscle weakness and a lack of coordination. Typically, patients with PPMA are treated on an outpatient basis with supportive care. There is no cure at this time.

During the acute stage of polio, treatment is palliative and supportive. After the primary illness has resolved, treatment is based on rehabilitation with a strong emphasis on physical and occupational therapy. To increase mobility, patients are fitted for mechanical supports (eg, braces and splints). Some patients may need to wear these devices indefinitely. Emotional support is important for these patients, particularly those with PPMA. They often require counseling to reconcile themselves to body image changes caused by the deformities and to allay fear of dependency and loss of autonomy.

Activities aimed at preventing polio are essential. As a medical assistant, you may be responsible for patient education regarding immunizations and the importance of keeping these current. (Polio immunizations are currently given at 2, 4, 6, and 15 months and repeated at 4–6 years of age.) The polio immunization is usually an oral weakened or attenuated vaccine. Persons on chemotherapy or steroidal therapy, transplant recipients, and those who are immunocompromised have been known to contract polio through contact with stools and saliva of recently immunized children. Therefore, children living with immunosuppressed individuals should receive a killed injectable form of the vaccine to avoid shedding the live, weakened virus through their digestive system.

Tetanus

This disorder, commonly called lockjaw, is an infection of nervous tissue caused by the tetanus bacilli *Clostridium tetani,* which live in the intestinal tract of animals and are excreted in their feces. The organisms are found in almost all soil. The bacilli enter the body through puncture wounds or open areas in the skin. Wounds caused by farm equipment in which manure is present are at very high risk for developing tetanus. All deep, dirty wounds should be treated as high risk for tetanus.

Tetanus has a very slow incubation period; it may be present in the body for up to 14 weeks before signs and symptoms occur. Initial symptoms include spasms of the voluntary muscles, restlessness, and stiff neck. As the disease progresses, seizures and **dysphagia** (difficulty swallowing) occur. The facial and oral muscles contract, leaving the mouth sealed with the teeth clenched tightly. The respiratory muscles become paralyzed. The disease is typically fatal.

Prevention is the best defense against tetanus. Wounds should be properly cleaned immediately. Dead tissue around the wound must be removed, and antibiotics should be given if the wound is contaminated with bacteria. Immunizations against tetanus are given prophylactically in infancy at 2, 4, 6, and 15 months, and repeated at age 4 to 6 years and every 10 years for life. If the infection is caused by an animal bite, and the tetanus immunizations are not current, tetanus immune globulin is given. Patients who develop tetanus require rapid hospitalization and aggressive antibiotic therapy with supportive care. The prognosis is guarded when tetanus has fully developed.

Rabies

Rabies is transmitted by infected animal saliva through a bite wound. Animals that most commonly transmit rabies are skunks, squirrels, raccoons, bats, dogs, cats, and foxes.

The incubation period for rabies ranges from 10 days to many months. Initial symptoms include fever, general malaise, and body aches. As the disease progresses, mental derangement, paralysis, and photophobia develop. The patient's saliva becomes extremely profuse and sticky, and the throat muscles begin to spasm, making swallowing difficult or impossible and causing profuse drooling. (The phrase "foaming at the mouth" has been used to describe this.) Muscle spasms of the throat occur at the sight of water, resulting in hydrophobia. If rabies reaches the brain, it is fatal.

Treatment for bite wounds must be aggressive. After the wound is cleaned, the patient should receive antibiotics and prophylactic vaccine therapy consisting of the human diploid cell vaccine and a rabies immune globulin vaccine.

All animal bites must be reported to the city or county animal control center. If possible, the animal should be quarantined and evaluated for behavioral changes. If the animal is domestic, a complete veterinary history must be obtained. A copy of the animal's rabies tag and certificate, if available, should be placed in the patient's chart.

Reye's Syndrome

This devastating nervous system illness is seen in children after a typical viral illness, most frequently varicella (chickenpox). Studies have found that the use of aspirin in combination with a viral illness increases the risk of developing Reye's syndrome. No other antifebrile agents have been implicated in this disorder.

Typical symptoms are vomiting and lethargy. A small red macular rash may occur. Later symptoms include seizures and coma. Diagnosis is made through a variety of blood testing.

Patients with Reye's syndrome require rapid hospitalization with aggressive antibiotic therapy and supportive care. The prognosis is good if the diagnosis is made early.

Degenerative Disorders

Multiple Sclerosis (MS)

In MS, the myelin sheaths degenerate and are replaced with plaques, which impair nerve impulse conduction. The cause of MS is unknown, although possible origins include a viral infection, autoimmunity, immunologic responses, or genetic predisposition.

Multiple sclerosis is more commonly seen in women between the ages of 20 and 40. The disease is characterized by remissions and exacerbations. The rate of progression varies greatly among patients.

Typically, patients present with complaints of progressive loss of muscle control. They may also complain of loss of balance, shaking tremors, and poor muscle coordination. Tingling and numbness can also be first signs. **Dysphasia** (difficulty speaking) may be another symptom. As the disease progresses, bladder dysfunction and complaints of visual disturbances are common. Patients may also develop nystagmus (involuntary rapid movement of the eyeball in all directions).

Treatment for MS is palliative. Physical therapy is critical to maintain mobility; its goal is to limit the extent of muscle deterioration and to promote existing muscle strength. As the disease progresses, the patient will be fitted for prosthetic appliances, such as crutches, to assist with ambulation. Drug therapy includes muscle relaxants and steroids.

A large part of caring for patients with MS involves providing psychological support. This disease affects persons in the "prime of life." Patients may have young children at home and so must struggle with emotional concerns regarding long-term welfare for the family. Eventually, sexual dysfunction occurs, and spouses may have difficulty dealing with this symptom. Many support groups and counselors specialize in providing therapy for persons affected by debilitating diseases; share this information with patients as appropriate.

Amyotrophic Lateral Sclerosis (ALS)

Commonly known as Lou Gehrig's disease, ALS causes the progressive loss of motor neurons. It is a terminal disease with no known etiology. There is a strong familial connection. Typically, ALS is seen most often in middle-aged men. It begins with loss of muscle mobility in the forearms, hands, and legs, then progresses to the facial muscles, causing dysphasia and dysphagia that worsen over time. Death usually occurs 3 to 5 years after the onset of symptoms.

Treatment of ALS involves instituting patient comfort measures and providing family education. As the disease progresses, it becomes increasingly difficult to maintain a patent airway. The family must be instructed in preventing and managing choking. Often, advance directives will be discussed with the family and patient.

Seizure Disorders

Seizures are involuntary contractions of voluntary muscles. (They are commonly called **convulsions** by the lay public.) Seizures have many causes, including chemical imbalances, trauma, pregnancy-induced hypertension, tumors, and withdrawal from drugs or alcohol. However, many seizures prove to be idiopathic (resulting from no known cause).

Epilepsy is the most common form of seizure disorder. The onset of epilepsy may appear in early childhood or at any life stage. Diagnosis is made through **electroencephalogram** (EEG) studies, blood tests, and radiologic tests.

Epileptic seizures are characterized as either petit mal or grand mal. Petit mal seizures, also called "ab-

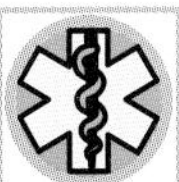

Action STAT!

Seizure Disorder

Scenario: Mrs. Rosa is waiting in the reception area to see the physician. She has a 10-year medical history of seizure disorder, which is currently being treated with phenytoin (Dilantin). Suddenly, she cries out to you. As you run to her, she begins to exhibit grand mal seizure (tonic-clonic) activity. What should you do?

1. Help Mrs. Rosa to the floor, and remove nearby objects (table, chairs, electrical cords) to help prevent injuries.
2. Call for the physician immediately, and have other staff members clear the room of other patients or screen the area from view.
3. Guard Mrs. Rosa's head and limbs from injury. Do not try to restrain her limbs, but protect them from striking nearby objects.
4. Do not put anything into Mrs. Rosa's mouth during the seizure. She will not "swallow her tongue," but her teeth may be broken or her airway obstructed if objects are forced into her mouth. Help her maintain a patent airway by using the head-tilt, chin-lift procedure.
5. Assist the physician as needed. In certain situations, medications may need to be administered to control the seizure.
6. Immediately postseizure, place Mrs. Rosa in the side-lying recovery position. Certain patients may vomit or may have trouble swallowing; the recovery position helps prevent aspiration.
7. Document the incident, including Mrs. Rosa's actions before, during, and after the seizure. Assess her vital signs and level of consciousness in the postseizure state. Be aware that incontinence may follow a seizure and will be very embarrassing for the patient. Provide for privacy as needed.

Note: The physician will decide if the patient requires transportation to the hospital. Patients with a long history of seizures may not be transferred to the hospital but may be evaluated in the office and have blood work done to check medication levels.

12

sence seizures" or "partial seizures," are briefer in duration than grand mal seizures and usually occur only in childhood. The child may appear to "fall asleep" or drift away momentarily. Some muscle twitching may occur. The child awakes and continues the interrupted activities without delay. Petit mal seizures may go undetected for many years.

Grand mal seizures or generalized tonic-clonic seizures, are more involved than petit mal seizures. Generally, the patient will go through three phases:

1. The first phase involves an aura or warning that a seizure is impending. The aura may include tingling in the extremities, visual signs (such as flashing lights), or perception of a particular taste or odor. Not all patients have auras, but those who do usually experience the same aural phenomena each time.
2. The second phase is the complete loss of consciousness with extensive muscle twitching or contractions, which may be violent. The patient falls to the ground and usually loses control of bladder and bowel functions.
3. The third phase is the postictal (postseizure) state. During this phase, the patient slowly regains consciousness but remains drowsy for an extended time.

The primary treatment during the actual seizure involves preventing injury to the patient. Epilepsy is treated with various pharmacologic agents. When providing patient teaching, instruct patients to take these medications every day as prescribed, never missing a dose. Many seizure patients who become stabilized and seizure free on medication feel they no longer need the medication. Remind these patients that stopping the medication may lead to the recurrence of seizures.

A patient who has seizures is allowed to have a driver's license; however, each state has specific regulations requiring that patients be seizure free for a particular length of time (eg, 2 years) to qualify.

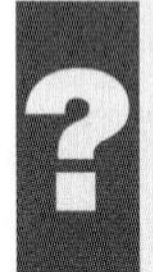

Checkpoint Question

5. *How do petit mal seizures differ from grand mal seizures? Describe the typical progression of a grand mal seizure.*

Febrile Seizures

These kinds of seizures occur in a small number of children, most commonly between the ages of 6 months and 3 years. Children suffering febrile seizures must have a complete physical and neurologic examination to rule out the possibility of an organic origin for the seizures. Children generally outgrow febrile seizures by age 6 or 7, with no other seizure activity after this time.

Treatment involves gently returning the body temperature to a more manageable level. Cool compresses are preferable to ice baths or alcohol sponges, which may cause hypothermia. To avoid Reye's syndrome, salicylates should not be given.

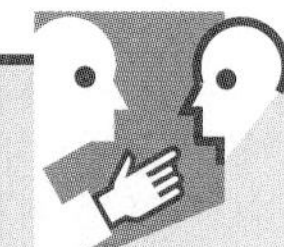

Advice and Tips

Coping With Febrile Seizures

Febrile seizures can be frightening for parents of small children. Here's how you can help parents cope:

- Reassure the parents that febrile seizures are common in young children and that they generally are not chronic in nature.
- Allow the parents to be involved in the care of the child. Once the child is stabilized, urge the parents to hold and comfort the child.
- Provide easy-to-understand explanations for all procedures.
- Encourage parents to verbalize their fears.

You, too, will probably be very anxious in this situation; however, you must remain calm and demonstrate confidence in handling the situation.

Focal (Jacksonian) Seizures

This type of seizure begins as a small localized seizure that spreads to adjacent areas. For instance, the small seizure may begin in the fingers and spread to the hand and arm. The cause of focal seizures must be researched to prevent the progression to generalized seizures.

Developmental Disorders

Neural Tube Defects

Many abnormalities may occur during the embryonic and fetal stages of development. As the neural tube develops in the embryo, it grows and expands as the embryo matures to the fetal stage. Tissue closes over the tube and evolves into the components of the CNS. If a developmental failure occurs on the proximal (upper) portion, anencephaly, or absence of a brain, results.

An abnormality in development in the distal, or caudal, end of the neural tube results in spina bifida. **Spina bifida occulta** is the most benign form. In this condition, the posterior laminae of the vertebrae fail to close, typically at L-5 or S-1. There are usually no external signs of a deformity; only a skin dimple or dark tufts of hair may be present. A **meningocele** occurs when the meninges protrude through the spina bifida. In spina bifida with **myelomeningocele,** the most severe form, the spinal cord and meninges protrude externally (Fig. 12-10). The main treatment is surgical intervention. Prognosis is based on the extent of spinal cord involvement.

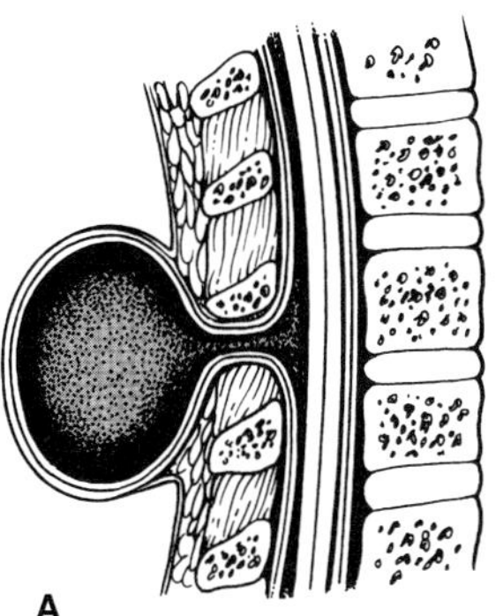
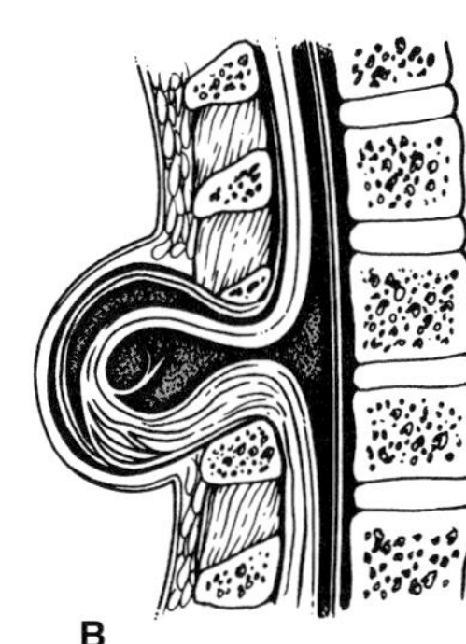

Figure 12-10 Types of spina bifida. (**A**) Meningocele. (**B**) Meningomyelocele.

Hydrocephalus

Hydrocephalus occurs when excessive CSF is present in the arachnoid and ventricular spaces of the brain. Although it occurs more commonly in children as the result of a defect in CSF production or absorption, hydrocephalus sometimes occurs in adults as a result of tumors or trauma. Treatment involves surgical insertion of a shunt, which reroutes the excessive CSF from the brain to the right atrium of the heart or the peritoneal cavity. The prognosis is usually good if treated aggressively in the early stages before CNS damage has occurred.

Cerebral Palsy

Cerebral palsy is the term used to describe a group of neuromuscular disorders that result from CNS damage sustained during the prenatal, neonatal, or postnatal periods. Although cerebral palsy is not progressive, the damage may become more obvious as developmental delays are discovered. Impairment may range from slight motor dysfunction to catastrophic physical and mental disabilities. Prognosis varies with the site of the damage and its severity. Treatment is supportive and rehabilitative. Currently, no cure exists.

Trauma

Traumatic injuries are the most common among the young to middle-age groups. Traumatic injuries are the number-one killer for individuals between ages 1 and 24.

Traumatic Brain Injuries

The pediatric population is particularly at risk for head trauma. A child's head is large in proportion to the rest of the body. Therefore, when children fall (as they do frequently), gravity pulls the head to the ground first. Children are also more prone to traumatic injuries because their reflex systems are immature.

Traumatic injuries to the brain include **concussions**, contusions, or intracranial hemorrhages. A concussion is a nonlethal brain injury that results from blunt trauma. The patient may experience a momentary loss of consciousness but returns to an awake and alert status promptly. A contusion is more serious and involves a focal alteration of cerebral circulation. Hemorrhages and extravasation of blood and fluid can result. Loss of consciousness results, and brain damage may occur. Intracranial hemorrhages involve the bleeding of a vessel inside the skull due to trauma, congenital abnormalities, or aneurysms. (See Chap. 15, Assisting With Diagnostic and Therapeutic Procedures Associated With the Cardiovascular System, for more information about aneurysms.)

Traumatic brain injuries are diagnosed through radiographic studies. Treatment for contusions and hemorrhages can involve surgery, drug therapy, and supportive care. The prognosis for all brain injuries depends on the extent of damage and the location of the injury.

Spinal Cord Injuries

Spinal cord injuries are most common among individuals 15 to 35 years of age. Most often, spinal cord injuries are due to trauma from motor vehicle accidents, diving accidents, or falls. Spinal cord injuries may be either complete, in which the cord is transected and no neurologic abilities remain below the point of injury, or incomplete, in which the cord is spared with minor to severe neurologic disabilities below the point of injury (Table 12-3). The higher in the spinal cord the in-

Table 12-3 **Spinal Cord Injuries**

Level of Injury	*Resulting Disabilities*
Cervical 1–2	Unable to breathe on own No neck muscle control
Cervical 3–4	May be able to manipulate electric wheelchair with mouth piece Some neck control possible
Cervical 5	Uses wheelchair with hand controls Self-feeds with hand splints Good elbow flexion
Cervical 6	Transfers to wheelchair and bed with little or no assistance Good shoulder control
Cervical 7	Transfers independently to wheelchair and bed Self-feeds with no special devices
Thoracic 1–4	Able to move from wheelchair to floor with little or no assistance Normal upper extremity function
Thoracic 5–Lumbar 2	Total wheelchair independence Limited ambulation with bilateral leg braces and crutches
Lumbar 3–4	Ambulation with short leg braces with or without crutches
Lumbar 5–Sacral 3	Able to ambulate on own with no equipment, if good foot strength is present

12

Table 12-4 **Types of Paralysis**

Type	*Causes*	*Result*
Hemiplegia	Cerebrovascular accident, trauma to one side of the brain, tumors	Paralysis on side of body opposite involvement
Paraplegia	Spinal cord trauma, spinal tumors	Paralysis of any part of the body below the point of involvement
Quadriplegia	Spinal cord trauma, spinal tumors	Paralysis of all limbs (usually cervical or high thoracic vertebra involvement)

jury is, the more serious the complications for the patient (Table 12-4). There is no cure at this time.

When caring for patients with spinal cord injuries, the initial consideration is to prevent further damage. Accident victims with suspected spinal cord injuries must be kept immobile until proper emergency medical services personnel are present. Treatment in the emergency department is focused on stabilization.

In the physician's office, patients in the post-trauma period receive follow-up treatment and evaluation. These patients are continuously monitored for changes in their reflexes and evaluated for physical therapy. The goal of long-term care is to prevent complications, which can include skin ulcerations (pressure ulcers), hypostatic pneumonia, bladder infections, contractures, and depression. Most of the physical complications are treated with physical therapy and good care; the mental and emotional complications require intensive therapy by counselors who specialize in treating patients with debilitating disorders.

Checkpoint Question

6. *How does a complete spinal cord injury differ from an incomplete one?*

Brain Tumors

Brain tumors may be either malignant or benign; many are secondary or metastatic sites. If the brain tumor is the primary site, it is named for the site of origin (eg, glioma, meningioma, medulloblastoma). Both malignant and benign tumors can produce serious complications for the patient because of the limited space inside the cranium.

Generally, the patient presents with vague complaints of headaches, blurred vision, personality changes, or memory loss. In more advanced cases, seizures, blindness, and dysphagia may be evident. The type of tumor and its location affect the presenting symptoms, their severity and onset, and the prognosis.

Diagnosis is made primarily through radiologic studies. The treatment can include surgery, radiation therapy, chemotherapy, or a combination of radiation and chemotherapy.

Headaches

It is estimated that 70% of the population experiences headaches. Headaches may have a variety of origins, including stress, trauma, bone pathology, infections (eg, sinus), or vascular disturbances. In many instances, the etiology will never be known.

Migraine headaches are one of the most common types of headaches. These can be triggered by stress, high altitudes, smoking, certain smells, or ingested chemicals (caffeine, alcohol, certain food additives), but in many situations the cause is unknown. Pa-

Patient Education

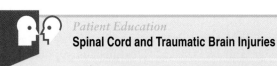

Spinal Cord and Traumatic Brain Injuries

Spinal cord and traumatic brain injuries are very common among young people. Both types of injuries can produce serious and even fatal results. As a medical assistant, you must take an active role in educating your community, patients, and friends about the prevention of these injuries. Education may include instructions such as:

- Use seat belts for all passengers.
- Secure infants and young children in approved car seats.
- Avoid alcohol when participating in sporting activities and driving.
- Obey traffic signs and speed limits.
- Avoid illicit drug use or any medication that impairs awareness.
- Wear helmets while bicycling and riding motorcycles.

tients who have migraines may complain of an aura before the onset. Symptoms usually include a unilateral temporal headache, photophobia, diplopia, and nausea. Generally, headaches are treated with analgesics, and the patient may be instructed to rest in a dark, quiet room. Propranolol (Inderal), ergotamine derivatives, and antidepressants have shown promise in headache prevention for patients with frequent, debilitating migraines. Sumatriptan succinate (Imitrex) is a specific drug therapy for migraines and is available in various dosage forms. Teaching a patient how to keep a headache diary can be an important part of therapy. The key to treatment is prevention; the diary will help the patient become aware of headache triggers.

Other common types of headaches include:

- *Tension headaches.* These are associated with contraction of the muscles of the neck and scalp due to stress. The treatment involves muscle relaxants, analgesics, and reversing the precipitating factors.
- *Cluster headaches.* These are similar to migraine headaches but typically occur at night. They are usually of short duration but may recur as often as four or five times a night for several weeks and then not again for weeks or months. They are associated with stress and tension. Treatment requires muscle relaxants, analgesics, and relieving the stressful situation.

COMMON DIAGNOSTIC PROCEDURES AND THE MEDICAL ASSISTANT'S ROLE

The physician may perform a variety of tests to evaluate a patient's neurologic status. These tests may be invasive or noninvasive and may include radiologic and electrical tests as well as physical examinations.

Physical Examination

The physical examination is a key component in diagnosing nervous system disorders and includes the following evaluations:

- Mental status and orientation
- Cranial nerve assessment
- Sensory and motor functions
- Reflex assessment

The patient's mental status is evaluated by routine questioning to establish mental alertness and orientation. For example, the examiner may ask the patient to count to 10 and to state the president's name and the current year.

Cranial nerves are assessed according to the methods discussed in Table 12-1. For example, visual acuity may be tested on a chart such as the Snellen eye chart.

Sensory function is tested with the pin versus soft brush method for spinal nerves and cranial nerves. The instrument commonly used is the Buck neurologic hammer (see Fig. 4-1 in Chap. 4, Physical Examination). With the patient's eyes closed, the physician uses the pin or brush to determine the patient's ability to distinguish between sensations. The physician evaluates sensory reception and determines if there is a reception difference on either side of the body.

Motor functioning is tested by watching the patient walk. Many disorders can be detected by observing a patient's gait. Part of this assessment will include the **Romberg test.** The patient is asked to stand with feet together and with eyes closed. A positive Romberg sign is noted if the patient sways or is unsteady.

The last part of the examination includes reflex testing (Table 12-5). Figure 12-11 depicts the correct method for tendon reflex testing. Reflexes are scored using this scale:

0—No response
1+—Diminished response

Table 12-5 **Reflex Testing**

Reflex	*Method of Testing*	*Expected Response*	*Localization*
Brachioradialis	Tapping the styloid process of radius	Flexion of elbow	C-5 and C-6
Biceps	Tapping biceps tendon	Flexion of elbow	C-5 and C-6
Triceps	Tapping triceps tendon	Extension of elbow	C-7
Patellar	Tapping patellar tendon	Extension of leg	L-2 and L-4
Achilles	Tapping Achilles tendon	Plantar flexion of foot	S-1
Corneal	Light touch on the corneoscleral corner	Closure of eyelid	Cranial nerves V and VII

C, cervical; L, lumbar; S, sacral

12

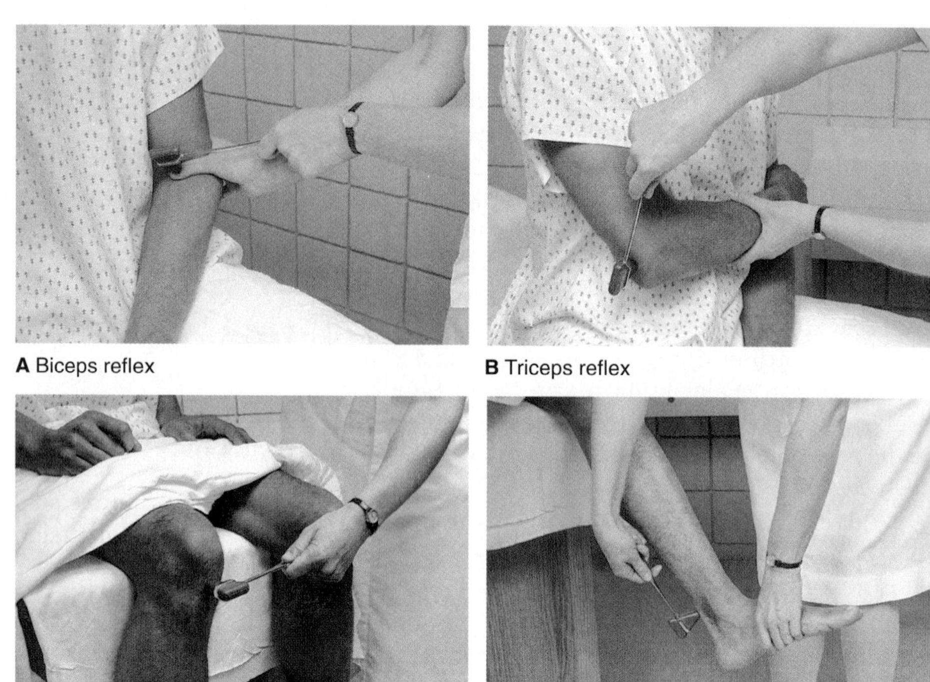

Figure 12-11 Techniques for eliciting major tendon reflexes.

2+—Normal
3+—Brisker than normal
4+—Hyperactive with clonus, which is the repetitive jerking of a muscle and indicates a neurologic disorder

Radiologic Tests

The most common examples of noninvasive radiologic tests include computed tomography scan and magnetic resonance imaging. These tests may also be done with a contrast medium or dye. The contrast medium helps differentiate between the soft tissue areas of the nervous system and the tumors, lesions, or hemorrhages that may blend in with their supporting tissues (see Chap. 24, Diagnostic Imaging).

A **myelogram** is an invasive form of radiologic test in which dye is injected into the CSF. The spinal cord is then filmed, and various abnormalities can be detected. The blood vessels of the brain can be visualized on x-ray by injecting a dye through a femoral artery catheter threaded up to the carotid artery in a test called a cerebral angiogram.

Radiography of the skull may be used to rule out many possible disorders and is diagnostic for fractures and malformations.

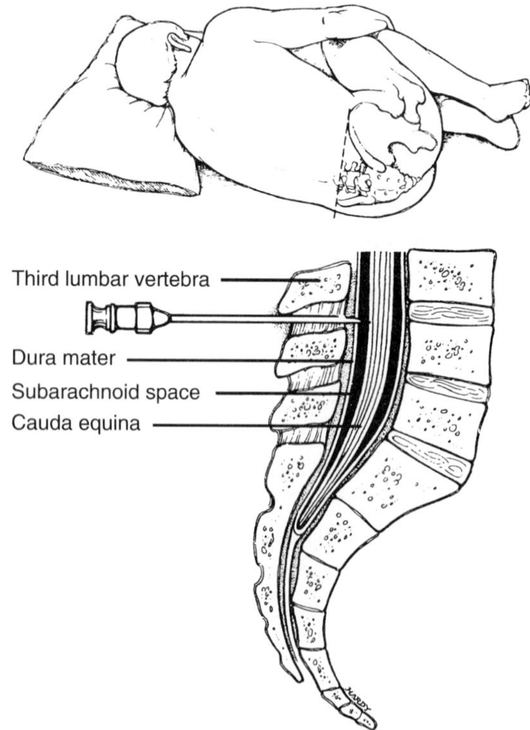

Figure 12-12 Technique for lumbar puncture. The interspaces between L-3 and L-5 and just below the line connecting the anterior-superior iliac spines.

Procedure 12-1 Assisting With a Lumbar Puncture

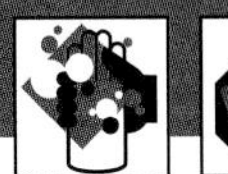

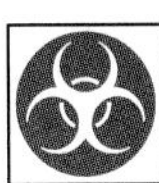

PURPOSE:

To obtain CSF specimen for analysis
To assess spinal fluid pressure readings

EQUIPMENT/SUPPLIES

On the sterile field

- 3–5-inch lumbar needle with a stylet (physician will specify gauge and length)
- gloves for the physician
- gauze sponges
- specimen tubes for transport
- spinal fluid manometer with a 3-way stopcock adapted (if CSF pressure is to be measured)
- fenestrated drape
- sterile drape
- antiseptic

On the side

- local anesthetic and syringe
- adhesive bandages
- sterile gloves (if not included on the field)
- examination gloves for the assistant
- skin preparation supplies
- blood pressure cuff (if Queckenstedt test is to be performed)
- completed lab slips for CSF

STEPS

1. Wash your hands.
2. Assemble the equipment. (Most offices stock the equipment in a purchased disposable tray or a site-prepared setup.)
3. Gather personal protective equipment (eg, gloves) as needed.
4. Identify the patient.
5. Check that the consent form is signed and posted on the chart.
6. Explain that the puncture will be made below the level of the spinal cord and should present no danger to the patient. Warn the patient not to move during the procedure. Tell the patient that the area will be numbed but that pressure may still be felt after the local anesthetic is administered.
   Although there is little chance of damage to the cord, movement may cause the patient injury and will probably contaminate the field.
7. Have the patient void.
   This will decrease the level of discomfort during the procedure.
8. Direct the patient to disrobe and put on a gown with the opening in the back.
   The back must be exposed for the procedure.
9. Determine and record the vital signs.
   Initial vital signs provide a baseline for comparison at completion of the procedure.
10. When the physician is ready, open the field (follow the steps described in Procedure 6-1, Opening Sterile Surgical Packs, in Chap. 6, Assisting With Minor Office Surgery), and assist with the initial preparations.
11. Prepare the skin if this is not done as part of the sterile preparation. Many physicians prefer to prepare the skin using a sterile forceps after gloving. If this is the preferred procedure, you may be required to add sterile solutions to the field (follow the steps in Procedure 6-3, Adding Sterile Solution to a Sterile Field in Chap. 6, Assisting With Minor Office Surgery).
12. Assist as needed with administration of the anesthetic.
13. Assist the patient into the appropriate position.
    For the side-lying position:
    - Stand in front and help by holding the knees and top shoulder. Have the patient move so the back is close to the edge of the table.

    For the forward-leaning, supported position:
    - Stand in front and rest your hands on the patient's shoulders as a reminder to remain still. Have the patient breathe slowly and deeply.

    These positions widen the space between the vertebrae to allow entrance of the needle. Your presence will help ensure that there is no movement during the procedure.
14. Throughout the procedure, observe the patient closely for signs such as dyspnea or cyanosis. Monitor the pulse at intervals.
15. When the physician has the needle securely in place, help the patient to straighten slightly to ease tension and to allow a more normal CSF flow. The physician may now use the stopcock and spinal fluid manometer to determine the intracranial pressure.
16. If specimens are to be taken, assist as follows:
    a. Put on gloves to receive the potentially hazardous body fluid.
    b. As you receive the tubes, label them in sequence and with the patient's identification.
    c. Place the tubes in biohazard specimen bags.

    Note: The first tube may be more likely to contain contaminants.

continued

12

Procedure 12-1 Continued Assisting With a Lumbar Puncture

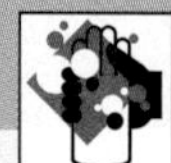
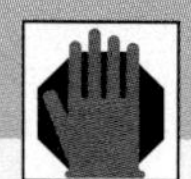

17. If the Queckenstedt test is to be performed, assist as follows:
    Method one:
    - Press the veins of the patient's neck with your hands, first the right, then the left, then both sides, each for 10 seconds, while the physician measures the pressure with the stopcock and manometer.

    Method two:
    - Before gloving for the procedure, the physician will place a blood pressure cuff around the patient's neck. According to the physician's instructions, inflate the cuff to 22 mmHg for 10 seconds while the physician measures the pressure with the manometer.

      The Queckenstedt test helps determine the presence of an obstruction in the CSF flow. Normally, the pressure rises and drops dramatically during the procedure. If an obstruction is present, the rise and return to normal may be very slow, or there may be no response to the external application of pressure.
18. At the completion of the procedure, perform these measures:
    a. Cover the site with an adhesive bandage.
    b. Assist the patient to a supine position.
    c. Record the patient's vital signs. Note mental alertness, any leakage at the site, nausea, and vomiting. Assess lower limb mobility. *Note:* The physician will determine when the patient is ready to leave the examining room and the office.

       Many patients experience severe headaches after the procedure and must be monitored during the recovery period.
19. Route the specimens as required.
20. Clean the room and care for or dispose of the equipment as needed. Wash your hands.

DOCUMENTATION GUIDELINES

- Date and time
- Vital signs before and after procedure; include the temperature, particularly if the procedure is for a fever of unknown origin
- Patient's tolerance of the procedure, complaints/concerns
- Patient education/instructions
- Your signature

Charting Example

DATE	TIME Pt positioned and draped for
	lumbar puncture. BP 120/80, P-86, R-18.
	Dr. Alexander performed LP.
	0900 LP completed. Pt tolerated
	procedure well. CSF sent to the lab.
	PostLP vitals: 114/74, P-76, R-16.
	Pt resting comfortably.
	0930 Pt denies discomfort. No n/v.
	No leakage at LP site. Pt and wife were
	given d/c instructions. Verbalized
	understanding. Pt d/c by Dr. Alexander.
	—Your signature

Note: Before beginning, assess the lumbar region. If the site is very hairy, it may be necessary to shave the skin before the procedure. (Follow the steps for skin preparation and hair removal in Procedure 6-4 in Chap. 6, Assisting With Minor Office Surgery.) Strict asepsis must be observed to reduce the risk of introducing microorganisms into the nervous system.

Electrical Tests

An EEG is a noninvasive test that records electrical impulses in the brain. A variety of electrodes are placed on the patient's scalp and tracings of brain wave activity are recorded. Typically, the patient is given a mild sedative to induce a quiet state.

Checkpoint Question

7. *What are the differences between a myelogram and an EEG?*

Lumbar Puncture

A lumbar puncture is used to diagnose infectious, inflammatory, or bleeding disorders. A needle is inserted into the subarachnoid space at the level of L-4 to L-5, below the level of the spinal cord (Fig. 12-12). CSF is removed and may be tested for glucose, protein, bacteria, cell counts, and the presence of red blood cells to indicate intracranial bleeding. It may also be evaluated to determine intracranial pressure. In addition, the presence of an obstruction in the CSF flow can be determined through the **Queckenstedt test.**

If a lumbar puncture is performed in the medical office, the medical assistant's responsibility includes assisting the patient into a side-lying, curled position or a supported, forward-bending sitting position. These are difficult and uncomfortable positions to maintain. You may help the patient to relax in these positions by encouraging slow, deep breathing. Procedure 12-1 describes the steps for assisting the physician with a lumbar puncture.

Patients may rest lying flat for 6 to 12 hours after a lumbar puncture and may require intravenous fluids and pain medications for the severe headaches that are often experienced. For these reasons, the lumbar puncture is more commonly performed in outpatient clinics than in the medical office.

Prenatal Screening

Great strides have been made in diagnosing fetal abnormalities early in gestation. During the first trimester, a procedure called chorionic villus sampling may be performed to detect chromosomal abnormalities. In this test, a small tissue sample is taken from the embryonic implantation site for analysis.

At 16 to 18 weeks of gestation, a routine blood test for **alpha-fetoprotein** (AFP) is done to assess development of the neural tube, which will evolve into the brain and spinal cord. AFP is a substance produced by the embryonic yolk sac and later by the fetal liver. Elevated AFP levels *may* indicate nervous system deformities. Falsely elevated samples can be caused by more than one fetus or incorrect gestational dates. A positive AFP result is often followed by an **amniocentesis.** In this invasive procedure, a needle is inserted through the abdomen into the gravid uterus to remove fluid from the amniotic sac. The fluid is analyzed for a variety of nervous system and sex-linked disorders.

An ultrasound allows the physician to see the brain and spinal cord of the developing fetus. Many CNS disorders can be detected by this method, including spina bifida and anencephaly.

What If?

You are working in an obstetrician's office and have been asked to draw a blood sample from a pregnant patient to test for AFP. What if the patient seems anxious about the test?

Allow the patient to voice any concerns and encourage her to ask questions about the test. Explain that AFP is a test to determine abnormalities of the CNS in the developing fetus. If the test results are positive, an amniocentesis likely will be performed to obtain additional information.

Pediatric Tests

The nervous system is immature at birth. Cortical function develops slowly and cannot be completely tested until early childhood. During regular visits to the pediatrician, the infant is tested for infantile automatisms—reflexes found in the newborn that disappear later in childhood. Examples include the Moro (or startle) reflex and the rooting reflex (see Chap. 22, Pediatric Patients). The absence of infantile automatisms, or the continuation of these reflexes beyond infancy, suggests potential CNS dysfunction and requires further testing.

Specific gross and fine motor coordination can be tested from birth through childhood by the Denver Developmental Screening Tests (DDST), which evaluate motor, sensory, and language development and social skills. DDST are usually performed at routine intervals throughout early childhood at well-child visits. The DDST do not measure intelligence levels.

Answers to Checkpoint Questions

1. *Communication between two neurons occurs when a message released by one axon jumps across the synapse to the next dendrite.*
2. *The frontal lobe is responsible for motor functions, reasoning, thinking, and speech. The parietal lobe is responsible for touch, pain, temperature, and interpretation of spatial concepts. The temporal lobe is responsible for interpreting sounds and smells. The occipital lobe is responsible for interpreting visual stimuli.*
3. *The specific function of each cranial nerve is as follows:*
   I. Olfactory—sensory—sense of smell
   II. Optic—sensory—vision
   III. Oculomotor—motor—eye muscles
   IV. Trochlear—motor—eye muscles

V. *Trigeminal—mixed—facial sensations, jaw muscles*
VI. *Abducens—motor—eye movements*
VII. *Facial—motor—expressions, sense of taste*
VIII. *Acoustic—sensory—hearing and balance*
IX. *Glossopharyngeal—mixed—taste, swallowing, salivation*
X. *Vagus—mixed—visceral functions and respirations*
XI. *Accessory—motor—neck and shoulder muscles*
XII. *Hypoglossal—motor—tongue movements*

4. *For viral meningitis, fluids and bed rest are encouraged. For bacterial meningitis, antibiotics are prescribed, and hospitalization may be required.*

5. *Petit mal or absence seizures are briefer in duration than grand mal seizures and usually occur only in childhood. Grand mal or generalized tonic-clonic seizures are more involved than petit mal seizures and encompass three phases. The first phase involves an* aura, *or warning that a seizure is impending. The second phase is the complete loss of consciousness. During the third phase, the* postictal state, *the patient slowly regains consciousness.*

6. *A complete spinal cord injury involves total transection of the spinal cord; no neurologic abilities remain below the point of injury. An incomplete spinal cord injury is one in which the cord is spared, with minor to severe neurologic disabilities below the point of injury.*

7. *An EEG is a noninvasive, electrical test of brain waves. A myelogram is an invasive, radiologic test in which dye is injected into the CSF to help detect abnormalities.*

Critical Thinking Challenges

1. Your patient has a spinal cord injury below C-5. Describe the functions of the spinal nerves above and below that point of injury. Explain what symptoms this patient might experience.
2. A 3-year-old girl comes into the office with varicella zoster (chickenpox). She has a fever, and the physician orders acetaminophen. The child's mother asks, "Why can't she have aspirin instead?" How would you respond?

Suggestions for Further Reading

Adams, R. D., & Victor, M. (1993). *Principles of Neurology,* 5th ed. New York: McGraw-Hill.

Bullock, B. L., & Rosendahl, P. P. (1996). *Pathophysiology,* 4th ed. Philadelphia: Lippincott-Raven.

Craven, R. F., & Hirnle, C. J. (1996). *Fundamentals of Nursing,* 2nd ed. Philadelphia: Lippincott-Raven.

Greenberg, D. A., Aminoff, M. J., & Simon, R. P. (1993). *Clinical Neurology,* 2nd ed. East Norwalk, CT: Appleton & Lange.

Memmler, R. L., Cohen, B. J., & Wood, D. L. (1996). *Structure and Function of the Human Body,* 6th ed. Philadelphia: Lippincott-Raven.

Memmler, R. L., Cohen, B. J., & Wood, D. (1996). *The Human Body in Health and Disease,* 8th ed. Philadelphia: Lippincott-Raven.

Porth, C. M. (1998). *Pathophysiology: Concepts of Altered Health States,* 5th ed. Philadelphia: Lippincott-Raven.

Professional Guide to Diseases, 4th ed. (1992). Springhouse, PA: Springhouse.

Rosdahl, C. B. (1995). *Textbook of Basic Nursing,* 6th ed. Philadelphia: J.B. Lippincott.

13

Assisting With Diagnostic and Therapeutic Procedures Associated With the Sensory System

Chapter Outline

Role Delineation

CLINICAL

Fundamental Principles

- Apply principles of aseptic technique and infection control.

Diagnostic Orders

- Collect and process specimens.

Patient Care

- Prepare patients for examinations, procedures, and treatments.
- Assist with examinations, procedures, and treatments.
- Prepare and administer medications and immunizations.

GENERAL

Professionalism

- Project a professional manner and image.
- Work as a team member.
- Prioritize and perform multiple tasks.

Communication Skills

- Treat all patients with compassion and empathy.
- Adapt communications to individual's ability to understand.

Legal Concepts

- Practice within the scope of education, training, and personal capabilities.
- Document accurately.

Instruction

- Instruct individuals according to their needs.
- Teach methods of health promotion and disease prevention.

Chapter Competencies

Learning Objectives

Upon successfully completing this chapter, you will be able to:

1. Spell and define the Key Terms.
2. Locate and describe the anatomic structures of eye, ear, and nose.
3. Describe the function of the organs associated with each structure.
4. List and define several diseases associated with the eye, ear, and nose.
5. Identify common diagnostic procedures associated with the eye, ear, and nose.
6. Describe patient education procedures associated with the eye, ear, and nose.
7. Identify other senses and give their importance in assessing patient wellness.

Performance Objectives

Upon successfully completing this chapter, you will be able to:

1. Prepare a diagnostic set for use in the examination of the eye, ear, and nose (Procedure 13-1).
2. Measure distance visual acuity with a Snellen chart (Procedure 13-2).
3. Measure close (or near) visual acuity with a Jaeger chart (Procedure 13-3).
4. Measure color perception with an Ishihara color book (Procedure 13-4).
5. Assist with tonometry.
6. Instill eye medication (Procedure 13-5).
7. Irrigate the eye (Procedure 13-6).
8. Assist with corneal lavage (Procedure 13-7).
9. Remove a foreign object from the eye (Procedure 13-8).
10. Perform audiometry (Procedure 13-9).
11. Irrigate the ear (Procedure 13-10).
12. Instill ear medication (Procedure 13-11).
13. Instill nasal medication (Procedure 13-12).

Key Terms

(See Glossary for definitions.)

adnexa
astigmatism
cerumen
decibel (db)
hyperopia
intraocular pressure
myopia
ophthalmologist
ophthalmoscope
optician
optometrist
otoscope
presbyopia
refract, refraction
retinal degeneration
tactile
tinnitus
upper respiratory infection (URI)

The sensory organs maintain our contact with the environment. They add richness and pleasure to our lives and warn us of danger. The main external senses include sight, hearing, taste, smell, and touch. The various stimuli are transmitted by the afferent nerves to their designated destinations in the brain for interpretation.

THE EYE

Basic Structure and Function

The eye is the organ of sight. The right and left eyes individually imprint an image on the optic center of the brain located in the occipital area. These singular images are then combined into one overlapping image by the brain to provide three-dimensional sight.

Approximately five-sixths of the eyeball fits into a bony orbit, by which it is protected. The eyeball is hollow and consists of three layers: the scleral–corneal layer, the choroid layer, and the retina (Fig. 13-1).

13

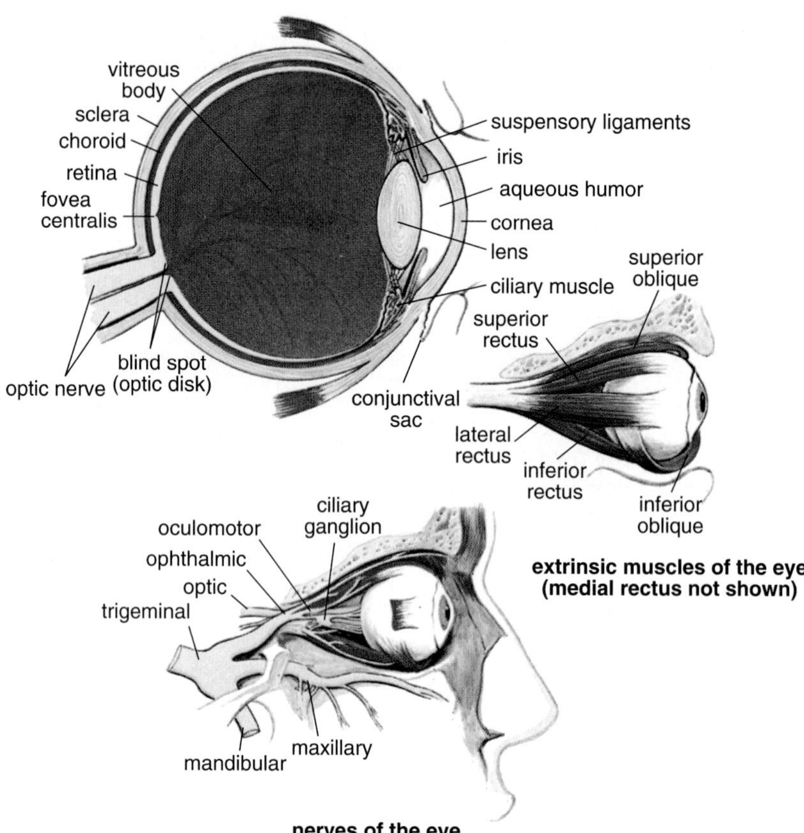

Figure 13-1 The eye.

The sclera, also known as the "white of the eye," makes up the majority of the outer cover of the eye and is connected to the cornea to form the fibrous tunic of the eye. The cornea is transparent and covers the iris and pupil. It has a greater curvature than the sclera to **refract** (bend) the light as it enters. Both the sclera and cornea are very sensitive and vascular and are covered with a mucous membrane called the conjunctiva that continues to the edges of the lids. What we see in a normal opened eye is the anterior one-sixth of the eyeball.

Between the scleral–corneal layer and the retina lies the choroid layer. This middle layer is highly vascular and extends to the ciliary body, which controls the shape of the lens. The lens lies directly behind the iris and changes shape to assist in the focusing process. The iris is the pigmented section of the eyeball. It contains a black center known as the pupil, actually just an empty space, which regulates the amount of light allowed to enter the eye. The iris is a smooth muscle that adjusts automatically to control the amount of light reflected onto the retina. The vascularity of the choroid layer makes it dark, like the lining of a camera, to absorb rather than reflect the entering light.

The retina, the innermost layer of the eye, functions primarily to form images. The rods and cones are nerve cells contained in the retina. Rods are responsible for shadings of light and dark but form no clear images. Cones are for color reception and require bright light. Cones record the colors red, blue, and green. Variations of colors are registered when the cones perceive bits of color on more than one receptor. For instance, violet may be recorded in part on the red receptors and on the blue receptors, then perceived by the brain as a combination of both colors.

The rods and cones are most concentrated in the fovea centralis, a small depression with great sensitivity exactly at the posterior of the eye opposite the lens. All receptive nerve fibers and vessels enter and exit just medial of the fovea at the optic disk, also known as the blind spot. The disk has no receptors of its own.

There are two main chambers containing fluid within the eye. *Aqueous humor* is a liquid similar to cerebrospinal fluid and is formed from the blood that circulates through the eye. This fluid passes back and forth through the pupil anterior to the lens to maintain the curvature of the sclera and to nourish the structure of the anterior eye. It drains from there back into the bloodstream through the canal of Schlemm. The **intraocular pressure** (pressure within the eyeball) is produced mainly by the aqueous humor.

Vitreous humor, a jelly-like substance, fills the large chamber behind the lens. Vitreous humor maintains the shape of the eye and helps with image refraction. This fluid also is produced by special cells within the eye from plasma fluid and is returned to general circulation as needed to maintain a homeostatic intraocular environment.

The optic nerve transmits impulses from the rods and cones to the brain's visual centers located in the cerebral cortex.

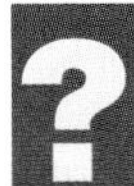

Checkpoint Question

1. *Where are the rods and cones located and what are their functions?*

The Adnexa

In addition to the eye itself, visual accessory structures (**adnexa**) include the lids, the lashes, and the lacrimal apparatus. The lids blink reflexively and are a protective device. Normally the blink reflex is triggered about 25 times a minute. Blinking increases with the need for moisture from tears.

The lacrima helps keep the conjunctivae moist as tears wash across from the excretory gland at the upper, outer rim of the bony orbit. Tears flow across the eye as the lids blink and deliver them to the puncti in the inner canthus (corner) of the upper and lower lids. The puncti drain into the lacrimal canaliculi, then to the lacrimal sac, then into the nasolacrimal ducts, and empty into the nasal passages through the turbinates. If the lacrimal glands produce more tears than the apparatus can channel away, the tears are shed onto the cheeks. Tears are salty and are slightly bactericidal as a protection against microorganisms. Figure 13-2 shows the lacrimal apparatus.

Musculature

The eye requires the intrinsic (inside) muscles to change the shape of the lens for refraction and the pupil for the entrance of light. This is controlled by the autonomic nervous system.

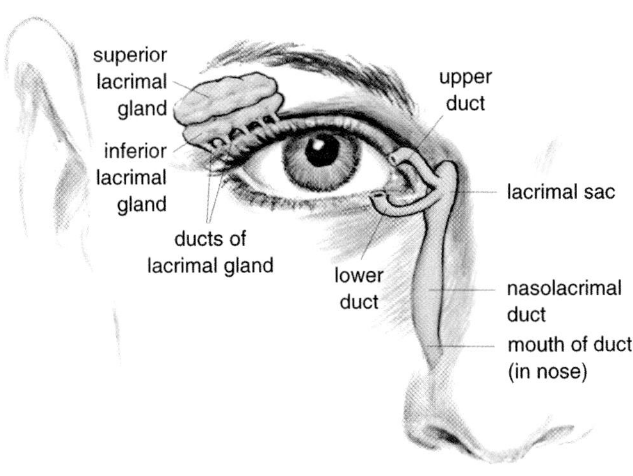

Figure 13-2 Lacrimal apparatus.

The extrinsic (outside) muscles are responsible for eye movement and must coordinate movements in the field of vision. There are six muscles per eye, and each is responsible for moving the eye into position very quickly. The initial movement to fix on an object is voluntary, then the involuntary focusing takes over on command of the optic center to define the image.

Paralysis or dysfunction of any of the intrinsic or extrinsic muscles causes focus to be poor and may result in diplopia (double vision) with an eventual loss of vision.

13

Process of Sight

Light waves are given off by all objects and are transmitted through the cornea, aqueous humor, lens, vitreous humor, and to the retina, then through the optic nerve to the occipital lobe of the cerebral cortex. The rays are bent, or refracted, by the curvature of the cornea and lens to reduce the image to a fine point on the fovea centralis. If the object is out of focus to the occiput, efferent impulses change the shape of the lens or the position of the extrinsic muscles to sharpen the image.

Common Disorders

The eye is a complex, highly developed organ. Any of its many components may malfunction or be the object of infection or disease. A few of the many eye disorders that you may encounter in the medical office are described below.

Cataract

A cataract is an opacity of the lens that leads to a decrease in visual acuity. Cataracts are usually bilateral and are more commonly seen in the elderly. Some infants are born with congenital cataracts, sometimes as a result of first-trimester maternal rubella. Occasionally, trauma to the lens or chemical toxicity causes clouding of the lens.

The symptoms are a gradual blurring and loss of vision. A sign for the observer is a milky opacity at the pupil rather than the normal black opening. Ophthalmoscopy reveals the white area behind the pupil if it is not fully advanced enough to be seen by the observer without diagnostic aids.

Surgery is beneficial in 95% of the patients and is usually an outpatient procedure. The opaque lens is removed by any of several effective methods, such as emulsification or capsular extraction. In some cases, an intraocular lens is implanted where the lens has been removed; in other instances the vision is corrected by contact lenses or special glasses.

Sty or Hordeolum

A sty or hordeolum is a staphylococcal infection of any of the glands of the eyelids, particularly the oil-producing follicles that contain the lashes. Patients present with redness, swelling, and pain. Warm compresses will hasten suppuration; topical drops or ointments attack the microorganism. You may be responsible for teaching the patient the procedure for applying warm compresses and instilling drops or ointment.

Conjunctivitis

Conjunctivitis is a common infectious disease of the conjunctiva caused by several forms of bacteria, Chlamydia, or viruses. It also may be caused by allergens or irritants without an infectious process. Many of the pathogens cause unilateral conjunctivitis; allergic conjunctivitis almost always is bilateral.

Signs and symptoms include tearing and occasionally exudate and pain. Bacterial conjunctivitis, or "pink eye," is highly contagious and spreads through schools and day-care centers quickly. It is spread by contact as the host child rubs the itching eyes, handles toys and books, and passes them and the disease to the next child who comes in contact with the pathogen. Treatment must address the specific pathogen. The patient, parents, and day care providers must be taught good hygiene to prevent the spread of the disease.

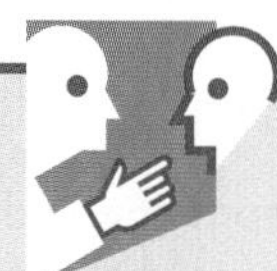

Advice and Tips

Assisting the Sight-Impaired Patient

Follow these tips to assist a sight-impaired patient.

- Ask the patient how you can help, and follow the patient's requests and suggestions. Many sight-impaired patients know best what they need.
- When escorting the patient, offer your arm. Tell the patient the approximate length of the hallway and advise the patient of any turns (eg, *"It should be about 20 steps and then we'll take a right"*). Avoid steps if possible, but if you must assist a sight-impaired patient up or down stairs, advise the individual of the number of steps. Many patients prefer to hold the railings for balance.
- If the patient has a guide dog, do not approach the dog without first speaking to the patient and receiving approval.
- If the patient needs extensive teaching on a particular subject, suggest using a tape recorder to record the instructions.

Checkpoint Question

2. *What is the difference between a sty and conjunctivitis?*

Corneal Ulcers and Abrasions

A corneal ulcer is the eroding away of the corneal surface, leaving scar tissue that may lead to visual disturbances or blindness. Corneal abrasions are scratches to the cornea that may or may not lead to visual disturbances. Corneal ulcers are caused by several types of bacteria, fungi, viruses, and protozoa or by trauma, allergens, or toxins. Signs and symptoms include tearing, pain on blinking, and sensitivity to light. A visual examination with a penlight will show an irregular corneal surface. A fluorescein dye will stain the perimeter of the lesion to confirm the diagnosis. Treatment includes rest to the eyeball and antibiotic therapy.

Retinopathy

Retinopathy refers to any disease or disorder affecting the retina. A decrease in the blood supply to the highly vascular retina will cause **retinal degeneration,** pathologic changes in the cell structure that impair or destroy the retina's function. The causes include atherosclerosis that impedes the blood flow to the retina, the microcirculatory changes associated with diabetes or sickling disease, or vascular changes from long-term hypertension. Depending on the cause, the loss of vision may be sudden or gradual. The loss of vision may be preceded by small intraocular hemorrhages, night blindness, or loss of central visual fields. If small vessels rupture and scar, they may pull against the retina and cause retinal detachment. Treatment depends on the cause. Some forms of retinopathy respond well to treatments; others progress to full blindness.

Glaucoma

Glaucoma is actually a group of disorders that results in increased intraocular pressure. As aqueous humor is formed in the chamber just in front of the lens, it flows through the pupil to the anterior portion of the chamber, just behind the cornea. It eventually is filtered into the canal of Schlemm and is returned to the general circulation. Any pathology that impedes the outflow of aqueous humor will cause the pressure to increase, either very gradually or quite suddenly. The gradual form may present with mild pain, halos around lights, and loss of peripheral vision (Fig. 13-3). The acute form presents with pain and inflammation, eye pressure, and even nausea and vomiting. Blindness may result within days of the onset of acute glaucoma.

Treatment for chronic glaucoma includes parasympathomimetics or diuretics. Acute glaucoma may require an iridectomy to remove part of the iris to increase the outflow of the humor.

Refractive Errors

These comprise the most common of all eye problems, resulting in either hyperopia, myopia, astigmatism, or presbyopia.

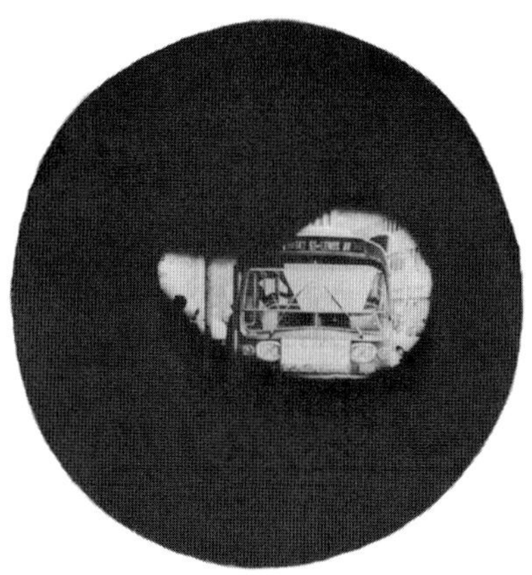

Figure 13-3 Glaucoma. Advanced glaucoma involves loss of peripheral vision, but the individual still retains most of his central vision.

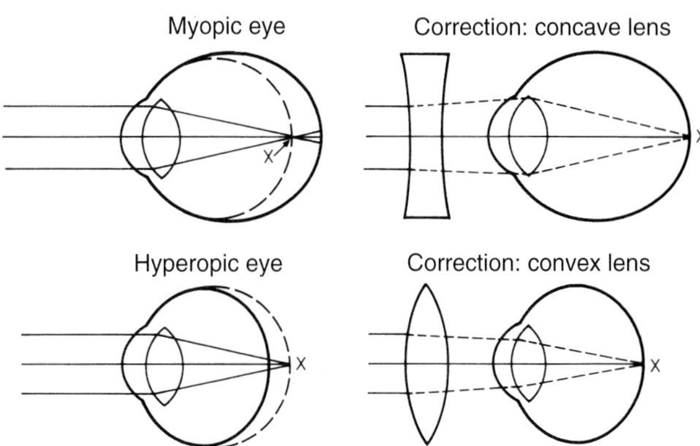

Figure 13-4 The myopic eye with concave corrective lens. The hyperopic eye with convex corrective lens.

13

Hyperopia, also known as farsightedness, is the result of an eyeball that is too short from front to back to allow the lines of vision to reflect distinctly on the fovea centralis. Objects must be held far from the face to focus the image on the retina.

Myopia, also known as nearsightedness, results when the eyeball is too long. The lines of vision converge before they reach the fovea centralis and begin to diverge again at the fovea. Objects must be held close to the face to focus the image far back on to the retina.

Astigmatism is unfocused refraction of light rays on the retina. It results from lens or corneal irregularities. If the cornea is not smooth, images refracted through it will not project sharply onto the retina but will look much like peering through wavy glass.

Presbyopia refers to vision changes resulting from age. It does not involve the length of the eyeball but is the result of loss of lens elasticity. The lens must be made to adjust thicker or thinner to refract light from near or far on to the retina. As the eye grows older, the ciliary bodies that hold and adjust the lens and the lens themselves all lose youthful elasticity and will no longer accommodate near vision; far vision may be unaffected. Symptoms usually begin gradually around age 40. Most adults are affected to some degree by age 50.

All refractive errors are treated with corrective lenses (Fig. 13-4). An **optometrist** is a trained specialist who can measure for errors of refraction and prescribe lenses. An **optician** is a trained specialist who grinds lenses to fit refraction corrective lens prescriptions written by either an optometrist or an **ophthalmologist,** a medical doctor who treats eye disorders.

Checkpoint Question

3. *List four common refractive errors. Briefly explain each.*

Strabismus

Strabismus is a misalignment of the eye movements, usually caused by muscle incoordination. Strabismus may be:

- Esotropic (also known as cross eye or convergent)
- Exotropic (also known as wall eye or divergent)
- Hypotropic (deviation downward)
- Hypertropic (deviation upward)

Strabismus may be concomitant if both eyes move together or nonconcomitant if they move independently. Treatment depends on the cause and may only require patching, or covering, the good eye to require the affected eye muscles to strengthen. In some cases, surgery may be required to correct the deviant muscle.

Color Deficit

Color deficit is an absence of or defect in color perception. Red, green, or blue perception or any combination of colors may be impaired or absent. The term color deficient or color deficit is commonly used rather than referring to the disorder as a type of blindness.

The disorder is usually inherited on the X chromosome and affects more men than women. Occasionally, chemically induced color deficit results from damage to the cones due to medications or other substances that are toxic to the color receptive nerve cells. Color deficit has no cure or correction.

Dacryocystitis

Dacryocystitis refers to an infection of the tear sac. In adults, dacryocystitis usually results from an obstruction of the nasolacrimal duct. Infants may present with an atresia (closing off) or an infection. Because the duct is closed, the normal flow of tears cannot drain into the puncta and through to the nose, causing constant tearing. The area may be swollen and tender; a purulent discharge from the puncta may develop.

Cultures are ordered if infection is suspected. Treatment includes palliative soaks and local or systemic antibiotics. If atresia is the cause, dilation or probing may open the sac.

Common Diagnostic Studies and Therapeutic Procedures and the Medical Assistant's Role

Almost all offices use **ophthalmoscopes** and **otoscopes.** An ophthalmoscope is a lighted instrument used to examine the inner surfaces of the eye (Fig. 13-5). It often is referred to as the "eye to the heart" of the patient. In many instances its use can alert the physician to a number of vascular and prehypertensive conditions and to many intraocular conditions. It is an important part of the everyday "diagnostic set" used in the office. The otoscope, an instrument used to examine the ear, is another part of the diagnostic set. Otoscopes have probe covers, which may be reusable or disposable.

Commonly, the base of the diagnostic set is one instrument, which houses a rechargeable battery with interchangeable heads (Fig. 13-6). Some offices are equipped with electrical, wall-mounted instruments. Procedure 13-1 describes preparation of the diagnostic set for use by the physician.

Visual Acuity Testing

Far vision is tested using the Snellen chart or any other of the far vision testing devices available. These charts are hung 20 feet away from the patient at eye level in an area with good lighting and few distractions (Procedure 13-2). Normal vision (20/20) means that the patient can read at 20 feet what the normal eye should see from that distance.

The figures on the chart—letters, numbers, or a series of Es—are progressively smaller to test levels of perception. For patients who cannot read or who are not English-speaking, an "E" chart, also called the tumbling E chart, may be used. A picture chart is often used for children (Fig. 13-7).

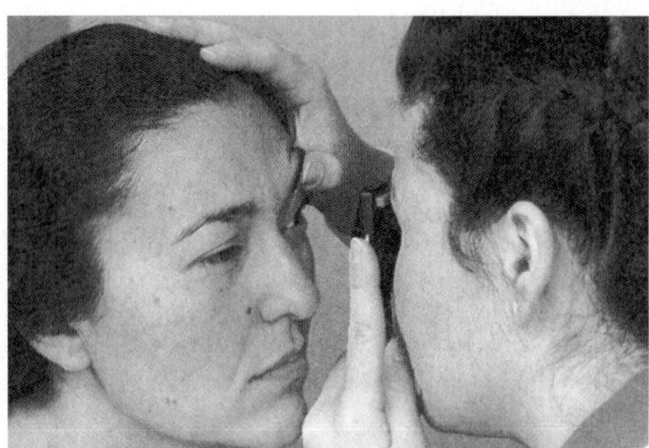

Figure 13-5 Ophthalmic examination.

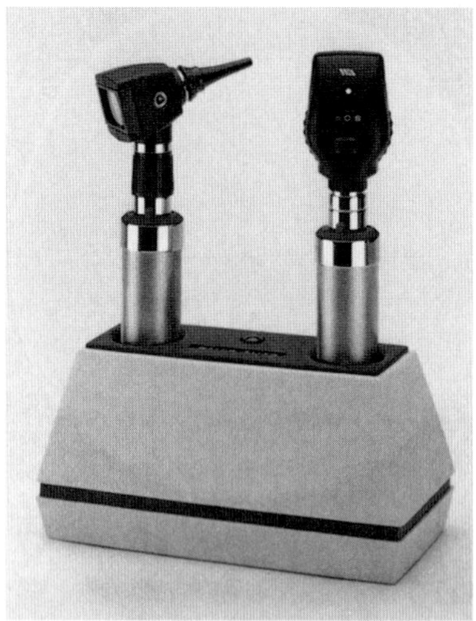

Figure 13-6 The diagnostic set includes an ophthalmoscope and an otoscope in a recharging base. The heads are interchangeable. Many physicians use one base and change heads as needed. The pictured otoscope has a reuseable speculum cover in place. (Courtesy of Welch Allyn.)

If a child is to be tested, spend a few moments familiarizing the child with the objects pictured on the chart. Some children may have no point of reference for some of the objects. For example, if the picture is of a Collie dog and the child has never seen one, the illustration may not be recognized as a dog. Children frequently are tested at 10 feet rather than at 20 feet because they do not focus well at distances and are easily distracted within the line of vision. Enlist a parent or coworker to help with the eye cover.

Near vision is tested by using the Jaeger system. The Jaeger is a series of ever smaller lines to test at what point the patient can no longer discern the letters. Rather than checking for the ability to distinguish objects at a distance, the Jaeger tests for difficulties at a near reading level. The Jaeger is usually used for patients over age 40 and suspected of presbyopia or for those with hyperopia. The steps are described in Procedure 13-3.

Checkpoint Question

4. *When is the tumbling E chart used to test visual acuity?*

Color Perception

The Ishihara method is used to test for color perception (Procedure 13-4). It consists of a series of color plates with many four-colored dots forming a number, a letter, or a pattern of contrasting color within the

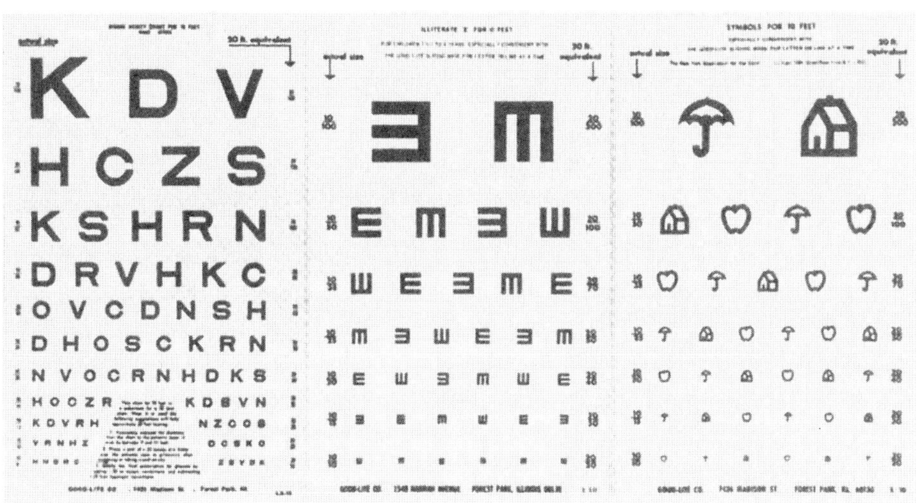

Figure 13-7 These are various Snellen charts used to test distant vision. The charts in the center and at far right are used for very young children and non-reading adults.

arrangement of dots (Fig. 13-8). Patients with deficient color perception will be unable to find the design within the plates.

Tonometry

Using a tonometer, such as the Schiotz or the applanation, the physician measures tension or pressure within a site—in this case, intraocular pressure. The anterior eye is anesthetized with drops, and the instrument is moved against the cornea to measure how much pressure is required to produce an indentation (tonometer) or to flatten a small area of the cornea (applanation) (Fig. 13-9).

Gonioscopy

Using the gonioscope, the physician measures the angle formed by the anterior chamber of the eye between the iris and the cornea. This method is used to diagnose the cause of glaucoma.

Instilling Eye Medications

The medical assistant frequently has the responsibility of instilling ophthalmic medications in the office and educating the patient about the procedure for home use. Instillations treat infection or irritation, dilate the pupil for retinal examination, and apply anesthetic for treatment or testing (Procedure 13-5).

Other Ophthalmic Procedures

To remove exudates and debris and relieve inflammation, eye irrigations are performed (Procedure 13-6). This procedure may be performed by the medical assistant using a syringe system or by the physician using a corneal lavage kit (Procedure 13-7). Sometimes, foreign objects lodge in the eye. The physician must remove objects that are embedded, but the medical assistant can remove loose debris (Procedure 13-8).

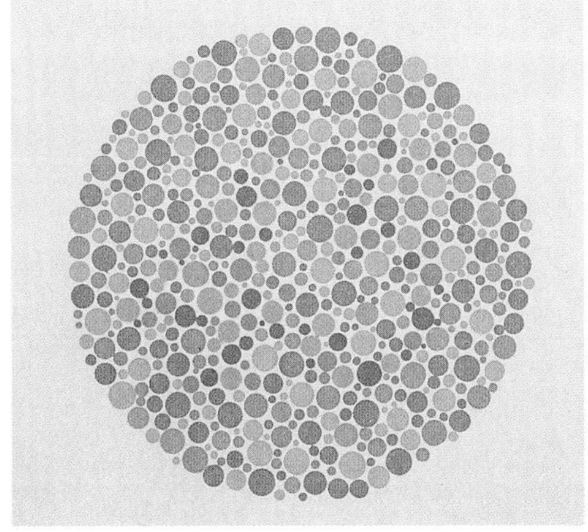

Figure 13-8 Ishihara color plate. (© B. Proud.)

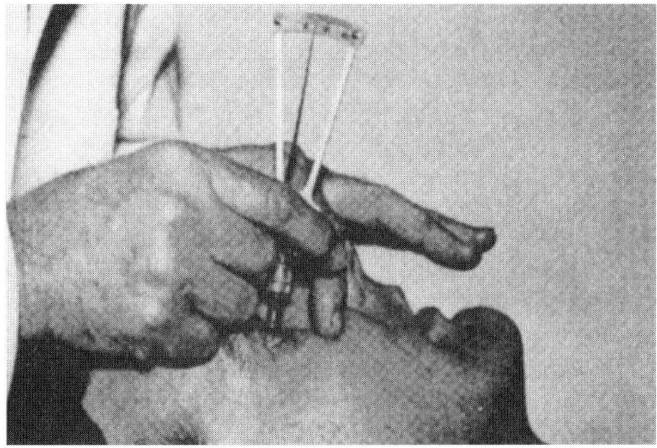

Figure 13-9 Tonometry. After a local anesthetic is instilled into the eye, the Schiotz tonometer is gently rested on the eyeball. The indicator measures the ocular tension in millimeters of mercury. (Courtesy of F. H. Rofy, M.D.)

13

Procedure 13-1 Preparing the Diagnostic Set

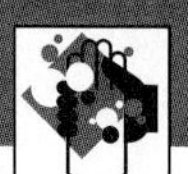

PURPOSE:

To ensure that all equipment is in operative order for the assessment of the eye and ear

EQUIPMENT/SUPPLIES

- an operative otoscope, ophthalmoscope, and tongue blade holder (optional)
- power source, such as an electrical charger or fresh battery

STEPS

1. Wash your hands.
2. Assemble the equipment.
3. Check to determine that the lights in the instrument are functioning by illuminating them.
   Function should be established before performing the procedure.
4. Place and remove the otoscope, ophthalmoscope, and illuminated tongue blade holder, if used, to check the readiness of each. Press firmly and twist to place or remove the head. The small red button at the connection is held down as the rim is rotated to keep the light on. Reverse the procedure to turn it off.
   Each item must be checked for function.
5. Place tongue blades and disposable ear specula on a covered tray for the physician's use.
   Items should be close at hand for the physician before the examination.
6. Have extra light bulbs available for replacement during the examination if needed.
   The examination cannot be completed if a light source is not available.

THE EAR

Basic Structure and Function

The ear is the organ of hearing. It is divided into three sections: external ear, middle ear, and inner ear (Fig. 13-10). The inner ear also functions to maintain balance.

The pinna or auricle also is known as the external ear. It is made of cartilage and is shaped to collect and channel sound waves through the auditory canal to the eardrum, or tympanic membrane. The lining of the auditory canal is made of modified sweat glands that are referred to as ceruminous glands. Earwax, or **cerumen,** is a protective mechanism for the ear.

The tympanic membrane separates the external and middle ear sections. The middle ear contains three

text continues on page 304

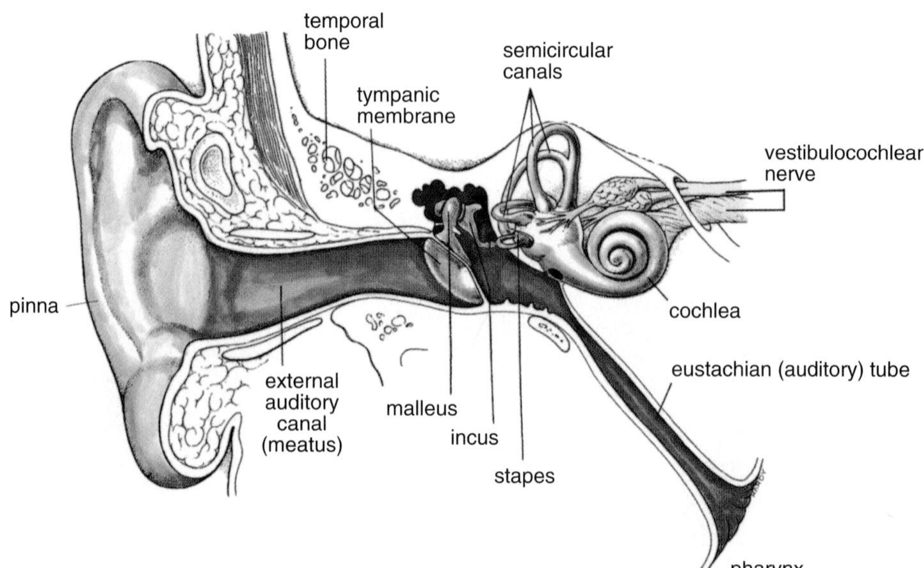

Figure 13-10 The ear, showing the external, middle, and internal subdivisions. (Chaffee, E. E., & Lytle, I. M. *Basic Physiology and Anatomy.* 4th ed., p 227. Philadelphia: J.B. Lippincott. [1980])

Procedure 13-2 Measuring Distance Visual Acuity

PURPOSE:

To assess the presence or degree of refraction errors in far vision

EQUIPMENT/SUPPLIES

- eye chart
- paper cup or eye paddle

STEPS

1. Wash your hands.

2. Prepare the examination room. Make sure the area is well lighted. A distance marker should be measured 20 feet from the chart; the chart must be at eye level.

The room must be well lighted to elicit the best response. All visual acuity tests require a distance of 20 feet for consistency of results.

3. Greet and identify the patient. Explain the procedure.

4. Position the patient in a standing or sitting position at the 20-foot marker.

The patient may stand or sit, if necessary, as long as the chart is at eye level, and the patient is 20 feet from the chart.

5. Ask if the patient wears glasses or contact lenses. Mark the record accordingly.

Office policy will state whether examinations will include corrective lenses. The patient record should indicate if the patient wore corrective lenses for the test.

6. Have the patient cover the left eye with the eye paddle. Instruct the patient to keep both eyes open.

The testing routinely starts with the left eye covered for consistency in testing. The eyes must be covered alternately by an opaque object. The hand may not be used to avoid pressure against the eye or peeking through the fingers. Squinting to close one eye changes the vision.

7. Stand beside the chart and point to each row as the patient reads aloud the indicated lines, starting with the 20/200 line.

It is generally best to start at about the second or third row to judge the patient's response. If these lines are read easily, move down to smaller figures. If the patient has trouble reading the larger lines, the physician should be notified.

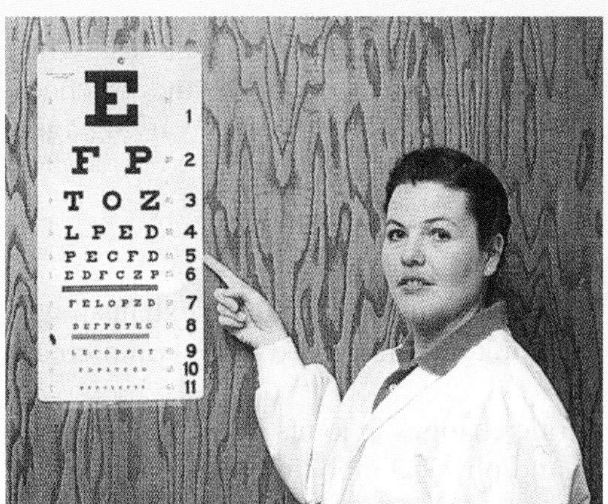

8. Record the smallest line the patient can read error free and note as OD (ocularis dexter). The numbers are listed on the side of the chart. For instance, if the patient reads line five (or the line marked 40) with one error for the right eye, record as OD 20/40−1. Your physician may prefer that only those lines read without error be counted as correct.

9. Repeat the procedure with the right eye covered and record as in step 8, using OS (ocularis sinistra). If the patient squints or leans forward, record this observation on the patient record.

10. Wash your hands.

DOCUMENTATION GUIDELINES

- Date and time
- Patient complaints/concerns
- Observations of patient during testing (include with or without visual aids)
- Test results—OD, OS, OU (ocularis unis)
- Your signature

Charting Example

DATE	TIME Pt arrived in the office c/o
	occasional blurred vision in the left eye.
	Pt does not wear eyeglasses. Last eye
	exam was 5 years ago. Visual acuity:
	OD 20/60−1, OS 20/40−2, OU 20/50.
	Pt squinting throughout procedure.
	—Your signature

13

Procedure 13-3 Measuring Near Visual Acuity

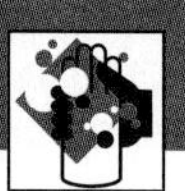

PURPOSE:

To assess the presence and degree of refraction errors in the near vision field

EQUIPMENT/SUPPLIES

- Jaeger near visual acuity testing card
- paper cup or eye paddle

STEPS

1. Wash your hands.
2. Assemble the equipment.
3. Greet and identify the patient. Explain the procedure. Ask for and answer any questions.
4. Hold the card containing lines of text or pictures of Es to be evaluated about 14 to 16 inches from the patient's face at a comfortable reading level.
   This distance provides a normal reading range for testing.
5. Start by covering the patient's left eye.
   Starting with the right eye ensures consistency of testing.
6. Record the last line read with no errors.
7. Repeat the procedure to test the left eye.
   Following this protocol continues to ensure consistency of testing.

DOCUMENTATION GUIDELINES

- Date and time
- Patient complaints/concerns
- Observations of patient during assessment, include with or without visual aids
- Jaeger results
- Your signature

Charting Example

DATE	TIME Pt c/o gradual onset of blurred
	near vision. States she holds objects
	at arm's length to focus. Does not wear
	glasses. Jaeger exam revealed last line
	read with no errors = #7 OD, #6 OS.
	—Your signature

Procedure 13-4 Measuring Color Perception

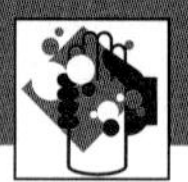
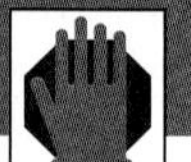

PURPOSE:

To assess the proper functioning of the color receptors (cones)
To assess the presence and degree of color perception deficit

EQUIPMENT/SUPPLIES

- Ishihara color plates
- gloves

STEPS

1. Wash your hands and put on gloves.
   Gloves in this case are not for the protection of the patient or worker, but for the protection of the color plates. Oils from the hands can cause the colors to deteriorate and interfere with testing.
2. Identify the patient, and explain the procedure by the first plate. Hold the plate about 30 inches from the patient.
   The first plate should be obvious to all patients and serves as an example.
3. Ensure that the patient is in a comfortable sitting position in a quiet, well lighted room. Indirect sunlight gives the best illumination. (Sunlight should not shine against the plates; the colors fade with bright lights.)
4. Be aware that patients who wear glasses or contact lenses may keep them on.
   The Ishihara is testing color acuity, not visual acuity. Corrective lenses will not interfere with accurate test results.
5. Follow directions on the chart with the right eye, then the left eye.
6. Record the results of the test by noting what the patient reports as being seen on each plate, using the plate number and the answer given by the patient. If the patient cannot distinguish the pattern, record as Plate #3 = X. It is not necessary to record those read correctly. Record any squinting or tearing or any hesitation or guesses indicating that the patient was not sure of what was being perceived.

continued

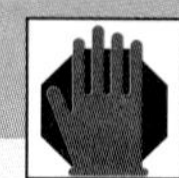

7. Store the book in a closed, protected area in its protective jacket to protect the integrity of the colors.

DOCUMENTATION GUIDELINES

- Date and time
- Observations of patient during testing
- Results of testing
- Your signature

Charting Example

DATE	TIME Color perception measured by
	Ishihara method. Pt stated he under-
	stood the procedure and successfully
	identified Plate #1. Pt identified all plates
	except Plate #9 = X. Dr. Barker notified.
	—Your signature

Procedure 13-5 Instilling Eye Medications

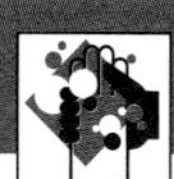

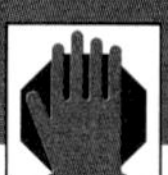

PURPOSE:

To provide medication by the route most appropriate for the optimum response
To treat infection or inflammation or to prepare for testing

EQUIPMENT/SUPPLIES

- physician's order
- medication
- sterile gauze
- tissues

STEPS

1. Wash your hands and put on gloves.
2. Obtain the physician's order, the correct medication (check the label three times as directed in Chap. 8, Preparing and Administering Medications), and all needed supplies.

   The medication must specify ophthalmic use. Medications formulated for other uses may be harmful if used in the eye.
3. Greet and identify the patient. Explain the procedure. Ask the patient about allergies not recorded in the chart.
4. Position the patient comfortably.

   The patient may be lying or sitting with the head tilted slightly back and positioned with the affected eye slightly downward to avoid the medication running into the unaffected eye.
5. Pull down the lower eyelid with sterile gauze and have the patient look upward.

   Pulling down the lower lid exposes the conjunctival sac to receive the medication. If the patient is looking up and away from the medication, the blink reflex may not be triggered.
6. Instill the medication.

   a. *Ointment:* Discard the first bead of ointment. Place a thin line of ointment across the inside of the lower eyelid, moving from the inner canthus outward. Release the line of ointment by twisting slightly. Do not touch the tube to the eye.

      The first bead is considered contaminated. Placing the ointment into the sac avoids touching the eye with the tip of the ointment tube. Twisting the tube releases the line of ointment.

   b. *Drops:* Hold the dropper close to the conjunctival sac (about ½ inch away), but do not touch the patient. Release the proper number of drops into the sac. Discard any medication left in the dropper.

      Discarding the remaining medication avoids contaminating the remainder of a multiple dose container.

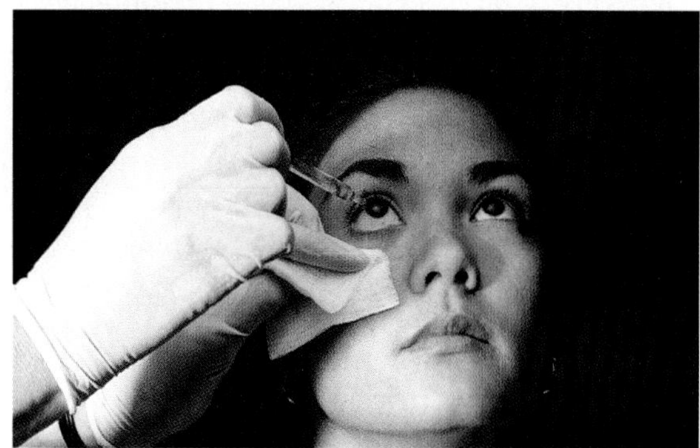

continued

Procedure 13-5 Continued **Instilling Eye Medications**

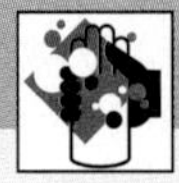
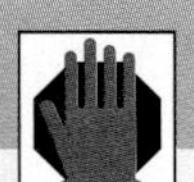

7. Have the patient gently close the eyelid and roll the eye to disperse the medication.
8. Wipe away any excess medication with the tissue. Instruct the patient to apply light pressure on the puncta for several minutes.

   Pressing the puncta prevents the medication from running to the nasolacrimal sac and duct.
9. Properly care for or dispose of equipment and supplies. Clean the work area. Wash your hands.

DOCUMENTATION GUIDELINES

- Date and time
- Patient complaints/concerns
- Medication (include type, ie, drops, ointment)
- Dose
- Location (which eye, ie, OD, OS, OU)
- Patient education/instructions
- Your signature

Charting Example

DATE	TIME Dr. Howser ordered Cortisporin
	eye drops to OD. Pt has NKA. Cortisporin
	2 gtt administered into OD. Pt instructed
	to close lids and roll eye to disperse
	medication. Pt educated in proper
	procedure for instilling eye medication.
	Pt verbalized understanding.
	—Your signature

Procedure 13-6 **Irrigating the Eye**

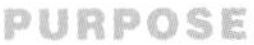

PURPOSE:

To remove foreign objects
To provide relief of symptoms

EQUIPMENT/SUPPLIES

- small sterile basin
- towels
- emesis basin
- sterile irrigating solution at about 100°F
- sterile syringe
- tissues

STEPS

1. Wash your hands.
2. Assemble the equipment and supplies. Check the solution label three times as recommended for medication administration. Make sure the preparation is for ophthalmic purposes. *Note:* If both eyes are to be treated, use separate equipment for each to avoid cross-contamination.

   Solutions used for the eye must be sterile, must be formulated for ophthalmic use, and should be just above body temperature to avoid patient discomfort.
3. Greet and identify the patient. Explain the procedure.
4. Position the patient comfortably, either sitting with head tilted with the affected eye downward or lying with the affected eye downward.

   With the affected eye downward, there is less chance of contamination running into the unaffected eye.
5. Drape the patient with a protective barrier to avoid wetting the clothing.
6. Have the patient hold the emesis basin against the upper cheek near the eye with the towel under the basin. Glove now. With clean gauze, wipe from the inner canthus outward to remove debris from the lashes.

   Gloves must be worn to prevent exposure to body fluid. Debris from the lashes might be washed into the eye.
7. Separate the lids with the thumb and forefinger of the nondominant hand. The dominant hand holding the syringe with solution may be lightly supported on the bridge of the patient's nose parallel to the eye to steady the hand.

continued

Procedure 13-6 *Continued* Irrigating the Eye

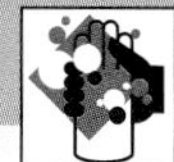
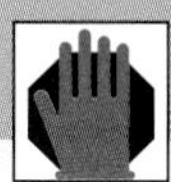

8. Gently irrigate from the inner to the outer canthus, holding the syringe 1 inch above the eye. Use gentle pressure and do not touch the eye. The physician will order the period of time required for the irrigation.

   The solution must flow across from the inner to the outer canthus to avoid washing pathogens into the puncta. With the syringe 1 inch above the eye there is little chance of touching the eye and causing patient discomfort.

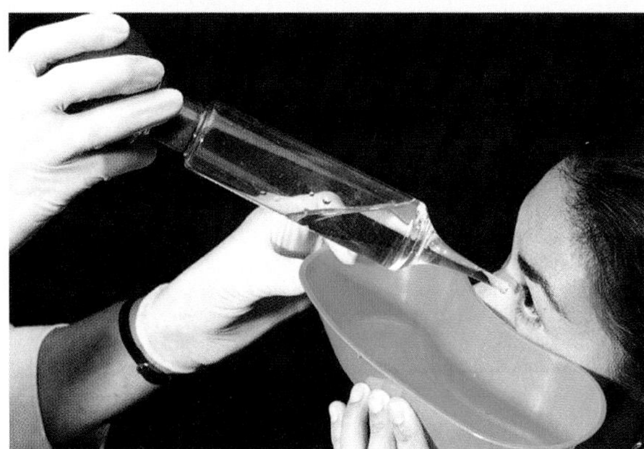

9. Use tissue to wipe away any excess solution from the patient's face.
10. Properly dispose of equipment or sanitize as recommended and remove the gloves. Wash your hands.

DOCUMENTATION GUIDELINES

- Date and time
- Medication or type of solution
- Amount of irrigation (optional for situation)
- Length of time of irrigation
- Which eye (OD, OS, OU)
- Patient complaints/concerns
- Patient education/instructions
- Your signature

Charting Example

DATE	TIME
	S: "I got some laundry detergent in my
	eyes about 45 minutes ago."
	O: 22-year-old woman. Both eyes appear
	red and teary. Dr. Burns in to see pt.
	Eye irrigation ordered.
	A: Chemical irritation both eyes.
	P: 1. Both eyes irrigated with 1000 mL
	normal saline. Tolerated procedure well
	2. Preventive education instructions
	given to pt. Pt verbalized
	understanding. —Your signature

Note: Eye irrigations can be performed using a Morgan lens, which consists of a plastic applicator that is placed directly on the eyeball (similar to a contact lens). An attachment to the lens connects to an irrigating solution, which runs in and irrigates the eye. One advantage to the system is that it prevents blinking during irrigation. Before using a Morgan lens, carefully read the manufacturer's instructions.

Procedure 13-7 Assisting With Corneal Lavage

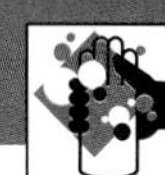
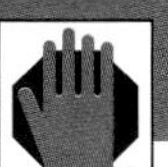

PURPOSE:

To remove foreign substances from the eye
To ensure that medication is delivered to the cornea and conjunctiva in the most efficient manner

EQUIPMENT/SUPPLIES

- corneal lavage equipment (Morgan Lens, prescribed solution, fluid management system to receive outflow)
- topical ophthalmic anesthetic
- sterile gloves

STEPS

1. Wash your hands.
2. Assemble equipment.
3. Greet and identify the patient. Explain the procedure. Ask about known allergies.

   Allergies may exist that are not noted on the chart.

4. Help to position the patient, generally in a supine position with the affected eye downward.

   This position prevents excess solution running into unaffected eye.

continued

Procedure 13-7 Continued Assisting With Corneal Lavage

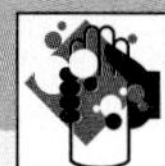
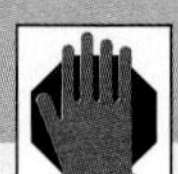

13

5. Assist the physician as needed to administer the anesthetic drops.
   a. Attach the irrigating solution to the lens apparatus.

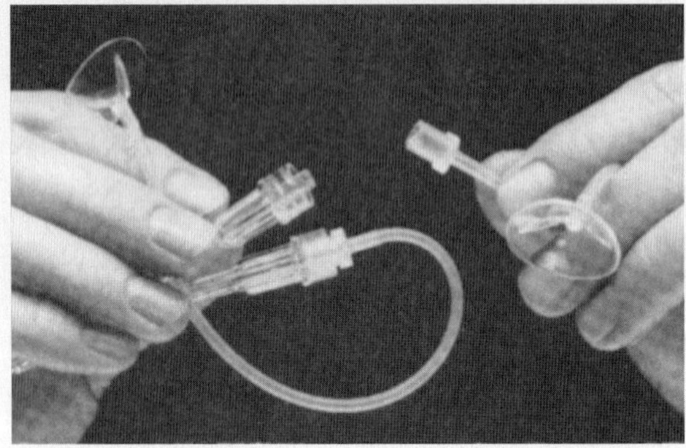

   b. Adjust the flow as the physician inserts the lens into the conjunctival sac.
      Anesthetic drops alleviate pain and permit the lens to be placed against the cornea. Starting the solution flow before inserting the lens facilitates insertion.
6. Tape the tubing to the patient's forehead to prevent tension on the lens and accidental displacement. Attach the outflow device to collect the solution as it exits the eye.
   The outflow device helps prevent wetting the patient's clothing.

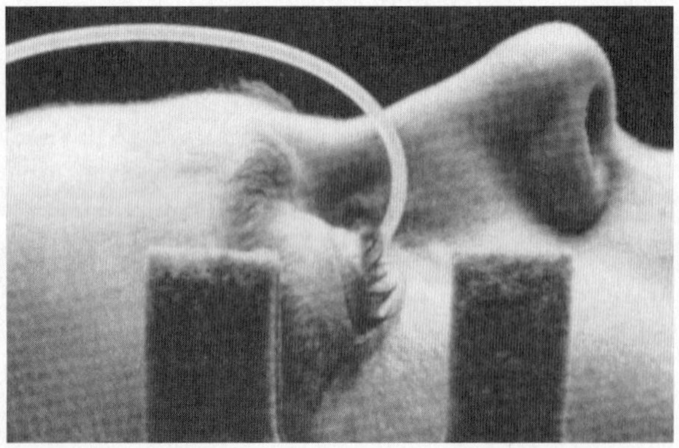

7. As the physician removes the lens at the completion of the procedure, you may be required to stop the flow of solution after the removal.
   Continuing the flow during removal of the lens provides for patient comfort by making the device easier to remove.
8. Assist the patient to clean away excess fluid. Allow the patient to rest for a few moments before trying to stand.
   Excess fluid will be uncomfortable for the patient. Having the patient rest will prevent dizziness and promote patient safety.
9. Wash your hands. Care for or dispose of equipment as needed.

DOCUMENTATION GUIDELINES

- Date and time
- Type of solution and amount
- Administration of anesthetic
- Which eye (OD, OS, OU)
- Patient complaints/concerns
- Patient education/instructions
- Your signature

Charting Example

DATE	TIME Pt arrived c/o caustic cleaning
	solution in OS. Ringer's Lactate solution
	by Morgan Lens ordered stat by
	Dr. Jacobs. Ocular anesthetic adminis-
	tered in OS as ordered. Pt positioned.
	1000 mL of Ringer's administered as
	ordered. Dr. Jacobs discontinued
	treatment, eye exam normal at comple-
	tion of procedure. Pt educated regarding
	eye safety. Verbalized understanding.
	—Your signature

(Photos courtesy of MorTan Inc., Missoula, MT)

Procedure 13-8 Removing a Foreign Object From the Eye

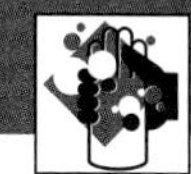
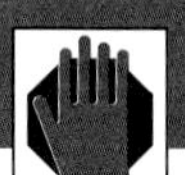

PURPOSE:

To free the eye safely of a foreign body

EQUIPMENT/SUPPLIES

- sterile, cotton-tipped applicator
- sterile water or saline
- sterile medicine dropper or small bulb syringe
- tissues
- sterile gauze

13

STEPS

1. Wash your hands.
2. Assemble the equipment and supplies.
3. Greet and identify the patient. Explain the procedure.
4. Glove now. With the gauze against the cheek, pull down the lower eyelid and check for the object. If it is seen, moisten the applicator with the water or saline and gently try to remove the object.
5. If the object is not found on the lower lid, grasp the lashes of the upper lid and pull gently upward, checking the upper surfaces of the eye for the object.
6. Perform an eye irrigation if necessary, following the steps in Procedure 13-6.
7. Wipe away any excess liquid with the tissue. Remove and dispose of the gloves.
8. Properly care for or dispose of equipment and supplies. Clean the work area. Wash your hands.

DOCUMENTATION GUIDELINES

- Date and time
- Removal of the foreign body
- Description of the foreign body, including size
- Patient complaints/concerns
- Results of any eye tests performed to determine extent of damage, as needed
- Full documentation of irrigation, if performed
- Full documentation of medication, if administered
- Notification of physician
- Patient education/instructions
- Your signature

Charting Example

DATE	TIME Pt arrived in office c/o metal chip
	in his OD. Occurred on the job at 0900.
	Dr. Spruce removed the foreign object.
	Neosporin ointment instilled in OD. Eye
	patch applied. Pt instructed to wear gog-
	gles on job site as needed. Pt verbalized
	understanding of teaching.
	—Your signature

Note: Imbedded objects must be removed by a physician, but loose debris may be removed by the medical assistant.

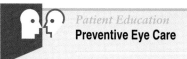

Patient Education

Preventive Eye Care

Preventive care of the eye is a vital component of patient education. Regular eye checkups, proper care of contact lenses, control of diabetes and hypertension, annual tonometer or "puff-of-air" checks for glaucoma each year after age 40, and proper attention to eye injuries are important aspects of eye health maintenance.

Patients should be advised to wear sunglasses with ultraviolet protection during any sun exposure to protect against ultraviolet ray damage to the eyes. Children should also be fitted for sunglasses to protect immature eyes from sun damage.

Rubbing the eyes should be avoided. This spreads infection from person to person and can damage the cornea if small foreign objects are introduced into the eye. Wearing eye goggles during procedures can prevent disease transmission and injury from foreign bodies.

small bones known collectively as the ossicles. The first is the malleus or hammer. Sound waves from the eardrum initiate a reaction in the attached malleus and are then transmitted to the next tiny bone, the incus or anvil. Vibrations from the anvil move the third bone, the stapes or stirrup, so named for its recognizable shape.

The auditory or eustachian tube connects the middle ear with the nasopharynx. This tube opens during swallowing and equalizes pressure in the middle ear.

The third section is divided into two parts called the cochlea and the semicircular canals. The two send the impulses for hearing (cochlea) and motion (semicircular canals) to the brain. The cochlea is attached to the stapes at the oval window, a thin membrane that moves as the stapes vibrate with transmitted waves. These sound waves are translated into nerve impulses by tiny hairlike processes in the cochlea that act as receptors for the organ of Corti, which sends the impulses through the acoustic nerve to the brain.

The semicircular canals, also known as the vestibular apparatus, are three half-circles set at right angles to each other. They are filled with a fluid called endolymph and lined with microscopic hairs. As the body position changes, the endolymph moves back and forth in the canals. This movement bends the hairs, which send a message to the brain regarding its current position. This function works closely with the visual images projected by the eyes. If the eyes perceive the horizon to be slanted and the semicircular canals transmit the message that the body is upright, the disorientation may lead to nausea; this is the reason many people experience motion sickness. If the vestibular apparatus is impaired or if an inner ear disorder is present, the patient will experience vertigo (moving sensation).

Checkpoint Question

5. *What are the functions of the cochlea and the semicirular canals?*

Transmission of Sound

Sound waves are produced by vibrations, such as the movement of air across the larynx, plucking the strings of a guitar, or slamming a door. The waves are caught by the pinna and channeled through the auditory canal to the tympanic membrane, which vibrates as the waves strike against it. The vibrations move the malleus, then the incus, then the stapes. The stapes move with the waves and transmit the impulse to the oval window, which moves the endolymph within the cochlea. The movement of the fluid is picked up by the tiny hairs of the organ of Corti. The waves are transmitted as impulses through the auditory nerve to the temporal lobe of the brain for interpretation.

Common Disorders

Hearing loss is a frequent outcome of diseases and disorders of the ear and can occur at any age. Congenital disorders, trauma, disease, and environmental noise can all result in hearing loss.

Ceruminosis

Also known as impacted earwax, ceruminosis is a frequent reason for diminished hearing. Cerumen is usually soft and moist and leaks out in such small amounts that it is unnoticed. Occasionally the cerumen may be hard and dry, or excess hair within the ear canal may hold the wax in, causing it to build up against the eardrum.

The presenting symptoms may be a gradual hearing loss or **tinnitus**, an extraneous noise heard in one or both ears. Otoscopy shows the obvious reason. The wax may be softened by warm oil ear drops or a commercial ceruminous softening agent and may be removed by an ear curet (refer to Chap. 5, Instruments and Equipment, for an illustration of a Buck ear curet) or by gently washing with an irrigating device (Fig. 13-11).

Conductive and Perceptual Hearing Loss

These disorders are the two categories of hearing impairment. In conductive loss, sound waves are not appropriately transmitted to the oval window and to the cochlear level. Perceptual, or sensorineural, loss in-

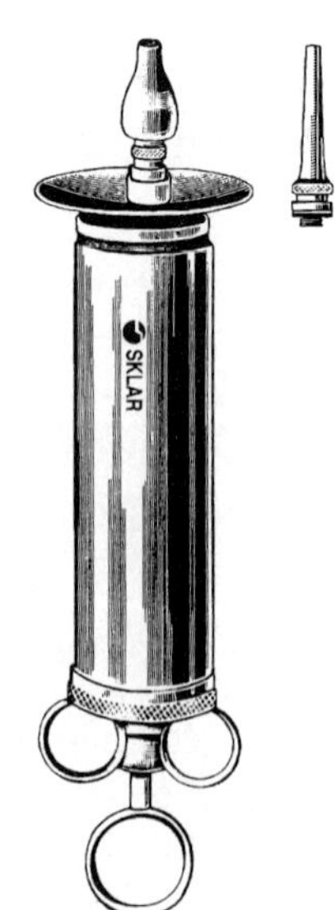

Figure 13-11 The ear syringe is used to irrigate the external auditory canal gently. Devices used to irrigate interdental spaces also are used to flush the canal. (Sklar Instruments, West Chester, PA.)

volves transmission from the oval window through to the receptors in the brain. Many patients present with a combination of both, called mixed deafness.

Causes of hearing loss may include heredity with predisposing factors to deafness; infections, particularly of the middle and inner ear; trauma; ototoxic drugs that affect the eighth cranial nerve; some neurologic diseases; exposure to loud noises; and presbycusis, also known as "old ear," which usually results from otosclerosis or a hardening of the joints between the ossicles.

Diagnosis involves the various audiometric tests as described below. Treatment addresses the underlying cause. A stapedectomy may be performed for otosclerosis with a replacement for the impaired joint. Cochlear implants are gaining favor for those whose loss involves impairment in the cochlear receptors. Cochlear implants are relatively new; the next few years will probably see as much improvement in this resource for the hearing impaired as has been made in the quality of hearing aids since their invention.

Conductive hearing loss can be treated successfully in most instances with hearing aids; however, perceptual loss is far more difficult to correct. If perceptual loss is due to tumor on the eighth cranial nerve, surgical removal of the tumor may be required. These tumors, although usually benign, tend to recur and often occur bilaterally.

What If?
What if your patient asks you if a hearing aid could help her? What would you tell her?

A hearing aid improves hearing ability, but it does not completely restore the ability to hear. The purpose of the device is to amplify sound waves. Given this fact, not every hearing-impaired patient is a good candidate for a hearing aid. For example, a patient who has permanent nerve damage generally will not experience significant improvement with a standard hearing aid.

There are two basic types of aids: bone conduction receivers sit behind the ear and press against the skull; air conduction receivers fit into the auditory canal. The size and type of hearing aid is based on the patient's specific condition and need. Binaural (both ear) aids are available and often can be fitted into eyeglasses for a less conspicuous appearance.

Have the patient discuss any concerns about the purchase and use of a hearing aid with the physician. If the patient does purchase a hearing aid, teach her how to maintain the device and adjust the volume control.

Checkpoint Question

6. *How would you differentiate between conductive and perceptual hearing loss?*

Meniere's Disease

Meniere's disease, a degenerative condition, affects the inner ear and upsets the body's ability to maintain equilibrium in addition to a loss of hearing. The symptoms include vertigo, sensorineural hearing loss, and tinnitus. Severe symptoms may lead to nausea and vomiting. Caution the patient to avoid situations that could cause falls.

Periods of remission are followed by periods of exacerbation. Many of the symptoms can be treated with palliative medication. If the symptoms persist and increase or become incapacitating, it may be necessary to destroy the organs of the inner ear. A cure is usually immediate, but the patient will be irreversibly deaf.

Otitis Externa

Also known as swimmer's ear, otitis externa is an inflammation or infection of the external ear. It is common in the summer and is caused by any number of pathogens that grow in the warm, moist ear canal. It is best treated by antibiotics, either topical or systemic, warm compresses, and pain relief medication.

The presenting symptom is pain on movement of any of the adjoining structures around the ear, jaw, auricle, and so on. Otoscopy reveals a red, swollen ear canal. Debris must be gently washed from the area using the procedure outlined. Preventive therapy of applying an alcohol solution after swimming can help avoid this problem. Encourage patients who are prone to otitis externa to wear earplugs while swimming and to avoid using any objects to clean the ears, such as swabs or hairpins.

Otitis Media

Otitis media, an inflammation or infection of the middle ear, frequently results from an **upper respiratory in-**

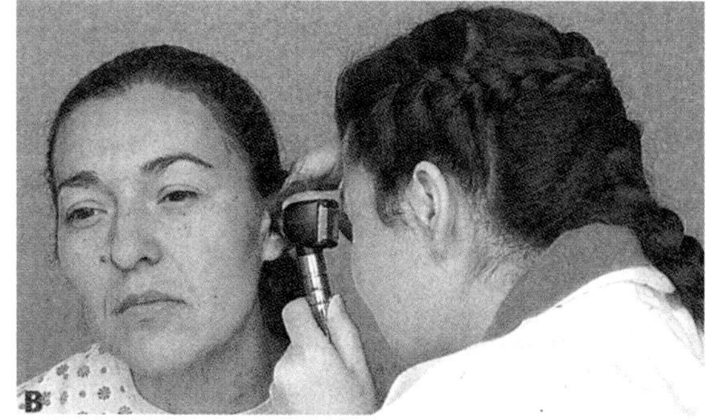

Figure 13-12 Visual otoscopic examination.

13

fection (URI). Pathogens responsible for pharyngitis, nasopharyngitis, and the common cold frequently travel through the warm, moist eustachian tube to the hospitable middle ear. As infection increases, the mucous membranes of the eustachian tubes swell, closing off the opening to the middle ear. With no way to drain, fluid builds up as a response to the infection and causes pain and pressure on the flexible tympanic membrane. If pressure is sufficient, the membrane may tear or perforate to relieve the pressure.

Symptoms include severe pain, fever of varying degrees, and mild hearing loss. Infants may be fussy and tug at their ears. Any elevation in a child's temperature should be a warning to check for otitis media. Diagnosis usually is made by otoscopy, which may reveal a reddened, bulging tympanic membrane. Bubbles can sometimes be seen behind the thin membrane. Treatment requires antibiotics to subdue the infection and analgesics for the pain. Decongestants may reduce some of the swelling. In severe chronic cases, a myringotomy may be performed to relieve pressure. Tubes may be inserted through the tympanic membrane and remain several months to equalize pressure if the problem persists.

Children have very short, almost horizontal eustachian tubes. For some children, virtually every cold and cough forces microorganisms into the middle ear, causing seemingly endless infections. The problem is compounded for children who are put to bed with a bottle of milk or formula. The milk acts as a hospitable medium for bacteria to grow.

Otosclerosis

Otosclerosis affects all of the ossicles, but most particularly the stapes bone and is thought to be hereditary. It causes loss of hearing in the low tones and is treatable with use of hearing aids. A stapedial prosthesis may also be implanted through microscopic surgery to replace the sclerotic joint and allow movement.

Common Diagnostic Studies and Therapeutic Procedures and the Medical Assistant's Role

Visual Examination

By using an otoscope that you prepare, the physician can view the auditory canal and the eardrum (Fig. 13-12). Disposable specula or specula covers are used most often. The otoscopic attachment is frequently used interchangeably with the base used for the ophthalmoscope.

Audiometry

An audiometer can be used to detect hearing loss by producing pure tones of various **decibel (db)** levels and various frequencies. (Decibel is a unit for measuring the intensity of sound.) The results of the test may be recorded by the audiometer on a special graph (Procedure 13-9). Speech audiometry uses voice tones rather than pure tones to assess hearing. Impedance audiometry evaluates tympanic membrane and ossicle mobility. A probe is inserted into the auditory meatus and emits tones of various intensity that bounce back to the probe receiver. If the tympanic membrane and ossicles are normal, the movement is transmitted and rebound is picked up by the receiver to produce a curve on the graph. If the tympanic membrane and ossicles are less mobile than normal, much of the sound transmitted bounces back and is reflected back to the instrument to produce a distinct curve on the graph.

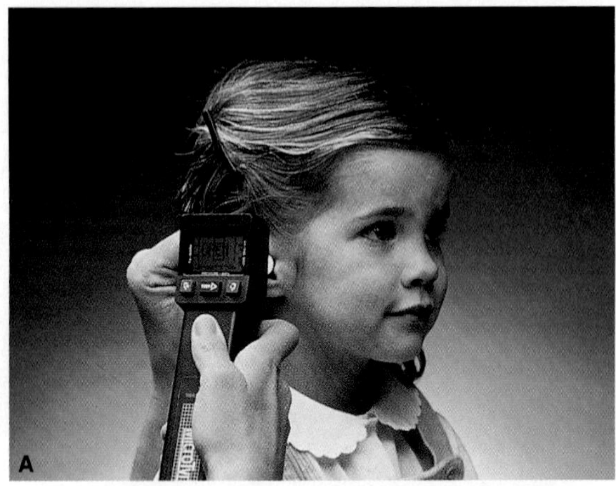

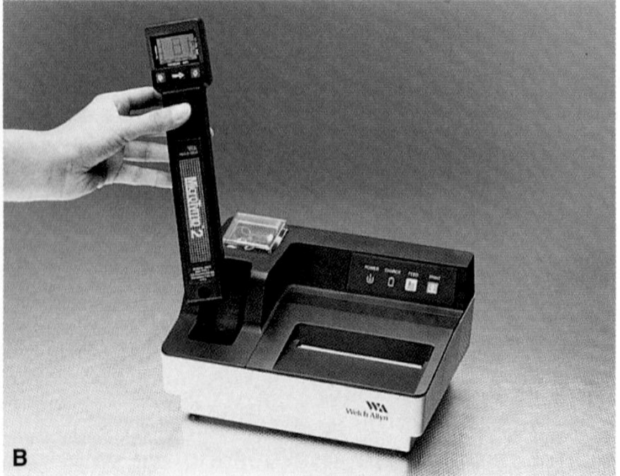

Figure 13-13 Microtymp 2 Tympanic Instrument. This tympanometric instrument is lightweight and portable and provides a hard copy printout of many middle ear disorders. (**A**) Press the button, then insert the probe tip in the ear. Watch the LCD screen as it completes the tympanogram in about 1 second. (**B**) Return the handle to the printer/charger and a printout appears in 5 seconds. (Courtesy of Welch Allyn.)

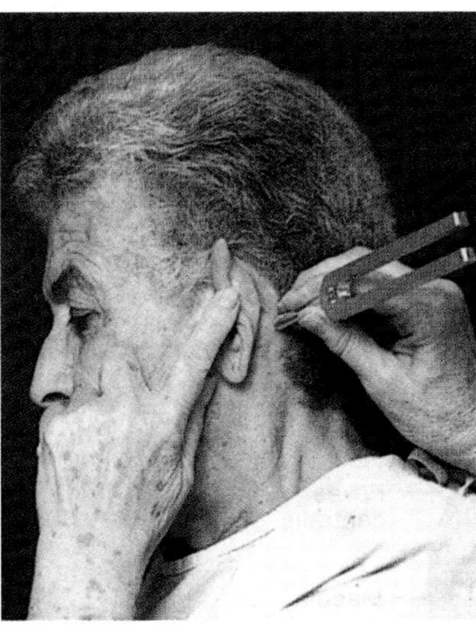

Figure 13-14 In the Rinne test, the base of the lightly vibrating tuning fork is placed on the mastoid bone.

Tympanometry

This works like the impedance audiometer but uses air pressure rather than tones to produce the graph. Figure 13-13 illustrates the steps for performing tympanometry. Tympanic mobility is measured to determine pressure behind the membrane or to assess ossicle mobility. With training the medical assistant may perform tympanometry.

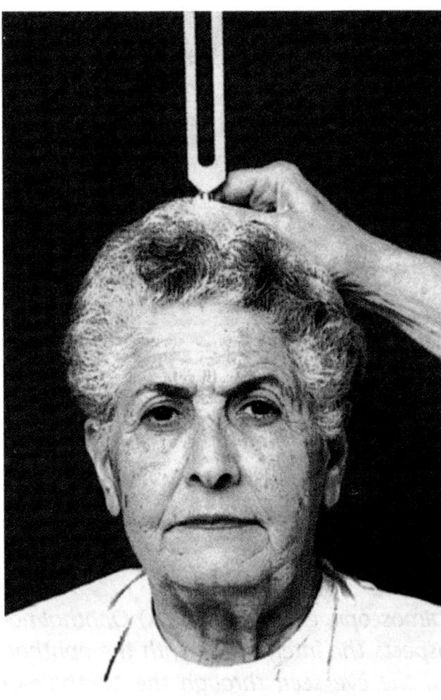

Figure 13-15 In the Weber test, the base of the lightly vibrating tuning fork is placed on the patient's head (or mid-forehead).

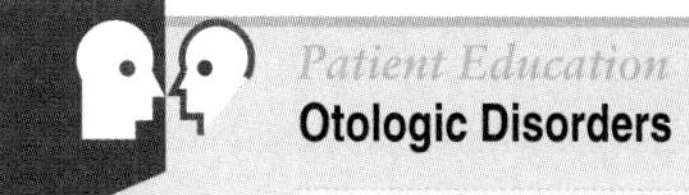

Patient Education

Otologic Disorders

Teach patients to recognize symptoms of otologic disorders and to report them promptly to the physician. Proper attention at the early stage of an infection or injury can often prevent serious or irreversible damage.

Instruct patients to avoid trying to clean the ears with cotton applicators or any other device. This drives cerumen deeper into the ear and creates more of an impaction than is already present.

Children should be instructed not to place small objects, such as beans, peas, or small parts of toys, into their ears because they may become lodged and require surgical removal.

Caution parents to complete all antibiotic treatment for children's ear infections even though the symptoms may subside. The infection may be present for awhile after the patient is asymptomatic. Ear recheck appointments should be kept as scheduled to ensure that the child is free of infection.

Rinne Test

By using a tuning fork against the mastoid bone then moving it to the external auditory meatus, testing for a conductive hearing loss is performed (Fig. 13-14).

Weber Test

This test uses a tuning fork on the midline of the forehead to differentiate between conductive and sensorineural loss (Fig. 13-15). Your only responsibility for the Rinne or Weber is to make the tuning fork available to the physician.

Irrigations and Instillations

Ear irrigations (Procedure 13-10) are performed to relieve pain, to remove debris or foreign objects, or to apply topical solutions. Ear instillations (Procedure 13-11) are usually in the form of local anesthetics for the pain of otitis externa or otitis media or topical antibiotics for otitis externa.

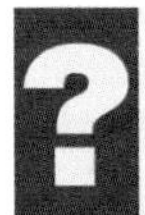

Checkpoint Question

7. *What is an audiometer used for and how does it work?*

THE NOSE

Basic Structure and Function

The nose is the primary organ of intake for oxygen and output for carbon dioxide. The external nares are the

13

Procedure 13-9 Performing Audiometry

PURPOSE:

To assess levels of hearing acuity

EQUIPMENT/SUPPLIES

- audiometer
- disposable scope cover

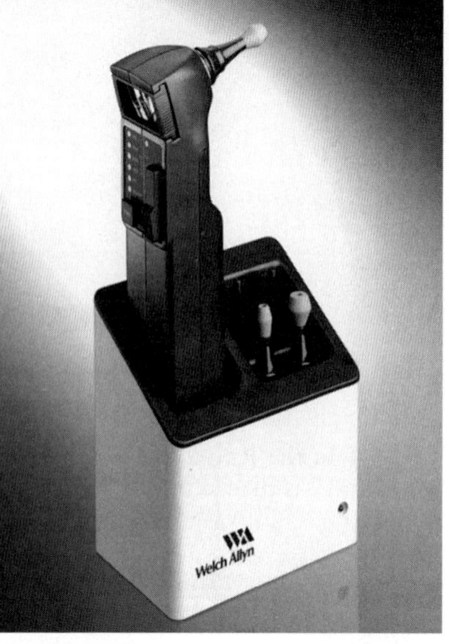

STEPS

1. Wash your hands.
2. Assemble the equipment.
3. Greet and identify the patient. Escort the patient to a quiet room free of distractions. Explain the procedure.
4. Cover the probe with the disposable scope cover.
   A disposable cover prevents the spread of microorganisms.
5. Position the auricle and canal by gently pulling up and back on the pinna for adults and down and back for small children to straighten the canal.
   Proper placement facilitates testing and helps ensure accurate test results.

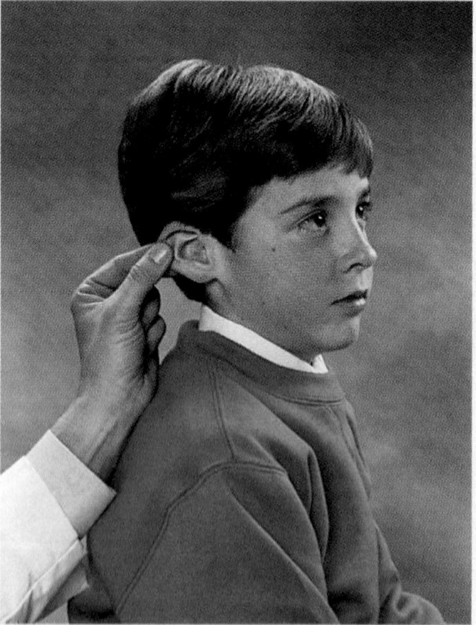

6. Insert the probe into the patient's ear. Visualize the tympanic membrane. Turn on the machine.

continued

Procedure 13-9 Continued Performing Audiometry

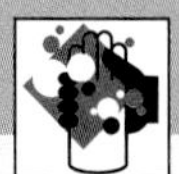

7. Practice with the patient using the pretone.
   Practicing helps ensure that the patient understands the instructions for testing.

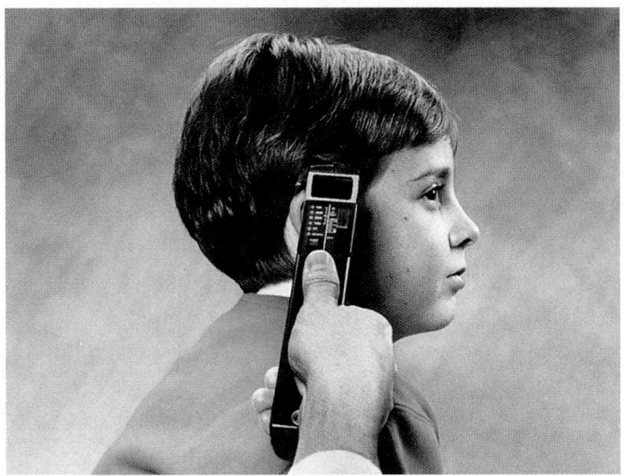

8. Select the testing level for the patient. Depress the "start" button. Observe the tone indicators and the patient's response.

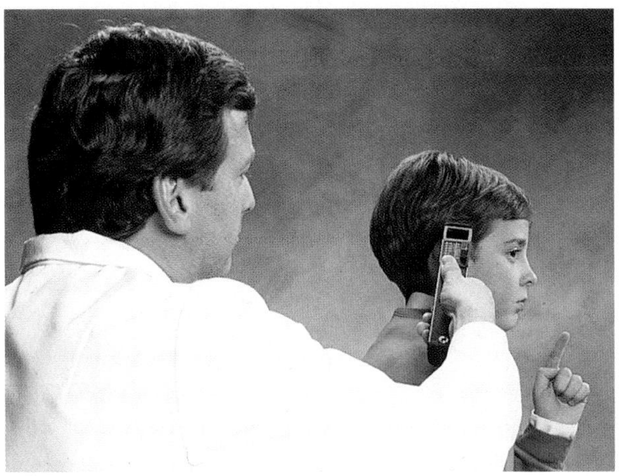

9. Screen the opposite ear.
   In most instances, assessment of hearing requires bilateral testing.
10. If the patient fails to respond at any frequency, retest through the procedure.
   Failure to respond must be assessed to ensure that directions for the testing were understood properly.
11. Remove and dispose of the probe cover. Wash your hands. Care for the equipment, and return the instrument to its charging base.

13

DOCUMENTATION GUIDELINES

- Date and time
- Patient complaints/concerns
- Physical findings
- Performance of procedure
- Testing results
- Patient education/instructions
- Your signature

Charting Example

DATE	TIME 7/y/o with extensive Hx of otitis
	media. Mother c/o apparent hearing loss
	noted recently. Child plays music very loud
	and does not readily respond to voices.
	Dr. Day ordered audiometry testing. Pt
	responded to midlevel and low tones but
	failed to respond to upper level tones.
	Test repeated with same results. Dr. Day
	notified. —Your signature

(Photos courtesy of Welch Allyn, Skaneateles Falls, NY.)

openings through which oxygen is inhaled and carbon dioxide is exhaled. Cartilage gives the nose its shape and makes the external structures flexible. The nasal cavity is separated by a nasal septum into right and left cavities.

Small hairlike projections covering virtually all surfaces of the nasal structures are called cilia and move secretions along to the throat for swallowing. The nasal surface area is increased by the presence of turbinates on the lateral surfaces of the nasal cavities. The mucous membranes of the turbinates cover the bones called conchae. This area moistens, warms, and filters the air that enters the nares.

The four sinuses—frontal, ethmoidal, sphenoidal, and maxillary sinuses—open into the nasal cavities within the folds of the turbinates. They make the skull lighter and help give the voice its resonance.

Process of Smell

The olfactory nerves are contained in the olfactory bulbs at the uppermost surface of the nasal cavity (Fig.

text continues on page 312

13

Procedure 13-10 Irrigating the Ear

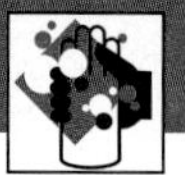

PURPOSE:

To clean the external ear of cerumen or a foreign body

EQUIPMENT/SUPPLIES

- irrigation solution of the physician's choice at no more than 100°F (about 37°C)
- basin for solution
- ear irrigation syringe or irrigating device
- waterproof barrier
- otoscope
- emesis basin or ear basin for outflow
- unsterile gauze

STEPS

1. Wash your hands.

2. Assemble the equipment and supplies.

3. Greet and identify the patient. Explain the procedure.

Ear irrigations usually are not painful, but the flow of the solution may be uncomfortable. The patient will be more cooperative if this is understood.

4. Position the patient comfortably in an erect position.

5. View the affected ear with an otoscope to locate the problem.

Adults: Gently pull up and slightly back to straighten the auditory canal.

Children: Gently pull slightly down and back to straighten the auditory canal.

Note: Do not irrigate if the tympanic membrane appears to be perforated without checking with the physician; solution may be forced into the middle ear through the perforation. Remove any obvious debris at the entrance of the canal before beginning the irrigation.

The area of treatment must be visualized before irrigation begins. If debris from the external auricle is not removed, it may be washed into the canal.

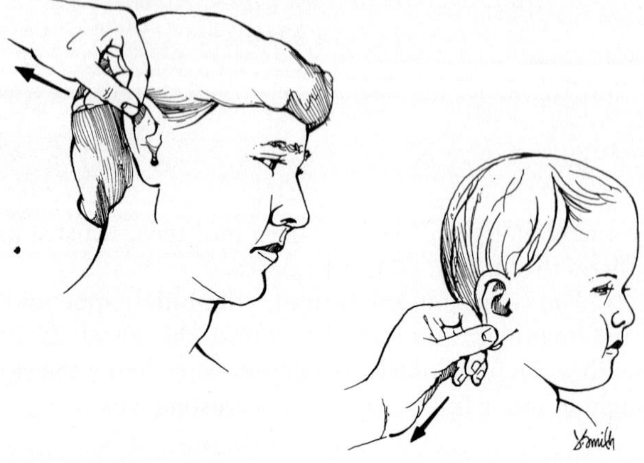

6. Drape the patient with a waterproof barrier.

Wet clothing would be uncomfortable for the patient.

7. Tilt the patient's head toward the affected side.

Tilting the head downward will facilitate the flow of solution.

8. Place the drainage basin beneath the affected ear.

9. Fill the syringe, or turn on the irrigating device.

10. Gently position the auricle as described above with the nondominant hand.

The canal must be straightened for either visualization or treatment.

11. With the dominant hand, place the tip of the syringe into the auditory meatus, and direct the flow of solution gently upward toward the roof of the canal.

Directing the flow against the upper surface will avoid pressure against the tympanic membrane and will facilitate the outflow of solution.

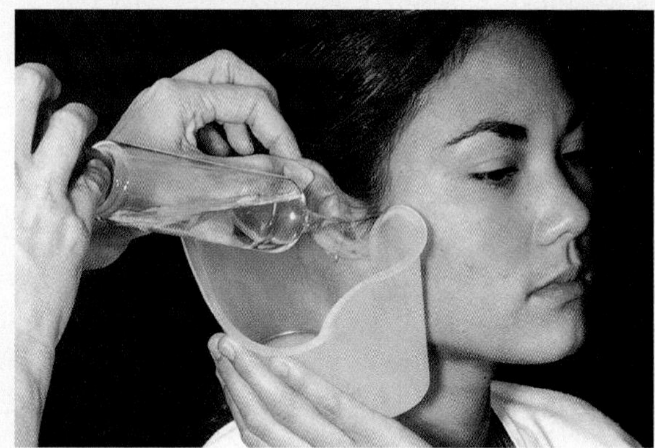

12. Continue irrigating for the prescribed period of time.

13. Dry the patient's external ear with gauze. Have the patient sit for awhile with the affected ear downward to drain the solution.

Allowing the solution to remain in the ear will be uncomfortable.

14. Inspect the ear with the otoscope to determine the results.

It may be necessary to repeat the procedure, and it is always necessary to inspect the area to record the results.

15. Properly care for or dispose of equipment and supplies. Clean the work area. Wash your hands.

continued

Procedure 13-10 Continued Irrigating the Ear

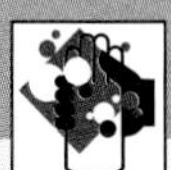

13

DOCUMENTATION GUIDELINES

- Date and time
- Type of solution or medication
- Which ear (AD, AS, AU)
- Description of outflow, if used to remove debris or foreign objects
- Patient complaints/concerns
- Patient education/instructions
- Your signature

Charting Example

DATE	TIME
	S: "I put a piece of corn in my ear."
	O: 30-month-old boy tugging on left ear.
	Mother states this occurred
	20 minutes ago. Kernel observed with
	otoscope. Tympanic membrane intact.
	A: Foreign object in left ear.
	P: 1. Left ear irrigated with 500 mL
	normal saline. One kernel of corn
	removed. Pt tolerated procedure well.
	Postirrigation ear canal clear. Tympanic
	membrane intact.
	2. Mother and child educated on
	prevention techniques.
	3. Dr. Rogers d/c pt to home.
	—Your signature

Procedure 13-11 Instilling Ear Medication

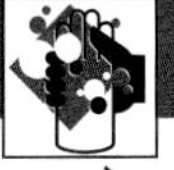

PURPOSE:

To soften cerumen for easier removal
To provide local comfort
To relieve otic pain

EQUIPMENT/SUPPLIES

- medication formulated for otic purposes, with dropper
- cotton balls

STEPS

1. Wash your hands.
2. Assemble the equipment.
3. Check the medication three times as specified for medication administration. It must specify otic preparation.

   Medication for otic instillation must be formulated for that purpose.

continued

13

Procedure 13-11 Continued **Instilling Ear Medication**

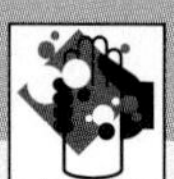

4. Greet and identify the patient. Explain the procedure.
5. Have the patient seated with the affected ear tilted upward.
   The medication must be allowed to flow through the canal to the area of concern.
6. Draw up the ordered amount of medication.
7. Position the auricle:
   a. *Adults:* Pull the auricle slightly up and back to straighten the S-shaped canal.
   b. *Children:* Pull the auricle slightly down and back to straighten the S-shaped canal.
8. Insert the tip of the dropper without touching the patient's skin, and let the medication flow along the side of the canal.
   Touching the patient will contaminate the dropper. The medication should flow gently to avoid patient discomfort.

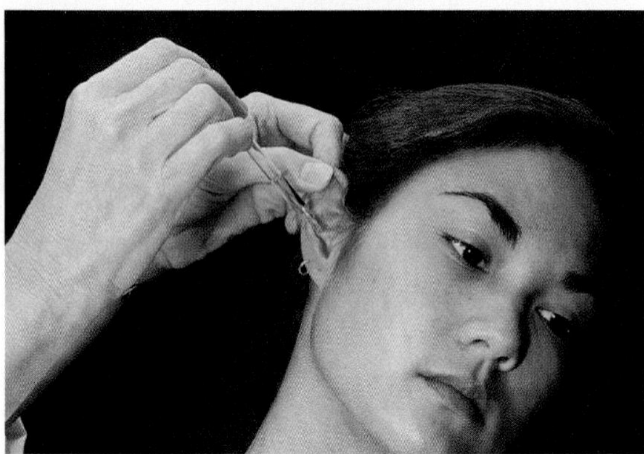

9. Have the patient sit or lie with the affected ear upward for a short while.
   The medication should rest against the tympanic membrane for as long as possible.
10. If the medication is to be retained, insert the cotton ball slightly into the external auditory meatus without force.
   A wick will help keep the medication in the canal. Force could be painful to the patient.
11. Properly care for or dispose of equipment and supplies. Clean the work area. Wash your hands.

DOCUMENTATION GUIDELINES

- Date and time
- Medication
- Dose
- Location (which ear, ie, AD, AS, AU)
- Patient complaints/concerns
- Patient education/instructions
- Your signature

Charting Example

DATE	TIME Pt presents with ceruminosis.
	Debrox ear drops ordered by Dr. Gleason
	for AD. Pt's auricle was pulled up and
	back. 10 drops of Debrox instilled into AD.
	Pt kept head tilted with AD up for
	5 minutes. Pt tolerated procedure well.
	Educated on procedure to instill ear
	drops. Pt verbalized understanding of
	teaching. —Your signature

13-16). Free olfactory nerve endings project into the mucous membranes and are specific for various types of smells. All scents or chemicals must be moistened by mucus to be perceived by the nerve endings. The impulses caused by the chemicals against the specific nerve endings travel by the olfactory tract to the thalamic and olfactory centers for interpretation. This area of the brain through which the nerve tract passes is so vital to associative memory and thought processes that smells can trigger an array of emotions from fear to joy and can stimulate appetite or cause nausea.

Loss of the sense of smell has an adverse effect on appetite and consequently on nutrition for patients with disease processes involving the nose or the transmission or perception of olfactory nerve impulses. The sense of smell tires easily; the initial perception of an odor diminishes as much as 50% within several minutes. The ability to discern odors is lost with age and plays an important part in the loss of appetite for the elderly.

Checkpoint Question

8. *What are cilia and what do they do?*

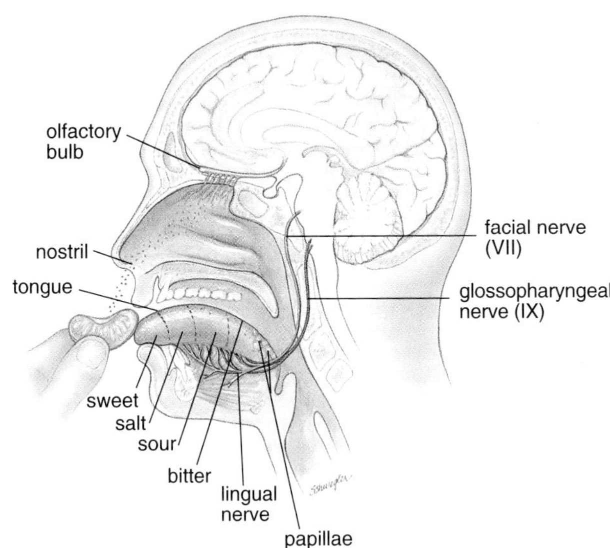

Figure 13-16 Organs of taste and smell.

Common Disorders

Allergic Rhinitis

Allergic rhinitis involves inflammation of the mucous membranes of the nasal passages and usually results from exposure to allergens. Symptomatic treatment is usually offered during peak pollen seasons. It also is known as hay fever or seasonal allergic rhinitis when it appears in response to seasonal plant pollens. If the symptoms are present year round, it is referred to as perennial allergic rhinitis and is usually a reaction to household irritants, such as dust mites and pet dander. The signs are obvious with paroxysmal sneezing, intense rhinorrhea, congestion, and watery, reddened eyes.

Diagnosis usually involves history and differential diagnosis. Mucous secretions may reveal an increase in immunoglobulin E in response to the allergens. An allergist may isolate the offending protein by skin testing. Allergy treatment involves exposure to the allergen in minute doses to desensitize the immune reaction. Nasal steroids and oral antihistamines are also effective.

Cleft Palate

Cleft palate is a separation of the palatine bones that divide the internal nose from the mouth. It is a congenital condition that requires surgery to correct. The abnormality occurs during the second embryonic month as the face is forming. Although a predisposition is present in some families, it is not strictly a familial pattern.

Cleft palate may or may not involve the entire palate area. If the defect involves only the posterior palate, surgery may be simple and will not require facial plastic surgery. The defect also may involve the anterior palate and may extend into the facial structure. If the lip is involved, the defect is referred to as "hare lip" and may be unilateral or bilateral. The defect may be complete and extend from the oral cavity to the nasal cavity all the way from the anterior surfaces to the posterior surfaces. Such defects will require extensive surgery over a period of years.

Epistaxis

Commonly known as nosebleed, epistaxis generally occurs as a result of trauma, but it may be secondary to other disorders. Hypertension, malignancies, polyps, and the fragile capillaries associated with pregnancy are other contributing factors. Bleeding beyond 10 minutes after treatment begins is considered severe. Diagnosis requires a history and inspection with a nasal speculum. History of severe epistaxis requires nasal packing or a balloon catheter that may remain from several hours to days. If the bleeding is secondary to anticoagu-

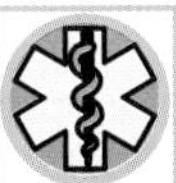

Action **STAT!**

Epistaxis

Scenario: Mr. Combe comes into the office complaining of intermittent nose bleeding for the past 2 days. While sitting in the reception area, his nose starts bleeding heavily. What should you do?

1. Remember to follow Standard Precautions. Quickly don gloves, then help Mr. Combe.
2. Compress Mr. Combe's nares against the septum using moderate pressure. Apply ice or cold, moist gauze sponges to help control the bleeding.
3. Assist Mr. Combe to an examining room. If he feels too weak to walk, place him in a wheelchair. Patients who are actively bleeding should not remain in the reception area.
4. Help Mr. Combe to sit upright with his head slightly forward. This position will help to decrease the amount of blood swallowed.
5. Notify the physician.
6. Check Mr. Combe's blood pressure and pulse. An elevated blood pressure may have contributed to the bleeding. A low blood pressure with a fast, rapid pulse may indicate significant blood loss.
7. After the bleeding has stopped, instruct Mr. Combe not to blow his nose until the physician has determined that the epistaxis is controlled.
8. Dispose of blood-soaked items and gloves following Standard Precautions. Wash your hands.
9. Document the incident in Mr. Combe's chart.

Procedure 13-12 Instilling Nasal Medication

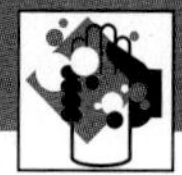
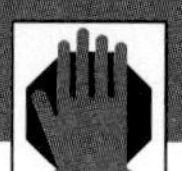

PURPOSE:

To relieve nasal congestion
To improve compromised respirations
To treat infection or inflammation of the nasal passages

EQUIPMENT/SUPPLIES

- medication (drops or spray)
- nonsterile tissues

13

STEPS

1. Wash your hands.
2. Assemble the equipment and supplies. Check the medication label three times.
   Preparations for use in the nasal passages must be formulated for these surfaces.
3. Greet and identify the patient. Explain the procedure. Ask the patient about allergies not documented.
   Nasal instillations are uncomfortable but should not be painful; patients will be more cooperative if they understand the procedure.
4. Position the patient in a comfortable recumbent position. Extend the patient's head beyond the edge of the examination table, or place a pillow under the patient's shoulders. Support the patient's neck to avoid strain as the head is tilted back.
   The patient must be properly positioned to reach the upper nasal passages.
5. Glove now. Administer the medication.
   Gloves must be worn to avoid contact with potentially hazardous material.
   a. Administer nose drops by holding the dropper upright just above each nostril and dropping the medication one drop at a time without touching the nares. Keep the patient in the recumbent position for 5 minutes.
      Touching the dropper to the nostril will contaminate the dropper. For effective treatment, the patient must allow the medication to reach the upper nasal passages.
   b. Administer nasal spray by having the patient sit. Place the tip of the dispenser at the nare opening without touching the patient's skin or nasal tissues, and spray as the patient takes a deep breath.
      The medication must reach the upper passages; if the patient breathes out, much of the medication will be exhaled.
6. Wipe away any excess medication from the patient's skin with tissues.
   Excess medication around the nares will be uncomfortable.
7. Properly care for or dispose of equipment and supplies. Clean the work area. Remove gloves. Wash your hands.

DOCUMENTATION GUIDELINES

- Date and time
- Medication (include form, such as drops or spray)
- Dose
- Location (which nostril or nare)
- Patient complaints/concerns
- Patient education/instructions
- Your signature

Charting Example

DATE	TIME Pt c/o dry, itching nares. Pt uses
	hot air for home heating. Saline nasal
	spray ordered by Dr. Thomas. Both
	nostrils were sprayed while the pt took
	deep breaths. Pt was instructed in the
	need to keep nasal passages open and
	clear. Home humidification was sug-
	gested. Pt verbalized understanding of
	teachings. —Your signature

lant therapy, adjustment of the medication may be required. Cautery to an exposed vessel helps if that is the only cause.

Immediate therapy involves having the patient sit upright with the head slightly forward to avoid postnasal drainage that may lead to nausea. Compress the nares against the septum for 5 to 10 minutes with either ice or a cold, wet compress. Advise the patient to remain still and not to blow the nose until the physician feels that all danger is past.

Nasal Polyps

Nasal polyps are small hanging pendulous tissues that obstruct breathing. They are easily treated by surgery, including laser treatments. Polyps are usually produced in the mucous membranes of the nasal passages as a response to long-term allergies. Symptoms include a feeling of fullness or congestion and occasionally a nasal discharge. Diagnosis requires direct examination with a nasal speculum or x-ray of the nasal structures. Treatment may involve corticosteroids by topical application or injection into the polyps. The underlying allergy must be treated as well to prevent recurrence. If conservative treatment is not effective, surgery is required.

Sinusitis

Sinusitis is the inflammation of one or more of the sinus cavities. It can be either acute or chronic. Acute sinusitis is usually the result of an upper respiratory infection and is fairly easily resolved. Chronic sinusitis is more persistent and more difficult to control. Either form is more common when bacteria are forced into the warm moist sinus during nose blowing.

Symptoms include the obvious signs of upper respiratory infection with the addition of a purulent nasal discharge and face pain. Diagnosis may be made by history alone or may require direct visualization, x-rays of the sinuses, punctures of the sinuses to withdraw a specimen for culture, and ultrasound.

Serious complications of brain and middle ear infection may occur if the condition is not treated promptly with antibiotics to kill the infecting agent. Total blockage may result if the disorder is not treated and may require surgical procedures, such as a Caldwell-Luc, or a nasal window procedure, to puncture the wall between the nose and the involved sinus cavity to allow drainage. Ephedrine nose drops are often used to shrink the mucosal tissue. (Procedure 13-12 describes the steps for instilling nasal medication.) A newer treatment is the use of steroidal nasal sprays. Acute sinusitis responds to antibiotic therapy within 7 to 10 days. For chronic sinusitis, therapy may have to be instituted for 4 to 6 weeks.

Checkpoint Question

9. *What factors contribute to epistaxis?*

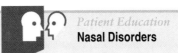

Patient Education

Nasal Disorders

Patients need to be aware of any changes in normal breathing patterns. It is imperative to have early symptoms of any nasal disorder treated as soon as possible to prevent complications. Children should be instructed never to place small pieces of toys or items, such as dried beans or peas, into the nares. These can be aspirated into the lungs and cause respiratory distress or aspiration pneumonia.

Instruct patients about the rebound phenomena of nasal sprays and drops. If used without the advice of a physician, these medications may become addictive. The nasal mucosa responds to the withdrawal by becoming congested if not routinely treated with the offending chemicals. Nasal preparations should never be used more than four times a day for 3 days unless specified by the physician.

Common Diagnostic Studies and Therapeutic Procedures and the Medical Assistant's Role

Many tests for the nose require direct visualization with a nasal speculum that you may prepare, including gross inspection and use of the illuminated otoscope (part of the diagnostic set). Diagnostic imaging (radiography and computed tomography scanning) may be used for the nasal sinuses, for traumatic injuries, and for congenital problems. Nose and throat cultures may also be ordered for you to perform or to route for differential diagnosis. (See Chap. 17, Assisting With Diagnostic and Therapeutic Procedures Associated With the Respiratory System, for the procedure for obtaining a throat culture.) Allergy testing may be performed for chronic rhinitis. A noninvasive procedure with a fiberoptic sinus endoscope may be performed after numbing the patient's nose with a light anesthetic spray. Rhinoplasty is the surgical repair of the nose either to correct actual structural damage or for cosmetic purposes.

OTHER SENSES

Taste

Taste receptors are located all across the tongue, through the mouth, and into the pharynx and larynx (see Fig. 13-16). The receptors require that food be moistened with saliva to be perceived. (Think of how tasteless food becomes when the mouth is dry.) The various chemical components of food are picked up by specific areas of the tongue:

- Sweet—tip of the tongue
- Sour—sides of the tongue
- Salt—edges of the tongue
- Bitter—back of the tongue

Some of the receptors pick up painful stimuli also, as in highly caustic foods, such as certain peppers and ginger. The receptors tire quickly, which explains why we frequently move bits of hard candy from side to side to renew the taste. The gustatory center of the brain is in the center of the parietal lobe. Lesions in the brain can be traced by assessing a patient's taste perception.

Smell

13

Taste perception is closely associated with the sense of smell. Foods that have no odor have less taste than those that are also perceived by smell. The perception of both smell and taste diminishes with age and interferes with nutrition for the elderly.

Touch

Specialized receptors are scattered throughout the body to receive impulses for heat or cold, pressure, vibration, pain, touch, or position (Fig. 13-17). Each receptor is designed to register and transmit just that particular sensation. For instance, the pacinian corpuscles are **tactile** organs that are specific for deep pressure and vibrations but do not transmit heat or cold (Table 13-1). Nerves in the muscles, joints, and tendons transmit the position of our body parts: *Is my arm by my side or over my head? Am I standing or lying?* These nerves are called proprioceptors and help coordinate our movements.

Pain Perception

Although we may learn to accept the perception of pain, we never adapt as we do to scents or tastes. The last painful stimulus is frequently as intolerable as the first, unlike some of our other perceptions. Pain is one of our most important protective devices. If we did not feel pain, we would be less aware of injury or disease. Pain receptors are found everywhere in our body but somewhat less viscerally.

Pain may be physiologic, implying that it is actually caused by an organic disorder, or it may be psychological, referring to pain that is perceived without the presence of an identifiable source. Whether or not pain has an organic basis, it is no less real to the patient and must be treated with the same care and compassion.

Referred Pain

It is sometimes difficult for the physician to determine the source of pain by the symptoms reported by the patients. Many patients who are experiencing a myocardial infarction complain of pain in the arms, shoulders, back, or jaw, rather than around the heart. Patients experiencing gallbladder attacks may complain of shoulder pain. These two examples are called referred pain. Theories suggest that the brain does not expect pain to be felt viscerally, so it assigns the origin of the pain to a body part fairly close to the source. The medical assis-

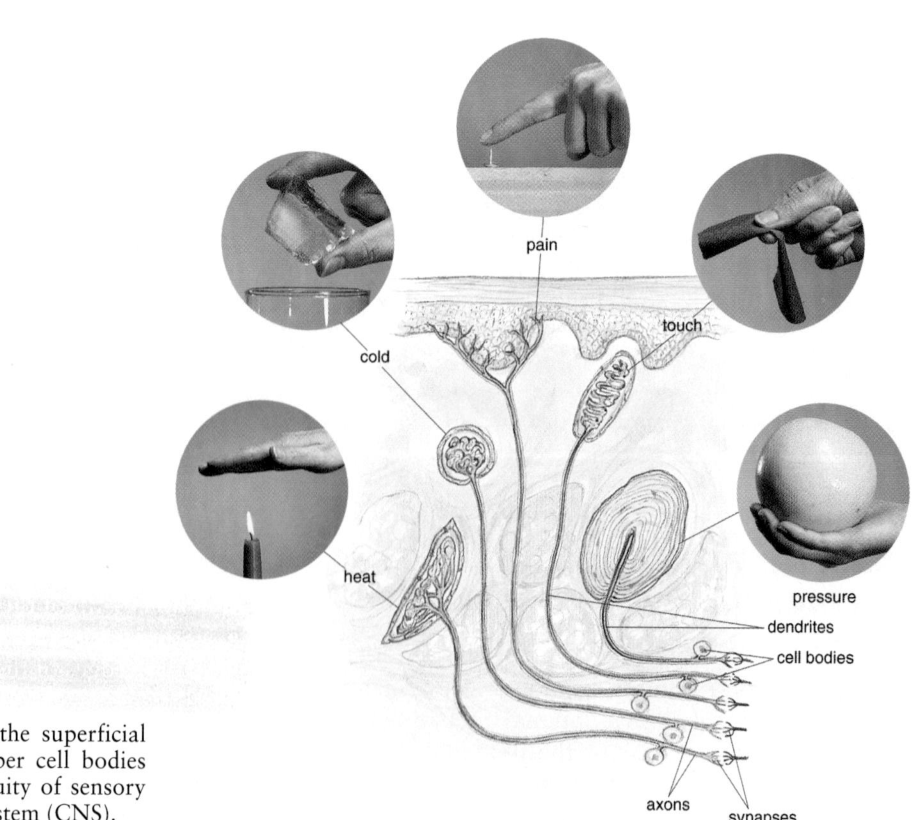

Figure 13-17 Diagram showing the superficial receptors (end-organs) and the deeper cell bodies and synapses, suggesting the continuity of sensory pathways into the central nervous system (CNS).

Table 13-1 **Tactile Organs**

Receptor	*Location*	*Sensation*
Pacinian corpuscles	Scattered throughout most of the surface of the body, including beneath the skin, mucous membranes, and serous tissues and around joints	Deep pressure and vibrations
Ruffini's corpuscles	Dermal layers of the skin and subcutaneously in the fingertips	Touch and pressure
Meissner's corpuscles	Upper layers of the skin, concentrated in the lips and fingertips	Fine touch
Krause's end bulbs	Dermal layer and subcutaneous tissues and lips	Touch and cold

Note: Many free nerve endings present throughout the skin and mucosa register pain, gross touch, heat, or cold.

tant must record and report all symptoms of pain exactly as the patient describes them. Open-ended questions must be pursued, such as: *"How long have you felt this pain?" "Describe how it feels. What makes it better or worse?"* The physician will correlate the pain with the physical and laboratory findings to arrive at a diagnosis.

Pain Treatment

Pain may be treated by many means. Some of the accepted methods mask the perception of pain, others deaden the source area, and some are used to confuse the brain into feeling something other than pain.

Pain medications mask the pain but do not usually relieve the source pathology. Surgery may help to remove the source of the pain. If removal is not possible, nerves to the area may be severed.

Transcutaneous electrical nerve stimulation, cold, and pressure are used to override the transmission of pain and confuse the pain receptors but will not treat the source of pain. Music, hypnosis or autohypnosis, imaging, and so on distract the patient from the pain but will not cure the source.

Checkpoint Question

10. *What is the difference between physiologic and psychological pain?*

Answers to Checkpoint Questions

1. *The rods and cones are nerve cells contained in the retina. Rods are responsible for light and dark shadings. Cones are responsible for color reception.*
2. *A sty is an infection of the glands of the eyelids; conjunctivitis is an inflammation of the conjunctiva, the mucous membrane that covers the sclera and cornea.*
3. *Four common refractive errors are hyperopia (farsightedness), myopia (nearsightedness), astigmatism (unfocused refraction of light rays on the retina), and presbyopia (age-related vision changes).*
4. *The tumbling E chart is used for patients who cannot read or who do not speak English.*
5. *The cochlea transmits sounds waves into nerve impulses and the semicircular canals aid balance and coordination.*
6. *Conductive hearing loss stops the flow of sound wave vibrations in the area before the cochlea. Perceptual hearing loss stops the flow of nerve impulses from the cochlea to the brain.*
7. *An audiometer is used to detect hearing loss. The patient listens for pure tones of various decibel levels and various frequencies. The results of the test are recorded by the audiometer on a special graph.*
8. *Cilia are small, hairlike projections covering virtually all surfaces of the nasal structures. They move secretions along to the throat for swallowing.*
9. *Hypertension, malignancies, polyps, and the fragile capillaries associated with pregnancy are factors that contribute to epistaxis.*
10. *Physiologic pain is caused by an organic disorder; psychological pain is perceived by the patient without the presence of an identifiable source.*

Critical Thinking Challenges

Pamela Martin calls your general practice office on Monday regarding her son Brian, age 8. She states that on Saturday, he began having a runny nose and sore throat. His temperature was only 99.4°F, so she has been giving him acetaminophen every 4 hours. This morning he awoke screaming and tugging at his right ear and has a temperature of 102.4°F.

As you decide how to handle this call, consider the following questions:

1. Would you see the child today or schedule him on Tuesday because Mondays are extremely busy?
2. On what facts would you base your decision?
3. Would you seat the child in the waiting room with other patients? What factors would influence this decision?
4. What pieces of equipment would you have prepared for the child's examination and why?

Suggestions for Further Reading

Memmler, R. L., Cohen, B. J., & Wood, D. L. (1996). *The Human Body in Health and Disease,* 8th ed. Philadelphia: Lippincott-Raven.

Professional Guide to Diseases, 4th ed. (1992). Springhouse, PA: Springhouse.

Rosdahl, C. B. (1995). *Textbook of Basic Nursing,* 6th ed. Philadelphia: J.B. Lippincott.

Scherer, J. C., & Timby, B. K. (1995). *Introductory Medical-Surgical Nursing,* 6th ed. Philadelphia: J.B. Lippincott.

Smeltzer, S., & Bare, B. (1996). *Brunner and Suddarth's Textbook of Medical-Surgical Nursing,* 8th ed. Philadelphia: Lippincott-Raven.

Timby, B. K. (1996). *Fundamental Skills and Concepts in Patient Care,* 6th ed. Philadelphia: Lippincott-Raven.

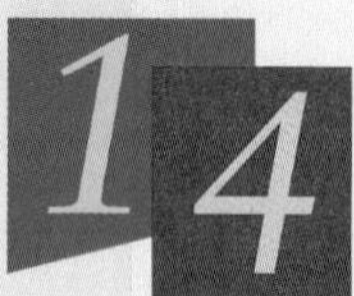

Assisting With Diagnostic and Therapeutic Procedures Associated With the Endocrine System

Chapter Outline

Role Delineation

CLINICAL

Fundamental Principles

- Apply principles of aseptic technique and infection control.

Diagnostic Orders

- Collect and process specimens.
- Perform diagnostic tests.

Patient Care

- Assist with examinations, procedures, and treatments.

GENERAL

Professionalism

- Project a professional manner and image.

Communication Skills

- Treat all patients with compassion and empathy.

Legal Concepts

- Practice within the scope of education, training, and personal capabilities.

Instruction

- Teach methods of health promotion and disease prevention.

Chapter Competencies

Learning Objectives

Upon successfully completing this chapter, you will be able to:

1. Spell and define the Key Terms.
2. Locate and identify the glands of the endocrine system.
3. State the hormones secreted by each gland, their actions, and their target tissues.
4. Identify abnormal conditions resulting from deficient and excessive hormone secretions.
5. Identify abbreviations, laboratory tests, and clinical procedures related to endocrinology.
6. State current treatments for common endocrine disorders.

Key Terms

(See Glossary for definitions.)

Addison's disease
corticoids
cretinism
diabetes insipidus
dwarfism
endemic
eunuchoidism
exophthalmic goiter
gigantism
goiter
glucocorticoids
glycosuria
Graves' disease
hormones
hypercalcemia
hyperglycemia
hyperplasia
hypoglycemia
insulin-dependent diabetes mellitus (IDDM)
ketoacidosis
ketones
myxedema
non–insulin-dependent diabetes mellitus (NIDDM)
polydipsia
polyphagia
polyuria
pruritus
radioimmunoassay
tetany
thyrotoxicosis
vasopressin

Together with the nervous system, the endocrine system regulates body functions. Although the control exerted by the nervous system is immediate and directed at a particular (usually short-term) response, the endocrine system regulates chemical metabolism for a longer-acting, more widespread response. **Hormones** are the chemical regulators, or messengers, of the endocrine glands. Some hormones stimulate system-wide metabolic processes; others are specific for a particular tissue.

The endocrine glands differ from the body's other glands (exocrine glands) because they are ductless, secreting hormones directly into the bloodstream for transmission rather than requiring direct access to the target tissue. Hormones circulate through the bloodstream to act on target tissues and exert specific regulatory effects.

Homeostatic regulation keeps hormone levels within certain ranges. Negative feedback alerts endocrine glands to the need for increased or decreased secretion. Some glands operate within a limited range to maintain almost constant hormonal levels; other glands function by cyclic or rhythmic fluctuations, as exemplified by estrogen and progesterone release during the menstrual cycle.

STRUCTURE AND FUNCTION OF THE ENDOCRINE SYSTEM

The glands of the endocrine system include:

- Pituitary
- Thyroid
- Parathyroids
- Thymus
- Adrenals
- Pancreas
- Gonads

The pineal body is also included in the endocrine system, although some sources do not consider it technically a gland (Fig. 14-1).

A description of each gland and its particular regulatory role follows. Table 14-1 lists the glands and provides a summary of their principal functions.

Pituitary

The pituitary gland (also known as the hypophysis) is the master gland and is responsible for controlling many components of the endocrine system. It is located at the base of the brain, protected in a saddle-like bone structure called the sella turcica, just beneath the hypothalamus. It is a small, bilobed gland, with the anterior lobe forming the largest portion of the gland.

The pituitary is controlled by the hypothalamus through a connection called the infundibulum. The anterior lobe of the pituitary is responsible for the majority of the body's hormonal control. The posterior lobe is a storage area for two hormones that are produced in the hypothalamus and retained within the lobe until needed. Several pituitary hormones act directly on target tissue or organs to produce the necessary reaction. Others, called tropic hormones, stimulate the target tissue or organs to secrete hormones from within the local tissues (Fig. 14-2).

Anterior Lobe

The pituitary's anterior lobe secretes a number of hormones. Human growth hormone (GH or HGH), also known as somatotropin hormone, stimulates growth by promoting protein metabolism. Growth is stimulated until the epiphyseal ends of the long bones have sealed. (See Chap 11, Assisting With Procedures Associated With the Musculoskeletal System, for more information on long bones and bone growth.) The hormone then acts to ensure proper tissue replacement and repair.

Gonadotropic hormones include luteinizing hormone (LH), interstitial cell-stimulating hormone (ICSH), and follicle-stimulating hormone (FSH). LH acts on ovarian tissue to stimulate ovulation, to develop the corpus luteum, and to liberate progesterone in the female. ICSH stimulates the interstitial cells of the testes to produce testosterone. In females, FSH acts on the ovarian follicles to stimulate the production of estrogen and growth of the ova. In males, FSH acts on the tissue of the testes to initiate sperm production.

Thyroid-stimulating hormone (TSH) functions to maintain the thyroid gland and stimulates it to produce the thyroid hormones.

Adrenocorticotropic hormone (ACTH or corticotropin) stimulates the secretion of adrenal corticosteroids by the adrenal cortex.

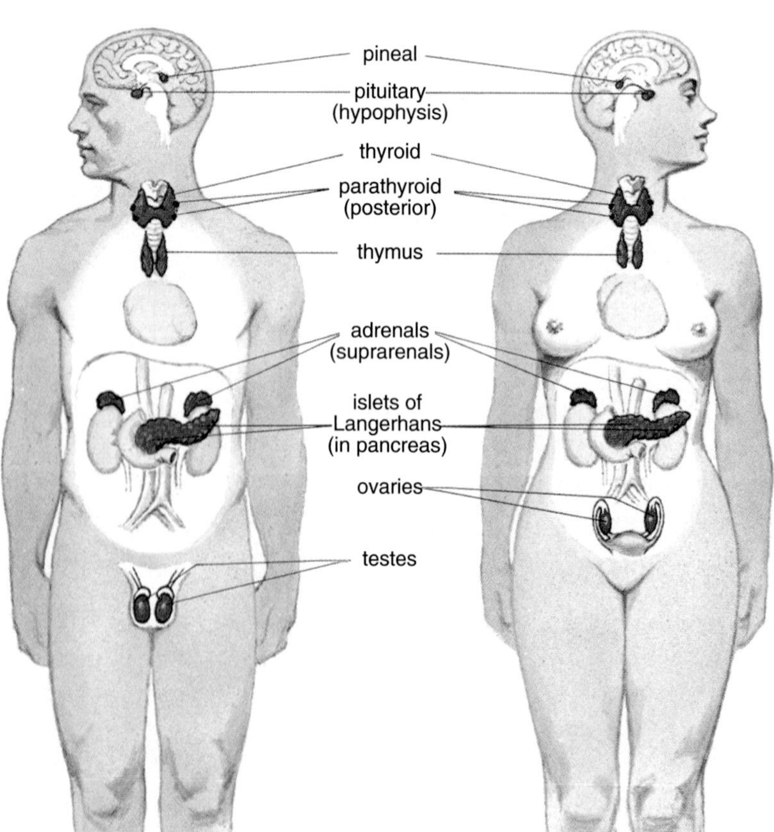

Figure 14-1 The main hormone-secreting organs.

Table 14-1 **The Major Endocrine Glands and Their Hormones**

Gland	*Hormone*	*Principal Functions*
Anterior pituitary	growth hormone (GH)	Promotes growth of all body tissues
	thyroid-stimulating hormone (TSH)	Stimulates thyroid gland to produce thyroid hormones
	adrenocorticotropic hormone (ACTH)	Stimulates adrenal cortex to produce cortical hormones; aids in protecting body in stress situations (injury, pain)
	prolactin (PRL)	Stimulates secretion of milk by mammary glands
	follicle-stimulating hormone (FSH)	Stimulates growth and hormone activity of ovarian follicles; stimulates growth of testes; promotes development of sperm cells
	luteinizing hormone (LH); interstitial cell-stimulating hormone (ICSH) in males	Causes development of corpus luteum at site of ruptured ovarian follicle in female; stimulates secretion of testosterone in male
Posterior pituitary	antidiuretic hormone; vasopressin (ADH)	Promotes reabsorption of water in kidney tubules; stimulates smooth muscle tissue of blood vessels to constrict
	Oxytocin	Causes contraction of muscle of uterus; causes ejection of milk from mammary glands
Thyroid	Thyroid hormone (thyroxine and triiodothyronine)	Increases metabolic rate, influencing both physical and mental activities; required for normal growth
	Calcitonin	Decreases calcium level in blood
Parathyroids	Parathyroid hormone	Regulates exchange of calcium between blood and bones; increases calcium level in blood
Adrenal medulla	Epinephrine and norepinephrine	Increases blood pressure and heart rate; activates cells influenced by sympathetic nervous system plus many not affected by sympathetic nerves
Adrenal cortex	Cortisol (95% of glucocorticoids)	Aids in metabolism of carbohydrates, proteins, and fats; active during stress
	Aldosterone (95% of mineralocorticoids)	Aids in regulating electrolytes and water balance
	Sex hormones	May influence secondary sexual characteristics in male
Pancreatic islets	Insulin	Aids transport of glucose into cells; required for cellular metabolism of foods, especially glucose; decreases blood sugar levels
	Glucagon	Stimulates liver to release glucose, thereby increasing blood sugar levels
Testes	Testosterone	Stimulates growth and development of male sexual organs (testes, penis, others) plus development of secondary sexual characteristics, such as hair growth on body and face and deepening of voice; stimulates maturation of sperm cells
Ovaries	Estrogens (eg, estradiol)	Stimulate growth of primary female sexual organs (eg, uterus, tubes) and development of secondary sexual organs, such as breasts, plus changes in pelvis to ovoid, broader shape
	Progesterone	Stimulates development of secretory parts of mammary glands; prepares uterine lining for implantation of fertilized ovum; aids in maintaining pregnancy

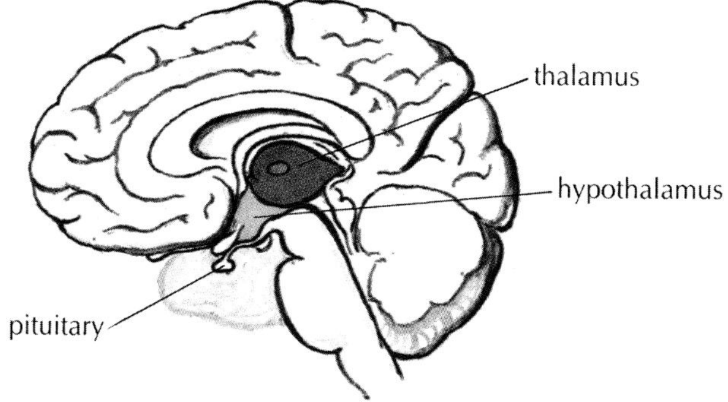

Figure 14-2 Diagram showing the relationship among the thalamus, hypothalamus, and pituitary (hypophysis).

Prolactin controls proliferation of the mammary glands and stimulates milk production.

Melanocyte-stimulating hormone controls the intensity of skin pigmentation.

Posterior Lobe

The two hormones stored in the pituitary's posterior lobe are oxytocin and antidiuretic hormone (ADH) (Fig. 14-3).

Oxytocin promotes contractions of the uterine muscle during labor and involution (the return to a pre-pregnancy state after delivery). In the postpartum period, oxytocin also affects the mammary glands and causes the "let down" reflex or ejection of milk.

14

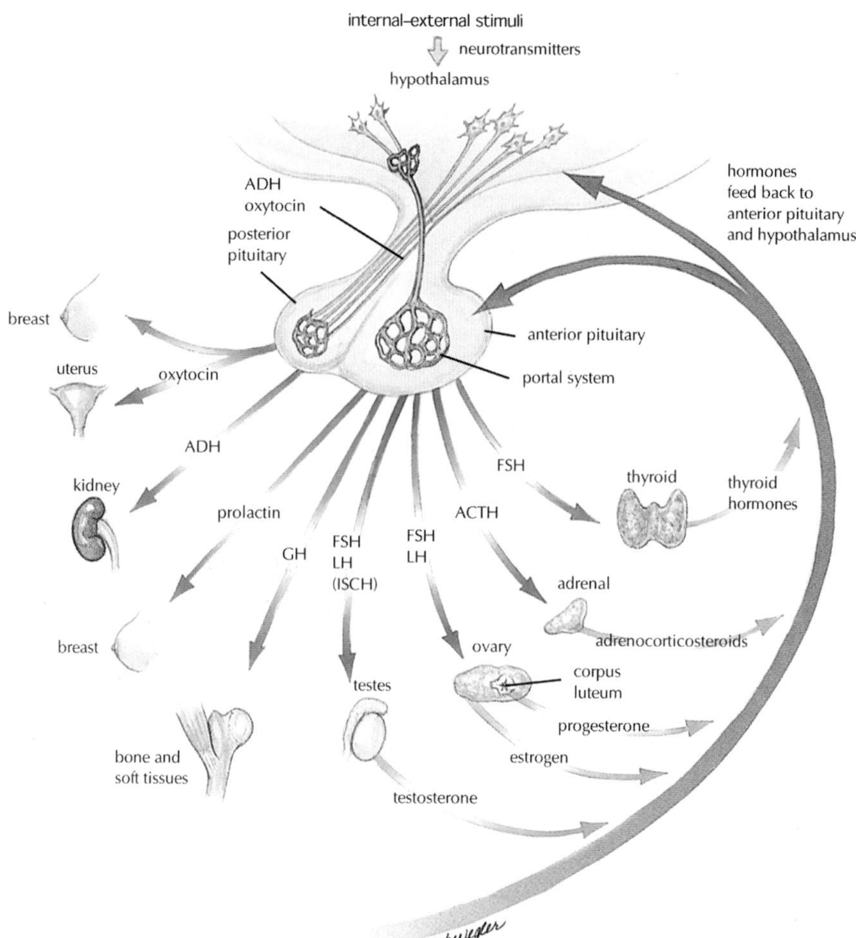

Figure 14-3 Pituitary gland and its relations with the brain and target tissues. Hypothalamic-releasing hormones influence the anterior pituitary gland through a portal system. Tropic hormones from the anterior pituitary affect the working of various other glands. The hypothalamus communicates with the posterior pituitary through tracts.

Also known as **vasopressin,** ADH increases reabsorption of water by the kidneys.

Checkpoint Question

1. *What are the responsibilities of the anterior and posterior lobes of the pituitary gland?*

Thyroid

The thyroid is a yellowish or amber-red shield-shaped organ located in the neck near the junction of the larynx and trachea. It consists of two lateral lobes that lie on either side of the trachea and are connected by an isthmus (narrow connection) that crosses anterior to the second and third tracheal rings. The blood supply to the thyroid is extremely rich; more blood flows through this gland in proportion to its size than through any of the body's other organs.

Iodine is essential to the production of the three thyroid hormones:

- Thyroxine (T_4)
- Triiodothyronine (T_3)
- Calcitonin

The thyroid hormones T_4 and T_3 are iodine-containing amino acids that stimulate cellular metabolism and promote growth. Their primary action is regulating the metabolic rate. They directly increase the rate of oxidation of foodstuffs within the cells, accelerating the rate of sugar absorption and directing the liver to convert glycogen to glucose as needed for energy. They also regulate mineral and protein metabolism to supply energy needed for cell growth and maintenance of life functions.

Calcitonin inhibits the release of calcium and phosphates from the bones to the blood, thereby decreasing the circulating calcium. In balance with the parathyroid hormone (see below), calcitonin maintains blood and bone calcium composition. Calcitonin is essential for normal bone development, for maintaining the balance of calcium available for impulse transmission in the nervous and muscular systems, and for clot development in the circulatory system.

Checkpoint Question

2. *How does the thyroid affect blood calcium levels? Name the hormone involved.*

Parathyroids

There are usually four parathyroids, two on each side, situated on and more or less intimately connected with the posterior thyroid. (The actual number of parathyroids can range from 2 to 10.) The parathyroids produce parathormone, also known as the parathyroid hormone (PTH).

Parathyroid hormone has a vital role in metabolizing calcium and phosphorus and regulating calcium in blood and tissues. It has two target sites:

1. Kidneys—PTH promotes the renal excretion of phosphate by decreasing reabsorption, thereby causing the serum phosphorus levels to decrease.
2. Bone tissue—PTH causes bone tissue to break down through increased osteoclastic activity. This breaking down of bone cells is necessary to return stored calcium to the general circulation when blood calcium levels are low.

It is vital that the parathyroids work together with the thyroid (calcitonin) to maintain bone strength. If either gland malfunctions, bone health and available calcium will be compromised.

Checkpoint Question

3. *What does PTH do at its two target sites?*

Thymus

The thymus is composed of two elongated, flask-shaped lobes, which occupy a region just above the heart where the chest cavity narrows at the base of the neck. The two glands are joined to one another by connective tissue, which also covers each gland, forming a distinct capsule around the inner mass of lymphoid tissue.

The thymus is a prominent organ at birth and reaches its greatest size at puberty, after which it undergoes a gradual regression. During regression, the thymic tissue is usually replaced by fat, so that the adult thymus is composed largely of fat and connective tissue. The thymus is believed to be vital to the development of the immune response in children. It produces thymosin, which is most important in the production and maturation of lymphocytes and the development of immunity.

Adrenals

The adrenals, also referred to as the suprarenal glands, are two pyramid-shaped structures lying close to the upper pole of the kidneys. The two glands usually differ somewhat in size, and there is also a difference in size between the glands in men and women. Each gland consists of two functionally distinct parts:

- Medulla—the central portion of the gland, which is closely associated with the central nervous system
- Cortex—a surrounding zone of tissue, which comprises eight to nine times the volume of the medulla

The functions of the adrenal medulla and adrenal cortex are completely unrelated.

Adrenal Medulla

The only function of the adrenal medulla is the secretion of epinephrine (adrenaline) and norepinephrine (noradrenaline) in response to sympathetic nervous system stimulation. Epinephrine is secreted in response to need, as in the fright-flight-fight syndrome. (See Chap. 12, Assisting With Diagnostic and Therapeutic Procedures Associated With the Neurologic System, for more information.) It has cardiovascular effects, exerting a constricting action on arteries, veins, and capillaries. The vasomotor effect, however, is not the same in all areas. For example, the blood vessels of the brain and muscles react only slightly to epinephrine, whereas those of the adrenal glands, thyroid, and placenta do not react at all.

Epinephrine's effects include:

- Contraction of arterioles, which increases blood pressure
- Conversion of glycogen stored in the liver to glucose, which is rushed to muscle tissue for energy
- Increased heart rate, which results in more blood for emergency response
- Increased cellular metabolism, which boosts energy output
- Dilation of the bronchi, which supplies more oxygen for metabolism
- Decreased intestinal movement and activity and contraction of the cardiac, pyloric, ileocecal, and anal sphincters
- Increased numbers of blood components and lymphocytes.

Because epinephrine mimics the effect of the sympathetic nervous system, it is often referred to as a sympathomimetic substance. Norepinephrine is also a product of the adrenal medulla and is produced in response to stressors.

Adrenal Cortex

The adrenal cortex affects almost all body systems and is necessary to maintain life. Excision of the adrenal medulla is not fatal. However, complete removal of both adrenals, with loss of the cortical hormones, leads to death in a short time. Approximately 28 steroid hormones have been separated from cortical extracts, but only 6 or 7 have been identified by their physiologic activity. These are called **corticoids** and their effects are called "corticoid effects."

Glucocorticoids regulate conversion of amino acids to maintain a carbohydrate reserve for energy. These hormones use sugar in times of stress for immediate energy and rely on carbohydrates for longer-term energy needs. They help suppress inflammation and may be used to treat acute or chronic inflammatory processes. Hydrocortisone made from the glucocorticoid cortisol is widely used for this purpose.

Mineralocorticoids help regulate electrolyte balance. They target the kidneys to control the sodium reabsorption and potassium secretion. Aldosterone is this group's major hormone.

The sex hormones arise from the adrenal cortex and assist estrogen and testosterone in establishing secondary sexual characteristics.

Checkpoint Question

4. *How do the functions of the adrenal medulla and adrenal cortex differ?*

Pancreas

The pancreas is located in the upper left quadrant of the abdominal cavity, extending from the curve of the duodenum to the spleen. The pancreas functions in both the gastrointestinal and endocrine systems. The bulk of the pancreas produces an external secretion, or enzyme, concerned with digestion. Within the pancreas are groups of cells—called the islets of Langerhans—that produce two endocrine hormones. The islets of Langerhans contain alpha and beta cells. Alpha cells produce glucagon, and beta cells produce insulin.

Glucagon stimulates the liver to change glycogen to glucose and to increase fat conversion and amino acid production for use as energy. The process, called gluconeogenesis, is the conversion of excess amino acids into simple carbohydrates that may aid cell respiration. The overall effect of glucagon is to raise the blood glucose level and to make energy stores available for metabolic needs. Glucagon secretion is stimulated by **hypoglycemia** (low blood glucose level).

Insulin production is stimulated by **hyperglycemia** (high blood glucose level). Insulin secretion removes glucose from the circulation and facilitates its transfer through cell membranes. Insulin increases the liver's ability to convert excess sugar into fatty acids for storage as fat cells. The effect of insulin is to lower blood glucose levels.

Checkpoint Question

5. *How is glucagon secretion stimulated, and what are its effects?*

Pineal Body

Situated within the brain, this glandlike structure is fairly large in children but, like the thymus, diminishes with age. The main purpose of the pineal body seems to be the production of the hormone melatonin, which is thought to play a part in the onset of puberty. Melatonin levels decrease in the presence of daylight and increase at night. This fluctuation is thought to be responsible for our diurnal rhythms that urge us to sleep at night and to awaken with daylight.

Gonads

The gonads include the ovaries and the testes. The ovaries are located in the pelvic cavity on each side of the uterus. The testes are located in the scrotum, a sac of skin between the upper thighs. (See Chap. 20, Male Reproductive System, and Chap. 21, Female Reproductive System, for more information about these organs.)

In the ovaries, estrogen (estradiol) is produced by the follicle cells. Estrogen stimulates:

- Maturation of the ova
- Proliferation of blood vessels in the endometrium
- Development of secondary sexual characteristics
- Growth of the duct system of the mammary glands
- Growth of the uterus
- Disposition of fat subcutaneously in the hips and thighs

Estrogen also promotes the closure of the epiphyses of the long bones and is believed to lower blood levels of cholesterol and triglycerides. Estrogen gets its stimulus from the anterior pituitary's FSH. Progesterone prepares and maintains the uterus during pregnancy.

In the testes, testosterone is produced by the interstitial cells in response to the anterior pituitary's ICSH. Testosterone promotes maturation of sperm in the testes. Testosterone stimulates:

- Development of secondary sexual characteristics
- Growth of the reproductive organs
- Production of facial and body hair
- Lengthening of the larynx and the deepening of the voice
- Development of the skeletal muscles

Testosterone also brings about closure of the epiphyses of the long bones.

Table 14-2 classifies the many hormones produced by the endocrine glands according to their various functions.

Table 14-2 **Functional Classification of Hormones**

Function	*Hormone*	*Major Source*
Control of water and electrolyte metabolism	Aldosterone	Adrenal cortex
	Antidiuretic hormone (ADH)	Posterior pituitary
	Calcitonin	C cells, thyroid
	Parathyroid hormone	Parathyroid
	Angiotensin	Kidney
Control of gastrointestinal function	Cholecystokinin	Gastrointestinal tract
	Gastrin	Gastrointestinal tract
	Secretin	Gastrointestinal tract
Regulation of energy, metabolism, and growth	Glucagon	Alpha cells, pancreatic islets
	Insulin	Beta cells, pancreatic islets
	Growth hormone	Anterior pituitary
	Thyroid hormones	Thyroid gland
Neurotransmitters	Dopamine	Central nervous system
	Epinephrine	Adrenal medulla
	Norepinephrine	Adrenal medulla and nervous system
Reproductive function	Chorionic gonadotropins	Placenta
	Estrogens	Ovary
	Oxytocin	Posterior pituitary
	Progesterone	Ovary
	Prolactin	Anterior pituitary
	Testosterone	Testes
Stress and control of inflammation	Glucocorticoids	Adrenal cortex
Tropic hormones (regulation of other hormone levels)	Adrenocorticotropic hormone (ACTH)	Anterior pituitary
	Follicle-stimulating hormone (FSH)	Anterior pituitary
	Luteinizing hormone (LH)	Anterior pituitary
	Thyroid-stimulating hormone (TSH)	Anterior pituitary

14

COMMON ENDOCRINE DISORDERS

Because many normal body processes depend on appropriate hormone levels, either a deficiency (hyposecretion) or excess (hypersecretion) of hormones can result in altered functioning.

Hypopituitarism

Hypopituitarism is a deficiency of the anterior pituitary hormones. It may be caused by injury or atrophy of the gland, or it may result from certain types of tumors.

Hypopituitarism that occurs before puberty is manifested chiefly by a retarded growth rate. If it begins very early in life, the patient will be extremely short but will retain normal body proportions. This condition is termed pituitary **dwarfism** and is not to be confused with achondroplastic dwarfism, an incurable genetic abnormality that results in very short limbs, a large head, and a long trunk. Because GH can be produced using genetic engineering, it can be used to stimulate growth in children with pituitary dwarfism.

Other hormonal deficiencies caused by hyposecretion of the pituitary can be treated with specific replacement therapy.

Adult hypopituitarism may be classified according to whether the various anterior pituitary hormones are selectively or completely deficient. If all the hormones are deficient, for example, the condition is called panhypopituitarism. If a selective deficiency exists, the condition is named for the specific deficiency. For instance, a deficiency in the gonadotropic hormones will lead to **eunuchoidism** (loss of secondary sexual characteristics) in the male. These deficiencies will respond to replacement therapy.

Hyperpituitarism

Hyperpituitarism is marked by excess production of HGH. If this occurs during childhood or adolescence, the result is a form of hyperpituitarism called **gigan-**

tism (excessive size and stature). Normally, HGH is active only up to the time of maturity, when the epiphyseal lines on the long bones seal. Oversecretion of HGH increases bone length, and sometimes width, in excess of normal growth before closure of the epiphyses. In some instances, a suppression of gonadotropic hormones occurs. If this happens, the testes and adrenals in the male or the adrenals in the female do not develop as in normal puberty. Consequently, epiphyseal closure, which is dependent on the male hormone, fails to occur. The result is that the individual reaches a height of 7 or 8 feet.

Associated metabolic changes are attributed to a generalized pituitary hyperfunction. If the pituitary malfunctions in any of its responsibilities, it may malfunction in all areas, causing widespread pathology. If pituitary hyperfunction occurs near the end of puberty or in adulthood, after the epiphyseal closure, bone length does not change, but bone width increases; this is called acromegaly (Fig. 14-4). This form of hyperpituitarism results in a prominent jaw, enlargement of the nose, and unusual thickening of the hands, feet, and skin. Unusual hyperactivity of the pituitary gland is associated with a tumor of the gland. Treatment of acromegaly requires surgical removal of the tumor or its destruction by radiation.

Checkpoint Question

6. *How does hypopituitarism differ from hyperpituitarism?*

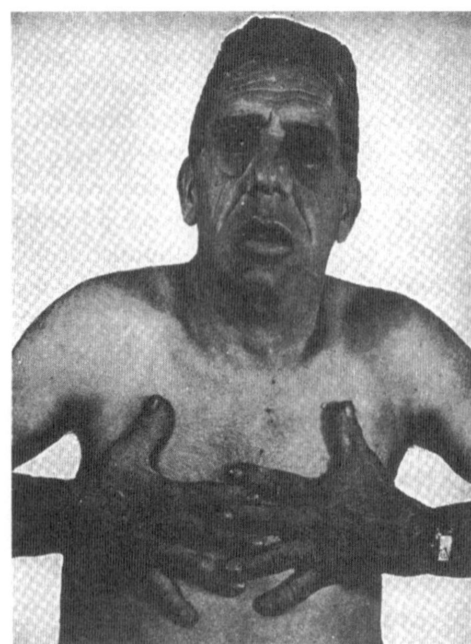

Figure 14-4 A patient with acromegaly.

Diabetes Insipidus

Diabetes insipidus results from hyposecretion (deficiency) of ADH in the posterior pituitary. Deficient ADH causes the renal tubules to reabsorb little of the water and salts, resulting in as much as 5 to 10 L of urine output a day (**polyuria**). Clinical symptoms also include **polydipsia** (excessive thirst) as the body tries to restore fluid balance. The cause is not usually known but may be due to head trauma or tumor formation. Treatment involves correction of the causative factor and the administration of synthetic ADH by injection or by nasal spray for vascular absorption.

Goiter

A dietary deficiency of iodine and certain other thyroid disorders are frequently accompanied by an enlargement of the gland, known as a **goiter.** Simple goiter is caused by insufficient dietary iodine. **Hyperplasia** (increased number of cells) is present, but there is neither inflammation nor malignancy. The condition does not lead to the thyrotoxic conditions associated with other thyroid pathologies. Simple goiter is **endemic,** occurring in areas in which the available supply of iodine in the drinking water and in the soil is low. In the United States, the areas of greatest concern are the Pacific Northwest, the Great Plains, the basin of the St. Lawrence River, and the Great Lakes region.

In simple goiter, there is no clinical syndrome because there is no hyposecretion or hypersecretion of the gland. The gland is essentially normal, capable of manufacturing a normal concentration of hormone if iodine is supplied in the diet. However, the gland may become so enlarged that it compresses the trachea and other structures located in the neck. Under these conditions, the goiter must be surgically removed. Generally, in the early stages of goiter development, supplemental iodine can reverse the glandular enlargement. The value of iodine used prophylactically against goiter is now generally accepted and recommended for all areas low in natural iodine. The most feasible method of administration has been the addition of sodium or potassium iodide to table salt.

Hypothyroidism

Hypothyroidism results from a deficiency of thyroid hormone secretion. It produces a number of symptoms depending on the degree of deficiency and the age at which it occurs.

In very early childhood, thyroid hormone deficiency leads to **cretinism,** a condition characterized by a low basal metabolic rate, slowed or retarded mental and physical development, slow heart rate, poor appetite, and constipation. The face is usually puffy with a characteristic apathetic expression (Fig. 14-5). The skin is dry, coarse, and pale yellow. Cretinism follows the incomplete development or congenital absence of the thyroid gland. It can be treated successfully if thyroid supplements are administered early in infancy. Treatment may be lifelong in many cases.

In later childhood, thyroid hormone deficiency results in childhood hypothyroidism or juvenile myxedema. This condition differs from cretinism in that it is not apparent as early in development. The severity of the symptoms depends primarily on the degree of thyroid activity and on the age at which the deficiency occurs. In general, the most characteristic symptoms are short, squatty stature; a head proportionately larger than normal for the child's age; a short, thick neck; puffiness and bloating around the face and eyes; a dull expression; dry, flaky skin; and a large tongue accompanied by drooling.

Treatment of childhood myxedema with thyroid supplements gives remarkable results. The outcome, however, depends on the degree of thyroid deficiency, the age at which treatment is begun, and the regularity with which it is continued.

In adults, hypothyroidism usually results from atrophy of the thyroid gland. Its progression may lead to **myxedema**, a condition characterized by expressionless, puffy, and pallid face; slowed mental and physical processes; dry, thick skin; and loss of hair and teeth. Sometimes, obesity and an undue sensitivity to cold are other signs. If not corrected, severe myxedema may lead to coma and death. The administration of adequate amounts of thyroid hormone usually results in a dramatic relief of all symptoms within 10 days of the start of treatment. With adequate continuous therapy, symptoms do not return.

If hypothyroidism is mild, a state of hypothyroidism without myxedema may exist. This is characterized chiefly by a lowered metabolic rate of variable degree.

Hyperthyroidism

The most common form of hyperthyroidism (hypersecretion of thyroid hormone) may also be known as Graves' disease (Fig. 14-6). The most characteristic symptoms are **exophthalmic goiter** (abnormal protrusion of the eyeballs accompanied by goiter), nervousness, irritability, purposeless movements, fatigue, loss of weight, increased heart rate, elevated metabolic rate, emotional instability, and increased body temperature with excessive perspiration. A severe form of hyperthyroidism is known as **thyrotoxicosis.** Treatment consists of medications that decrease thyroxine (T_4) secretion or administration of radioactive iodine. When radioactive iodine becomes concentrated in the gland, it depresses glandular activity and decreases the output of pituitary thyrotrophic hormone.

Checkpoint Question

7. *What are the characteristic symptoms of cretinism and Graves' disease?*

Hypoparathyroidism

This deficiency disorder is caused most commonly by accidental removal or injury of the parathyroid glands as a result of surgery on the thyroid. Degenerative disease of the glands may also occur. The symptoms most commonly associated with this condition are muscle weakness, irritability, and **tetany**—an abnormally in-

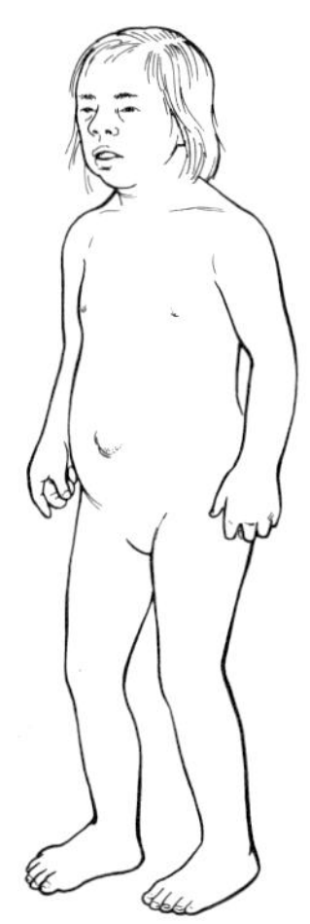

Figure 14-5 A patient with cretinism.

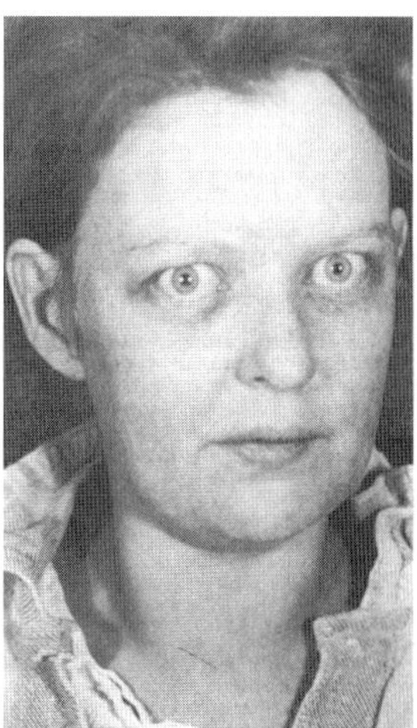

Figure 14-6 A woman with Graves' disease. Note the exophthalmos and enlarged thyroid gland.

creased sensitivity of the nervous system to external stimuli, resulting in painful muscle spasms. Tetany requires prompt injection of calcium salts, either intramuscularly or intravenously. Generally, hypoparathyroidism is treated by administration of calcium lactate.

Hyperparathyroidism

Excess PTH secretion is called hyperparathyroidism. It is usually due to a tumor of the gland. Hyperparathyroidism causes **hypercalcemia,** a release of excessive amounts of stored calcium into the bloodstream. As a result, polyuria usually occurs and may be the first and sometimes the only symptom of increased parathyroid activity. Kidney stones may form, and the decalcification of bones that usually occurs causes pain, deformities, and spontaneous fractures. The long bones and ribs may soften and bend. Occasionally, alterations in muscular function occur, including weakness and decreased response to stimulation.

Treatment of hyperparathyroidism usually involves surgical removal of the parathyroid tumor. After the surgery, the parathyroid deficiency that usually occurs requires calcium and vitamin D supplements.

14

What If?

A patient with Addison's disease is prescribed a course of hydrocortisone. What if you must assess the patient's understanding of the potential long-term effects of this medication?

Long-term cortisone therapy has many adverse effects, including increased risk for the development of cataracts and osteoporosis. The patient also is at high risk for developing secondary infection and must take care to minimize exposure to infectious diseases. Ensure that the patient has a clear understanding of dietary needs because long-term therapy may result in hypocalcemia, hypokalemia, and hypernatremia. Also assess the patient's understanding of signs and symptoms of gastric ulcers; steroid therapy is contraindicated for patients with existing gastric ulcers. Additionally, the patient should be cautioned against abruptly stopping this medication, but instead should follow the physician's orders to taper the dosage until the treatment has run its course.

Thymic Abnormalities

Pathology of the thymus gland is usually congenital. There is usually accompanying hypocalcemia with facial dysplasia, cardiac abnormalities, and early death. The only cure at this time is fetal thymic transplant.

Hypoadrenocorticalism

Degeneration of the adrenal cortex resulting in hypoadrenocorticalism (adrenal deficiency) is called **Addison's disease.** The symptoms of Addison's disease are skin hyperpigmentation, appetite loss, weight loss, weakness, hypotension, and anemia. Sodium loss due to decreased renal reabsorption occurs. Chloride and bicarbonate are lost, and potassium is retained. Changes in the ion concentration of the circulation cause water loss from the blood and the tissue spaces, resulting in severe dehydration and hemoconcentration. Addison's disease is treated with high doses of hydrocortisone.

Hyperadrenocorticalism

Hyperadrenocorticalism may be caused by hyperplasia of the adrenal cortex resulting from increased production of ACTH from the pituitary or by tumors of the cortex. Hyperadrenocorticalism is known as Cushing's syndrome. Excessive cortisol promotes fat deposits in the trunk of the body, with the extremities remaining thin. The skin is fragile and thin, and healing after injuries is slow. Osteoporosis is accelerated. The face is characteristically rounded. Cushing's syndrome may also be present in patients who are receiving corticosteroids for medical reasons. These patients may include transplant recipients and patients with severe asthma or rheumatoid arthritis. Treatment for hyperadrenocorticalism requires removal of the cause of the hypersecretion, which could be either a pituitary or an adrenal tumor.

Diabetes Mellitus

In the pancreas, dysfunction of the islets of Langerhans results in diabetes mellitus, a disorder of carbohydrate metabolism. It is characterized by hyperglycemia and **glycosuria** (glucose in the urine) resulting from inadequate insulin production or utilization.

The exact cause of diabetes mellitus is unknown, but it arises from failure of the beta cells in the islets of Langerhans to secrete adequate insulin. Some cases of diabetes mellitus can be attributed to a genetic predisposition, but it may also result from a deficiency of beta cells caused by inflammation, pancreatic cancer, or surgery. It is also thought to be an autoimmune disorder perhaps triggered by a virus.

There are two types of diabetes mellitus—**type I, insulin-dependent diabetes mellitus (IDDM)**, and **type II, non–insulin-dependent diabetes mellitus (NIDDM).**

Type I occurs most often in children and young adults. Onset of type I is abrupt, with symptoms such as polyuria, polydipsia, **polyphagia** (abnormal hunger),

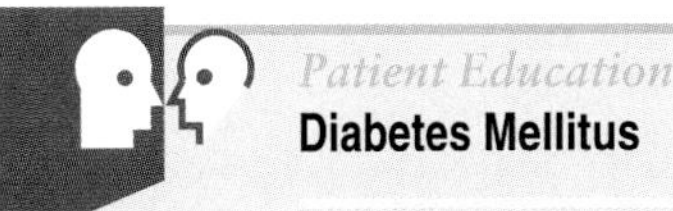

Patient Education

Diabetes Mellitus

All patients with diabetes mellitus should understand:

- The need for good hygiene (Opportunistic diseases are attracted to the high levels of sugar in the body.)
- Dietary management (Calorie intake must be regulated.)
- Proper foot care (Peripheral circulation is poor, and injuries or lesions heal slowly.)
- Proper dosage administration of insulin or an oral agent (Inaccuracies may result in shock or coma.)
- Proper disposal of insulin syringes (State laws regulate hazardous waste disposal.)
- How to test the blood correctly by a capillary puncture finger stick or the urine for glucose or ketones (Insulin is sometimes calibrated by the results of patient self-testing.)
- Signs and symptoms of insulin shock and diabetic ketoacidosis, and the procedure to follow if symptoms occur

Without insulin, the patient's blood glucose levels will remain high, and glucose will be lost in the urine. More water will be lost as well, resulting in polyuria and polydipsia. Ensure that patients recognize that although diabetes can be controlled, the long-term effects of hyperglycemia produce vascular changes. The capillary walls thicken, and the exchange of gases and nutrients diminishes. The effects of these circulatory changes can be seen in the retina, the kidneys, and the skin, particularly the feet. Uncontrolled diabetes can lead to blindness, dry gangrene, and severe kidney damage. Atherosclerosis is also common in non–insulin-dependent diabetes mellitus.

There are various support groups for diabetics. The American Diabetes Association has a broad selection of printed materials to help diabetic patients adjust to lifestyle changes. Type I diabetic individuals may need a support group to learn to incorporate medical compliance into their lives with as little disruption as possible.

weight loss, and **ketoacidosis**—acidosis accompanied by an accumulation of **ketones** (end products of fat metabolism) in the body. Insulin must be administered parenterally to control type I diabetes.

Type II occurs most often in adults over age 40. Onset of type II is gradual, with symptoms such as polyuria, polydipsia, **pruritus** (severe itching), and peripheral neuropathy. In this condition, insulin is produced but cannot exert its effect on cells because of a deficiency of insulin receptors on cell membranes. Risk factors are obesity and a family history of diabetes.

Control of type II diabetes may not require insulin. The patient is usually placed on a well-balanced diet, adequate in all basic essentials: carbohydrates, proteins, fats, vitamins, minerals, and fluids. Obese patients must be placed on a diet that will enable them to lose weight. Controlling diabetes is difficult in an obese person. When the patient is given an adequate diet and glucose still appears in the urine, insulin may be required. Oral drugs that enable insulin to react with the remaining cell membrane receptors have been used successfully in middle-aged and older patients.

As the medical assistant, you must help patients understand their disease by instructing them about possible complications and treatments available.

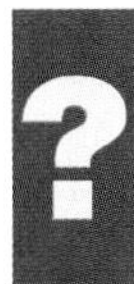

Checkpoint Question

8. *How would you describe the difference between diabetes mellitus and diabetes insipidus?*

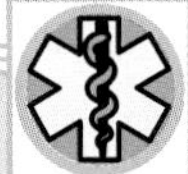

Action **STAT!**

Insulin Shock

Scenario: At 11:30 AM, Ms. Maria Sefferin arrives at the office for her routine monthly examination. You know that she was diagnosed with insulin-dependent diabetes fairly recently. She tells you that she feels shaky, weak, and lightheaded. She appears pale and is sweating. What should you do?

1. Recognize that these are signs of insulin shock, and quickly place Ms. Sefferin in an examining room.
2. Notify the physician immediately.
3. Instruct a coworker to get a glass of orange juice, sugar packet, or an instant glucose tube for Ms. Sefferin.
4. Obtain a quick glucose meter reading of her blood sugar. However, if this cannot be done promptly, administer the sugar immediately and obtain the glucose reading as quickly as possible. Enlist a coworker to help manage this crisis.
5. As you assess Ms. Sefferin's blood sugar and administer sugar, ask her exactly when she last took insulin, the amount and type of insulin she took, and the last time she ate and the amount consumed.
6. After Ms. Sefferin is stabilized, instruct her on ways to prevent future episodes and how to respond if this happens again.
7. Document the incident and all patient education in Ms. Sefferin's chart.

Diabetic Ketoacidosis

Ketoacidosis is a serious problem for patients with IDDM. When glucose cannot be used for energy, the body turns to fats and proteins, which the liver converts to ketones. Ketones accumulate in the blood because the cells cannot use them rapidly; as these organic acids build up, they lower the pH of the blood. The kidneys will excrete excess ketones, but in doing so, will excrete more water. This excess secretion of water will lead to dehydration, worsening the acidosis.

14

The administration of insulin is necessary to permit the use of glucose for energy. Intravenous fluids are used to restore blood volume to normal. If left untreated, ketoacidosis will progress to coma and death.

Checkpoint Question

9. *In diabetic ketoacidosis, what happens when the kidneys excrete excess ketones?*

Diabetic Coma and Insulin Shock

Diabetic coma results from lack of insulin. This condition causes metabolic changes with excess production of ketone bodies. Insulin shock occurs from an overdose or overproduction of insulin. This results in blood sugar levels well below normal. Skipping a meal without adjusting insulin levels will also result in insulin shock. Table 14-3 provides a comparison of these two disorders.

Table 14-3 **Comparison of Diabetic Coma and Insulin Shock**

	Diabetic Coma	*Insulin Shock*
Onset	Gradual	Sudden
Skin	Flushed, dry	Pale, moist
Tongue	Dry or furred	Moist
Breath	Smell of acetone	No change
Thirst	Intense	Absent
Respiration	Deep	Shallow
Vomiting	Common	Rare
Pulse	Rapid, feeble	Rapid, bounding
Urine	Glucose and acetone present	No glucose or acetone
Blood glucose	Elevated (>200 mg/dL)	Subnormal (20–50 mg/dL)
Blood pressure	Low	Normal
Abdominal pain	Common, often acute	Absent

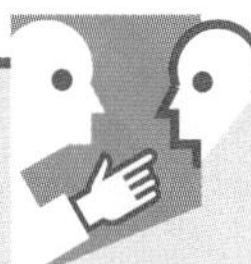

Advice and Tips

Monitoring Elderly Diabetic Patients

Frail, elderly diabetic patients who live alone require special attention. These patients are at high risk for insulin shock or coma. They may tend to measure their insulin incorrectly due to poor vision, forget to take their insulin, or forget to eat after taking their insulin.

Assess each patient's ability with each office visit because conditions may deteriorate between scheduled visits. For example, ask the patient what time of day insulin is taken, how much is taken, how it is administered, when food is eaten, and how often blood sugar levels are checked. To determine the patient's ability to self-administer insulin, ask the patient to demonstrate how medications are drawn up. Look at the amount of medication in the syringe; it is not uncommon to see errors.

Home health nurses may be able to help monitor compliance. Often, home health services will prefill and label syringes for patients for each day until the next visit. Some forms of insulin can be administered in special syringes that allow only a preset amount of insulin to be injected. Diabetic patients may benefit from installation of Lifeline boxes in the home. Check with your local hospital or pharmacy for your community resources.

Gonadal Abnormalities

Pathologies of the gonads occur in malignancies, in pituitary malfunctions, and in genetic anomalies. Sexual dysfunction is the usual result in cases of nonmalignant gonadal pathology. Specific disorders of the gonads are discussed in Chapter 20, Male Reproductive System, and Chapter 21, Female Reproductive System.

COMMON LABORATORY TESTS AND DIAGNOSTIC PROCEDURES AND THE MEDICAL ASSISTANT'S ROLE

Through various laboratory tests and diagnostic procedures, the physician can identify endocrine disorders so that treatment may be initiated.

Tests of blood and urine can be used to measure hormone levels (Table 14-4). For example, a glucose tolerance test (GTT) measures the glucose levels in a blood sample from a fasting patient and in specimens taken at intervals of 30 minutes, 1 hour, 2 hours, and 3 hours after the ingestion of a measured dose of glucose. Delayed return of blood glucose to normal levels indicates diabetes mellitus.

Table 14-4 **Serum Tests for Diagnosing Endocrine Disorders**

Serum tests for	*Help Diagnose Disorders of the*
Follicle-stimulating hormone (FSH), growth hormone (GH), thyroid-stimulating hormone (TSH), luteinizing hormone (LH), and prolactin	Anterior pituitary
T_3, T_4	Thyroid
Calcium, parathyroid hormone (PTH)	Parathyroids
Corticoids	Adrenal cortex
Glucose, insulin	Pancreas
Estradiol	Ovaries

Urinary hormone excretion can be measured using a 24-hour urine sample. (Because of fluctuations in hormonal activity, STAT specimens or one-time specimens may not contain the substances necessary for a diagnosis of the presenting condition.)

As the medical assistant, you may be responsible for obtaining the blood and urine samples necessary for these two tests and for actually performing the procedures. Chapter 28, Urinalysis, includes the procedure for obtaining a 24-hour urine specimen and performing various urine tests. Chapter 29, Phlebotomy, explains the procedure for obtaining a blood specimen. Chapter 32, Clinical Chemistry, discusses the steps for performing a GTT.

Thyroid function tests measure the levels of thyroxine (T_4), triiodothyronine (T_3), and TSH in the blood. Table 14-5 shows thyroid hormone levels for several abnormal conditions. During a thyroid scan, a radioactive compound is administered and localizes in the thyroid gland. The gland is then visualized with a scanner device to detect tumors or nodules. Radioactive iodine uptake is a procedure in which iodine is administered orally, and its absorption into the thyroid gland is measured as evidence of thyroid function.

Radioimmunoassay measures hormone levels in plasma by introducing radioactive substances into the body. The test is based on the ability of antibodies to bind specifically to radioactively labeled hormone molecules and to nonradioactive molecules.

Computed tomography scans provide transverse views of the pituitary and other endocrine glands and are used in the diagnosis of pathologic conditions. Ultrasonography is used to identify pancreatic, adrenal, and thyroid masses.

Table 14-5 **Thyroid Hormone Levels in Abnormal Conditions**

	T_3	T_4	*TSH*
Hyperthyroidism			
Hyperthyroidism or thyrotoxicosis	↑	↓	Normal/↑/↓
Graves' disease	↑	↑	Normal/↑/↓
Hypothyroidism			
Cretinism	↓	↓	Normal/↓
Endemic goiter	Normal/↑	Normal/↓	Normal/↑
Myxedema	↓	↓	↑

↓, decreased hormone levels; ↑, increased hormone levels; T_3, triiodothyronine; T_4, thyroxine.

Answers to Checkpoint Questions

1. *The anterior lobe of the pituitary is responsible for most of the body's hormonal control. The posterior lobe stores two hormones that are produced in the hypothalamus.*
2. *The thyroid gland produces calcitonin, a hormone that inhibits the release of calcium and phosphates from the bones to the blood, thereby decreasing the amount of calcium in the circulation.*
3. *In the kidneys, PTH promotes the renal excretion of phosphate by decreasing reabsorption, thereby causing the serum phosphorus levels to decrease. In bone tissue, PTH causes bone cells to break down through increased osteoclastic activity.*
4. *The adrenal medulla has only one function: to secrete epinephrine and norepinephrine in response to sympathetic nervous system stimulation. In contrast, the adrenal cortex affects nearly all body systems and is essential for life.*
5. *Hypoglycemia (low blood glucose level) stimulates the secretion of glucagon, which raises the blood glucose level and makes energy stores available for metabolic needs.*
6. *Hypopituitarism is an undersecretion of the anterior pituitary hormones; hyperpituitarism is marked by excess secretion of growth hormone.*
7. *Cretinism is characterized by low basal metabolic rate, slowed or retarded mental and physical development, slow heart rate, poor appetite, and constipation. In Graves' disease, the most characteristic symptoms are exophthalmic goiter, nervousness, irritability, purposeless movements, fatigue, weight loss, increased heart rate, elevated metabolic rate, emotional instability, and increased body temperature.*
8. *Diabetes mellitus involves dysfunction of the islets of Langerhans in the pancreas and is a metabolic disorder. Diabetes insipidus involves dysfunction of ADH in the posterior pituitary.*
9. *When the kidneys excrete excess ketones, more water also is excreted. This excess secretion of water will lead to dehydration, worsening the acidosis.*

Critical Thinking Challenges

1. While performing a complete physical examination, the physician will palpate the patient's neck. Identify the gland that is located here, then explain why the physician would palpate it.
2. Your patient has recently been diagnosed with asthma and will need to use an inhaler. Consider the sympathomimetic effects of epinephrine. What symptoms might you expect the patient to exhibit?

Suggestions for Further Reading

Burke, S. (1992). *Human Anatomy in Health and Disease,* 3rd ed. Albany, NY: Delmar.

Memmler, R., Cohen, B., & Wood, D. (1996). *The Human Body in Health and Disease,* 8th ed. Philadelphia: Lippincott-Raven.

Memmler, R. L., Cohen, B. J., & Wood, D. L. (1996). *Structure and Function of the Human Body,* 6th ed. Philadelphia: Lippincott-Raven.

Porth, C. M. (1998). *Pathophysiology: Concepts of Altered Health Status,* 5th ed. Philadelphia: Lippincott-Raven.

Professional Guide to Diseases, 4th ed. (1992). Springhouse, PA: Springhouse.

Rosdahl, C. B. (1995). *Textbook of Basic Nursing,* 6th ed. Philadelphia: J.B. Lippincott.

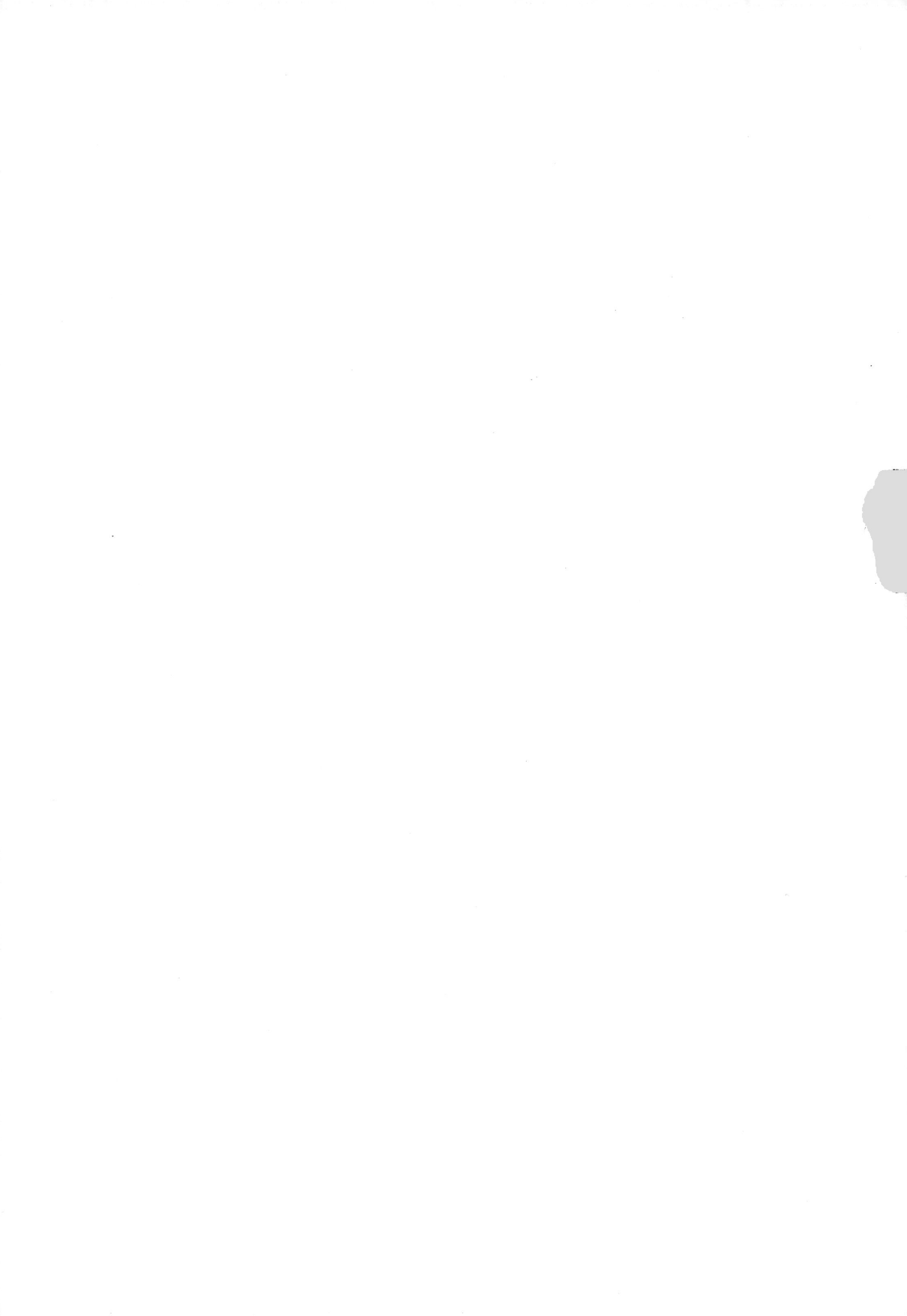

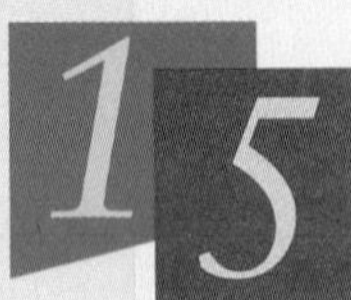

Assisting With Diagnostic and Therapeutic Procedures Associated With the Cardiovascular System

Chapter Outline

Role Delineation

CLINICAL

Fundamental Principles

- Apply principles of aseptic technique and infection control.

Diagnostic Orders

- Perform diagnostic tests.

Patient Care

- Prepare and maintain examination and treatment areas.
- Prepare patients for examinations, procedures, and treatments.
- Assist with examinations, procedures, and treatments.

GENERAL

Professionalism

- Project a professional manner and image.
- Work as a team member.
- Prioritize and perform multiple tasks.

Communication Skills

- Treat all patients with compassion and empathy.
- Adapt communications to individual's ability to understand.

Legal Concepts

- Practice within the scope of education, training, and personal capabilities.
- Document accurately.

Instruction

- Instruct individuals according to their needs.
- Teach methods of health promotion and disease prevention.

Chapter Competencies

Learning Objectives

Upon successfully completing this chapter, you will be able to:

1. Spell and define the Key Terms.
2. Understand the basic structure and function of the cardiovascular system.
3. Trace a drop of blood through the circulatory system.
4. Describe the blood components and state their functions.
5. Trace the conduction of an electrical impulse through the heart.
6. List and describe common cardiovascular disorders.
7. Identify and explain common cardiovascular procedures and tests.
8. Describe the roles and responsibilities of a medical assistant during a cardiovascular examination.
9. Explain the information recorded on a basic 12-lead electrocardiogram.
10. Explain the purpose for a Holter monitor.

Performance Objectives

Upon successfully completing this chapter, you will be able to:

1. Perform a basic 12-lead electrocardiogram (Procedure 15-1).
2. Mount an electrocardiogram strip for reading (Procedure 15-2).
3. Apply a Holter monitor for a 24-hour test (Procedure 15-3).

Key Terms

(See Glossary for definitions.)

aneurysm
angina pectoris
artifacts
atria
atrioventricular node
bundle of His
depolarization
dextrocardia
endocardium
epicardium
leads
mediastinum
myocardium
pericardium
Purkinje fibers
repolarization
sinoatrial node
ventricles

Cardiovascular disease is a major cause of illness and death in today's society. Because medical assistants often work with patients who have cardiovascular disorders that require frequent monitoring through the physician's office, you must understand the cardiovascular system, associated disorders, and the common tests and procedures that are ordered for diagnosis and treatment. This chapter will help you to understand cardiovascular function and dysfunction. It will also help you to work independently and confidently in performing a 12-lead electrocardiogram and applying a Holter monitor.

STRUCTURE AND FUNCTION OF THE CARDIOVASCULAR SYSTEM

Heart

The heart is a hollow, muscular organ that by rhythmic contractions pumps oxygen-rich blood throughout the body to oxygenate and nourish the tissues and return wastes to the points of elimination. It is located between the lungs in the part of the thoracic cavity known as the **mediastinum.** It is triangular, with the tip, or apex, extending toward the left in the chest cavity and resting on the diaphragm. The bulk of the heart is located behind the sternum and extends from the second rib to the fifth intercostal space distally. The heart itself weighs less than 1 lb (about 250–350 g) and is approximately the size of a closed fist (Fig. 15-1).

The heart is enclosed within a double sac of serous membrane called the **pericardium.** The pericardium has two layers: a fibrous layer and a serous layer. The fibrous layer, which is composed of tough, white connective tissue, protects the heart and anchors it to surrounding structures, such as the diaphragm, sternum, and great vessels issuing from the heart base. The

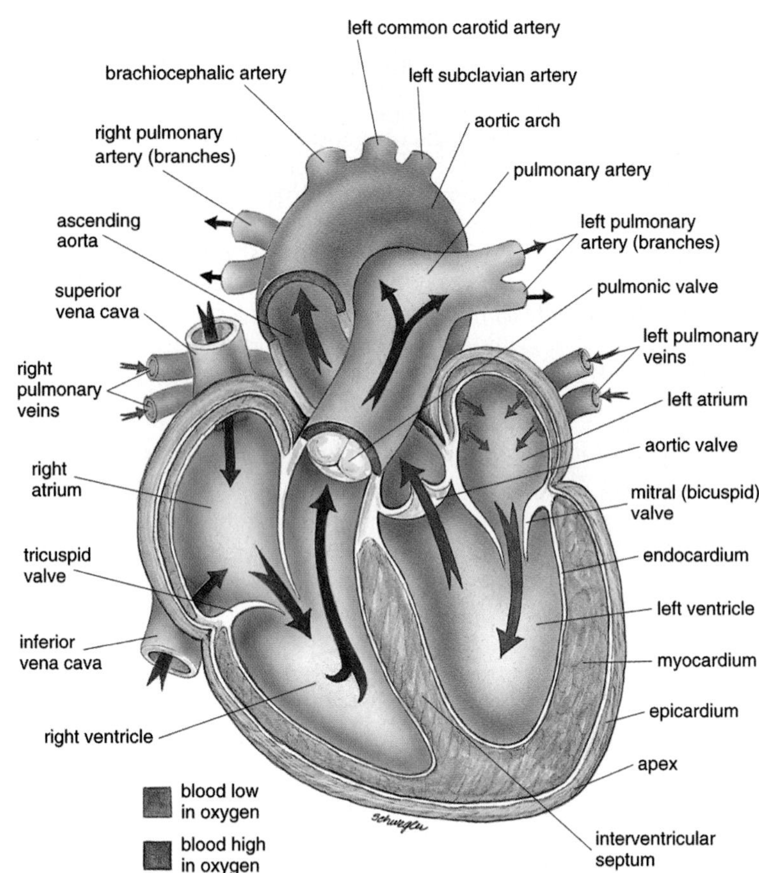

Figure 15-1 Heart and great vessels.

15

serous layer, which lines the fibrous layer, is composed of serous membrane and connective tissue. Between the serous and the fibrous layers is serous fluid that cushions and protects the heart.

The serous layer turns downward at the heart base and continues over the heart surface as the visceral pericardium, also called the **epicardium.** The epicardium is an essential part of the heart wall; it adheres closely and forms the outermost layer of the heart wall.

The **myocardium** (middle layer) is composed of cardiac muscle and forms the bulk of the heart. It is this layer that actually contracts. Within the myocardium, the branching cardiac muscles are bonded to each other by connective tissue fibers and arranged in spiral or circular bundles. The bundles link all parts of the heart together. The connective fibers form a dense network, called the fibrous skeleton or the skeleton of the heart. This network reinforces the heart internally. The **endocardium** or innermost part of the heart wall lines the heart chamber and covers the connective tissue skeleton of the heart valves.

The inner portion of the heart is made up of four chambers. Two upper chambers, the right and left **atria,** receive the blood pumped into the heart. The two lower chambers, the right and left **ventricles,** are the pumping chambers (see Fig. 15-1).

Blood Vessels

Arteries, capillaries, and veins are the three major types of blood vessels that form the transportation path of the blood in the cardiovascular system (Fig. 15-2).

Arteries (Fig. 15-3) transport blood away from the heart by the pumping action of the ventricles. Arterial blood leaves the heart for the periphery by way of the aorta and is under relatively high pressure. Arteries have thick walls to withstand this pressure. Blood is transported by the initial pumping action of the heart and then by an inner muscular wall in the arteries that helps maintain the blood flow. Blood flows through the arteries, which become progressively smaller and divide into small arteries called arterioles. These arterioles feed into the capillary beds of the body organs and tissues (Fig. 15-4).

Capillaries provide contact with tissue cells and interstitial fluid to serve cellular needs directly. Capillary walls are one cell thick to allow the exchange of oxy-

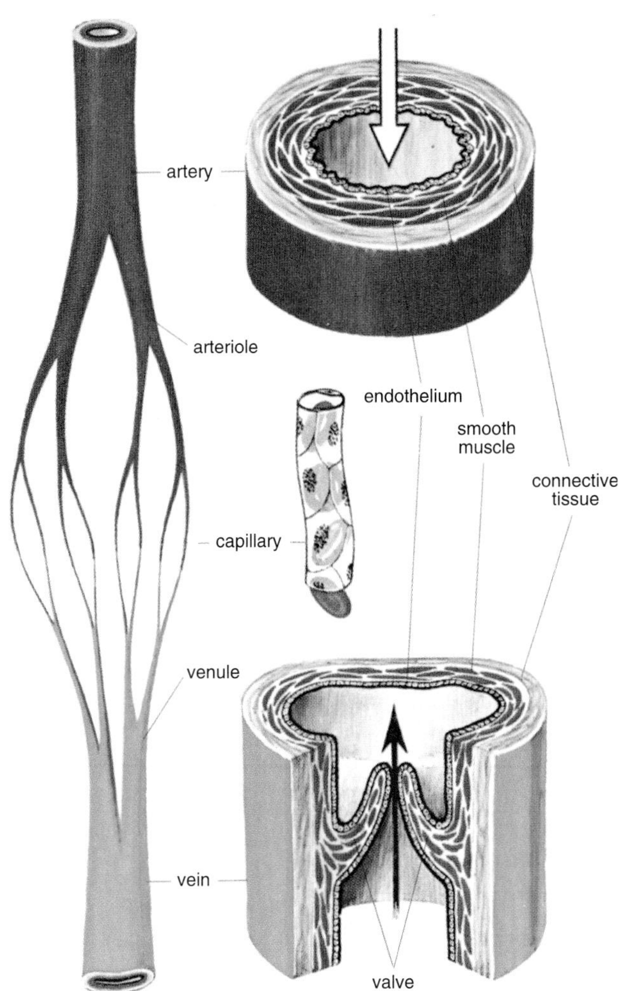

Figure 15-2 Sections of blood vessels showing the thick arterial walls and the thin walls of veins and capillaries are illustrated. Venous valves also are shown. The arrows indicate the direction of blood flow.

gen, nutrients, and waste products, which occurs in the capillary bed.

From the tiny capillaries, blood then flows into small *veins* called venules, which merge into larger veins for the return of the blood to the heart. The blood return is aided by skeletal muscle contractions and by valves within the veins that prevent the backflow of blood and keep it moving in the direction of the heart. The large veins combine into the largest vein at the heart entrance called the vena cava, which returns the blood to the heart. Although the walls of the veins increase in thickness as the vessels increase in size, they are never as thick as the walls of arteries (Fig. 15-5).

Checkpoint Question

1. *Where does the exchange of nutrients and oxygen occur?*

Circulation

The heart is actually two pumps, and although physically joined, each pump controls the flow of blood into one of the two loops of the blood's circulatory paths. The two routes that blood must travel are the pulmonary and the systemic circuits (Fig. 15-6).

In the pulmonary circuit, the right side of the heart receives deoxygenated blood from the vena cava into the right atrium and sends it by way of the right ventricle and pulmonary arteries to the lungs. In the lungs, blood is reoxygenated and returned to the left side of the heart. The oxygen-rich blood is pumped by the left ventricle into the systemic circuit. The equivalent of about 4000 to 5000 gallons of blood is pumped through this circuit each day.

Each pump consists of a receiving chamber (the right and left atria) and an ejection chamber (the right and left ventricles). The ventricles must develop enough pressure to drive the blood through the entire circuit and back to the proper receiving chamber. Because there is more resistance in the systemic circuit to move blood through, a greater force is required. Therefore, the left ventricle and the larger systemic arteries have thicker walls than the right ventricle and the pulmonary artery.

Blood flows through the heart in one direction—from the atria (receiving chambers) to the ventricles (ejection chambers) and out of the great arteries leaving the base of the heart. The forward path of circulation is enforced by four heart valves that prevent the backflow of blood. There are two atrioventricular (AV) and two semilunar valves (Fig. 15-7).

The two AV valves are located at the junction of the atrial and ventricular chambers of the heart and prevent the backflow of blood into the atria when the ventricles are contracting. The right AV valve, or tricuspid valve, has three flexible valve flaps or cusps. The left AV valve has two valve flaps or cusps and is called the bicuspid valve or mitral valve.

When the heart is relaxed, the AV valve flaps hang limply into the ventricular chambers below; blood flows into the atria and then through the open AV valves into the ventricles. When the ventricles begin to contract, compressing the blood in their chambers, the blood is forced superiorly against the valve flaps, causing their edges to meet and close the valve. The chordae tendinae and the papillary muscles anchor the valve flaps and help them to remain in their closed position.

The two semilunar valves guard the bases of the large arteries leading from the heart and prevent backflow of blood into the ventricles. The aortic semilunar valve is at the junction of the aorta and the left ventricle and prevents the blood in the aorta from flowing

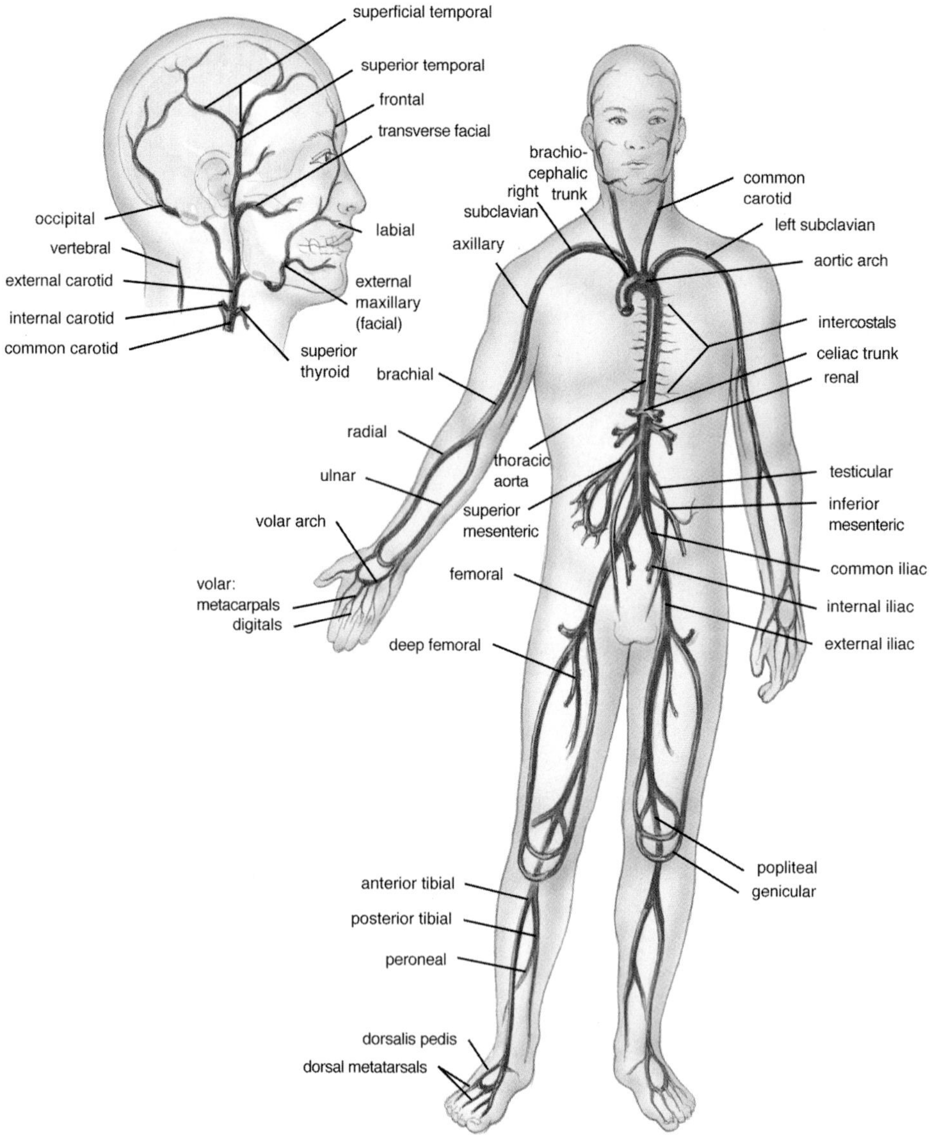

Figure 15-3 Principal arteries.

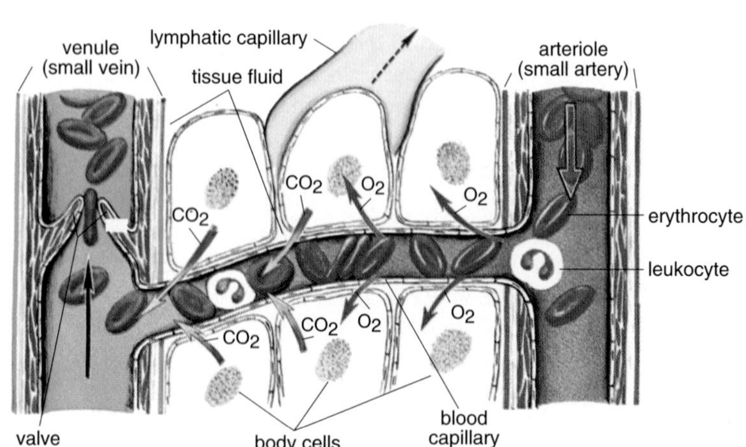

Figure 15-4 Diagram showing the connection between the small blood vessels through capillaries. Note the lymph capillary, which assists in returning excess tissue fluid to the general circulation.

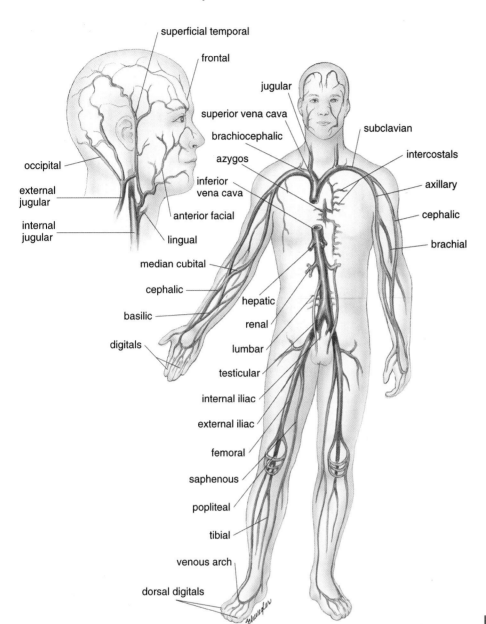

Figure 15-5 Principal veins.

back into the left ventricle. The pulmonary semilunar valve protects the opening between the right ventricle and the pulmonary artery.

Each semilunar valve is similar in structure. Their mechanism of action differs from that of the AV valves. When the ventricles are at their peak of contraction, the semilunar valves are forced open, and the cusps flatten against the arterial walls as the blood flows past them. When the ventricles relax, the blood (no longer propelled forward by the pressure of the ventricular contraction) begins to flow backward toward the heart, fills the cusps, and closes the valve.

The blood supply to the heart is provided by the coronary arteries. They arise from the aorta, just above the aortic semilunar valve, and encircle the heart, passing to the right and to the left in an indentation known as the atrioventricular groove, marking the junction between the atria and the ventricles. Blood from the coronary circulation is returned to the heart by the right and left coronary veins, which empty into the coronary sinus, then into the right atrium (Fig. 15-8).

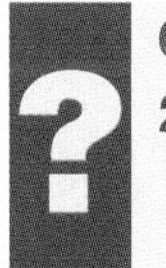

Checkpoint Question

2. *How many chambers are in the heart? What are the upper chambers called? The lower chambers?*

Conduction System

The pumping action of the heart is regulated by the electrical activity of the cardiac muscle cells in the myocardium. These impulses follow a specific pathway known as the conduction system of the heart (Fig. 15-9).

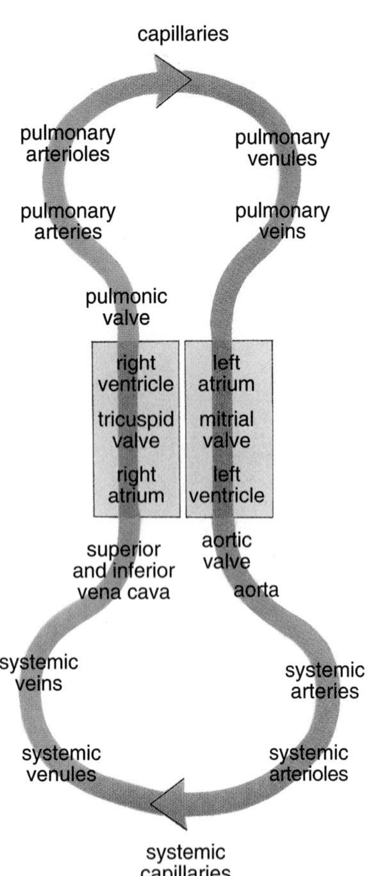

Figure 15-6 Blood vessels constitute a closed system for the flow of blood. Note that changes in oxygen content occur as blood flows through the capillaries.

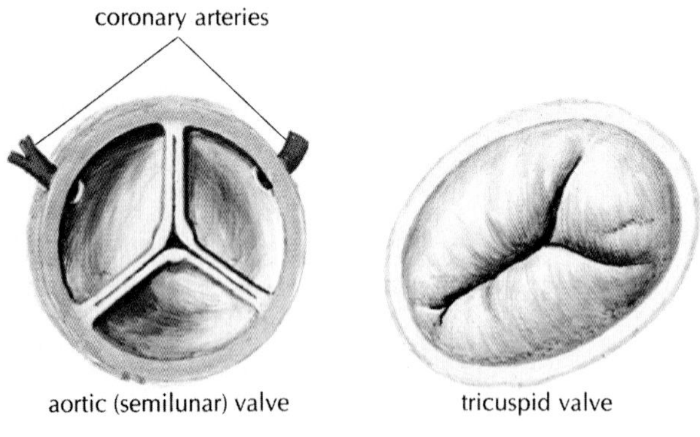

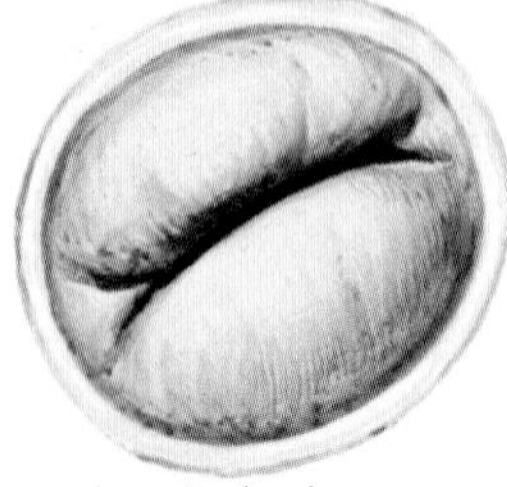

Figure 15-7 Valves of the heart, seen from above, in the closed position.

The components of the conduction system are the sinoatrial (SA) node, the atrioventricular (AV) node, the bundle of His, the right and left bundle branches, and the Purkinje fibers.

The **sinoatrial node** is referred to as the pacemaker of the heart. This node, a group of specialized cells, is located in the right atrial wall, just inferior to the entrance of the inferior vena cava. The cells depolarize (send an impulse) spontaneously at a rate of 70 to 80 times per minute. The SA node initiates each **depolarization** wave that travels across the heart causing the heart to contract (or beat). It sets the pace for the heart as a whole. Its characteristic rhythm is called the normal sinus rhythm.

From the SA node, the depolarization wave spreads across both atria causing them to contract, and reaches the **atrioventricular node,** located in the inferior portion of the interatrial septum. This action takes approximately 0.04 second. The impulse is delayed a moment at the AV node, approximately 0.1 second, which allows the atria to complete their contraction. It then passes rapidly into and through the AV **bundle of His** (specialized cardiac muscle fibers) and the bundle branches in the interventricular septum and continues to the **Purkinje fibers,** which penetrate the ventricular myocardium, causing the ventricles to contract. The pumping action of the heart depends on the proper sequence of events in this transmission (Box 15-1).

The normal rhythm may be altered by extrinsic factors that initiate sympathetic nervous system activation (eg, when the body needs the heart to beat faster to deliver more blood to meet the demands of the fright-flight-fight syndrome). During times of normal circulatory need, the parasympathetic nervous system allows the SA node to control the pace of the heart.

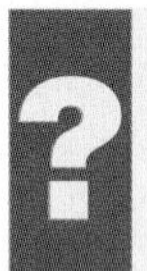

Checkpoint Question

3. *What are the five components of the conduction system? Which component is the pacemaker?*

Blood

Blood consists of erythrocytes (red blood cells), leukocytes (white blood cells), and thrombocytes (platelets) suspended in plasma. A 150-lb adult has about 5 to 6 quarts of blood.

Cells are formed in the red marrow of long bones and in the centers of smaller bones. All of the formed elements of blood develop from stem cells called *hemocytoblasts*. As the body signals the need for a certain type of cell, the available stem cells differentiate into the needed cell. If infection is present, more stem cells become leukocytes; if the number of red blood cells is low, more cells differentiate into erythrocytes. (See

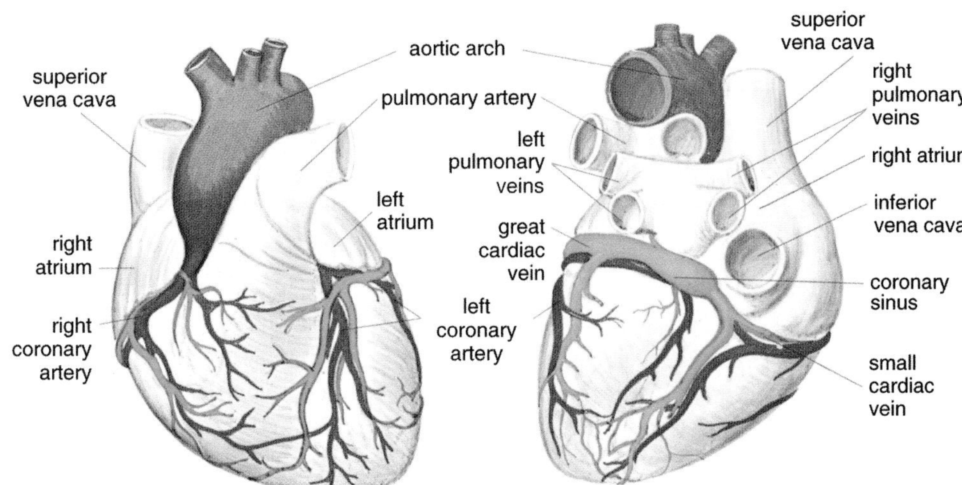

Figure 15-8 Coronary arteries and cardiac veins. (*Left*) Anterior view. (*Right*) Posterior view.

15

Chap. 30, Hematology, for further discussion and illustrations of blood components.)

Plasma accounts for about 55% of the blood, and about 90% of plasma is water. The other components vary because of the plasma functions but remain a fairly constant mix of protein, salts, oxygen, nutrients, wastes, and hormones.

Erythrocytes, or red blood cells, are the most numerous and are specialized for packaging hemoglobin, an iron-containing protein, for transporting oxygen to the cells. As the red cell matures, the nucleus disintegrates to allow more room for oxygen transport. Without a nucleus, the red blood cell is unable to reproduce itself and dies within a short time, usually about 120 days. Dead red blood cells are filtered by the liver and the spleen. The iron content is recycled to the marrow where it is used for new cells. The waste products of dead red blood cells become bile and give feces their characteristic color.

Leukocytes, or white blood cells, are much larger than erythrocytes and are designed to fight infection. They come in various sizes and shapes, use the bloodstream for transport to tissues, and may live for years in the tissues as they wait to be needed.

There are two types of leukocytes: granulocytes and agranulocytes. Granulocytes contain granules within the cytoplasm, agranulocytes do not. The granules are actually the sacs of digestive enzymes (lysosomes) common to all cells but are specially designed in leukocytes to aid in phagocytosis of any cell per-

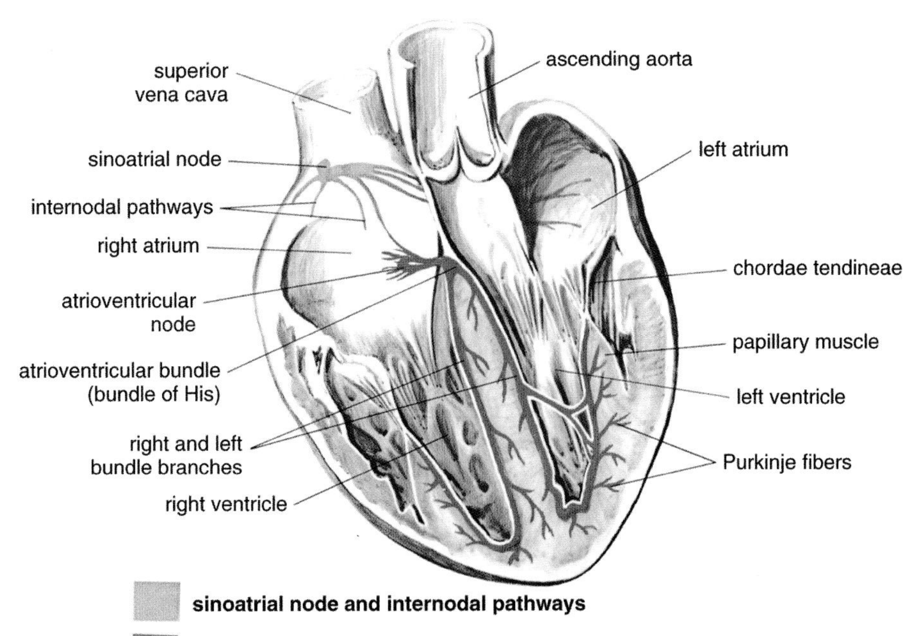

Figure 15-9 Conduction system of the heart.

Box 15-1
Artificial Pacemakers

When a patient's conduction system can no longer maintain normal sinus rhythm without assistance, an electrical source can be implanted to assist or to replace the sinoatrial node function. Artificial pacemakers are surgically implanted either between the chest wall and the rib cage or within the chest cavity. They are battery operated and usually are manufactured to retain their charge for up to 20 years. They may be permanent or temporary and may work constantly to ensure electrical activity or may be calibrated to override the sinoatrial node only when the heart slows below a certain rate.

Pacemaker programming is frequently conducted by transtelephone monitoring, using a special remote surveillance device. At any properly outfitted site, such as a long-term care facility, remote health care center, or physician's office, the patient will insert moistened fingertips (usually bilateral index fingers) into the devices connected to a telephone modem. A tone is transmitted to a receiving system at a centrally located pacemaker clinic. The pacemaker rate and function are obtained and evaluated by a cardiologist at the receiving site.

If battery function is failing and replacement is not possible or advisable, batteries can be recharged transdermally. A charging unit is placed over the implantation site and plugged into an ordinary electrical outlet. The power cell is then recharged through the skin with no discomfort to the patient.

ceived as a threat to the body. Granulocytes are named for the dyes that will stain the granules within the cytoplasm. This concept is discussed in Chap. 27, Microbiology. Table 15-1 lists types of white blood cells and their functions. (See Chap. 30, Hematology, for more information.)

Thrombocytes (platelets) are fragments of megakaryocytes, the portion of the stem cell that is used for platelet formation rather than a red or white blood cell. Platelets are important in clot formation. The numbers and significance of all types of blood cells are discussed in detail in Chap. 30, Hematology.

Table 15-1 **Types of White Blood Cells**

Granulocytes	• Neutrophils: increased in bacterial infections • Eosinophils: increased in parasitic infections and allergies • Basophils: thought to play a role in clot production
Agranulocytes	• Monocytes: enter the tissue to become macrophages • Lymphocytes: increased in the immune response

COMMON CARDIOVASCULAR DISORDERS

The lifestyles and diets of the American public contribute to the increase in premature death by cardiovascular causes, making heart disease the leading cause of death in the United States.

Symptoms of cardiovascular disorders can include:

- Chest pain
- Dyspnea
- Fatigue
- Diaphoresis (excessive sweating)
- Nausea and vomiting with chest pain
- Irregular heartbeat

Other less obvious symptoms might include:

- Changes in peripheral circulation, such as aching in the extremities
- Edema
- Skin ulcers that do not heal
- Pain that increases with ambulation and decreases during rest
- Changes in skin color and symptoms associated with inflammation

Below are descriptions of cardiovascular disorders that you may see in the medical office.

Atherosclerotic Coronary Heart Disease or Coronary Artery Disease

Diseases of the coronary arteries are caused initially by the collection of fatty plaques and other material inside the walls of the coronary arteries. These plaques nar-

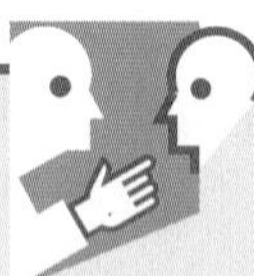

Advice and Tips
Handling Cardiovascular Complaints

A patient reporting cardiovascular symptoms typically will have a high level of anxiety. You must be aware of and attentive to the patient's needs and concerns. It is vital that you listen carefully to complaints and provide accurate data related to the duration and type of symptoms experienced by the patient. This attention to detail is especially important during telephone calls, when decisions must be made regarding directions for evaluation or treatment of the presenting problem. The information you obtain assists the physician in determining the best method of caring for the patient.

row the lumen (opening) of the arteries and constrict normal blood flow through the arteries that serve the heart. The plaques are rougher than the walls of a normal artery and may cause a thrombus (blood clot) to form (Fig. 15-10).

Common symptoms of atherosclerotic coronary heart disease are:

- **Angina pectoris** (pain radiating to the arm, jaw, shoulder, back, or neck, usually felt on exertion and relieved by rest)
- A pressure or fullness in the chest, felt more severely during exertion and relieved by rest
- Syncope (fainting)
- Edema
- Unexplained cough, generally without respiratory symptoms
- Hemoptysis (coughing up blood from the respiratory tract)
- Excessive fatigue

Predisposing conditions for coronary artery disease (CAD) include either a high intake of cholesterol or saturated fats or a familial hypercholesterolemia. A history of high cholesterol and triglyceride levels, cigarette smoking, diabetes mellitus, or hypertension is also likely to precede CAD. It may be controlled by a diet low in cholesterol and saturated fats, exercise, maintaining normal body weight, blood pressure control, and not smoking. If these methods are not successful, medication may be necessary. Atherosclerosis contributes to many other cardiovascular diseases.

Checkpoint Question

4. *List four predisposing factors for heart disease.*

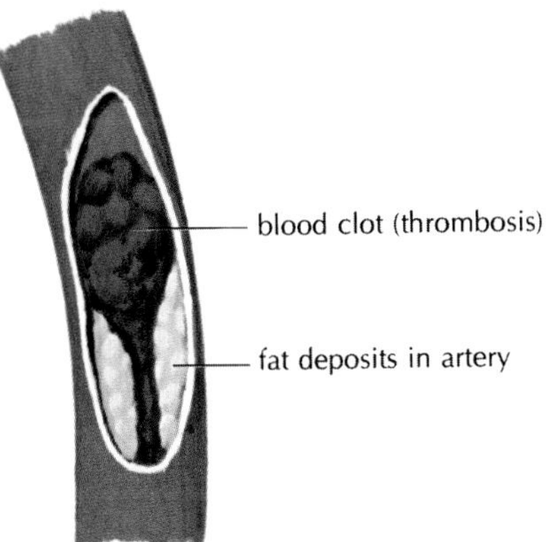

Figure 15-10 Development of coronary thrombosis.

Arterial Occlusive Disease

This disease is caused by an obstruction or narrowing of an arterial lumen in areas other than the coronary arteries. Occlusions may occur in any artery and may be acute or chronic. They are caused by atherosclerotic plaques that may remain stationary as a thrombus or break away to become an embolus.

Signs and symptoms usually indicate decreased blood supply to a part, such as pain or numbness, loss of normal blood flow, or loss of palpatory pulse. Diagnosis is made by arteriography to locate the occlusion and evaluate the degree of obstruction. Doppler ultrasonography is a noninvasive but less diagnostic method of evaluating peripheral circulation for occlusion.

Treatment for mild chronic occlusions requires a lifestyle change to reverse atherosclerotic formations. If the condition is moderately severe, drug therapy may be initiated. If the occlusion is severe, the clot may be removed by embolectomy using various and constantly improving methods of treatment. If the clot cannot be removed, a bypass graft may be performed.

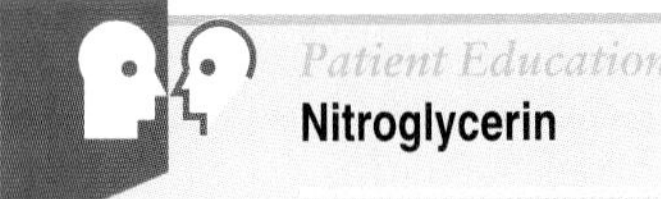

Patient Education

Nitroglycerin

A medication commonly prescribed for cardiac patients is nitroglycerin, a vasodilator. Vasodilators open the lumen of vessels, resulting in increased blood supply to the heart muscle. Patient education should include the following instructions:

- Keep the medication in the dark bottle supplied by the pharmacy because nitroglycerin can become deactivated in sunlight.
- Be alert for any side effects, such as lightheadedness, syncope, and hypotension.
- Be aware that the nitroglycerin may be prescribed as tablets or a spray, to use on an as-needed basis. (The spray is often easier for patients with poor dexterity or with poor eyesight.) The usual administration guidelines are for three doses at 5-minute intervals. If pain persists, call emergency medical services. Check with the physician for dosage instructions. (Nitroglycerin can also be prescribed as a skin patch to be used on a daily basis to maintain vasodilation.)
- Check the expiration date of the medication frequently and always have an adequate supply available.
- Ensure that the medication is kept out of the reach of children.

Myocardial Infarction

Death of the heart muscle, called myocardial infarction (MI), occurs when the coronary artery becomes totally occluded (blocked), usually by atherosclerotic plaques or by an embolism. An MI may occur suddenly, without prior symptoms, or in patients with diagnosed atherosclerotic coronary heart disease. Studies by the American Heart Association reveal that in the United States alone, approximately 1,500,000 people develop MIs annually, with approximately 500,000 deaths or one fourth of all deaths attributed to the killer disease.

Symptoms of myocardial infarction may be similar to those felt during angina pectoris, but this disorder is distinguished by pain that lasts longer than 20 to 30 minutes and is unrelieved by rest or nitroglycerin (Box 15-2). Other symptoms may include nausea, diaphoresis, weakness, vomiting, or abdominal cramps. The patient may complain of a viselike grip around the chest wall. The skin is cool, clammy, and pale, and there may be a feeling of impending doom. Some patients only experience nonspecific symptoms of indigestion and do not seek medical attention. In 20% of patients, and particularly in diabetic patients, the MI may be silent, diagnosed only by routine electrocardiography (ECG) and later blood work when complications develop. It is imperative not to ignore or dismiss complaints by patients with symptoms of MI because this is a life-threatening condition. If the patient is found to have coronary occlusion, surgery may be performed before MI occurs or afterward to prevent further damage (Box 15-3).

15

Hypertension

Patients with a resting systolic blood pressure above 140 mmHg (millimeters of mercury) and a diastolic pressure above 90 mmHg are said to be hypertensive.

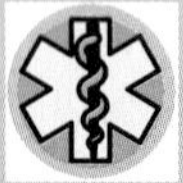

Action STAT!

Myocardial Infarction

Scenario: Mr. Rodriquez, a 52-year-old man, comes into the office complaining of nausea, left arm pain, and tightness in his chest. He states that the pain started about an hour ago, after he shoveled snow. While standing at the reception desk, he grabs his chest and falls to the floor. What should you do?

Summon help and notify the physician immediately. Then do the following:

1. Establish unresponsiveness.
2. Alert a coworker to call emergency medical services (EMS).
3. Place Mr. Rodriguez in a supine position with his head level with his body, and kneel by his shoulders.
4. Open the airway, using the head-tilt/chin-lift maneuver.
5. Determine breathlessness (look, listen, and feel).
6. If Mr. Rodriguez is breathing but is unresponsive, place him in the side-lying recovery position until the EMS arrives. If he is not breathing, maintain the head-tilt/chin-lift position and give two slow breaths while watching for his chest to rise. Use an Ambu bag or resuscitation device for this procedure.
7. Check for a carotid pulse for a full 15 seconds. If there is no pulse, locate the proper hand position (two fingerbreadths above the xiphocostal notch on the sternum) and start cardiopulmonary resuscitation (CPR) (15 compressions to two breaths for a one-rescuer response). If there is a pulse, but the patient is not breathing, start rescue breathing (1 breath every 5 seconds). After four cycles (about 1 minute), recheck his pulse.

***Note:* It is important to keep your CPR training and certification up to date and to follow the current recommended guidelines. CPR should be done by properly trained persons to help ensure a favorable patient recovery and to minimize patient complications.**

If you are called by a coworker to assist with the procedure, you should:

- Call EMS or your local ambulance service.
- Bring the crash cart or code cart to the rescuer. The Ambu bag or other ventilation device should be used rather than mouth-to-mouth resuscitation. If a defibrillator is available, bring it to the area to be used by the physician or other trained personnel.
- Escort bystanders in the reception area to another part of the office.
- Assist the rescuer with the procedure for two-rescuer CPR.

After the patient has been stabilized or transported to the hospital, carefully document the incident and related issues, and clean and organize the emergency cart.

Your role and responsibility during a patient's cardiac arrest will vary greatly based on the medical specialty in which you work and the personnel employed at your facility. It is important to remember that this scenario can occur at any medical office and at any time. The patient's survival depends on your quick and calm response.

Box 15-2
Is It Angina or MI?

The pain felt with angina and myocardial infarction is brought about by myocardial anoxia, which may be caused by an increased need for oxygen to the heart muscle due to exertion, stress, or temperature extremes of heat or cold. Typically, angina may be relieved by rest or nitroglycerin. However, pain from a myocardial infarction will not be relieved by these measures. Below is a brief comparison of these two disorders:

	Angina	*Myocardial Infarction*
Description	Moderate pressure felt deeply in the chest; a squeezing, suffocating feeling	Severe deep pressure not relieved by reducing stressors; a crushing pressure
Onset	Pain may occur gradually or suddenly and subsides quickly, usually in less than 30 minutes. It can be relieved by reducing the stressors, by rest, and by nitroglycerin protocol.	Pain occurs suddenly and remains even after stressors are reduced or relieved. Pain will not be relieved by nitroglycerin, which may be given up to three times, one dose every 5 minutes for a total of three doses in 15 minutes.
Location	Mid-anterior chest, usually diffuse, radiates to the back, neck, arms, jaw, and epigastric area	Mid-anterior chest with the same radiating patterns
Signs and Symptoms	Dyspnea, nausea, signs of indigestion (eg, burping), profuse sweating	Nausea and vomiting, fear, diaphoresis, pounding heart, palpitations (possible)

Any patient who calls the medical office complaining of chest pain must be examined immediately. The office should have an established protocol for handling these calls. The physician will need to be consulted to decide if the patient should be directed to the nearest emergency room, if emergency medical services should be dispatched, or if the patient should come directly to the office. This is not a decision that medical assistants should make.

15

Hypertension cannot be diagnosed on the basis of one blood pressure measurement alone. A physician will often require several readings before making the diagnosis of hypertension.

Hypertension is a major cause of stroke and renal failure and is a major consequence of atherosclerosis anywhere in the circulatory system. The long-term effects of hypertension cause weakening of the arteries and enlargement of the left ventricle, which results from overwork as the ventricle works harder to overcome the higher pressure in the arteries. The disease itself frequently produces no symptoms. The cause usually is unknown, but a correlation between hypertension and an elevated cholesterol level has been shown. Hypertension can strike anyone, regardless of age, race, sex, or ethnic origin.

Some high blood pressure (usually mild or borderline) may be controlled with a low-sodium diet, an exercise program, or weight reduction if needed. If hypertension cannot be controlled by these measures, a diuretic medication may be prescribed. Diuretics reduce the amount of sodium in the body, which in turn reduces the total fluid volume. The decrease in fluid volume reduces strain on the heart and blood vessels. Patients with high blood pressure should be advised to eliminate stressors in their lives, to limit the intake of alcohol, to stop smoking, and to lower their levels of cholesterol and triglycerides.

It should be emphasized to hypertensive patients that medication should be taken as prescribed. Often patients feel that because their blood pressure has reached a manageable level, they do not need to continue the prescribed medication. Explain that the medication is the cause of the lowered pressure and that discontinuing the treatment will jeopardize recovery.

Checkpoint Question

5. *Which two disorders may result from untreated hypertension?*

Box 15-3
Corrective Cardiac Surgery

The least traumatic form of cardiac surgery is the *percutaneous transluminal coronary angioplasty* (PCTA). A double-lumen catheter with a balloon surrounding the upper portion is inserted into a vessel in the groin or axilla. This catheter is threaded into the coronary vessels by watching a fluoroscopic screen as the procedure is performed. When the occlusion is found, the balloon is inflated to press the atherosclerotic plaque against the arterial walls and relieve the occlusion. Lasers may be used to remove the plaque. Springs or mesh (called a stent) may be inserted and left in place within the vessel to maintain patency. This procedure is less invasive than bypass surgery, but occasionally the artery will rebuild plaque at the site or the stent may fill with plaque and support occlusion.

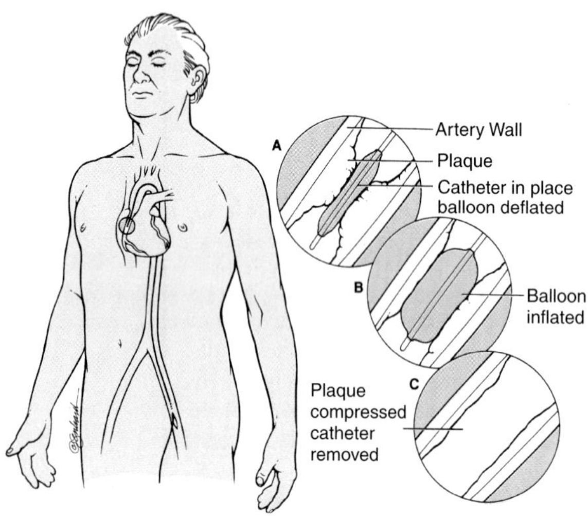

Percutaneous transluminal coronary angioplasty. (**A**) A balloon-tipped catheter is passed into the affected coronary artery and placed within the atherosclerotic lesion. (**B**) The balloon is then rapidly inflated and deflated with controlled pressure. (**C**) After the plaque is cracked, the catheter is removed, allowing improved blood flow through the vessel.

Coronary artery bypass graft (CABG) surgery is performed by grafting a piece of vessel from another part of the body to the area beyond the occlusion and to the ascending aorta, providing a patent passage for the blood supply. The surgery requires a still field of surgery, so the heart must be stopped and the patient supported by a cardiopulmonary bypass machine for the length of the operation. The saphenous vein may be used if multiple bypasses will be performed, or the internal mammary artery will be used if the surgery is not extensive. Hospitalization may be as long as 5 to 7 days. As many as 20% of patients will develop a repeat thrombus within 1 year.

Valvular Heart Disease/ Rheumatic Heart Disease

Disease of the heart valves is an acquired or congenital abnormality of any of the four cardiac valves. It is characterized by stenosis (narrowing) and obstructed blood flow or by valvular degeneration and backflow of the blood against the course of the circulatory pathway. Isolated stenosis and regurgitation of one or more valves may also be present, although the left heart valves are more often involved.

Rheumatic heart disease, an acquired valvular disease, presents clinically as a generalized inflammatory disease occurring 10 to 21 days after an upper respiratory infection caused by group A β-hemolytic streptococci. It is characterized by inflammatory lesions of the connective tissues, particularly in the heart, joints, and subcutaneous tissues. The heart valves are damaged by an abnormal response of the immune system caused by the turbulence of the bacterially infected blood. This damage results in a systolic murmur. The disease usually attacks young people between the ages of 5 and 15.

Since the 1940s, when there were an estimated 200,000 to 250,000 cases of rheumatic fever per year in the United States, incidence has dropped significantly. Today, rheumatic heart disease is considered rare in North America and Western Europe. The decline is due to improved health care and the availability of antimicrobial agents.

Mitral stenosis is most commonly a manifestation of rheumatic heart disease. Congenital forms of mitral stenosis may occur but are rare. Stenosis occurs when the mitral valve leaflet cusps fuse and thicken, resulting in an abnormally narrow valve. In addition, scarring of the free margins of the anterior and posterior leaflets occurs with shortening and thickening of the chordae tendinae. This may contribute to mitral regurgitation, which is a backflow of blood from the left ventricle into the left atrium across the mitral valve. Patients with mitral stenosis present with symptoms of dyspnea, and their ability to exert themselves physically may be limited. Pulmonary edema may also develop.

Treatment of valvular disease depends on the type and severity of the abnormality. Severe cases may require medication, sodium-restricted diets, and prophylactic antibiotics before surgery or dental work. If medication is not successful, replacement valves may be necessary.

Aortic Stenosis

Aortic stenosis results from the narrowing of the aortic valve leaflets or a narrowing anywhere in the aortic arch. Because blood cannot easily pass out of the left ventricle into or through the aorta, the ventricle has to work harder to pump blood through the narrow opening. This causes a turbulence of the blood as it flows past the stricture and is heard as a systolic murmur. If aortic stenosis progresses, the valve will become inflexible, reducing the opening of the valve to a small slit. Symptoms seen with aortic stenosis include angina, syncope, and heart failure. Treatment may require dilatation of the aortic arch or, in severe cases, replacement of the stenosed area.

Congestive Heart Failure

Congestive heart failure (CHF) is a condition in which the heart is unable to pump a sufficient blood volume through the body to meet the metabolic needs of the tissues (called forward failure) or cannot distend sufficiently during diastole, leading to cardiac and pulmonary congestion (called backward failure). Coronary artery disease, myocardial disease, valvular heart disease, and hypertension are among the causes of CHF.

As a result of impaired cardiac function, pressure increases in the atria. Symptoms include reduced exercise tolerance and ventricular arrhythmias. Patients with CHF have a shortened life expectancy. CHF affects about 3 million Americans or about 1% of the population. It is one of the most common hospital discharge diagnoses for patients over the age of 65, and each year approximately 400,000 people develop CHF.

Cardiac Arrhythmia

Cardiac arrhythmia or dysrhythmia is an abnormal heart rhythm. It may occur as a primary disorder or as a secondary response to a systemic problem. It may also be a reaction to a drug toxicity or an electrolyte imbalance.

The SA node is considered the pacemaker of the heart. If the SA node is damaged, or a blockage occurs in the conduction pathway, the heart will beat too slowly to meet the body's demands. This type of arrhythmia is called bradycardia, which is a heart rate less than 60 beats/min.

More serious arrhythmias occur when the ventricles beat too fast, a condition known as ventricular tachycardia (VT). VT occurs when some of the electrical signals originate in the ventricles, rather than in the SA node. Once the ventricles begin to beat at a very rapid rate, less blood is pumped out of the heart with each contraction. This occurs because the heart's chambers do not have time to fill with blood adequately before the next contraction begins. Because less blood is being pumped into the circulation, less oxygen is being carried to the tissues. This lack of adequate blood and oxygen may cause dizziness, unconsciousness, or even cardiac arrest. Ventricular fibrillation is a medical emergency that occurs when the heart is quivering rather than contracting in an organized fashion. Very little blood is pumped out of the heart, and the blood pressure may fall to 0. A patient in ventricular fibrillation will become unconscious and die very quickly unless an electrical shock with a cardiac defibrillator is administered immediately to restore normal cardiac electrical activity.

What If?
What if your patient asks you to explain a defibrillator?

A defibrillator is used to correct ventricular fibrillation. Defibrillators work by releasing an electrical current that is aimed at the conduction system in the heart. The goal of the defibrillator is to restore a normal rhythm in the heart. The current is released into the body by placing two paddles on the anterior aspect of the chest wall and delivering a preset number of joules (an electrical current measurement). Defibrillators are used in hospitals, ambulatory care centers, physicians' offices, and ambulances. Special training is needed to operate this machine. Patients may have surgically "implanted defibrillators" in the chest wall. The implant releases "shocks" as needed to keep the heart rhythm regular.

Varicose Veins

Varicosities, the most common circulatory disease of the lower extremities, occur when the superficial veins of the legs become swollen and distended. Eventually the valves fail to close properly, allowing blood to pool and stretch the walls of the veins. People who sit or stand for long periods without moving or contracting their leg muscles are predisposed to developing varicose veins. A hereditary weakness in the vein walls is also a predisposing factor. Varicosities may also be secondary to deep-vein thrombosis. Symptoms of varicose veins are swelling, aching, or a feeling of heaviness in the legs. Varicosities may also be totally asymptomatic. Treatment is usually conservative with instructions to avoid standing or sitting for long periods. Other helpful measures include wrapping the legs with elastic bandages, using sturdy support hose, and elevating the legs for specified periods. Surgery to remove the vein is usually the last approach. Newer treatment techniques involve the injection of a sclerosing agent into small varicose vein segments but is not suggested for large areas.

Stasis Ulcers

Peripheral vascular occlusion leads to stasis ulcers. Signs and symptoms include deep red discolorations, itching, pitting edema, and large areas of scaling skin leading to fissures and ulcers. Diagnosis is obvious by observation of the peripheral venous insufficiency but may be confirmed by Doppler ultrasonography. Treatment is directed at prevention by weight reduction, support stockings, and elevation of the affected limbs. If ulcers develop, measures to aid healing are instituted, such as wet dressings and pressure dressings.

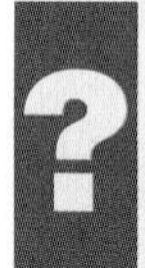

Checkpoint Question

6. *What disorder occurs when the superficial veins in the legs become swollen and distended?*

Venous Thrombosis and Pulmonary Embolism

Deep-vein thrombosis and pulmonary embolism are common cardiovascular illnesses, accounting for thousands of hospitalizations annually. Risk factors are either primary (inherited), which include the sickling diseases and hemolytic anemias, or secondary (acquired), which include long-term immobility, chronic pulmonary disease, thrombophlebitis, varicosities, and defibrillation after cardiac arrest. Oral contraceptives have been implicated in young women with none of the usual predisposing factors.

Symptoms include dyspnea, syncope, lightheadedness, or severe pleuritic chest pain. Testing for venous thrombosis or pulmonary embolism requires a chest x-ray or an electrocardiogram. Doppler studies are also used to diagnose deep-vein thrombosis. If the diagnosis is still uncertain, a lung scan and a pulmonary arteriogram may be ordered. Depending on severity, treatment may include bed rest with elevation of the affected extremity, anticoagulant therapy, or surgery.

Cerebrovascular Accident

Cerebrovascular accidents (CVAs), sometimes called strokes, result when damage occurs to the blood vessels in the brain. The damage blocks the circulation, resulting in ischemia (lack of oxygen) to that part of the brain. Death of the brain tissue will occur without adequate oxygen. Common causes of CVA are blockage of a cerebral artery by a thrombus or embolus and hemorrhage. Atherosclerotic heart disease and hypertension also contribute to CVAs. CVAs are the most common nervous system disorder in the elderly and one of the leading causes of death in the United States.

If a CVA occurs on the right side of the brain, the left side of the body is affected and vice versa. Patients who suffer CVAs usually exhibit varying degrees of weakness or paralysis of one side of the body, with possible involvement of language and comprehension. Symptoms vary according to which artery and which part of the brain is affected. CVAs are fatal when vital centers of the brain are damaged. Treatment involves rehabilitation of these deficiencies after recovery from the acute phase. Therapy includes occupational and physical rehabilitation. Support may be offered to the patient in the form of counseling and a strong post-CVA support group.

Transient ischemic attacks (TIAs), or "mini-strokes," should be considered a warning sign for a major CVA. TIAs signal that small areas of the brain are without oxygen for short periods of time. The symptoms will vary, as those of a true stroke, according to the arteries affected, but will usually include:

- Mild numbness or tingling in the face or a limb
- Difficulty swallowing
- Coughing and choking
- Slurred speech
- Unilateral visual disturbances
- Dizziness

As many as 50% to 80% of patients who exhibit symptoms of TIAs will progress to a stroke. A major stroke may begin as a TIA but will progress to loss of consciousness, hyperpnea (deep, gasping breaths), anisocoria (unequal pupils), and hemiplegia (unilateral paralysis).

Carotid endartectomy, the removal of atherosclerotic plaques from an occluded carotid artery, has proven to be beneficial in reducing the number of TIAs experienced by some persons. The procedure is still being studied as a prevention for CVA.

Carditis

Inflammation may affect any of the layers of the heart muscle, and although other factors may be cited, it is usually the result of a systemic infection.

Pericarditis

Pericarditis is caused by pathogens, neoplasias, autoimmunity (as in lupus erythematosus and rheumatoid arthritis), certain chemicals, radiation, and uremia. It may be acute or chronic.

Signs and symptoms include a sharp pain in the same location expected with a myocardial infarction with the exception that pain increases on inspiration and on lying down but decreases on sitting up and leaning forward. Dyspnea, tachycardia, neck venous distention, pallor, and hypertension are warning signs that serous fluid is compressing the heart and interfering with cardiac function.

Diagnosis is made by eliminating the other disorders with similar presenting signs and symptoms. There is a characteristic pericardial rubbing sound caused by friction within the sac as the heart contracts and relaxes. Chronic pericarditis may not produce the rubbing sound. White blood cell counts, erythrocyte sedimentation rates, and cardiac enzymes may or may not be elevated. Cardiocentesis will aid in diagnosis if the causative agent is a pathogen. An ECG or echocardiogram may show changes consistent with effusion.

Treatment involves relieving the symptoms and correcting the underlying cause. Treatment during recovery is usually directed toward pain relief and reducing inflammation.

Myocarditis

Myocarditis may be chronic or acute and may be diffused through the heart muscle or may be localized at a focal point. Causes include radiation, chemicals, or infections, such as a virus, bacteria, parasites, or helminths (worms).

Signs and symptoms of early acute episodes are usually nonspecific, such as fatigue, fever, and mild chest pain. Chronic cases may lead to heart failure with cardiomegaly, arrhythmias, and valvulitis.

Diagnosis is made by patient history, which usually reveals a recent upper respiratory infection with fever. On auscultation, a murmur may be heard, and arrhythmias are usually present during acute episodes.

Myocarditis has no conclusive laboratory studies, although cardiac enzymes may be elevated and ECG tracings may be atypical. If bacteria are suspected, stool or throat cultures may identify the pathogen.

Treatment includes antibiotics if a pathogen has been identified. Recovery is usually good and is frequently spontaneous. Supportive care during resolution hastens a return to health.

Endocarditis

Endocarditis may be chronic or acute and is caused by a systemic bacterial or fungal invasion. The lining of the heart and its valves may gather clusters of platelets, fibrin, and white blood cells to trap the pathogens. These clusters are called vegetations and may break away to become emboli that travel to the spleen, kidneys, lungs, or nervous system. These formations may also cause scarring of the valves and erosion of the chordae tendinea with resulting valvular reflux.

Signs and symptoms are general to many infectious disorders and include fatigue, low-grade fever, joint pain, and anorexia. Auscultation may reveal a murmur during febrile episodes. If the vegetations become emboli, evidence of occlusion will be seen wherever the clot lodges, such as central nervous system signs of ischemia or an infarction, or signs of a pulmonary infarction.

Diagnosis requires a blood culture to identify the causative agent. Treatment is directed toward eliminating the infecting organism.

Checkpoint Question

7. *How does the pain in pericarditis differ from pain with a myocardial infarction?*

Aneurysm

Weakened vessel walls are predisposed to abnormal dilatation. Dilatation in the form of an **aneurysm** may occur in any vessel, but arteries are most often affected. Because of the high pressure so close to the heart, the aorta is the most common site. The normal elastic vessel wall develops a ballooning effect in many different forms, all of them dangerous:

- A *dissecting aneurysm* tears the inner walls of the artery and allows blood to leak into the lining of the vessel; the wall will eventually die and tear.
- A *sacculated aneurysm* balloons from the wall into a sac, which may burst.
- A *berry aneurysm* is usually a congenital defect in a cerebral vessel.

15

Causes of aneurysms include trauma, hypertension, atherosclerosis, certain fungal infections, syphilis, and congenital defects. Symptoms include pain or pressure at the site. An abdominal aneurysm may be asymptomatic; the pain becomes sharp and tearing if it bursts. Death may occur quickly if the tear is not repaired. If an aneurysm is suggested by the presence of pain or discovered on a routine physical examination, diagnosis is confirmed by an arteriogram, or an aortogram; computed tomography scan; or magnetic resonance imaging. Surgical resection is the only option.

Anemia

Deficiencies in hemoglobin or in the numbers of red blood cells are called anemia. Anemia is not considered a disease but a symptom of an underlying disorder. Anemia can result from:

- Blood loss due to hemorrhage or slow internal bleeding
- A diet low in iron or a malabsorption condition (nutritional anemia)
- Suppressed or diseased marrow, resulting in decreased blood cell formation (aplastic anemia)
- Vitamin B_{12} deficiency (pernicious anemia)
- Genetic abnormalities (sickle cell anemia [Fig. 15-11] or thalassemia)
- Destruction of functioning red blood cells by various means, such as liver or spleen dysfunction or toxins (hemolytic anemia)

Symptoms may include cardiovascular alterations, anorexia and weight loss, dyspnea on exertion, and fa-

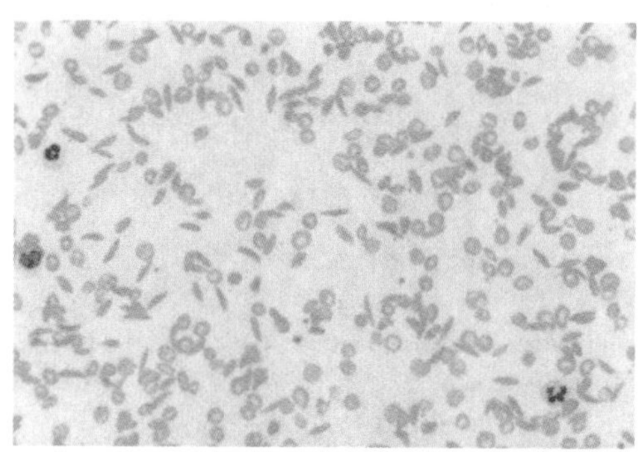

Figure 15-11 Abnormal red cells showing sickled cells.

15

tigue. Laboratory tests reveal decreased hemoglobin and hematocrit levels.

Treatment of anemia must address the cause. Nutritional or malabsorption anemias respond to diets rich in iron, iron supplements, folic acid, or ascorbic acid and replacement of vitamin B_{12}, if these substances are deficient. If anemia is due to blood loss, the cause must be found and corrected and blood volume restored. If erythrocytes are destroyed by premature hemolysis, the cause must be found and corrected. Aplastic anemia may require marrow transplant or supportive therapy. Genetic abnormalities cannot be corrected at this time.

COMMON DIAGNOSTIC PROCEDURES AND THE MEDICAL ASSISTANT'S ROLE

Testing for cardiovascular disorders is either noninvasive, which does not require entering the body or puncturing the skin, or invasive, which requires entering the body cavity by use of a tube, needle, or other device. Depending on the patient's symptoms, testing may be basic (eg, auscultation of the heart and chest cavity

Table 15-2 **Common Cardiovascular Tests**

Diagnostic Test	*Description*	*Indications*
Chest x-ray or chest roentgenogram	Noninvasive diagnostic tool using high-energy electromagnetic waves	Used to detect and follow the advancement of cardiovascular and other diseases and to evaluate the patient's response to therapy. Posterior and lateral views are generally used to assess normal radiographic findings.
12-lead electrocardiogram (ECG)	Graphic recording of the electrical activity of the heart from different angles, using leads uniquely placed on the chest and extremities	May be done to obtain a baseline during a physical examination or in acute situations as seen in patients with myocardial infarctions. Also used to eliminate or complete a potential diagnosis in patients with cardiovascular symptoms.
Holter monitor	Continuous cardiac monitoring of heart rhythm using a portable device worn by patients for 12, 24, or 48 h	Used for patients with symptoms of rhythm disturbances not shown on ECGs or during physical examinations. Holter monitors are also used to show effectiveness of antiarrhythmic drugs or proper pacemaker function.
Cardiac stress test	ECG recording of heart rhythm while patient is exercising on a graded treadmill or stationary bicycle	May be ordered with or without isotopes to help diagnose patients with known or suspected heart problems. Stress testing may also be used to obtain a baseline in healthy adults who are at high risk for cardiovascular disease or in patients starting an exercise program.
Echocardiogram (also known as echo)	Ultrasound of the heart using harmless sound waves generated from a small device known as a transducer	Used to diagnose suspected or known valvular disease. Also used in diagnosing the severity of heart failure and cardiomyopathy. May be indicated in patients with trauma to diagnose injury to the heart or in situations involving possible harvest of the heart for transplant.
Cardiac catheterization	Common nonsurgical procedure involving insertion of a catheter into the heart	Used to help diagnose or determine severity of heart disease. Often indicated after a preliminary stress test or echocardiogram reveals an abnormality or indications of a heart problem.
Coronary arteriography	Injection of a contrast medium into the coronary arteries, allowing visualization	Used to assess congenital or acquired heart disease and to assess damage after myocardial infarction.

done during the physical examination) or intensive and extensive. For instance, a simple chest x-ray or 12-lead ECG may give the cardiologist (a physician who specializes in the treatment of heart disease) enough information to make the proper diagnosis. Sometimes, however, the initial findings may indicate the need for more sophisticated procedures (eg, cardiac catheterization). The most commonly performed cardiovascular tests are discussed below and summarized in Table 15-2.

Cardiovascular Examination

The cardiovascular examination is the most basic, noninvasive procedure. When preparing a patient for cardiovascular examination, you are responsible for obtaining vital information (Box 15-4). Data collected may include an accurate weight (without shoes), blood pressure in one or both arms (depending on physician preference), resting apical pulse when indicated, respirations, and temperature. (See Chap 2, Medical History and Patient Interview, and Chap. 3, Anthropometric Measurements and Vital Signs, for a more detailed discussion.) You may also be responsible for obtaining a complete list of the patient's medications and current dosage, including over-the-counter drugs.

The physician or cardiologist usually begins the examination with a review of the patient's history and reason for the office visit. The physician also reviews vitals signs and medications, noting allergies to medications and other substances or, if no allergies are present, noting NKA (no known allergies). A brief social history may be taken, noting risk factors for cardiovascular disorders, such as smoking, drinking, family history of heart disease, or hypercholesterolemia. The physician then examines the eyes, ears, nose, throat, neck, lungs, heart, and extremities. The circulatory system is examined by use of inspection, palpation, percussion, and auscultation. (See Chap. 4, Physical Examination, for more information.)

The physician uses visual inspection to evaluate the general appearance of the body, noting the circulation to extremities, configuration of the chest, facial expression, color, respiratory patterns, jugular venous distention, circumoral cyanosis, clubbed nails, and so on.

Palpation is used to detect vibrations produced by the cardiac cycle. Thrills may be felt over the cardiac area in some diseases of the circulatory system. Palpation of peripheral pulses evaluates the efficiency of the circulatory pathways.

Percussion helps to determine the areas of dullness outlining the heart and aids the physician in the diagnosis of cardiac enlargement.

By auscultating with a stethoscope, the physician can evaluate the sounds made by blood coursing through the heart, the carotid arteries, or the peripheral vessels. During auscultation, abnormal heart sounds (bruits or murmurs) may be detected (Box 15-5).

After completing the examination of the heart, the physician examines the abdomen. The neurologic system is then reviewed. Lastly, in no specific order, a re-

Box 15-4
Obtaining a Cardiovascular Patient's History: Key Questions to Ask

By asking the following questions, you can elicit important information from a patient with cardiovascular problems.

- Why are you seeing the cardiologist today?
- What symptoms have you been having?
- How long have you been experiencing the pain, discomfort, distress, or unusual sensation? (Patients may not associate chest discomfort as a cardiac symptom.)
- Where is the pain located? Does it stay in one place or does it radiate in any direction?
- Rate the pain on a scale of 1 to 10.
- Is the pain associated with any other symptoms, such as shortness of breath, nausea, weakness, sweating, dizziness?
- If you have been experiencing shortness of breath, does it restrict any of your activities or require you to sleep on additional pillows at night?
- Are you a smoker?
- Do you drink alcoholic beverages?
- Have you noticed any additional problems?

As you proceed with the interview, keep in mind that patients with cardiovascular problems are usually understandably anxious and concerned. They may bring with them family members who also are concerned or anxious. It is your responsibility to help ease apprehension and to offer reassurance and support when appropriate.

Box 15-5
Abnormal Heart Sounds

Abnormal heart sounds, called *murmurs,* are the sounds the blood makes as it courses through the heart. The sounds will vary. For instance, they may blow, rasp, rub, bubble, whistle, whoosh, click, or may be a combination of these. A murmur is not a disease; however, it may indicate organic heart disease. *Functional murmurs* may occur only during elevations in body temperature or during times of physical stress and are not usually cause for great concern. *Organic murmurs* indicate structural abnormalities of varying degrees and are always present. A cardiologist evaluates the murmur by noting its location within the heart, when it occurs in the cardiac cycle, how long it lasts, and its characteristic sound.

view of the peripheral vascular system is performed. The physician then makes recommendations and comments.

During the examination, your role is to provide proper gowning and physical support as necessary. (See Chap. 4, Physical Examination, for more information.) Either before or after the examination, the physician may order an ECG. Depending on the size of the clinic, this test may be performed either by a technician in the ECG department or by a medical assistant (see below).

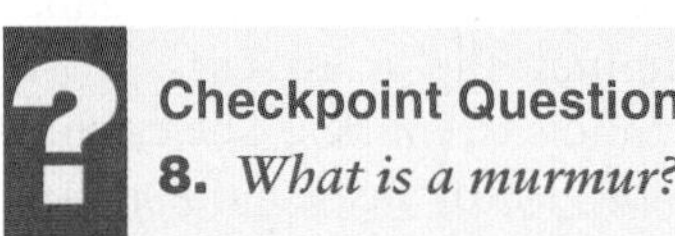

Electrocardiogram

One of the most valuable diagnostic tools for the cardiologist is the electrocardiogram, known by the acronym ECG or EKG. The ECG is the graphic record of the electrical current as it progresses through the heart. Patients with symptoms of chest heaviness or pain, jaw or arm pain, or feelings of skipped heartbeats may undergo an ECG to eliminate or complete a potential diagnosis. Combinations of electrodes, called **leads,** are placed on the patient's limbs and in the precordium (the area anterior to the heart) to measure the electrical impulses. ECGs are used to assist in diagnosing ischemia, delays in impulse conduction, hypertrophy of the chambers, and arrhythmias. They are not considered

15

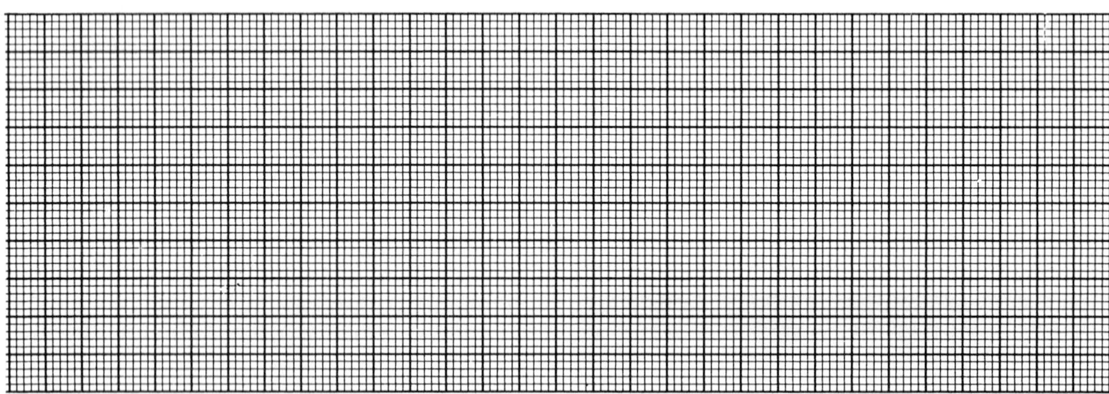

A
On standard ECG paper, each small block is 1 millimeter by 1 millimeter. The large blocks are 5 millimeters by 5 millimeters. (actual size)

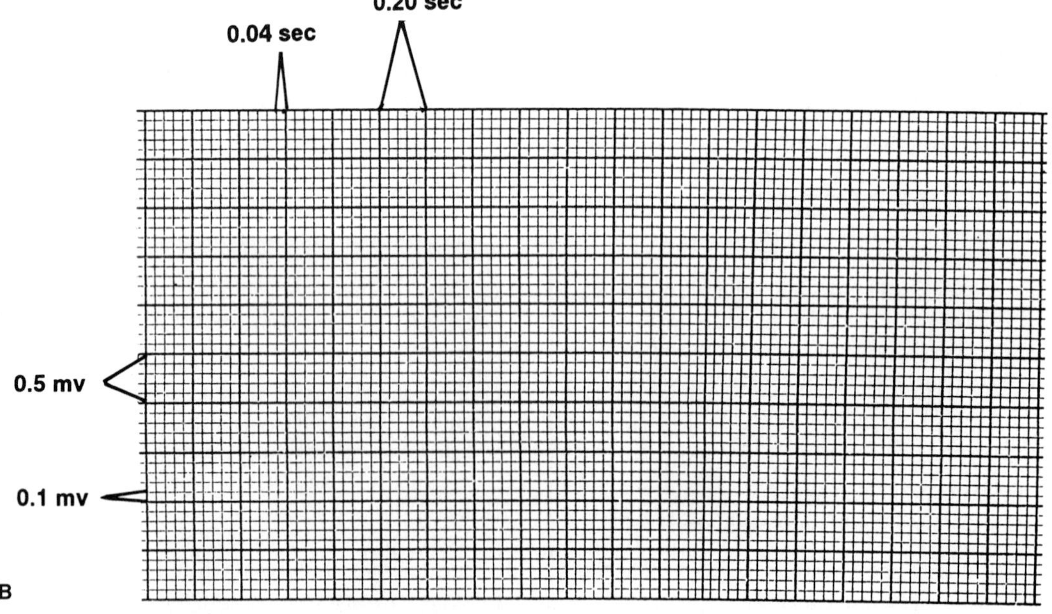

Figure 15-12 Electrocardiogram (ECG) graph paper. (**A**) Each small square is 1 × 1 mm. Each fifth line is marked darker to make a cube of 5 × 5 mm. (**B**) Time in seconds. Each small square is 0.04 second in duration and each large square is 0.20 second in duration. Five large squares = 1 second (5 × 0.20).

reliable for predicting an impending myocardial infarction.

ECG Paper

The ECG tracing is printed on graph paper at a standard speed of 25 mm/s (millimeters per second), with a 0.1 mV (millivolt) electric impulse. The ECG graph paper, although it appears white, is either blue or black with a white, heat-labile coating. A graph is printed over the white coating. The stylus of the ECG machine is heated to melt the white coating, exposing the dark background to record the movement of the stylus. The ECG paper is affected by pressure and heat and should be handled carefully to prevent extraneous markings. Newer ECG machines have controlled stylus temperatures; older machines may require adjustment of the temperature. If the stylus is too hot, the plastic coating will melt irregularly. If the stylus is not hot enough, the mark may be too light to read.

The voltage of the heart's impulse is measured in millimeters on a vertical axis. Each small square on the graph paper is 1 × 1 mm. Each fifth line is marked darker to make a cube of 5 × 5 mm, or 25 small cubes. These measurements are standard, and all physicians use them to interpret the length and strength of the electricity generated during each phase of the impulse transmission (Fig. 15-12).

The Cardiac Cycle

The electrical wave called depolarization begins in the SA node, then spreads across the atria causing the atria to contract and producing the P wave on the ECG. The time required for the impulse to travel through the atria is called the PR interval. The wave then pauses about 0.1 second before stimulating the AV node. The pause allows blood to enter the ventricles. The wave proceeds down the AV bundle, into the bundle branches, to the Purkinje fibers, and into the myocardial cells, causing the ventricles to contract. This phase of transmission is displayed on the ECG as the QRS complex. The R wave represents the moment of greatest electrical charge and should rise in a sharp peak as the ventricles receive the charge and contract in response.

The QRS complex normally is followed by a flat portion, a pause (the ST segment). The T wave then follows, which represents **repolarization** of the ventricles. Repolarization is a resting state and occurs so that the heart can regain the negative charge within each cell to prepare for the next wave of depolarization.

Together, the P wave (atrial contraction), QRS wave (ventricular contraction or depolarization), and T wave (resting stage or repolarization between beats) represents a cardiac cycle (Fig. 15-13).

PR Interval. The time from the beginning of the P wave to the beginning of the QRS complex is called the *PR interval*. This time interval represents depolarization of the atria and the spread of the depolarization wave up to and including the AV node.

PR Segment. The PR segment represents the period of time between the P wave and the QRS complex.

ST Segment. The distance between the QRS complex and the T wave from the point where the QRS complex ends (J-point) to the onset of the ascending limb of the T wave is called the *ST segment*. On the ECG, this segment is a sensitive indicator of myocardial ischemia or injury.

QT Interval. The time from the beginning of the QRS complex to the end of the T wave is called the *QT interval*. This interval represents both ventricular depolarization and repolarization.

Ventricular Activation Time. The time from the beginning of the QRS complex to the peak of the R wave is called the *ventricular activation time* and represents the time necessary for the depolarization wave to travel from the inner surface of the heart (endocardium) to the outer surface of the heart (epicardium).

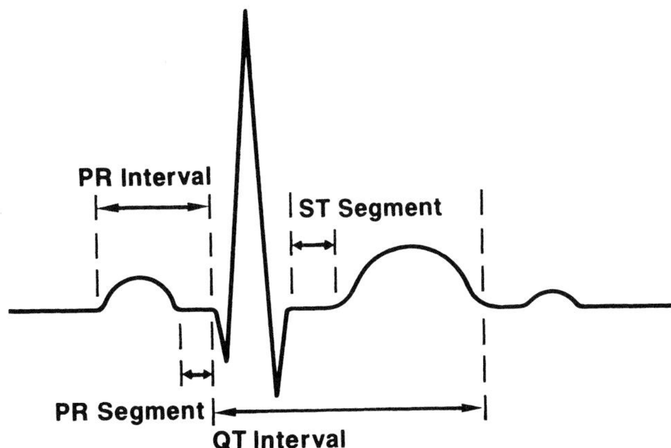

Figure 15-13 Intervals and segments.

ECG Leads

Over the years, a standard system of electrode placement has evolved, and a nomenclature has been developed for the recordings made from different electrode combinations. Each combination is known as a lead. Each lead records the electrical impulse through the heart from a different angle. The standard ECG has 12 leads that produce a three-dimensional record of the impulse wave.

There are four wires with connectors labeled for the patient limbs (Box 15-6). The four limb electrodes

Box 15-6
Abbreviations Used in Performing ECGs

RA—right arm
LA—left arm
LL—left leg
RL—right leg
V_1–V_6—chest lead
aVR—augmented voltage right arm
aVL—augmented voltage left arm
aVF—augmented voltage left foot or leg

should be positioned away from bony areas and onto more muscular areas, such as the calves, outer thighs, and above the elbow. The leads may be placed in any position on the patient's limbs for recording, but the best results are obtained by proper placement. Adjustments may be necessary for amputees, patients who have had limb surgery, or trauma patients.

The right leg electrode is the grounding lead to reduce alternating current interference. It keeps the average voltage of the patient the same as that of the recording instrument and is the "referencing" electrode. The first three combinations derived from the other three limb electrodes are standard bipolar limb leads or Einthoven leads. These leads also allow a frontal visualization of the heart's electrical activity from side to side. Figure 15-14 shows 12-lead ECG electrode placement.

Each lead provides a specific measurement:

- Lead I measures the difference in electrical potential between the right arm (RA) to left arm (LA).
- Lead II measures the difference in electrical potential between the RA and the left leg (LL).
- Lead III measures the difference in electrical potential between the LA and the LL.

Using the same three electrodes, measurements can be made of the signal between one electrode and the average of the remaining two. These second three combinations are the augmented unipolar limb leads and allow visualization from a frontal view top to bottom:

- Lead aVR = (LL + LA) to RA measures the potential at the right arm.
- Lead aVL = (LL + RA) to LA measures the potential at the left arm.
- Lead aVF = (RA + LA) to LL measures the potential at the left foot (see Fig. 15-14).

To take a closer look at the heart, electrodes are placed directly on the chest wall. The limb electrodes must remain attached to the patient. Six chest positions are universally defined. Positioning of these electrodes must be precise to record the chest leads accurately. These leads show the comparison of the chest electrode potential to the average of the three limb electrodes and are called the unipolar precordial (chest) leads (Box 15-7).

All electrodes must connect to the wires of the ECG machine. Specific codes are used to mark each lead (Table 15-3). The production of the ECG recording onto paper varies from one ECG machine to another, but the principle and technique are universal.

Checkpoint Question

9. *Which three waves represent a cardiac cycle on an ECG?*

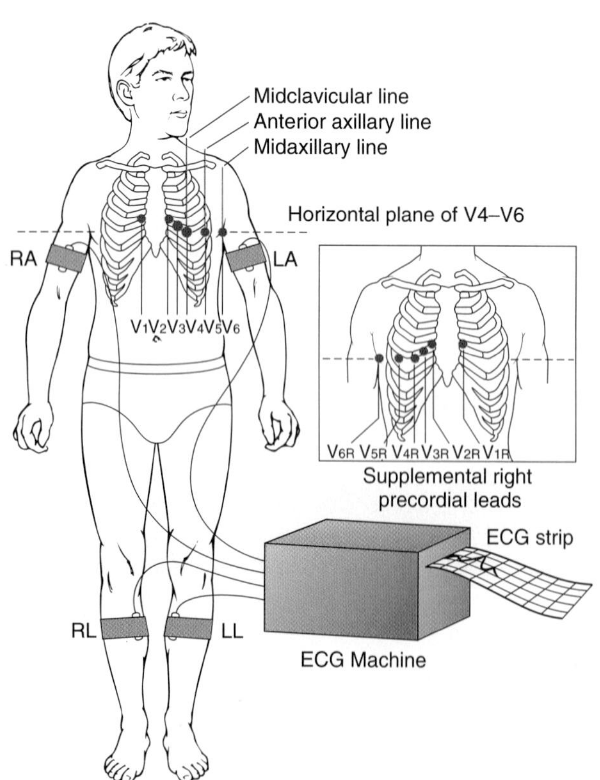

Figure 15-14 Twelve-lead ECG-electrode placement.

Preparing for the ECG

Many offices are equipped with ECG machines that are designed to interpret the readings as they are recorded. These machines will also alert you on the printout if any of the various attachments are not in the correct order or are placed incorrectly. Most offices now use three-channel machines that automatically progress from one lead to the next and mark each lead on the graph paper as it moves through the standard

Box 15-7

Positioning of Unipolar Precordial (Chest) Leads

- Lead V_1: Fourth intercostal space at right margin of sternum
- Lead V_2: Fourth intercostal space at left margin of sternum
- Lead V_3: Midway between position V_2 and position V_4
- Lead V_4: Fifth intercostal space at junction of midclavicular line
- Lead V_5: At horizontal level of position V_4 at left anterior axillary line
- Lead V_6: At horizontal level of position V_4 and position V_5 at midaxillary line

Table 15-3 **Coding ECG Leads**

Lead	*Code*	*Lead*	*Code*
I	.	V_1	-.
II	..	V_2	-..
III	...	V_3	-...
aVR	-	V_4	-....
aVL	--	V_5	-.....
aVF	---	V_6	-......

order of recording. Some offices still use older machines that must be advanced by hand and marked with standardized lead indicators. You must become familiar with the particular machine used where you work by reading the manuals provided by the manufacturer and by asking questions to clarify points of concern.

The area in which an ECG is recorded should be comfortable, warm, and private. Lighting should be indirect and restful. A small pillow or cushion should be placed under the patient's head and perhaps also under the knees and shoulders to provide comfort. Tables should be long and wide enough to support the patient's body and limbs comfortably.

To calm and comfort a frightened patient, give friendly smiles, offer assistance when needed, and provide reassurance that the ECG is harmless. A frightened patient is not as likely to be compliant with instructions and may interfere with the quality of the recording by moving about or actually trembling in fear. Procedures 15-1 and 15-2 describe the steps for performing a 12-lead ECG and mounting the strip for reading.

ECG Interpretation

Interpretation of the standard 12-lead ECG is done by the physician, who takes the following elements into consideration:

- Rate: how fast the heart is beating
- Rhythm: regularity of recurring amplitudes and intervals
- Axis: position of the heart and direction of depolarization
- Hypertrophy: size of the heart
- Ischemia: decrease in the blood supply to an area
- Infarction: death of heart muscle resulting in loss of function

Under usual diagnostic conditions, the 12-lead ECG demonstrates sufficient data. As the medical assistant, you are responsible for obtaining an ECG that is of good quality without avoidable **artifacts.** An artifact is the appearance of an abnormal signal that does not reflect electrical activity of the heart during the cardiac cycle. It can be attributed to patient movement, mechanical problems with the ECG machine, or improper technique. Table 15-4 describes three types of artifacts and how to prevent them. To avoid artifacts due to improper technique, review and practice the procedure. It is your responsibility to feel comfortable with the ECG and to ensure good technical quality and attain the proper ECG tracing.

Sometimes the physician may request a rhythm strip along with the ECG. A rhythm strip is a long strip of QRS complexes of a certain lead or combinations of leads; it may be used to define certain cardiac arrhythmias. The physician may also request that chest electrodes be positioned on the right side of the chest, instead of the left, for cases of true **dextrocardia** (right-sided heart placement) or in pediatric patients (the heart of a young child is not angled as sharply to the left as an adult's).

Holter Monitor

In many instances, cardiac problems will not be apparent during a brief ECG. For diagnosis of intermittent cardiac arrhythmias and dysfunctions, a monitor that records for at least a 24-hour period is used. The Holter monitor is small and portable and can be worn comfortably for long periods of time without interfering with daily activities. It may be set to record continuously, or it may be programmed to record when the patient presses a record button at the onset of symptoms. This is also known as an incident or event button. As part of this test, the patient must also keep a diary of daily activities (Box 15-8). Frequently, the medical assistant will be responsible for applying the monitor and instructing the patient in its purpose and use (Procedure 15-3).

Not all Holter monitors record on graph paper. Newer, less bulky Holter monitors have computer memory and print the reading at the end of testing. The physician will receive the computerized synopsis of the diary and the cardiac events for the testing period.

A 30-day event monitor is designed for use during a longer period than is possible with the Holter monitor. Two leads are used rather than six, and the machine is very small and light. The recorder must be activated whenever symptoms are perceived by the patient and will not record unless the marker is pressed (Fig. 15-15).

Chest X-ray or Chest Roentgenogram

A chest x-ray provides valuable basic information about the anatomic location and gross structures of the heart, great vessels, and lungs. Chest x-rays aid in the

15

Table 15-4 Types of Artifacts

Artifact	Possible Causes	How to Prevent Problems
Wandering baseline 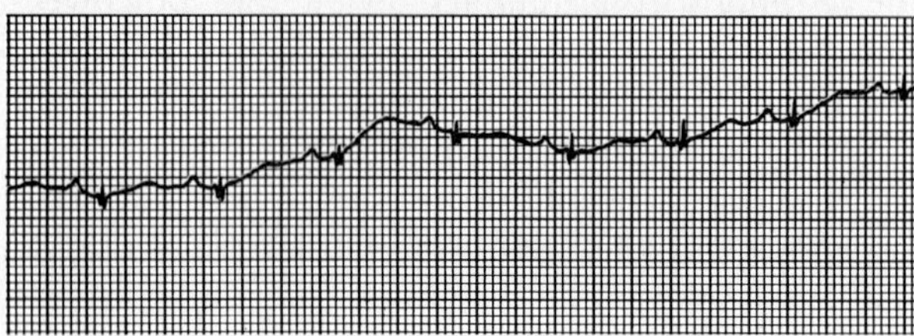 Wandering Baseline	• Electrodes are too tight or too loose. • Electrolyte gel may have built up on electrodes. • Patient's skin may not have been cleaned of oil, lotion, or excess hair.	• Apply electrodes properly. • Thoroughly remove old gel before applying new gel. • Prepare the patient's skin before performing the test.
Muscle or somatic artifact 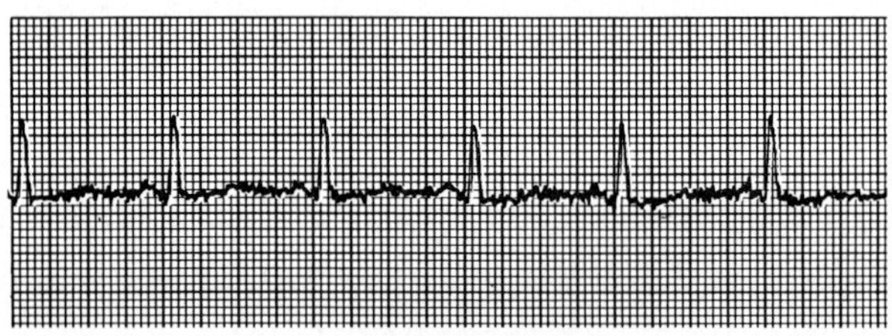 Somatic Muscle Tremor	• Patient cannot remain still due to involuntary tremors or fear.	• Reassure the patient about the test and stress the need to keep still, but be aware that patients with diseases that cause tremors may not be able to remain motionless.
Alternating current artifact 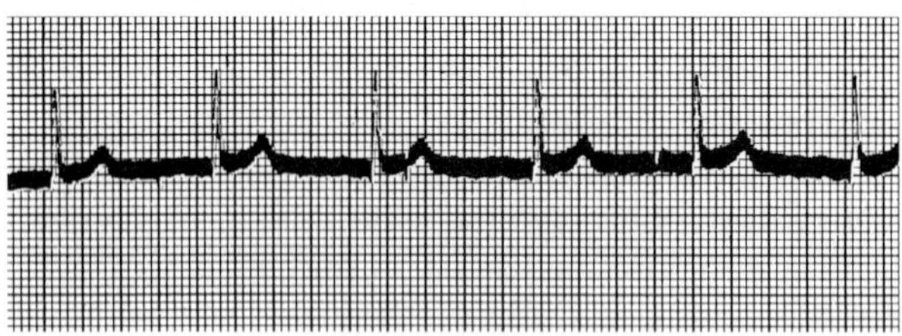 AC Interference	• The ECG machine is improperly grounded. • Electrical interference exists in the room. • Lead wires are dangling.	• Check cables to ensure the machine is properly grounded before beginning the test. • Move the patient to an area that is free of interference, or unplug any appliances in the immediate area for the duration of the test. If possible, set aside one room that is completely free of electrical appliances other than the ECG machine. • Arrange the leads along the contours of the patient's body, and neatly support them on the table.

> *Box 15-8*
> **Patient Diary for Holter Monitoring**
>
> A patient with a Holter monitor must keep a diary of daily activities. When symptoms are experienced, the patient depresses an incident (or event) button on the machine, then records in the diary the activity that caused the incident and the resulting symptoms. At intervals, the patient also records daily activities, such as working quietly at a desk, driving a car, eating a meal, watching television, or sleeping. All activities must be noted, including elimination, sexual intercourse, anger, laughter, and so on. Some monitors are equipped with small tape recorders so the patient can keep an audio diary instead of a written one.

evaluation of such cardiovascular disorders as congestive heart failure and pericardial effusions.

Cardiac Stress Test

To measure the body's response to increased demands made on the myocardium, the physician may request a cardiac stress test. This is usually done on a treadmill, but it may also be done on a stationary bicycle (Fig. 15-16). The patient will be attached to an ECG monitor for a constant tracing. The medical assistant should never perform a cardiac stress test without the physician on site. The test is performed according to the physician's orders, and the ECG strip is mounted for the patient's record. Based on a positive or negative reading, this test may indicate the need for further cardiac testing.

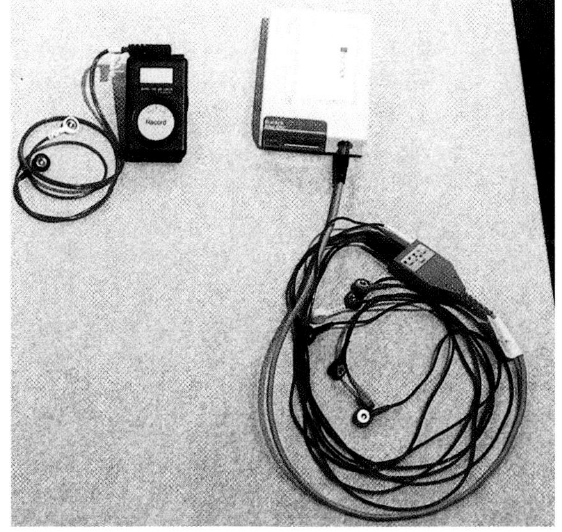

Figure 15-15 Monitors. (*Left*) A 30-day event monitor. (*Right*) A 24-hour Holter monitor.

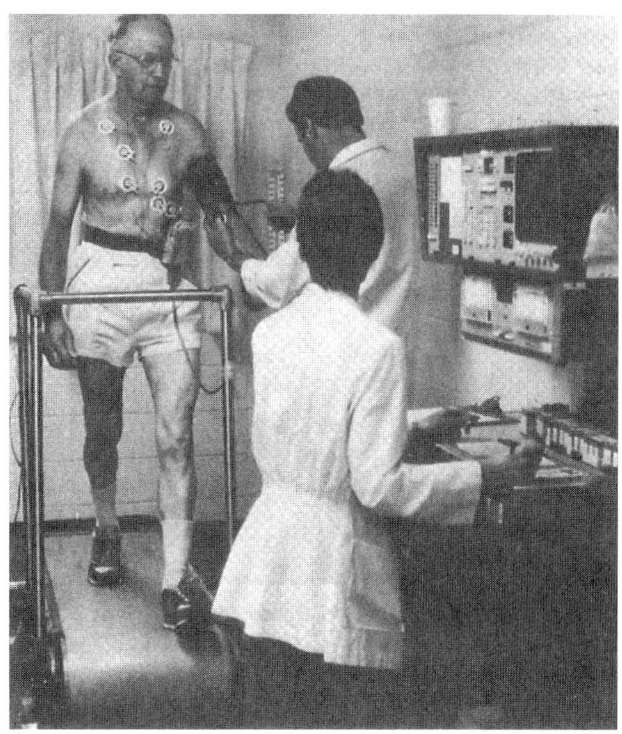

Figure 15-16 Walking a treadmill that moves at a progressively faster pace while the heart's activity is recorded is a way of determining the heart's ability to adapt to increased work during exercise. (Courtesy of Borgess Medical Center, Kalamazoo, MI.)

In some instances, the physician may order a thallium scan to be performed with the stress test. Thallium 201, an isotope, is administered intravenously and localizes in the myocardium. A scintigraphy machine (a device to show distribution and intensity of radioactivity in a body part) produces two-dimensional images of radioactivity in the tissues of the myocardium, instantly showing areas of decreased perfusion or "cold spots." These areas are diagnostic for occlusion of coronary arteries when a regular ECG or stress test may not be as exact. This is frequently the test of choice for patients who are unable to perform a standard stress test.

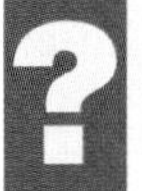

Checkpoint Question

10. *What is the purpose of a cardiac stress test?*

Echocardiography

An echocardiogram, or echo, uses harmless sound waves generated from a small device called a transducer. These waves travel through the cardiac cham-

text continues on page 363

Procedure 15-1 Performing a 12-Lead Electrocardiogram

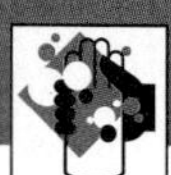

PURPOSE:

To assess cardiac dysrhythmias
To evaluate cardiac medication therapy

EQUIPMENT/SUPPLIES

- equipment for measuring vital signs
- ECG machine
- ECG paper
- coupling gel or pads
- electrodes
- gown or cape
- razor (if necessary)
- comfortable table

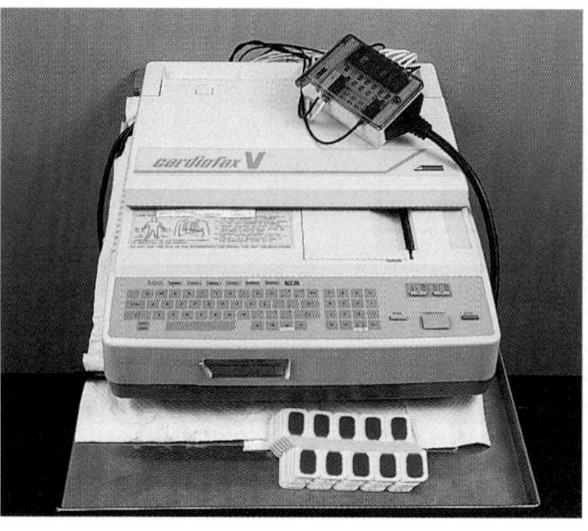

ECG machine.

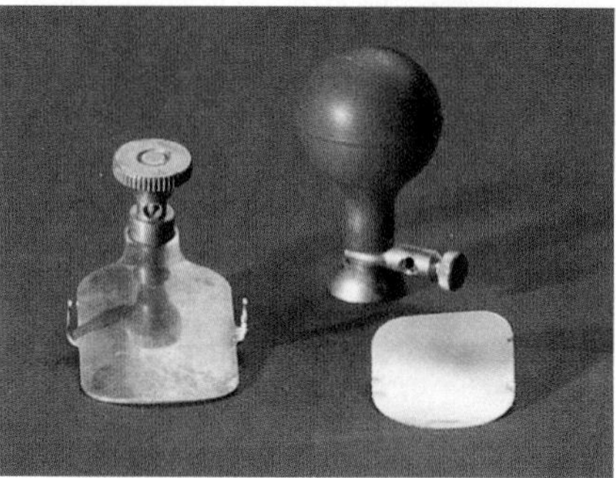

(From left to right) A metal electrode, a welch cup, a disposable adhesive electrode.

STEPS

1. Wash your hands.
2. Assemble the equipment.
3. Greet and identify the patient. Explain the procedure, noting that the machine will pick up tremors or muscle movement and instructing the patient to lie still for the usually brief duration of the test. Ask for and answer any questions.
4. Before beginning the ECG, record the patient's data base: name, age, sex, height, weight, vital signs, symptoms, and medications. Note the time and date of the recording.

   This information is needed for proper diagnosis.
5. Note any preparation required for the test. Generally, no preparation is needed. However, the physician may request that the patient exercise for a prescribed time before the test to record changes brought about by physical stress. Also, skin preparation (eg, slight skin abrading or shaving) may be necessary for patients with extremely dry or oily skin, or for those with coarse arm or chest hair.

   Skin preparation ensures properly attached leads and helps avoid improper readings and lost time repeating the test.
6. Instruct the patient to disrobe above the waist and provide a gown for privacy. Nylons or tights should be removed also.

   Clothing may interfere with the proper placement of leads.
7. Position the patient comfortably in a supine position with pillows as needed for comfort. Drape for warmth and privacy.

   If the patient is uncomfortable, too cool, or improperly draped, movement is likely, resulting in artifacts (see Table 15-4).
8. Check the machine for safety of grounding. Position it with the power cord away from the patient. Turn the machine on to warm the stylus.

   With the cord away from the patient, electrical current artifacts are less likely. The warmth of the stylus melts the white coated surface of the ECG paper, exposing the dark background to record the movement of the stylus.

continued

Procedure 15-1 Continued **Performing a 12-Lead Electrocardiogram**

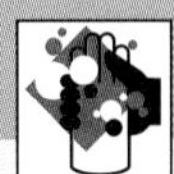

9. Apply the electrodes according to the manufacturer's directions.

For metal electrodes:

a. Apply a small amount of gel evenly and equally to all electrodes, or use a pad impregnated with electrolyte gel.

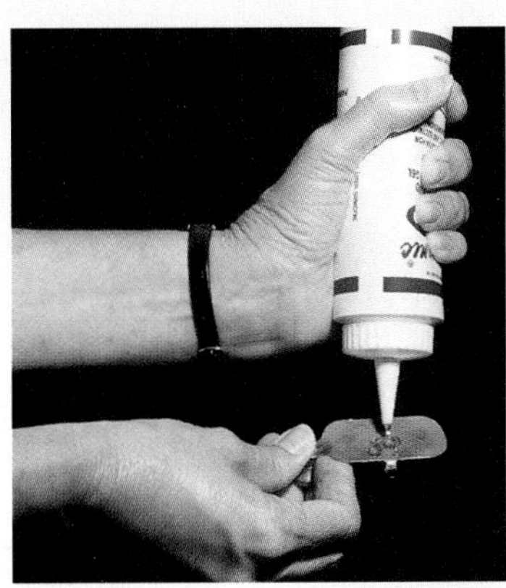

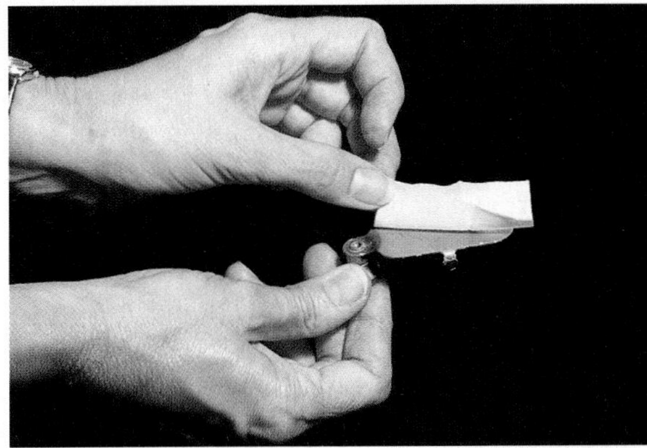

b. Rub the gel into the skin using the side of the electrode to redden the skin slightly for increased conduction.

c. Apply rubber straps to the prongs of the metal electrodes and attach snugly to the limbs.

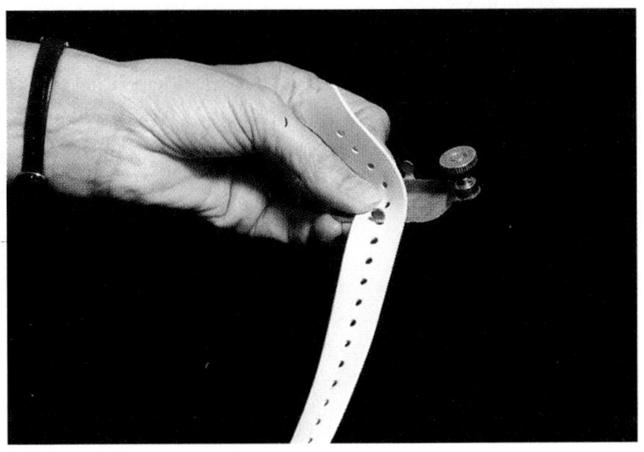

For disposable electrodes:

Be aware that disposable electrodes have electrolyte gel already applied equally and adequately. Place the electrodes on the skin. (*Note:* Disposable electrodes adhere to the skin without straps.)

An electrolyte-conducting gel transmits electrical impulses from the skin to the electrodes. Unequal amounts of gel on electrodes will lead to artifacts. If leads are not snug against the skin, an improper reading will result.

10. Be sure to place electrodes on the fleshy, muscular parts of the upper arms and lower legs. The attachments will point to the hands and feet of the patient.

Conduction will be impaired if attachments are placed on bony prominences. Attachments pointing toward the lower portion of the patient's body will offer better connections and follow the patient's contours.

11. If using Welch electrode cups for the chest leads, apply a small amount of electrolyte gel, compress the bulb to create a suction, press it against the patient's chest at first position, V_1, and release the bulb. Some chest leads may be attached with a rubber strap around the patient's chest, and others may be weighted with a metal strip.

12. Connect the leads securely. They will be coded RA, LA, LL, RL, and C-V. Some are color coded. Untangle the leads before applying to decrease electrical artifacts. Be sure that each lead lies unencumbered along the contours of the patient's body to decrease the incidence of artifacts. Double check the placement.

Improperly placed leads will result in time lost to an inaccurate reading and retesting.

13. Plug in the cable and arrange it along the side of the patient on the table.

This placement will decrease pressure and tugging on the lead attachments.

continued

15

Procedure 15-1 Continued **Performing a 12-Lead Electrocardiogram**

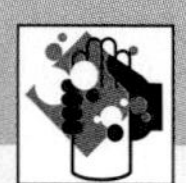

14. Center the stylus and press the standardization button (STD). Set on RUN 25. The mark should be 2 × 10 mm, or 2 small squares wide by 10 small squares high. Adjust appropriately within those parameters. Check at this time for artifacts.

The standardization mark documents accuracy of operation and provides a reference point for reading impulses.

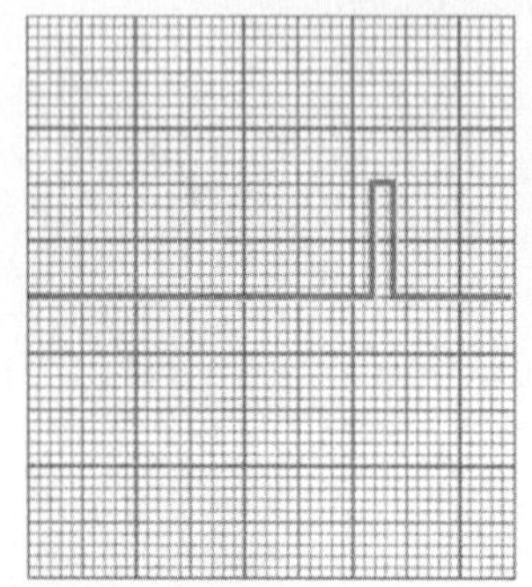

Normal Standard
Standardization mark
is 10 mm high

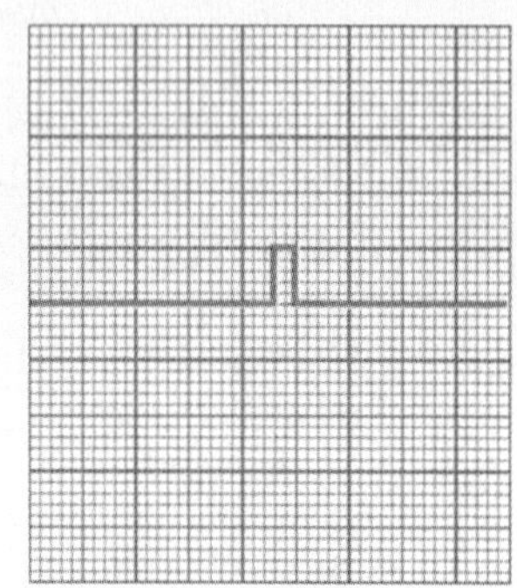

One-Half Standard
Standardization mark
is 5 mm high

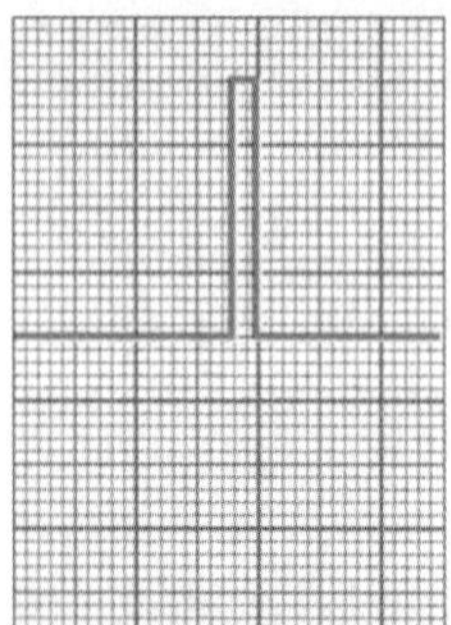

Double Standard
Standardization mark
is 20 mm high

15. Center the stylus on the paper and run 8–10 inches of leads I, II, III. If the R wave is too large for the reading, reduce the standardization to 1/2. If the reading is too small to be accurately read, increase the standardization × 2. If you must move the stylus from the position of the standardization mark, make another mark for reference. If any of the leads are not properly attached, it will be apparent at this time.

16. If the leads were accurately placed and the stylus was appropriately centered for correct readings of leads I, II, III, then proceed manually to aVR, aVL, and aVF, if the machine does not progress automatically. Check the standardization each time a progression is made.

17. Switch to V_1 through V_6 for 5–6 inches of paper. If the instrument is not automatic, you will need to mark each lead as it is run (see Table 15-3 for standard marks).

The physician will need these markings to identify the leads that are being recorded for interpretation.

18. If the machine does not progress automatically, and chest leads must be manually moved to the next position, turn off the machine before disconnecting the leads and restandardize each time. *Note:* If disposable electrode patches are used or if a myocardial infarction is suspected, the physician may want to check the reading before the electrodes are removed to avoid removing them and then replacing them for a repeat ECG run.

If the leads are removed from the patient or from an electrode, the stylus will thrash across the paper. Each time the machine is turned off or leads are moved, the machine must be restandardized.

19. Turn off and unplug the machine at the completion of the reading.

20. Remove the electrodes and clean the patient's skin. Assist the patient from the table and help with dressing, as needed.

Some patients may become dizzy from lying supine.

21. Carefully roll the ECG strip. Do not use clips to secure the roll.

Creases and clips may remove some of the coating and mar or mark the surface, obscuring the reading.

22. Store the equipment by carefully coiling the leads. Clean the electrodes with kitchen cleanser if reusable.

Coiling the leads reduces tangling and damage to the wires. Cleaning the electrodes will prevent build up of electrolyte gel, which would cause artifacts.

continued

Procedure 15-1 Continued Performing a 12-Lead Electrocardiogram

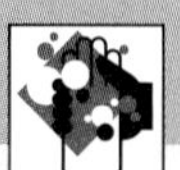

DOCUMENTATION GUIDELINES

- Date and time
- Performance of procedure
- Ordering physician or physician who will evaluate the reading
- Patient complaints/concerns
- Patient education/instructions
- Your signature

Charting Example

DATE	TIME 12-lead ECG done. Pt tolerated
	procedure well. No complaints of chest
	pain during the ECG. ECG mounted and
	given to Dr. Bruno to evaluate. Pt was
	discharged by Dr. Bruno. —Your signature

15

bers, walls, and valves and are then transmitted back to a screen where they can be viewed and interpreted. Echocardiograms help the physician to diagnose patients with suspected or known valvular disease. Echoes also aid in diagnosing the severity of heart failure and cardiomyopathy. In addition, this test can be used to detect injuries to the heart in patients with trauma or in situations involving possible harvest of the heart for transplant after a fatal accident.

Cardiac Catheterization

Cardiac catheterization is a common invasive procedure used to help diagnose or treat a heart condition. It

Procedure 15-2 Mounting the ECG Strip for Reading

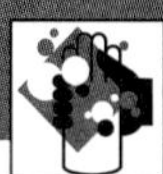

PURPOSE:

To present the reading in a manner most accessible to the physician for interpretation

EQUIPMENT/SUPPLIES

- physician-preferred mounting device
- clean, flat surface
- scissors

STEPS

1. Label the mounting paper with the patient's data.
   This information is important for interpretation of the reading.
2. Unroll the strip on a clean, flat surface, and identify the area of lead I with the standardization mark. Cut this strip with scissors to the length preferred by the physician.
   A soiled strip may be illegible. The standardization mark will be used as a reference. Physicians have set opinions regarding the proper length for various types of readings.
3. If the mounting device has protective sleeves, carefully open the sleeve as far as possible and insert the strip. If the mounting papers have adhesive strips and clear plastic covers, use care to prevent marring the surface of the strip.
   A scratch may mar the surface and make it unreadable.
4. Repeat the procedure until all of the leads are in their proper places on the sheet.
5. File the report in the area the physician has designated for reports pending review.

Procedure 15-3 Applying a Holter Monitor

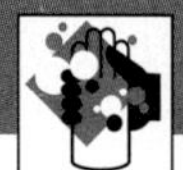 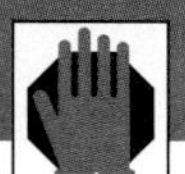

PURPOSE:

To provide an extended assessment of cardiac function

EQUIPMENT/SUPPLIES

- monitor
- fresh batteries
- roll of blank tape
- carrying case with strap
- electrodes
- skin swabs
- gauze
- razor (as needed)
- patient diary
- gloves, if skin must be shaved

STEPS

1. Assemble the equipment.

   Fresh batteries and a whole roll of monitor tape will avoid battery failure and prevent the patient from running out of tape during the test.

2. Greet and identify the patient. Explain the procedure. Remind the patient that it is important to carry out all normal activities for the duration of the test.

   Avoiding a normal routine will not allow the physician to identify areas of concern.

3. Explain the purpose for the incident diary, emphasizing the need for the patient to carry it at all times during the test.

4. Prepare the patient's skin for electrode attachment. Provide privacy and have the patient sit. Expose the chest, then shave the areas of attachment as needed. Glove, if shaving is required. Clean with the approved de-fatting agent to remove skin oils. Abrade the area with the gauze.

   The chest must be exposed for proper placement of the electrodes. Shaving and abrading will improve adherence of the adhesive on the electrodes.

5. Apply the special Holter electrodes at the specified sites:

   a. The right manubrium border
   b. The left manubrium border
   c. The right sternal border at the fifth rib level
   d. The fifth rib at the anterior axillary line
   e. The right lower rib cage over the cartilage as a ground lead. To do this, expose the adhesive backing of the electrodes and follow manufacturer's instructions to attach firmly. Check for security of attachment.

   Electrodes may also be placed at the left manubrium border at the level of the second rib and at the left sternal border at the fifth intercostal space.

   Products will vary, but all will require moist electrolyte and secure adhesive to ensure a full 24 hours of operation.

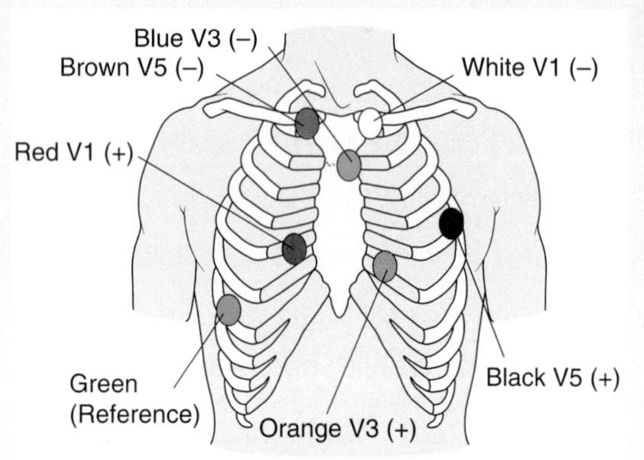

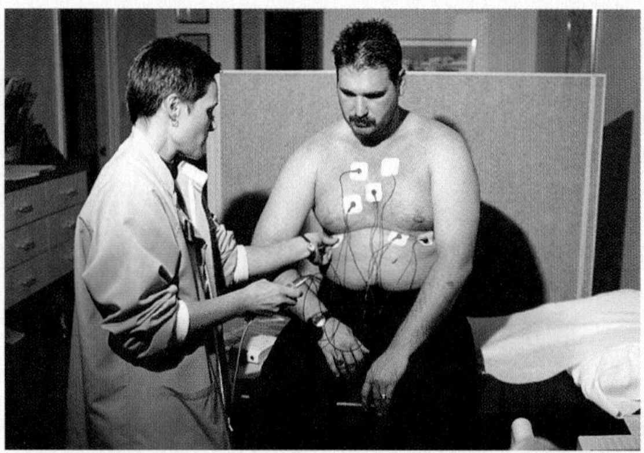

continued

Procedure 15-3 *Continued* Applying a Holter Monitor

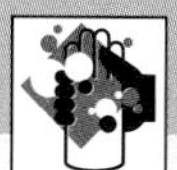
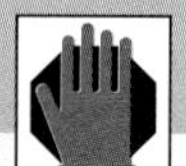

6. Position electrode connectors downward toward the patient's feet. Attach the leads and secure with adhesive tape.

The addition of adhesive tape over the connections will help ensure that the leads do not work loose during the day.

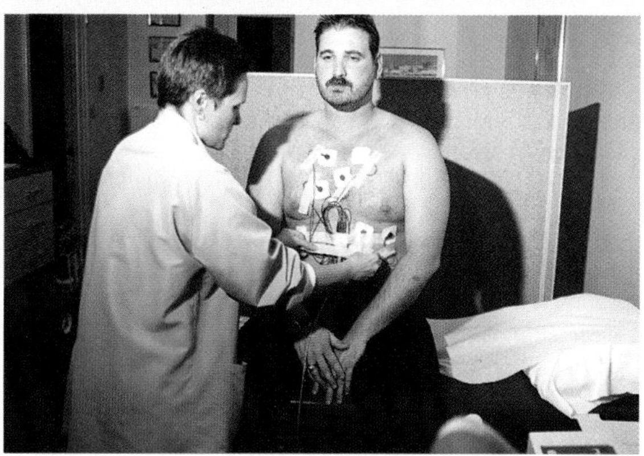

7. Connect the cable and run a baseline ECG by hooking the Holter to the ECG with the cable hookup.

Do this to check for accurate function of the Holter.

8. Assist the patient to redress carefully with the cable extending through the garment opening. Clothing that buttons down the front is more convenient.

This prevents pulling and strain on the leads.

9. Plug the cable into the recorder and mark the diary. If needed, explain the purpose of the diary to the patient again. Give instructions for a return appointment to evaluate the recording and the diary.

DOCUMENTATION GUIDELINES

- Date and time
- Application of monitor
- Patient education/instructions
- Date and time scheduled for return
- Your signature

Charting Example

DATE	TIME
	S: "I had three spells with my monitor
	on."
	O: Pt reported and recorded three
	episodes.
	A: Holter removed. Strip mounted.
	P: Dr. Royal notified. —Your signature

15

may be performed on patients with shortness of breath, angina, dizziness, palpitations, fluttering in the chest, rapid heartbeat, and other cardiovascular symptoms to determine the severity of the problem. It is often indicated after a cardiac stress test or echocardiogram reveals an abnormality.

The cardiologist inserts a flexible tube called a catheter into a blood vessel in either the arm or groin, then guides it gently toward the heart. When the catheter is in place, contrast medium is injected, allowing the heart's chambers, valves, great vessels, and coronary arteries to be visualized. If atherosclerotic plaques are found at this time, angioplasty may be performed (see Box 15-3).

Coronary Arteriography

This invasive procedure involves injecting a contrast medium into the coronary arteries located on the outer surface of the heart, allowing visualization of any lesions that may be present. It provides enough data for an accurate assessment of possible congenital or acquired heart disease. It also is frequently used to assess heart damage after myocardial infarction.

Answers to Checkpoint Questions

1. *The exchange of nutrients and oxygen occurs in the capillary beds.*
2. *There are four chambers in the heart. The upper chambers are the atria; the lower chambers are the ventricles.*
3. *The five components of the conduction system are sinoatrial node, atrioventricular node, bundle of His, right and left bundle branches, and the Purkinje fibers. The sinoatrial node is the pacemaker.*

4. *Four predisposing factors for heart disease are history of elevated cholesterol, smoking, diabetes mellitus, and hypertension.*
5. *Stroke and renal failure may result from untreated hypertension.*
6. *Varicose veins occur when the superficial veins in the legs become swollen and distended.*
7. *With pericarditis, pain increases with inspiration and movement; pain in a myocardial infarction will not change with patient positioning.*
8. *A murmur is an abnormal heart sound.*
9. *P, QRS, and T waves represent a cardiac cycle on an ECG.*
10. *A cardiac stress test measures the response of the myocardium to increased demands for oxygen.*

Critical Thinking Challenges

1. Draw a diagram of the heart. Draw a cardiac cycle as seen by the ECG. Connect the ECG waves to the appropriate areas of the heart. How would you explain an ECG to a patient? How would you assist the patient in relaxing for this procedure?
2. Compare and contrast the signs and symptoms of a cerebrovascular accident and a transient ischemic attack. Make a list of questions that you would ask a patient to determine if he or she is having a stroke. What kind of help would a patient need at home after experiencing a stroke?
3. Explain anemia and identify the symptoms seen with it. Why does anemia cause these symptoms? What dietary instructions should be given to a patient with iron deficiency anemia?

Suggestions for Further Reading

Akhtar, M. (1994). *Examination of the Heart—The Electrocardiogram.* Dallas, TX: American Heart Association.

Canobbio, M. M. (1990). *Cardiovascular Disorders—Mosby's Clinical Nursing Series.* St. Louis: C.V. Mosby.

Catalano, J. T. (1993). *Guide to ECG Analysis.* Philadelphia: J.B. Lippincott.

Davis, D. (1992). *How to Quickly and Accurately Master ECG Interpretation.* Philadelphia: J.B. Lippincott.

Memmler, R. L., Cohen, B. J., & Wood, D. L. (1996). *The Human Body in Health and Disease,* 8th ed. Philadelphia: Lippincott-Raven.

Professional Guide to Diseases, 4th ed. (1992). Springhouse, PA: Springhouse.

Smeltzer, S., & Bare, B. (1996). *Brunner and Suddarth's Textbook of Medical-Surgical Nursing,* 8th ed. Philadelphia: Lippincott-Raven.

Thaler, M. S. (1995). *The Only EKG Book You'll Ever Need,* 2nd ed. Philadelphia: J.B. Lippincott.

Chapter Competencies

Learning Objectives

Upon successfully completing this chapter, you will be able to:

1. Spell and define the Key Terms.
2. Describe the circulation of the lymph fluid through the lymphatic system from the capillaries to the return of fluid to the circulatory system.
3. State the location and functions of the lymph nodes and nodules.
4. Explain the role of the thymus in immunity.
5. State the location and functions of the spleen.
6. List and describe disorders of the lymphatic and immune systems.
7. Identify laboratory tests and clinical procedures related to the lymphatic and immune systems.
8. Describe what is meant by the term immunity.
9. Describe and compare the types of immunity.
10. Describe the function of T cells and B cells in immunity.
11. Explain what a vaccine is, and identify some of the common vaccines in use today.
12. Define HIV and AIDS.
13. Explain the methods of transmission and the impact of HIV and AIDS on the body.

Key Terms

(See Glossary for definitions.)

acquired immunodeficiency syndrome (AIDS)
allergy
antibodies
antigens
antihistamine
attenuated
B cells
complement
didanosine (formerly dideoxyinosine, ddI)
dideoxycytidine (ddC)
ELISA
histamine
immune globulins
interferon
Kaposi's sarcoma
macrophages
opportunistic infection
phagocytes
phagocytosis
retrovirus
septicemia
T cells
titer
toxoid
vaccine
Western blot
zalcitabine
zidovudine (formerly azidothymidine, AZT)

Our environment contains a large variety of infectious agents, such as viruses, bacteria, fungi, and parasites. Any of these agents can cause pathologic damage, and if they are allowed to multiply unchecked, they may eventually kill their host. In a normal individual with an intact immune system, the majority of infections are of limited duration and rarely result in permanent damage. The lymphatic system and certain specifically designed blood cells make up the immune system and are responsible for protecting us from the pathogens in our environment. The lymphatic system is considered part of the circulatory system, and although its functions are different from those of the circulatory system, all of the functions of both systems are interdependent.

STRUCTURE AND FUNCTION OF THE LYMPHATIC SYSTEM

Lymph

Clear, watery fluid filtered from the blood in the capillaries exchanges with fluid found in the interstitial spaces. Most of this fluid is reabsorbed by osmosis back into the blood in the capillaries. Some tissue fluid, however, remains in interstitial spaces and must be returned to the circulation by the lymphatic system. As soon as the tissue fluid enters the lymphatic system through a lymphatic capillary, it is referred to as lymph. Lymph is similar to plasma and may contain a few erythrocytes, electrolytes, proteins, and variable numbers of lymphocytes, the white blood cells that function in immunity. The milky, fatty fluid brought to the system by the lymphatic vessels that surround the intestines is called chyle.

16

Lymph Vessels

The lymphatic system is a network of vessels to convey the excess fluid from the tissue spaces back to the general circulation (Fig. 16-1). These vessels begin as fine, blind-ended lymphatic capillaries made from one layer of flat epithelial cells. The capillaries act as wicks to absorb and filter fluid from around the cells. They do not join corresponding veins and arteries, like the capillaries of the circulatory system, but begin in pools of tissue fluid and join with larger lymphatic vessels.

Lymph vessels have thicker walls than those of the lymph capillaries. Like veins, lymph vessels contain valves so that lymph flows in one direction—toward the thoracic cavity. Lymphatic vessels include superficial and deep sets. The superficial vessels are immediately below the skin, often accompanying the superficial veins. The deep vessels are usually larger and accompany the deep veins. Lymphatic vessels carry lymph away from the regional nodes, eventually draining it into one of two terminal vessels: the right lymphatic duct or the thoracic duct.

The right lymphatic duct receives lymph from the right side of the head, neck, and thorax and from the right upper extremity and empties into the right subclavian vein. The rest of the body is drained by the thoracic duct, which receives lymph from all parts of the body except those above the diaphragm on the right side. The thoracic duct empties into the left subclavian vein. Both ducts are separated from the general circulation by semilunar valves that prevent blood from entering the lymphatic system and prevent the backflow of lymph.

Lymphatic vessels are usually named according to their locations. For example, those in the breast are

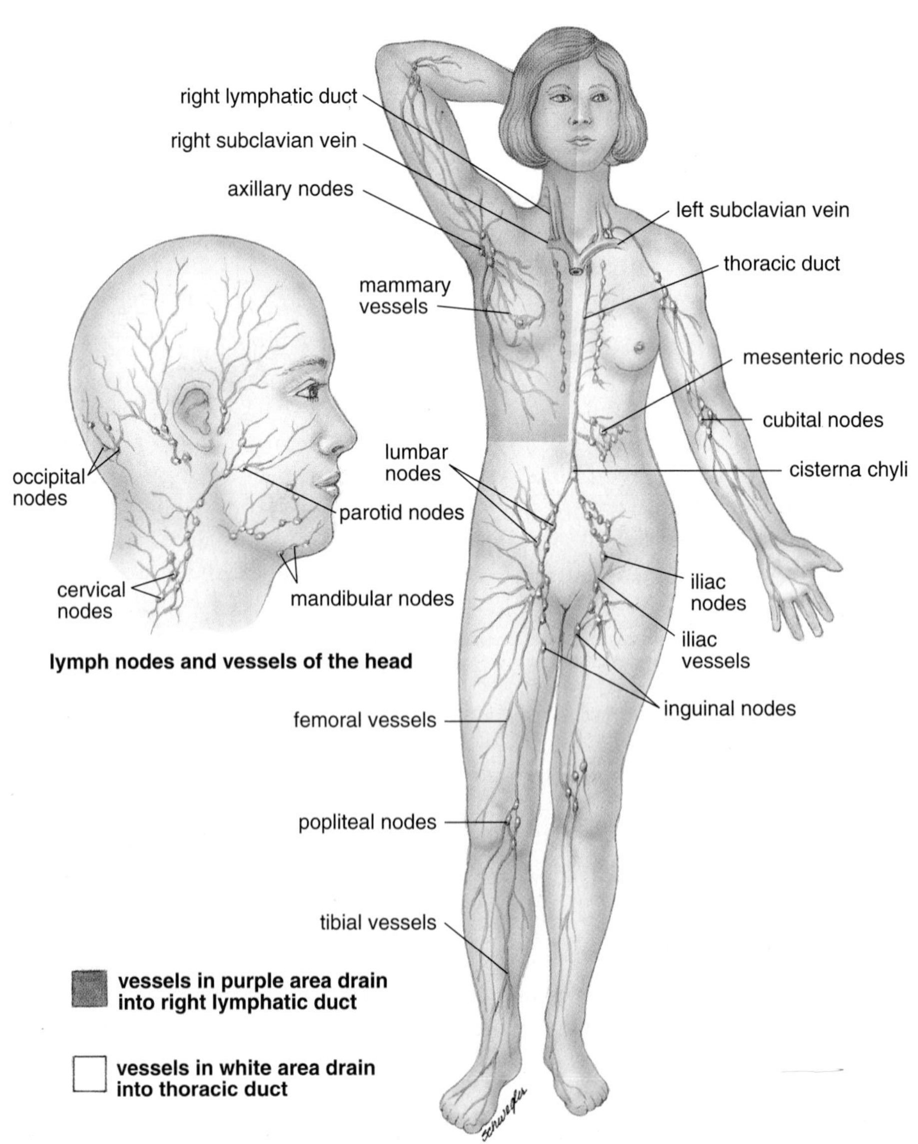

Figure 16-1 The lymphatic system.

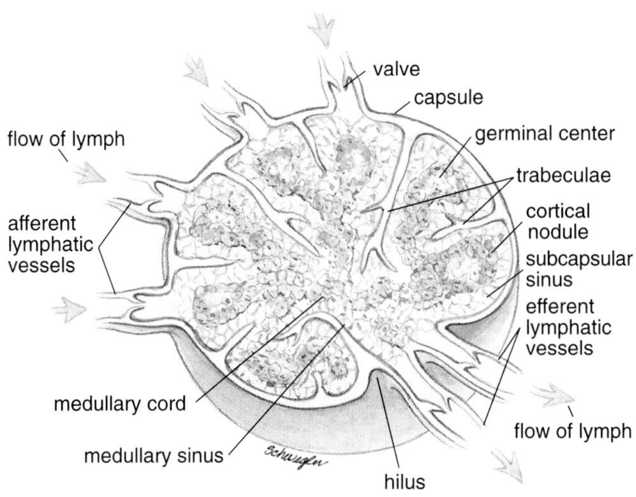

Figure 16-2 Structure of a lymph node.

called mammary lymphatic vessels, those in the thigh are called femoral lymphatic vessels, and those in the lower leg are called tibial lymphatic vessels. The vessels that drain fatty chyle from the intestinal area are called lacteals because of the milky appearance of the fluid from this area.

Lymph Nodes and Nodules

Collections of stationary lymphatic tissue are called lymph nodes and nodules.

Lymph nodes (Fig. 16-2), sometimes incorrectly called lymph glands, are located along the path of the lymphatic vessels (Table 16-1). Afferent vessels bring fluid in; efferent vessels carry it away. Lymph nodes are designed to filter the lymph once it is drained from the tissues. They are rounded masses of lymph tissue varying in size from a pinhead to about 1 inch and occur from one or two to hundreds at a site. Inside the nodes are masses of lymphatic tissue with spaces designated for the production of lymphocytes and partitioned into compartments that bring the lymph fluid into contact with **macrophages,** cells that are responsible for **phagocytosis** of pathogens. Phagocytosis is the process by which cells engulf and digest microorganisms.

Lymph nodules are small masses of lymphatic tissue found just beneath the epithelium of all mucous membranes of the respiratory, digestive, urinary, and reproductive tracts. They bring macrophages and lymphocytes as close as possible to these barrier surfaces.

Checkpoint Question

1. *What is the purpose of the lymphatic vessel system and the lymph nodes?*

Tonsils

Tonsils are the lymph nodules of the pharynx. The palatine tonsils are located on each side of the soft palate at the oropharynx. Pharyngeal tonsils are commonly referred to as adenoids and are located in the nasopharyngeal space on the back wall of the upper pharynx. The linqual tonsils are located at the base of the tongue. Any or all of these tonsils may become so loaded with bacteria (tonsillitis) that their removal is necessary. However, because the tonsils appear to function in immunity during early childhood, efforts are made to remove them only if absolutely necessary. (See Chap. 17, Assisting With Diagnostic and Therapeutic

Table 16-1 **Important Lymph Nodes, Locations, and Immune Responses**

Nodes	*Location*	*Immune Response*
Cervical	Neck	Become enlarged during upper respiratory, facial, and scalp infections
Axillary	Axillae (armpits)	May become enlarged after infections of the upper extremities and breasts; cancer cells from the breasts often metastasize to axillary nodes
Tracheobronchial	Near the trachea and the larger bronchial tubes	May become solid masses of blackened tissue in patients who live or work in severely polluted areas
Mesenteric	Between the layers of the peritoneum that form the mesentery	Filter lymph from the abdominal and pelvic organs
Inguinal	Groin	Receive drainage from the lower extremities and external genitalia; when they become enlarged, they are referred to as buboes (as in bubonic plague)

Procedures Associated With the Respiratory System, for a discussion of tonsillitis.)

Spleen

The spleen is located in the upper left quadrant of the abdominal cavity, just below the diaphragm and behind the stomach. The lower rib cage protects the spleen from physical trauma. The spleen contains lymphoid tissue designed to filter blood.

The spleen has several functions:

1. Destroys old red blood cells. As hemoglobin from the red blood cells is broken down, iron is salvaged and liberated into the bloodstream for reuse by the body.
2. Cleanses the blood by filtration and phagocytosis.
3. Produces all types of blood cells before birth and lymphocytes and monocytes in adulthood.
4. Serves as a reservoir for blood, which can be returned to the bloodstream in case of hemorrhage or other emergency.

Although the spleen is the largest mass of lymphoid tissue in the body, splenectomy is not ordinarily life-threatening; other lymphoid tissues can take over the spleen's function.

Thymus

The thymus is located in the upper thorax above the heart and behind the sternum. The thymus is thought to play a key role in the development of the immune system before birth and during the first few months of infancy. Certain lymphocytes (T cells) mature in the thymus gland before they can perform their functions in the immune system (see below). Usually by the age of 2 years, the immune system matures and becomes fully functional. By adolescence, the thymus undergoes involution and is replaced with adipose and connective tissue. It is insignificant in the adult.

All of the lymphoid tissues:

- Remove impurities, such as carbon particles, certain cancer cells, pathogenic organisms, and dead blood cells, through filtration and phagocytosis.
- Process lymphocytes. Some of these lymphocytes produce **antibodies,** which are substances in the blood that aid in combating infection; other lymphocytes attack foreign substances directly. This is explained later in this chapter.

Checkpoint Question

2. *List four functions of the spleen.*

COMMON LYMPHATIC DISORDERS

Any disease of the lymphatic system is referred to as lymphadenopathy. Listed below are several of the more common diseases affecting the organs of the lymph system.

Lymphangitis

Lymphangitis is an inflammation of the lymphatic vessels. Red streaks may be seen extending along an extremity following the course of a lymph vessel, usually beginning in the region of an infected or neglected injury. If the infection is not treated by antibiotics, the lymph nodes may not be able to stop a serious infection and may allow pathogens to enter the bloodstream, causing **septicemia,** or blood poisoning. Streptococci are often the invading organisms in these infections. The disease is usually treated with antibiotics, such as penicillin and the cephalosporins.

Elephantiasis

Elephantiasis is characterized by enormous swelling of the legs and, in men, the scrotum. It is caused by small worms called filariae. These parasites, which are carried by insects such as flies and mosquitoes, invade the tissue as embryos then grow in the lymph channels, thus blocking the flow of lymph. The excessive swelling may cause affected individuals to become incapacitated. Elephantiasis is common in certain parts of Asia and the Pacific Islands. Diagnosis of filariasis can sometimes be made by observing the microfilariae in wet mounts or in Wright-stained smears of blood. There is no known cure.

Elephantiasis without an infectious process is sometimes seen as the result of metastasis into lymph nodes that block the return of fluid and cause swelling in the limb distal to the nodes.

Lymphadenitis

Lymphadenitis is an inflammatory condition that commonly results from an infection (eg, measles, septic sore throat, scarlet fever, diphtheria, common cold) or sometimes cancer. Symptoms include enlarged, tender lymph nodes. This enlargement is caused by increased drainage of bacteria or toxins from the infection into the nodes. The infection's site of origin often can be determined by the location of the affected node. For example, enlarged inguinal lymph nodes typically result from infections of the external genitalia; enlarged axillary nodes are caused by infections in the upper extremities or breast. Treatment is directed at eliminating the primary cause.

16

Mononucleosis

Mononucleosis is caused by the Epstein-Barr virus and affects the entire lymphatic system. Symptoms include fatigue, asthenia (weakness), sore throat, and enlarged tender nodes in the cervical region and sometimes in the axillary and inguinal regions. Mononucleosis is usually transmitted by direct contact with infected saliva and primarily affects young adults. The diagnosis is usually made by blood test. The presence of more than 10% atypical T lymphocytes in the blood, and a total white blood cell count of 15,000 to 20,000 cells/mm are further signs of the disease. Recovery usually takes 4 to 8 weeks. As with most viruses, treatment is symptomatic and palliative.

What If?
What if a mother voices concern over her teenage daughter's diagnosis of mononucleosis?

The mother may be concerned because mononucleosis has sometimes been referred to as the "kissing" disease. However, it is important to note that the virus is spread through contact with contaminated saliva, which can occur through other activities besides kissing (eg, sharing drinking cups).

Splenomegaly

Splenomegaly is an enlargement of the spleen. It is often associated with the destruction of blood cells and accompanies acute infections and diseases, including scarlet fever, typhus fever, typhoid fever, and syphilis. It is considered a sign of disease rather than a distinct disease process.

Hodgkin's Disease

Hodgkin's disease is a malignancy characterized by lymphadenopathy, splenomegaly, fever, weakness, anorexia, and weight loss. It can originate in any lymphoid tissue but usually begins in the lymph nodes of the supraclavicular, high cervical, or mediastinal areas. It commonly affects young men. The diagnosis is often made by identifying a malignant cell (Reed-Sternberg cell) in the lymph nodes. If the disease is localized, the treatment of choice is radiotherapy using high-dose radiation. If the disease is more widespread, chemotherapy is given alone or in combination with radiotherapy. There is a high probability of cure with available treatments.

Lymphosarcoma

Lymphosarcoma, a malignant disease affecting lymphoid tissue, usually leads quickly to death. There is no known cause, but it is more common in men than in women. Symptoms include swelling of the affected nodes, usually painless, progressing to weight loss, fatigue, and malaise. Currently, the only cure is early surgery with radiotherapy. Diagnosis of lymphosarcoma is made by biopsy.

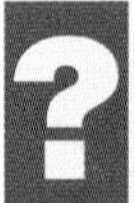

Checkpoint Question

3. *In lymphadenitis, why do the lymph nodes become enlarged and tender?*

FUNCTIONS OF THE IMMUNE SYSTEM

The body is protected from the microorganisms around it by two types of defenses. These defenses can work against any invading pathogen (nonspecific defenses), or they may work against only a particular pathogen (specific defenses).

Nonspecific Defenses

The body's first line of protection involves the barrier defenses (as noted in Chap. 1, Asepsis and Infection Control). These can be mechanical or chemical in nature and include:

- Intact skin and mucous membranes
- Respiratory barriers (eg, nostril hairs, cilia, and mucus)
- Enzymes of the digestive tract and acidity of the genitourinary tract
- Tears (which are slightly bactericidal)
- Protective reflexes (eg, coughing, sneezing, vomiting, and diarrhea)

After the barrier defenses, the next line of defense includes phagocytosis. When the body's immune surveillance system finds pathogenic organisms, **phagocytes** (cells that ingest and destroy microorganisms) go to the site to ingest the pathogens. The phagocytes release proteins that attract other immune cells and cause a local inflammatory process. Macrophages from local tissue and from the bloodstream move in to clear away the dead cells and debris as the infection subsides.

When bacteria or viruses enter the body in sufficient numbers and overcome these phagocytic cells, the next line of defense consists of lymphocytes, known as natural killer cells, which can destroy invading microorganisms.

16

Fever is another of the body's nonspecific defenses. Certain pathogens affect the heat-regulating mechanism of the hypothalamus causing it to reset itself higher than normal for the patient. Most pathogens prefer a body temperature of 97° to 100°F (about 36°–37°C) and find a higher temperature inhospitable for replication.

Inflammation is the body's effort to protect itself by limiting the effect of the disease process. Blood vessels in the area dilate, increasing the blood flow to the area and bringing with it extra phagocytes, oxygen, nutrients, and immunoglobulins. This increase in blood flow causes the skin to appear red. Vasodilation opens the walls of the capillaries, allowing plasma fluid to escape and causing edema (swelling). The edema presses against the nerve endings in the skin, causing discomfort. Extra blood to the area causes the skin to feel warm to the touch. This reaction is called the inflammatory process.

Interferon, another nonspecific defense, is produced by cells infected with viruses. Viruses must be inside a living cell to reproduce, and although interferon cannot prevent the entry of viruses into cells, it does block the reproduction of infected cells. When this happens, viruses cannot replicate themselves and therefore the disease will not spread. Interferon is thought to be the self-limiting factor of many viral diseases and certain tumor cells (Box 16-1).

Antigens and Antibodies

Antigens are chemical markers that identify cells. Human cells have their own antigens that identify all the cells in an individual as "self" (autoantigen). When antigens are foreign, or other than "self," they must be recognized as such during immune surveillance and destroyed. Bacteria, viruses, fungi, protozoa, malignant cells, and organ transplants are all foreign antigens that activate immune responses.

Antibodies, also called **immune globulins** or gamma globulins, are proteins produced by plasma cells in response to foreign antigens. Antibodies do not themselves destroy foreign antigens, but rather become attached to such antigens to label them for destruction. Each antibody produced is specific for only one antigen. It is estimated that as many as one million different antigen-specific antibodies can be produced (Fig. 16-3).

Several laboratory tests involving antibodies are useful in confirming a diagnosis, as described in Table 16-2.

Specific Defenses

Immunity is the body's specific defense against invading pathogens. Two types of lymphocytes—B cells and T cells—play a major role in immunity.

B Cells

B cells are lymphoid stem cells from the bone marrow that migrate to and become mature antigen-specific

Box 16-1
Types of Interferon

There are three types of human interferon: alpha (α), beta (β), and gamma (γ). These were first produced in amounts sufficient for clinical research in the 1970s. At that time, there was hope that interferon would be an effective anticancer therapy, but results proved disappointing. Alpha interferon is effective, however, in the treatment of a rare form of leukemia called hairy cell leukemia and has been approved for use in cases of genital warts and Kaposi's sarcoma.

Studies have shown that alpha interferon may be useful in the treatment of AIDS. When given in small doses and in combination with zidovudine (AZT), alpha interferon seems to block the reproduction of HIV, the virus that causes AIDS. This may prove to be useful in people who are infected with HIV but who have no symptoms and might slow the progress of the infection.

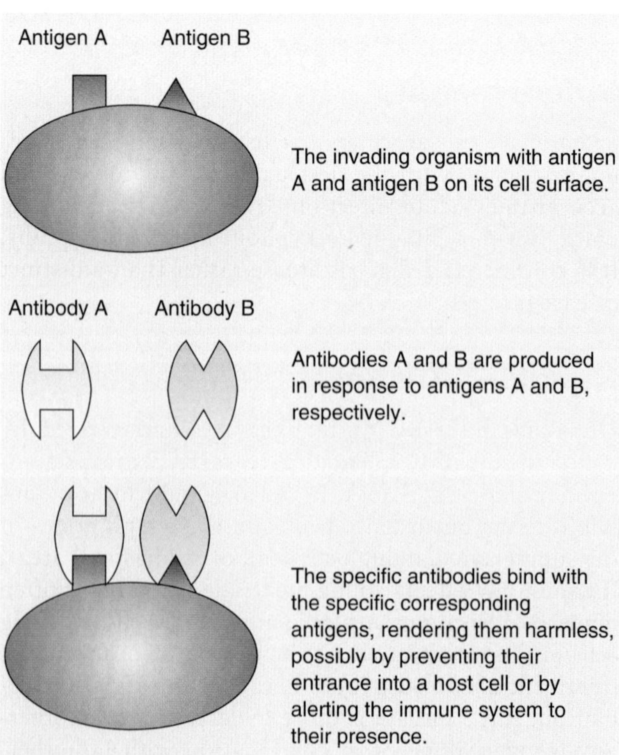

Antigen A
Antigen B
The invading organism with antigen A and antigen B on its cell surface.
Antibody A
Antibody B
Antibodies A and B are produced in response to antigens A and B, respectively.
The specific antibodies bind with the specific corresponding antigens, rendering them harmless, possibly by preventing their entrance into a host cell or by alerting the immune system to their presence.

Figure 16-3 Antibody specificity. Antibodies are produced by B-cell lymphocytes to bind with specific antigens.

Table 16-2 **Antibody-Specific Laboratory Tests**

Test	*Purpose*
Complement Fixation Test	Measures the severity of an infection and helps indicate the extent and effectiveness of antigen–antibody reactions occurring in the body.
Antibody Titer	Measures the amount of a specific antibody in the blood. If in several weeks there is an increase in the antibody level, the infection is identified as a current one.
Fluorescent Antibody Test	Antibodies are stained or marked by a fluorescent material, permitting rapid diagnosis of various kinds of infections.

Table 16-3 **Immunoglobulins**

Immunoglobulin	*Properties/Functions*
IgA	Found in exocrine secretions, such as milk, tears, mucous secretions Probably a protective device for mucosa
IgD	Plasma preparation from persons with a high concentration of Rh antibodies Given to an Rh-negative mother soon after delivery of an Rh-positive infant to prevent hemolytic disease of the newborn in subsequent pregnancies
IgE	Found in the mast cells of the respiratory and gastrointestinal tracts Important in allergic responses Elevated in the presence of an allergic response
IgG	Main immunoglobulin in human serum Produces antibodies for various pathogens Elevated in the presence of infection Activates complement to complete the immune response Frequently given to provide immediate, but temporary, immunity
IgM	Formed in the early stages of almost all immune reactions Controls the ABO blood group antibodies Helps to stimulate the production of complement

cells in the spleen and lymph nodes. Many immature B cells are found in the spleen, which, because of the large amount of blood passing through it, provides many chances for the B cells to become exposed to new antigens. When a B cell is confronted with a specific type of antigen, it transforms into an antibody-producing cell called a plasma cell or a memory cell. Plasma cells produce antibodies that aid in the destruction of the invading cell. Memory cells are available to produce antibodies quickly if the same antigen appears again. The antibodies that are made by plasma cells are known as immunoglobulins, such as IgA, IgD, IgE, IgG, and IgM (Table 16-3). The type of immunity dependent on B cells is called ***humoral immunity***.

Sometimes, in addition to destroying antigens in the way described previously, antibodies can activate a complex series of nine proteins in the blood. These proteins, called **complement,** aid the antibodies in destroying antigens by prompting the inflammatory process. They are responsible for the components of inflammation, such as promoting vasodilation, attracting white blood cells to the area, destroying antigens, and preventing the spread of pathogens.

T Cells

T cells are lymphoid cells from the bone marrow that migrate to the thymus gland, where they develop into mature differentiated lymphocytes that circulate between blood and lymph. T cells are antigen specific, meaning that each one responds usually to only one antigen.

A type of immunity called ***cell-mediated immunity*** depends on T lymphocytes. If a T cell encounters an antigen, usually brought to it by a macrophage that has ingested it, the T cell can multiply rapidly and, in some instances, destroy the antigen, such as cancer cells, viruses, fungi, or bacteria. T cells also, unfortunately, react to beneficial foreign tissues, such as skin grafts and transplanted organs.

Activated T-helper cells secrete interleukin, a chemical that stimulates B cells and other T lymphocytes to destroy the invading antigen. T-helper cells also stimulate the production of interferon. Two other types of T cells are cytotoxic (killer) T cells and suppressor T cells. Cytotoxic T cells destroy cells bearing antigens, such as tumor cells and tissue transplanted from an organ donor as noted above. Suppressor T cells regulate the amount of antibody produced by inhibiting the activity of B cells once the need for their production no longer exists.

Checkpoint Question

4. *What are antigens? What does the body form in response to foreign antigens?*

16

Types of Immunity

Genetic Immunity

Genetic, or natural, immunity does not involve antibodies. Genetic immunity is programmed in the DNA. Some individuals are born with a natural, inherent immunity to certain diseases. Some pathogens invade certain host species but not others; this is called species immunity. For example, infections such as measles, scarlet fever, diphtheria, and influenza do not affect animals in contact with humans who have these illnesses. In the same way, many animal infections do not affect humans in contact with the animals that have these disorders (eg, chicken cholera, distemper).

Acquired Immunity

Acquired immunity involves antibodies. It may be natural or artificial and may be acquired either passively or actively.

- *Passive acquired natural immunity* is acquired from another source, such as transplacentally from mother to fetus or through breast milk to a nursing infant from a mother who has immune factors.
- *Passive acquired artificial immunity* is acquired through the injection of gamma globulins after presumed exposure. Gamma globulins are NOT **vaccines.** (A vaccine is a suspension of infectious agents given to establish resistance to an infectious disease.) Gamma globulins do not stimulate immune mechanisms but provide immediate antibody protection. Passive acquired artificial immunity is always temporary, lasting a few weeks to a few months. Some examples of gamma globulins are noted in Table 16-4.
- *Active acquired natural immunity* is acquired through contracting a specific disease with production of antibodies and memory cells. Memory cells survive in the body for a long time and are ready to respond immediately when they encounter that same antigen again.

Table 16-4 **Gamma Globulins**

Globulin	*Function*
Tetanus immune globulin	Prevents tetanus in patients not currently immunized
Immune serum globulin	May prevent infectious hepatitis
Immune globulin Rh_0 (concentrated human antibody)	Prevents the formation of antibodies against the Rh factor in an Rh-negative mother after the birth of an Rh-positive fetus
Rabies antiserum (from humans or horses)	Used to treat victims of rabid animal bites

- *Active acquired artificial immunity* is acquired through administration of a vaccine, which stimulates production of antibodies and memory cells to prevent specific diseases. A vaccine contains an antigen to which the immune system will respond just as it would to the actual pathogen. Vaccines take the place of the first exposure to a disease. Types of vaccines are described in Table 16-5.

Vaccines may be made with live organisms or with organisms killed by heat. If live organisms are used, they must be nonvirulent for humans, or the organisms must be treated in the laboratory to weaken them. An organism weakened for use in vaccines is described as **attenuated.** A third type of vaccine is made from a form of the toxin produced by a disease organism. The toxin is altered with heat or chemicals to reduce its ability to harm, but it can still function as an antigen to induce immunity. Such an altered toxin is called a **toxoid.**

"Booster" shots are administered at intervals to maintain a high level (**titer**) of antibodies in the blood. In some cases, active immunity acquired by artificial means does not last a lifetime, making it necessary to "boost" the body's production of antibodies against a specific disease.

Checkpoint Question

5. *List three types of vaccines.*

COMMON IMMUNE DISORDERS

Allergies

An **allergy** is a hypersensitivity reaction (exaggerated response) to a particular foreign antigen, called an allergen. The reactions may be as mild as seasonal rhinitis (hay fever) or as severe as anaphylaxis (a total system collapse). Allergens include plant pollens, foods, chemicals, antibiotics, pet dander, and mold spores. They may be inhaled, ingested, injected, or absorbed into the skin. Because of the complexity of the antibody response, the first contact builds the memory cells that wait for the next contact with the allergen to produce a reaction.

In sensitive individuals, the antigen–antibody reaction may cause the release of excessive amounts of **histamine,** a substance found normally in the body in response to injured cells. The histamine causes an inflammatory reaction, including vasodilation, increased capillary permeability, resulting in edema. It may also cause contraction of involuntary muscles, particularly those in the bronchial tree. **Antihistamines** (medications that oppose the action of histamine such as Bena-

Table 16-5 **The Importance of Vaccines**

Disease	*Vaccine*
Pertussis	Protects against whooping cough; is given in conjunction with diphtheria toxoid and tetanus toxoid, all in one mixture referred to as DPT
Hepatitis B	Protects high-risk individuals, such as health care workers and emergency personnel; now administered to infants as part of routine immunization
Measles, mumps, and rubella (MMR)	Protects against all three viruses; although each vaccine can be administered separately, immunity is conferred just as effectively with the triple vaccine. This vaccine should not be administered before 15 months of age
Influenza	Given annually to high-risk groups but has limited effectiveness in influenza epidemics because of the new strains of the virus that develop periodically
Haemophilus B (HiB)	Produces an immunity to *Haemophilus influenzae* and prevents *Haemophilus* B influenza meningitis; administered routinely during pediatric immunizations
Poliomyelitis	Usually given in live oral form, except in instances when a member of the patient's family is receiving immunosuppressive medication or is on antineoplastic (cancer) drugs; such individuals are at risk from the shedding of live poliovirus in the stool that occurs for several weeks after the administration of the oral polio form

Without vaccines, infant mortality in the United States would be high, and death from childhood diseases would occur much more frequently. In certain parts of the world, however, this is still the case. Many developing countries still cannot afford extensive vaccination programs for their children. Although some of the diseases listed above may rarely be seen in general practice today, many still pose significant threats to the lives of millions of people throughout the world.

dryl or Claritin) are sometimes effective in reducing the allergic reaction.

Autoimmunity

Normally the body is able to recognize those proteins that belong to its "self" and only produces antibodies when "foreign" proteins invade. Autoimmune diseases are conditions in which the body fails to recognize its own proteins and produces antibodies that destroy its own cells and tissues. Some examples of autoimmune diseases include rheumatoid arthritis, chronic thyroiditis, lupus erythematosus, and pernicious anemia. Diabetes mellitus, colitis, and multiple sclerosis are thought to be caused by autoimmune processes. At this time there is no cure for autoimmunity.

Immunodeficiency Diseases

Failure of any of the components of the immune system results in an immune deficiency. This may be genetic and may be apparent soon after birth, or it may be acquired as the result of a disease process. The deficiency may involve any part of the immune system and will vary in its severity.

Infantile Hypogammaglobulinemia

Infantile hypogammaglobulinemia, an inherited disorder, is passed by a carrier mother usually to a son. The immunoglobulins and B cells may be either absent or deficient, but the T cells are usually not affected. Infants with this disorder may retain transplacental immunity for several months but will then exhibit chronic, devastating infections. Diagnosis requires testing for immunoglobulins after about 9 months when inherited immunity is no longer a factor. Treatment involves injections and transfusions of immunoglobulins. Prognosis is mixed and depends on the severity of the deficiency.

Acquired Immunodeficiency Syndrome (AIDS)

Acquired immunodeficiency syndrome (AIDS) is an example of an infectious disease that overwhelms the body's immune system. The human immunodeficiency virus (HIV) is the pathogen that causes AIDS by destroying T-helper cells and suppressing the body's cell-

16

Box 16-2
History of AIDS

No other disease has ever generated such negative stereotyping as AIDS. Once thought of as a male homosexual disease, AIDS is now identified as a disease that can affect anyone. In fact, from 1990 to 1995, the number of reported AIDS cases among men who have sex with men fell, but the number of AIDS cases among heterosexuals increased.

AIDS was first diagnosed in the early 1980s. The Centers for Disease Control and Prevention (CDC) began officially recording cases of AIDS in 1981, but not by the name AIDS. (At that time, it was called "Gay-Related Immune Deficiency.") In 1982, the CDC designated a new condition called AIDS and began formal surveillance.

In 1984, French researchers isolated what is now known as the human immunodeficiency virus (HIV); they called it lymphadenopathy-associated virus (LAV). At the same time, U.S. researchers isolated the same virus; they called it human T-cell lymphotropic virus type III (HTLV-III). The virus was officially called HIV in 1985.

As of June 1997, the CDC recorded 612,078 cases of AIDS in the United States. (This number included all cases starting from June 1981.) The CDC estimates that over 1 million individuals in the U.S. are currently infected with HIV.

mediated immune response. HIV is a **retrovirus,** which means that it enters the cell, infiltrates the cell's RNA, and transfers its own DNA to the cell's DNA by means of an enzyme called transcriptase. The change in DNA prevents the affected cell from functioning normally; it can only function to nourish and incubate more HIV. The patient is predisposed to life-threatening infections and malignancies. Box 16-2 provides a brief overview of the history of AIDS.

The infectious diseases associated with AIDS are called **opportunistic infections** because HIV lowers resistance and allows opportunity for infections by bacteria, parasites, and abnormal cell development that are usually contained by normal defenses. Table 16-6 lists a number of opportunistic infections associated with AIDS.

Although a direct result of HIV infection, AIDS is a combination of several disease processes. Alone, none is considered to be specific to AIDS, but each of the signs and symptoms carries a reason for serious concern. Box 16-3 describes some of the signs and symptoms frequently associated with AIDS.

The incubation period for HIV infection can range from a few months to several years. An infected person may unknowingly spread HIV to others before any symptoms appear. HIV is not spread by casual contact. Transmission of HIV most often occurs through an ex-

Table 16-6 **Opportunistic Infections Associated with AIDS (AIDS-OI)**

Infection	*Description*
Candidiasis	Yeast-like fungus that overgrows, causing infections of the mouth (thrush), respiratory tract, and skin
Cryptococcus	Yeast-like fungus causing lung, brain, and blood infections
Cryptosporidiosis	One-celled parasitic infection of the gastrointestinal tract, causing diarrhea, fever, and weight loss
Cytomegalovirus (CMV)	Virus causing colitis, pneumonitis, and retinitis
Herpes simplex	Viral infection causing small, painful blisters on the skin of the lips, nose, or genitalia
Histoplasmosis	Fungal infection from inhalation of dust contaminated with *Histoplasma capsulatum;* causes fever, chills, and lung infections
Mycobacterium avium-intracellulare	Bacterial disease with fever, malaise, night sweats, anorexia, diarrhea, weight loss, and lung and blood infections
Pneumocystis carinii pneumonia (PCP)	One-celled organism causing lung infection with fever, cough, chest pain, and sputum production
Toxoplasmosis	Parasitic infection involving the brain, lungs, and other organs and causing fever, chills, visual disturbances, confusion, hemiparesis, and seizures

Box 16-3

Signs and Symptoms Frequently Associated with AIDS

Malignancies: One of the malignancies associated with HIV is called **Kaposi's sarcoma,** a cancer arising from the lining cells of capillaries. Kaposi's sarcoma produces bluish red nodules on the skin, particularly on the lower limbs. Cancer of the lymph nodes, called lymphoma, is also associated with HIV infection.

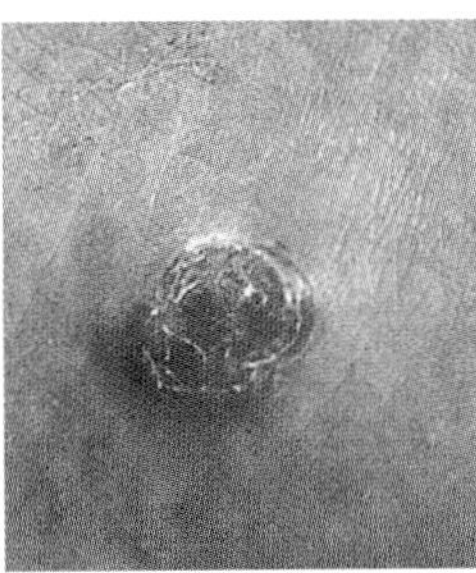

Periods of severe fatigue: Even though everyone experiences periods of some fatigue, these periods should not be prolonged or unexplained. Periods of extreme fatigue that last for more than several weeks should be considered a warning sign.

Sudden, unexplained weight loss: As a general rule, an unexplained weight loss of 10 lb or more in less than 60 days should be cause for concern.

Night sweats or fever: Drenching night sweats and chills with fever often occur with AIDS and with tuberculosis and other serious illnesses.

Diarrhea: Diarrhea that persists for more than a week is common among AIDS patients.

Bruising or bleeding: The blood of an HIV-positive person has an unusually delayed clotting time. The HIV-positive patient will have a tendency to bleed or bruise easily; even minor injuries can result in severe bruising. The mucous membranes may bleed with no evidence or history of trauma or injury.

Coughing, shortness of breath, and other respiratory symptoms: Pneumocystis carinii pneumonia is a type of pneumonia associated closely with HIV infection. It begins as a cough, either dry or productive. If the patient is HIV positive, the cough will persist for weeks and lead to severe shortness of breath. The persistent cough may be accompanied by chills, fever, tightness in the chest, increased pulse, and increased respirations. *P. carinii* pneumonia is considered to be the most frequent life-threatening opportunistic infection in persons with HIV.

Persistent generalized lymphadenopathy: When a person has AIDS, the lymph system is unable to process the infections associated with the disease. The lymph glands and nodes become enlarged in an effort to control the disease. Lymphadenopathy is manifested as enlarged, hard, painful nodes in various parts of the body.

Oral thrush: Candida albicans thrives in the suppressed immune system. Although AIDS patients frequently present with thrush, esophageal thrush is the most significant indicator of HIV infection. A condition called hairy leukoplakia often is observed in HIV-positive patients. This symptom presents as lesions on each side of the tongue with grayish white patchy discolorations.

Neurologic problems: Patients who are HIV positive often experience a variety of nervous system disorders, including headaches, stiff neck, generalized pain, and weakness or numbness of the extremities. They have also experienced depression, delusions, hallucinations, paranoia, and dementia.

change of blood or body fluids that may result from sexual contact, sharing contaminated needles, transfusions of contaminated blood, or accidental injury from sharp instruments used in invasive procedures. It also may be spread transplacentally from an infected mother to her infant.

A person with HIV may experience the following stages as the infection progresses to AIDS.

1. Acute infectious stage, with generally mild flulike symptoms
2. Latent period, without symptoms
3. Complaints of weight loss, lymphadenopathy, fever, diarrhea, anorexia, fatigue, and skin rashes
4. Onset of immunodeficiency disorders, such as Kaposi's sarcoma and *Pneumocystis carinii* pneumonia (possibly the initial stages of full-blown AIDS)

Patients who are HIV positive are treated prophylactically based on laboratory data. One parameter that is continuously monitored is the CD4 count. The CD4 is a surface molecule on the T cell. When HIV enters the body, it attaches to these molecules and destroys them, causing the CD4 count to fall. Treatment begins as the CD4 count falls, whether or not the patient has symptoms. As the CD4 count falls further, prophylactic antibiotic therapy may be started.

Three primary drugs are used to treat HIV and AIDS: **zidovudine (formerly Azidothymide [AZT]), zalcitadine and didanosine (formerly dideoxysine [ddI], and dideoxycytidime [ddC]).** These drugs work by blocking the growth of the virus after it enters the T cell. D4t and 3TC are new medications that work by preventing the virus from entering the T cell. Other new drugs include protease inhibitors (ritonavir, indinavir, and nevirapine), which block the ac-

16

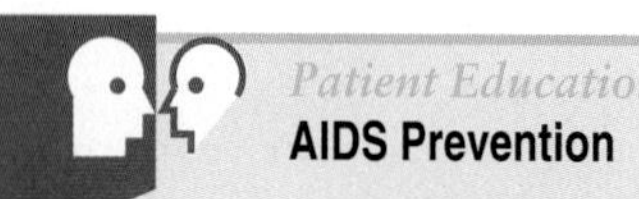

Patient Education
AIDS Prevention

When providing instructions about AIDS prevention, explain to your patient that it is safest, of course, to abstain from sex. However, if that is not feasible, instruct your patient to have sex only with a partner who is known not to be infected, who has sex with no one but the patient, and who does not use needles or syringes. Also tell the patient to use a latex condom and a spermicide if it is not known whether the sexual partner is infected.

Generally, instruct patients to:

- Avoid contact with another person's blood, body fluids, semen, or vaginal secretions.
- Avoid sharing needles or syringes, or any objects that come in contact with blood or body fluids.
- Avoid using alcohol or drugs. Use of these substances can hinder clear thinking, lead to unwise decision making and will suppress your immune response.
- Ask about the sexual history of current and prospective sexual partners.
- Always use latex condoms for any type of sex (vaginal, anal, or oral). Latex offers the greatest protection against all sexually transmitted diseases, including HIV.
- Never use oil-based lubricants with a condom; use only water-soluble lubricants.
- Avoid any sexual practice that may cause tears in the vaginal, anal, or oral mucosa.
- Avoid deep "French" kissing or any contact with saliva of an infected person. It is considered safe to dry kiss your partner, and cuddling is always safe.
- Do not share personal hygiene items, such as toothbrushes or razors, with an infected person.

tion of enzymes and may prove to be effective against AIDS. These drugs are given in combination and are known as a "cocktail." Other drugs in stages of development, such as MKC-442, show promise in the treatment of HIV. It is important to note that although these medications can help the patient, they also have significant side effects. Therefore, the physician will continuously monitor T-cell counts and other laboratory values.

As a medical assistant, you must be knowledgeable about AIDS, especially its transmission, both for your own protection and for the protection of your patients. In accordance with guidelines issued by the Centers for Disease Control and Prevention (CDC), you must follow Standard Precautions when caring for all patients, regardless of their known or suspected infection status. (See Chap. 1, Asepsis and Infection Control, for a detailed discussion of Standard Precautions.)

A good understanding of this disease and methods for preventing its transmission will help prevent misinformation, rumor, apathy, and fear (Box 16-4). Additionally, obtaining an accurate medical history from patients at risk for HIV or AIDS is important. Table 16-7 offers some suggestions for interview questions.

Besides being informed about AIDS, you must also be aware of AIDS patients' need for compassion. Patients are sometimes abandoned by family and friends and shunned at work. You and other health care workers may provide the only personal contacts these individuals may have on a regular basis. You will need to foster a caring attitude that puts aside prejudices and value judgments. Special care should be given to individuals with organic brain damage who will need instructions and treatment information.

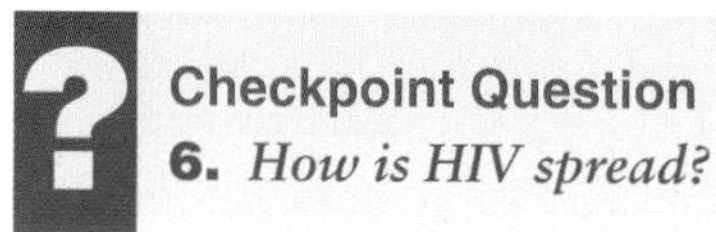

Checkpoint Question

6. *How is HIV spread?*

COMMON DIAGNOSTIC PROCEDURES AND THE MEDICAL ASSISTANT'S ROLE

Allergy Testing

As a medical assistant, your responsibility for allergy testing will vary with the practice. However, it will

Box 16-4
AIDS Facts

1. AIDS is caused by a virus called HIV.
2. People infected with HIV may look and feel healthy long before symptoms appear.
3. When symptoms do appear, they vary from person to person.
4. Most people who are HIV positive or who have AIDS became infected by having sex or sharing needles with someone who was infected.
5. You cannot "catch" HIV as you do a cold or the flu.
6. It is impossible for a donor to get HIV from giving blood or plasma.
7. The chances of contracting AIDS from a blood transfusion in the United States are now very low.
8. There are reliable blood tests for HIV.
9. So far, there is no vaccine for HIV or a cure for AIDS.
10. You can protect yourself from the virus by observing Standard Precautions.
11. Latex condoms can help prevent the spread of HIV.
12. People with HIV and AIDS need you to show them love and understanding.

16

Table 16-7 **Obtaining an Accurate History from a Patient at Risk for HIV or AIDS**

A patient who is at risk for HIV or AIDS may be reluctant to provide you with an accurate social history. Here are some helpful hints for obtaining an accurate history.

Instead of asking . . .	*Ask . . .*	*Rationale*
Do you have sex with prostitutes?	Have you ever paid for sexual activities?	Some patients may not admit to using a prostitute, but may acknowledge paying for sexual favors.
Do you do IV drugs?	Do you do skin popping? Steroid injections?	Some patients do not perceive skin popping or steroid injections as IV drug use.
Do you practice safe sex?	What method of safe sex do you use? Do you use a condom? Do you reuse condoms?	Some patients perceive using birth control as practicing safe sex; birth control offers no protection against HIV.
Are you a homosexual?	What is your sexual preference? Do you have sex with members of your same sex?	Some patients may not perceive themselves as homosexuals or do not want to be labeled.

probably include obtaining a careful history of allergic episodes, setting up the allergens as ordered by the physician, and following up with patient education. Because of the potential for anaphylaxis, the administration of the test is usually done by the physician or a trained technician. An emergency setup must be close at hand during the complete process.

As noted in Chapter 10, Assisting With Diagnostic and Therapeutic Procedures Associated With the Integumentary System, allergy skin testing methods include scratch tests, intradermal injections, and patch tests. Diagnosis for the scratch, intradermal, and patch will be made by comparing the response to the specific allergen with a control substance administered in the same manner. Reactions are usually graded according to comparison with guides supplied by the manufacturers of the allergens.

Laboratory blood tests, which are more expensive and invasive, test for specific antibodies in the blood, usually ingestants. You may be responsible for collection and transportation of blood specimens.

Laboratory Testing for Human Immunodeficiency Virus (HIV)

ELISA, or enzyme-linked immunosorbent assay, is used to screen blood for antibodies to the AIDS virus. A positive result indicates probable exposure to the virus and the possibility that the virus is in the blood. Because false-positive results can occur with the ELISA test, the Western blot test is used to confirm positive findings and is considered to be diagnostic. Your responsibility in this testing is usually confined to collecting the specimen by phlebotomy and routing it to the proper laboratory.

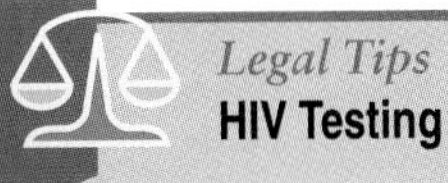

Legal Tips
HIV Testing

Testing for HIV has many legal implications. The laws vary from state to state, but they generally hold that:

- Patients must sign an informed consent form before being tested.
- Pretest and post-test counseling (usually by a state-approved HIV counselor) is required, regardless of the test results.
- Results cannot be given over the telephone. Most states have specific laws that state who can give test results and when and how those results can be given.
- Utmost care must be given to ensure patient confidentiality. Most laboratory settings will use a patient coding system rather than the patient's name on the requisition slip to ensure privacy.
- Laboratories that test for HIV must be approved by the state for this testing.

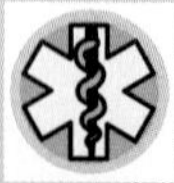

Action STAT!

Needle Stick

Scenario: You are drawing blood from a 26-year-old male patient who has a history of drug abuse and is HIV positive. While withdrawing the needle, you accidentally stick yourself. What should you do?

1. Remain calm. Your first priority is to take care of your patient. Remove his tourniquet, and properly care for his venipuncture site and the blood tubes.
2. Dispose of the venipuncture equipment properly, and remove your gloves.
3. Immediately wash your hands in the examining room sink. Clean the puncture wound site thoroughly as outlined in your office protocol for postexposure procedure.
4. Put on gloves, and if the bleeding has stopped, apply an adhesive dressing to the patient's venipuncture site.
5. Label the blood tubes, and place them in the appropriate area.
6. Report to the physician regarding your needlestick. Complete an incident report, and follow your office policy for needlesticks.

Note: Be aware that state laws vary regarding your rights to require that a patient be tested for blood-borne pathogens when there is no documentation regarding his or her status. Also, keep in mind that you can receive immune globulin therapy to prevent hepatitis B virus (HBV) infections from needlesticks. This consists of a series of injections and must be given free of charge by your employer. The HBV vaccine series is thought to be sufficient to prevent hepatitis B virus in properly immunized persons. Immune globulin injections are not effective against HIV infections.

Answers to Checkpoint Questions

1. *The lymphatic vessels return excess fluid from the tissues back to circulation. The lymph nodes filter the lymph once it is drained from the tissues.*
2. *The spleen destroys old red blood cells, cleanses the blood, produces blood cells, and serves as a reservoir for blood.*
3. *Lymphadenitis usually results from an infection. The enlarged lymph nodes are caused by increased drainage of bacteria or toxins from the infection into the nodes.*
4. *Antigens are chemical markers that identify cells. Foreign antigens must be destroyed. The body forms antibodies that attach to these antigens, marking them for destruction.*
5. *Three types of vaccines are live, attenuated, and altered toxin (toxoid).*
6. *HIV is transmitted through an exchange of blood or body fluids that may result from sexual contact, sharing contaminated needles, transfusions, or accidental injury from sharp instruments used in invasive procedures. It also can be transmitted transplacentally from infected mother to infant.*

Critical Thinking Challenges

1. Your patient has been diagnosed with breast cancer. Why would it be important to biopsy lymph nodes in the axillary area?
2. Why might the removal of lymph vessels from a region, such as the axillary area, cause edema of the area drained by those nodes? How might you help your patient understand this concept?
3. The mother of your pediatric patient questions the need for booster shots for her son. How would you impress on her the importance of immunization boosters? Explain in terms that a lay person would understand.

Suggestions for Further Reading

American Red Cross. (1992). *HIV and AIDS.*

Blood Borne Pathogens, OSHA Inst. 29CFR 1910.1030.

Bullock, B. L., & Rosendahl, P. P. (1996). *Pathophysiology,* 4th ed. Philadelphia: Lippincott-Raven.

Centers for Disease Control and Prevention. (1998). Recommendations for prevention of HIV transmission in the health care setting. *MMWR*

Fischbach, F. (1992). *A Manual of Laboratory and Diagnostic Tests,* 4th ed. Philadelphia: Lippincott-Raven.

Fischbach, F. (1995). *Quick Reference for Laboratory and Diagnostic Tests.* Philadelphia: Lippincott-Raven.

Hamann, B. (1994). *Disease: Identification, Prevention and Control.* St. Louis: Mosby–Year Book.

Memmler, R., Cohen, B., & Wood, D. (1996). *The Human Body in Health and Disease,* 8th ed. Philadelphia: Lippincott-Raven.

Porth, C. M. (1998). *Pathophysiology: Concepts of Altered Health States,* 5th ed. Philadelphia: Lippincott-Raven.

Professional Guide to Diseases, 4th ed. (1992). Springhouse, PA: Springhouse Corporation.

Staines, N., Brostoff, J., & James, K. (1993). *Introducing Immunology.* London: Mosby–Year Book.

17

Assisting With Diagnostic and Therapeutic Procedures Associated With the Respiratory System

Chapter Outline

Role Delineation

CLINICAL

Fundamental Principles

- Apply principles of aseptic technique and infection control.

Diagnostic Orders

- Collect and process specimens.

Patient Care

- Prepare patients for examinations, procedures, and treatments.

GENERAL

Professionalism

- Project a professional manner and image.
- Work as a team member.
- Prioritize and perform multiple tasks.

Communication Skills

- Treat all patients with compassion and empathy.
- Adapt communications to individual's ability to understand.

Legal Concepts

- Practice within the scope of education, training, and personal capabilities.
- Document accurately.

Instruction

- Instruct individuals according to their needs.

Chapter Competencies

Learning Objectives

Upon successfully completing this chapter, you will be able to:

1. Spell and define the Key Terms.
2. List and explain the primary functions of the respiratory system.
3. Label a diagram of the organs of the respiratory system.
4. List and discuss the function of each part of the airways, from the nares to the alveoli.
5. Discuss the structure and function of the lungs.
6. Explain the process of ventilation in relation to Boyle's law.
7. Discuss and explain the processes of external and internal respiration.
8. List the primary defense mechanisms of the respiratory system.
9. List and describe disorders of the respiratory system.
10. Identify and explain diagnostic procedures of the respiratory system, and state the medical assistant's responsibilities where applicable.
11. Describe the physician's examination of the respiratory system, and state the medical assistant's responsibilities in assisting with this procedure.

Performance Objectives

Upon successfully completing this chapter, you will be able to:

1. Collect a specimen for throat culture (Procedure 17-1).
2. Collect a sputum specimen for culture or cytologic examination (Procedure 17-2).

Key Terms

(See Glossary for definitions.)

alveolar-capillary membrane
aspiration
atelectasis
carina
cilia
chronic obstructive pulmonary disease (COPD)
diaphragmatic excursion
dyspnea
endotracheal tube
epiglottis
eustachian tubes
hemoptysis
iatrogenic
laryngectomy
mediastinum
palliative
pleura
respiration
status asthmaticus
stoma
thoracentesis
tonsils
tracheostomy
tracheotomy
turbinates

The respiratory system provides the body with the oxygen that every cell needs to perform its designated function. It also eliminates from the body one of the waste products of cellular metabolism, carbon dioxide (CO_2). The respiratory system works closely with the cardiovascular system in performing this function. Oxygen is carried by the blood, which is pumped by the heart through the blood vessels to reach every cell. When a cell is deprived of oxygen for a period of time, it dies. The processes involved in getting oxygen to the cells include ventilation and **respiration** (gas exchange), which can be external and internal. These processes are discussed later in this chapter.

STRUCTURE AND FUNCTION OF THE RESPIRATORY SYSTEM

Figure 17-1 shows the major organs of the respiratory system. These include the nose, sinuses, mouth, pharynx (the mouth and pharynx are shared with the digestive system), larynx, trachea, airways, and the lungs. The mouth, nose, pharynx, larynx, trachea, and conducting airways serve simply as a passageway for fresh air that is warmed and filtered to enter the lungs and for exhaled air, rich in carbon dioxide, to leave the body. Within the lungs, the exchange of gases occurs between the lung fields and the blood. These processes are described in more detail below.

17

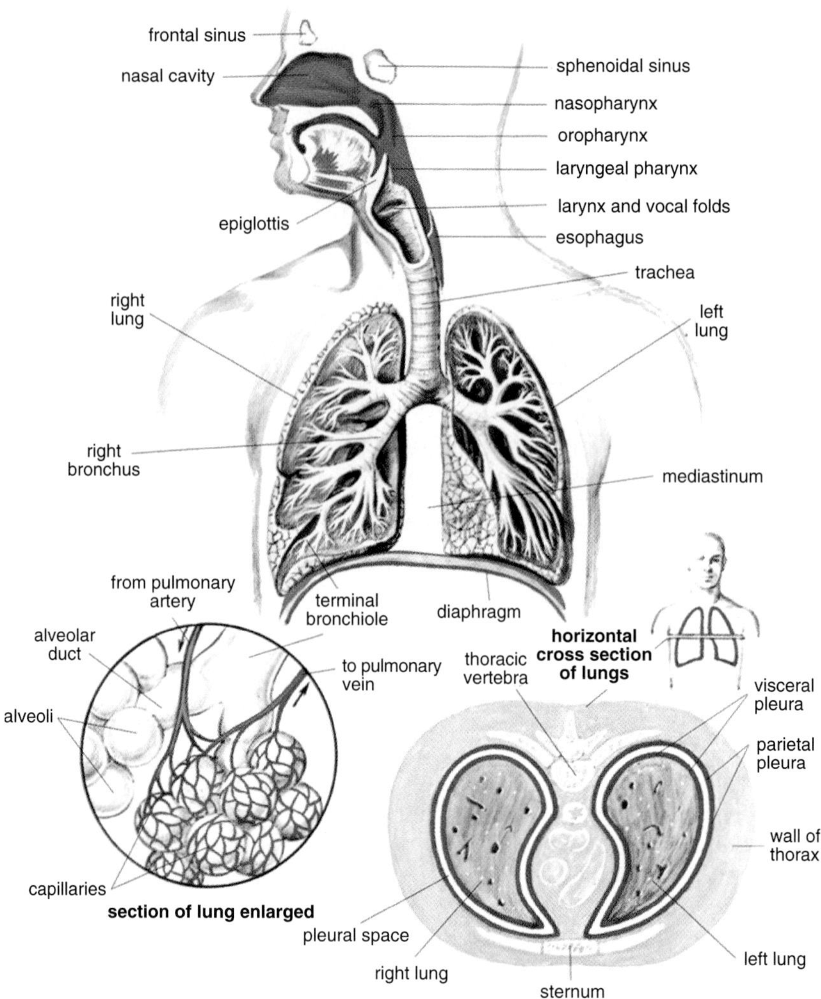

Figure 17-1 The respiratory system.

The major function of the respiratory system is to supply oxygen to the bloodstream for delivery to the cells and to eliminate carbon dioxide from the body. The respiratory system also helps eliminate water from the body. In addition, parts of the system are involved in the sense of smell and in speech.

Checkpoint Question

1. *Describe the functions of the respiratory system.*

ORGANS OF THE RESPIRATORY SYSTEM

Airways

Using the illustration of the respiratory system (see Fig. 17-1), follow the path of the air as it enters and passes the structures on its way to the lung fields. The mechanism of air movement is discussed later.

Nose

Usually, air enters the body through the nose. The external nose is formed by bone and cartilage and has two openings in its anterior surface called nares or nostrils. As the air enters, it is filtered by hairs within the nasal cavity. The walls of the nasal cavity contain bony projections called **turbinates,** which increase the surface area and whirl the air around to allow it to be warmed and humidified by the mucous membranes that line the cavity.

Paranasal Sinuses

The paranasal sinuses are hollow cavities in the bones around the nose lined with mucous membrane (Fig. 17-2). There are four pairs of paranasal sinuses (Table 17-1). The paranasal sinuses have several functions, including providing mucus that drains through a duct to the nasal cavity, acting as a resonating chamber for speech, and lightening the bones of the skull. The sinus ducts are somewhat narrow and, if they swell shut because of infection, can cause pain and pressure in the

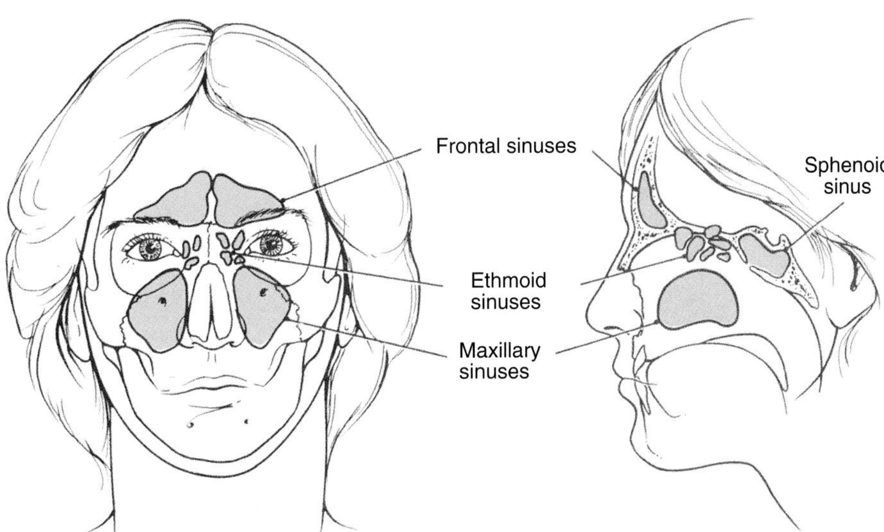

Figure 17-2 Location of paranasal sinuses.

areas around the eyes, nose, cheeks, and forehead. The paranasal sinuses do not conduct air to the lungs but are important accessory structures.

Mouth

The structures of the mouth are discussed in detail in Chapter 18, Assisting With Diagnostic and Therapeutic Procedures Associated With the Gastrointestinal System, and therefore are not included here. The mouth provides an alternate passageway for air if the nose is blocked for some reason. Some people breathe through their mouths out of habit.

Pharynx

The pharynx (throat) serves the dual purpose of providing a passageway for food and drink to the digestive tract via the esophagus and air to the respiratory tract via the larynx. It can be divided into three sections: the nasopharynx (posterior to the nasal cavity), the oropharynx (posterior to the oral cavity), and the laryngopharynx (the most inferior section).

Table 17-1 **Paranasal Sinuses**

Name	*Location*
Frontal	Located just above the brow ridge on each side of the nasal bridge
Sphenoid	Within the sphenoid bone at the base of the skull, between the occipital and ethmoid bones in front and the parietal and temporal around its sides
Ethmoid	Within the spongy bone that forms the roof of the nasal cavity and part of the floor of the skull
Maxillary	Paired sinuses within the bones that form the floor of the orbits and the sides of the nasal cavities

The pharynx contains several important structures. The **eustachian tubes**, which connect the nasopharynx with the middle ear, allow the pressure between the atmosphere and the area between the eardrum and the inner ear to equalize. These tubes also provide a route for infection to spread from the throat to the middle ear. These infections are more common in young children whose eustachian tubes are more horizontal than those of adults. Also within the pharynx are three sets of **tonsils** (lymphoid tissue). These include:

- Pharyngeal tonsils (also known as adenoids)
- Palatine tonsils (at the back of the oral cavity; commonly referred to as tonsils)
- Lingual tonsils (at the base of the tongue)

The tonsils are made of lymphoid tissue and are designed to prevent infection from spreading to the lower respiratory tract. If the tonsils are overwhelmed by the virulence of the infection they are trying to contain, they also may become a site of infection, especially in children.

Checkpoint Question

2. *Name the two functions of the pharynx.*

Larynx

The larynx or voice box is located below the pharynx and is made up of cartilage and muscles. This is the next structure through which air passes on its way to the lungs. One of the cartilages that makes up the larynx is the **epiglottis.** The epiglottis is a leaflike flap that closes down over the opening of the larynx during swallowing, thus preventing solids or liquids from entering the airway.

Besides providing a passage for air and preventing **aspiration** (solids or liquids entering the airway), the larynx is important in the production of speech. Within the larynx are the vocal cords. These are tendons that are tightly stretched across the opening of the airway in the shape of a V. They can vibrate like the strings of a violin, producing sound as air passes over them. The pitch of the sound produced is regulated by tightening the vocal cords (for a higher pitch) or relaxing them (for a lower pitch). The loudness of the sounds produced is regulated by how fast or hard air is forced through the vocal cords.

Another of the large cartilages of the larynx is the thyroid cartilage or Adam's apple. You can feel this cartilage moving up and down as you swallow. This is due to the movement of the epiglottis as it closes over the larynx.

Trachea

The trachea (sometimes referred to as the windpipe) is a tube that extends from the larynx in the neck down into the chest. The trachea conducts air down to the bronchi, which then take it into the lungs. It is about 1 inch wide and 5 inches long and is anterior to the esophagus. It is rigid on three sides due to the presence of many C-shaped cartilage rings that are placed with the open end of the C facing posteriorly, toward the esophagus. The rings are connected to each other by bits of soft tissue to allow the neck to bend in all directions. The front of the trachea is rigid so that the airway stays open, even when the neck is struck or bumped. The back is more flexible to allow a large bolus of food to pass down the esophagus without catching.

The trachea is lined with a mucous membrane containing special cells and glands that produce mucus. This mucus is designed to trap any dust or other particles inhaled on its sticky surface. The innermost layer of this membrane is made up of specialized cells that are covered with tiny hairs called **cilia.** These cilia beat together to cause the mucus, containing dust and debris, to be moved toward the pharynx where about a quart a day is swallowed. Many inhaled pathogens are neutralized by the digestive tract in this manner.

The trachea marks the beginning of the tracheobronchial tree, which is known by this name because it looks like an inverted tree with the trachea as its trunk. This "tree" is actually made up of a branching series of tubes that conduct air to the working parts of the lungs.

Sometimes a patient may require a **tracheotomy,** the procedure of making a surgical incision into the trachea. The resulting opening is called a **tracheostomy** (Fig. 17-3). Tracheotomies are performed for various reasons:

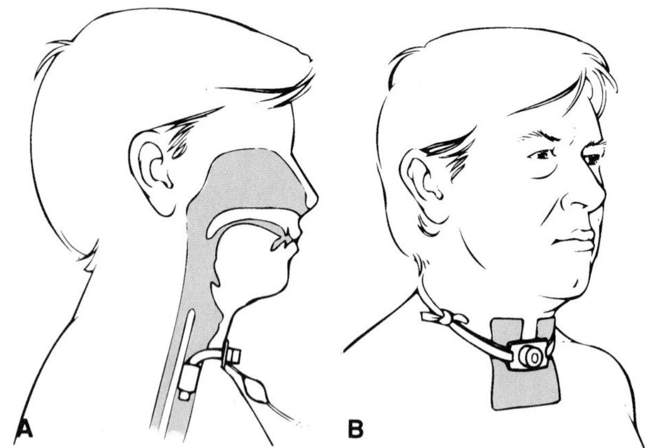

Figure 17-3 Pictured are a sagittal view (**A**) and a frontal view (**B**) of a tracheostomy tube in place.

- Facilitate long-term ventilation
- Relieve upper airway obstruction
- Provide an airway after a **laryngectomy** (removal of the larynx) has been performed
- Facilitate suctioning in a patient who is unable to cough effectively
- Decrease "dead space ventilation" in patients with **chronic obstructive pulmonary disease (COPD),** a progressive disorder of diminished respiratory capacity

Tracheostomies may be temporary or permanent, and the patient may or may not have a tracheostomy tube in the **stoma,** or opening. The area around a tracheostomy needs to be kept very clean, and tracheostomy tubes need to be changed or cleaned regularly. This complex procedure is not normally within the scope of practice for a medical assistant without additional specialized training under a physician's preceptorship.

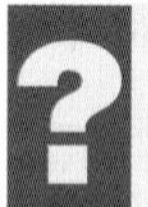

Checkpoint Question

3. *How are inhaled particles trapped in the trachea and then neutralized?*

Bronchi and Bronchioles

The trachea splits at about the level of the second ribs into two large tubes called the right and left mainstem bronchi. These bronchi enter the right and left lungs and continue to branch again and again, with the tubes getting narrower each time they branch. The larger tubes are called bronchi and contain smooth muscle and some cartilage. As the tubes get smaller, the cartilage diminishes, but they still have the smooth muscle. When something irritates the airways, this smooth muscle constricts, narrowing the opening to prevent the irritant from traveling any further in the airway.

This is the same type of constriction (bronchoconstriction) that is partly responsible for asthma attacks.

The airways branch approximately 27 times. When the tubes reach about 1 mm or less in diameter, they are called bronchioles. Bronchioles also have smooth muscle in their walls and conduct air down to the tiny grapelike sacs called alveoli.

Alveoli

Alveoli are tiny sacs whose thin walls are only one cell thick. They are covered with thin-walled capillaries and are the site of gas exchange in the lungs. Oxygen diffuses through the wall of the alveolus (singular) into the blood, and carbon dioxide diffuses out of the blood into the alveolus where it can be exhaled. The bulk of the lung tissue is made up of these little air sacs, which gives the lungs their spongelike appearance. There are approximately 300 million alveoli in the lungs of an adult. Their shape makes them specialized to provide as much area as possible for gas exchange. If all the alveoli in a pair of lungs were flattened out, they would cover a tennis court!

The alveoli also contain specialized cells that produce a substance called surfactant, which lines the alveoli and keeps them from collapsing with every expiration. Premature infants frequently lack surfactant in their lungs. This is the major cause of the respiratory distress syndrome often seen in these infants.

Checkpoint Question

4. *After air enters the nose, what other structures must it pass through before oxygen can be diffused into the blood?*

Lungs

The lungs are large, spongy organs located in the chest or thoracic cavity. They are somewhat cone shaped, with the broad base of each cone resting on the diaphragm (the dome-shaped muscle that separates the thoracic and abdominal cavities) and the apex (point) extending up above the clavicles. The heart is nestled between the lungs, in a cavity called the **mediastinum.**

The right lung is broader and thicker than the left, due to the presence of the liver below the diaphragm on the right side. This causes the right diaphragm to be somewhat higher than the left. The right lung is divided into three lobes or sections; the left lung has only two lobes to allow space for the heart, which is angled toward the left. Each lobe of the lung is separate from the other and is attached by a separate bronchus to the tracheobronchial tree. If one lobe of the lung is severely damaged or diseased (eg, with cancer), it can be surgically removed without affecting the other lobes.

The lungs are enclosed in a serous membrane called the **pleura.** The visceral pleura covers the surface of the lungs; the parietal pleura lines the internal surface of the chest cavity and the top of the diaphragm. These two membranes normally are stuck together with a thin layer of fluid between them, just as two flat pieces of glass will stick together if there is a layer of water between them. (Try this with two glass slides. There is a negative pressure between the slides that makes them stick together.) These two membranes are important in the process of ventilation.

17

VENTILATION

Ventilation is the movement of gases from the atmosphere to the alveoli and from the alveoli back into the atmosphere. The path these gases take as they move through the upper airways and lungs is discussed above, but what makes these gases move? To understand the forces that cause this movement of gas, it is necessary to understand one of the basic physical laws governing gas, Boyle's law.

Boyle's law states that when gases are kept at the same temperature, if the volume holding the gas is increased, the pressure of the gas will decrease. Conversely, if the volume is decreased, the pressure will increase. Consider how this law can be applied to the process of ventilation as it is divided into two phases, inspiration and expiration (Fig. 17-4). Note that the terms inspiration and inhalation have the same meaning and can be used interchangeably. Expiration and exhalation have the same meaning as well.

Inspiration

Inspiration involves the movement of air from the atmosphere into the lungs. In the medulla of the brain stem is a respiratory center, which periodically sends a signal by way of the nerves to the muscles of inspiration as the level of carbon dioxide builds up in the blood. The major muscle of inspiration is the diaphragm, which is innervated by the phrenic nerve. When the diaphragm gets a signal from the respiratory center, it contracts, which causes it to flatten out and pull downward. At the same time, the external intercostal muscles (located between the ribs) also contract, causing the ribs to move outward. Both of these movements enlarge the chest cavity. Because the lungs are "stuck" to the chest wall and diaphragm by the forces between the visceral and parietal pleura, as the chest expands, the lungs expand as well. Thus, the volume in the lungs increases and (according to Boyle's law), the pressure within the lungs decreases.

17

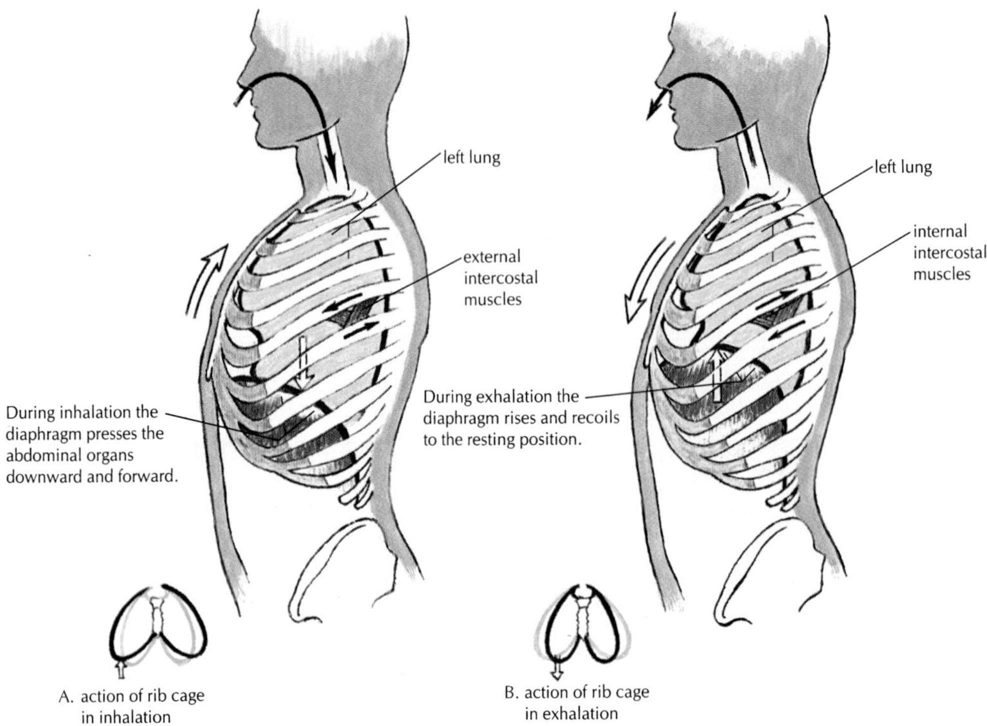

Figure 17-4 Diagram showing (**A**) inhalation and (**B**) exhalation.

Remember that the alveoli are directly connected to the atmosphere by the tracheobronchial tree and the upper airways. Thus, when the pressure drops in the lungs, the pressure in the atmosphere is higher than the pressure in the alveoli. Gases will always flow from higher to lower pressures, thus gas flows from the atmosphere into the lungs until the pressures within the lungs equal the atmospheric pressure. The more the muscles of inspiration (the diaphragm and external intercostals) are contracted, the more air will flow in and the deeper the breath will be.

Notice that inspiration is an active process; in other words, energy is used to produce the contraction of the inspiratory muscles. When the diaphragm and external intercostals are unable to meet the ventilatory needs of the body, accessory muscles of inspiration may be called on to try to expand the chest cavity even more. This can occur when someone with normal lungs is trying to breathe very rapidly and deeply, or when someone has a respiratory disease and is unable to move enough air with the diaphragm and external intercostals alone.

Expiration

The process of expiration, or movement of gas out of the lungs into the atmosphere, is normally a passive process. This means that no muscles need to contract to remove the air from the lungs, so no energy is used. When inspiration has ended, the diaphragm and external intercostals automatically relax and the chest wall and diaphragm recoil to their resting position. As they do this, the volume within the lungs is decreased, which (again according to Boyle's law) causes the gas pressure within the lungs to increase. The pressure of the gas within the lungs becomes higher than that in the atmosphere, and, once again, gas flows from higher to lower pressure until the pressures are equalized. When the pressure within the lungs is equal to that in the atmosphere, expiration stops.

Expiration is normally a passive process. However, when someone with normal lungs wants to exhale forcefully, or when someone has a disease that makes it difficult to get air out of the lungs, such as asthma or emphysema, accessory muscles of expiration may be used.

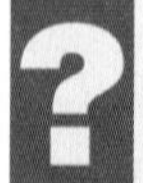

Checkpoint Question

5. *How would you contrast the processes of inspiration and expiration?*

RESPIRATION

External Respiration

External respiration is the exchange of gases between the alveoli and the pulmonary capillaries within the lungs. The wall of the alveolus is only one cell thick, as

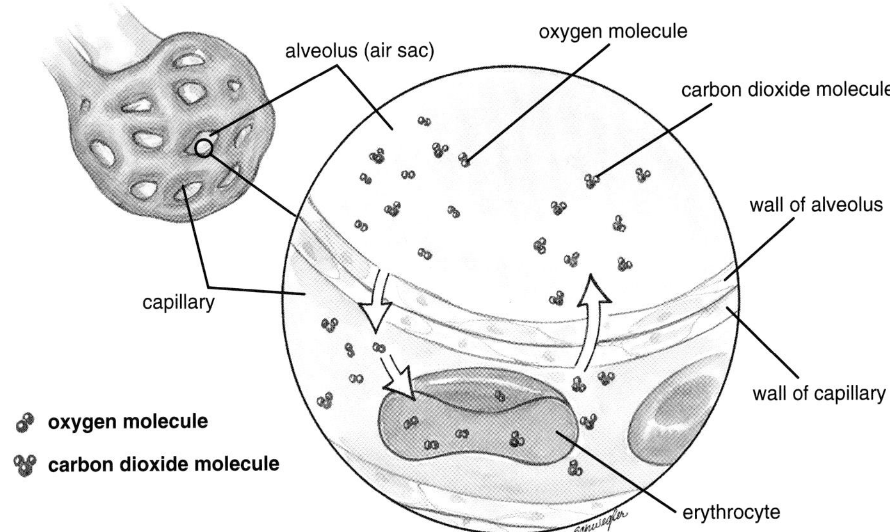

Figure 17-5 Diagram showing the diffusion of gas molecules through the cell membranes and throughout the capillary blood and air in the alveolus.

are the walls of the capillaries that surround the alveoli. The respiratory gases (oxygen and carbon dioxide) must pass through the **alveolar-capillary membrane** (Fig. 17-5). This membrane is only about 0.5 μm thick to make it easy for these gases to pass through.

The blood entering the pulmonary capillaries is high in carbon dioxide and low in oxygen. The alveolus contains a large quantity of oxygen and small amounts of carbon dioxide. As the blood passes through the pulmonary capillaries, oxygen diffuses from the alveolus into the blood, and carbon dioxide diffuses from the blood into the alveolus. When the lungs are not diseased, equilibration is complete—that is, the blood leaving the pulmonary capillary has the same oxygen pressure and carbon dioxide pressure as the alveolus it just passed.

Certain respiratory and cardiac diseases can interfere with the process of external respiration by thickening the alveolar capillary membrane, thus interfering with diffusion (as seen in pulmonary edema), by decreasing the surface area available for external respiration (as seen in emphysema), or by decreasing the amount of oxygen that reaches the alveolus (as seen in pneumonia). These diseases are discussed later in this chapter.

Table 17-2 **Defenses of the Respiratory System**

Defense	*Function*
Hairs (vibrissae) at entrance to nose	Filter large dust particles from air
Mucous membranes in nose	Trap dust and other particles, add moisture
Turbinates in nose	Whirl air around to increase warming, humidifying, and filtering
Epiglottis	Closes over airway to prevent aspiration of liquids and solids
Airway reflexes	Trigger a cough when irritation occurs to pharynx, larynx, trachea, or **carina** (ridgelike structure) to help clear airway
Mucous membranes of trachea and airways	Trap particles of dust and debris in air
Airway smooth muscle	Constricts when irritation occurs to prevent entry of foreign substances
Macrophage in alveoli	Phagocytize ("eat") bacteria or other foreign cells or debris that reach the respiratory zone
Tonsils (palatine, pharyngeal, lingual)	Act as filters for air moving through passageways to protect against bacterial invasion; aid in the formation of white blood cells

17

Internal Respiration

Internal respiration is the exchange of gases between the systemic capillaries, located throughout the body, and the cells of the body. Every cell in the body is located near enough to a capillary so that internal respiration may occur. In internal respiration, oxygen in the systemic capillaries diffuses out of the blood and into the cells to fuel the cell's work. Carbon dioxide, a waste product of cellular metabolism, diffuses out of the cell and into the blood of the systemic capillaries. The blood from the systemic capillaries enters the venous system, returns to the right side of the heart, and is circulated through the lungs where external respiration occurs again.

DEFENSE MECHANISMS OF THE RESPIRATORY SYSTEM

The respiratory system has a series of defense mechanisms designed to protect it from disease. Remember that the upper airways, tracheobronchial tree, and alveoli are all directly connected to the atmosphere, which can contain dust, pathogenic bacteria and viruses, and other irritants.

Table 17-2 summarizes the major defense mechanisms of the respiratory system. Without these defenses, infections and other diseases of these organs would be more common than they already are. Diseases of the respiratory system can occur when defenses are overwhelmed by cigarette smoking (Box 17-1), air pollution, infectious organisms, or other irritants.

Box 17-1
Effects of Smoking on the Airways

Cigarette smoking has many harmful effects on the body. The normal functioning of the mucous membrane lining the trachea and other airways is described in the text. Smoke from a cigarette irritates the airways and causes the membrane to produce more mucus. This increased production of mucus, as well as the increase in dust and debris that collects in the mucus, slows down the clearing process. The smoke anesthetizes the cilia so they stop waving the debris away. Over time, large amounts of thick, sticky mucus are retained in the lungs, blackening the lung tissue and sealing the alveolar sacs. This thick, tarry mucus causes the patient to cough frequently (especially in the morning) and to be prone to bronchitis (both acute and chronic).

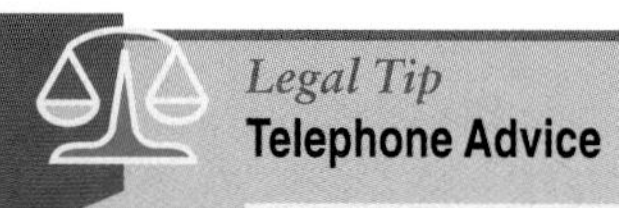

Legal Tip
Telephone Advice

A patient calls the office at 4:45 PM complaining of a sore throat. Scheduled appointments are running 1 to 2 hours behind. Because it is the middle of the flu season, you assume that the patient has a viral sore throat and can be seen in the morning. During the night, the patient's throat closes due to the infection and obstructs his airway. The patient is rushed to the hospital and is pronounced brain dead from anoxia. After his death, an autopsy shows the patient had a tonsillar abscess. Could you be sued? Yes! As a medical assistant, you cannot presume to diagnose medical conditions. Only the physician can make a diagnosis. Many symptoms may seem minor but may be warning signs of a more serious condition. Always follow your office policy regarding telephone advice. Document all phone conversations, and bring them to the physician's attention.

COMMON RESPIRATORY DISORDERS

Because it is open to the atmosphere, the respiratory system is susceptible to many diseases. These diseases can be divided into diseases of the upper respiratory tract and those of the lower respiratory tract. Cancers of the respiratory system are discussed separately. Table 17-3 describes respiratory disorders that commonly affect pediatric patients.

Upper Respiratory Disorders

The most common problems associated with the upper respiratory tract are caused by infectious organisms or allergic reactions that produce inflammation.

Acute Rhinitis

Acute rhinitis is an inflammation of the mucous membranes of the nose. It produces sneezing, nasal discharge, swelling of the mucous membranes (which may make it difficult to breathe through the nose), and tearing of the eyes. If the problem is an infection, it is usually caused by a virus and is called a "common cold." It may also be caused by allergens, in which case it is called "hay fever." Treatment is symptomatic rather than curative and usually includes over-the-counter antihistamine medication, rest, and fluids, or nasal steroid sprays if symptoms are chronic.

Table 17-3 **Common Pediatric Respiratory Disorders**

Disorder	*Description*
Infant respiratory distress syndrome (IRDS)	IRDS occurs in premature infants whose lungs have not fully developed. The alveolar-capillary membrane is thickened, and mature surfactant is insufficient to keep the alveoli open. These infants often need assistance with their breathing for several days to a week, until the lungs mature.
Bronchopulmonary dysplasia	This disease is seen in infants who have suffered from IRDS and still require assisted ventilation after a week. It is thought to be caused by the treatment (high pressures of ventilation and high oxygen concentrations) and is therefore an **iatrogenic** (resulting from medical treatment) disease. The infant's lungs are damaged and require prolonged treatment with ventilation, oxygen, or medication. Some children have residual damage from this disease; others outgrow all signs and symptoms.
Bronchiolitis	This disorder is characterized by inflammation of the bronchioles, wheezing, and congestion. It is most serious in children under 6 months old, although it is commonly seen in children up to 3 years old. The most common causative virus is respiratory syncytial virus. Very young infants and those with other respiratory or cardiac problems often require hospitalization and even mechanical ventilation.
Croup (laryngotracheobronchitis)	Croup is a disease seen primarily in children 3 months to 3 years of age. It is caused by a viral infection of the larynx, resulting in swelling and narrowing of the airway. This causes difficulty in breathing, characterized by a high-pitched crowing wheeze (stridor) on inspiration and a sharp barking cough. Treatment may include hospitalization, mist tents, and medications to decrease the swelling.
Epiglottitis	Swelling of the epiglottis may present similarly to croup but is usually more serious and may be life threatening if it progresses to complete obstruction of the airway. It occurs most frequently in children aged 2–6 y, although it can be seen in all age groups. It is caused by a bacterial infection, usually *Haemophilus influenzae.* A child with epiglottitis must be treated in the hospital. The first priority is establishing an airway, usually by inserting an **endotracheal tube** (tube in the trachea).
Cystic fibrosis	Cystic fibrosis is an inherited disease that affects the exocrine glands of the body, changing their secretions and causing mucus to be extremely thick and sticky. Although it affects several areas of the body, the most serious complications of cystic fibrosis are usually respiratory. Children with this disease are prone to repeated respiratory infections because of the difficulty in clearing the mucus from their airways. Many new treatments are being developed for this disease, and much exciting research into prevention and cure is ongoing.

Sinusitis

Sinusitis is inflammation of the mucous membrane of the sinuses. It can produce pain and pressure over the upper facial area, headache, and fever. The problem may be acute or chronic, and treatment may include symptomatic over-the-counter remedies and antibiotics (for bacterial infection), heat application, irrigation, and occasionally surgery. Patients should be cautioned to seek medical attention if symptoms linger or become worse or if a severe headache is present.

Pharyngitis/Tonsillitis

Inflammation of the epithelial tissues of the throat or of the tonsils produces similar symptoms of sore throat and difficulty swallowing. Throat examination will reveal red, swollen tissues and possibly pustules on the tonsils or in the throat. The medical assistant may be asked to obtain a throat culture from these patients. Treatment of sore throat may include antibiotics (especially if the throat culture reveals streptococcal infection), gargles, and analgesics. Tonsillitis may be treated with antibiotics if the causative agent is bacterial, or if the problem is chronic, the tonsils may be surgically removed. This procedure usually includes removal of the pharyngeal tonsils (adenoids) and the palatine tonsils.

Laryngitis

Inflammation of the larynx can result from an infection, irritation (as from cigarette smoke), or from overuse of the voice. The result is hoarseness, a cough, and difficulty speaking. Laryngitis may be treated with antibiotics if it is thought to be caused by a bacterial infection, but more often it is left to resolve on its own. The patient is told to rest the voice and speak as little as possible. Cool mist humidifiers may help soothe the throat.

Checkpoint Question

6. *Name five diseases of the upper respiratory tract.*

Lower Respiratory Disorders

Diseases of the lower respiratory tract may be acute (sudden in onset with relatively short duration) or chronic (progressing over time or appearing frequently). Acute diseases of the lower respiratory tract include bronchitis and pneumonia. Chronic diseases include asthma, chronic bronchitis, and emphysema. The latter two diseases are usually grouped together as COPD. Because most patients with COPD have elements of both emphysema and chronic bronchitis, these are discussed together.

Bronchitis

Bronchitis is an inflammation of the mucous membranes of the bronchi, which causes an increased production of mucus. This inflammation can be produced by infection or irritation of the mucous membrane. The most prominent symptom of bronchitis is a productive cough. If infection is present, the sputum produced may change color from the normal white or clear to yellow, green, gray, or tan. The medical assistant may be asked to obtain a sterile sputum specimen for culture and sensitivity from these patients. Treatment generally includes antibiotics (if bacterial infection is suspected), smoking cessation, and rest and fluids. Cough suppressants may be prescribed, especially for nighttime use, but their use is controversial because of the need to clear secretions from the airways. Retained secretions can become infected and lead to pneumonia.

Pneumonia

Pneumonia is an infection of the working areas of the lungs, or alveoli, that prevents effective gas exchange (external respiration) in the affected area. It may be bacterial or viral in origin. Diagnostic testing usually includes a sputum specimen and a chest x-ray. Bacterial pneumonias tend to be more sudden and severe in onset, presenting with fever, cough, chills, and **dyspnea** (difficulty breathing). They also tend to be localized to one lobe or area of the lung.

Treatment primarily involves appropriate antibiotics, bed rest, and symptomatic medications. Bacterial pneumonias often require hospitalization for administration of intravenous antibiotics and oxygen, especially in elderly or debilitated patients. Viral pneumonia is usually more gradual in onset but can be just as serious; antibiotics are generally ineffective. Viral pneumonia tends to be spread throughout the lung fields, instead of being localized, and may present with fever and a hacking cough. Treatment may include bed rest or hospitalization.

Checkpoint Question

7. *List the characteristic symptoms of bacterial and viral pneumonia.*

Asthma

Asthma is a reversible inflammatory process involving primarily the small airways. It is manifested by constriction of the smooth muscle lining the airways (bronchospasm), increased mucus production with a productive cough, and swelling of the mucous membranes of the airways. All three of these manifestations narrow the airways, which makes it difficult to move air into and out of the lungs.

The person having an asthma attack may present with dyspnea, coughing, wheezing, and, in a severe attack, cyanosis (bluish discoloration of the skin caused by lack of oxygen). Patients with asthma usually have periods when they are experiencing an attack (exacerbations) and other periods when they are relatively symptom free (remissions). Attacks may be brought on by allergens in the environment, irritants, infection, psychological stress, rapid breathing, cold air, or unknown causes. Many medications are available to treat asthma, but it is important that they be used properly.

A peak flowmeter may be used by the patient to assess his or her breathing each day and to determine

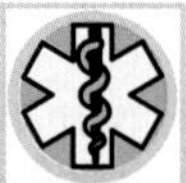

Action **STAT!**

Asthma Attack

Scenario: Barbara Richards arrives at the clinic in obvious respiratory distress. She has audible wheezing and labored breathing with pursed lips. She tells you that she has asthma and states that she has had a chest cold for 3 days. What should you do?

1. Place Ms. Richards in a wheelchair, and take her to an examining room.
2. Notify the physician immediately.
3. Assist Ms. Richards to remove her shirt, and have her put on a gown.
4. Obtain her pulse rate, respiratory rate, and blood pressure. Question her regarding her medication profile, and complete a brief health history. If you have been trained in the procedure, obtain a baseline peak flowmeter reading.
5. Assist the physician in administering medications as ordered. The most common procedures include epinephrine injections, bronchodilators, and nebulizer treatments. Oxygen may be administered if directed by the physician.
6. Recheck and document Ms. Richards' pulse and respiratory rate after administering respiratory medications or treatments. Repeat a peak flowmeter reading after the treatments to document her improvement.
7. If Ms. Richards is transferred to the hospital, assist the ambulance technicians as directed.
8. Document the incident in her chart.

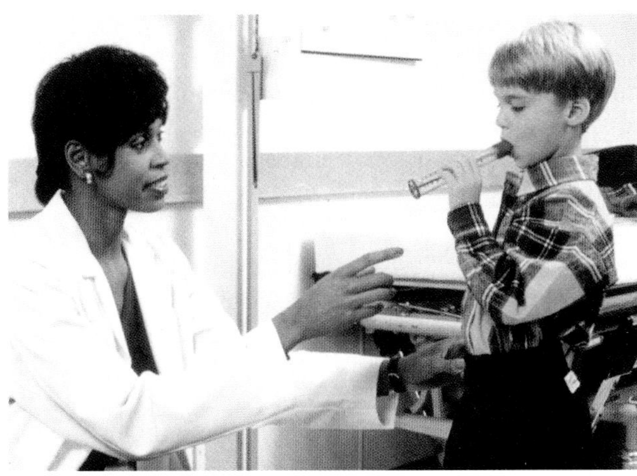

Figure 17-6 Using a peak flowmeter. (Courtesy of Monoghan Medical Corporation, Plattsburgh, PA.)

what medication regimen to use that day (Fig. 17-6). To use the peak flowmeter, the patient blows as hard as possible into the device during a period when breathing is at its best to establish a "personal best." The physician then devises a medication protocol based on this information.

Medical practices that evaluate and treat patients with respiratory disorders such as asthma usually establish a baseline pulmonary function using a spirometer, an instrument designed to measure the air capacity of the lungs at various stages of respiration. These include inspiratory reserve volume (how much more air can be inhaled with special effort), residual air (the amount left in the lungs after a complete exhalation), and expiratory reserve volume (how much more can be exhaled after normal exhalation).

These and other function parameters are assessed after treatment is initiated and then as needed or on an annual physical examination. Comparing the assessments to the daily peak expiratory flow measurements kept by the patient helps to establish a treatment protocol.

Patients are usually tested for response to allergens to identify those most likely to trigger an asthma attack. This may be difficult to establish if the allergens are present year round or if the trigger is psychological (intrinsic) rather than extrinsic.

Initially, treatment usually is limited to daily inhaled inflammatory therapy to maintain optimum respiratory function. Mild intermittent asthma may be treated with prescribed bronchodilators on an as-needed basis.

A patient who is having an asthma attack that does not respond to medications is said to be in status asthmaticus. Because such asthma attacks can be fatal, the patient needs to be taken to a hospital immediately. In recent years, with increased levels of air pollution, the mortality rate from asthma has been increasing despite new and improved diagnostic techniques and medications.

As with most chronic illnesses, the goal of asthma management is self-management. The strategy is to guide the patient through education and support toward asthma control to prevent the attacks or to restore function quickly if an attack occurs.

Checkpoint Question

8. *List six factors that may trigger an asthma attack.*

Chronic Obstructive Pulmonary Disease

Both chronic bronchitis and emphysema are most commonly caused by cigarette smoking. Thus, patients who have smoked for a long time often exhibit signs and symptoms of both of these disorders.

Chronic bronchitis is a chronic inflammation and swelling of the airways, with excessive mucus production, obstruction of the bronchi, and trapping of air behind mucous plugs, which causes alveoli to become overinflated. During inspiration, as the chest expands, the airways are stretched open and air enters the alveoli. However, during expiration, as the chest closes down, the airways also close, and the air is trapped and cannot be exhaled. This produces alveoli that are stretched and overinflated. Chronic bronchitis is not usually an infectious process but is produced by chronic irritation of the airways by cigarette smoke or other pollutants. However, because of the increased sputum produced and the difficulty these patients have in clearing their sputum, they are prone to develop respiratory infections.

Emphysema is a disease process affecting primarily the alveoli. Remember that normally alveoli exist in small clusters like bunches of grapes. In emphysema, the walls of the alveoli become stretched and break down. The pulmonary capillaries also break down, and the tiny airways leading to each grapelike cluster weaken and collapse. The result is that there is much less surface area for gas exchange, and, once again, air is trapped in the enlarged "sacs" that were once clusters of tiny alveoli.

The combination of these two diseases in the COPD patient produces characteristic symptoms. COPD should be suspected whenever a patient with a history of smoking presents with complaints of shortness of breath (especially with exercise), chronic cough and sputum production (especially in the morning), and wheezing. The onset of these symptoms is usually slow and gradual, and the patient may go a long time without realizing that he or she is experiencing symptoms of a disease. People with COPD often experience

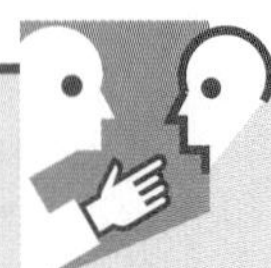

Advice and Tips
Patients Living With COPD

To help improve the quality of life, encourage a patient with COPD to follow these suggestions:

1. If you have not already done it, QUIT SMOKING! Even if you have permanent damage to your lungs, their deterioration will slow if you stop smoking now. Avoid second-hand smoke.
2. Have the current flu vaccine each fall, and be sure to get a pneumococcal pneumonia vaccine.
3. Avoid being out in crowds whenever possible, especially in the winter when colds and influenza are prevalent. If you live in an area with high air pollution, you may want to wear a respiratory mask outside on days when the pollution level is high.
4. When you breathe, inspire through your nose, then exhale slowly through pursed lips. Do not puff your cheeks or blow—allow your expiration to be passive.
5. Use your abdominal muscles instead of your shoulder and neck muscles to help you breathe. On inspiration, allow your abdominal muscles to relax and your abdominal wall to move outward to give the diaphragm room to move downward. On expiration, tighten your abdominal muscles to push upward on your diaphragm and help get a more complete expiration.
6. Drink a lot of fluids all day long (unless your physician has limited your fluid intake). Water is the best fluid. Avoid drinking too many caffeinated drinks or alcohol. Good fluid intake is the best way to keep the mucus in your airways thinned so that it is easier to cough up.
7. Follow a healthy, balanced diet.
8. Avoid doing several difficult physical tasks (eg, vacuuming or mowing the lawn) all in one day. If you must do these chores, do them in short periods spaced throughout the day, with frequent rest periods.
9. Organize your home to minimize the amount of standing, reaching, and lifting you have to do. For example, put a high stool in your kitchen. Keep frequently used items at waist level (on the counter), rather than in high or low cabinets. Have a rolling basket in your home that you can push around to take items (such as laundry) from one room to another.

some of the symptoms of asthma as well, especially bronchospasm, and therefore often take many of the same medications that an asthmatic would take.

Once a patient has COPD, the process is not usually reversible. Many patients have a hard time accepting that fact and insist that their physician must be able to provide a "cure." Although the disease is not curable, the progression of COPD can be slowed, and the quality of life for the patient may be improved significantly through thorough patient education about the disease, a supervised exercise regimen, proper use of medications, good nutrition, home oxygen therapy, and so on.

What If?
What if a patient requires home oxygen therapy?

Many patients with severe COPD or end-stage lung cancer are discharged from the hospital with oxygen to use in the home. Most surgical supply companies and pharmacies can arrange to have oxygen therapy equipment delivered to the home. The oxygen usually is supplied by a machine called a concentrator, which runs on electricity. The concentrator separates oxygen out of room air for use by the patient. Attached to the cylinder is a flowmeter that indicates the amount of oxygen being delivered. A cannula (plastic tube with pronged openings that fit into the nares) is attached to the flowmeter and delivers the oxygen. Instruct the patient to leave the oxygen at the setting prescribed by the physician. In some cases, too much oxygen can be toxic. The company supplying the oxygen also should instruct the patient regarding safe home oxygen administration. In addition, the supplier should be available 24 hours a day for emergency oxygen maintenance. It is usually the supplier's responsibility to notify the local power company about patients in the area who require supportive oxygen therapy. In the event of a power outage, emergency service is supplied to these patients' homes as quickly as possible.

Common Cancers

Laryngeal Cancer

Cancer of the larynx is seen most commonly in heavy smokers and alcoholics. The presenting symptoms are usually hoarseness for longer than 3 weeks, a "lump" in the throat, or pain and burning in the throat when drinking citrus juice or hot liquid. The patient with laryngeal cancer may be treated with radiation or surgery or both. Surgery usually involves removal of the larynx and formation of a permanent tracheostomy stoma. Patients who have had a laryngectomy are unable to speak normally, but they can be trained to speak using esophageal speech or a prosthetic device.

Lung Cancer

Lung cancer is one of the most common causes of death in both men and women. Cigarette smoking is believed to be the most common cause; 80% of lung cancer patients are smokers. Prognosis is generally poor for patients with lung cancer, with only 8% of men and 12% of women surviving for 5 years. One of the reasons for this is that symptoms tend to present rather late in the disease when it has already had a chance to spread. Also, many of the symptoms are nonspecific and are seen in most heavy smokers. These symptoms include chronic cough, wheezing, dyspnea, **hemoptysis** (coughing up blood), and chest pain.

Diagnosis is made by chest x-ray, sputum cytology, bronchoscopy, biopsy, or **thoracentesis** (surgical puncture and drainage of the thoracic cavity). Treatment is generally **palliative** (giving relief but not assuring a cure) and usually includes some combination of surgery, radiation, and chemotherapy. These treatments may improve the patient's prognosis and prolong survival.

COMMON DIAGNOSTIC PROCEDURES AND THE MEDICAL ASSISTANT'S ROLE

Many different studies, procedures, and examinations are performed to detect and diagnose the previously mentioned disorders and other respiratory problems. Some of these studies can be performed in the physician's office, whereas others need to be done in the hospital.

Physical Examination of the Respiratory System

You may be responsible for preparing the patient for an examination of the respiratory system by the physician or you may assist in the examination. It is important to maintain a calm, reassuring attitude while you prepare the patient for the examination. If the physician is performing a chest assessment, the patient will have to remove all clothing from the waist up and put on a gown.

Upper Airway Examination

When the physician examines the patient's nose, ears, and throat, you may be required to prepare the equipment for the examination. Because the ears open into the pharynx through the eustachian tubes, they are usually assessed as part of the upper airway examination. An otoscope is the instrument used for this examination and must be prepared with the correct size earpiece (speculum) for the patient. The nose and sinuses are then assessed, using a nasal speculum, followed by a visual inspection of the throat, using a tongue depressor and small light (Fig. 17-7). The physician also

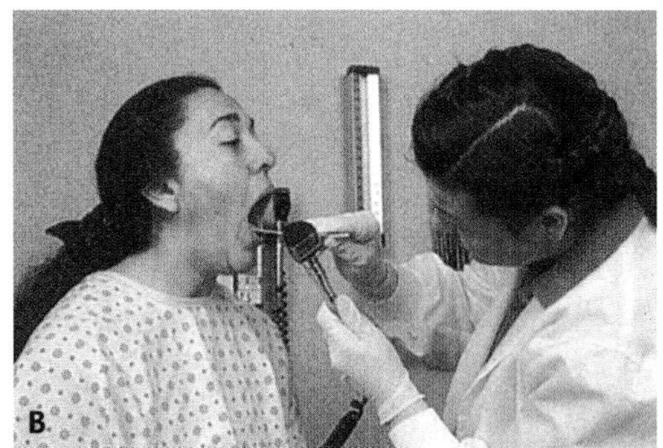

Figure 17-7 The physician visually inspects the throat.

palpates the lymph nodes in the neck and the other neck structures that relate to the upper airway

Lower Airway Examination (Chest Examination)

The traditional examination of the chest consists of four parts: inspection, palpation, percussion, and auscultation. Each is briefly described below. To allow the physician to perform this examination, the patient should be sitting and all clothing should be removed above the waist, except for a hospital gown for female patients. You may be asked to help adjust the gown to allow the physician adequate access to all areas of the chest and back.

INSPECTION. This part of the examination consists of a visual inspection of the chest and the patient's respiratory pattern (Table 17-4). During inspection, the physician looks for abnormal shape of the thorax, use of accessory muscles for ventilation, respiratory pattern, surgical scars, cyanosis, or any other visual signs of previous or current respiratory disease.

PALPATION. In the palpation segment of the examination, the physician uses his or her hands to feel the pa-

Table 17-4 **Abnormal Respiratory Patterns**

Pattern	*Description*
Apnea	No respirations
Bradypnea	Slow respirations
Cheyne-Stokes	Rhythmic cycles of dyspnea or hyperpnea subsiding gradually into periods of apnea
Dyspnea	Difficult or labored respirations
Hypopnea	Shallow respirations
Hyperpnea	Deep respirations
Kussmaul	Fast and deep respirations
Orthopnea	Inability to breathe in other than a sitting or standing position
Tachypnea	Fast respirations

17

tient's throat for lumps, areas of tenderness, and location of the trachea. The patient may be asked to say "99" while the physician feels the chest wall in different places to assess the vibrations produced. Solid masses (such as tumors) or fluids (as in pneumonia) will produce an increase in vibrations, whereas increased air (as seen in emphysema) will produce a decrease in vibrations.

PERCUSSION. Percussion is performed by placing a finger or fingers on the chest and striking it with the fingers of the other hand. During percussion, the physician listens for the sound produced to determine if it is a normal (resonant) sound, like that produced by a drum; dull or flat, which would be seen in consolidation of pulmonary tissue as in **atelectasis** (collapse of alveoli), pneumonia, or tumor; or hyperresonant (more hollow in sound), which would be seen in emphysema. The physician may also use percussion to assess **diaphragmatic excursion,** or how far the diaphragm moves during a deep inspiration.

AUSCULTATION. Auscultation involves listening to the patient's lungs with a stethoscope. The physician systematically listens to each side of the chest in each area to compare the sounds bilaterally. The patient should breathe somewhat deeply, with an open mouth and the head turned away from the physician's face. Make sure the patient does not breathe too rapidly to avoid hyperventilation, which could cause dizziness. During auscultation, the physician listens for abnormal or adventitious sounds, such as crackles and wheezes, which could indicate a disease process (Table 17-5). The physician may also wish to assess vocal sounds and may ask the patient to say "e," "1, 2, 3," or "99" while auscultating.

Table 17-5 **Abnormal Breath Sounds**

Breath Sound	*Description*
Bubbling	Gurgling sounds as the air passes moist secretions in the airways
Crackles (rales)	Crackling sound, usually inspiratory, as air passes moist secretions in the airways. Fine to medium crackles indicate secretions in the small airways and alveoli. Medium to coarse crackles indicate secretions in the larger airways.
Friction rub	Dry, rubbing or grating sound; may indicate pericarditis or pleuritis
Rhonchi	Low-pitched, continuous sound as air moves past thick mucus or narrowed air passages
Stertorous	Snoring sound on inspiration or expiration, indicates a partial airway obstruction
Stridor	Shrill, harsh inspiratory sound; indicates a laryngeal obstruction
Wheeze	High-pitched musical sound, either inspiratory or expiratory; indicates partial airway obstruction

Checkpoint Question

9. *Describe the four parts of the chest examination.*

Throat Culture

A throat culture is done in cases of suspected pharyngitis or tonsillitis to help determine which microorganism is causing the problem. The patient's throat is gently swabbed with a sterile culture stick to obtain the specimen (Procedure 17-1).

Sputum Culture or Cytology

Sputum cultures are obtained to aid with diagnosis and treatment decisions in patients with suspected pneumonia, tuberculosis, or other infectious diseases of the lower airway. A microbiology laboratory cultures and incubates the specimen to identify any pathogenic microorganisms. Sputum is obtained for cytology to search for abnormal cells that might indicate cancer or a precancerous condition of the lung or airway. In either case, it is important to obtain a specimen that has been coughed up and expectorated from the lower airways, with minimal contamination by oral and pharyngeal secretions. The patient must be asked to cough deeply, and the specimen is collected in a sterile container (Procedure 17-2).

Sputum collection for suspected cancer or for tuberculosis may be required for three consecutive mornings. The specimens should be brought to the office as soon as possible to avoid deterioration of the material.

Most diagnostic specimens are obtained early in the morning when the greatest volume of secretion has had a chance to accumulate. If this is not possible, specimens may also be collected after respiratory treatments or therapy.

It is vitally important that the patient understand that the specimen must be collected from the lung fields and not from the mouth. The difference between saliva and sputum may need to be explained on the patient's level of understanding. Before the collection, encourage the patient to increase fluid intake to decrease the viscosity (thickness) of the secretions. The patient may be weak from illness, and thick mucus will be hard to bring up, causing the patient to be even more exhausted. A cool mist humidifier may help also.

Procedure 17-1 Collecting a Specimen for a Throat Culture

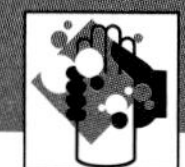
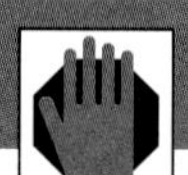
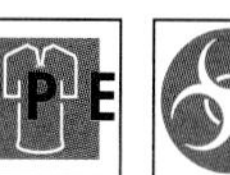

PURPOSE

To provide a specimen to determine the presence and type of microorganisms in the oropharynx

EQUIPMENT/SUPPLIES

- tongue blade (depressor)
- sterile specimen container
- sterile swab (if one is not supplied with the specimen container)
- completed laboratory request slip

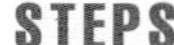

17

STEPS

1. Wash your hands.
2. Assemble the equipment and supplies.
3. Greet and identify the patient. Explain the procedure.
4. Have the patient sit with a light source directed at the throat.
   Good visibility is vital to collection from the areas of concern.
5. Put on gloves and face mask or shield.
6. Carefully remove the sterile swab from the container.
7. Have the patient say "AHHH" as you press on the midpoint of the tongue with the tongue depressor.
   Saying "AHHH" raises the uvula out of the way and decreases the urge to gag. If the depressor is placed too far forward, it will not be effective; if it is placed too far back, it will gag the patient unnecessarily.
8. Swab the areas of concern on the mucous membranes, especially the tonsillar area, the crypts, and the posterior pharynx. Turn the swab to expose all of its surfaces. Avoid touching areas other than those suspected of infection.
   Pathogens must be collected from sites of concern with a twisting motion for maximum collection. Touching other areas will alter the substances on the swab.
9. Maintain the tongue depressor position while withdrawing the swab.
   Keeping the tongue down avoids contaminating the swab unnecessarily.
10. Follow the instructions on the specimen container for transferring the swab. Some require that the wooden swab stick be broken after dropping into the culture; others may have a special swab that is contained within the cap and is secured when the container is sealed.
    Improper handling of the specimen will alter the results.
11. Properly dispose of the equipment and supplies. Remove gloves and wash your hands.
12. Route the specimen or store it appropriately until routing can be completed.

DOCUMENTATION GUIDELINES

- Date and time
- Collection of throat culture
- Routing of specimen
- Patient complaints/concerns
- Patient education/instructions
- Your signature

Charting Example

DATE	TIME Pt arrived in office c/o sore
	throat × 2 days. T-103 oral. Throat cul-
	ture to PGH Lab. —Your signature

Chest X-rays

Chest x-rays can help in the diagnosis of a large variety of pulmonary problems, including pneumonia, lung cancer, emphysema, pulmonary edema, and many others. When performed in a radiology department, usually two views are ordered: a posterior to anterior view and a lateral view. This gives the radiologist a more three-dimensional perspective of the chest. X-rays may also be taken of the sinuses in cases of sinusitis.

Bronchoscopy

Bronchoscopy is an endoscopic procedure in which a lighted scope is inserted into the trachea and large air-

17

Procedure 17-2 Collecting a Sputum Specimen

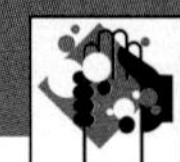
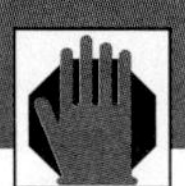

PPE

PURPOSE

To obtain a specimen to determine the presence and type of microorganisms in the respiratory tract.

EQUIPMENT/SUPPLIES

- labeled sterile specimen container
- cover bag

STEPS

1. Wash your hands.
2. Assemble the equipment.
3. Greet and identify the patient. Explain the procedure.
4. Put on gloves and, if necessary, face shield and impervious gown (if you are assisting the patient with sputum collection).
   Standard Precautions must be followed when handling blood and body fluids. If the patient will be coughing in your presence, a face shield and impervious gown provide protection.
5. Have the patient brush his or her teeth or rinse his or her mouth well.
   Food particles will contaminate the specimen.
6. Have the patient cough deeply, using the abdominal muscles and the accessory muscles to bring secretions from the lung fields and not just the upper airways.
   The specimen needs to reflect the pathogens at the lower levels rather than from the upper throat.
7. Have the patient expectorate directly into the specimen container without touching the inside and without getting sputum on the sides of the container. About 5–10 mL is usually needed.
   Touching the inside will contaminate the container. Sputum on the outside of the container is potentially hazardous.
8. Handle the specimen observing Standard Precautions. Cap the container immediately, and drop it into the cover container.
   The specimen is potentially hazardous. Capping it immediately will eliminate the danger of spreading microorganisms, and covering it will contain microorganisms that may have settled on the outside of the container.
9. Assist the patient to rinse his or her mouth after collecting the specimen.
   The procedure may be upsetting to some patients. Some patients may become nauseated during the procedure.
10. Properly care for or dispose of equipment and supplies. Clean the work area. Remove gloves, gown, and face shield and wash your hands.
11. Process the specimen immediately, or within 2 hours, to avoid compromising the studies.
    The pathogens may either proliferate, causing overgrowth, or die, causing a false-negative result.

DOCUMENTATION GUIDELINES

- Date and time
- Collection of sputum specimen
- Routing of specimen
- Patient complaints/concerns
- Patient education/instructions
- Your signature

Charting Example

DATE	TIME
	S: "I have an awful cough."
	O: 80/y/o COPD pt c/o dyspnea
	× 3 days and a productive cough.
	Sputum Greenish-yellow in color.
	Crackles in (L) lower lung field. T-102 oral
	A: Productive cough
	P: 1. Sputum collected per order
	Dr. Raymond. Pt instructed in collec-
	tion procedure. Approximately 10 mL
	of dark yellow, thick mucus obtained.
	2. Specimen routed to CGH Lab.
	3. Pt ed. Re: need to stop smoking.
	Hygiene instructions re: covering
	nose and mouth when coughing. Pt
	verbalized understanding of all
	instructions and pt ed brochure.
	4. Dr. Raymond ordered CXR. Pt given
	directions to Radiology Dept. at
	CGH —Your signature

ways for direct visualization. Bronchoscopy can be used for many diagnostic purposes, such as obtaining sputum specimens, obtaining tissue for biopsy, removing foreign objects, or visually assessing airway changes. It can also be used therapeutically, for example, to clear out mucous plugs or remove foreign bodies. Bronchoscopy is an invasive procedure, and written consent must be obtained from the patient.

Pulmonary Function Tests

Pulmonary function tests are done using a spirometer that measures the amount of air a patient can move in and out and how fast he or she can process it. The patient breathes into a mouthpiece and performs several different breathing maneuvers that are explained by the technician performing the test. By measuring the patient's airflow and comparing the results with predicted values for each patient's height, weight, age, and gender, valuable information can be obtained concerning whether the patient has mild, moderate, or severe obstructive or restrictive lung disease. (See "Asthma")

Arterial Blood Gases

Arterial blood gases (ABGs) measure the pH and pressures of oxygen and carbon dioxide in arterial blood. By this test, the physician can tell whether the lungs are adequately exchanging gases. ABGs can also give information about metabolic acid–base problems, such as diabetic ketoacidosis. Drawing blood from an artery takes special training and is not considered a medical assisting procedure. The site most commonly used is the radial artery in the wrist. Instead of visualizing the vessel as is commonly done in phlebotomy (drawing blood from a vein), the pulse is palpated and the needle is inserted where the pulse is felt. Due to the higher pressures in an artery, after arterial puncture the site must be held tightly with sterile gauze for at least 5 minutes or until all signs of bleeding stop.

Checkpoint Question

10. *List seven ways the physician can obtain information to help diagnose respiratory disorders.*

Answers to Checkpoint Questions

1. *The respiratory system supplies oxygen to the blood, eliminates carbon dioxide, assists with the sense of smell, and assists with speech.*
2. *Functions of the pharynx include passage of food into the digestive tract and passage of air into the respiratory tract.*
3. *Special cells and glands in the trachea produce mucus, which traps any inhaled particles on its sticky surface. Tiny hairs called cilia beat together to move the mucus toward the pharynx, where it is swallowed. Once in the digestive tract, pathogens in the mucus are neutralized.*
4. *After air enters the nose, it must pass through the pharynx, larynx, trachea, bronchi, bronchioles, and alveoli.*
5. *Inspiration is the process by which air is drawn into the lungs from the atmosphere; it is an active process (requires energy). Expiration involves the movement of gas out of the lungs and into the atmosphere; normally, it is a passive process (requires no energy).*
6. *Five upper respiratory tract disorders are rhinitis, sinusitis, pharyngitis, tonsillitis, and laryngitis.*
7. *The onset of bacterial pneumonia is usually sudden and severe; symptoms include fever, cough, chills, and dyspnea. This type of pneumonia is typically localized. In contrast, the onset of viral pneumonia is usually gradual; symptoms include fever and a hacking cough. Unlike bacterial pneumonia, viral pneumonia tends to be spread throughout the lung fields.*
8. *Six factors that may trigger an asthma attack are environmental allergens, irritants, infections, stress, cold air, or rapid breathing.*
9. *Four parts of the chest examination are inspection, percussion, palpation, and auscultation.*
10. *Seven methods for diagnosing respiratory disorders include physical examination, throat culture, sputum culture, chest x-ray, bronchoscopy, pulmonary function tests, and arterial blood gases.*

17

Critical Thinking Challenges

1. Describe the structures of the nose. Why do you think it is better to inhale through the nose than through the mouth?
2. Mr. Gardner, age 55, has been diagnosed with COPD and has many questions about his condition. Identify the characteristics of COPD. How would you explain the disease to Mr. Gardner? Develop educational materials on COPD that can be given to all patients with this disorder.

Suggestions for Further Reading

Burton, G. G., Hodgkin, J. E., & Ward, J. J. (1991). *Respiratory Care: A Guide to Clinical Practice.* Philadelphia: J.B. Lippincott.

Des Jardins, T. (1993). *Cardiopulmonary Anatomy and Physiology.* Albany, NY: Delmar.

Hodgkin, J. E., Connors, G. L., & Bell, C. W. *Pulmonary Rehabilitation: Guidelines to Success.* Philadelphia: J.B. Lippincott.

James, T. C. (1997). Key points of the new asthma diseases. *The Journal of Respiratory Diseases* 18(9).

Miller, B. F., & Keane, C. B. (1992). *Encyclopedia of Medicine, Nursing and Allied Health,* 5th ed. Philadelphia: W. B. Saunders.

Professional Guide to Diseases, 4th ed. (1992). Springhouse, PA: Springhouse.

Whitaker, K. (1992). *Comprehensive Perinatal and Pediatric Respiratory Care.* Albany, NY: Delmar.

Assisting With Diagnostic and Therapeutic Procedures Associated With the Gastrointestinal System

Chapter Outline

Structure and Function of the Gastrointestinal System
- Construction of the Transport System
- Digestion
- Metabolism

Organs of the Gastrointestinal System
- Mouth
- Oropharynx
- Esophagus
- Stomach
- Small Intestine
- Large Intestine

Accessory Organs
- Liver
- Gallbladder
- Pancreas

Common Gastrointestinal Disorders
- Mouth Disorders
- Esophageal Disorders
- Stomach Disorders
- Intestinal Disorders
- Colon Disorders
- Functional Disorders
- Liver Disorders
- Gallbladder Disorders
- Pancreatic Disorders

Common Diagnostic Procedures and the Medical Assistant's Role
- History and Assessment
- Blood Tests
- Radiologic Studies
- Endoscopic Examinations
- Stool Specimens
- Screening for Occult Blood

Role Delineation

CLINICAL

Fundamental Principles

- Apply principles of aseptic technique and infection control.
- Screen and follow up patient test results.

Diagnostic Orders

- Collect and process specimens.
- Perform diagnostic tests.

Patient Care

- Prepare and maintain examination and treatment areas.
- Prepare patients for examinations, procedures, and treatments.
- Assist with examinations, procedures, and treatments.

GENERAL

Professionalism

- Project a professional manner and image.
- Work as a team member.
- Prioritize and perform multiple tasks.

Communication Skills

- Treat all patients with compassion and empathy.
- Adapt communications to individual's ability to understand.

Legal Concepts

- Practice within the scope of education, training, and personal capabilities.
- Document accurately.

Instruction

- Instruct individuals according to their needs.
- Teach methods of health promotion and disease prevention.

Chapter Competencies

Learning Objectives

Upon successfully completing this chapter, you will be able to:

1. Spell and define the Key Terms.
2. Describe the action of anabolism and catabolism.
3. Describe the process of digestion.
4. List and describe the structures of the digestive system.
5. List and locate the primary and accessory organs of the gastrointestinal system.
6. Describe the function of the primary and accessory organs of the gastrointestinal system.
7. List and describe disorders of the gastrointestinal system.
8. Identify and explain the purpose of diagnostic procedures of the gastrointestinal system.

Performance Objectives

Upon successfully completing this chapter, you will be able to:

1. Prepare a patient for procedures pertaining to the colon (Procedure 18-1).
2. Collect a stool specimen (Procedure 18-2).
3. Perform testing on stools for occult blood (Procedure 18-3).

Key Terms

(See Glossary for definitions.)

ascites
bolus
chyle
chyme
deciduous
defecation
deglutition
dentin
emulsify
enzymes
gingiva
guaiac
hematemesis
hepatomegaly
hepatotoxic
hiatus
insufflator
malocclusion
mastication
melena
metabolism
obstipation
papilla (pl. papillae)
papillae lingua
peristalsis
reflux
rugae
turgor
villus (pl. villi)

The gastrointestinal (GI) system, or tract, is responsible for the ingestion, digestion, transportation, and elimination of the food we eat. Nutrients are broken down by the action of digestive **enzymes** (proteins that start a chemical reaction) into units that can be absorbed through the walls of the GI system into the circulatory and lymphatic systems. The nutrients are transported to the cells to supply fuel for all metabolic processes. The solid waste products are eliminated as feces.

STRUCTURE AND FUNCTION OF THE GASTROINTESTINAL SYSTEM

The GI system of organs includes the mouth, oropharynx, esophagus, stomach, small intestine, and large intestine. Accessory organs include the liver, the gallbladder, and the pancreas (Fig. 18-1).

Construction of the Transport System

The entire GI tract is lined with mucous membranes from the lips to the anus. The properties of the membranes change at intervals to accommodate the digestive action at that point. For instance, the gastric mucosa is able to withstand the hydrochloric acid (HCl) present for digestion, but the esophagus, just above the stomach, can be seriously damaged by this same acid.

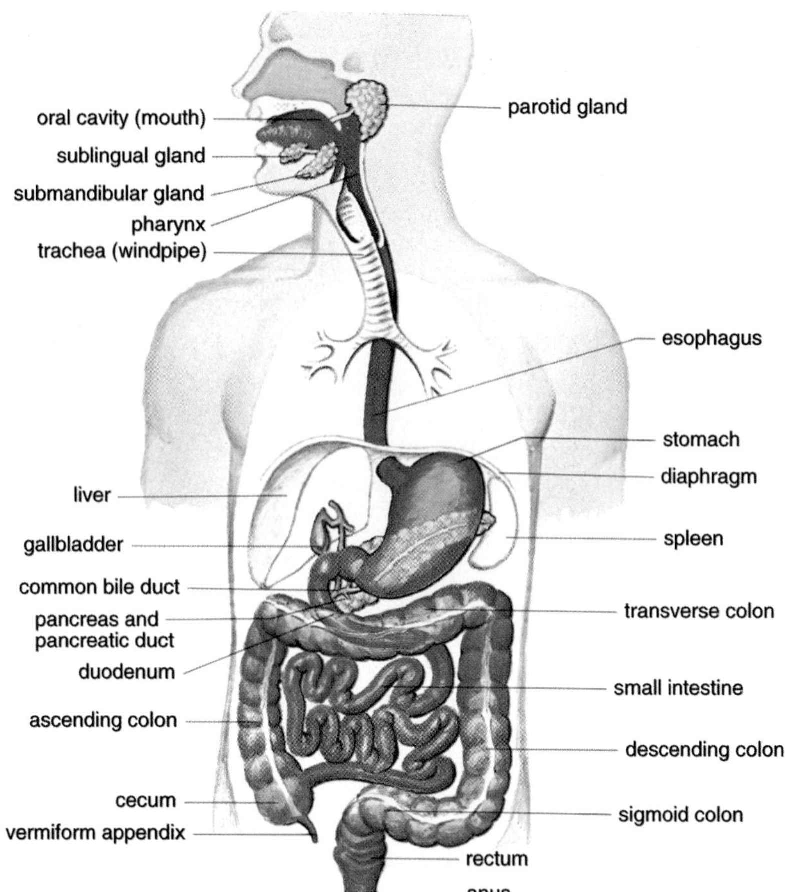

Figure 18-1 The gastrointestinal system.

Little absorption occurs within the stomach because of its protective membranes, but just beyond the stomach, the membranes of the small intestines are designed for great absorption of nutrients and fluids and become progressively less resistant to digestive enzymes through their length.

Most of the length of the GI tract beyond the mouth consists of four layers.

1. The inner mucosa keeps the **bolus** (mass) of food moving. It is composed of epithelium throughout its length. It changes characteristics from the relatively smooth inner surface of the mouth and esophagus to the velvety **villi** (tiny projections) of the intestines.
2. The submucosa is highly vascular with a strong nerve supply.
3. The smooth muscle layer has an inner circular lumen to dilate and constrict and an outer longitudinal layer that shortens with contractions. The food is pushed along by squeezing the inner lumen and shortening the outer layer in rhythmic waves of **peristalsis.** This movement continues to break the bolus into segments and mix it with enzymes to hasten the digestive breakdown.
4. The outer wall connects the tract to the peritoneum, which supports, insulates, and cushions the organs within its highly vascular connective tissue (Fig. 18-2).

Digestion

Digestion starts in the mouth with the intake, or ingestion, of food. The teeth and tongue break the food into small pieces and mix it with saliva for swallowing. Saliva begins the process of digestion by breaking down some of the carbohydrates into sugars. Food flows through the esophagus by peristalsis and enters the stomach to be mixed with the gastric enzymes (Table 18-1). Wavelike motions of the stomach press this thick liquid, called **chyme,** through the pyloric sphincter into the duodenum. Bile from the liver and gallbladder and pancreatic enzymes continue to break the food into molecules that can be absorbed through the lining of the small intestines into the bloodstream and lymph system. Liquid portions of the chyme are reabsorbed in the large intestines, and the solid waste is eliminated as feces.

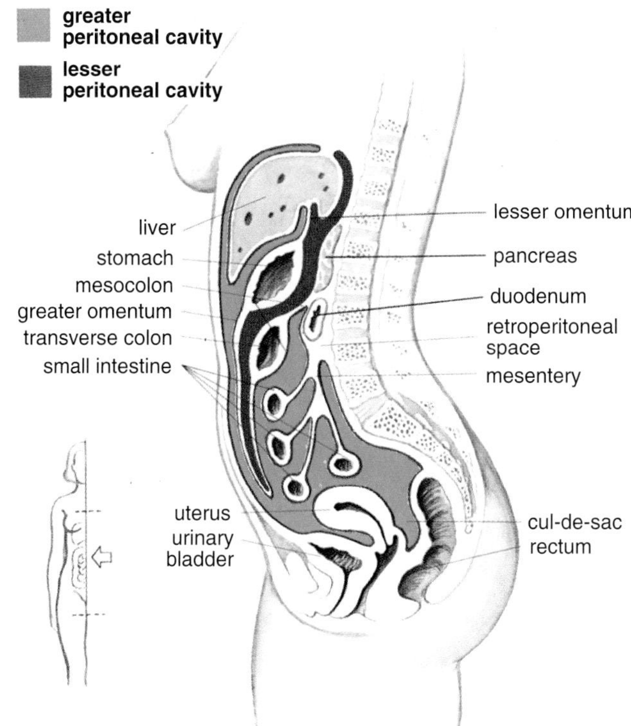

Figure 18-2 Diagram of the abdominal cavity showing the peritoneum.

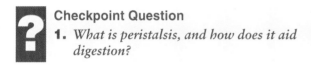

Checkpoint Question

1. *What is peristalsis, and how does it aid digestion?*

Metabolism

Food is broken down into usable units by a process of physical and chemical changes called **metabolism.** There are two phases of metabolism: anabolism and catabolism. As part of the anabolic or constructive phase, digested nutrients are converted into units that can be absorbed and used by the cells for growth, repair, and each cell's specific functions. As part of the catabolic or destructive phase, these chemical units are broken down to release the energy stored within the compounds.

Table 18-1 **Digestive Enzymes**

Enzyme	*Source*	*Action Target*
Amylase	Salivary glands and pancreas	Starch
Hydrochloric acid	Gastric glands	Protein, sucrose, collagen
Pepsin	Gastric glands	Protein
Bile	Liver (stored in gallbladder)	Fats
Trypsin	Pancreas	Protein
Lipase	Pancreas	Fats
Lactose	Duodenal mucosa	Glucose
Maltase	Intestinal villi	Maltose (sugar)

ORGANS OF THE GASTROINTESTINAL SYSTEM

18

Mouth

The oral cavity begins at the lips, which help to move the food into the mouth during ingestion and aid in speech formation. The cheeks are formed by the buccal muscles and help push the food from side to side for more efficient chewing. The tongue is composed of skeletal muscle and covered with mucous membranes. Within the mucous membranes of the tongue are several sizes and shapes of **papillae,** or taste buds, called **papillae lingua.** They provide friction for moving the food about and are part of the sensory system that provides us with the sense of taste. The tongue moves the food back and forth to aid in chewing and helps mix the food particles with saliva for swallowing.

The teeth break the food into manageable pieces in a process called **mastication,** or chewing. The teeth are fixed in the **gingiva,** or gums, with a root below the gum line, firmly attached in the mandible and maxilla. They are composed internally of **dentin,** which surrounds the inner pulp and lies just below the enamel and are covered with enamel above the gum line. The exposed portion is called the crown. The 20 **deciduous** teeth (baby teeth) begin to erupt at about 6 months. As the roots are absorbed, these teeth are shed; 36 permanent teeth begin to replace the deciduous teeth by about age 6. The replacement teeth consist of central and lateral incisors for cutting, canines for tearing and grasping, and premolars and molars for grinding.

The salivary glands secrete saliva to moisten the ground food particles and bind them for swallowing. The three main pairs of salivary glands are:

- *Parotid,* just below and in front of the ears; ducts open into the cheeks
- *Submandibular,* in the floor of the mouth; ducts open near the frenulum
- *Sublingual,* under the tongue with several small ducts

Saliva is usually neutral (6.5–7.5 pH) to protect the teeth. Its production is easily affected by olfactory stimuli, emotions, visual impulses, and even by memories. Digestion begins with saliva production and the breakdown of some of the carbohydrates into sugars.

The palate consists of the mucous membrane-covered palatine bone anteriorly and soft tissue posteriorly. When the bolus of food reaches the pharynx, the soft palate rises, lifting the uvula, and closes the nasopharynx to keep food from entering the nasal cavity.

Oropharynx

The oropharynx, or throat, is common to both the GI and respiratory systems. Just above the oropharynx is the nasopharynx, posterior to the nasal cavity. Just below the oropharynx is the laryngopharynx, which opens into the larynx and the trachea. When the bolus of food is ready to be swallowed, it is lifted by the tongue and moved to the oropharynx, a process called **deglutition**, or swallowing. Smooth muscles and peristalsis transport it to and through the esophagus.

Checkpoint Question

2. *Explain the difference between mastication and deglutition.*

Esophagus

The esophagus is located behind the trachea. (See Chap. 17, Assisting With Diagnostic and Therapeutic Procedures Associated With the Respiratory System.) Except during the act of swallowing, the esophagus remains closed. When a bolus of food passes through the laryngopharynx into the esophagus, the epiglottis closes over the larynx and seals the airway. The esophagus expands into the thin, membranous area at the posterior of the tracheal cartilages.

The esophagus is about 10 inches long and descends through the mediastinum, penetrates the diaphragm, and empties into the stomach. No digestive action occurs in the esophagus. The lower esophageal, or cardiac, sphincter separates the esophagus from the stomach at the **hiatus** (opening or gap). The esophagus is not protected from the stomach's digestive enzymes and can be damaged if acids **reflux** (flow backward) through the cardiac sphincter.

Stomach

The stomach is a J-shaped muscular pouch located under the diaphragm in the left upper quadrant and extends to the inner curve of the underside of the liver. The stomach has a three-tiered muscular structure consisting of circular, longitudinal, and oblique smooth muscle. The function of the muscle layers of the stomach is to churn the food and mix it with gastric enzymes. The inner layers are composed of a mucosa and submucosa layer to protect the underlying muscular structure from the acids necessary for digestion (Fig. 18-3).

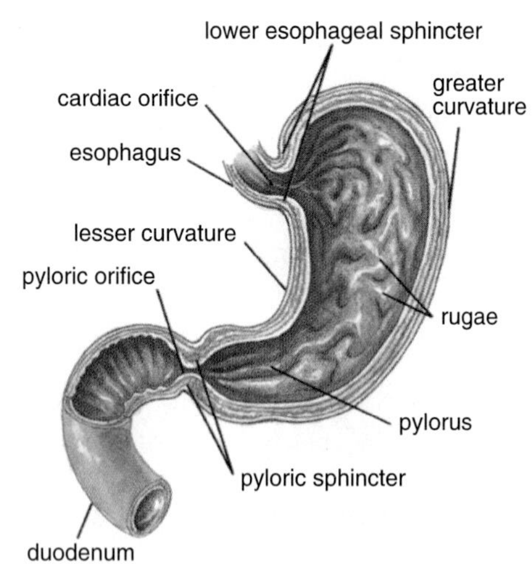

Figure 18-3 Longitudinal section of the stomach and a portion of the duodenum showing the interior.

The stomach is divided into four main regions:

1. Cardiac region (the upper curve of the stomach near the heart)
2. Fundus (balloons above the cardiac region)
3. Body (middle or main portion)
4. Antrum or pylorus (narrows to the pyloric sphincter)

The pyloric sphincter guards the opening between the stomach and the first portion of the small bowel.

The cells that make up the inner lining of the stomach produce HCl to help dissolve the food and kill ingested bacteria. The pH of HCl is approximately 2. The presence of HCl stimulates the production of pepsin from cells in the mucous membrane lining of the stomach walls. The mixing, churning action of the muscular walls of the stomach aid the enzymes in liquefying the food into chyme. The chyme is then pressed in small amounts (5–15 mL at a time) through the pyloric sphincter and passes into the small intestine.

Very few substances are absorbed through the gastric mucosa. These substances may include limited amounts of water, alcohol, and certain drugs. Food that is absorbed through the stomach walls has been ingested as simple molecules, such as the simple sugars.

When the stomach is empty, it folds into **rugae** to allow for expansion. The stomach can hold about one quart of food or liquid and completes its part of the digestive process in about 3 to 4 hours.

Small Intestine

The small intestine is the longest portion of the GI system and is divided into three sections: duodenum, jejunum, and ileum. The divisions of these sections are marked only by microscopic structural differences. The total small bowel can stretch to 23 to 26 feet long. In its usual compressed configuration, its length is about 10 to 12 feet. The final stages of digestion occur in the small intestine.

The upper section, the *duodenum,* is about 12 inches long. It is located in front of the right kidney and just below the liver. It is connected to the gallbladder for bile and to the pancreas for enzymes to begin the digestion of the chyme pressed from the stomach. Bile breaks down the fats into small globules that can be digested. The pancreatic enzymes break down carbohydrates, fats, and proteins. The middle section, the *jejunum,* is the longest section, measuring about 6 to 8 feet. Digestion and absorption continue throughout its length and are completed in the *ileum,* the remaining 1- to 2-foot section.

The entire inner surface of the small intestine has a soft, velvet-like covering of villi that slows the chyme and increases the surface area for greatest absorption (Fig. 18-4). Each projection of villi is also covered with microvilli, which further increase the opportunities for absorption. Most of the digestion occurs in the duodenum by the action of the bile and pancreatic enzymes; absorption occurs further into the jejunum and ileum. Passage through the small intestine usually takes from 3 to 10 hours, with peristalsis pushing the food slowly through. The bowel sounds that can be heard are produced by the relaxation and contraction of the intestinal walls against the mass of food as it moves toward the large intestine.

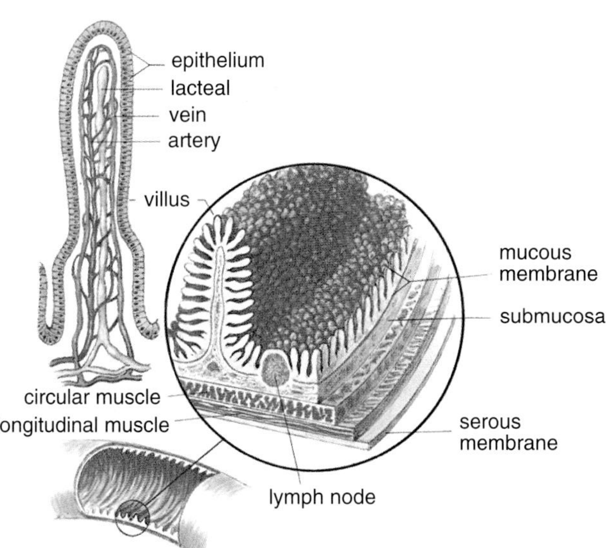

Figure 18-4 Diagram of the wall of the small intestine showing numerous villi. At the left is an enlarged drawing of a single villus.

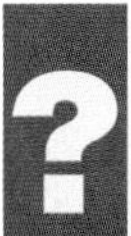

Checkpoint Question

3. *Name the three sections of the small intestine. In which sections do digestion and absorption occur?*

Large Intestine

The ileocecal valve divides the ileum from the first part of the large intestine, called the *cecum.* The large intestine stores the digested material while fluids are reabsorbed into the bloodstream, and the indigestible particles are passed along for elimination. The large intestine is about 6 to 8 feet long.

From the cecum in the right lower quadrant, the intestine rises as the ascending colon toward the liver in the right upper quadrant. It turns at the hepatic flexure and crosses the abdominal cavity toward the left upper quadrant as the transverse colon. At the gastric, or splenic, flexure, it turns downward toward the left lower quadrant as the descending colon. In the extreme lower left quadrant, it turns toward the midline as the sigmoid colon and joins the rectum. The rectum ends at the anus.

Little is absorbed in the colon except water, minerals, and certain vitamins. A normally present bacteria, *Escherichia coli,* synthesizes vitamin K and some of the B-complex vitamins and devours the last of the nutrients. As the undigested material fills the sigmoid colon and rectum and presses against the inner rectal sphincter, the urge to defecate builds. Expelling the feces (the products of digestion) is called **defecation.**

ACCESSORY ORGANS

The accessory organs of the gastrointestinal system include the liver, gallbladder, and pancreas (Fig. 18-5).

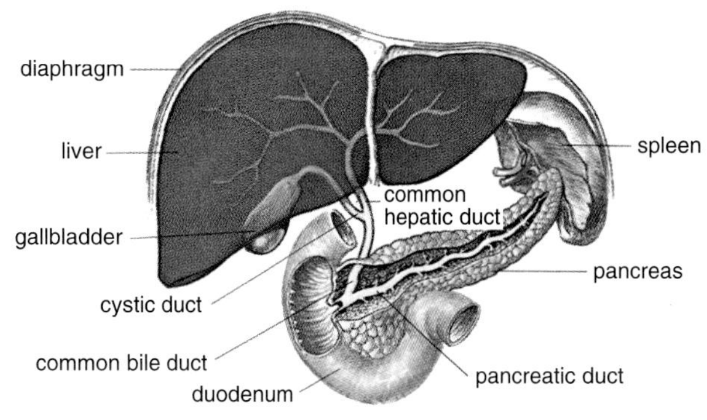

Figure 18-5 Accessory organs of digestion.

18

18

Liver

The liver lies just below the diaphragm in the right upper quadrant. This complex organ has two main lobes, a large right lobe further divided into smaller partitions and a smaller left lobe that stretches toward the top of the stomach.

The liver has a double blood supply. The hepatic artery carries oxygen-rich blood to the liver to maintain its functions. Blood is received from the intestinal vessels into the portal vein and is shunted to the liver to be processed before rerouting to the general circulation.

The liver removes glucose and converts it to glycogen for storage. Excess glucose is changed to fatty acids, carbon dioxide, and water. Amino acids are broken down for cellular use, and the ammonia that results from the chemical conversion is transported as urea to the kidneys for elimination. The liver manufactures and metabolizes many of the proteins, fats, and carbohydrates used by the body. It removes and stores vitamins A, D, B_{12}, K, and the mineral iron. The liver destroys old red blood cells and manufactures bile to **emulsify** (disperse) fats for digestion. Special phagocytic cells, called Kupffer cells, remove toxins, bacteria, and foreign agents to clean the blood before returning it to the heart by way of the hepatic veins.

Checkpoint Question
4. *List several functions of the liver.*

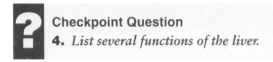

Gallbladder

The liver constantly manufactures the enzyme bile, even though bile is only needed during digestion. Bile flows from the liver through the cystic duct to the gallbladder for storage until needed. As chyme leaves the stomach in small 5- to 15-mL portions, bile is added to the mixture to break the fat particles into globules that can be absorbed through the intestinal walls into the lymph system. This milky, fatty substance is called **chyle** and is carried to the thoracic lymphatic duct and added to the general circulation.

Pancreas

The pancreas is a large, long organ that stretches behind the stomach from the duodenum to the spleen. The spleen has several functions, such as filtering old red blood cells for the lymphatic system and storing blood for emergencies. The pancreas functions in both the endocrine and the exocrine systems. As an endocrine gland, the pancreas secretes insulin and glucagon from the islets of Langerhans to regulate blood sugar levels. As an exocrine gland, it excretes pancreatic enzymes for the digestion of fats, proteins, and carbohydrates. The pancreatic enzymes are very alkaline to counteract the acidity of the gastric enzymes as they pass through the duodenum. The pancreas empties into the duodenum through a duct that it shares with the gallbladder called the common bile duct.

COMMON GASTROINTESTINAL DISORDERS

Mouth Disorders

Caries

Dental caries (tooth decay) is the most widespread disease of the oral cavity. Bacteria allowed to remain on the tooth surfaces erode the enamel and allow infection to reach the inner portions of the tooth. There are many reasons for a susceptibility to tooth decay. These include diet, hygiene, **malocclusion** (abnormal contact between the teeth), and the prenatal diet. The treatment includes a proper diet low in sugars, good oral hygiene as prescribed by the dentist, and frequent professional dental care.

Stomatitis

The most common disease of the mouth tissues is stomatitis or inflammation of the oral mucosa. It may be caused by a virus or a bacteria. The two most common forms are herpetic stomatitis, caused by the herpes simplex virus, and candidiasis, caused by the fungus *Candida albicans.*

Herpes simplex usually is self-limiting after the initial exposure to the virus. The exposure is usually hand to mouth, mouth to mouth, or by vector (eg, shared drinking glasses or eating utensils). It presents as a painful sore in the mouth or on the lips. The virus lies dormant for long periods with exacerbations during periods of illness, stress, and overexposure to the sun. There is no cure; palliative measures relieve discomfort until the ulcers heal.

Formerly called *Monilia albicans, C. albicans* is an opportunistic yeast or fungus. It always is present in the mouth but is kept in check by other normal oral bacteria. When the normal bacterial balance in the mouth is altered, *C. albicans* organisms multiply. Broad-spectrum antibiotics kill many different bacteria, upsetting the balance and allowing the opportunistic organisms to grow without control. In babies, the disease is called thrush. It occurs because milk has changed the pH in the mouth, establishing a more favorable environment for the growth of the *C. albicans.* Oral treatments with antifungal agents are usually effective at relieving the disorder.

When *Candida* spreads to the esophagus, it is usually caused by a breakdown in the immune system, as seen in immune suppression.

Gingivitis

Gingivitis is inflammation of the gingiva or gums. It may lead to periodontitis and destruction of the support structures of the teeth. In Americans, more teeth are lost to gum disease than to tooth decay. Good oral hygiene and frequent dental care will prevent premature loss of teeth. Vincent's angina is a severe form of gum infection with systemic symptoms. It is usually treated by antibiotics.

Oral Cancers

Oral cancers are common, especially among individuals who use tobacco products. The constant irritation of the tobacco causes white spots or patches, called leukoplakia, to form on the oral mucosa, particularly the lips and tongue. These lesions frequently become malignant and are treated by surgery or chemical agents. Cancer of the lips usually responds well to radiation or surgery. Cancer of the margins of the tongue metastasize quickly and are hard to treat.

Checkpoint Question

5. *Name four common mouth disorders.*

Esophageal Disorders

Hiatal Hernia

Hiatal hernia is a common condition that frequently affects people over age 40. Weight gain can be a contributing factor. A hiatal hernia is caused by a defect in the diaphragm that allows a portion of the stomach to slide up into the chest cavity. Normally, the stomach's cardiac sphincter and the tone of the diaphragm muscle prevent reflux of gastric acids into the unprotected esophagus. This barrier loss enables the stomach acid to invade the esophagus, causing considerable discomfort (Fig. 18-6).

Diagnosis is made by chest x-ray, barium swallow, or endoscopy. Because surgically corrected hiatal hernias frequently recur, medical treatment is usually the first choice. This includes diet modification (eg, small, frequent meals with no food at least 2 hours before bedtime), antacid treatments, weight loss, elevating the head of the bed, and drug therapy to increase the tone of the lower esophageal sphincter.

Constant exposure to gastric acid from a hiatal hernia or gastroesophageal reflux can lead to esophagitis, a condition that resembles abraded skin along the lining of the esophagus. Constant irritation of the lining of the esophagus may lead to malignancy. This condition is called Barrett's esophagus. Patients with Barrett's esophagus have a 30% to 40% chance of developing adenocarcinomas. If the source of irritation is gastroesophageal reflux, it will be diagnosed and treated much the same as a hiatal hernia (Box 18-1).

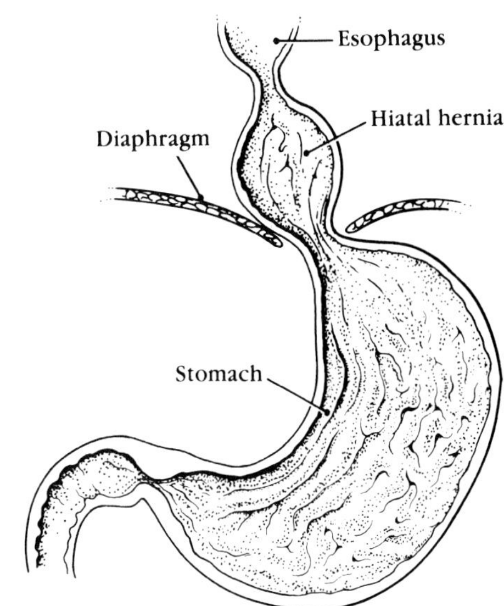

Figure 18-6 Location and appearance of hiatal hernia.

Esophageal Varices

Varicose veins of the esophagus result from pressure within the esophageal veins. This is common with cirrhosis of the liver because the damaged liver structure impedes the drainage of the portal vein. Hemorrhage is the most common and dangerous possibility. Pressure tubes are applied in the esophagus as an emergency procedure. Endoscopic procedures, such as chemical sclerosis, are the treatment of choice when the patient is able to tolerate the procedure.

Box 18-1
Avoiding Gastric Reflux

1. Avoid acidic or spicy foods and chocolate, especially in the evening.
2. Limit caffeine.
3. Maintain optimum weight.
4. Avoid overeating.
5. Wait 1 hour after meals before exercising.
6. Do not eat just before going to bed.
7. Do not lie down just after eating.
8. Stop smoking.
9. Raise the head of the bed with blocks, bricks, or stacks of books.
10. See the physician if symptoms persist.

Esophageal Cancer

Cancer of the esophagus is most common among older men and is usually fatal. Gastric reflux, smoking, and alcohol use are predisposing factors.

The malignancy narrows the lumen of the esophagus and causes dysphagia. As the mass enlarges, swallowing solid food may become extremely painful. Vomiting and weight loss occur as the symptoms progress. This cancer usually spreads to the mediastinal organs. A barium swallow fluoroscopy outlines the lesion, and esophagoscopy with biopsy confirms the diagnosis. If the disease is localized, surgical resection is the treatment of choice. Radiation and chemotherapy also are used. No treatment has proven satisfactory, and survival rates are very low.

Checkpoint Question

6. *Describe a hiatal hernia and how it can affect the esophagus.*

Stomach Disorders

Gastritis

Gastritis is an inflammation of the stomach lining. The most common causes are irritants, such as alcohol, and the excessive intake of aspirin and nonsteroidal anti-inflammatory drugs (NSAIDs). The organism *Helicobacter pylori* is also frequently implicated. The ingestion or presence of any sufficiently irritating substance can erode the mucosal lining and cause inflammation. The condition may be acute or chronic.

Gastritis can cause significant oozing of blood and may result in a positive test for occult (hidden) blood. In elderly patients, sufficient blood loss can cause anemia. Symptoms include GI bleeding, epigastric discomfort, nausea, and vomiting. Diagnosis usually includes gastroscopy. Treatment usually involves eliminating the irritant and restoring the proper gastric acidity. Chronic atrophic gastritis is seen frequently with types of severe anemia. Vitamin B_{12} must be given by injection to combat the anemia.

Ulcers

Ulcers are sloughed tissues that leave erosions or sores. Within the GI tract, these erosions can expose small blood vessels and produce bleeding and pain. The exposure of subsurface areas of the gastric mucosa to HCl causes pain that is intensified by the action of peristalsis. The acids flow in abundance through the pylorus and may also erode the duodenum. The bleeding ranges from oozing to massive, life-threatening hemorrhage. Slight seepage can be detected by a test for occult blood. Heavier bleeding will lead to **melena** (black, tarry stools) or a "coffee-ground" appearance in **hematemesis** (vomiting blood). Ulcers in the GI tract may perforate into the abdominal cavity with life-threatening consequences. Ulcerative conditions may progress to malignancies.

Peptic or gastric ulcers frequently are caused by the use of salicylates, NSAIDs, and alcohol. It has recently been discovered that many gastric ulcers are caused by a chronic *H. pylori* infection.

H. pylori is a bacteria presumed to enter the body either by the fecal/oral route or the oral/oral route. It resides in the mucous lining of the stomach and through its metabolism secretes enzymes that attack the mucous membrane. A small tissue sample is obtained by endoscopy and placed on a gel that will indicate if *H. pylori* is present.

H. pylori is treated with antibiotics and bismuth subsalicylate. The prescribed treatment for ulcers caused by hyperacidity involves limiting the production of hydrogen by the gastric cells to neutralize the acid in the stomach. The gastric acids produced by the stomach are under nerve and hormonal control and are increased in stressful situations. Severing the vagus nerve (vagotomy) reduces the secretion of HCl. Pyloroplasty to open the lumen of the pyloric sphincter eases gastric emptying to reduce the gastric load and reduces the length of mucosal exposure to the gastric enzymes.

Pyloric Stenosis

Pyloric stenosis occurs when an abnormally narrow pylorus delays or obstructs the emptying of the gastric contents. Vomiting (sometimes projectile) occurs as peristalsis pushes against the stricture. There is no known cause. A pyloroplasty relaxes the lumen (see Fig. 18-3).

What If?

What if your pediatric patient's mother complains that her baby vomits everything he eats?

If the vomiting is projectile, the child might have pyloric stenosis. This disorder is usually seen in infants and young children from several days to several months of age. Diagnosis is usually made by parental history, physical examination, and radiologic examination. The physician is often able to palpate an olive-shaped lump in the right upper quadrant while the child is in a supine position. Surgery (pyloroplasty) is the treatment. Although pyloric stenosis is not an emergency, surgery is usually scheduled promptly to prevent dehydration. Educate the parents about the disorder, reassure them, and offer supportive counseling.

Gastric Cancer

Gastric cancer has no known cause, although smoking, high alcohol intake, and genetic predisposition have been implicated. Populations consuming foods high in preservatives, such as smoked, pickled, and salted foods, have a high incidence of gastric cancer.

Gastric cancer spreads rapidly to the adjacent organs and throughout the peritoneal cavity. Symptoms include chronic indigestion, weight loss, anorexia, anemia, and fatigue. The patient may have hematemesis with bright blood or "coffee-ground" vomitus with dark blood. There may also be dark, bloody stools.

Diagnosis requires an upper GI series with fluoroscopy and fiberoptic gastroscopy. The extent of the disease can be determined by computed tomography (CT) scans and by biopsy of the suspected metastatic sites. Surgery to remove the lesion may range from a subtotal gastric resection to a total gastrectomy. If the cancer has metastasized, other organs may be removed, and radiation and chemotherapy may be necessary.

Intestinal Disorders

Gastroenteritis

Gastroenteritis is the inflammation of the stomach, small intestine, or colon. It can include one organ or all three. It is caused by ingesting food or water that contains bacteria, viruses, parasites, or irritating agents. It can be provoked by food allergies or a reaction to medication, such as antibiotics. Symptoms include abdominal pain and cramping, nausea, vomiting, and diarrhea; sometimes fever is present.

Gastroenteritis usually is self-limiting, but in the elderly, young children, or persons with diabetes mellitus, the dehydration that can accompany the diarrhea and vomiting could be life-threatening. Bacteria and parasites are treated with medication if the condition persists. Fluids and electrolytes are restored intravenously as needed.

Duodenal Ulcers

Ulcers formed in the duodenum are caused by the highly corrosive gastric acid. Unlike the stomach, the pH of the duodenum is more alkaline, and the mucosa is not as well protected as the gastric mucosa. The lining of the duodenum may tolerate bile, but it does not tolerate concentrated gastric juices. When the food material passes through the pylorus and brings with it excessive acid, an ulcer forms.

Treatment for duodenal ulcers involves lowering the stomach acid by reducing the gastric acidity and limiting the irritating factors. If these measures are not successful, surgery is an option. If left untreated, ulcers both in the stomach and the duodenum may perforate or may progress to cancer.

Malabsorption Syndromes

Malabsorption syndromes prevent absorption of certain substances through the walls of the small intestines. Fat is a common substance at risk. Stools associated with fat malabsorption are frothy and pale. Because fat is necessary for the metabolism of vitamins A, D, E, and K, patients with this disorder require supplemental vitamin therapy. Celiac sprue is a malabsorption syndrome with an intolerance of gluten. Gluten is a protein found in wheat and wheat byproducts. Celiac sprue can develop at any stage of life and many times presents with diarrhea high in fat. The treatment is usually a gluten-free diet. The cause of sprue is not known, but it runs in families, so a genetic factor may be involved.

Malabsorption syndromes are treated by addressing the suspected causes and replacing the substances at risk.

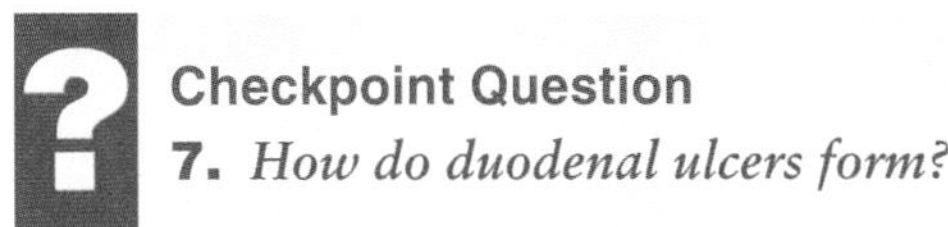

Checkpoint Question

7. *How do duodenal ulcers form?*

Colon Disorders

Crohn's Disease

Crohn's disease is an inflammation of the bowel, ranging from very mild to severe and debilitating. The cause of Crohn's disease is unclear; it is thought to be an autoimmune disorder with a possible genetic link. Crohn's disease can affect the small bowel and the colon but is more common in the area of the ileocecal valve. The bowel walls become inflamed, and the lymph nodes become enlarged; this in turn leads to edema of the bowel wall. When the lining of the bowel is swollen, the fluid from the intestinal contents cannot be absorbed, causing diarrhea and cramping, and may lead to more irritation and bleeding.

Each episode of inflammation causes scarring. The scarring may lead to narrowing of the colon, causing an obstruction of the bowel. Bowel obstruction, no matter what its cause, can be life-threatening and is a medical emergency. Laboratory tests reveal an increase in white blood cells (WBCs) and the erythrocyte sedimentation rate (ESR). A barium enema (BE or BaE) shows strictures alternating with normal bowel (the "string sign"). Sigmoidoscopy and colonoscopy show patchy areas of inflammation.

The treatment is symptomatic and involves restoration of electrolytes, administration of corticosteroids for the inflammation, rest, and a low-fiber diet. Surgery is performed for perforation or hemorrhage. If the situation is severe, a colectomy with an ileostomy may be performed (Fig. 18-7).

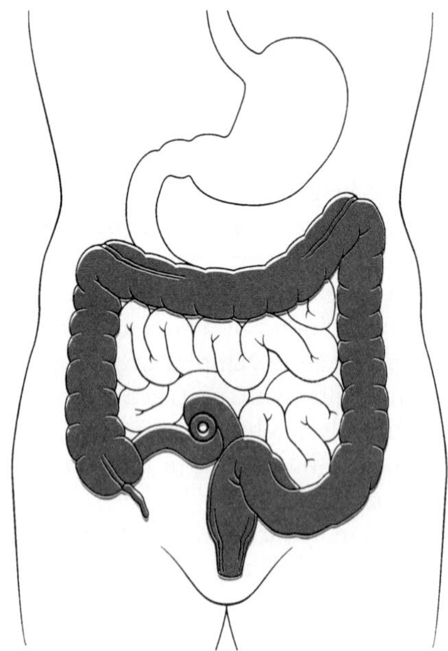

Figure 18-7 An ileostomy. The shaded portion, the entire colon, is removed as a colectomy. Waste is eliminated by the distal portion of the ileum into a bag attached to the abdominal wall.

Ulcerative Colitis

Ulcerative colitis is a chronic inflammatory disease of the lining of the colon. It occurs most often in young women but may occur at any age and may affect men also. The cause is not known but is thought to be an abnormal GI immune reaction to foods or microorganisms. Like Crohn's disease, it can be mild or severe.

The tissue that lines the colon becomes congested and edematous and sloughs off, leading to ulcers and bloody diarrhea. Sometimes pus and mucus are present in the diarrhea. Malabsorption of fluids causes weakness, anorexia, and nausea and vomiting. Scarring can occur as the ulcers heal. The colon may produce pseudopolyps, which can be precancerous. Diagnosis may be made by sigmoidoscopy, which shows a fragile mucosa with inflammation or by BE, which shows areas of edema and ulceration. Biopsy confirms the diagnosis. Colonoscopy evaluates strictures caused by scarring and assesses the risk of cancer.

Treatment requires controlling the inflammation and preventing debilitating loss of fluids and nutrients. If the disease is severe, corticosteroids will be used to relieve the inflammation. Surgery is a last resort and usually involves a proctocolectomy with an ileostomy (see Fig. 18-7).

Irritable Bowel Syndrome

Patients with irritable bowel syndrome frequently complain of bouts of constipation alternating with diarrhea. Although it presents with symptoms resembling mild Crohn's disease or ulcerative colitis it usually does not result in weight loss, and the prognosis is good. It can be debilitating because there is no warning for the bouts of diarrhea. It has a range of symptoms from mild to severe. Women are more likely than men to experience spastic colon. Its origin is thought to be psychogenic, but food irritants may precipitate an attack. Diagnosis requires a careful history, both physical and emotional. Other diseases are ruled out by testing. Treatment requires stress management and identifying the offending food irritants.

Checkpoint Question

8. ***Which inflammatory bowel disorder can lead to life-threatening bowel obstruction? How?***

Diverticulosis

Diverticulosis results from the thinning of the bowel wall, causing small out-pouches. It usually occurs in the sigmoid colon but may occur anywhere in the GI tract. The cause has been attributed to a diet deficient in roughage. Diverticulosis becomes serious when the bowel wall becomes so thin that it exposes veins and arteries. When nicked by a piece of stool, bleeding can occur. The bleeding can be so severe that surgery is required to stop the hemorrhage.

Diverticulosis may progress to diverticulitis or inflammation of these areas of weakness in the bowel wall. The inflammation usually is caused by fecal material becoming lodged in the thin pockets. The symptoms are fever and abdominal pain. As the bowel becomes swollen and distended, the diseased areas may rupture, exposing the peritoneum to fecal material and resulting in peritonitis. The pouches usually show on BE or other radiologic studies.

During the acute phase, treatment includes a bland diet and stool softeners. When the initial inflammation has subsided, a high-fiber diet is ordered.

Polyps

Colon polyps are masses of mucous membrane tissue. Polyps are usually slow growing but over a period of years may become cancerous. They may be discovered by a BE or during a colonoscopy performed to evaluate a change in bowel habits or after occult blood is found in the stool. If the polyps are discovered at an early stage and removed, cancer of the colon can be prevented. Cancer of the colon may invade the muscle of the bowel and metastasize through the lymph system to other organs.

Hemorrhoids

Hemorrhoids are dilated veins (varicosities) in the rectum. They may be external or internal. Internal hemorrhoids may become enlarged and may bleed during defecation. External hemorrhoids may become very painful and itchy and may also bleed. The bleeding may range from a stain on the toilet paper to massive hemorrhage. The blood is bright red rather than the darker blood expected from sites higher in the GI tract. External hemorrhoids are obvious on inspection. Internal hemorrhoids are diagnosed by anoscopy or proctoscopy. Hemorrhoids are caused by poor muscle tone, poor dietary habits, and constipation.

Treatment involves regulating the diet to control constipation, providing local pain relief, using stool softeners, administering chemical sclerosing agents, and surgical or rubber band ligation.

Colorectal Cancers

Cancer of the colon and rectum usually spreads slowly with good survival rates with early diagnosis and treatment. The cause is unknown, but its incidence has been linked to diets high in animal fats and low in fiber. It is commonly seen in patients with a history of ulcerative colitis or colorectal polyps (Fig. 18-8).

Early signs are vague pains with occasional bloody stools. Later signs depend on the section of the colon involved and the degree of metastasis. These signs usually include anemia, weakness, diarrhea or **obstipation** (extreme constipation), anorexia, and weight loss. Many rectal cancers are discovered by a digital examination or an anoscopy. Sigmoidoscopy or colonoscopy is suggested to determine the extent of involvement and are recommended for screening beginning at 50 years of age and then every 3 to 5 years. BE with contrast air aids in diagnosis. Laboratory tests include **guaiac** (reagent) tests, such as the Hemoccult, which test for occult blood in the stool. Surgery to remove the affected area is the treatment of choice and usually is followed by chemotherapy and radiation.

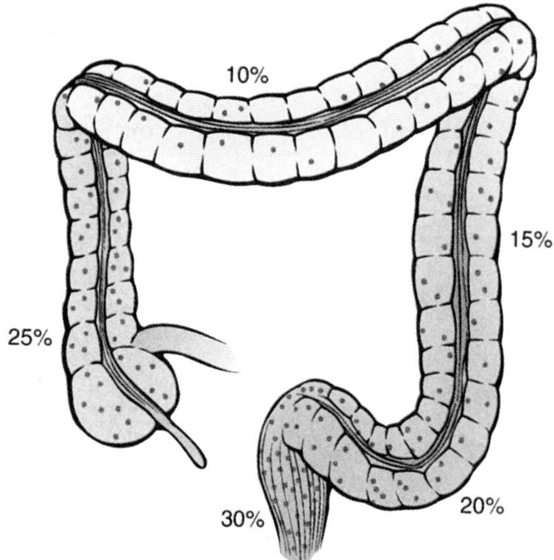

Figure 18-8 Percentage distribution of cancer sites in the colon and rectum.

Functional Disorders

Constipation

When the lower colon is full of fecal material, nerve endings send impulses to the brain that in turn tell the pelvic and rectal muscles to expel the accumulated material. If the nerve endings have been injured or paralyzed, these impulses are not transmitted. Most constipation, however, is caused by poor bowel habits, low-fiber diets, and inadequate fluid intake. The solid material stays in the colon too long and becomes progressively dryer and harder. The normal interval between bowel movements varies with the individual. Infrequent but easy-to-pass stools are not considered constipation. The quality of the stool is more important than the quantity.

Constipation that is not attributed to poor dietary and bowel habits may be due to spasticity of the intestinal walls. The walls clamp against the stool and will not allow it to pass. Several intestinal disorders result in spasticity and constipation. The underlying cause must be treated.

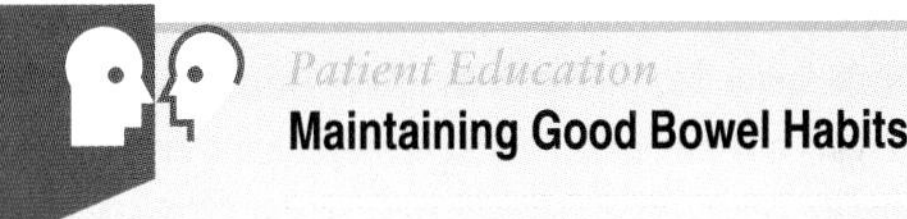

Maintaining Good Bowel Habits

By following the guidelines below, patients can avoid problems of elimination.

1. Eat a wide variety of foods, especially fresh fruits, vegetables, and whole grains. Limit intake of highly processed foods.
2. Drink eight glasses of water a day to help keep the stools moist and easy to pass and to hydrate the tissues.
3. Participate in some form of exercise daily. Even a walk around the block will aid muscle tone and help prevent a sluggish metabolism.
4. Make time for bowel movements when the stimulus is felt. Avoiding or delaying defecation will result in loss of moisture from the stool and may make the bowel insensitive to the stimulus.
5. Avoid laxative or enema use. Frequent use may result in a "lazy bowel."
6. Recognize that the frequency of bowel elimination is an individual characteristic. If stools are passed only several times a week but are soft formed and passed with little effort, there should be no concern about constipation. However, constipation may be a problem even if stools are passed daily but are hard, dry, and difficult to pass.

Atonic or flaccid constipation is the opposite of spasticity and is considered a lazy colon. The causes include poor dietary habits, low fluid intake, lack of exercise, chronic laxative use, and reliance on enemas. Reversing the causes usually corrects the situation in time.

Diarrhea

Normal peristalsis allows the products of digestion to move at a speed that allows fluid reabsorption. When the fluid contents of the bowel are rushed through, as in diarrhea, the water and minerals are not reabsorbed into the system. Infections (bacterial or viral) or GI irritants cause the smooth muscles and the mucous membranes to work to flush out the bowel as quickly as possible. The treatment for diarrhea includes medication to slow peristalsis, a bland diet, and increased fluids. Diarrhea usually is self-limiting. Any significant or prolonged changes in bowel habits should be evaluated by a physician.

Gas

Bacterial decomposition of proteins in the digestive process produces gas that can lead to abdominal discomfort. Gas causes a feeling of fullness that can be expelled by erupting the gas from the stomach through the mouth (eructation) or from the intestines through the rectum (flatulence). The causes include an intolerance of milk products, swallowing air, chewing gum, eating gas-producing or fatty foods, or slow emptying of the stomach and bowels. The problem can usually be relieved by avoiding the offending foods. Various over-the-counter preparations and prescription medications can be used if the problem persists.

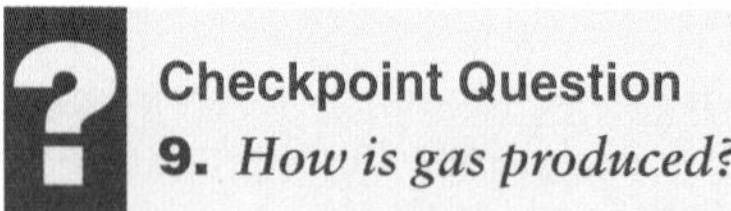

Checkpoint Question

9. *How is gas produced?*

Liver Disorders

Liver disorders are assessed by observing the cardinal signs of liver dysfunction: jaundice, **ascites** (fluid accumulation in the peritoneal cavity), and **hepatomegaly** (liver enlargement). It is vital to obtain a complete medical history from an individual with suspected liver disorder; focus particularly on the history of prior jaundice, anemia, splenectomy, past alcohol use, travel to third-world countries, blood transfusions, use of **hepatotoxic** medications (drugs that are damaging to the liver), or controlled substance abuse. Diagnostic tests for liver disorders include:

- liver function tests, a panel that includes levels of bilirubin, alkaline phosphatase, albumin, prothrombin times, and cholesterol
- x-rays, barium studies, and ultrasound
- radioisotope liver scans
- biopsy
- percutaneous peritoneoscopy
- surgical laparotomy

Hepatitis

Hepatitis is an inflammatory process that causes liver destruction and necrosis. Its cause can be viral, bacterial, or toxic.

Five types of viral hepatitis exist. Table 18-2 summarizes the detailed descriptions of each type listed below:

- *Hepatitis A (HAV),* the most common type of viral hepatitis, also is known as infectious hepatitis. HAV is spread through fecal/oral contamination, from contaminated food and water, or from seafood high in coliform bacteria. It is highly contagious and will spread through closely confined communities. The prognosis for recovery is good.
- *Hepatitis B (HBV),* also known as serum hepatitis, can be transmitted by contaminated sera and other body fluids. The disease may be so severe that death results. Use of Standard Precautions will prevent its spread. Hepatitis B vaccine is recommended for health care workers at risk for contact with blood or body fluids.
- *Hepatitis C (HCV),* also known as non-A, non-B hepatitis, can be transmitted by blood transfusion or percutaneous contamination. It frequently progresses to chronic hepatitis. As with HBV, use of Standard Precautions prevents its spread.
- *Hepatitis D (HDV)* occurs only in patients who have had HBV; it cannot survive without the HBV.
- *Hepatitis E (HEV)* is spread through fecal/oral routes or through dirty water. It is self-limiting.

For all types of viral hepatitis, the symptoms may include fatigue, joint pain, flulike symptoms with fever,

Table 18-2 **Types of Viral Hepatitis**

Type of Virus	*Mode(s) of Transmission*	*Precautions*
HAV	Fecal/oral route	Handwashing
HBV	Sera and body fluids	Standard Precautions HBV vaccine
HCV	Blood transfusions Percutaneous contamination	Standard Precautions
HDV	Coinfector of HBV	Standard Precautions HBV vaccine
HEV	Fecal/oral route	Handwashing Standard Precautions

jaundice, dark urine, and light stools. Complications include impaired liver function, chronic hepatitis, liver cancer, and death.

Diagnosis is made through medical history (eg, past transfusions or exposure to hepatotoxic drugs or chemicals), blood work for hepatitis antibodies, and liver function studies. There is no cure at this time except rest and supportive diet. Interferon-A studies are currently in clinical trials to assist the immune system in responding to viral forms of hepatitis. Standard Precautions must be observed to protect caregivers and health care workers from viral hepatitis.

Toxic hepatitis may result from exposure to chemical toxicants or hepatotoxic substances, including certain medications and alcohol. If the offending toxicant is eliminated early enough, the prognosis for recovery is good. The symptoms of toxic hepatitis resemble viral hepatitis, and the diagnosis is similar. A liver biopsy may identify underlying pathology.

Checkpoint Question

10. *How does the cause of viral hepatitis differ from that of toxic hepatitis?*

Cirrhosis or Fibrosis

Cirrhosis is a chronic inflammatory disease characterized by destruction of liver cells and the formation of fibers throughout the liver, altering its function and efficiency. It occurs most often in men. Causes include a history of alcoholism, prolonged biliary obstruction, or posthepatitis sequela.

In the early stages of cirrhosis, symptoms include vague GI discomfort. In the late stages, diminished respiratory efficiency occurs as ascites force the abdominal contents against the diaphragm. Bleeding tendencies result from the loss of clotting factors formed in the liver. Dermal pruritus (itching), jaundice, and hepatomegaly are usually present. Diagnosis is made by liver biopsy, liver scan, and blood work. Treatment includes removing the cause of the damage (such as abstinence from alcohol), a good diet, vitamin supplements, and supportive care.

Liver Cancer

The liver is rarely a primary site for cancer but is frequently the target site for metastasis. It is more common in men and is rapidly fatal. There is no known cause, but primary liver cancers are thought to be due to exposure to carcinogens. Patients who have cirrhosis or who have hepatitis B are more likely than the general population to develop liver cancer.

Patients usually complain of weight loss, weakness, and right upper quadrant pain. Jaundice may be present in the early stages and will definitely develop as the disease progresses. Diagnosis is confirmed by biopsy, liver function tests, and CT scan or magnetic resonance imaging (MRI). If the lesion is small and localized, resection is possible. Chemotherapy may be used in some instances. If there is no metastasis, transplantation may be a possibility.

Gallbladder Disorders

Cholelithiasis and Cholecystitis

18

Cholelithiasis is the formation of gallstones (Fig. 18-9). Gallstones are made of cholesterol and bilirubin. When the peristaltic action of the gallbladder is sluggish and the bile is allowed to pool in the sac, fluid is absorbed, leaving the solids to concentrate and solidify into stones. Cholecystitis is an acute or chronic inflammation of the gallbladder, usually resulting from an impacted stone in the duct.

Cholecystitis or cholelithiasis usually causes pain as peristalsis presses bile against the blockage, especially after a fatty meal. Acute right upper quadrant pain may radiate to the shoulders, back, or chest. Later in the illness, jaundice may appear. Treatment requires removal of the stones, usually by endoscopic laparotomy. Diet modification may prevent recurrence.

Choledocholithiasis is a stone lodged in the duct system. Cholangitis is an infection of the bile ducts.

Signs and symptoms of any gallbladder disorder include pain, indigestion, nausea, and an intolerance for fatty foods. Tests to determine the cause include cholecystography after the ingestion of a radiopaque dye, percutaneous transhepatic cholangiography, endoscopic retrograde cholangiopancreatography (ERCP), and duodenal endoscopy. Noninvasive procedures include ultrasound and CT scans. Flat plate x-rays are not especially accurate for evaluating gallbladder disorders.

Gallbladder Cancer

Cancer of the gallbladder is rare and difficult to diagnose. It usually is discovered during gallbladder se-

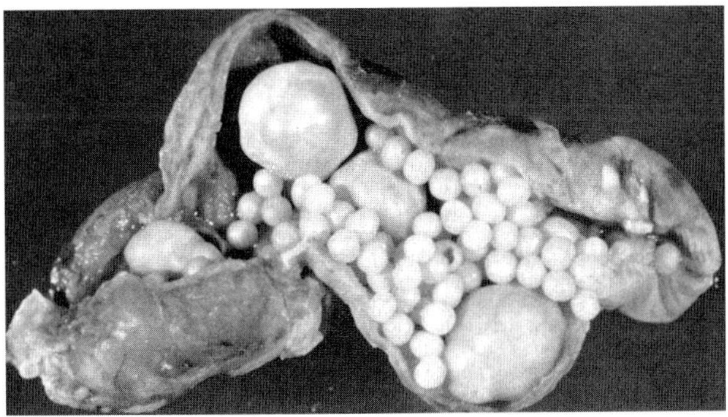

Figure 18-9 Multiple gallstones in a gallbladder. (Courtesy of National Institute of Diabetes and Digestive and Kidney Diseases.)

18

ries to diagnose cholelithiasis. It is more common in older women and is rapidly fatal. The cause is not known, but theory suggests that cholelithiasis is a predisposing factor. The signs and symptoms are indistinguishable from cholecystitis: right upper quadrant pain, nausea and vomiting, weight loss, and anorexia. However, cholecystitis pain usually is sporadic, and pain due to malignancy usually is chronic and severe. The gallbladder may be palpable, and jaundice may be present. Diagnosis includes liver function tests, CT scan, MRI, and cholecystography. Cholecystectomy is the treatment, but survival rates are low.

Checkpoint Question

11. *What is cholelithiasis and how does it occur?*

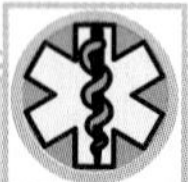

Action STAT!

Hematemesis

Scenario: Mr. Williams is sitting in an examining room. His chief complaint is epigastric pain and vomiting for 2 days. While you are helping him change into an examination gown, he vomits bright red blood. What should you do?

1. Call for help, then quickly put on nonsterile gloves and hand Mr. Williams an emesis basin.
2. Reassure Mr. Williams. If he feels dizzy or weak, place him on the examining table, and have him assume the recovery position. (This will help prevent aspirating vomitus if he should vomit again.)
3. Assist the physician as directed. The plan of care depends on the amount of blood and the physician's specialty. Mr. Williams probably will be transferred to the hospital emergency department for further testing.
4. Monitor Mr. Williams' pulse and blood pressure frequently for signs of shock.
5. Document the incident carefully, and assist with the patient transfer to the ambulance.
6. Remove any blood from the area that was not contained in the basin. Put on gloves and sprinkle liquid absorbing gel on the spill. Using paper towels, remove the liquid and the gel. Place the towels in a biohazard bag. Next, flood the area with a 1:10 bleach solution. Wipe the bleach solution with more paper towels until the area is completely free of blood. Remove and properly discard your gloves. Wash your hands.

Pancreatic Disorders

Pancreatitis

Pancreatitis is an inflammation of the pancreas that may be related to alcoholism, trauma, gastric ulcer, and biliary tract disease. Symptoms include vomiting and steady epigastric pain radiating to the spine; signs of progressive disease include abdominal rigidity and decreased bowel activity. Complications include diabetes mellitus, hemorrhage, shock, coma, and death as the digestive enzymes cause the organ to digest itself. Diagnostic blood work will show an increase in serum amylase and glucose levels. Ultrasound and CT scans are useful in diagnosing the disorder. Treatment includes pain relief medication to reduce pancreatic secretions while the organ recovers.

Pancreatic Cancer

One of the deadliest malignancies is pancreatic cancer. Most patients die within a year of diagnosis. There is no definitive cause, but it occurs most often in middle-aged African American men who smoke, have diets high in fats and proteins, or who are exposed to industrial chemicals for long periods.

Patients complain of weight loss, back and abdominal pain, and diarrhea. They are frequently jaundiced. Diagnosis is made by laparoscopic biopsy, CT scan, MRI, ERCP, and pancreatic enzyme studies. Pancreatectomy is an operative option; chemotherapy and radiation therapy are used also, but the survival rate is very low with current therapies.

COMMON DIAGNOSTIC PROCEDURES AND THE MEDICAL ASSISTANT'S ROLE

History and Assessment

Before beginning any patient's care, an adequate history must be obtained. The patient presenting with GI concerns will be assessed for signs (eg, vomiting) and symptoms (eg, nausea). From that base, the physician determines the direction of the diagnostic testing to rule out or to confirm possible diagnoses. The history must include occupation, family history, diet and alcohol use, recent travel to third-world countries, and current medications. You may be required to assist the patient in completing a checklist of concerns, which might include heartburn, GI bleeding, weight gain or loss, social history of alcohol use, and laxative and enema use.

The physician will assess skin **turgor** (tension), jaundice, edema, bruising, breath odor, size and shape

Box 18-2
Patient Preparation for Bowel Studies

Many bowel studies, such as barium enema and flexible sigmoidoscopy, require that the bowel be completely clear of fecal matter for the test to be considered diagnostic. With minor variations as directed by the physician, the bowel preparation will include the following:

- Liquid diet without dairy products for the full day before the procedure or a clear liquid evening meal
- A laxative the evening preceding the procedure; enemas also may be ordered
- NPO except water after midnight through the time of the procedure
- Rectal suppository, Fleet's enema, or cleansing enema the morning of the procedure

If inflammatory processes or ulcerations are suspected, only gentle cleansing will be used to avoid undue discomfort or possible perforation of lesions.

of the abdomen, and presence and quality of bowel sounds and will palpate the abdominal contents.

Blood Tests

Blood work may include hemoglobin or hematocrit to assess possible anemia as the result of GI bleeding. WBC counts can help detect the presence of infection. The ESR is used to assess inflammatory processes. (See Chap. 30, Hematology, for a detailed discussion of these specific tests.)

Radiologic Studies

Radiologic studies of the stomach and bowels consist of instilling barium, a radiopaque substance, to outline the organs. Barium swallows are used to test for abnormal narrowing or masses in the esophagus. Fluoroscopy is used to watch the chalky liquid as it fills the esophagus.

The upper GI (UGI) shows abnormal constrictions, masses, and obstruction in the esophagus, stomach, and duodenum. This examination requires that the client have nothing by mouth (NPO) after midnight. A small bowel series is an extension of the UGI that visualizes the barium flowing through the small intestines.

A BE provides an outline of the colon. It can reveal a blockage, cancerous growth, polyps, and diverticula. A BE requires that the colon be empty of stool. Box 18-2 outlines the standard patient preparation for a BE.

Flat plate x-rays of the abdomen may be ordered without contrast media but are not as diagnostic as contrast x-rays.

Endoscopic Examinations

The definitive test for the hollow organs of the GI system is an endoscopy examination. Fiberoptic technology has enabled physicians to pass soft, flexible tubes down the esophagus into the stomach and small bowel or up into the colon for direct visualization of these organs. Supplemental laboratory specimens can be obtained, such as tissue biopsies, samples for gastric analysis, fluids to check for bacteria, bile for crystals, and cells for cytology to diagnose malignancies.

Endoscopic examinations also are used to diagnose biliary disorders. ERCP is used to visualize the esophagus, the stomach, the proximal duodenum, and the pancreas. Dye is injected directly into the ducts of the gallbladder and the pancreas to establish patency and function.

Anoscopy involves inserting a metal or plastic instrument into the rectal canal for visual inspection of the anus and the rectum and to obtain swabs for cultures. The sigmoidoscopy examination is a visualization of the sigmoid colon using either a rigid sigmoidoscope or the more widely accepted flexible fiberoptic sigmoidoscope.

The rigid sigmoidoscope is about 10 inches (25 cm) long. This instrument is supplied as reusable metal or disposable plastic and is calibrated in centimeters. An obturator in the lumen allows the instrument to be inserted with minimal discomfort. The lens at the end is magnified for closer observation of the intestinal mucosa and can be moved aside to allow the physician to swab, suction, or biopsy the mucosa. The handle contains the light source. The scope may be equipped with a hand bulb **insufflator** (a device for blowing air, gases, or powders into a cavity) or a powered source of air to expand the walls of the colon for easier visualization to diagnose hemorrhoids, polyps, and diverticula.

The flexible fiberoptic sigmoidoscope is rapidly gaining favor. It offers better visualization and is more acceptable and less uncomfortable to patients. The scope is very thin, can bend and maneuver curves, and can be inserted much farther than the rigid scope (Fig. 18-10). The instrument is supplied as 35 cm (about 14 inches) or 65 cm (about 26 inches). The electrical source of the instrument usually includes an insufflator and suction in addition to the light source. Though smaller than the rigid scope, it also can be used to obtain samples and cultures.

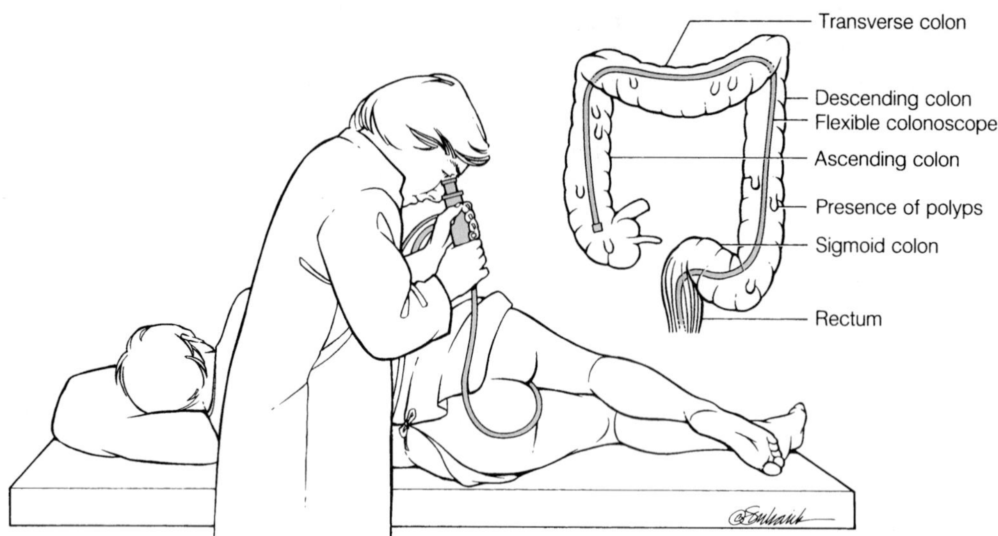

Figure 18-10 Colonoscopy. Flexible scope passes through the rectum and sigmoid colon into the descending, transverse, and ascending colon.

Some physicians prefer that the bowel be as free of feces as possible and may order a light, low-residue meal the evening before the endoscopic examination. An evening laxative also may be ordered to be followed by a cleansing enema in the morning before the procedure. A light breakfast may be allowed. Other physicians, however, prefer to view the mucosa as it normally appears without preparation. Most medical offices will note the preferred preparation in a policy and procedure manual (see Box 18-2).

Procedure 18-1 describes the specific steps for preparing the patient for the above-mentioned colon procedures.

Checkpoint Question

12. *What is involved in anoscopy, and how does it differ from sigmoidoscopy?*

Stool Specimens

As a part of the routine examination for patients over a certain age, many physicians order a stool specimen to test for occult blood. Stool specimens to test for ova and parasites are ordered if an infestation is suspected. Stool specimens also are collected to test for bile, fat, pus, or mucus (Box 18-3). Standard Precautions must be followed when collecting stool specimens for any purpose.

As a medical assistant, you may be responsible for instructing the patient in the procedure, or you may assist in the collection of a stool specimen. A stool specimen may be collected in the office in situations in which the patient may not understand directions for appropriate collection or if test results require a fresh specimen. Appointments for stool specimens should be scheduled early in the morning. Most people move their bowels shortly after awakening; delaying the appointment may cause the patient discomfort or may result in loss of the specimen. Some specimens may be collected and transported in containers with preservatives. All specimens should be transported as quickly as possible. Procedure 18-2 describes the specific steps for collecting a stool specimen.

Screening for Occult Blood

Testing stool for occult blood using a test pack or kit is convenient, quick and easy, and readily acceptable to most patients. This method is used widely for screening purposes to detect the presence of disorders that cause GI bleeding: hemorrhoids, polyps, diverticula, ulcers, or cancers. Most physicians routinely screen patients over age 50 for occult blood. Testing may be done for younger patients if the history suggests a need. Testing for the presence of occult blood will not diagnose the cause but will alert the physician to the need for further testing.

Several pharmaceutical companies manufacture test packs or kits to detect fecal occult blood. Beckman Coulter Inc. supplies three methods: Hemoccult I, a simple slide for a single, simple test; Hemoccult II,

Box 18-3
Special Stool Examinations

Follow the tips below when collecting stool specimens to test for pinworms or parasites or to obtain a swab for culture. Keep in mind that Standard Precautions must be followed.

- *Pinworms:* Schedule the appointment very early in the morning, preferably before a bowel movement or bath. Pinworms tend to leave the rectum and lay eggs around the anus during the night. Use clear adhesive tape to press against the perineal area. Remove it quickly and place it sticky side down on a glass slide for the physician's inspection.
- *Parasites:* Caution the patient not to use a laxative or enema before the test to avoid destroying the evidence of parasites. If the stool contains blood or mucus, include as much as possible in the specimen container; these substances are most likely to contain the suspected organism.
- *Stool culture:* A sterile cotton-tipped swab is passed into the rectal canal beyond the sphincter and rotated carefully. Place it into the appropriate culture container, or process as directed for smear preparation. (See Chap. 27, Microbiology, for specific procedure.)

with three test areas for collection from separate sites from three separate stools if intermittent bleeding is suspected; Hemoccult Tape, for quick testing during rectal examinations.

These tests use the guaiac reagent to indicate the presence of blood. Developers are added to the combination of stool and guaiac to turn the test site an indicated color. Laboratory quality control monitors are supplied on each test pack. Read the package inserts to be familiar with the procedure. Store packs, reagents, and developers properly. Follow the directions for the exact amount of reagent or developer to add and the specific period of time to elapse before reading the results (Fig. 18-11).

Avoid having the patient collect a specimen during menses or when there is obvious rectal bleeding. Patients usually are cautioned to avoid certain foods or medications that may interfere with testing. Red meat and certain vegetables and fruits (especially those high in vitamin C) interfere with test results. Aspirin and NSAIDs usually are avoided for a week before testing.

The physician may perform a quick test during a routine physical examination (Box 18-4), or the patient may take the test kit home to perform the more extensive testing and bring in or mail the completed pack (Procedure 18-3).

text continues on page 423

Box 18-4
Simple Screening for Occult Blood

The simplest methods used to screen for occult blood are either the test tape or the specimen card. These methods are commonly used by the physician during a routine physical examination. A test card is used, or a measure of tape is removed from the dispenser and held by the gloved medical assistant. After the physician has completed the digital rectal examination with the gloved hand, the gloved finger is swiped across the tape or the test area of the card to make a smear of the contents of the rectal canal. Developer is dropped onto the specified test area, and the results are read within a specified time frame, usually about 60 seconds. These methods are considered to be screening tools and must be followed up with more extensive testing if the test is positive.

Negative Smears*

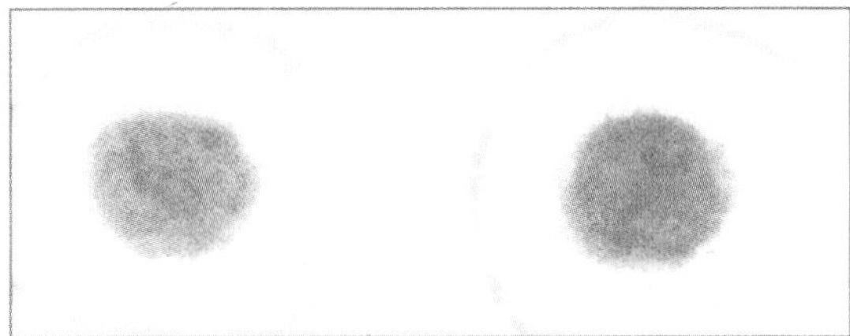

Negative and Positive Smears*

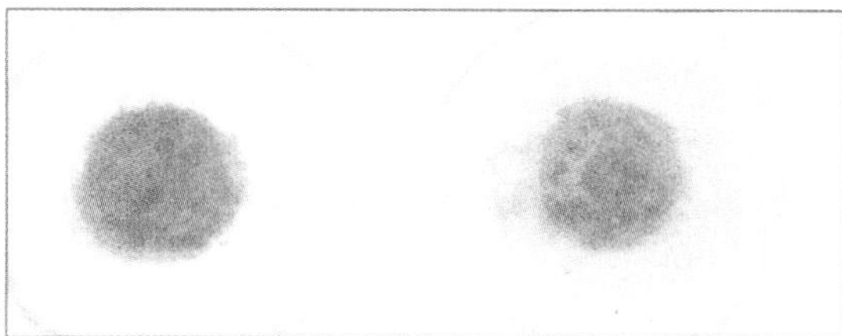

Positive Smears*

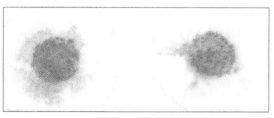

Figure 18-11 Test results for fecal occult blood using the Hemoccult routine screening test. Two samples from the specimen are included on each slide. No detectable blue on or at the edge of the smears indicates the test is negative for occult blood. Any trace of blue on or at the edge of one or more of the smears indicates the test is positive for occult blood. (Courtesy of Beckman Coulter, Inc.)

18

Procedure 18-1 Preparing the Patient for Colon Procedures

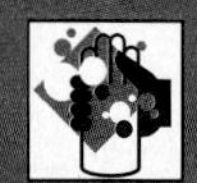
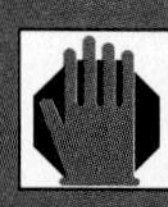
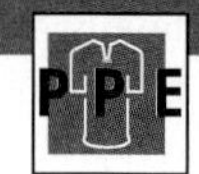

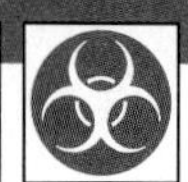

18

PURPOSE

To ensure proper testing and diagnostic results with a minimum of patient discomfort

EQUIPMENT/SUPPLIES

- appropriate instrument (flexible or rigid sigmoidoscope, anoscope, or proctoscope)
- water-soluble lubricant
- fenestrated drape or gown
- cotton swabs
- suction source (if not part of the scope)
- biopsy forceps
- specimen container with preservative
- completed laboratory requests
- personal wipes
- equipment for assessing vital signs

STEPS

1. Wash your hands.
2. Assemble the equipment.
3. Check the illumination of the light source. Turn off the power to avoid a buildup of heat.

   This ensures that all equipment is in proper working condition.
4. Greet and identify the patient. Explain the procedure. The patient will feel pressure and may have the urge to defecate. Tell the patient that the pressure is from the instrument and that the feeling will ease. The patient also may experience gas pressure when air is insufflated. *Note:* Some patients are ordered a mild sedative before the procedure.
5. Instruct the patient to empty the bladder.

   Pressure from the instrument may injure a full bladder. Urine in the bladder may increase discomfort.
6. Assess the vital signs and record.

   Colon examination procedures may cause cardiac arrhythmias and a change in blood pressure in some patients. Baseline vital signs allow you to detect variations from the patient's normal signs.
7. Have the patient undress from the waist down or undress completely and put on a gown.
8. Assist the patient onto the table. If the instrument of choice is an anoscope or a fiberoptic device, Sims' position or a left-lying position is most comfortable for the patient. If a rigid instrument is used, the patient will assume a knee-chest position or be placed on a proctologic table that supports the patient in a knee-chest position. *Note:* Do not ask the patient to assume the knee-chest position until the physician is ready to begin. The position is difficult to maintain, and the patient may become faint.

   The suggested positions reposition the abdominal contents into the abdominal cavity rather than the pelvis to facilitate the procedure.
9. When the patient is in position, drape properly. A fenestrated drape usually is used.
10. Continually monitor the patient's response and offer reassurance during the examination. Instruct the patient to breathe slowly through pursed lips to aid in relaxation.
11. Assist the physician as needed with lubricants, instruments, power sources, swabs, biopsy equipment, and specimen containers. Glove before receiving biohazardous specimens.
12. Following the procedure, assist the patient into a comfortable position and allow a rest period. Offer personal cleaning wipes, and assist with cleaning as needed. Monitor the vital signs before allowing the patient to stand. Assist the patient from the table, and remain close at hand to avoid falls.

    A drop in blood pressure on standing is common after any of these procedures and may cause fainting.
13. Have the patient dress.
14. Clean the room. Route the specimens to the proper laboratory. Clean or dispose of the supplies and equipment as appropriate, and wash your hands.

continued

Procedure 18-1 Continued Preparing the Patient for Colon Procedures

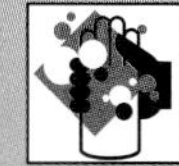
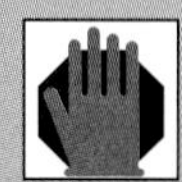
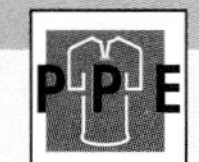

DOCUMENTATION GUIDELINES

- Date and time
- Colon preparation and adherence to protocol
- Patient complaints/concerns
- Patient education/instructions
- Your signature

Charting Example

DATE	TIME Pt scheduled for colonoscopy;
	states he followed bowel prep protocol as
	outlined in pt ed brochure and instruc-
	tions. P-100 regular, BP-120/86.
	Pt instructed to empty bladder and put
	on pt gown. Pt assisted into position on
	exam table. Colon exam by Dr. Jacobs.
	Pt tolerated procedure well, d/c by
	Dr. Jacobs. —Your signature

Procedure 18-2 Collecting a Stool Specimen

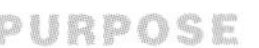
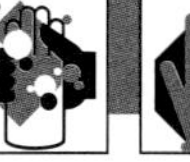
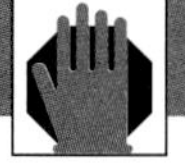
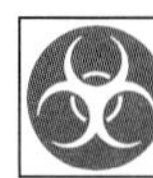

PURPOSE

To determine the presence and type of abnormal constituents in the feces or gastrointestinal tract

EQUIPMENT/SUPPLIES

- stool specimen container (usually waxed cardboard or plastic to avoid the transfer of pathogens through a moist container)
- wooden spatula or tongue blade
- bedpan with cover or toilet collection container (popularly called a "nun's cap" or "Mexican hat") with cover
- personal wipes for the patient

STEPS

1. Wash your hands.
2. Assemble the equipment.
3. Greet and identify the patient. Explain the procedure. Tell the patient to defecate in the bedpan or toilet collection container, not the toilet. The patient must void separately. Make sure the patient discards toilet tissue in the toilet and not in the bedpan or collection container.

   Water, urine, or toilet tissue mixed with the stool may interfere with test results.
4. Put on gloves, and obtain the bedpan or collection container from the patient.

   Standard Precautions must be followed when handling stool.
5. Using a tongue blade or wooden spatula, remove small portions of the stool from the bedpan or collection container. Take the specimens from the first and final portions of the stool. Transfer the stool to the specimen container. Do not allow feces to soil the outer surface of the specimen container.

   The first and last portions of the stool usually contain concentrations of the substances most often required for testing.

continued

Procedure 18-2 *Continued* Collecting a Stool Specimen

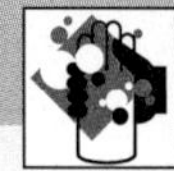
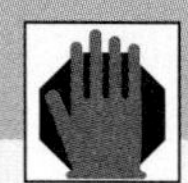

6. Discard the supplies in biohazard containers, and flush the remaining stool.
7. Cap the specimen quickly and tightly.
   This prevents loss of moisture, which may alter the results.
8. Assist the patient with cleaning the rectal area. Have the patient wash his or her hands.
   This provides comfort and promotes infection control.
9. Clean, disinfect, and store or properly dispose of the bedpan or collection container. Remove gloves and wash hands after handling the specimen and supplies.
10. Label the specimen, and attach the laboratory requests.
11. Store the specimen as directed. Some require refrigeration, others are kept at room temperature, and some must be incubated. Check the office policy and procedure manual for recommendations for storage and routing of all specimens.

18

DOCUMENTATION GUIDELINES

- Date and time
- Collection of specimen and time received (if to be routed)
- Description of specimen as needed
- Routing of specimen
- Occult blood test results if done prior to routing specimen
- Your signature

(Note: See Procedure 18-3 for charting example.)

Procedure 18-3 Testing for Occult Blood

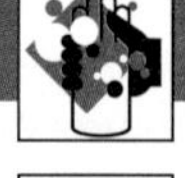
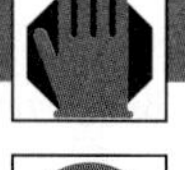
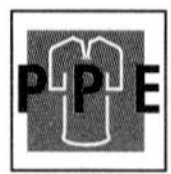
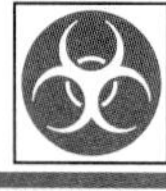

PURPOSE

To determine the presence of abnormal amounts of red blood cells in the gastrointestinal tract

EQUIPMENT/SUPPLIES

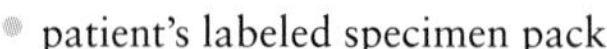

- patient's labeled specimen pack
- developers or reagents

STEPS

1. Wash hands and put on gloves before receiving the specimen.
2. Identify the patient pack or the specimen from the physician. Depending on the testing method, the specimen may be tested as quickly as 3 to 5 minutes after collection or up to 14 days later if properly stored.
3. Open the window on the back of the pack, and apply the testing reagent or developer.

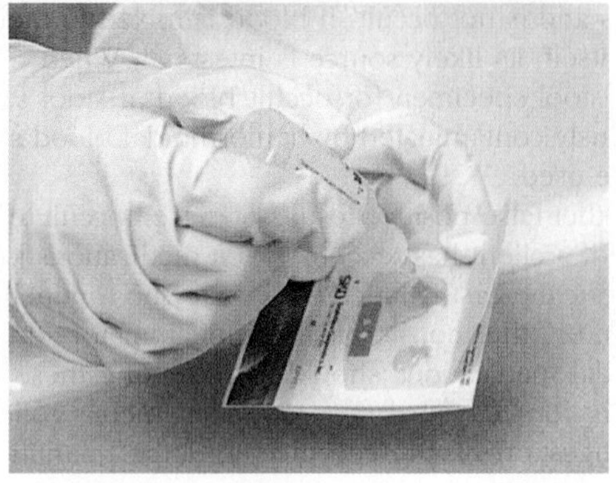

4. Read the color change in the specified time frame, usually 60 seconds.
   This ensures accurate results.

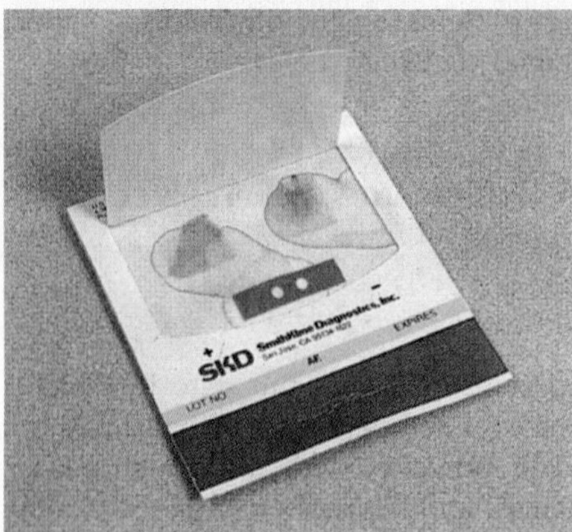

5. Apply developers as directed onto the control monitor section of the pack. Wait the specified time.
   Running a control confirms testing accuracy.
6. Properly dispose of the pack, gloves, and supplies. Wash your hands.

continued

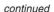

Procedure 18-3 Continued Testing for Occult Blood

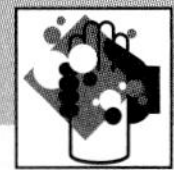
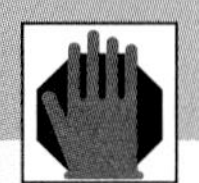
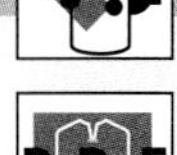

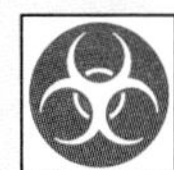

DOCUMENTATION GUIDELINES

- Date and time
- Testing results
- Notification of physician
- Patient complaints/concerns
- Patient education/instructions
- Your signature

Charting Example

6-13-99	1030 Pt given Hemoccult container with
	instructions re: diet and collection
	procedures.
6-19-99	930 Pt returned with Hemoccult test
	pack. Guaiac positive. Dr. Franklin notified
	of test results. —Your signature

18

Answers to Checkpoint Questions

1. *Peristalsis is rhythmic waves of smooth muscle contractions that move food through the GI tract. The motion helps break the food bolus into pieces and mix it with digestive enzymes to accelerate digestion.*
2. *Mastication is the process of chewing. Deglutition is the process of swallowing.*
3. *The small intestine is divided into the duodenum, jejunum, and ileum. Most of the digestion occurs in the duodenum by the action of the bile and pancreatic enzymes. Absorption occurs further into the jejunum and ileum.*
4. *The liver is responsible for glucose and glycogen metabolism and storage; breakdown of amino acids; manufacture and metabolism of protein, fats, and carbohydrates; storage of vitamins and minerals; destruction of old red blood cells; manufacture of bile; and removal of toxins.*
5. *Four common mouth disorders are caries, stomatitis, gingivitis, and oral cancer.*
6. *A hiatal hernia is caused by a defect in the diaphragm that lets part of the stomach slide up into the chest cavity. The stomach's cardiac sphincter and the diaphragmatic muscle tone normally prevent gastric acid reflux into the esophagus. Hiatal hernia permits the stomach acid to invade the esophagus, causing irritation.*
7. *Because the lining of the duodenum cannot tolerate concentrated gastric juices, ulcers form when food material containing excessive gastric acid passes through the pylorus.*
8. *Crohn's disease can lead to bowel obstruction. With each episode of inflammation, the scarring that occurs may lead to narrowing of the colon, which may cause an obstruction.*
9. *Gas is produced from the bacterial decomposition of proteins during digestion.*
10. *Viral hepatitis is caused by a virus; toxic hepatitis results from toxic reactions to chemical toxicants, certain medications, or alcohol.*
11. *Cholelithiasis is the formation of stones in the gallbladder. It occurs when slowed peristalsis allows bile to pool in the sac; fluid is absorbed and the solids are left to concentrate and solidify into stones.*
12. *Anoscopy involves the insertion of an instrument into the rectal canal for visualization of the anus and rectum and to obtain swabs for culture. Sigmoidoscopy involves visualization of the sigmoid colon using either a rigid or flexible sigmoidoscope.*

Critical Thinking Challenges

1. Review the patient preparations needed for an upper GI series and a barium enema. Create a patient education handout that includes:
   - A description of the procedure
   - A list of reasons for the procedure
   - Preparations required to ensure reliable test results

   (Hint: Refer to Chap. 24, Diagnostic Imaging.)
2. Trace a bolus of food through the GI tract. Describe the metabolic process occurring at each step. (Review Chap.

12, Assisting With Diagnostic and Therapeutic Procedures Associated With the Neurologic System.) How does the autonomic nervous system affect the process of digestion?

3. Many endoscopic examinations require the patient to be in an uncomfortable and embarrassing position. How can you help alleviate the stress and anxiety that a patient may experience?

18

Suggestions for Further Reading

Bates, B., Bickley, L. S., & Hockelman, R. A. (1995). *A Guide to Physical Examination and History Taking,* 6th ed. Philadelphia: Lippincott-Raven.

Bullock, B. L., & Rosendahl, P. P. (1996). *Pathophysiology,* 4th ed. Philadelphia: Lippincott-Raven.

Fischbach, F. (1996). *A Manual of Laboratory and Diagnostic Tests,* 5th ed. Philadelphia: Lippincott-Raven.

Fischbach, F. (1995). *Quick Reference for Common Laboratory and Diagnostic Tests.* Philadelphia: Lippincott-Raven.

Memmler, R. L., Cohen, B. J., & Wood, D. L. (1996). *The Human Body in Health and Disease,* 8th ed. Philadelphia: Lippincott-Raven.

Porth, C. M. (1998). *Pathophysiology: Concepts of Altered Health States,* 5th ed. Philadelphia: Lippincott-Raven.

Professional Guide to Diseases, 4th ed. (1992). Springhouse, PA: Springhouse.

Smeltzer, S. C., & Bare, B. G. (1996). *Brunner and Suddarth's Textbook of Medical and Surgical Nursing,* 8th ed. Philadelphia: Lippincott-Raven.

Timby, B. K., & Lewis, L. W. (1996). *Fundamental Skills and Concepts in Patient Care,* 6th ed. Philadelphia: Lippincott-Raven.

19

Assisting With Diagnostic and Therapeutic Procedures Associated With the Urinary System

Chapter Outline

Role Delineation

CLINICAL

Fundamental Principles

- Apply principles of aseptic technique and infection control.

Patient Care

- Prepare patients for examinations, procedures, and treatments.
- Assist with examinations, procedures, and treatments.

GENERAL

Professionalism

- Project a professional manner and image.

Communication Skills

- Treat all patients with compassion and empathy.

Legal Concepts

- Practice within the scope of education, training, and personal capabilities.

Instruction

- Teach methods of health promotion and disease prevention.

Chapter Competencies

Learning Objectives

Upon successfully completing this chapter, you will be able to:

1. Spell and define the Key Terms.
2. List and describe the primary functions of the urinary system.
3. Label a diagram of the organs of the urinary system.
4. Describe the gross and microscopic anatomy of the kidney.
5. Differentiate between the structures within a nephron, and give the functions of each.
6. Identify and describe the functions of the organs of the urinary system below the level of the kidney.
7. Describe the way that wastes are formed and transported to the urinary system.
8. Name other systems involved in the excretion of wastes and the types of wastes usually managed by those systems.
9. Trace a drop of liquid waste in the bloodstream through the urinary system to its eventual elimination as urine.
10. List and describe disorders of the urinary system.
11. Identify and explain diagnostic procedures of the urinary system and the medical assistant's responsibilities.

Key Terms

(See Glossary for definitions.)

angiotensin
anuria
blood urea nitrogen (BUN)
calyces (singular, calyx)
catheterization
convoluted tubules
cystoscopy
dialysis
enuresis
erythropoietin
filtration
glomerulus
hematuria
incontinence
intravenous pyelogram (IVP)
lithotripsy
loop of Henle
micturition
nephron
nephrostomy
nitrogenous
nocturia
oliguria
pH
proteinuria
pyuria
renal cortex
renal medulla
renal pelvis
renal pyramids
renin
retrograde pyelogram
retroperitoneal
specific gravity
staghorn
trigone
urea
uremic frost
ureterostomy
ureters
urethra
uric acid
urinalysis

Nutrients and substances required for metabolism create waste products that must be eliminated from the body. Several systems are responsible for helping to prevent a buildup of these end-products of metabolism. Solid waste, water, bile, and some salts are eliminated by the gastrointestinal system. Products of respiration, such as carbon dioxide and water, are excreted by the respiratory system. Even the integumentary system is responsible for its share of excretion of water, salts, and some nitrogen in the form of perspiration. The body rids itself of most liquid wastes by way of the urinary system. The urinary system also aids the regulation of fluid volume, electrolytes, red blood cell production, blood pressure, and **pH** (acid–base) balance.

STRUCTURE AND FUNCTION OF THE URINARY SYSTEM

The urinary system consists of six distinct organs: two kidneys, two **ureters,** the bladder, and the **urethra** (Fig. 19-1). The kidneys remove the products of cellular metabolism from the bloodstream and aid in homeostasis. The ureters are a pair of tubes that transport the urine from the kidneys. The bladder is a hollow sac that holds the urine until **micturition** (voiding or urination). The urethra is a tube that transports the urine to the outside of the body.

The urinary system is involved in multiple functions to maintain the homeostasis of the body. In cooperation with chemoreceptors throughout the body, various functions turn on and off as indicated by rising and falling levels of those substances necessary for the maintenance of life.

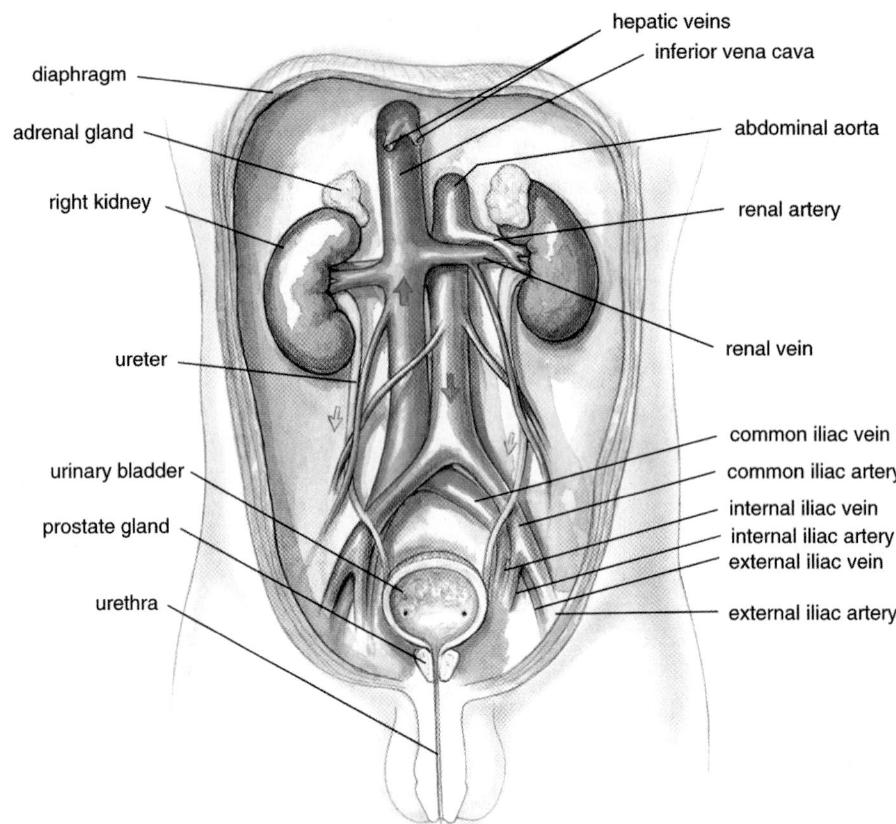

Figure 19-1 Urinary system, with blood vessels.

Formation and Transportation of Metabolic Wastes

As the body uses the available nutrients for metabolism, wastes accumulate at the cellular level. Initially, the breakdown of amino acids, the building blocks of protein, yields ammonia, which is then converted to **urea,** the final product of protein metabolism. In addition, the breakdown of nucleic acids, found in all cells, is somewhat similar to urea and is excreted by the urinary system as **uric acid,** also a by-product of protein metabolism. Creatinine, a by-product of the catabolism of creatine in muscle activity, is the third major waste product eliminated by the urinary system.

These wastes are filtered from the blood by the liver and are transported to the kidney by the renal arteries, which are short branches of the abdominal aorta. The cleansed blood leaves the kidney by way of small vessels that connect with the renal vein, which empties into the vena cava for recirculation through the bloodstream.

Excretion of Wastes

The capillary system of the kidney is specially designed to retain or reabsorb substances needed for normal blood levels and to eliminate substances in abundance or no longer needed. As these levels fluctuate, the kidneys receive signals to excrete more or less of these substances as indicated. Waste products are generally small enough to fit between the walls of the renal capillary cells. They are squeezed out to be filtered into the waste water that will become urine. Protein, fats, blood cells, and other components coursing through the kidneys are generally too large to fit between the walls of the capillaries unless there is an imbalance of these substances or an impairment of the **filtration** system. (Filtration involves removal of particles from a solution by passing the solution through a membrane.) Some toxins and expendable salts are also excreted by the kidneys. Metallic salts, such as lead and mercury, can be detected in the urine in cases of poisoning.

Checkpoint Question

1. *What main products of metabolism are filtered by the kidneys?*

Maintaining Fluid Balance

When the volume of blood decreases because of fluid loss or inadequate fluid intake, levels of dissolved salts in the blood increase, causing a change in the osmotic pressure of the blood. Chemoreceptors in the brain and several large vessels signal the posterior lobe of the pituitary to release antidiuretic hormone (ADH). ADH in turn passes the signal to the distal **convoluted tubules** (the twisted portion of the nephron connecting the glomerulus to the collecting tubules) and collecting ducts of the kidneys to allow more water to be reabsorbed into the bloodstream, thereby increasing the fluid level of the blood. Conversely, when too much fluid is circulating, blood becomes diluted, causing sensors in the brain and large vessels to decrease the ADH levels, reducing the amount of water reabsorbed by the filtering system so that urine production is increased and fluid balance is restored.

Regulation of pH Balance

Cell metabolism produces acids that must be excreted by the body to maintain a fairly constant blood pH of about 7.4. The ingestion of bases, such as too many antacids, will alter the pH of the blood. If the sensitive monitoring devices throughout the body detect levels of acid that are becoming dangerously high, extra hydrogen ions are combined with either ammonia or phosphates in the distal tubules to be excreted in the urine. If these sensors detect acid levels too low and base levels too high, the distal tubules hold back hydrogen ions to increase the blood acid level to normal limits.

Maintenance of Blood Pressure

When oxygen levels in the kidney are low because of a decrease in blood pressure that slows blood flow to the vessels of the kidneys, the enzyme **renin** is released by the kidney tissues to activate the production of **angiotensin,** a powerful vasoconstrictor. Vasoconstriction causes blood pressure to rise, which in turn signals the adrenal cortex to release aldosterone to retain the sodium and water flowing through the kidney. This increases the blood volume and raises the blood pressure to increase the blood and oxygen flow through the sensors in the kidneys. When the kidneys are satisfied by the increase in oxygen levels, the whole process is reversed.

Production of Erythropoietin

If oxygen levels are low because of decreased production of oxygen-bearing red blood cells rather than decreased blood pressure, the kidneys release the hormone **erythropoietin** to act on the red bone marrow to increase the production of red blood cells.

Metabolism and Retention of Calcium and Vitamin D

In conjunction with the parathyroid hormone, the kidneys regulate the blood levels of calcium. This is done by activating vitamin D molecules, which control the mechanism by which calcium is absorbed by the intestines.

Checkpoint Question

2. *How does the pituitary affect fluid balance?*

19

ORGANS OF THE URINARY SYSTEM

Kidneys

The kidneys excrete wastes and aid in the maintenance of homeostasis. They are located in the **retroperitoneal** area, near the back body wall at about thoracic 12 to lumbar 3. They are just below the diaphragm and are protected by the lower rib cage. The left kidney is slightly higher than the right because of the position of the liver. Encased in a capsule of renal fat, the kidneys are held in position by renal fascia. They are reddish brown, bean-shaped, fist-sized, and approximately 4 inches by 2 inches by 1 inch. The inner curve has a notch called the hilus where nerves and the blood and lymph vessels enter and exit and the renal pelves (singular, pelvis) are attached. An adrenal gland covers the top of each kidney (see Fig. 19-1).

The kidneys are surrounded by heavy fibrous connective tissue called the renal capsule. There is an outer **renal cortex** and an inner **renal medulla.** The renal cortex is the shell that surrounds the medulla and is made up of the microscopic **nephron** units that do most of the work for the kidney (see the section "Nephrons," below). The renal medulla contains the conical structures, called **renal pyramids,** that collect the urine from the nephrons for transport to the **renal pelvis** (Fig. 19-2).

The renal pelvis is a funnel-shaped collecting basin formed from a dozen or more minor calyces embedded in the medulla. The minor **calyces** (cuplike collecting structures) empty into several major calyces (singular, calyx). The distal end of the renal pelvis is continuous with its ureter.

Nephrons

Each kidney is composed of about one million nephrons (Fig. 19-3), each consisting of a renal corpuscle and a renal tubule. The renal corpuscle is made up of a twisted mass of capillaries, called the **glomerulus,**

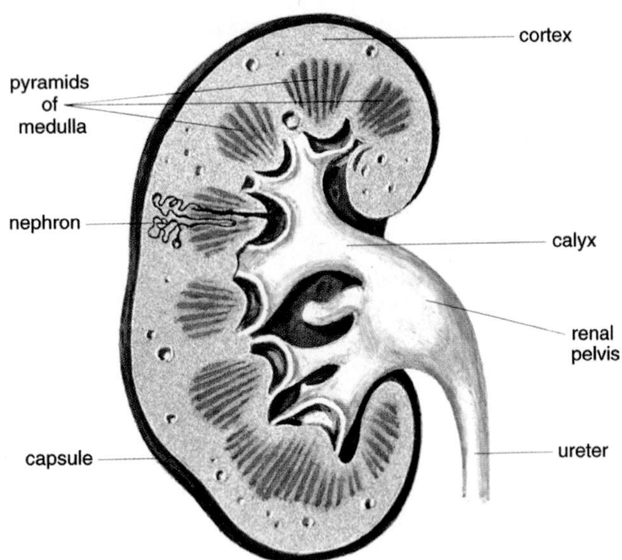

Figure 19-2 Longitudinal section through the kidney showing its internal structure and a much enlarged diagram of a nephron. There are more than one million nephrons in each kidney.

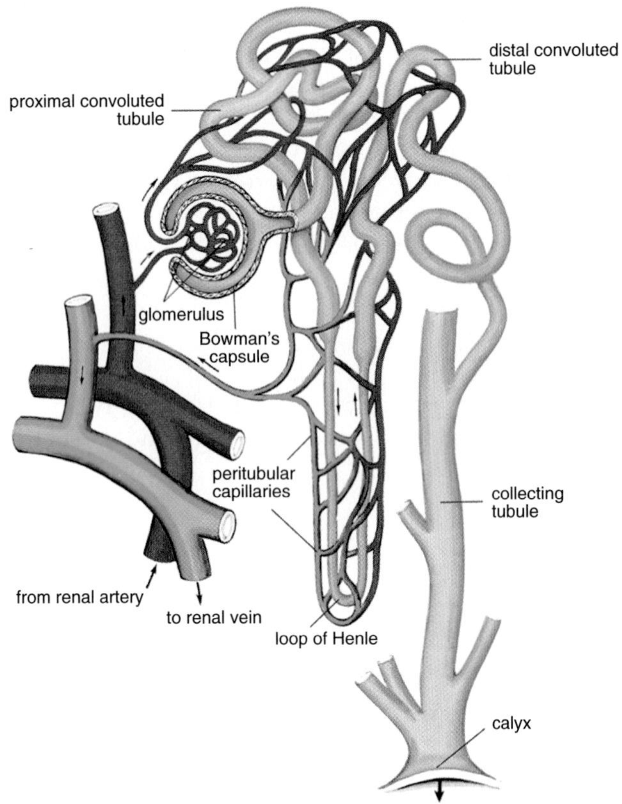

Figure 19-3 Simplified diagram of a nephron.

surrounded by a double-walled, funnel-shaped structure called Bowman's capsule. The renal tubule is an extension of Bowman's capsule that twists and turns on its way to transport the filtrate that will become urine.

The purpose of the nephron is to filter the blood through the glomerulus and produce a filtrate to be passed on to the renal tubule. As the body works to maintain its balance, substances needed for homeostasis are returned by reabsorption to the circulatory system by the mechanisms described above. Waste products and excess water are passed on to the collecting tubules and eliminated as urine.

Urine Formation

Blood is brought to the kidney by the renal arteries that arise from the abdominal aorta. In a 24-hour period, 160 to 180 L (about 45 gallons) of filtrate pass through the kidneys to become approximately 1 to 1.5 L (about 1–1.5 quarts) of urine. The rest of the filtrate returns to the circulation. About 25% of the cardiac output from each heartbeat goes to and through the kidneys. About every 4 minutes, all of the blood in the body is filtered by the kidneys and sent back to the heart as clean blood. Follow a drop of fluid as it becomes a drop of urine on the illustration of a nephron.

Blood enters the renal corpuscle, where filtration begins, by way of a wide-diameter renal arteriole. This initial vessel is called an afferent arteriole. Once within Bowman's capsule, the afferent arteriole branches to become the glomerulus, a dense network of capillaries, which are compressed by the walls of the surrounding chamber. The efferent arteriole exiting Bowman's capsule has a smaller diameter than the afferent, or entering, arteriole. This change in the exiting diameter and the small size of the glomerular capillaries raise the pressure within these capillaries. The backup of pressure forces the fluid from the blood through the capillary walls, rather like squeezing a sponge. Blood components are generally too large to pass between the capillary cells, but salts (such as electrolytes), glucose, and other small dissolved molecules are pressed out with the plasma.

From the collecting basin of Bowman's capsule, the filtrate begins a twisting, turning journey through the proximal convoluted tubule. This tubule eventually descends to become the **loop of Henle,** a much narrower and straighter tube. At this point, more plasma and wastes are pressed out to enter the tissue fluid around the nephron. By the process of filtration, some of this fluid that has been pressed out is reabsorbed by the distal convoluted tubule as it widens just past the loop of Henle and begins to twist and turn toward the collecting tubule. Some of the fluid is reabsorbed by the peritubular capillaries. These capillaries are extensions of the efferent arteriole that has been winding its way around the various portions of the tubular system and are most dense at the loop of Henle. The blood within the peritubular capillaries is very concentrated and absorbs much of the double-filtered fluid in the tissue surrounding the loop of Henle to dilute its components to a homeostatic level. These capillaries become renal venules that drain into the renal veins to take the filtered blood away from the kidney and back to general circulation.

If all of the checks and balances of the mechanisms that make up homeostasis are in place and the body does not require that the nephron reabsorb the filtrate, it makes its way through the collecting tubule to the minor calyx, the major calyx, the renal pelvis, the ureter, the bladder, and the urethra and is voided.

Checkpoint Question

3. *What is the glomerulus, and where is it located?*

Ureters

The ureters are two long, slender tubes reaching from the kidney basin, or renal pelvis, through the lower posterior portion of the bladder (see Fig. 19-1). They are about 10 to 13 inches long and are lined with epithelial cells that are continuous with the kidney and the bladder. They contract rhythmically with peristalsis triggered by the presence of urine in the renal pelvis. The entry of the ureters into the bladder at its posterior and inferior surface is covered by flaplike folds of mucous membrane, which act as valves to prevent reflux when the bladder is full.

Urinary Bladder

The bladder is a temporary urine storage and collecting sac below the parietal peritoneum and behind the pubis (see Fig. 19-1). When it is full, it may rise above the pubis into the abdominal cavity. It is highly expandable, although the urge to urinate is usually felt when it contains about 5 ounces. Discomfort is usually triggered when it contains about 10 ounces.

The inner layer is mucous membrane, which becomes rugae when the bladder is empty. The outer layers are very elastic and are interlaced in many directions.

The inferior and posterior portion of the bladder, in an area formed as a triangle by the openings of the ureters and the urethra, is called the **trigone.** This area does not expand when the bladder is filled.

Urethra

The urethra is a tube that reaches from the bladder to the outside of the body (see Fig. 19-1). In the female, the tube is about 1½ inches long. It passes anteriorly from the bladder, behind the symphysis pubis, and terminates between the labia minora, anterior to the vaginal meatus and posterior to the clitoris. In the male, the urethra is part of both the urinary and reproductive systems. It is about 8 inches long and is S shaped. It passes from the bladder through the prostate gland just below the bladder and is joined by various ducts arising from the reproductive system. The urethra exits at the tip of the penis.

Checkpoint Question

4. *Explain the difference between the ureters and the urethra.*

THE VOIDING REFLEX

When the bladder begins to fill with urine, stretch receptors transmit the signal to the sacral section of the spinal cord, which releases the internal sphincter at the base of the bladder. If timing is not appropriate, it is possible to override the impulse to void by inhibiting the external sphincter through control by nerve centers in the cerebral cortex and midbrain. The urge to void will subside and return in waves. If the timing is right to void, the parasympathetic nervous system takes control and releases the external sphincter. The bladder muscles begin to contract, and urine is expelled.

COMMON URINARY DISORDERS

Renal Failure

Renal failure is a sudden drop in kidney function manifested by inability of the kidney to excrete wastes, concentrate urine, and aid in homeostatic electrolyte conservation.

In acute renal failure, there will be **oliguria** (scant urine formation) and a corresponding rise in **nitrogenous** (nitrogen-containing) wastes in the blood, dehydration, and an electrolyte imbalance. Causes include a grave loss of fluid due to burns or hemorrhage, trauma, toxic injury to the kidney (as in nephrotoxic drugs or poisons), acute pyelonephritis or glomerulonephritis, or an obstruction beyond the level of the collecting tubules.

Chronic renal failure is a gradual loss of the nephrons with a corresponding inability of the kidney to complete its functions. It may result from other disease processes, such as lupus erythematosus, diabetes, radiation, or renal tuberculosis. There will be general weakness, edema of the lungs and the tissues in general, and neurologic symptoms, such as clouding or dullness progressing to seizures and coma. If **dialysis** (removal of urine wastes) is not performed, the patient will likely exhibit pale or white crystals on the skin called **uremic frost.** This is formed by the urea and waste products as they exit the skin.

Treatment for both acute and chronic renal failure may involve dialysis (Box 19-1). Chronic failure frequently involves other systems as well as the urinary system and requires treatment to reflect the level of involvement.

Box 19-1
Renal Dialysis

Patients whose kidneys are not functioning need the assistance of dialysis to remove nitrogenous waste products and excess fluid from the body. Dialysis dependence may be short term in acute illness or long term in end-stage renal disease (ESRD). In the absence of functional nephrons, wastes must be filtered through membranes other than those in the renal tissues. Two methods are currently used for dialysis. These are hemodialysis and peritoneal dialysis.

Hemodialysis

Toxins are removed from the blood by routing the patient's blood through a dialysis machine containing synthetic filters and a dialysate (a substance used to balance the electrolyte concentration in the blood). The machine can be regulated to remove or retain substances as needed for the individual patient.

The patient's circulatory system must be accessed as many as three times a week for 3–4 hours. Therefore, most patients receive a surgically created fistula (an opening or passage) or a graft between an artery and a vein to make entry easier for the patient.

Hemodialysis is confining and life changing. Maintaining employment is difficult. Many complications, such as nausea and vomiting, chest pains, cramping, seizures, and air embolus, are possible with hemodialysis.

Peritoneal Dialysis

The peritoneal membranes can also be used to filter wastes. An appropriately balanced dialysate is administered through a catheter into the abdominal cavity, then after a period of time allowed to flow out into a collecting bag, bringing with it the wastes and excess fluid that must be removed. Patients who have had extensive abdominal surgery with disruption of the peritoneal membranes are not good candidates for peritoneal dialysis. Systemic inflammatory disease and immunosuppression are also contraindications for this method.

Peritoneal dialysis allows the patient the freedom to move about and continue a more normal life-style than hemodialysis. However, the presence of an abdominal catheter may result in an altered body image, leading to depression. The access to the peritoneal cavity as a source of infection is always a consideration.

Neither of these methods is a cure for the underlying renal dysfunction but both can prolong life almost indefinitely if properly performed.

Glomerulonephritis

Glomerulonephritis is an inflammation of the glomerulus of the kidney. Symptoms range from very mild edema, **proteinuria, hematuria,** and oliguria to complete renal failure. It may be seen in children several weeks after a streptococcal infection as the strep antibodies attack and injure the glomeruli. It may be chronic in adults with scarring and hardening of the glomeruli and eventual renal failure. Symptoms of the chronic form include proteinuria (excessive protein in the urine), casts in the urine, and hematuria (bloody urine). Treatment is usually symptomatic. If bacterial infection is involved, antibiotics will be prescribed.

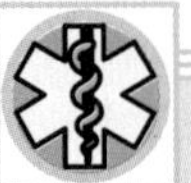

Action **STAT!**

Kidney Stones

Scenario: Mrs. Hood arrives at the clinic complaining of severe flank pain and blood in her urine. You escort her into an examining room and help her to change into a gown. She begins vomiting and appears very uncomfortable. She tells you that she thinks she has a "kidney stone." What should you do?

1. Assist Mrs. Hood onto the examination table, put on examining gloves, and give her an emesis basin.
2. Notify the physician.
3. Check Mrs. Hood's vital signs, and assist her to the recovery position to prevent aspiration of vomitus if she begins vomiting again.
4. Assist the physician in administering any medications for pain or for vomiting.
5. Monitor Mrs. Hood's blood pressure and pulse carefully. Be aware that she may experience severe pain with kidney stones and may require admission into the emergency department for hydration and pain management.
6. Document the incident, and assist with the transfer into the ambulance if necessary.
7. Remove vomitus not contained in the emesis basin. Put on gloves, flood the area with liquid absorbing gel, then remove as much of the liquid and gel as possible with paper towels. Dispose of the towels in a biohazard bag. When you have removed all of the visible vomitus, flood the area with a 1:10 bleach solution, and wipe the area again with paper towels. Discard these in the biohazard bag. Remove your gloves, discard them properly, and wash your hands.

Calculi

Calculi are stonelike formations. These may be found anywhere in the urinary system and may range from a sandlike consistency to **staghorn** structures that fill the renal pelvis and assume the shape of the calyces, or huge stones that fill the bladder. Stones seem more likely to form if the urine is alkaline; acidity frequently discourages this formation. Symptoms vary with the size and location of the stone. Hematuria may be present if the rough edges abrade the mucous membrane of the system. The patient will have flank pain if the stone lodges in a ureter.

Treatment may not be needed if the stones are small enough to flush with increased fluid intake. Large stones may require surgery or **lithotripsy** (crushing the stone in situ, usually using ultrasound). In either case, the chemistry of the stones will need to be evaluated for the forming components, and the patient's diet will need to be adjusted to prevent recurrence.

Checkpoint Question

5. *What are calculi, and when are they more likely to form?*

Pyelonephritis

Pyelonephritis is an inflammation of the renal pelvis and the body of the kidney. It usually results from an infection ascending the ureters and may be acute or chronic. Symptoms include those of any infection, such as chills and fever, nausea, and vomiting but with the addition of flank pain and **pyuria** (pus in the urine).

Medication to acidify the urine, making the system less hospitable to bacteria, may be the treatment of choice. In addition, antibiotics may also be prescribed.

Hydronephrosis

Hydronephrosis is a distention of the renal pelvis and calyces from an obstruction that causes a backup of urine. The symptoms include flank pain, hematuria, pyuria, fever, and chills.

To restore the flow of urine, the stricture must be removed. If it is not possible to restore the flow to the bladder, it may be necessary to perform a **nephrostomy** (opening into the kidney) or **ureterostomy** (opening into a ureter).

Cystitis

Cystitis is inflammation of the bladder. Because of the short length of the urethra, cystitis is far more common in women than in men. Symptoms begin with frequency, dysuria, and urgency and progress to chills, fever, nausea and vomiting, and flank pain.

Identification of the organism will precede the decision for treatment, which usually involves antibiotics. Educating the patient about personal hygiene is also important to prevent recurrence.

Urethritis

Urethritis is inflammation of the urethra. This may be a prelude to simple cystitis, or it may be symptomatic of a sexually transmitted disease, such as gonorrhea or nongonococcal urethritis. The treatment for cystitis, noted above, is also effective for urethritis.

19

What If?

What if a mother brings her 5-year-old daughter to the office with complaints of burning on urination? What questions might you ask? How might you educate the mother and child?

First, ask if the child urinates when she feels the urge or if she holds her urine for long periods. Some young girls are inclined to hold their urine long past the time to void, setting up a perfect situation for bacterial growth. Caution the child to void when the need arises, making sure to use terms she can understand. Next, ask the mother if she uses bubble bath in the child's bath water. Young girls have a very short urethra and are prone to urethritis if they bathe in water with certain types of bubble bath. Finally, explain that the child must learn to wipe from front to back when cleaning herself to avoid urinary tract infections.

Tumors

The urinary system may be the primary or the secondary site for tumors. Tumors are more common in the bladder but may also occur in the kidney. Symptoms will vary but usually include hematuria and an unexplained abdominal mass. Treatment, which will be dictated by the extent and type of tumor, may include surgery, chemotherapy, radiation, or a combination of these.

Table 19-1 summarizes the symptoms of urinary tract disorders and their possible causes.

Checkpoint Question

6. *Why are women more likely than men to experience cystitis?*

19

Table 19-1 **Symptoms of Urinary Tract Disorders and Possible Causes**

Symptom	*Possible Cause(s)*
Anuria (lack of urine production)	Renal failure, acute nephritis, metal poisoning (lead, mercury), complete obstruction of the urinary tract
Burning during voiding	Urethritis
Burning during and after voiding	Cystitis
Dribbling	Prostatic hypertrophy, infection, neurogenic bladder
Dysuria	Infection
Edema	Renal failure, nephrosis
Enuresis (bed wetting)	Normal to age 3; thereafter, functional or symptomatic of disease
Frequency	Infection, diabetes
Hematuria	Diseases of the glomeruli, trauma, neoplasms, calculi
Hesitancy	Prostatic hypertrophy
Incontinence (inability to control elimination)	Infections, uterine prolapse, nerve damage, neoplasms, senility, neurogenic bladder
Stress incontinence	Impaired sphincter control
Nocturia (voiding at night)	Infection, prostatic hypertrophy, pressure (eg, pregnancy), diabetes, inability to concentrate urine
Oliguria	Acute nephritis, heart disease, dehydration, inadequate intake, fever, obstructions, renal insufficiency, neoplasms
Polyuria	Diabetes mellitus, diabetes insipidus, neurologic diseases, diuretics, increased fluid intake
Proteinuria	Diseases of the glomeruli, infection, nephrotic syndrome, diseases of protein metabolism
Pyuria	Infection
Renal colic	Calculi
Urgency	Infection, diseases of the prostate

COMMON DIAGNOSTIC PROCEDURES AND THE MEDICAL ASSISTANT'S ROLE

Urine Tests

The single most important step in diagnosing urinary system diseases begins with the examination of the patient's urine, or **urinalysis.** This should be performed routinely on all patients but particularly on those presenting with urinary system symptoms. Tests should always be on fresh urine specimens and on the first morning specimen when a more concentrated specimen is needed. Tests performed on the obtained urine may involve a chemical evaluation, **specific gravity** (relative density), microscopic examination, and cultures. (See Chap. 28, Urinalysis, for more detailed information.)

If infection is suspected, it may be necessary to obtain either a clean-catch, midstream urine specimen or a specimen obtained through **catheterization,** which involves introducing a tube into the bladder to remove urine. The physician is more likely to choose the first procedure, rather than catheterization, because there is far less chance of introducing bladder infection, and no patient discomfort is involved. (Box 19-2 presents information about catheterization.) With proper precautions, there is little chance that surface contaminants will interfere with diagnostic procedures ordered for the urine. You may be responsible for collecting the urine in some cases. (See Chap. 28, Urinalysis, for the procedure for obtaining a clean-catch, midstream urine specimen.) However, the patient is generally instructed to do this in the restroom alone.

Blood Tests

Serum levels of uric acid, **blood urea nitrogen (BUN),** or creatinine may be indicated in some disease processes. It will likely be your responsibility to draw the blood and process it on site or direct it to the proper testing facility. (See Chap. 29, Phlebotomy, and Chap. 30, Hematology, for more information.)

Cystoscopy or Cystourethroscopy

Cystoscopy is direct visualization of the bladder and the urethra with a lighted instrument called a cystoscope. Cystoscopy allows the physician to diagnose many diseases common to the lower urinary tract. You may be responsible for providing preoperative instruction to the patient, as outlined by the physician. This will probably include instructing the patient to increase fluid intake preoperatively and postoperatively and alerting the patient to the probability of some hematuria. Be sure to caution patients to report gross hematuria. These procedures are usually done under local anesthesia but may require hospitalization and general anesthesia.

Intravenous Pyelogram (IVP)

An **intravenous pyelogram (IVP)** is an x-ray examination of the kidneys and urinary tract requiring the injection of a radiopaque dye into the circulatory system. The dye is filtered by the kidneys to enhance visualization of the renal structures. The patient is required to cleanse the bowels with a laxative the night before the test and to administer an enema the morning of the procedure to prevent the presence of feces from obscuring the film. The patient will be NPO (nothing by mouth) for at least 8 hours before the dye is injected to

Box 19-2
Principles of Catheterization

In most cases, catheterization is a last resort in the medical office. Even under the most aseptic conditions, the possibility of introducing infection into the urinary system exists. However, some patients require catheterization when there is no other alternative. For example, catheterization is required when:

- It is impossible to obtain a clean-catch, midstream specimen for urinalysis.
- Intake and output must be measured accurately (these patients usually will be hospitalized).
- Other methods of bladder retraining have failed and the patient is incontinent and in danger of decubiti formation (this may be avoided with good skin care).
- The residual urine must be measured.
- Medication must be instilled into the bladder.

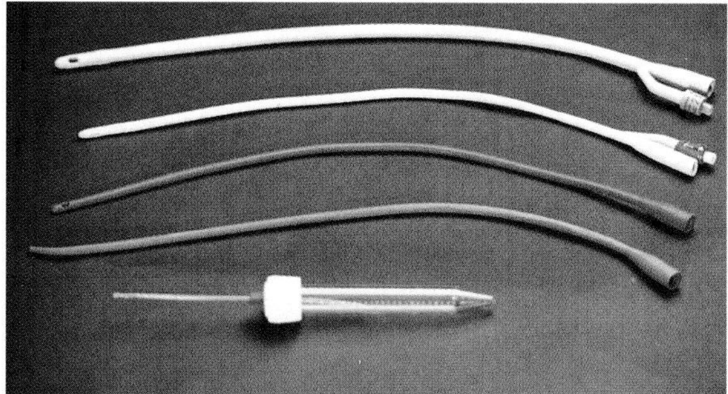

Types of catheters. From the top: #24 Foley catheter, #16 Foley catheter, #16 straight catheter, coudé catheter, self-contained catheterized specimen collection unit.

The catheter types and sizes vary. They may be plastic or rubber and occasionally metal or woven silk. The catheters may be straight, to use immediately and remove, or retention (usually called a Foley catheter) to inflate and leave in. The Foley catheter is a double-lumen tube with a second, smaller tube inside with a balloon near the tip to inflate to hold in place within the bladder.

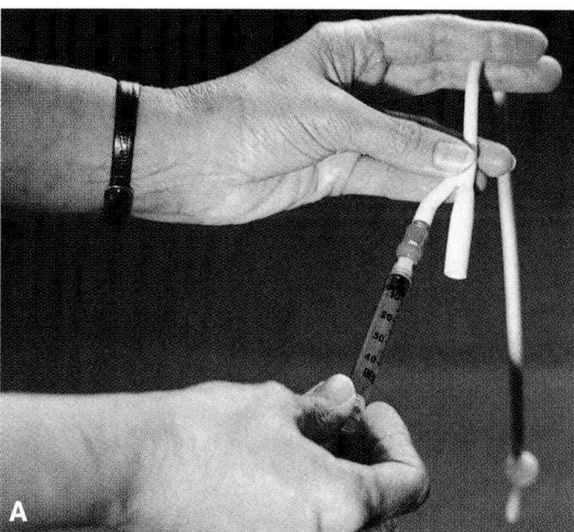

(A) Sterile water is inserted into the indicated lumen to inflate the balloon of the catheter.

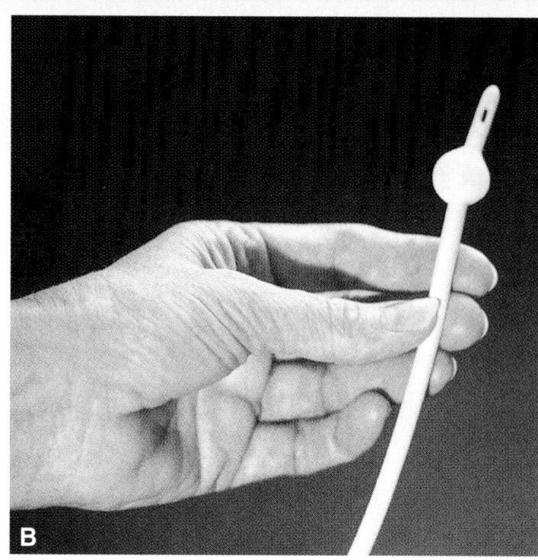

(B) When the balloon is inflated, the catheter will remain within the bladder.

If the patient has prostatic hypertrophy, the physician may use a coudé, which is slightly curved and a bit stiffer than the others mentioned, making it easier to advance beyond the obstructing prostate.

Catheters are sized from 8–10 for children and 14–20 for adults. Larger catheters are also available. Sterile disposable kits with a wide array of options are available; many contain everything needed to perform a successful catheterization. It will likely be the responsibility of the medical assistant to order these kits and to set them up for the physician before the procedure.

Some states do not allow medical assistants to perform urinary catheterization. If your state allows catheterization, you will need to observe catheterization several times before attempting it without supervision. You must be precepted by your physician for the first few times that you attempt to catheterize and thereafter must be authorized by the physician to perform the procedure.

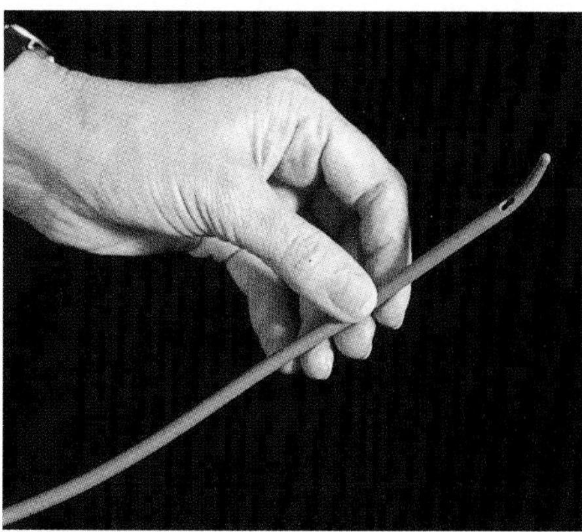

The coudé is firm and slightly curved for easier insertion past prostatic hypertrophy.

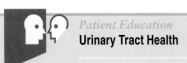

Patient Education

Urinary Tract Health

Frequently it will be your responsibility as the medical assistant to educate patients in everyday habits that will ensure good general health. Encourage patients presenting with urinary system symptoms to follow the suggestions below to avoid problems in the future.

FOR ALL PATIENTS

- Ensure adequate fluid intake, which helps remove waste products from the fluid compartments. There is wisdom in the "old wives' tale" advising 8 glasses of water a day. Tissues will be well hydrated, feces will be softer, and infections will be less likely in the lower urinary system.
- Empty your bladder when you feel the need. Urine held for periods beyond comfort causes bladder stress and irritation. Allowing urine to stagnate in the bladder increases the risk of infection.
- Keep in mind that cranberry juice and vitamin C help acidify the urine and make the urinary system less attractive to bacteria.

ESPECIALLY FOR WOMEN

- Avoid using perfumed products in the perineal area. The female urinary meatus is very short and prone to irritation. Urethral infections quickly become bladder infections without proper precautions.
- Avoid tight-fitting lower garments, especially nylon underwear. Loose-fitting cotton underwear absorbs moisture and allows for an air flow, making both bladder and vaginal infections less likely.
- Wipe carefully from front to back after using the toilet, particularly after defecating. Wash with soap and water and rinse well if infections are a recurrent problem.
- If you are prone to urinary tract infections, void immediately after intercourse to free the area of bacteria that might have intruded into the urethra. Avoid tub baths, particularly bubble baths; showers are less likely to contribute to infections.

19

increase the blood concentration and the visibility of the dye. The patient must be questioned closely about iodine allergies and may require a skin test for sensitivity. Fluids must be increased after the test to flush the dye and counteract dehydration from the preliminary cleansing.

Retrograde Pyelogram

A **retrograde pyelogram** is similar to the IVP except that dye is not injected intravenously but is introduced through a catheter inserted into the ureters through a cystoscope. This test is commonly used when the IVP procedure is contraindicated because of poor kidney function.

Ultrasound

Similar to other uses of ultrasound, this noninvasive use of sound waves will show the presence of stones and obstructions and the tissue involved. No special preparation is required other than explanation to the patient.

Checkpoint Question

7. *How does a retrograde pyelogram differ from an intravenous pyelogram?*

Answers to Checkpoint Questions

1. *The kidney filters urea, uric acid, and creatinine.*
2. *The pituitary secretes antidiuretic hormone (ADH), which helps regulate the amount of urine produced, thereby maintaining fluid balance.*
3. *The glomerulus is the twisted mass of capillaries located within Bowman's capsule.*
4. *The ureters are a pair of tubes that transport urine from the kidneys to the bladder. The urethra is a tube that transports urine from the bladder to outside the body.*
5. *Calculi are stonelike formations that are more likely to form when the urine is alkaline.*
6. *In women, the urethra is shorter, allowing more bacteria to reach the bladder. Also, the urethra is contained within the labia, a site that can harbor bacteria.*
7. *With a retrograde pyelogram, dye is introduced through a catheter inserted into the ureters, not injected intravenously.*

Critical Thinking Challenges

1. Analyze how a breakdown in any body system will affect the urinary system. What would happen if the liver failed? How would severe anemia, heart failure, or bone marrow suppression affect the kidney? Describe the effects.
2. What do you think has happened if the capillary walls allow the escape of large components, such as red blood cells, white blood cells, or protein? Justify your response.
3. What is a neutral pH? Why are ammonia and phosphates good transportation devices for hydrogen ions?
4. Differentiate between hemodialysis and peritoneal dialysis. Why are some patients poor risks for peritoneal dialysis?

Suggestions for Further Reading

Bullock, B. L., & Rosendahl, P. P. (1996). *Pathophysiology,* 4th ed. Philadelphia: Lippincott-Raven.

Craven, R. F., & Hirnle, C. J. (1996). *Fundamentals of Nursing: Human Health and Function,* 2nd ed. Philadelphia: Lippincott-Raven.

Memmler, R. L., Cohen, B. J., & Wood, D. L. (1996). *The Human Body in Health and Disease,* 8th ed. Philadelphia: Lippincott-Raven.

Porth, C. M. (1998). *Pathophysiology: Concepts of Altered Health States,* 5th ed. Philadelphia: Lippincott-Raven.

Professional Guide to Diseases, 4th ed. (1992). Springhouse, PA: Springhouse Corporation.

Smeltzer, S. C., & Bare, B. G. (1996). *Brunner and Suddarth's Textbook of Medical-Surgical Nursing,* 8th ed. Philadelphia: Lippincott-Raven.

Taylor, C., Lillis, C., & LeMone, P. (1997). *Fundamentals of Nursing: The Art and Science of Nursing Care,* 3rd ed. Philadelphia: Lippincott-Raven.

Timby, B. K., & Lewis, L. W. (1996). *Fundamental Skills and Concepts in Patient Care,* 6th ed. Philadelphia: Lippincott-Raven.

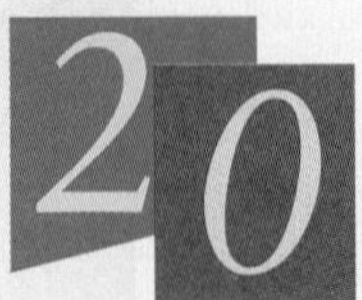

Assisting With Diagnostic and Therapeutic Procedures Associated With the Male Reproductive System

Chapter Outline

Evolution and Differentiation of the Male Reproductive System
Organs of the Male Reproductive System
- Testes
- Epididymis
- Vas Deferens
- Seminal Vesicles
- Prostate
- Cowper's Glands
- Penis
- Spermatozoa
- Composition of Semen

Common Disorders of the Male Reproductive System
- Prostatic Hypertrophy
- Hydrocele
- Cryptorchidism
- Inguinal Hernia
- Infections
- Impotence
- Sexually Transmitted Diseases
- Phimosis
- Infertility
- Testicular Cancer

Common Diagnostic Procedures and the Medical Assistant's Role
- Urinalysis
- Blood Work
- Cultures
- Rectal and Scrotal Examinations
- X-rays
- Cystoscopy

Preparing the Patient for Procedures
- Vasectomy

Role Delineation

CLINICAL

Fundamental Principles

- Apply principles of aseptic technique and infection control.

Patient Care

- Prepare patients for examinations, procedures, and treatments.
- Assist with examinations, procedures, and treatments.

GENERAL

Professionalism

- Project a professional manner and image.

Communication Skills

- Treat all patients with compassion and empathy.

Legal Concepts

- Practice within the scope of education, training, and personal capabilities.

Instruction

- Teach methods of health promotion and disease prevention.

Chapter Competencies

Learning Objectives

Upon successfully completing this chapter, you will be able to:

1. Spell and define the Key Terms.
2. State the purpose of the male reproductive system.
3. Explain how the male embryo differentiates from the female and how the union of the gametes determines the eventual gender.
4. Describe the descent of the male organs into the pelvic region and the scrotal sac.
5. Name and describe the organs of the male reproductive system.
6. Explain the function of each component of the system.
7. Trace the maturation process of a sperm cell from mitosis to ejaculation.
8. Describe a sperm cell.
9. List the components of semen, their approximate percentages, and their function in the fertilization process.
10. Name and describe common diseases of the male reproductive system, giving their symptoms and possible treatments.
11. List diagnostic procedures the medical assistant may encounter, and explain the responsibilities for proper preparation and completion.

Key Terms

(See Glossary for definitions.)

acrosome
Bartholin glands
chancre
circumcision
corpora cavernosa
corpus spongiosum
flagellum
fructose
gonads
impotence
interstitial
meiosis
monosaccharide
nocturia
phimosis
prepuce
prostate-specific antigen
psychogenic
smegma
truss
urinary frequency

Many lower life forms reproduce without a partner or a sexual contact. The cells simply divide, and the primary cell ceases to exist and instead becomes two daughter cells. Higher life forms require sexual reproduction with specialized cells from both parents to perpetuate the characteristics of each in the offspring. The male contributes the spermatozoon and the female contributes the ovum; both are called gametes. These combine to become a zygote, a fertilized egg.

The purpose of the reproductive system in the male is the formation and transportation of gametes necessary for reproduction, the physiology of intercourse, and fertilization of the egg. Cooperation between the hypothalamus, the pituitary glands, and the **gonads** (sex glands) is vital to reproductive success.

Checkpoint Question

1. *How does reproduction in higher life forms differ from that of one-celled organisms?*

EVOLUTION AND DIFFERENTIATION OF THE MALE REPRODUCTIVE SYSTEM

20

Every system in the body is identical in the male and female except for components of the reproductive system. By the 12th week of pregnancy, the reproductive organs of the embryo have begun to evolve as male or female. The testes have differentiated within the medulla of the gonad that is common to both the male and female embryo, whereas the ovaries have evolved from the cortex of the gonad.

Early in gestation, the genitalia and internal organs are indistinguishable between male and female. As the embryo becomes a fetus, it gradually becomes clearly defined as one sex or the other, and gender is evident by the fourth month. This definition is decided by the presence of the Y chromosome carried by the sperm at the time of conception. If the male gamete carries an X chromosome to the egg, which always brings with it its own X chromosome, the embryo will evolve into a female. A Y chromosome combined with the egg's X chromosome will yield a male.

The testes, which have developed from the gonads, are carried high in the abdominal cavity during development. During the last months of gestation, the testes normally begin to descend through the inguinal canal into the scrotum, bringing with them their supplying nerves and vessels. The canal then closes behind the testes to prevent other organs from protruding through this structure. At this time, all organs of the male reproductive system are in place and include:

- Two testes, contained in an external sac called the scrotum
- Two epididymides (singular, epididymis)
- Two vasa deferentia (singular, vas deferens)
- Two seminal vesicles
- Prostate gland
- Two Cowper's (or bulbourethral) glands
- Penis, containing the urethra, dual-purpose organ serving both the urinary system and the reproductive system (Fig. 20-1).

ORGANS OF THE MALE REPRODUCTIVE SYSTEM

Testes

Located outside of the body between the thighs in a sac called the scrotum, the testes are small, egg-shaped organs about 1½ to 2 inches long by about 1 inch in diameter. In their protective pouch, they are kept at a fairly constant temperature about 2°C lower than the body temperature. To maintain this constant environment, the scrotum contracts and relaxes reflexively to bring it closer to the body for warmth or lower it away if the body is too warm. The scrotum is also rich in blood vessels and sweat glands that aid in keeping the testes at the temperature that is ideal for the production of viable sperm.

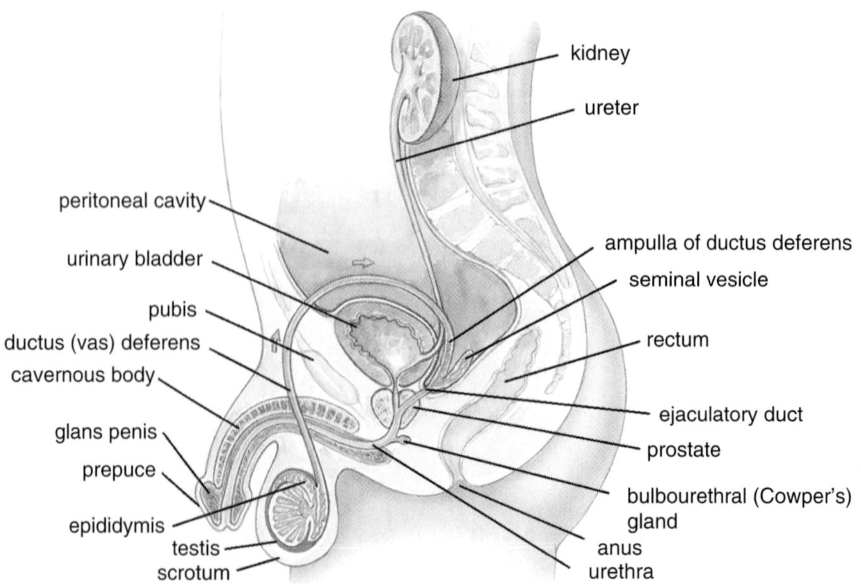

Figure 20-1 Male genitourinary system. The arrows indicate the course of sperm cells through the duct system.

Most of the tissue of the testes is made up of tightly coiled seminiferous tubules, which produce the spermatozoa. Between the tubules lie the **interstitial** cells that produce the male hormone testosterone in response to the interstitial cell-stimulating hormone from the anterior pituitary. Testosterone is essential for the maintenance of the reproductive functions and for the development of the masculine secondary sexual characteristics. Testosterone is also responsible for the male distribution of hair, deeper voice, larger and heavier bone structure, greater muscle mass, and a generally higher production of red blood cells (possibly due to larger bones).

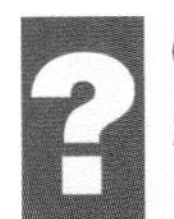

Checkpoint Question

2. *Name the male hormone, where it is formed, and its main functions.*

Within the testes, spermatogenesis (sperm formation) begins. Spermatogenesis is a continuous process, beginning with a cell containing a full component of 46 chromosomes. This then divides by **meiosis** (cell division specific to sperm and ova), rather than mitosis, and will contain only 23 chromosomes after division. As they mature, the sperm are passed from the seminiferous tubules to the epididymis. As these are passed on, more sperm are in the process of maturation within the various compartments of the system. This process takes 70 to 75 days. However, because excess formation is stored for future use, there is rarely a shortage. Those sperm not used are simply absorbed by the system. The average ejaculate contains 3 to 5 mL of semen, with approximately 120 million sperm per milliliter, all of which will need to be replaced by the supply that has been gradually working its way to full maturity.

Epididymis

Still within the scrotum, each epididymis is a tightly coiled thin cord that attaches to the ducts of its testes. It wraps around from the top of the testes down the posterior surfaces then turns upward to become the vas deferens. The epididymis serves as a resting place for the sperm as they mature and are slowly moved along by mild peristalsis. Sperm cells gradually become capable of independent movement during this phase of their journey.

Vas Deferens

The vas deferens, or ductus deferens, is continuous with its epididymis at the lower edge of the testes and travels upward through the inguinal canal into the abdominal cavity and curves up and over to the posterior aspect of the urinary bladder. It is primarily an organ of transport.

Seminal Vesicles

Situated just below the posterior bladder, the seminal vesicles are convoluted tubes that connect with the vas deferens and are responsible for producing part of the seminal fluid. The seminal fluid is slightly alkaline and is thought to help neutralize the acid environment in the vagina during ejaculation. It also contains **fructose,** a **monosaccharide** (simple sugar), and several nutrients to provide an energy source for the sperm. This fluid is the largest component of semen.

Prostate

The prostate completely encircles the urethra at the base of the bladder and is about 1½ inches across and about 1 inch thick. This gland includes a passageway for the seminal vesicles and the vas deferens to join at the ejaculatory duct. The prostate produces secretions that add to the volume of semen. This fluid is also alkaline to aid the fluid from the seminal vesicles in altering the vaginal pH for a less hostile environment for sperm. The prostate empties its fluid into the urethra through many small ducts during the smooth muscle contractions of ejaculation along with the products of the vas deferens and seminal vesicles.

Cowper's Glands

The Cowper's, or bulbourethral, glands are mucus-producing organs lying on the pelvic floor and connecting with the urethra below the prostate. Sexual stimulation causes this fluid to release to act mainly as a lubricant. It has little other purpose and is comparable to the female's **Bartholin glands,** small mucous glands that actually produce most of the lubrication needed during intercourse.

Penis

The penis is common to both the urinary and the reproductive systems. It contains three columns of cavernous, spongelike erectile tissue. There are two **corpora cavernosa** (erectile bodies) along each side of the penis. The **corpus spongiosum,** which contains the urethra, is at the anterior surface. It is attached with ligaments to the pubic arch. At the distal end is a cone-shaped surface called the glans penis that contains the urinary meatus. The glans is normally covered with a fold of loose skin called the **prepuce** or the foreskin. This is frequently removed during infancy as a religious ritual or as an aid to hygiene in a procedure called **circumcision,** which is surgical removal of the prepuce.

During sexual stimulation, nerve impulses cause the arteries supplying the penis to enlarge. This in turn fills the cavernous spaces with blood and compresses the venous spaces, impeding the outflow of blood. The penis elongates and becomes firm, creating an organ capable of vaginal penetration. With sufficient stimulation of the glans penis, sexual satisfaction results in an orgasm. Peristaltic contractions begin throughout the reproductive system, resulting in emission, emptying each of the transporting tubes and storage compartments in turn, and ejaculation, expelling the combined contents with great force. After this event, engorgement subsides with a decrease in the pressure within the supplying arteries, allowing the cavernous spaces to empty and reducing the pressure on the venous outflow.

Checkpoint Question

3. *Describe the sequence of ejaculation.*

Spermatozoa

The spermatozoon (pl. spermatozoa) is a small cell, shaped like a tadpole, with an oval head containing 23 chromosomes within the nucleus (Fig. 20-2). At the tip of the head, like a cap, is an area called the **acrosome,** which contains an enzyme that is capable of penetrating the barrier wall of the ovum. The body of the spermatozoon is made up of a concentration of mitochondria wrapped around just under the head, providing a ready source of energy needed for the high degree of motility required for the sperm to reach its destination.

The **flagellum** (pl. flagella) is a long, whiplike, fiber-filled tail. It is an extension of the cell wall with a store of adenosine triphosphate for energy. Only one cell will succeed in fertilizing the egg, but an abundance of spermatozoa is needed to help that one cell dissolve the barrier wall of the ovum. All others will usually die within a few hours, but some may live up to 3 days.

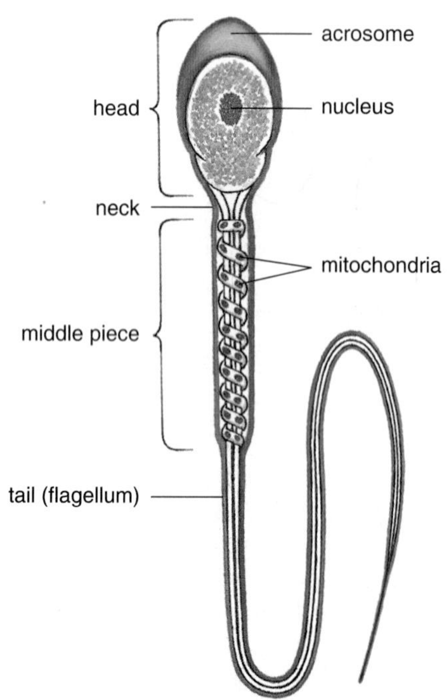

Figure 20-2 Diagram of a human spermatozoon showing major structural features. (Chaffee, E.E., & Lytle, I.M. [1980]. *Basic Physiology and Anatomy,* 4th ed, p. 549. Philadelphia: J.B. Lippincott.)

Composition of Semen

The accessory organs of the male reproductive system provide the secretions necessary for support and transport of the spermatozoa. The thick, white ejaculate is only about 1% to 5% spermatozoa, even though the 3 to 5 mL contains as many as 120 million sperm per milliliter. The primary contributing organ is the prostate, making up to 60% of the fluid. The seminal vesicles add about 30% and the bulbourethral glands about 5%.

Checkpoint Question

4. *How would you describe a sperm cell and its motility? Why must there be so many per ejaculate?*

COMMON DISORDERS OF THE MALE REPRODUCTIVE SYSTEM

The male reproductive system is so inextricably linked to the urinary system that disorders affecting one frequently affect the other. Listed below are several of the disorders that are most likely to be encountered in the medical office.

Prostatic Hypertrophy

As most men reach their middle years, the prostate begins to enlarge (hypertrophy); this disorder may be benign or malignant. The benign form of the disorder has no known cause, but it is presumed to be the result of decreasing hormonal levels. The malignant form of hypertrophy is the second most common form of cancer in men, either as a primary or secondary site.

Presenting symptoms are usually the same for both forms of the disorder. Complaints might include a

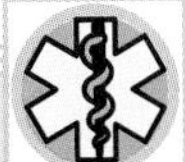

Action **STAT!**

Obstructed Catheter

Scenario: Three days ago, Mr. Dell had transurethral surgery for prostatic hypertrophy. He was sent home with a Foley catheter to drain his bladder during the recovery period. He arrives at the office complaining of severe pain in his lower abdomen. The urine in his drainage bag is bright red with several large clots. What should you do?

1. Assist Mr. Dell into an examining room.
2. Notify the physician. Assess and record Mr. Dell's vital signs.
3. Assist the physician. Because the catheter may be obstructed with blood clots, the physician probably will attempt to irrigate the catheter to remove the obstruction. If the physician is unable to dislodge the obstruction, the catheter may need to be replaced.
4. Monitor Mr. Dell's blood pressure and pulse as frequently as needed during the procedure.
5. Document the incident carefully. If the catheter can be irrigated, and urine can flow through the tube, Mr. Dell probably will be sent home with instructions regarding at-home care. He may be a good candidate for a visiting nurse program; discuss such a referral with the physician.

weak urinary stream, a feeling of urgency but with a hesitant start to the stream, dribbling, **nocturia** (excessive urination at night), and **urinary frequency** (frequent urge to urinate). Because the enlarged prostate compresses the internal urinary sphincter, residual urine frequently causes stagnation and urinary tract infections. Symptoms of the malignant form are late in appearing and are usually a sign that the malignancy is firmly entrenched.

Treatment in the early stages of the benign form is not usually aggressive, addressing the symptoms until such a time as the enlargement requires surgery. Surgery for either form will vary in the approach to the organ (Box 20-1). If cancer is present, radiation may be required to halt metastasis. A radical resection of the perineum may be required to remove the testes to reduce the production of testosterone, which seems to feed malignancies in this area.

Many patients with prostatic hypertrophy have other diseases common to the aging process and need to be evaluated to determine which type of treatment will be most beneficial without compromising fragile health. It is vitally important that all men, especially those over age 40, realize the importance of the digital rectal examination (DRE) performed during routine yearly physical examination. The DRE is the easiest and quickest way for the physician to check for prostatic hypertrophy. Although further testing will always be done for a suspiciously enlarged prostate, the physician will be alerted to malignancy by the consistency of the gland. Malignant hypertrophy is generally more

Box 20-1

Surgical Intervention for Prostatic Hypertrophy

Transurethral Resection

A type of cystoscope with an electrocautery wire cutting loop, called a resectoscope, is inserted through the urethra and rotated through the prostate to remove pieces of the gland. The pieces are washed out with irrigating fluid. There is no abdominal incision, making this a safer alternative for the high-risk patient. The whole organ usually is not removed in this surgery; therefore, the obstruction frequently returns, and strictures are likely to develop. This is not a choice for malignancies.

Suprapubic Prostatectomy

Performed from the abdomen and through the bladder, this procedure allows the surgeon to peel out the whole organ through a wide surgical field and to check the bladder for involvement. This approach is the choice for large organs or for malignancies. As in all surgeries, there are postoperative risks, particularly for the elderly. These include pain, hemorrhage, urinary leakage, and prolonged convalescence.

Perineal Resection

An incision between the scrotum and the anus is a short, direct route without interfering with the bladder and is preferred for some large malignancies. It appears to be less traumatic for the very old or infirm. Surgeons find that the field is more restrictive than that for the suprapubic, with less room to maneuver. It is not a good choice for young men because impotence and urinary and fecal incontinence are frequent postoperative complications. Because of the proximity to the anal area, infection is also a risk.

Retropubic Prostatectomy

A low abdominal incision that approaches above the pubis but below the bladder avoids trauma to the bladder and thereby allows a shorter convalescence than the suprapubic approach but better removal options than the transurethral. It is a good choice if pathology is limited to the prostate with no bladder involvement that requires attention.

20

firm than simple benign hypertrophy and may present in the early stages as prostatic nodules.

Blood testing is done to determine levels of serum acid phosphatase or **prostate-specific antigen** (PSA). PSA, a normal protein produced by the prostate, is usually elevated in men with prostatic cancer. PSA testing is done frequently as a screening device and is offered by many health departments as a public service. The American Cancer Society recommends a yearly PSA for men over age 50. Abnormal findings on the PSA and DRE are followed by an ultrasound. Definitive diagnosis requires a biopsy.

Checkpoint Question

5. *Describe what happens to the prostate in prostatic hypertrophy, and list common symptoms of this disorder.*

Hydrocele

Hydrocele, a collection of fluid within the scrotum and around the testes, may be the result of trauma or infection or may simply be due to the aging process (Fig. 20-3). If the condition is extremely uncomfortable, aspiration may be required. If it persists, surgical intervention may be the treatment of choice. In most cases, the fluid is reabsorbed by the body. Hydrocele is common in male infants and generally subsides gradually.

Differentiation between simple hydrocele, hematocele (a collection of blood within the scrotum), a tumor, or a hernia may be accomplished by transillumination, shining a bright light through the structure. The hydrocele transilluminates easily; hematoceles, tumors, and hernias obscure the light.

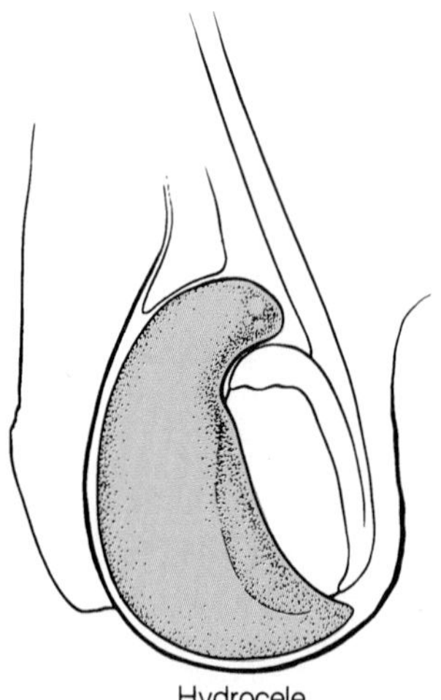

Figure 20-3 A hydrocele.

Cryptorchidism

Cryptorchidism refers to undescended testes (Fig. 20-4). Normally, the testes descend in the male fetus by the eighth month of gestation. In a small percentage of male infants, one or both testes fail to descend by time of delivery. Many of those descend spontaneously by the end of the first year. Those remaining in the abdomen, the inguinal canal, or at the perineal wall after this time need to be brought down surgically. If an undescended testis is not surgically corrected (orchiopexy), it results in sterility of the undescended organ and increases the risk of testicular malignancy. The abnormality also may increase the risk of inguinal hernia on the affected side if not corrected. Surgery is usually performed before age 4, preferably by age 1 or 2.

What If?

You are working in a surgeon's office. When the physician informs the mother of a 10-month-old boy that her son needs surgery for cryptorchidism, the mother starts to cry. What if you are asked by the surgeon to comfort her?

The most therapeutic response is to be supportive of the mother's feelings and to encourage her to verbalize these feelings. Never minimize the surgery or say anything such as, "It is a very simple operation" or "I know he will be just fine." Encourage the mother to ask questions regarding the surgery and relay these questions to the surgeon. Ask open-ended questions to elicit her concerns. Allow the mother to use the telephone to call friends and family. Offer tissues as needed. If the child senses the mother's anxiety, encourage her to hold and reassure her son.

Inguinal Hernia

After the descent of the testes, the inguinal canals close with small rings left open at the anterior base of the abdominal wall (the external ring) as a passage for the spermatic cord, which encloses the vas deferens and the vessels and nerves that supply the testes. There is no connection between this area and the abdominal contents because of the fascia that encloses the abdominal organs; however, this area remains a possible site for weakness to occur with age or exceptional exertion. Men are many times more likely than women to suffer this type of hernia.

Diagnosis is made in the early stages by having the patient bear down and cough while the physician inserts a finger into a pouch made by the scrotum up into the

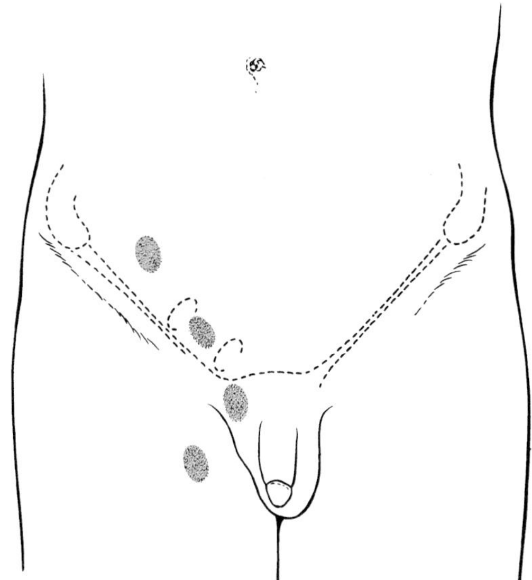

Figure 20-4 Possible locations of undescended testicles.

external and internal inguinal rings. Pressure against the finger indicates a weakness in this area. In later stages, visual examination will reveal an obvious swelling as loops of the bowel descend into the inguinal area.

Treatment will depend on the patient's physical condition. Elderly or infirm patients will benefit from a **truss,** a pressure device used to hold the hernia in place if surgery is not an option. Herniorrhaphy replaces the organ and repairs the opening. Hernioplasty not only returns the organ and repairs the opening, but also reinforces the area with wire or mesh.

Infections

Infections of the urinary tract are likely to become infections of the male reproductive system because they share many of the same organs and functions. The most common infections for the male reproductive system are listed below.

Epididymitis

Infection here usually results from an infected prostate or urinary tract. Agents include staphylococci, streptococci, *Escherichia coli, Chlamydia,* or *Neisseria gonorrhoeae.* Symptoms include pain, tenderness, fever, malaise, and a characteristic walk with the legs wide apart to protect the painful scrotum. Treatment includes antibiotics, bed rest with the scrotum elevated, fluids, and palliative measures for pain.

Orchitis

Many of the same organisms listed above are responsible for infections of the testes, with the addition of mumps as a causative agent. The symptoms and treatment are virtually the same. In mumps orchitis, sterility is a prime concern. Orchitis may result in hydrocele, which needs to be treated if it becomes a severe complication.

Prostatitis

Chronic prostatitis is common among the elderly and may be confused with prostatic hypertrophy if the repeated infections cause the organ to fibrose. The causative agents are much like those of other infections of the male reproductive system, with the leading cause being *E. coli.* It is frequently a result of catheterization or cystoscopy. Some pathogens reach the prostate by way of the bloodstream or the lymph system. Symptoms may include inguinal pain, fever, low back and joint pain, burning and dysuria, and urethral discharge. Urine specimens include blood and pus. Antibiotic treatment is required.

20

Impotence

Impotence, the inability to either achieve or maintain an erection capable of intercourse, may be **psychogenic** (psychological) or organic in origin. Psychogenic impotence may be caused by something as simple as exhaustion, anxiety, or depression and disappears with a resolution of the situational etiology. Deep-seated psychological problems require extensive psychotherapy. Organic impotence may be the result of disease in almost any other body system, such as endocrine imbalances, cardiovascular problems, nervous system impairment, or urinary diseases. Organic impotence also may be caused by injuries to the pelvic organs or to medications that impair any of the systems serving the reproductive system.

Diagnosis involves a detailed medical and sexual history with a holistic analysis of life-style and current emotional status. Blood studies and measurements of both penile arterial flow and nerve conduction to this area are usually required.

Treatment reflects the cause, for example, correction of endocrine imbalances, psychotherapy, or medication adjustment, if any of these are found to be the cause. If none of these are effective, penile implants are available after extensive counseling. Urethral inserts are rapidly gaining favor as a less intrusive treatment method.

Sexually Transmitted Diseases

Many of the diseases transmitted through sexual contact have serious consequences. The most deadly of these currently is acquired immunodeficiency syndrome (AIDS), which is discussed in Chapter 16, Diag-

Advice and Tips
Reducing Anxiety

A variety of diseases that affect the male reproductive system will produce anxiety and tension for the patient. The following tips can help ease stressful situations.

- Provide privacy by closing the examining room door when obtaining the patient history.
- Maintain a nonjudgmental manner when asking questions regarding sexual partners or life-style behaviors.
- Always knock on the examining room door before entering.
- Allow the patient to change into the examination gown in private.
- Supply a drape for the patient to cover himself while he is on the examining table.
- Uncover only the area being examined; keep the patient draped during all other aspects of the examination.
- Have all of the equipment ready for the physician to prevent delays while the patient is in an uncomfortable and exposed position.

20

nostic and Therapeutic Procedures Associated With the Immunologic System. However, the diseases listed below are no less a problem for the health care system. All sexually transmitted diseases (STDs) must be reported to the local health department.

Chlamydia

Chlamydia infections include urethritis in men, cervicitis in women, and lymphogranuloma venereum (LGV) in both, all caused by the organism *Chlamydia trachomatis*. These infections are the most common STDs in the United States.

Without treatment, men with chlamydia infections may develop epididymitis, prostatitis, and sterility. Transmission is by contact with the mucous membranes of infected persons. The disease may be asymptomatic in men. The primary lesion of LGV, a small vesicle or ulcer, may go unnoticed. In 1 to 4 weeks, lymphadenopathy near the site of infection occurs. Systemic symptoms include flulike myalgia, fever, and chills.

In men, the LGV lymph nodes may become very large and tender and spread to surrounding nodal sites. The nodes may become so enlarged they rupture and form sinus tracts to drain the affected nodes.

As the organism ascends the urethral tract, epididymitis may occur with painful scrotal swelling and penile discharge. Chlamydial prostatitis and urethritis will lead to dysuria, urinary frequency, and urethral discharge.

Diagnosis is made by a swab culture of the site. Aspiration of interstitial fluid is used to diagnose epididymitis or prostatitis. Blood tests will determine antibodies in men with previous exposure. Treatment includes courses of penicillin and tetracycline until the patient tests negative for the disease.

Gonorrhea

Gonorrhea is the second most common of the STDs, with an estimated 2 million cases a year in the United States. It is caused by a gram-negative diplococcus, *N. gonorrhoeae*. If left untreated, *N. gonorrhoeae* may ascend the reproductive tract and infect the organs located beyond the penis. Adhesions from the infection may cause sterility, and, if it enters the bloodstream, septicemia is a possibility. The symptoms are obvious within a few days to several weeks and exhibit as a purulent discharge from the urethra with pain and burning on urination. Diagnosis is established symptomatically and with a urethral culture. An initial dose of ceftriaxone intramuscularly followed by oral penicillin for 7 days is the treatment of choice. If the disease is penicillin resistant, spectinomycin is prescribed. The patient should be warned that, until the cultures are negative, he is considered infectious.

Syphilis

Syphilis first presents as a **chancre**, or ulcer, on the penis, in the genital area or at the point of entry. It is caused by a spirochete that spreads quickly through the bloodstream to become a systemic disease with far-reaching consequences. The disease has three stages:

- Primary, with the presenting chancre that may go totally unnoticed
- Secondary, with variable flu-type symptoms up to 8 weeks after exposure and rashes on the skin and mucous membranes, leading to a latency phase that may last for years.
- Tertiary, with systemic involvement that will frequently cause death as the spirochete invades virtually every body system

A battery of efficient and effective tests, such as the Venereal Disease Research Laboratory (VDRL) and Rapid Plasma Reagin (RPR), help to determine the presence of syphilis. Penicillin treatment is effective but must be ongoing with strict follow-up for compliance and cure.

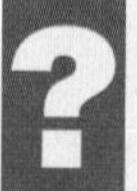

Checkpoint Question

6. *What is usually the first symptom of syphilis?*

Herpes Genitalis

Herpes genitalis is commonly caused by the herpesvirus 2, but may mutate with herpesvirus 1, which causes cold sores on the mouth. This disease has reached epidemic proportions and has no known cure. The patient presents with painful vesicles that rupture and leave equally painful ulcers. Lymph nodes are swollen and tender, and flulike symptoms are sometimes reported. Response to the disease is variable, with symptoms ranging from scarcely noticeable to excruciatingly painful; remissions may last for years, or the symptoms may recur with each stressful situation. Diagnosis is symptomatic, although tissue cultures may be used for a definitive diagnosis. Acyclovir has been effective as a palliative measure to reduce the severity of the symptoms of herpes genitalis, but it cannot be considered a cure.

Phimosis

Phimosis is a narrowing or tightening of the prepuce (foreskin) that prevents retraction over the glans penis. Uncircumcised males, or those with excessive prepuce covering the glans penis, may find that the skin adheres to the surface of the glans is the accumulation of **smegma** (an oily secretion from small glands under the foreskin) is not regularly washed free and the area of the glans kept clean. As a medical assistant, you may be responsible for educating caregivers of male infants in the proper cleaning techniques at bath time and diaper changes. For infants and adults, the foreskin should be retracted, the glans washed well and rinsed, and the foreskin returned to its natural position. It may be necessary to use petrolatum on the surface of the glans if it seems to adhere despite these efforts. Adults who experience this may need circumcision.

Infertility

Infertility is the inability to reproduce. Male infertility is easier to diagnose than female infertility. If pregnancy is not achieved after 1 year of regular, unprotected intercourse, infertility tests are initiated. Causes of male infertility include:

- Semen disorders, such as low volume (oligospermia), low motility, abnormal sperm, immature sperm
- Systemic disease, such as diabetes mellitus or renal or hepatic disease
- STDs, such as gonorrhea or herpes
- Testicular disorders, such as cryptorchidism or ductal obstructions
- Sexual dysfunction

A physical examination may reveal many of the above causes. A detailed patient history may direct the diagnosis to a history of prolonged fever, mumps, impaired nutritional status, or genital trauma. The most conclusive laboratory test is a semen analysis. Serum testosterone levels, gonadotropin assays, and a testicular biopsy may be performed.

If the cause is a correctable anatomic problem, surgery will be performed. Hormonal treatment may correct a diagnosed imbalance, and counseling may alleviate psychological dysfunction. If the accepted corrective measures do not result in pregnancy and the woman is fertile, options include artificial insemination or adoption.

Testicular Cancer

Testicular cancer accounts for only about 1% of all malignancies, but it involves extremely high metastatic and mortality rates. The cause is unknown, but the factors most often implicated include cryptorchidism, infection, genetics, and endocrine abnormalities. The symptoms are gradual and painless, involving initially only a vague feeling of scrotal heaviness. In fact, the most significant symptom is a painless enlargement of the testes. By the time a patient presents with back or abdominal pain, metastasis has usually occurred.

20

Testicular self-examination is the best method of early detection and should be performed as a matter of habit for all men. All suspicious areas of thickness or lumps should be reported immediately. Further testing by α-fetoprotein and human chorionic gonadotropin blood work will be ordered. A computed tomography (CT) scan is frequently ordered to determine the extent of the malignancy and possible metastasis.

Treatment is usually an orchiectomy through the inguinal approach, with lymph node resection if cancer cells are found in the local nodes. Radiation is added if metastasis is found.

The sequela is sterility if both testes are involved, but sexual function should not be impaired because the testes only provide semen, which is about 1% to 3% of the ejaculate. The other organs of the reproductive system will continue to produce their various secretions. However, the reduction in testosterone produced by the testes usually results in reduced sexual desire.

COMMON DIAGNOSTIC PROCEDURES AND THE MEDICAL ASSISTANT'S ROLE

In addition to the information gathered by diagnostic tests described below, establishing diagnoses for the male reproductive system often involves a detailed social and sexual history.

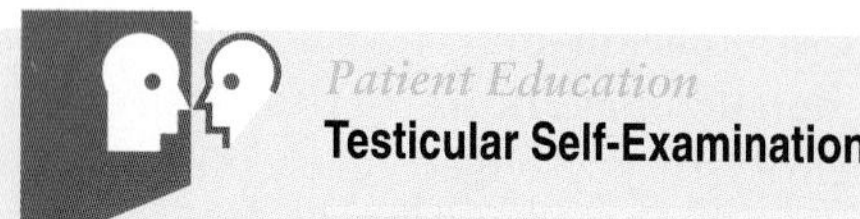

Patient Education

Testicular Self-Examination

Testicular cancer is commonly found between the ages of 15 and 34, at a time when many young men are not yet aware of health concerns. This cancer is highly treatable if found very early, making it imperative that men understand the importance of vigilance.

Men should be taught the signs of testicular cancer in addition to the procedure for the self-examination. They include the following:

- A feeling of heaviness in the scrotal area, generally without pain, although a dull ache may be present
- Fluid accumulation in the scrotal sac without a history of injury
- A change in the consistency of the testis or its surrounding sac
- Possible breast tenderness

Some physicians recommend that this examination be performed as often as weekly by all men 15 years old and older. The best time is after a warm bath or shower when the scrotal sac is most relaxed. Roll each testicle between the thumb and forefinger and feel for hard lumps or bumps or even a change in the consistency of the scrotal tissue. This procedure should not be hurried and typically takes about 3 minutes.

If there is any cause for concern, any change in the normal texture, size, shape, or consistency, an appointment should be made promptly for an examination by the physician. He may order certain x-rays after performing a complete physical examination. Surgery is usually the preferred treatment, possibly in addition to chemotherapy or radiation therapy.

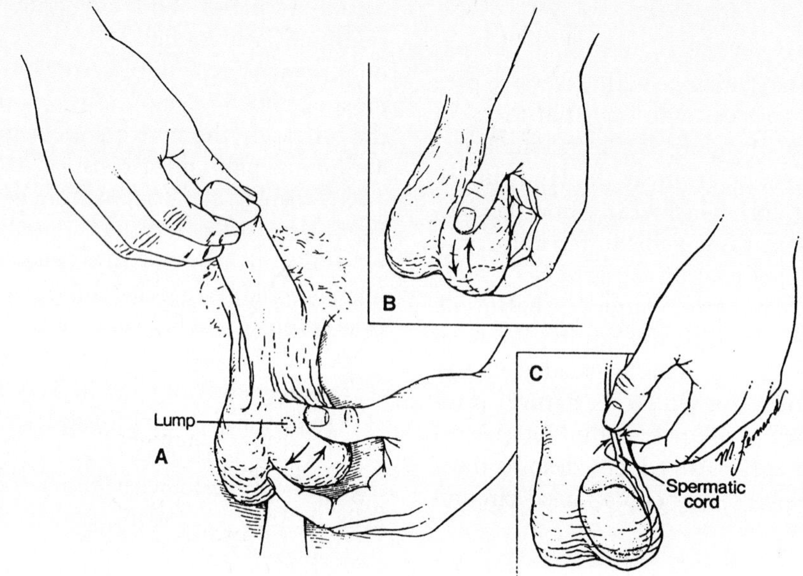

1. Use both hands to palpate the testis; the normal testicle is smooth and uniform in consistency.
2. With the index and middle fingers under the testis and the thumb on top, roll the testis gently in a horizontal plane between the thumb and fingers (*A*).
3. Feel for any evidence of a small lump or abnormality.
4. Follow the same procedure and palpate upward along the testis (*B*).
5. Locate the epididymis (*C*), a cordlike structure on the top and back of the testicle that stores and transports sperm.
6. Repeat the examination for the other testis. It is normal to find that one testis is larger than the other.
7. If you find any evidence of a small, pealike lump, consult your physician. It may be due to an infection or a tumor growth.

Urinalysis

A specifically directed urine workup differentiates between diseases of the urinary system and of the male reproductive system. They share many of the same symptoms and are difficult to distinguish without the tests that correspond with the presenting symptoms. Cultures and sensitivities are commonly ordered, which will require that you instruct the patient in the proper procedure for a clean-catch, midstream specimen (see Chap. 28, Urinalysis). For all tests, you will need to assemble the proper specimen containers, complete the required laboratory slips, instruct the patient in any special precautions, and route the specimen to the proper testing facility.

Blood Work

You may be required to draw blood specimens for a white blood count to determine infection, blood urea nitrogen (to determine urinary system involvement), or any of several diagnostic tests for syphilis. Standard Precautions for blood and body fluid must be followed as always, and the blood must be routed to the proper testing facility with all of the appropriate paperwork.

Cultures

Generally, medical assistants will not be responsible for performing a urethral swab for a culture, but the proper equipment must be provided for the physician. The equipment includes gloves for the physician, a culture tube with the proper medium and swab, and completed laboratory slips.

Rectal and Scrotal Examinations

You will be required to supply the physician with latex gloves and a water-soluble lubricant and to instruct the patient to disrobe appropriately. The physician inspects and palpates the scrotum as described for inguinal hernias. To determine if the patient has prostatic hypertrophy, the physician lubricates a gloved index finger and palpates the patient's prostate rectally for size, shape, and consistency. Female medical assistants may be asked to leave the examining room during this phase of the examination.

X-rays

To confirm diagnoses, the physician may order an intravenous pyelogram or CT scan. These allow the physician to determine the extent of involvement for disorders that are difficult to differentiate by palpation, inspection, or diagnostic laboratory studies.

Cystoscopy

Physicians diagnose and treat many of the diseases of the male reproductive system and urinary system by cystoscopy. A cystoscope is used to view the interior of the bladder by passing a lighted viewing instrument through the urethra. Fiberoptic scopes are used most frequently now, but rigid scopes are still in use.

Most patients are lightly sedated before the surgery, with local anesthetics administered just before the procedure. The patient is placed in a lithotomy position and covered with a fenestrated drape. The urethra and the surrounding area are prepped with an antiseptic solution. The physician then passes the scope through the urethral meatus. Urine may be collected for sampling by passing a catheter through the scope into the bladder, ureters, or kidneys. Fluoroscopic x-rays may be used to assess the patency of the urinary tract by injecting radiopaque dye through the scope into the area of concern. Stones may be removed during the procedure, and lesions may be viewed directly and treated through the scope.

After the procedure, have the patient rest in a supine position until he feels ready to stand. Pain and slight hematuria will usually be present after most of the procedures performed during cystoscopy.

PREPARING THE PATIENT FOR PROCEDURES

Few of the diagnostic procedures involving the male reproductive system require extensive or involved preparations. Equipment to be assembled will usually only include latex gloves, a water-soluble lubricant, and tissues for the patient's use. Laboratory tests will require the proper specimen containers or tubes and properly completed laboratory slips.

Vasectomy

An increasingly popular form of reproductive control is the vasectomy—bilateral removal of a segment of the vas deferens to prevent the passage of sperm from the testes. This procedure is frequently performed in the medical office.

The patient will receive a light preoperative sedative and may be NPO (nothing by mouth). He will be placed in the lithotomy position, covered with a fenestrated drape, and given a local anesthetic. Small incisions are made bilaterally near the scrotal sac. The vas deferens is pulled through the incision, clamped proximally and distally, and the connecting segment is removed. The clamped ends of the ducts are returned to the inguinal canal, and the site is sutured.

Ejaculation and sexual function are not affected by the surgery. The volume of sperm in the ejaculate is so minute that its absence will not be noticed. The sperm that are produced are absorbed by the body. Sterility may not be immediate. The patient is advised to return for sperm counts until the ejaculate is free of sperm. Although vasectomies can be reversed, studies report varied success rates.

Answers to Checkpoint Questions

1. *Higher species require a mate or a sexual contact to reproduce. Many lower life forms, such as one-celled organisms, simply divide.*
2. *The male hormone, testosterone, is produced in the interstitial spaces of the seminiferous tubules. It functions in reproduction and in the development of secondary sexual characteristics.*
3. *Nerve impulses cause the arteries to enlarge, fill the cavernous spaces, and entrap the venous blood within the penis. The penis enlarges and elongates, and peristaltic contractions empty the transfer tubes and storage compartments and result in ejaculation.*
4. *A sperm cell is a tadpole-shaped cell with a flagellum for motility. It is nourished by the mitochondria wrapped around the flagellum at the base of the cell. Many are required to dissolve the shell around the ovum.*
5. *The prostate enlarges and closes off the urethra, causing urgency, hesitation, dribbling, weak stream, nocturia, and frequency.*
6. *The first symptom of syphilis usually is a chancre at the site of infection.*

20

Critical Thinking Challenges

1. Review the chapter on the endocrine system. Explain the relationship between the hypothalamus, the pituitary, and the gonads.
2. You are caring for a patient with oligospermia-induced infertility. The physician recommends abstinence for prescribed periods. Why might the physician make this recommendation?
3. Research the available statistics regarding penile cancer rates among circumcised versus uncircumcised men. Compare statistics also for cervical cancer among the wives of both groups. Explain why there might be a difference.
4. Your patient is concerned that if he has a vasectomy, his ejaculate will be noticeably diminished. How would you explain to him why neither he nor his mate will discern any difference?

Suggestions for Further Reading

Bates, B., Bickley, L. S., & Hockelman, R. A. (1995). *A Guide to Physical Examination and History Taking,* 6th ed. Philadelphia: Lippincott-Raven.

Bullock, B. L., & Rosendahl, P. P. (1996). *Pathophysiology,* 4th ed. Philadelphia: Lippincott-Raven.

Memmler, R. L., Cohen, B. J., & Wood, D. L. (1996). *The Human Body in Health and Disease,* 8th ed. Philadelphia: Lippincott-Raven.

Miller, B. F., & Keane, C. B. (1992). *Encyclopedia and Dictionary of Medicine, Nursing and Allied Health.* Philadelphia: W.B. Saunders.

(1992). *Professional Guide to Diseases,* 4th ed. Springhouse, PA: Springhouse.

Rosdahl, C. B. (1995). *Textbook of Basic Nursing,* 6th ed. Philadelphia: Lippincott-Raven.

Smeltzer, S. C., & Bare, B. G. (1996). *Brunner and Suddarth's Textbook of Medical-Surgical Nursing,* 8th ed. Philadelphia: Lippincott-Raven.

21

Assisting With Diagnostic and Therapeutic Procedures Associated With the Female Reproductive System

Chapter Outline

Role Delineation

CLINICAL

Fundamental Principles

- Apply principles of aseptic technique and infection control.

Diagnostic Orders

- Collect and process specimens.

GENERAL

Professionalism

- Project a professional manner and image.
- Work as a team member.

Communication Skills

- Treat all patients with compassion and empathy.
- Adapt communications to individual's ability to understand.
- Serve as liaison.

Role Delineation *(continued)*

CLINICAL	GENERAL
Patient Care	*Legal Concepts*
• Obtain patient history and vital signs. • Prepare and maintain examination and treatment areas. • Prepare patient for examinations, procedures, and treatments. • Assist with examinations, procedures, and treatments.	• Practice within the scope of education, training, and personal capabilities. • Document accurately. • Maintain and dispose of regulated substances in compliance with government guidelines. • Comply with established risk management and safety procedures. *Instruction* • Instruct individuals according to their needs. • Teach methods of health promotion and disease prevention.

Chapter Competencies

Learning Objectives

Upon successfully completing this chapter, you will be able to:

1. Spell and define the Key Terms.
2. Identify and describe the organs of the female reproductive system.
3. Describe the menstrual cycle.
4. Describe menopause.
5. Describe the processes of fertilization, implantation, and gestation.
6. Explain the methods for determining a pregnant patient's estimated date of delivery.
7. Identify and explain fetotoxic and teratogenic factors.
8. Describe the components of prenatal and postpartum patient care.
9. Identify the various methods of contraception.
10. List and describe common gynecologic and obstetric disorders and outline the medical assistant's role as it relates to the disorders.
11. Identify and explain diagnostic tests and therapeutic procedures of the female reproductive system and state the medical assistant's role where applicable.

Performance Objectives

Upon successfully completing this chapter, you will be able to:

1. Assist with performance of a pelvic examination with Pap smear (Procedure 21-1).
2. Assist with performance of a colposcopy with cervical biopsy (Procedure 21-2).
3. Assist with the insertion of an intrauterine device (IUD) (Procedure 21-3).
4. Assist with the removal of an IUD (Procedure 21-4).
5. Assist with the insertion of subdermal hormonal implants (Procedure 21-5).
6. Assist with the first prenatal examination.
7. Assist with subsequent prenatal examinations.
8. Assist with the first postnatal examination.

Key Terms

(See Glossary for definitions.)

ablation
abortion
amenorrhea
anovulation
asymptomatic
Braxton Hicks
Chadwick's sign
climacteric period
colpocleisis
colporrhaphy
colposcopy
cul-de-sac
culdocentesis
curettage
cystocele
cytology
dysmenorrhea
dyspareunia
episiotomy
erythematous
etiology
fimbriae
gestation
Goodell's sign
gravid
gravida
gravidity
hirsutism

(continued)

21

Key Terms *(continued)*

(See Glossary for definitions.)

human chorionic gonadotropin (HCG)
hysterosalpingogram
hysteroscopy
idiopathic
intrauterine pregnancy (IUP)
introitus
labor
laparoscopy
laparotomy
leukocytosis
lightening
lyse
lochia
menorrhagia
menarche
menses
metrorrhagia
multigravida
multipara
nulligravida
nullipara
oophorectomy
ovulation
ovum
parity
pessary
polymenorrhea
primigravida
primipara
proteinuria
puerperium
pyosalpinx
rectocele
salpingo-oophorectomy
secundigravida

The female reproductive system is responsible for the development and maintenance of secondary sexual characteristics and for sexual reproduction of the species.

Secondary sexual characteristics are developed and maintained by the interaction of the follicle-stimulating hormone (FSH), luteinizing hormone (LH), estrogen, and progesterone. This hormonal interaction brings about the onset of puberty, which is characterized by budding of the breasts, an increase in body fat, growth of pubic and axillary hair, and **menarche** (beginning of menstruation).

Sexual reproduction requires the union of specialized sex cells (gametes) from the male and the female. The ovaries produce the female gamete, the **ovum,** which joins with the spermatozoon of the male during fertilization to form a zygote (a fertilized ovum).

Gynecology and obstetrics are the two medical specialties concerned with female sexual and reproductive functions. Gynecology concentrates on the care of female patients with disorders of the reproductive organs. Obstetrics is the branch of medicine that cares for female patients through pregnancy, childbirth, and the postpartum period.

ORGANS OF THE FEMALE REPRODUCTIVE SYSTEM

Ovaries

The primary gonads of the female are the ovaries (Fig. 21-1), which produce ova, the female reproductive cells. The ovaries have an estimated 400,000 follicles

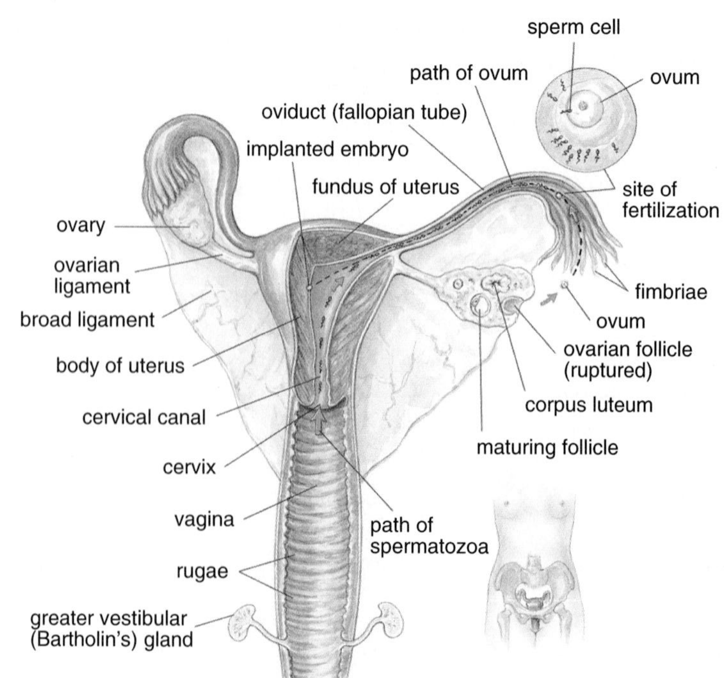

Figure 21-1 Female reproductive system.

present at birth, each containing an undeveloped ovum. Several follicles will begin to grow with each menstrual cycle, but usually only one will develop into a graafian follicle containing a mature ovum. **Ovulation** is the process by which the fully matured ovum ruptures from the graafian follicle and is released from the ovary. (This process is discussed further in the section "The Menstrual Cycle," below.)

Fallopian Tubes

The fallopian tubes, or oviducts, arise from the uterine fundus and extend to just above the ovaries. The fallopian tubes serve as a passageway for the ovum on its way to the uterus and for the sperm in its search for the ovum. At the distal ends of the tubes are many finger-like extensions called **fimbriae** that wave the released egg toward the duct and pass it to the cilia-lined interior of the tube for transport to the uterus.

Uterus

The uterus is a pear-shaped, muscular organ that is primarily responsible for housing and nourishing the developing fetus from conception to birth. The uterus is made up of three tissue layers.

1. The *endometrium,* the innermost lining, has a rich blood supply and a great ability to regenerate. It is the outermost part of the endometrium that is shed during menstruation.
2. The *myometrium,* the middle, muscular layer, is important in **labor** (the physiologic process necessary for expelling the fetus from the uterus) and delivery of the neonate. The myometrium also contracts during menses to assist in eliminating the necrotic endometrium.
3. The *perimetrium* is a layer of connective tissue that covers the outer walls of the uterus and attaches to the supportive ligaments that secure the uterus in place.

The uterus is actually a tube that has a cervix (neck), body (central portion), and a fundus (see Fig. 21-1). The cervix opens into the vaginal canal; this opening is called the external os. The cervical opening into the uterine cavity is called the internal os. The uterus as a whole may be viewed as a series of ducts because the fallopian tubes, uterine cavity, and the cervix are continuous with one another and are passageways for the functions specific to the female reproductive system.

Vagina

The vagina is a hollow, muscular tube lined with mucous membrane that extends from the cervix to the vulva. Although the vagina canal is generally narrow, the walls are capable of considerable expansion for the birth process.

Vulva

The vulva, or external genitalia, includes the labia majora, labia minora, clitoris, vaginal orifice, Bartholin's glands, Skene's glands, hymen, vestibule, and perineum. Bartholin's glands (one on each side of the vaginal opening) and Skene's glands (just inside the urethral opening) secrete substances that are important in providing lubrication and maintaining the acid–base balance in the vaginal and vulval areas. The clitoris is a small body that is similar to the male penis in that it is made of erectile tissue. It is located in the anterior portion of the labia minora. The labia minora are two small folds of tissue that lie between the labia majora. Between the labia minora is a triangular space called the vestibule that contains the openings of the glands and vaginal orifice, or **introitus.**

From the vestibule to the anus lies the perineum, which is a body of connective tissue that allows for the attachment of muscles and provides for pelvic support. During a vaginal delivery of the fetus, an **episiotomy** (incision of the perineum) may be performed to facilitate the delivery and reduce the risk of a perineal laceration (tear).

Breasts (Mammary Glands)

The breasts are located on the upper anterior portion of the chest and contain 15 to 20 lobes of glandular tissue that are capable of producing milk for nursing an infant (Fig. 21-2). The bulk of the breast is composed of fatty tissue. Following delivery, prolactin and oxytocin from the pituitary gland stimulate and maintain the production of milk.

Checkpoint Question

1. *The uterus is composed of what three layers? Briefly explain each.*

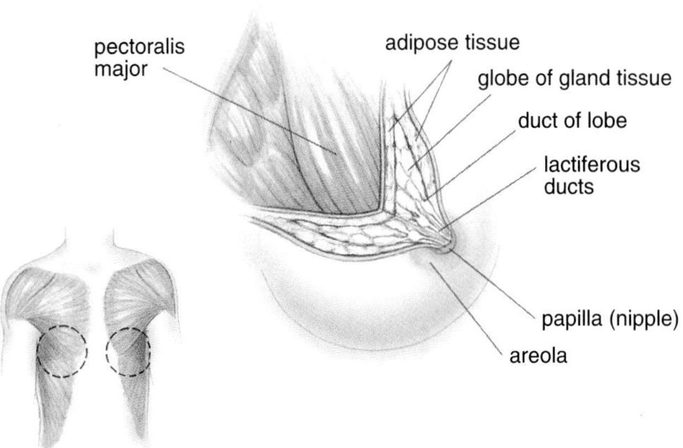

Figure 21-2 Section of the breast.

THE MENSTRUAL CYCLE

Menstruation is a normal body process involving the elimination of a bloody discharge from the uterus through the vagina. The age at which a girl begins **menses** is known as menarche and is one of the many signs of puberty. The cessation of menses marks the **climacteric period,** or menopause (see the section "Menopause," below). The menstrual cycle is about 28 days in length, counting the first day of the menstrual flow as day 1, and involves a series of complex events controlled by hormones secreted by the anterior pituitary and the ovaries (Fig. 21-3). It has three phases, which are described below.

Proliferative (Follicular) Phase

During the proliferative phase (days 5–14), the endometrium grows very rapidly, preparing for possible implantation of a fertilized ovum. The anterior pituitary begins secreting FSH, causing several follicles within the ovary to begin development. Although several follicles are growing, usually only one actually matures into a graafian follicle. The graafian follicle contains the ovum and also secretes estrogen, stimulating the growth of the endometrium.

At the end of the proliferative phase, the graafian follicle bulges against the ovarian wall and eventually ruptures from the ovary, releasing the ovum. This process of ovulation is triggered by the secretion of LH by the anterior pituitary gland and occurs on about day 15. Once the graafian follicle ruptures, the ovum is pulled into the fallopian tube by the waving action of the fimbriae. The tissue (corpus luteum) left behind begins to secrete progesterone (meaning pro pregnancy), further stimulating endometrial growth.

Ovulation is accompanied by an increase in the basal body temperature after the ovum is released. Some women notice pain, tenderness, or both over the ovary in which ovulation is occurring.

Secretory (Luteal) Phase

The secretory phase (days 15–28) begins immediately after ovulation and is influenced by the progesterone that is produced by the corpus luteum of the ovary. The primary characteristic of the secretory phase is the impact that the progesterone has on the endometrium, which undergoes tremendous growth as it prepares for a possible pregnancy. It becomes very vascular and rich in glycogen, creating an environment that is essential for fetal growth.

If implantation occurs, the corpus luteum will continue to secrete the progesterone until the pregnancy is well established and the placenta takes over the production of the progesterone. The placenta also secretes **human chorionic gonadotropin (HCG),** which supports the corpus luteum and is the hormone that is detected in the urine and serum of pregnant women. The HCG level is used to confirm suspected pregnancy and to estimate the **gestation,** or the period of time from conception to birth.

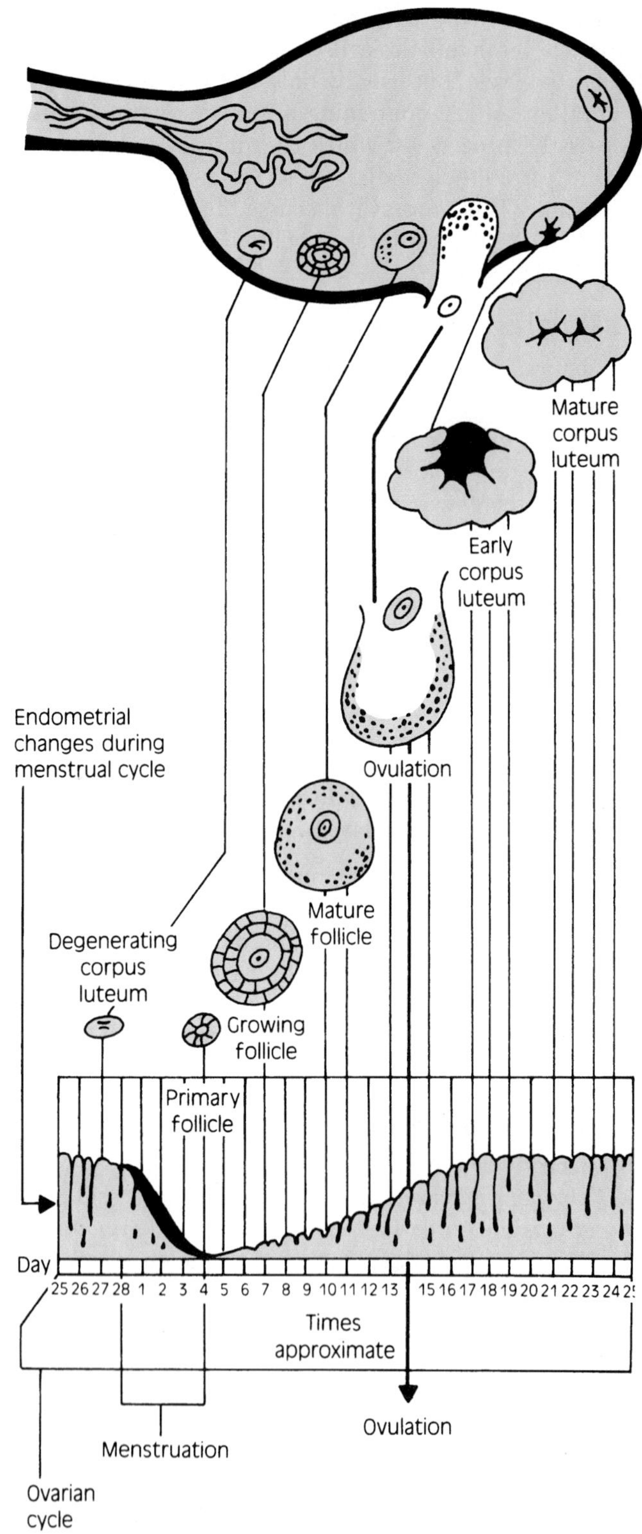

Figure 21-3 The menstrual cycle.

If implantation does not occur, then the HCG, which is necessary for the survival of the corpus luteum, is not produced. The corpus luteum will degenerate, and without the progesterone, there will be thinning of the endometrium with eventual necrosis and sloughing of the functional layer. The sloughing of the endometrium is the menstrual flow.

Menstruation

Menstruation itself usually lasts about 5 days (days 1–5). The discharge consists of pieces of the necrotic (dead) endometrium, mucus from the uterine walls, and blood. Often, this phase is accompanied by painful uterine cramps that result from the contractions of the myometrium to assist in eliminating the bloody discharge.

If, however, the ovum unites with the male sperm within 48 hours of ovulation, fertilization occurs. When this happens, the menstrual cycle is interrupted, and the endometrium grows and develops, creating an environment that will support the implantation and fetal growth.

The medical assistant should always remind and encourage patients, especially adolescents, to record on a calendar the days of menses. Instruct each patient to note the date of the first day of the last menstrual period (LMP) and to bring the information to the medical office. The regularity of the menstrual cycle is often critical to the physician's assessment of the patient's gynecologic health, the duration of pregnancy, and the estimated date of confinement (EDC) or estimated date of delivery (EDD).

Keep in mind that other conditions besides pregnancy (eg, dysfunctional uterine bleeding, leiomyomas) also can alter the normal menstrual cycle. Such conditions are described below.

Checkpoint Question

2. *What is the primary characteristic of the secretory phase of the menstrual cycle?*

GYNECOLOGIC DISORDERS

Vulvovaginitis

Vulvovaginitis is inflammation of the vulva and vagina. It is one of the more common complaints of female patients. Symptoms often include pruritus, burning of the vulva or the vagina (or both), and increased vaginal discharge. On examination, the vulva and vagina are **erythematous** (reddened). The type of discharge often indicates the **etiology** (cause) of the disorder. The most common etiologies include *Candida*, *Trichomonas*, and bacterial vaginosis or *Gardnerella vaginitis* (previously known as *Haemophilus vaginalis*). Confirmation of the causative agent is by a microscopic examination of a vaginal smear or by culture of the vaginal discharge. Effective treatment depends on the etiology (Box 21-1).

Dysfunctional Uterine Bleeding

Dysfunctional uterine bleeding (DUB), or abnormal uterine bleeding, is defined as abnormal or irregular uterine bleeding, including heavy, irregular, or light bleeding caused by an endocrine imbalance. DUB includes:

- **Menorrhagia** (excessive bleeding during menses)
- **Metrorrhagia** (irregular bleeding at times other than menses)
- **Polymenorrhea** (abnormally frequent menses)
- Postmenopausal bleeding not associated with tumor, inflammation, or pregnancy

Diagnosis is based on ruling out other causes for the bleeding. Treatment is with hormones, oral contraceptives, or **curettage** (scraping) of the uterine cavity, depending on the etiology. Hysterectomy may be the treatment of choice for those patients who do not respond to conservative therapy, who are at increased risk of adenocarcinoma, and who do not desire pregnancy.

Premenstrual Syndrome (PMS)

Premenstrual syndrome is characterized by a wide variety of physical, psychological, and behavioral symp-

Box 21-1
Infectious Agents in Vulvovaginitis

Trichomonas vaginalis: Known as "Trich," this disease is caused by a protozoa and is transmitted through sexual intercourse. The signs are a thin, frothy, greenish or gray discharge with an odor. The symptoms include dysuria with frequency and intense pruritus. Treatment requires that both partners be treated with oral metronidazole.

Candida albicans: Also known as monilia, this fungal disease grows best in the presence of glucose. The signs include a thick, curdlike discharge with white patches on the vaginal walls, usually with no odor. There is usually intense itching. The pathogen is found in the intestines and is more likely to affect the patient during the secretory phase of the menstrual cycle. It is very common during pregnancy and for those on antibiotic therapy. Treatment requires nystatin vaginal suppositories, which may be purchased without a prescription, or other antifungals. Oral fluconazole (Diflucan) is also frequently prescribed.

Gardnerella vaginitis: A gram-negative bacillus is responsible for this disease. There is a gray discharge with a foul odor. It is treated with metronidazole.

21

toms that occur on a regular, cyclic basis (Box 21-2). For diagnostic purposes, the patient must experience a complex of symptoms associated with PMS, the symptoms must occur during the 7 to 10 days before menses, and they must be severe enough to interfere with interpersonal relationships and routine activities.

Symptoms of PMS usually diminish a few hours after the onset of menses. The etiology is **idiopathic** (unknown). Diagnosis of PMS is based on the physician's assessment of the history and physical examination. Patients will need to chart their symptoms for several months on a calendar that includes the menstrual cycle.

As a medical assistant, you can have a dramatic impact on the patient's ability to cope with this syndrome by providing emotional support, educating the patient about the syndrome, and encouraging regular exercise and dietary restrictions of caffeine, salt, and animal fats. To minimize the effects of PMS, encourage patients to get adequate rest and avoid stressful situations.

Endometriosis

Endometriosis is a condition of unknown etiology in which endometrial tissue is found growing outside (ectopic) of the uterine cavity in such areas as the fallopian tubes, around the ovaries and uterosacral ligaments, and, in rare cases, in other parts of the abdominal cavity. The patient, who is most often of reproductive age, complains of infertility, **dysmenorrhea** (painful menstruation), pelvic pain, and **dyspareunia** (painful intercourse). The patient's symptoms and physical findings may indicate endometriosis, but the diagnosis and the severity must be confirmed by direct visualization, usually by way of **laparoscopy** (internal examination of the abdominal cavity). Treatment of endometriosis may relieve the pelvic pain but has a less desirable impact on fertility. The type of therapy depends on the age, symptoms, severity, and the patient's desire for pregnancy. Treatment includes hormone and drug therapy to suppress the growth and laparoscopic **ablation** (excision) by laser or cautery to **lyse** (destroy) the adhesions. For patients who have severe symptoms and who do not desire pregnancy, the treatment of choice may be a hysterectomy with bilateral **salpingo-oophorectomy** (excision of both ovaries and fallopian tubes).

Box 21-2

PMS Symptoms

The hormonal flux associated with the menstrual cycle affects other body systems in addition to the reproductive system. The cascade of events results in a series of symptoms that include:

- Hypoglycemia—A drop in blood sugar results in headaches, nausea, and fatigue and may explain the food cravings many women experience. Increasing carbohydrate intake will ensure a steady blood glucose level.
- Fluid retention—Fluid is retained in all parts of the body with edema, weight gain, mastalgia, sinusitis, backache, and headache. Reducing the intake of salt during this period will alleviate some of the edema.
- Sodium and potassium imbalance—the cyclical fluctuation of these chemotransmitters causes fatigue, irritability, and depression. Dietary forms of these minerals should be encouraged.
- Decreased immunity—At this time, the patient may experience rhinitis and other upper respiratory infections, acne, and herpes outbreaks.

Checkpoint Question

3. *Briefly explain each of the three types of dysfunctional uterine bleeding.*

Uterine Prolapse and Displacement

Prolapse of the uterus is an abnormal condition in which the uterus droops or protrudes downward into the vagina. Often the condition is accompanied by **cystocele, rectocele,** or both. Cystocele is the herniation of the urinary bladder into the vagina; rectocele is the herniation of the rectum into the vagina.

Different methods can be used to describe the degree of prolapse (mild, moderate, severe; grade I, II, III). A commonly used method involves classifying the degree of prolapse:

- First-degree prolapse occurs when the uterus has descended to the level of the vaginal orifice.
- Second-degree prolapse occurs when the uterine cervix protrudes through the vaginal orifice.
- Third-degree prolapse occurs when the entire cervix and uterus protrude beyond the vaginal orifice (Fig. 21-4).

Diagnosis is confirmed by pelvic examination, at which time the degree of prolapse can be determined. Surgical treatment includes hysteropexy (stitching the uterus back into place in first-degree prolapse), vaginal hysterectomy, **colporrhaphy** (stitching the vagina), and **colpocleisis** (surgery to occlude the vagina) in severe cases. Medical management for patients who are elderly or who are poor risks for surgery include hormone therapy to strengthen the muscular floor of the pelvis and the use of a **pessary.** A pessary is a device that fits around the cervix, usually into the **cul-de-sac.** The patient inserts the pessary into the vagina to support the uterus.

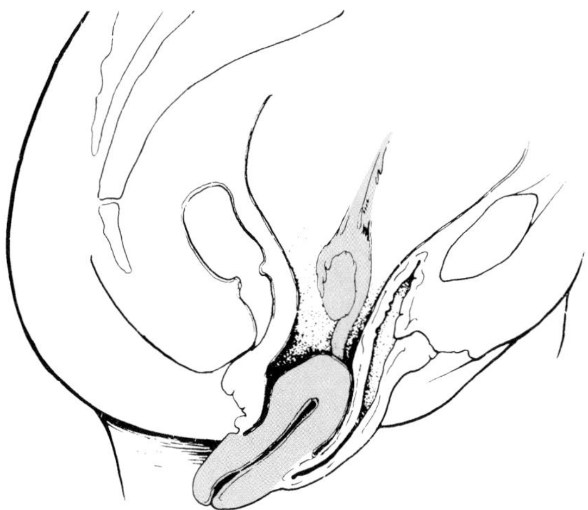

Figure 21-4 Complete prolapse of the uterus through the introitus.

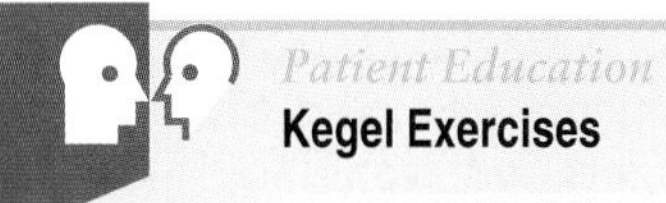

Kegel Exercises

Age, gravity, and childbearing take their toll on the muscles of the perineum. The Kegel exercises can increase the tone of this area. Stronger perineal tone helps eliminate stress incontinence and offers support to the vaginal walls to avoid uterine prolapse.

Explain to the patient that she can practice doing Kegel exercises at any time: standing in the grocery line, waiting at a stop light, sitting in class. Instruct her to tighten the vaginal opening and the buttocks as if she were stopping the flow of urine, then hold this position for about 3 seconds. The patient should work up to doing as many as 15 to 20 repetitions of the exercises four or five times a day.

You will need to educate the patient about the use of a pessary. The pessary should be changed every 2 to 3 months, and the patient should be advised to douche about once a week. The patient should be educated about the signs of vaginal infection because the pessary increases the risk of inflammation and infection.

The uterus is normally tilted slightly forward over the bladder with the cervix at a right angle to the direction of the vagina. The uterus is movable, and due to stress on the supporting ligaments, it occasionally tilts either anteriorly or posteriorly from its natural position. This is called uterine displacement (Fig. 21-5).

The symptoms may be simply pressure in the rectal area or against the bladder. The symptoms are not usually severe but are troublesome to the patient. Displacement may contribute to infertility and require correction to facilitate pregnancy. Treatment follows the same protocol as required for uterine prolapse. In most instances, the uterus may simply be stitched back into its original position (hysteropexy).

Sexually Transmitted Diseases

Acquired immunodeficiency syndrome (AIDS), the deadly sexually transmitted disease (STD), is discussed in detail in Chapter 16, Assisting With Diagnostic and Therapeutic Procedures Associated With the Immunologic System. However, it should be noted here that the incidence of AIDS is rising rapidly among young women in the United States and is frequently a coinfector with other STDs.

Chlamydia trachomatis

The STD caused by *Chlamydia trachomatis* may be **asymptomatic** (without symptoms) in the female patient or may present with vague, flulike symptoms that are difficult to diagnose without specific reason to suspect the infection. In severe cases, there may be extensive lymph gland involvement known as lymphogranuloma venereum. *Chlamydia* is one of the leading causes of pelvic inflammatory disease causing tubal scarring and eventual infertility. The disease is treated with azithromycin.

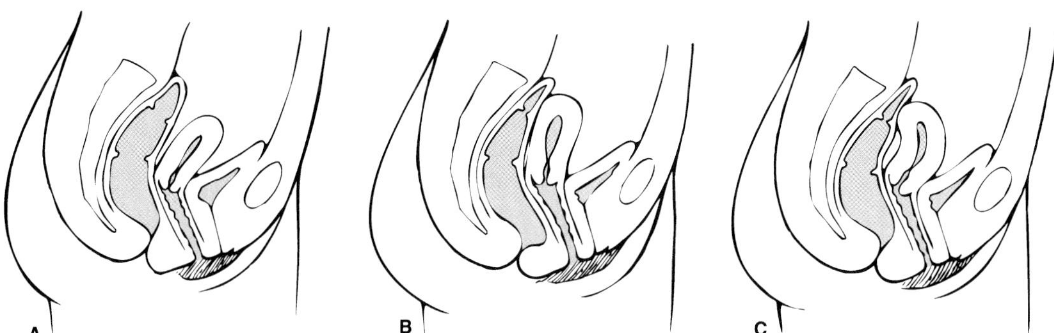

Figure 21-5 Retrodisplacements of the uterus. (A) The normal position of the uterus detected on palpation. (B) In *retroversion* the uterus turns posteriorly as a whole unit. (C) In *retroflexion* the fundus bends posteriorly above the cervical end.

Infants born to mothers with chlamydial infection may present with conjunctivitis and an intractable pneumonia. Many infants will spontaneously abort, deliver prematurely, or be stillborn.

Condylomata Acuminata

Condylomata acuminata is a viral infection of the genital area causing the growth of soft, papillary warts that appear in a wide variety of places, including the vulva, vagina, cervix, and perineum. The etiology is human papillomavirus (HPV). The genital warts usually appear about 3 months after exposure. Biopsy of the condyloma is appropriate to rule out the slight possibility of a malignancy. Although HPV is difficult to eradicate, treatment includes cryotherapy or laser ablation (tissue removal) with moderate success. Genital warts have been implicated in an increase in cervical cancer.

Gonorrhea

Gonorrhea is the second most common STD. The symptoms appear in the genitalia 2 to 8 days after exposure. Bartholin's and Skene's glands fill with pus; the infection also may spread to the cervix. Men develop urethritis with large amounts of pus, but women may be asymptomatic and unaware of the disease. Gonorrhea responds well to penicillin if detected early; however, penicillin-resistant strains are appearing. Intramuscular ceftriaxone sodium (Rocephin) is effective against gonococcus and is usually prescribed to avoid ineffective penicillin therapy. The disease may lead to salpingitis causing scarring and adhesions or pelvic inflammatory disease (see below).

Infants born to mothers infected with gonorrhea may develop a purulent conjunctivitis with corneal ulcerations that result in blindness. All infants are now treated prophylactically in the newborn nursery.

Syphilis

After AIDS, syphilis is the most serious STD. It is caused by a spirochete, *Treponema pallidum*. Symptoms develop with a chancre (an ulcerated skin lesion) at the primary site of infection several days to several weeks after infection. This chancre may not be noticed and heals fairly quickly. The second phase is expressed by a rash anywhere on the body. The patient is infectious at this stage but can be treated with penicillin. If left untreated, syphilis may lie dormant for years until it exacerbates into the third, or tertiary, phase with cardiovascular damage, central nervous system involvement, and death.

Infants born positive for syphilis by transplacental infection are frequently mentally retarded, deaf, blind, or deformed. Many will spontaneously abort or be stillborn.

Herpes Genitalis

Herpes genitalis is characterized by painful, vesicular lesions in the vaginal, vulvular, or anorectal area. This genital infection usually appears within 3 to 7 days after exposure. The vesicles ulcerate and form necrotic craters that eventually heal in about 10 days. The etiology is herpes simplex virus II (HSV II). The virus is almost always sexually transmitted and is diagnosed by obtaining scrapings for **cytology** (cell study). Patients with herpes genitalis should be advised to avoid sexual contact during episodes of vesiculation because the exudate is highly contagious. Although there is no cure, the condition is somewhat controlled with antiviral agents, such as acyclovir.

Infants born vaginally to mothers with active lesions may develop the disease within a few weeks of birth. The virus spreads rapidly to the organs and up to 90% of neonatally infected infants will die.

Salpingitis/Pelvic Inflammatory Disease

Salpingitis is a bacterial infection of the fallopian tubes that is most often transmitted by sexual intercourse. Young sexually active women, women with multiple sexual partners, and women with intrauterine devices are at increased risk of salpingitis. Numerous microorganisms may cause salpingitis, but the more common etiologies include *Neisseria gonorrhoeae, C. trachomatis,* genital mycoplasma, and normal flora bacteria.

Salpingitis is sometimes called pelvic inflammatory disease (PID) when the surrounding structures or tissues are inflamed. With PID, the infection may be found in areas such as the pelvic peritoneum, uterus, ovaries, and surrounding tissues. Symptoms include varying degrees of abdominal pain and tenderness, with or without fever, and **leukocytosis** (abnormal increase in the white blood cell count).

Cultures for gonorrhea and tests for chlamydia are essential for the antibiotic therapy. **Culdocentesis** for culture of purulent discharge may be necessary to determine the exact etiology. Culdocentesis involves the surgical puncture and aspiration of fluid from the vaginal cul-de-sac. A laparoscopy may be performed to determine the extent of the infection.

Treatment for mild infections includes antibiotic and analgesic therapy, bed rest, and removal of an intrauterine device, if present. In patients with **pyosalpinx** (pus in the fallopian tubes), tubal obstruction, abscess, and serious inflammation and edema, treatment may involve a hysterectomy with bilateral salpingo-oophorectomy or incision and drainage via **laparotomy** (incision into the abdominal cavity).

Checkpoint Question

4. *Which sexually transmitted disease is associated with a female reproductive cancer?*

Leiomyomas

Leiomyomas are benign tumors of the uterus, also called fibroids, myomas, or fibromyomas. The tumor may be located in any of the uterine tissue layers: endometrium, myometrium, or perimetrium. The tumors vary greatly in size. Most patients will be asymptomatic. Large tumors tend to distort the uterus, are palpable, and are more likely to be symptomatic. Symptoms may include abnormal bleeding (menorrhagia, metrorrhagia), pelvic pressure and discomfort, constipation, urinary frequency, and infertility.

A presumptive diagnosis is based on patient symptoms and physician assessment that initially includes bimanual examination and sounding of the uterus. Sounding of the uterus requires the physician to do a pelvic examination and insert a uterine sound into the uterine cavity (see Chap. 5, Instruments and Equipment). Obstruction or resistance can be detected that may be due to the tumor pressing in on the uterine cavity. A differential diagnosis to eliminate other conditions includes ruling out pregnancy by testing for HCG in the urine or serum, diagnostic curettage or **hysteroscopy** (visual examination of the uterus with magnification) to rule out a malignancy, and ultrasonography of the uterus.

Treatment of leiomyomas depends on the size of the tumors. Small asymptomatic tumors will need to be monitored for excessive growth. Depending on the patient's age and desire for pregnancy, myomectomy or hysterectomy may be indicated for large tumors or for those with symptoms.

Ovarian Cysts

There are numerous types of ovarian cysts that are benign, including the functional cysts and polycystic ovaries. Functional ovarian cysts are fairly common

Table 21-1 **Cancers of the Female Reproductive System**

Warning Signs	*Risk Factors*	*Early Detection*	*Treatment (Dependent on Involvement)*
Breast Cancer			
Breast changes: lump, pain, thickening, swelling, tenderness, distortion, retraction, dimpling, scaliness	Over age 40 (risk increases with age), history of breast cancer, early menarche, nulliparity, first birth at late age, family history	Monthly self-examination; mammogram by age 40, every 2 years between ages 40 and 49, and every year after age 50 in asymptomatic women	Lumpectomy, mastectomy, radiation therapy, chemotherapy, hormone manipulation therapy
Cervical Cancer			
Often asymptomatic; symptoms, if present, can include irregular bleeding or abnormal vaginal discharge	Intercourse at an early age, multiple sex partners, cigarette smoking, history of certain sexually transmitted diseases, such as human papillomavirus	Annual Pap smears for women over age 18 or who are sexually active; after three consecutive normal smears, Pap smears may be done less often at the physician's discretion	Carcinoma in situ: cryotherapy, electrocoagulation, local excision Metastatic cancer: surgery or radiation therapy or both
Endometrial Cancer			
Irregular bleeding outside of menses, unusual vaginal discharge, excessive bleeding during menstruation, postmenopausal bleeding	Obesity, early menarche, multiple sex partners, late menopause, history of infertility, **anovulation** (not ovulating), unopposed estrogen or tamoxifen therapy, family history of endometrial cancer	Endometrial biopsy at menopause (for high-risk women)	Precancerous changes: progesterone therapy Diagnosed cancer: surgery or radiation therapy or both
Ovarian Cancer			
Often asymptomatic; symptoms, if present, can include abdominal enlargement, vague digestive disorders, discomfort, gas distention	Risk increases with age (especially after age 60), nulliparity, history of breast cancer	Periodic, complete pelvic examination; cancer-related checkup every year after age 40	Surgery, including **oophorectomy** (excision of an ovary), hysterosalpingo-oophorectomy, salpingo-oophorectomy, excision of all intra-abdominal disease; radiation therapy; chemotherapy

and include several types of cysts, one of which is the follicular cyst. This type of cyst is a fluid-filled sac that causes few, if any, problems. The patient is most often asymptomatic unless the cyst is large or if it ruptures or hemorrhages. The functional cysts are usually detected during surgery, and treatment is simply puncture or excision.

In contrast, polycystic ovary syndrome (Stein-Leventhal syndrome) is a more troublesome and complex disorder. It affects both ovaries (bilateral) and is most often found in adolescent girls and young women who have numerous symptoms of an endocrine imbalance. The symptoms are manifested as anovulation, irregular menses or **amenorrhea** (no menses), and **hirsutism** (excessive hair growth). Diagnosis is based on pelvic examination, ultrasonography, laparoscopy, or exploratory laparotomy. Treatment is difficult and depends on the patient's symptoms and desire for pregnancy. Management of this disorder includes hormone therapy or oral contraceptives.

Gynecologic Cancers

The malignant tumors affecting the female reproductive system and their characteristics, diagnosis, and treatment are outlined in Table 21-1. For patient edu-

Why do the Breast Self-Exam?

There are many good reasons for doing a breast self-exam each month. One reason is that it is easy to do and the more you do it, the better you will get at it. When you get to know how your breasts normally feel, you will quickly be able to feel any change, and early detection is the key to successful treatment.

Remember: A breast self-exam could save your breast–and save your life. Most breast lumps are found by women themselves, but in fact, most lumps in the breast are not cancer. Be safe, be sure.

When to do Breast Self-Exam

The best time to do breast self-exam is right after your period, when breasts are not tender or swollen. If you do not have regular periods or sometimes skip a month, do it on the same day every month.

How to do Breast Self-Exam

1. Lie down and put a pillow under your right shoulder. Place your right arm behind your head.
2. Use the finger pads of your three middle fingers on your left hand to feel for lumps or thickening. Your finger pads are the top third of each finger.
3. Press firmly enough to know how your breast feels. If you're not sure how hard to press, ask your health care provider. Or try to copy the way your health care provider uses the finger pads during a breast exam. Learn what your breast feels like most of the time. A firm ridge in the lower curve of each breast is normal.
4. Move around the breast in a set way. You can choose either the circle (**A**), the up and down (**B**), or the wedge (**C**). Do it the same way every time. It will help you to make sure that you've gone over the entire breast area, and to remember how your breast feels.
5. Now examine your left breast using right hand finger pads.
6. Repeat the examination of both breasts while standing, with one arm behind your head. The upright position makes it easier to check the upper and outer part of the breasts (toward your armpit). You may want to do the standing part of the BSE while you are in the shower. Some breast changes can be felt more easily when your skin is wet and soapy.

For added safety, you can also check your breasts for any dimpling of the skin, changes in the nipple, redness, or swelling while standing in front of a mirror right after your BSE each month.

If you find any changes, see your doctor right away.

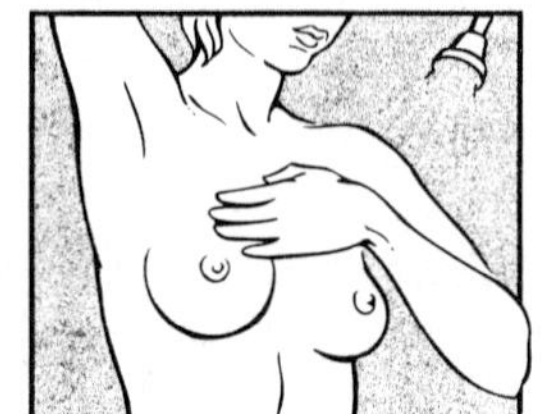

Figure 21-6 Following these steps, any woman can perform a breast self-examination. *Note:* Women should have regular mammograms in addition to performing monthly breast self-examinations. (Courtesy of the American Cancer Society.)

cation, medical assistants need to be aware of the American Cancer Society's recommendations regarding the frequency of pelvic and breast examinations and Pap smears. The prognosis of all cancers is directly related to early diagnosis and treatment.

Have available and accessible brochures and literature on the various types of cancers. This information can be obtained from the American Cancer Society, which is listed in your local telephone directory.

Cervical and breast cancers have an excellent prognosis when detected and treated early. Medical assistants should instruct patients on breast self-examination to be performed every month (Fig. 21-6).

Also encourage patients to schedule regular annual visits for a complete physical with a thorough pelvic examination that includes the Papanicolaou (Pap) smear. The Pap smear is a screening test for the early detection of cancer (Table 21-2). The procedure for the Pap smear involves scraping cells from the cervix, endocervix, or vagina for microscopic examination (see Procedure 21-1, Assisting With the Pelvic Examination With Pap Smear).

Initially the abnormal growth of the cancerous cells in the cervix is asymptomatic and therefore patients should be encouraged to come regularly for a Pap smear. The Pap smear grades the abnormal growth according to the tissue involvement. Abnormal growth patterns in the epithelium of the cervix is called cervical intraepithelial neoplasia (CIN). The degree of abnormal growth is graded (usually mild, moderate, severe, and carcinoma in situ or class I, II, III, IV, V; see Table 21-2). Carcinoma in situ means that the malignant cells have invaded the entire tissue, but have not become invasive to the surrounding structures. CIN is diagnosed by the Pap smear and further evaluated by **colposcopy** (visualization of the vagina and cervix under magnification) and biopsy.

Infertility

Female infertility is more difficult to diagnose than male infertility. Most testing begins by eliminating the man as the responsible party, then concentrates on the woman. Testing is not usually attempted until 1 year of unprotected intercourse without conception.

The causes may include uterine or cervical abnormalities, tubal occlusion or scarring, a hormonal imbalance that interferes with LH or FSH resulting in anovulation or poor ova production, or psychological factors. Diagnosis requires a complete history and physical examination. An endometrial biopsy will diagnose anovulation, progesterone blood levels may indicate hormonal deficiencies, and a hysterosalpingography will indicate tubal occlusion or uterine abnormalities. Treatment includes identifying and correcting the problem.

Table 21-2 **Classifications of Papanicolaou Tests**

Class	*Characteristics*
I	Normal test, no atypical cells
II	Atypical cells but no evidence of malignancy
III	Atypical cells, possible but not conclusive for malignancy
IV	Cells strongly suggestive of malignancy
V	Strong evidence of malignancy

Checkpoint Question

5. *What two factors greatly affect the prognosis of all cancers?*

COMMON GYNECOLOGIC TESTS AND THERAPEUTIC PROCEDURES AND THE MEDICAL ASSISTANT'S ROLE

The Gynecologic Examination

As part of the gynecologic examination, the physician will examine the patient's breasts, perform a pelvic examination, and obtain a Pap smear. Because of the risk of contracting infection from body fluids, especially blood, the medical assistant, the physician, and others having direct contact with the patient must observe Standard Precautions and wear protective barriers as appropriate.

Breast Examination

The physician usually begins the examination by examining the breasts with the patient in a sitting position to check for dimpling or size disparity. The patient will then lie back on the table. The physician then systematically palpates all breast tissue, including areas such as the axillae and the tissue up to the clavicle to assess the lymph nodes that lead from the mammary area.

Pelvic Examination With Pap Smear

The purpose of the pelvic examination with Pap smear is to assess the female genitalia and to identify or diagnose any abnormal conditions (see Procedure 21-1). When scheduling an appointment for a pelvic examination, instruct the patient not to douche, use vaginal medication, or have sexual intercourse within 24 hours before the examination. If a Pap smear is also to be performed, schedule the appointment for about 1 week after menses.

21

When preparing for the pelvic examination, ensure that the vaginal speculum is warm and is the correct size for the patient. Warm the speculum by running it under warm water or by storing it on an electric heating pad set on a low setting. Selecting an appropriate vaginal speculum is important to maintain the patient's comfort and to facilitate the examination. Although the patient's age and size are the primary factors, the largest speculum that is comfortable for the patient will provide the best visibility. Two different sizes may be set out to give the physician a choice. Vaginal specula come in pediatric, small, medium, and large sizes; the manufacturers of specula also vary in that some make longer, more narrow specula. A wide variety of sizes should be available in each examination room.

Try to allow plenty of time with the patient to establish rapport, especially with new patients and patients with special needs (young, elderly, adolescents, disabled, distressed). If the procedure is rushed or seems hurried to the patient, it will affect the professional image of the office and the patient's attitude toward the physician and staff.

What If?

The first Pap smear or gynecologic examination for young women may cause great anxiety. What if an 18-year-old is to have her first Pap smear today? How should you handle the situation?

Bring the patient into the room and encourage her to talk about her feelings. Do not have her change into an examining gown until she has had an opportunity to speak to the physician or practitioner about the procedure. If the patient's mother is present, ask her to follow her daughter's wishes about remaining in the room. (Some young women want their mothers present and others will not.) You are more likely to be given an accurate sexual history if the mother is not present. The physician will require the presence of another health care worker during the examination; this will give you an opportunity to provide reassurance and patient education.

Although the dorsal lithotomy position provides the best visibility for the physician, the position may be difficult for elderly and some disabled persons to maintain. Elevating the head of the table to 30 degrees may be easier for the patient and allows the physician to make eye contact. The elevation of the table does not seem to have any disadvantages, and often the patient finds the position more comfortable. If elevating the head of the table is not appropriate, then an alternative position, such as Sims', may be necessary. Consult with the physician about patient positioning if the lithotomy position is not possible or desirable.

Checkpoint Question

6. *What procedures does the physician perform as part of a complete gynecologic examination?*

Colposcopy

Colposcopy is the visual examination of the vaginal and cervical surfaces with the use of a stereoscopic microscope called the colposcope. It is often performed to evaluate patients with abnormal cell studies; to locate the origin of abnormal cells; to select areas for cervical, endocervical, or endometrial biopsy; to assess tissue with cervical lesions; for an atypical Pap smear; or for follow-up with history of cervical dysplasia or cervical cancer.

If a biopsy is to be done, be sure that a written, informed consent has been obtained. When possible, label specimen containers and complete laboratory request forms before the procedure. The completed forms and labeled containers should be retained in the patient examination room until the specimen is obtained.

Although there is usually very little, if any, bleeding, have available silver nitrate or Monsel's solution, either of which controls bleeding by chemical cautery. The patient preparation for colposcopy with cervical biopsy is similar to that required for the pelvic examination (Procedure 21-2).

Culdocentesis

Culdocentesis is the surgical puncture of the vaginal cul-de-sac and aspiration of fluid from the abdominal cavity. A culdocentesis is often done to diagnose PID or ruptured ectopic pregnancy.

Hysterosalpingography

The hysterosalpingography is a diagnostic procedure in which the uterus and uterine tubes are radiographed after the injection of a contrast medium. The radiograph is called a **hysterosalpingogram.** The test is often performed to determine the configuration of the uterus and the patency of the uterine tubes for fertility purposes.

Laparoscopy

Abdominal and pelvic structures can be visualized directly by inserting a lighted scope into the abdominal

text continues on page 469

21

Procedure 21-1 Assisting With a Pelvic Examination With a Pap Smear

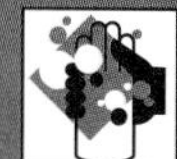
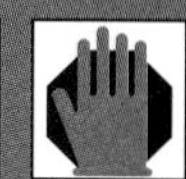
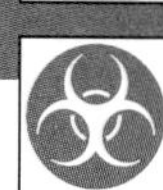

PURPOSE

To assess the health status of the internal female genitalia
To obtain a specimen for cytology study of the cervical and vaginal cells

EQUIPMENT/SUPPLIES

- patient drape
- vaginal speculum, appropriate size
- uterine sponge forceps
- cotton-tipped applicators, long
- water-soluble lubricant
- direct lighting
- cleansing tissues or personal wipes
- biohazard barrier devices, as appropriate
- materials for Pap smear—cervical spatula or cervical brush, glass slides, fixative solution (spray or liquid), laboratory request form, identification label

STEPS

1. Wash your hands.
2. Assemble the equipment and supplies.
3. Label and date each slide.
   Accurate identification of all specimens is critical to an accurate diagnosis.
4. Complete the laboratory request form for Pap smear with essential information, including the date, patient's name, age, first day of last menstrual period, relevant history, physician, and your signature.
   Complete and accurate patient information is essential to the interpretation of the laboratory report.
5. Greet and identify the patient. Explain the procedure.
6. Ask the patient to empty her bladder and if necessary collect a urine specimen.
   An empty bladder makes the examination more comfortable for the patient and helps her relax.
7. Provide the patient with a drape, and ask her to disrobe from the waist down.
   Providing concise instructions reduces anxiety because the patient knows exactly what is expected.
8. Position the patient in the dorsal lithotomy position with buttocks at the bottom edge of the table.
   Correct positioning facilitates the procedure.
9. Adjust the drape to cover the patient's abdomen and knees, exposing only the genitalia.
   Adequately draping the patient will help her relax and will ensure her privacy.
10. Adjust the light over the genitalia for maximum visibility.
    Good visibility is essential for a thorough examination.
11. Assist the physician with the examination by handing instruments and supplies as needed. Place the spatula firmly in the physician's hand in a functional position.
    Anticipating the physician's needs during the procedure will aid in a more thorough and efficient examination.

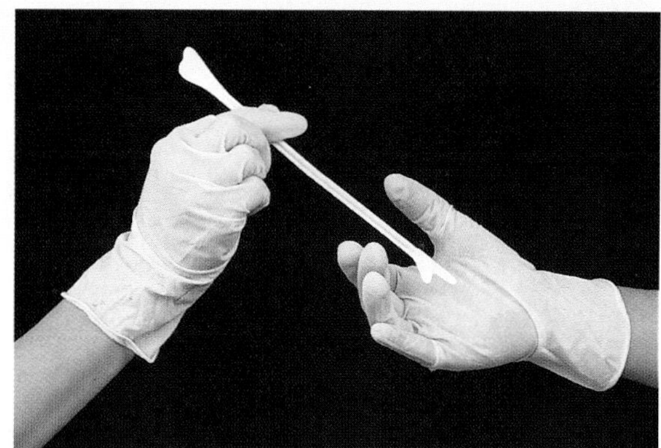

12. Hold the microscopic slides by the frosted ends while the physician is obtaining and making the vaginal and endocervical smears.

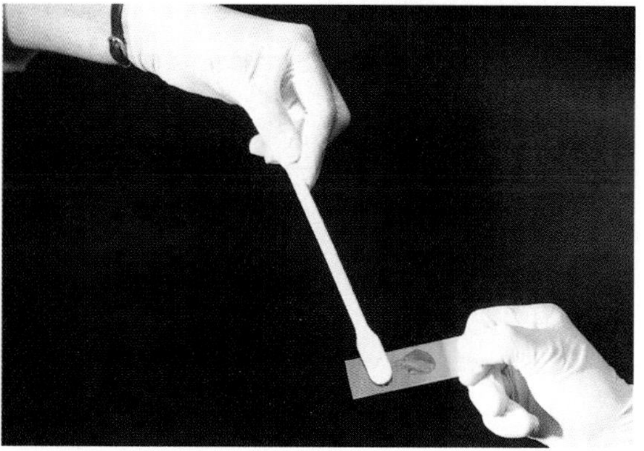

continued

21

Procedure 21-1 Continued Assisting With a Pelvic Examination With a Pap Smear

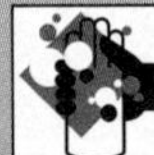
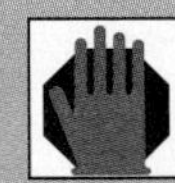

13. Spray each slide with fixative or immerse each slide in a fixative solution.

When performing a Pap smear, a fixative spray or solution is necessary to preserve the cervical and vaginal scrapings for cytology.

14. Explain to the patient that the physician will now remove the vaginal speculum and do a bimanual examination of the pelvis.

The patient will be more relaxed and cooperative if she is informed of each step.

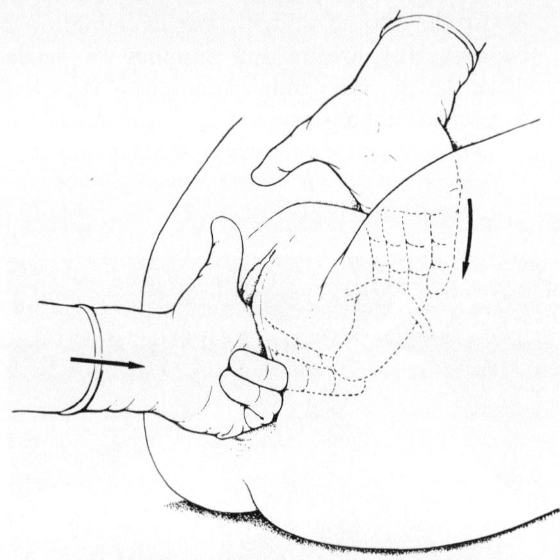

15. Hold a basin for receiving the now contaminated vaginal speculum. Place the speculum in a basin of cold water to begin sanitization.

All equipment must be cared for properly. Soaking the speculum now will make it easier to clean for sanitization.

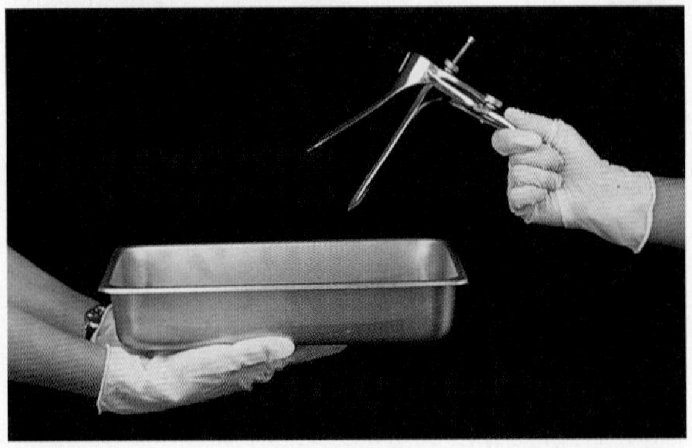

16. Apply about 1 to 2 inches of water-soluble lubricant across the physician's two gloved fingers.

Water-soluble lubricant helps make the manual examination more comfortable.

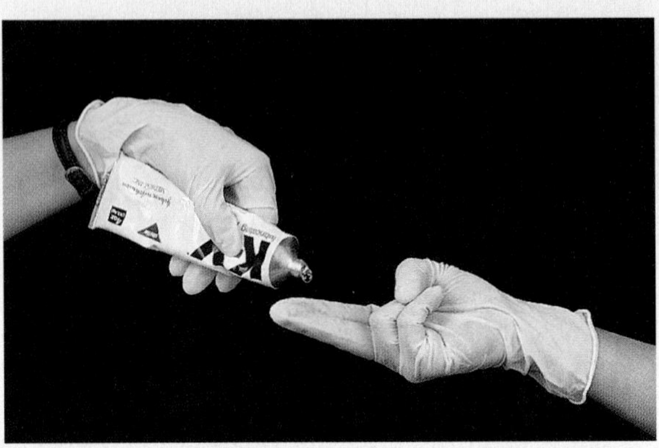

17. After completion of the examination, assist the patient in sliding up to the top of the examination table.

Patient injury can be avoided if the patient first moves back up the table before removing feet from the stirrups.

18. Assist the patient in removing both feet at the same time from the stirrups. Help the patient to remove excess lubricant by handing her a personal wipe or tissues.

Removing both feet at the same time puts less strain on the patient's back. Excess lubricant can be uncomfortable for the patient.

19. Package the specimen for transport to the laboratory.

Special packaging is required for safe transportation or mailing to the laboratory.

20. Provide for privacy while the patient is dressing.

The patient is entitled to respect and privacy.

21. Thank the patient. Reinforce the physician's instructions about follow-up. Address any concerns or questions.

Courtesy encourages the patient to have a positive attitude about the physician's office. For quality management, let the patient know when to schedule follow-ups and when and how laboratory results will be obtained.

22. Properly care for or dispose of equipment. Clean the examination room. Wash your hands.

continued

21

Procedure 21-1 Continued Assisting With a Pelvic Examination With Pap Smear

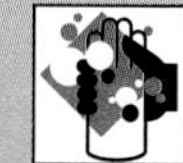
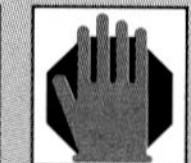
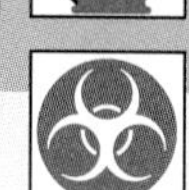

DOCUMENTATION GUIDELINES

- Date and time
- Patient preparation
- Patient complaints/concerns
- Patient education/instructions
- Routing of specimen
- Your signature

Charting Example

DATE	TIME
	S: "I am here to see Dr. Jacobs for my
	annual Pap smear."
	O: 36-year-old para 3, gravida 3. U/A neg.
	Pt positioned and draped for
	Dr. Jacobs.
	A: Routine Pap smear.
	P: Pap smear to laboratory. Pt educated
	regarding the result notification.
	—Your signature

Procedure 21-2 Assisting With Colposcopy With Cervical Biopsy

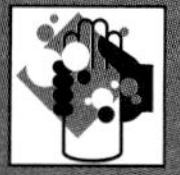
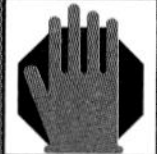
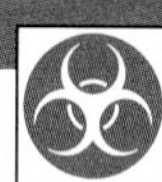

PURPOSE

To provide direct and magnified visual examination of the cervix
To facilitate biopsy of the cervix

EQUIPMENT/SUPPLIES

- setup for pelvic examination
- colposcope
- specimen container with preservative (10% formalin)
- sterile gloves
- povidone-iodine (Betadine)
- sanitary napkin, mini pad, or tampon
- biohazard barrier devices, as appropriate
- silver nitrate sticks or ferric subsulfate (Monsel's solution)

On the Sterile Field

- long cotton applicators, sterile
- normal saline solution
- 3% acetic acid or vinegar
- uterine dressing forceps
- sterile 4 × 4 gauze
- sterile towel

Sterile Materials for Cervical Biopsy

- biopsy forceps or punch
- uterine curet
- endocervical curet
- uterine tenaculum

STEPS

1. Verify that the patient has signed the consent form.
   Colposcopy with biopsy is an invasive procedure that requires written consent.
2. Wash your hands.
3. Assemble the equipment and supplies.

continued

21

Procedure 21-2 Continued **Assisting With Colposcopy With Cervical Biopsy**

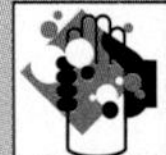
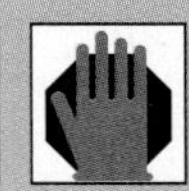
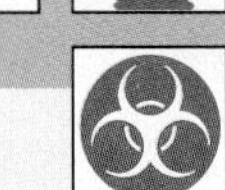

4. Check the light on the colposcope.
Properly functioning equipment is crucial to the quality of the examination.

5. Set up the sterile field.
A biopsy is an invasive procedure requiring surgical asepsis.

6. Pour normal saline and acetic acid into their respective sterile containers. Cover the field with a sterile drape.
These solutions are critical to the examination of the cervix. The field must be covered to maintain sterility as you prepare the patient.

7. Greet and identify the patient. Explain the procedure. Caution the patient that there may be a sharp cramp at the time of biopsy. Have the patient disrobe from the waist down and cover with a privacy drape.

8. Position the patient in the dorsal lithotomy position. *Note:* If you are to assist the physician from the sterile field, put on sterile gloves now and assist as follows.
Correct positioning is necessary to visualize the cervix properly.

9. Hand the physician the applicator immersed in normal saline, followed by the applicator immersed in acetic acid.
Acetic acid swabbed on the area improves visualization and aids in identifying suspicious tissue.

10. Hand the physician the applicator with the antiseptic solution (Betadine).
An antiseptic solution is used to prevent contaminating the area to be biopsied.

11. If you did not glove to assist the physician, put on nonsterile gloves before accepting the specimen.
The specimen is potentially hazardous; therefore, you must use Standard Precautions.

12. Receive the tissue specimen by holding the container of 10% formalin in which the specimen can be immersed.
For proper preservation, the specimen must be immediately immersed in a preservative.

13. Label the specimen container with the patient's name, date, and medical record number.
The specimen must be properly identified.

14. Prepare the specimen for transport to the laboratory/pathology.
The specimen must be transported in appropriate packaging to ensure its integrity.

15. Provide the physician with Monsel's solution or silver nitrate sticks, if necessary.
If bleeding occurs, a coagulant may need to be applied.

16. Explain to the patient that a small amount of bleeding may occur. Have a sanitary pad available.
Bleeding with a cervical biopsy is usually minimal, and a small sanitary pad should be sufficient.

17. Thank the patient. Reinforce the physician's instructions.
Courtesy encourages the patient to have a positive attitude about the physician's office. Instruct the patient regarding biopsy results and scheduling a follow-up visit.

18. Properly care for or dispose of equipment and supplies. Clean the examination room. Wash your hands.

DOCUMENTATION GUIDELINES

- Date and time
- Verification of consent
- Patient preparation
- Patient complaints/concerns
- Patient education/instructions
- Routing of specimen as needed
- Your signature

Charting Example

DATE	TIME Informed consent signed by pt.
	Pt positioned and draped for colposcopy.
	Colposcopy performed by Dr. Davis.
	Minimal bleeding. Cervical biopsy sent to
	Central Path Lab. —Your signature

cavity through a small incision. For better access to the pelvic organs, carbon dioxide or other gas is injected to expand the abdominal walls and intestines away from the organs. Endometriosis, ectopic pregnancies, and tumors are a few of the disorders that may be diagnosed by laparoscopy. This is the method of choice for tubal ligation, the female sterilization procedure. Figure 21-7 illustrates the laparoscopic procedure for tubal ligation covered later in this chapter.

The medical assistant would require extensive training in an outpatient surgical unit to assist with this procedure. In most instances, you are more likely to assist with patient preparation, such as signing consents or relaying preoperative and postoperative instructions.

Dilatation and Curettage (D & C)

A D & C may be performed to remove uterine tissue for diagnostic testing, to reduce endometrial tissue, to prevent or treat menorrhagia (excessive menstrual flow), or to remove retained products of conception. The cervical canal will be widened with a uterine sound, and the lining will be scraped with a curet (see Chap. 5, Instruments and Equipment). This procedure usually requires anesthesia and will be performed as an inpatient procedure or as an outpatient procedure in a day surgery unit. The patient must sign all preoperative consents, but no specific preoperative preparation is required. The patient will need a perineal pad, light postoperative analgesia, and instructions regarding signs of infection, hemorrhage, and follow-up care.

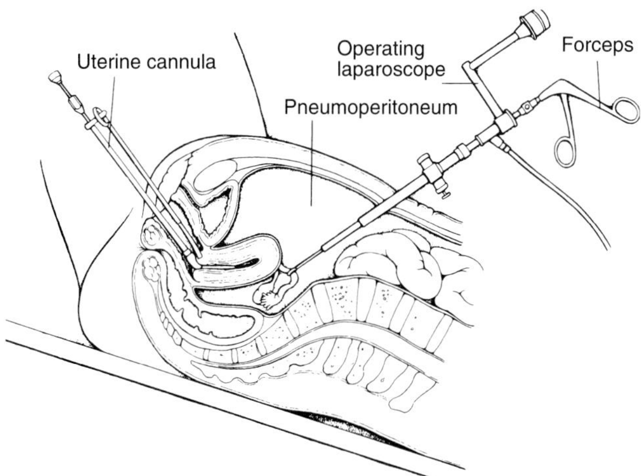

Figure 21-7 Laparoscopy. The laparoscope (*right*) is inserted through a small incision in the abdomen. A forceps is inserted through the scope to grasp the fallopian tube. To improve the view, a uterine cannula (*left*) is inserted into the vaginal to push the uterus upward. Insufflation of gas creates an air pocket (pneumoperitoneum), and the pelvis is raised (note the angle), which forces the intestines higher in the abdomen.

Your responsibility will probably be limited to patient preparation and patient education as directed by your physician.

OBSTETRIC CARE

Unlike other physicians, obstetricians are often at the hospital delivering infants during regular office hours. If you are assisting in an obstetric practice, you must use good judgment when pregnant patients present or call with questions and concerns. For instance, you will have to determine if the situation can wait for the physician's return, if another physician should be consulted, if the patient should go to the emergency room, or if you can, with the physician's permission, advise the patient on how to manage the problem. Protocol listed in the policy and procedure manual for action to be taken in specific situations will ensure that, in the physician's absence, safe procedures will be followed for your patients and will protect you and your physician from errors in treatment.

Diagnosis of Pregnancy

Many patients suspect that they are pregnant (**gravid**) because of the symptoms they are experiencing. However, these early symptoms of pregnancy may be indicative of other disorders, as noted above. Therefore, the early symptoms are called presumptive signs and symptoms of pregnancy, meaning that the pregnancy must still be confirmed by more conclusive diagnostic procedures. The presumptive symptoms include amenorrhea, nausea and vomiting, breast enlargement and tenderness, fatigue, and urinary frequency. Other more probable signs and symptoms of pregnancy include presence of HCG in the maternal urine or serum, enlargement of the abdomen, changes in the uterus and cervix, and occurrence of **Braxton Hicks** uterine contractions.

Early in pregnancy, the patient may notice irregular uterine contractions that occur fairly frequently. These contractions, called Braxton Hicks contractions, do not affect the cervix like the contractions of active labor and are normal for pregnancy. Although the patient may or may not be aware of the contractions, the physician can palpate the contractions during a bimanual examination or by palpating the uterus from the abdomen.

Cervical changes that occur during pregnancy include softening of the cervix (**Goodell's sign**); increased vascularity of the cervix causing the cervix, vulva, and vagina to develop a bluish violet color (**Chadwick's sign**); and formation of a mucous plug. The mucous plug forms in the cervical os and protects the developing fetus and the amniotic sac from the external envi-

21

Table 21-3 **Signs and Symptoms of Pregnancy**

Presumptive Signs	*Probable Signs*	*Conclusive Signs*
Cessation of menses	HCG present in urine and serum	Presence of fetal heart tones
Nausea and vomiting	Braxton Hicks contractions	Fetal movement detected by the examiner
Breast tenderness	Enlargement of abdomen	Visualization of the fetus
Breast enlargement	Uterine changes	
Quickening or fetal movement felt by the patient	Goodell's sign	
Fatigue	Chadwick's sign	
Urinary frequency		

ronment. With the onset of labor, the mucous plug is expelled with a small amount of blood and is often referred to as the "bloody show."

The diagnosis of pregnancy is actually confirmed by the presence of fetal heart tones and fetal movement detected by the physician or the visual image of a fetus on ultrasonography (Table 21-3). Box 21-3 describes the process of fertilization, implantation, and gestation.

Box 21-3
Fertilization, Implantation, and Gestation

Although only one ovum is needed for conception, many spermatozoa are required to erode the ovum cell membrane to allow the entry of one sperm for fertilization. Fertilization usually occurs in the fallopian tube. At that point, the male and female gametes become a zygote, or fertilized egg. Because sperm and ova each bring to the union 23 chromosomes, the zygote will have 46, or 23 pairs. Sex is determined at this union.

Cell division begins immediately. By the fifth or sixth day, the zygote has traveled by ciliary movement of the fallopian lining to the uterus, and implantation begins with the finger-like chorionic villi grasping and burrowing into the endometrium, resulting in a normal **intrauterine pregnancy (IUP).** Enzymes are secreted by the zygote to help gain access to the endometrial wall, which has been prepared by estrogen and progesterone to receive the egg. Estrogen and progesterone stay high to maintain the endometrium; no more follicles will mature during the pregnancy.

From the second to the eighth week of gestation, the developing offspring is called an embryo. From the eighth week to birth, it is referred to as a fetus. The amniotic sac is formed to protect and hydrate the fetus. The placenta acts as an organ of exchange for nutrients from the mother and wastes from the fetus. The umbilical cord attaches the placenta to the embryo. The average gestation takes between 266 and 280 days, which equals 38 to 40 weeks, or about 10 lunar months or 9 calendar months. (See the section "Obstetric Care.")

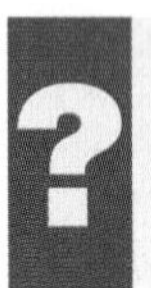

Checkpoint Question

7. *Why are presumptive signs and symptoms of pregnancy not considered to be conclusive?*

First Prenatal Visit

The pregnant patient's initial prenatal visit is extensive and critical to the ongoing assessment of the pregnancy. A thorough and detailed history of the patient must be obtained (Box 21-4). To elicit the most complete and accurate information, the health history interview should be conducted in a private room where there will be no interruptions.

The first prenatal visit includes the confirmation of pregnancy, complete history and physical, establishment of the EDC or EDD, assessment of gestational age, identifying risk factors, and patient education. The EDC or EDD is a prediction of the "due date," assuming the pregnancy progresses normally (Box 21-5). Normal gestation is 37 to 41 weeks. Infants born before the 37th week are considered to be premature; those born after the 41st week are postmature.

The complete physical examination includes a pelvic examination with Pap smear and cultures for gonorrhea and chlamydia, pregnancy test, clinical pelvimetry, complete blood count, blood glucose, blood type and Rh factor, antibody screen, urinalysis, human immunodeficiency virus (HIV) screen and serologic tests for syphilis and rubella and hepatitis B virus (HBV). The medical assistant should reinforce the physician's instructions to the patient and encourage patients to call the office if they have further questions or concerns.

Patients should be instructed to notify the physician or medical assistant if any of the following occur:

- Vaginal bleeding or spotting
- Persistent vomiting
- Fever or chills

Box 21-4
Parity Versus Gravidity

The prenatal history must include information regarding previous pregnancies to help predict the outcome of the current pregnancy.

The term **parity** refers to the number of live births, and **gravidity** refers to any pregnancy, regardless of its length and outcome. The pregnant, or **gravid,** woman is termed a **gravida,** usually with an indicator of the number, such as **primigravida** (first pregnancy), **secundigravida** (second pregnancy), and so forth to **multigravida** (many pregnancies). A woman who has never been pregnant is a **nulligravida.** The number of live births is also given a prefix indicator, such as **nullipara** (has never borne a living child), **primipara** (first living child), and so forth to **multipara** with many live births.

These numbers are listed for the physician's review as gr (or simply g), p, pret (preterm or premature), and ab (abortion, spontaneous or induced). For example, a woman who is pregnant for the third time, has lost no pregnancies, and carried her previous pregnancies to term is listed:

gr iii, pret 0, ab 0, p ii

(Arabic numbers are acceptable also.)

A woman who is pregnant for the fifth time and who has delivered one set of twins, two single infants, has had no premature infants, and has lost one pregnancy spontaneously would be listed:

gr v, pret 0, ab i, p iv

- Dysuria
- Abdominal or uterine cramping
- Leaking amniotic fluid
- Altered fetal movement
- Dizziness or blurred vision
- Other problems

Understanding Fetotoxic and Teratogenic Factors

Certain factors can put the developing fetus at risk for problems. Depending on the severity of the factor, fetal development may be so altered as to be incompatible with life; such factors are referred to as *fetotoxic.* Fetuses not spontaneously aborted are stillborn or die soon after birth in the event of fetotoxicity. Certain factors disrupt development, causing abnormalities but not death; these factors are referred to as *teratogenic* (*terato* is the word root for monster and *genic* means to form or begin). The stage of greatest danger ranges from about the 3rd to the 12th week of development, a time at which many women are not yet aware they are pregnant.

Advise the pregnant patient against taking any medications or drugs (even over-the-counter preparations) without consulting the physician. The patient also should avoid smoking cigarettes and drinking alcoholic beverages. Evidence indicates that nicotine, alcohol, certain medications (Box 21-6), and other factors (Box 21-7) are harmful to the developing fetus.

Box 21-5
Determining the Estimated Date of Confinement or the Expected Date of Delivery

The estimated date of confinement (EDC) is frequently referred to as the expected date of delivery (EDD). Because of the negative connotations of "confinement" and because women are no longer "confined" during pregnancy or the postpartum period, terminology for the due date is changing somewhat to reflect current maternity trends. Many methods are used for determining this projected date. Nägele's rule requires a mathematical calculation using the following formula:

The first day of the last menstrual period (LMP) + 7 days −3 months + 1 year. Example: LMP = May 3, 1996

5	3	96	(LMP)
−3	+7	+1	(Nägele's rule)
2	10	97	(EDD)

A simpler method involves adding 9 months and 7 days to the first day of the LMP. Try that method with the example above.

The third common method is to use one of the various gestational wheels available. Using the inner wheel, line up the first day of the LMP on the outer wheel with the appropriate arrow, and read around the wheel to the indicated milestones in the pregnancy. Many wheels will indicate the date of conception, times recommended for blood work and other testing, and all will work toward the date that delivery is expected.

More reliable dates are determined by quickening, uterine size and growth, and ultrasound.

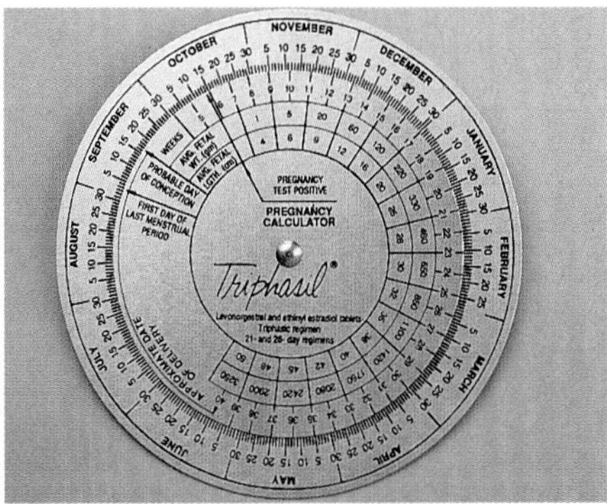

Gestational wheel

Box 21-6
Classifying Drugs That May Harm the Developing Fetus

Many of the medications that might be beneficial to the mother may be dangerous to the developing fetus. The Food and Drug Administration has issued a list of categories (A, B, C, D, and X) used for classifying drugs that are dangerous to the fetus. These categories are listed on sources of drug information (eg, the *Physician's Desk Reference,* package inserts) and are based on animal and human research during the development of the drug.

A—Research indicates that there is probably no risk at any point in the pregnancy.
B—Animal research indicates no fetal risk but human studies are not complete.
C—Research on animals shows this drug to be a danger. Human studies are inconclusive, or no studies are available.
D—There is clear precedence for risk, but the drug may be used if there is no substitute.
X—There is clear evidence of risk, and the drug should not be used by pregnant women.

Assisting With the First Prenatal Examination

The first prenatal examination establishes a detailed baseline of the patient's current physical condition. It includes a complete physical examination with a pelvic examination and additional screening tests.

In addition to the routine steps of a complete physical examination, the first prenatal visit will require:

- Blood work—Venereal Disease Research Laboratory (VDRL), Rapid Plasma Reagin (RPR), or other test for syphilis, complete blood count with hematocrit, hemoglobin, white blood cell count with differential, blood type with Rh factor, antibody screen, and other tests as necessary
- Tuberculosis screening—tine test or purified protein derivative injection
- Urinalysis—glucose, albumin, and acetone testing
- Smears for *Neisseria gonorrhoeae,* chlamydial infection, and cancer

Subsequent Prenatal Visits

If the pregnancy is progressing as expected and without complications (Fig. 21-8), the patient should be scheduled at 12, 16, 20, 24, and 28 weeks of gestation. The patient is usually seen every 2 weeks during the last 2 months and once a week after the 36th week of

Box 21-7
Other Risk Factors for Fetal Abnormalities

Factors other than medications may result in damage to the fetus. These include inadequate oxygen to the fetus, radiation, and disease processes. The effect on the fetus depends on the degree of exposure and fetal age at the time of exposure. A few of the more commonly encountered risk factors and their effects are listed below.

Risk Factor	*Effects*
Syphilis	Structural deformities, blindness, deafness, fetal death
Alcohol (fetal alcohol syndrome)	Craniofacial and limb defects, intrauterine growth retardation (IUGR), retarded development
Diethylstilbesterol (DES) (used to prevent threatened spontaneous abortions)	Implicated in reproductive cancers; children of DES mothers may present with ovarian and cervical cancer or testicular cancer
Heavy metals (eg, lead and mercury)	Potentially fetotoxic; both lead and mercury cause physical and mental retardation and a galaxy of related deformities and central nervous system disorders
Toxoplasmosis (protozoal infection spread by cat feces)	Fetotoxic to teratogenic with microcephaly, hydrocephaly, mental and growth retardation
Rubella	Central nervous system involvement, blindness, deafness, cardiac abnormalities
Cytomegalovirus	Fetotoxic to teratogenic with hydrocephaly, mental and growth retardation
Herpes	Infants delivered during active outbreak may develop central nervous system involvement that may lead to neonatal death.

(The last four risk factors, with the addition of "other," form a complex referred to as TORCH. Any of the group may cause many severe pregnancy and fetal difficulties. Testing will be done to evaluate TORCH titers to identify the causative agent.)

*Fetal Development**

1st Lunar Month

The embryo is 4 to 5mm in length.

Trophoblasts embed in decidua.

Chorionic villi form.

Foundations for nervous system, genitourinary system, skin, bones, and lungs are formed.

Buds of arms and legs begin to form.

Rudiments of eyes, ears, and nose appear.

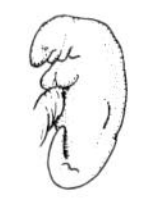

4 weeks

2nd Lunar Month

The fetus is 27 to 31 mm in length and weighs 2 to 4g.

Fetus is markedly bent.

Head is disproportionately large as a result of brain development.

Sex differentiation begins.

Centers of bone begin to ossify.

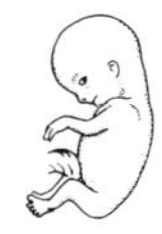

8 weeks

3rd Lunar Month

The fetus average length is 6 to 9 cm, and weight is 45 g.

Fingers and toes are distinct

Placenta is complete.

Fetal circulation is complete.

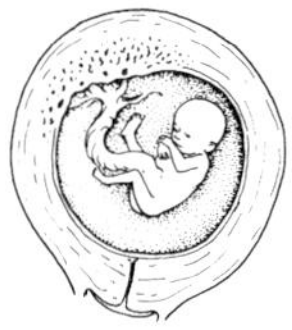

3 months

4th Lunar Month

The fetus is 12 cm in length and weighs 110 g.

Sex is differentiated.

Rudimentary kidneys secrete urine.

Heartbeat is present.

Nasal septum and palate close.

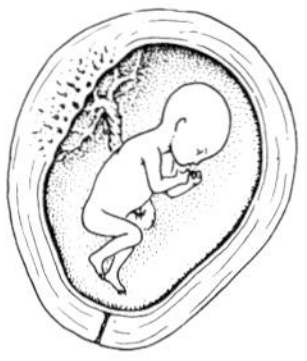

4 months

5th Lunar Month

The fetus is 19 cm in length and weighs approximately 300 g.

Lanugo covers entire body.

Fetal movements are felt by mother.

Heart sounds are perceptible by auscultation.

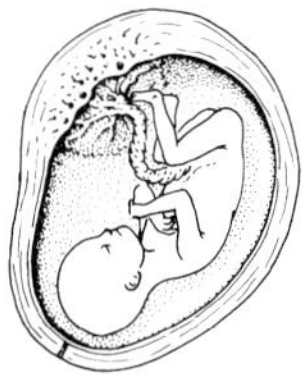

5 months

6th Lunar Month

The fetus is about 23 cm in length and weighs 630 g.

Skin appears wrinkled.

Vernix caseosa appears.

Eyebrows and fingernails develop.

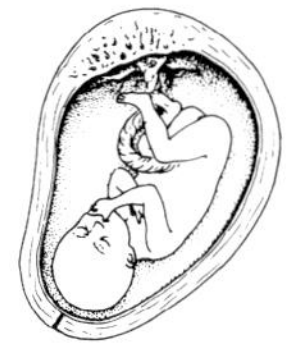

6 months

7th Lunar Month

The fetus is 27 cm in length and weighs about 1100 g.

Skin is red.

Pupillary membrane disappears from eyes.

The fetus has an excellent chance of survival.

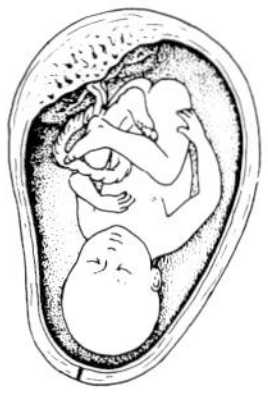

7 months

8th Lunar Month

The fetus is 28 to 30 cm in length and weighs 1.8 kg.

Fetus is viable.

Eyelids open.

Fingerprints are set.

Vigorous fetal movement occurs.

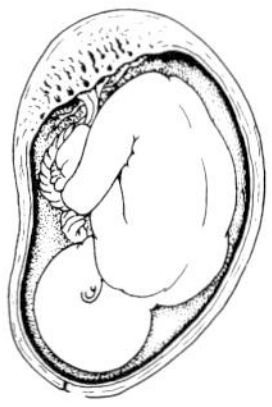

8 months

9th Lunar Month

The fetus' average length is 32 cm; weight is about 2500 g.

Face and body have a loose wrinkled appearance because of subcutaneous fat deposit.

Lanugo disappears.

Amniotic fluid decreases.

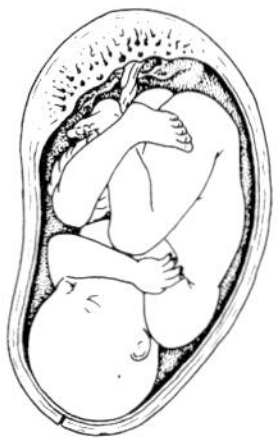

9 months

10th Lunar Month

The average fetus is 36 cm in length and weighs 3000 to 3600 g.

Skin is smooth.

Eyes are uniformly slate colored.

Bones of skull are ossified and nearly together at sutures.

* All lengths given are crown to rump.

Figure 21-8 Fetal development.

gestation. Of course, this schedule should be altered according to the patient's condition.

Table 21-4 outlines the specific examination and procedures to be performed during subsequent prenatal visits. This table is useful in knowing how to prepare the room and patient.

Assisting With Subsequent Prenatal Visits

Subsequent prenatal visits are scheduled to assess the fetal growth and development and the maternal health throughout the pregnancy. As the pregnancy progresses, the patient is always at risk of supine hypotension. Supine hypotension is the result of the fetus resting on the mother's aorta and vena cava when she is flat on her back. The weight of the uterus compresses these major vessels and restricts the blood flow, causing a drop in the maternal blood pressure. The patient may become pale, clammy, and breathless; the fetal heart rate may drop. Immediately turn the patient onto her left side to relieve the compression.

21

Table 21-4 **Schedule of Return Prenatal Visits**

First through sixth month—visits once per month
Seventh and eight months—visits every 2 weeks
Ninth month until delivery—visits once per week

Included in Visit	*When Done*
Weight	Each visit
Blood pressure	Each visit
Fundal height (McDonald's)	Each visit
Fetal heart rate	Each visit
Check for edema	Each visit
Pelvic examination	Middle of ninth month, then weekly as indicated
Other examination	As indicated by symptoms
Inquiry about symptoms, signs, or problems	Each visit
Prenatal education	Each visit
Nutrition and appetite	Each visit
Family and personal adjustment	Each visit
Urinalysis for glucose and albumin	Each visit
Hematocrit and hemoglobin	At 32–34 wk (more often if anemic)
Urine culture	As indicated by symptoms or signs
Rh titers	If initially negative, twice more during pregnancy; if positive, more often as indicated by titer levels
α-Fetoprotein	At 15–20 wk
Glucose (blood sugar)	At 24–28 wk
Ultrasonography	For fetal age, best between 8 and 16 wk
Other tests	As indicated by symptoms or signs

From Reeder, S. J., Martin, L. L., & Koniak, D. (1992). *Maternity Nursing,* 17th ed., p. 403. Philadelphia: J.B. Lippincott.

To prevent supine hypotension, have the patient rest in an upright position until the physician is ready to examine her. Also try elevating the head of the table about 30 degrees during the examination. If the patient's pregnancy is progressing normally, she may only be required to expose her abdomen to measure the fundal height (Fig. 21-9) and listen for fetal heart sounds. If she has had any problems since the last visit, have her disrobe from the waist down.

Checkpoint Question

8. *The pregnant patient should be advised to contact the physician when what problems occur?*

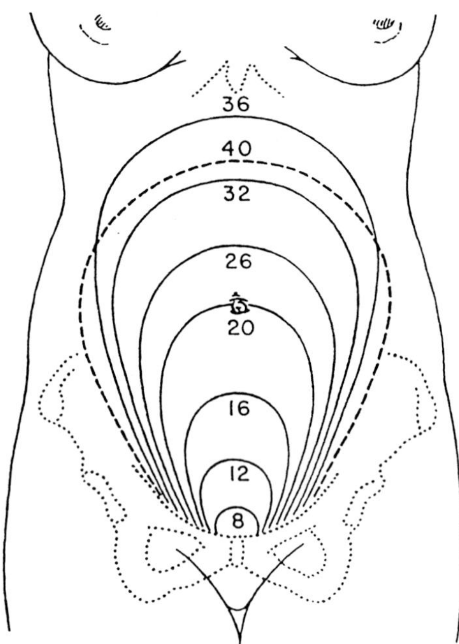

Figure 21-9 Height of the fundus at comparable gestational dates varies greatly from patient to patient. Those shown are most common. A convenient rule of thumb is that at 5 months' gestation, the fundus is usually at or slightly above the umbilicus.

OBSTETRIC DISORDERS

Ectopic Pregnancy

A gestation in which a fertilized ovum implants somewhere other than in the uterine cavity is an ectopic pregnancy. Usually the implantation of an ectopic pregnancy is in the fallopian tube; this may be referred to as a tubal pregnancy. Other sites include the abdomen, ovaries, and cervical os. The patient may present with signs of early pregnancy: breast enlargement or tenderness, nausea, late menses. Pelvic pain, syncope, abdominal symptoms, painful sexual intercourse, and irregular menstrual bleeding present fairly early in the pregnancy. If an ectopic pregnancy is not diagnosed early, there is the potential for rupture of the fallopian tube causing hemorrhage into the abdominal cavity and the possibility of shock and death. Diagnostic procedures include urine or serum human chorionic gonadotropin pregnancy test, ultrasound to determine the location of the pregnancy, laparoscopy to visualize the enlarged tube, and perhaps culdocentesis to confirm abdominal bleeding. Treatment is surgical excision of the ectopic pregnancy by either a laparoscopy or laparotomy.

Hyperemesis Gravidarum

Nausea and vomiting ("morning sickness") are expected during early pregnancy and are treated with small, frequent meals; adequate hydration; and patient reassurance. However, if the vomiting becomes unrelenting and leads to dehydration, electrolyte imbalance, and weight loss, then the diagnosis is hyperemesis gravidarum. Occasionally, the patient must be hospitalized. The medical assistant must be prepared to discern between the complaints of morning sickness and the more serious hyperemesis gravidarum.

Abortion

One of the more common disorders of pregnancy is the first trimester **abortion,** also called an early pregnancy loss or miscarriage. Because of early diagnosis of pregnancy, it is now known that the spontaneous abortion occurs with greater frequency than previously thought. Abortions may be either induced or spontaneous. The induced abortion is intentional and is a result of instrumentation. The spontaneous abortion occurs because of fetal or maternal conditions without outside interference in the pregnancy.

A spontaneous abortion is defined as the loss of pregnancy prior to the time that the fetus is viable in extrauterine life or prior to 20 weeks' gestation. You will need to be familiar with the early signs and symptoms of an impending abortion to advise the patient until the physician can be contacted. An office protocol should be established to ensure patient safety if the physician is not available. The patient may be instructed to come into the medical office, go to the emergency room, or remain at home on bed rest until the physician returns the call. The first symptom of the impending abortion is usually bleeding followed by uterine cramps and low back pain. Table 21-5 describes types of abortions and related symptoms.

Table 21-5 **Types of Abortions and Related Symptoms**

Threatened Abortion

Vaginal bleeding or spotting occurring in early pregnancy that may or may not be associated with mild cramps; closed cervix; the process may abate or result in an abortion.

Inevitable Abortion

The above process has progressed such that termination of the pregnancy cannot be prevented; bleeding is moderate to copious; uterine cramping is moderate to severe; the membranes may or may not have ruptured; the cervical canal is dilating.

Incomplete Abortion

Part of the products of conception has been passed, but part (usually the placenta) is retained in the uterus; heavy bleeding usually persists until the retained products of conception have been passed; uterine cramping is severe; the cervix is open, with tissue present.

Complete Abortion

All of the products of conception have been expelled; bleeding is slight; uterine cramping is mild.

Missed Abortion

The fetus dies in utero but is retained; regression in uterine growth and breast changes are present; if 6 weeks or more elapse between fetal death and expulsion, degenerative changes occur (eg, maceration [general softening], mummification [drying up into a leatherlike structure], and rarely, lithopedion formation [stony material]); symptoms, except for amenorrhea, are usually lacking; malaise, headache, and anorexia are occasionally present; hypofibrinogenemia may result; the condition may be discovered because fundal height fails to increase or fetal heart tones are absent.

Habitual Abortion

Spontaneous abortion occurs in successive pregnancies (three or more)

Illegal Abortion

Termination of pregnancy outside of appropriate medical facilities (eg, hospitals or clinics), generally by nonphysician abortionists; the frequency of such abortions is not precisely known but has dropped precipitously in the United States because of legalized abortion; the method may involve ingestion of drugs, such as quinine or castor oil, or the placement of a foreign body, such as a urethral catheter, into the uterus with or without the instillation of toxic substances; severe infection, often with shock and renal failure, may result.

From Reeder, S. J., Martin, L. L., & Koniak, D. (1992). *Maternity Nursing,* 17th ed., p. 774. Philadelphia: J.B. Lippincott.

Pregnancy-Induced Hypertension

Hypertension that is directly related to the pregnancy is termed pregnancy-induced hypertension (PIH). There are two types of PIH: preeclampsia and eclampsia.

Preeclampsia

Preeclampsia is characterized by **proteinuria** (protein in the urine), edema of lower extremities, and hypertension occurring after the 20th week of gestation. As the condition progresses, the patient may complain of blurred vision, headaches, edema, and vomiting. Medical management includes restricted activities, increased bed rest, sexual abstinence, antihypertensive therapy, and well balanced meals with an increase in proteins and decrease in sodium. Close monitoring of the patient is important and requires scheduling the patient for more frequent office visits. The risk of developing eclampsia increases with the advancing pregnancy.

Eclampsia

Eclampsia is almost always preceded by preeclampsia and its onset is sudden. In eclampsia, the clinical signs of preeclampsia are still present but exaggerated. However, eclampsia is always characterized by seizures that may be followed by coma, hypertensive crisis, and shock. The number and severity of the seizures vary. The progression from preeclampsia to eclampsia constitutes an emergency. Management of eclampsia includes stabilizing the patient and may require that delivery of the fetus be induced.

Placenta Previa

Placenta previa is a condition in which the placenta is implanted either partially or completely over the internal cervical os, making delivery of the fetus before the placenta difficult. During the second or third trimester of pregnancy the patient may have painless, vaginal bleeding. The vaginal bleeding may be minimal, as in spotting, or it may be profuse. Placenta previa is easily diagnosed by prenatal ultrasound. However, the placenta tends to migrate (move), and the ultrasounds need to be periodic if placenta previa is suspected or diagnosed. Medical management includes bed rest and drug therapy if the patient is preterm. If the patient is near term and if the bleeding is severe and poses a danger to mother or fetus, then delivery of the baby is essential and usually requires a cesarean delivery (Box 21-8).

Abruptio Placentae

The premature separation or detachment of the placenta from the uterus is known as abruptio placentae. Depending on the severity of the separation, symptoms include pain, uterine tenderness, bleeding and signs of impending shock, and fetal distress or even fetal death. If abruptio placentae is confirmed, the baby is usually delivered by cesarean section.

Checkpoint Question

9. *What is placenta previa, and how is it managed in a preterm patient?*

ONSET OF LABOR

Labor is the physiologic process necessary for expelling the fetus from the uterus. About 4 weeks before the onset of labor, **lightening** or dropping indicates that the fetus has descended further into the pelvis, and the patient will appear to be carrying the baby lower in the abdomen. The actual onset of labor is characterized by regular uterine contractions that become more intense and more frequent with time. True labor is distinguished from false labor by its effect (dilation and effacement [thinning]) on the cervix and the increased frequency and intensity of contractions. Another indication of true labor is the appearance of "bloody

Box 21-8
Cesarean Section

In some situations, a normal vaginal delivery is not possible or advisable. These include:

- Cephalopelvic disproportion (CPD)—the baby's head is too large for the pelvic outlet or birth canal
- Poor presentation—other than an occipital presentation, such as transverse (the baby lying across the cervix) or breech (a buttocks first presentation)
- Failure to progress—inefficient labor or the cervix will not dilate
- Infant or maternal distress

In these situations, the infant will be delivered by cesarean section. An incision is made through the abdominal wall into the uterus and the infant is removed. It was once believed that women who had delivered by cesarean must never be allowed to go into labor and delivery vaginally because it was feared that the uterine scar tissue might rupture. Current surgical techniques have lessened that fear, and many women now deliver vaginally after a cesarean delivery, referred to as vaginal birth after cesarean (VBAC).

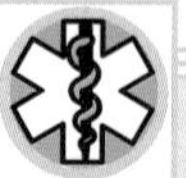

Action **STAT!**

Possible Abruptio Placentae

Scenario: Mrs. Baxter is at 31 weeks' gestation. She arrives at the physician's office complaining of severe lower abdominal pain and bright red vaginal bleeding. What should you do?

1. Immediately assist Mrs. Baxter into a wheelchair, and take her to an examining room. Provide her with a drape, and have her remove her lower garments.
2. Notify the physician. Mrs. Baxter may have an abruptio placentae—an obstetric emergency.
3. Place her on her left side—the position of choice because it increases blood flow to the vena cava and thus to the fetus. Monitor her blood pressure and pulse frequently.
4. Assist the physician. Put on gloves if exposure to blood or body fluid is possible. The obstetrician probably will complete a vaginal examination and listen to fetal heart tones.
5. Administer oxygen if ordered by the physician.
6. Document the incident carefully, and assist with Mrs. Baxter's transfer to an ambulance if necessary.

Note: Mrs. Baxter and her family will be very anxious. Offer emotional support throughout the procedures.

show," which is the mucous plug from the cervical os. The amniotic sac may break; the patient may call to say that "my bag of water broke."

Whatever signs or symptoms of labor occur, you need to know how to advise the patient. The physician will make the decision to send the patient to the hospital, schedule her to come to the medical office, or have her stay home and wait. However, you will need to relay the information from patient to physician, or decisions may need to be made in the physician's absence. A policy and procedure manual must be maintained in the office that includes specific instructions regarding how the physician wants the pregnant patient managed if the physician is not immediately available.

The onset of labor should be discussed with the patient so she knows what to expect and how to manage the situation. Always obtain the patient's medical record when talking with the patient or the physician; the patient's estimated date of delivery and physical condition are critical to the decision-making process.

POSTPARTUM CARE

The postpartum period involves the time frame, known as **puerperium,** from childbirth until the reproductive structures return to normal, referred to as involution, which may take as long as 6 weeks. Once the patient is discharged from the hospital after labor and delivery, her care is managed at the medical office. Reports received in the medical office from the hospital contain certain acronyms and abbreviations related to labor and delivery and the postpartum period. The information contained in Box 21-9 will help you become familiar with these special terms.

The appointment time for the first postpartum visit depends on the type of delivery and the patient's condition when discharged from the hospital. Today, the needs of the postpartum patient may be greater because the length of stay in the hospital is normally short, with some patients discharged within 24 hours. Patients who have no prenatal or postnatal complications or risks are scheduled for their first postnatal examination within 2 to 6 weeks of delivery.

First Postpartum Visit

At the first postnatal or postpartum visit, the physician performs a complete gynecologic and breast examination. Allow plenty of time for patient counseling regarding her new role as a parent. Many patients will have questions and concerns regarding breast-feeding (Box 21-10), birth control, menstruation, parenting, and so on. Before the physician's examination, the patient's weight and vital signs will need to be determined, and a urinalysis, hematocrit, and hemoglobin will be performed.

During the examination, the physician assesses any uterine discharge; **lochia** is usually still present at this stage. Lochia is a discharge from the uterus during puerperium and is composed of mucus, blood, and tissue shed from the uterine cavity.

Box 21-9

Acronyms and Abbreviations Used in Labor and Delivery and the Postpartum Period

Following is a brief list of terms frequently used in the medical record.

AROM	Artificial rupture of membranes
AVD	Assisted vaginal delivery
CPD	Cephalopelvic disproportion
L & D	Labor and delivery
NSVD	Normal spontaneous vaginal delivery
PROM	Premature rupture of membranes
SROM	Spontaneous rupture of membranes
VBAC	Vaginal birth after cesarean
Terms for presentations:	
LOA	Left occiput anterior
ROA	Right occiput anterior
LOP	Left occiput posterior
ROP	Right occiput posterior
Fetal descriptors:	
AGA	Appropriate for gestational age
LGA	Large for gestational age
SGA	Small for gestational age
LBW	Low birth weight

> *Box 21-10*
> **Breast-Feeding**
>
> Estrogen and progesterone stimulate the mammary glands and ducts to produce milk. Immediately postpartum, thin white fluid called colostrum is released. It is very high in proteins, antibodies, vitamins, and minerals. Several days postpartum, prolactin from the pituitary stimulates milk production, called lactation. Suckling or nursing stimulates the release of oxytocin to "let down" milk and encourages uterine contractions for involution.

- Lochia rubra—blood tinged discharge within first 6 days
- Lochia serosa—thin, brownish discharge lasting about 3 to 4 days after the lochia rubra
- Lochia alba—white postpartum discharge that has no evidence of blood

The amount of lochia should diminish considerably during puerperium. The physician should be notified if there is any abnormality of the lochial progression.

Postpartum Endometritis

Endometritis is an infection of the endometrium. In postpartum endometritis, the infection is directly related to puerperium. Usually the patient will complain of low back pain, bleeding, fever, chills, and foul-smelling lochia. Postpartum endometritis is treated with antibiotics.

Postpartum Depression

Postpartum depression occurs fairly frequently and usually within 2 to 3 days after delivery. There are varying degrees of depression, and you should always be alert to the more serious form. This discussion is limited to what the patient calls postpartum "blues" or "let down." The patient feels anxious or depressed, cries easily, has difficulty sleeping, or has a loss of appetite. As a medical assistant, you need to reassure the patient that her feelings probably are due to hormonal changes. Talk with her about her feelings, and let her know that the depression is normal and temporary. Encourage the patient to eat well, get adequate rest (including naps), and begin walking short distances daily. Usually the patient feels better just having someone to talk with and knowing that the depression is a normal extension of pregnancy and will subside.

If the patient expresses fear of harming herself or the baby or if she expresses anger regarding the baby, report this to the physician immediately. In some instances, severe parenting problems may be masked by postpartum depression. These cases must be referred to professionals trained to diagnose and treat potentially abusive parenting situations.

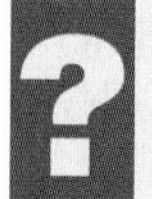

Checkpoint Question

10. *What is lochia? Name and describe the three types.*

COMMON OBSTETRIC TESTS AND THERAPEUTIC PROCEDURES AND THE MEDICAL ASSISTANT'S ROLE

Pregnancy Test

Many over-the-counter pregnancy tests are available for patients to use at home. If there are questions regarding the results, more reliable tests are available in the obstetrician's office. These are covered in Chapter 31, Serology and Immunohematology.

α-Fetoprotein

Levels of α-fetoprotein (AFP) are obtained from maternal serum to screen the fetus for possible neural tube defects. Maternal serum AFP levels vary according to numerous factors, including gestational age, number of fetuses, and patient weight. The test is used only for screening purposes and not for diagnostic purposes. The medical assistant's role usually is confined to drawing the specimen by phlebotomy to transfer to the proper laboratory. If the test is performed immediately, the specimen may be drawn in a serum separator tube; if it is to be routed to a regional laboratory, a red stopper tube is appropriate. As in all testing, the facility and testing site recommendations for sampling may vary and must be followed.

Amniocentesis

An amniocentesis is the transabdominal puncture of the amniotic sac and aspiration of amniotic fluid for study. Amniocentesis usually is done to diagnose genetic problems, estimate gestational age, or assess the lung maturity of the fetus.

Amniocentesis safety guidelines require that the procedure be performed in conjunction with a supporting concurrent ultrasound to avoid damage to the fetus. Many small obstetric offices are not equipped for this procedure. Larger offices with this capability will offer extensive training in assisting with the procedure and with patient education if this is considered within the scope of medical assisting practice for that office.

Contraction Stress Test

A contraction stress test (CST) is performed to determine how well the fetus will tolerate uterine contractions. The uterine contractions may be induced by the woman stimulating her nipples (nipple stimulation CST) or by administration of oxytocin (oxytocin-stimulated CST) to the patient. In both tests, the fetal heart tones and movement are monitored in relation to the uterine contractions. You may educate the patient about the procedure and set up the examination after instructions by your physician. This test should not be attempted without further training and should never be performed by a medical assistant without the physician in attendance.

Nonstress Test

The nonstress test (NST) is a noninvasive obstetric procedure used to evaluate the fetal heart tones and movement in relation to spontaneous uterine contractions. The NST may be safely performed in the medical office, whereas the CST is usually performed in an outpatient facility or in a labor and delivery unit of the hospital.

Doppler Ultrasonography

Doppler ultrasonography is a noninvasive procedure to detect fetal heart tones and measure the fetal heart rate (FHR). The Doppler, an ultrasonic transducer device, is positioned over the abdomen at a point where fetal heart tones are clearly audible. A coupling agent must be applied to facilitate the transfer of sound from the abdomen to the appliance. Dopplers are equipped with earpieces, such as those on a stethoscope that allow only the examiner to hear the sounds, and with an amplifier to broadcast the sound so that it can be heard by the mother and the examiner. The heart rate can be measured in much the same manner as counting a pulse.

Your responsibility may include checking the FHR as a part of the preliminary procedures done before the physician enters to complete the obstetric examination. You will need additional training in locating and identifying the heart sounds; without sufficient training, you may confuse these sounds with maternal and placental sounds. After the procedure, help the patient remove the coupling agent from the skin before reclothing.

Fetal Ultrasonography

An ultrasound of the fetus involves the use of high-frequency sound waves to create an image of internal structures. Fetal ultrasound is performed to assess the size, gestational age, position, and number of fetuses. Some abnormal maternal and fetal conditions, such as ectopic pregnancy, placenta previa, neural tube defects, and cardiac defects, can be diagnosed by ultrasound. The gender of the fetus may be identified; however, this is never a justification for performing ultrasound.

Your responsibility in this procedure is limited to assisting the patient onto the examining table after instructions for disrobing in the manner the physician prefers. You will probably assist in applying the coupling agent required to transfer the images through the transducer. After the procedure, help the patient clean her skin before reclothing.

CONTRACEPTION

Common Methods of Contraception

Numerous methods of contraception (birth control) are available for family planning (Table 21-6). The decision to practice contraception and the selection of the appropriate method involves many factors. The patient's religious, cultural, and personal beliefs as well as the health history, financial situation, and motivation are all important considerations for both the physician and patient.

To reinforce the physician's advice and instructions, the medical assistant must be knowledgeable about the various methods, including the indications, risk factors, cost, and effectiveness. Both the physician and medical assistant should be prepared to educate and advise the patient regarding the choice of contraception.

Certain methods of contraception require the patient to undergo an invasive procedure. These methods and procedures are discussed below.

Intrauterine Device

The intrauterine device (IUD) is a sterile device that is inserted into the uterine cavity to prevent pregnancy. The presence of the device causes a local inflammatory reaction that is possibly toxic to spermatozoa before they reach the ovum. Two IUDs currently are approved for consumer use in the United States, the Progestasert and the Paragard. The IUDs are highly effective (95%), and once inserted, the patient need only check the placement. Unless complications develop, the Progestasert can remain in place for 1 year and the Paragard can remain in place for 4 to 8 years. IUDs are only indicated for patients who are in monogamous relationships, are multiparous, and who have no history of PIDs.

The insertion of the IUD is recommended during menses because the uterine os is slightly dilated, which facilitates the procedure. The physician also can be as-

21

Table 21-6 **Main Methods of Contraception Currently in Use**

Method	*Description*	*Advantages*	*Disadvantages*
Surgical			
Vasectomy/tubal ligation	Cutting and tying of tubes carrying gametes	Nearly 100% effective; involves no chemical or mechanical devices	Not usually reversible; rare surgical complications
IUD	Small device inserted into uterus to prevent implantation	Requires no last-minute preparation or drugs	Has side effects; may cause uterine scarring; may be spontaneously expelled
Hormonal			
Birth control pill	Estrogen and progesterone or progesterone alone taken orally to prevent ovulation	Highly effective; requires no last-minute preparation	Alters physiology; possible serious side effects
Birth control injection	Injection of synthetic progesterone every 3 months to prevent ovulation	Highly effective, lasts for 3–4 mo	Alters physiology; possible side effects include menstrual irregularity, amenorrhea
Birth control implants	Devices containing synthetic progesterone implanted under the skin prevent ovulation	Highly effective; last for 5 y	Alter physiology; possible side effects include menstrual irregularity, amenorrhea; expensive
Barrier			
Male condom	Sheath that fits over erect penis and prevents release of semen	Easily available; does not affect physiology; protects against sexually transmitted disease (STD)	Must be applied just before intercourse, may slip or tear
Diaphragm (with spermicide)	Rubber cap that fits over cervix and prevents entrance of sperm	Does not affect physiology; some protection against STD	Must be inserted before intercourse; requires fitting by physician
Other			
Spermicide	Chemicals used to kill sperm; best when used in combination with a barrier method	Easily available, does not affect physiology; some protection against STD	Local irritation; must be used just before intercourse
Fertility awareness	Abstinence during fertile part of cycles as determined by menstrual history, basal body temperature, or quality of cervical mucus	Does not affect physiology; accepted by certain religions	High failure rate; requires careful record keeping

Adapted from Memmler, R. L., Cohen, B. J., & Wood, D. L. (1996). *The Human Body in Health and Disease,* 8th ed., p. 373. Philadelphia: Lippincott-Raven.

sured that the patient is not pregnant. Furthermore, slight cramping and bleeding, which is to be expected, will not be as alarming to the patient at the time of menses. Some physicians, on the other hand, prefer not to insert IUDs during menses because of increased risk of infection and because growing evidence indicates that the expulsion rate is higher right after menses.

The procedure is invasive; therefore, written, informed consent should be obtained from the patient. Federal regulations mandate that the patient be provided with product information and be counseled about the safety and effectiveness of the IUD. The package insert provides information to the patient on the risks, alternatives, and efficacy of the IUD. Once the patient reads the information and signs it, the documentation should be added to the patient record. A copy should be given to the patient.

Always reinforce the physician's instructions regarding expected and unexpected side effects. There is usually some increase in bleeding and cramping during menses; this usually subsides after the device has been in place for several months. The patient should be advised to notify the office if she misses a period; experi-

Procedure 21-3 Assisting With the Insertion of an Intrauterine Device

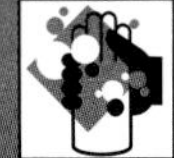
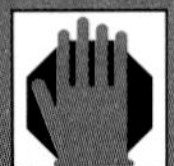

PURPOSE

To provide a means of birth control appropriate for selected patients

EQUIPMENT/SUPPLIES

- setup for pelvic examination
- sanitary pad
- cleansing tissues or personal wipes
- biohazard barrier devices, as appropriate
- sterile gloves for medical assistant or sterile transfer forceps
- scissors

On the Sterile Field

- uterine tenaculum
- uterine sound
- antiseptic solution (Betadine)
- container for solution
- 4 × 4 sterile gauze
- IUD insertion kit
- sterile gloves for physician (possibly at the side)

STEPS

1. Verify that the patient has signed the consent form.
   Federal regulations require an informed consent for IUD insertion.
2. Wash your hands.
3. Prepare equipment and supplies as needed for the pelvic examination (see Procedure 21-1).
4. Greet and identify the patient. Explain the procedure. Have the patient disrobe from the waist down and cover with a privacy drape.
5. Position and drape the patient in the dorsal lithotomy position, as you would for the pelvic examination.
   Proper positioning facilitates the examination.
6. Put on gloves or use sterile transfer forceps. Set up the sterile field using strict sterile technique.
   An invasive procedure mandates sterile technique to reduce the risk of infection.
7. Pour antiseptic solution into the sterile container on the sterile field.
   Antiseptic solution, such as Betadine, reduces the risk of infection.
8. Assist the physician as directed with gloving and gowning. Adjust the light source over the genitalia.
   This facilitates the procedure.
9. Open the IUD insertion kit with sterile technique. Drop it onto the sterile field, or allow the physician to grasp it from the opened package. The physician will insert the IUD at this point.
   Sterile technique must be maintained.
10. Have scissors available for the physician.
    Scissors are used to trim the string of the IUD so that it extends just beyond the external opening of the cervical os.
11. Assist the patient back up on the table, and help her remove her legs from the stirrups.
    Assisting the patient gives you the opportunity to assess her response to the procedure.
12. Provide the patient with cleansing tissues or personal wipes.
    These may be used to wipe away any secretions.
13. Instruct the patient on how and when to check for IUD placement.
    IUD placement must be checked after each menstrual period to be sure of correct position.
14. Have the patient check for the placement of the IUD before leaving the office.
    Patient compliance is increased with understanding of what is expected. If she has difficulty palpating the string in the office, it will be easier to give further instructions now than by phone later.
15. Offer the patient a sanitary pad for small amounts of bleeding that may occur.
    The procedure may cause slight bleeding with uterine cramps.
16. Thank the patient. Reinforce the physician's instructions regarding follow-up and side effects. (If there are no problems, a follow-up visit should be within 4–6 weeks.)
17. Properly care for or dispose of equipment and supplies. Clean the room. Wash your hands.

DOCUMENTATION GUIDELINES

- Date and time
- Verification of consent
- Performance of procedure
- Patient complaints/concerns
- Patient education/instructions
- Your signature

Charting Example

DATE	TIME Informed consent signed by pt.
	IUD inserted by Dr. Lang. Pt instructed in
	checking placement and post-insertion
	guidelines. No bleeding noted.
	—Your signature

Procedure 21-4 Assisting With the Removal of an Intrauterine Device

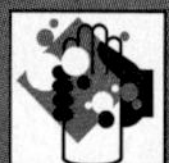
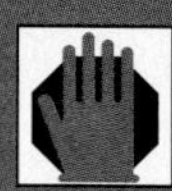

PURPOSE

To ensure that the removal of the device is accomplished with minimal discomfort and maximum safety for the patient

EQUIPMENT/SUPPLIES

- patient drape
- vaginal speculum
- uterine dressing forceps
- direct lighting
- cleansing tissues or personal wipes
- sanitary pad or tampon

STEPS

1. Wash your hands.
2. Set up equipment and supplies as for the pelvic examinations (see Procedure 21-1).
3. Greet and identify the patient. Explain the procedure. Have the patient disrobe from the waist down and cover with a privacy drape.
4. Position the patient in the dorsal lithotomy position.
   This position makes visualizing the string easier for the physician.
5. Glove and assist the physician as required—adjust the light source, hand the instruments, and receive the contaminated materials on tray or basin.
   Anticipating each step facilitates the procedure and increases the confidence of the physician and patient. Standard Precautions must be observed to avoid exposure to hazardous material.
6. Assist the patient back up on the table, and remove her legs from the stirrups.
   Assisting the patient protects her from injury and allows you time to assess her response to the procedure.
7. Offer the patient a sanitary pad or tampon.
   There may be a small amount of bleeding after IUD removal.
8. Thank the patient. Reinforce the physician's instructions.
9. Properly care for or dispose of equipment and supplies. Clean the examination room. Wash your hands.

DOCUMENTATION GUIDELINES

- Date and time
- Removal of the IUD
- Patient complaints/concerns
- Patient education/instructions
- Your signature

Charting Example

DATE	TIME IUD removed without incident by
	Dr. Williams. Pt advised re: birth control
	options. —Your signature

ences heavy bleeding, severe cramping, unusual vaginal discharge, or lower abdominal pain; has unexplained fever or chills; or is unable to locate the string or the string feels longer.

When setting up for the procedure, you will need first to prepare for the pelvic examination and assemble materials for the sterile field. To maintain strict sterile technique, the sterile field should be set up just before the procedure. Sterile transfer forceps or sterile gloves should be used while preparing the sterile field. When preparing the antiseptic, note that some physicians may prefer that the solution be poured directly onto the 4 × 4 gauze, which remains on top of the packaging as opposed to using sterile containers. If so, do not pour the solution until the physician is ready to cleanse the cervix (Procedure 21-3).

Removal of an IUD usually is accomplished in patients who do not tolerate the IUD or who desire pregnancy or when the IUD has expired. It is a simple procedure in which the physician grasps the string with a uterine dressing forceps or other instrument and gently retrieves the device (Procedure 21-4). The patient should be prepared for some temporary cramping and slight bleeding.

Checkpoint Question

11. *What are the benefits and drawbacks of IUD insertion during menses?*

Subdermal Hormone Implants

This form of birth control involves the subdermal implantation of six capsules that contain le-

Procedure 21-5 Assisting With the Insertion of Subdermal Hormonal Implants

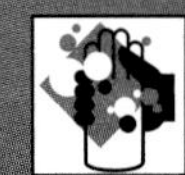
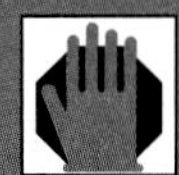
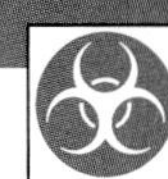

PURPOSE

To provide a means of birth control appropriate for selected patients

EQUIPMENT/SUPPLIES

- Norplant System Kit (completely self-contained with all essential materials)
- sterile gloves
- sterile towel
- light source
- local anesthetic

Additional Materials on Sterile Field

- antiseptic solution
- sterile container for antiseptic
- sterile syringe (3 or 5 mL)
- sterile needle (1 inch, 23–25 gauge)
- sterile 4 × 4 gauze

STEPS

1. Verify that the patient has signed the consent form. Make sure the patient understands all aspects of the procedure.
   Invasive procedures require written, informed consent. Patients will be more compliant if they understand the procedure.
2. Wash your hands.
3. Position the patient in the supine position with the chosen upper arm exposed.
   The position should be comfortable for the patient to enhance relaxation and should make insertion easier for the physician.
4. Assemble the equipment and supplies.
5. Set up the sterile field.
   a. Pour antiseptic solution. (*Note:* Antiseptic solution can be poured into the sterile container on the field *or* onto 4 × 4 sterile gauze that remains on top of the inside of the packaging.)
   b. Open and drop gauze, syringe, and needle onto the field.
   c. Open the Norplant System and drop onto the field.
6. Be aware that the physician may prefer to administer the local anesthetic before gloving. However, if he or she prefers to inject after gloving, follow these steps:
   a. Cleanse the top of the anesthetic vial with alcohol prep.
   The use of antiseptic reduces the risk of contamination.
   b. Hold the anesthetic vial in the physician's preferred position while the physician aspirates the anesthetic into the syringe.
   Assisting the physician maintains sterile technique.
7. Assist the physician as necessary during the implant insertion.
8. Help the patient into an upright position.
   Assisting the patient conveys a sincere, caring attitude. Some patients may become dizzy after procedures; assisting may prevent a fall.
9. Thank the patient. Reinforce the physician's instructions.
   Patient understanding of follow-up, side effects, and wound care will enhance compliance to therapy.
10. Properly care for or dispose of equipment and supplies. Clean the room. Wash your hands.

DOCUMENTATION GUIDELINES

- Date and time
- Verification of informed consent
- Location of subdermal implant
- Patient complaints/concerns
- Patient education/instructions
- Your signature

Charting Example

DATE	TIME Informed consent signed by pt.
	Subdermal hormonal implant inserted in
	upper right arm by Dr. York. No bleeding
	noted at site. Pt given written instruc-
	tions re: implant. —Your signature

vonorgestrel (Norplant System), which is a hormone that inhibits ovulation. The implants are usually inserted into the inner surface of the upper arm (Procedure 21-5). Removal of the implants may be necessary because of bleeding, headaches, weight gain, depression, acne, anxiety, nervousness, and breast pain or tenderness.

This is an invasive procedure and therefore requires a written consent. The Norplant System contains a product insert that the patient must read. Ask if she has questions about the implants or the procedure. The procedure for insertion can be performed within a short time, usually less than 10 minutes. However, the procedure for removal may take more time because fibrous tissue often forms a capsule around the implants, making retrieval more difficult. Occasionally, the devices must be removed by a surgeon. Let the patient know that contraception is achieved within 24 hours of the procedure.

MENOPAUSE

Menopause, or the climacteric period, is the developmental stage during which the ability of the woman to reproduce ceases because of decreasing ovarian function. The climacteric period is characterized by the cessation of the menstrual cycle and usually occurs around 45 to 50 years of age. Perimenopause occurs before menopause and includes changes in the menstrual cycle, such as oligomenorrhea, amenorrhea, dysfunctional uterine bleeding, and hot flashes, flushing, or perspiration.

The decrease in circulating estrogen has been implicated in an increase in the risk of atherosclerosis, coronary heart disease, and osteoporosis (brittle bones). Supplementary estrogen (hormonal replacement therapy or HRT) protects against the cardiovascular and skeletal disorders and decreases the menopausal symptoms, such as hot flashes, depression, and drying of the vaginal mucosa. Estrogen is given alone after a hysterectomy or estrogen and progesterone are given in combination if the woman still has her uterus. In addition to an active exercise program, dietary calcium, and a healthy and moderate life-style, HRT will help menopausal women retain optimum health and vitality. For those with only minor menopausal symptoms, weight-bearing exercises, a healthy diet, and vitamin and mineral supplements have eased the transition through the menopausal stage.

There is inconclusive and conflicting evidence regarding HRT and an increase in the risk of reproductive cancers. This concern can be alleviated by regular Pap smears and mammograms.

Answers to Checkpoint Questions

1. *The uterus is composed of the endometrium (the inner layer, which has a rich blood supply), the myometrium (the middle, muscular layer), and the perimetrium (connective tissue).*
2. *The primary characteristic of the secretory phase of the menstrual cycle is the impact of progesterone on the endometrium, which becomes highly vascular and rich in glycogen as it prepares for a possible pregnancy.*
3. *Dysfunctional uterine bleeding includes menorrhagia (excessive bleeding), metrorrhagia (irregular bleeding), polymenorrhea (abnormally frequent bleeding), and postmenopausal bleeding not associated with tumor, inflammation, or pregnancy.*
4. *Genital warts have been implicated in an increase in cervical cancer.*
5. *The prognosis of all cancers is much better with early diagnosis and treatment.*
6. *As part of a complete gynecologic examination, the physician examines the patient's breasts and performs a pelvic examination with Pap smear.*
7. *The presumptive signs and symptoms of pregnancy are not conclusive because they may indicate other disorders.*
8. *The pregnant patient should notify the physician if there is vaginal bleeding or spotting, persistent vomiting, fever or chills, dysuria, abdominal or uterine cramping, leaking amniotic fluid, altered fetal movement, dizziness, or blurred vision.*
9. *Placenta previa is a condition in which the placenta is implanted either partly or completely over the internal cervical os. In the preterm patient, the condition is managed with bed rest and drug therapy.*
10. *Lochia is a discharge from the uterus composed of mucus, blood, and tissue. Types include lochia rubra (blood tinged), lochia serosa (thin, brownish discharge), and lochia alba (white discharge with no evidence of blood).*
11. *During menses, the uterine os will be slightly dilated, facilitating insertion of the IUD. Also, the physician can be certain that the patient is not pregnant. Furthermore, slight cramping and bleeding will not be as alarming to the patient at the time of menses. However, some physicians prefer not to insert IUDs during menses because of increased risk of infection and because growing evidence indicates that the expulsion rate is higher right after menses.*

Critical Thinking Challenges

1. A multiparous patient who is married and has a history of cigarette smoking desires a highly effective method of contraception. What are her choices for contraception? Explain which choice is best and why.
2. A patient who has a scheduled appointment is complaining of painful blisters in the vaginal and vulvular area. For what type of examination would you prepare? Why?

3. Your patient has both genital herpes and condylomata acuminata. She wants to know if these disorders are contagious and how they can be cured. How would you respond to these questions?

Suggestions for Further Reading

Berkow, R., (Ed.). (1992). *The Merck Manual.* Rahway, NJ: Merck Sharp and Dohme Research Laboratories, Division of Merck and Co, Inc.

DeDona, N. A., & Marks, M. A. (1996). *Introducing Maternal-Newborn Nursing.* Philadelphia: Lippincott-Raven.

Glass, R. H., (Ed.). (1993). *Office Gynecology.* Baltimore: Williams & Wilkins.

Nettina, S. M. (1996). *The Lippincott Manual of Nursing Practice,* 6th ed. Philadelphia: Lippincott-Raven.

Pillitteri, A. (1995). *Maternal and Child-Health Nursing: Care of the Child-Bearing and Child-Rearing Family,* 2nd ed. Philadelphia: Lippincott-Raven.

Reeder, S. J., Martin, L. L., & Koniak, D. (1997). *Maternity Nursing: Family, Newborn and Women's Health Care,* 18th ed. Philadelphia: Lippincott-Raven.

Rosdahl, C. B. (1995). *Textbook of Basic Nursing,* 6th ed. Philadelphia: J.B. Lippincott.

Scott, J. R., DiSaia, P. J., Hammond, C. B., & Spellacy, W. N. (1994). *Danforth's Obstetrics and Gynecology,* 7th ed. Philadelphia: J.B. Lippincott.

Unit 3

Assisting With Special Patient Populations

22 Pediatric Patients

Chapter Outline

Role Delineation

CLINICAL

Fundamental Principles

- Apply principles of aseptic technique and infection control.

Diagnostic Orders

- Collect and process specimens.

Patient Care

- Obtain patient history and vital signs.
- Prepare and maintain examination and treatment areas.
- Prepare patient for examinations, procedures, and treatments.

GENERAL

Professionalism

- Project a professional manner and image.

Communication Skills

- Treat all patients with compassion and empathy.
- Adapt communications to individual's ability to understand.

Legal Concepts

- Practice within the scope of education, training, and personal capabilities.
- Document accurately.

Instruction

- Instruct individuals according to their needs.
- Teach methods of health promotion and disease prevention.

Chapter Competencies

Learning Objectives

Upon successfully completing this chapter, you will be able to:

1. Spell and define the Key Terms.
2. List safety precautions to use in the pediatrician's office.
3. Explain the differences between a well-child and a sick-child office visit.
4. List types and schedule of immunizations.
5. Describe the role of the parent during the office visit.
6. Describe the kinds of feelings a child might experience during an office visit.
7. List the anthropometric measurements obtained in preparation for a pediatric physical examination.
8. Explain how to record anthropometric measurements on a graphic chart.

Chapter Competencies *(continued)*

9. Identify two sites for intramuscular injections in an infant.
10. Identify two sites for intramuscular injections in a child.

Performance Objectives

Upon successfully completing this chapter, you will be able to:

1. Restrain a pediatric patient (Procedure 22-1).
2. Obtain measurements on an infant or child, including height (Procedure 22-2), length (Procedure 22-3), chest and head circumference (Procedure 22-4), and weight (Procedure 22-5).
3. Measure pediatric blood pressure (Procedure 22-6).
4. Apply a pediatric urine collection device (Procedure 22-7).

Key Terms

(See Glossary for definitions.)

aspiration
autonomous
congenital anomalies
humidifier
immunizations
malaise
neonatologists
pediatrician
pediatrics
psychosocial
restrains
sick-child visits
varicella zoster
well-child visits

Medical assistants who work in a pediatric practice must understand that the needs of children and adolescents are typically different from those of adult patients. This chapter discusses special considerations in caring for pediatric patients. It also addresses the particular skills needed by medical assistants working with this distinct patient population.

THE PEDIATRIC PRACTICE

Pediatrics is the medical specialty devoted to the care of infants, children, and adolescents. This care involves the diagnosis and treatment of childhood diseases as well as monitoring the physical and **psychosocial** (mental and emotional) development of the child.

Pediatric patients are not simply small adults; they are susceptible to a unique array of illnesses and problems generally not present in adults. The acute illnesses suffered by children typically are not encountered in adulthood. Some young patients will present with **congenital anomalies** (abnormalities present from birth) that are life-threatening or debilitating. Because of their increased metabolism, immature nervous systems, and accelerated growth patterns, pediatric patients often experience complications that may not occur in adult patients. There are few routine medical concerns related to infants and children that can be resolved with the same treatments used for adult patients.

A **pediatrician** is a physician who is specially trained to care for the well child and the diseases present in infants, children, and adolescents. Traditional pediatricians treat children of all ages, up to and through the teen years. Pediatric subspecialists include **neonatologists,** who treat only newborns, and other pediatricians who treat only adolescents.

THE OFFICE ENVIRONMENT

A pediatric office that is decorated and furnished in a manner appropriate to children's physical and psychosocial needs provides a nonthreatening and possibly even inviting environment. Child-size furniture allows pediatric patients to feel comfortable and welcome. Popular toys evoke happy associations. Safe toys allow for hands-on activity while the child is waiting to see the physician. All toys should be washable and should be cleaned frequently to reduce the risk

22

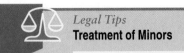

Legal Tips

Treatment of Minors

Before treating a minor (persons under age 18), parental permission must be obtained. The **exceptions** to this rule include treatment for:

- Pregnancy (testing or prenatal care)
- Birth control
- Sexually transmitted diseases
- Rape
- Life- or limb-threatening injuries

Emancipated minors (persons under 18 years who support themselves financially), minors enlisted in the armed services, or minors who are married may obtain treatment without parental consent. You are responsible for knowing your state's laws regarding treatment of minors.

of disease transmission. Popular storybooks and magazines give parents an opportunity to read quietly to a child who may not feel well enough to play. Many offices are designed with separate waiting areas for sick children and well children.

Safety

Medical assistants who care for children must always protect them from injury and accidents. Providing a "safe world" demands an awareness of children's insatiable curiosity and the need to explore their surroundings. Children must never be left unattended in any area of the medical office.

Safety is a prime concern when considering toys and equipment in a pediatric office. Toys should be examined frequently and replaced when damaged or soiled. Try to see the office from a child's viewpoint. If necessary, get down to a child's level to discover potential danger areas—sharp table corners or exposed electrical outlets—that an adult might overlook.

The examination room presents special concerns for children's safety. Keep all medical equipment out of a child's reach, and never leave a child alone in the examining room. Follow these tips to ensure your pediatric patient's safety:

- Place infant scales on a sturdy table, and never leave a child alone on a scale.
- Store any disinfection solutions away from patient care areas.
- Dispose of all sharps in proper containers.
- Practice stringent handwashing and Standard Precautions with every patient. Many childhood illnesses are highly contagious and can be transmitted by poor medical asepsis. These practices protect both the patient and the medical assistant from the spread of infection. (See Chap. 1, Asepsis and Infection Control, for more information.)

Types of Office Visits

The two types of pediatric patient office visits are the well-child visit and the sick-child visit. Well-child visits are regularly scheduled checkups designed to maintain the child's optimum health. **Sick-child visits** occur whenever the child requires medical treatment for symptoms or signs of illness or injury. (See Physiologic Aspects of Care, below, for more specific information about these types of visits.)

Checkpoint Question

1. *List three safety precautions that should be used in a pediatric practice.*

PSYCHOLOGICAL ASPECTS OF CARE

Psychosocial Development

Understanding a child's psychological needs and development will enable you to provide safe and effective care. During an office visit, the pediatric patient may experience many of the same feelings that adults do, depending on the child's age and ability to understand. These feelings might include:

- Fear that something painful and frightening might be done
- Anxiety that a previous bad experience may be repeated at the current visit
- Guilt and feelings of being punished for "being bad" or "misbehaving."
- Powerlessness and loss of physical autonomy
- Curiosity about new surroundings and experiences

Some children may be able to verbalize these feelings. Others may only be able to express them physically by crying and resisting the approach of the medical staff. As a medical assistant, you can reassure the pediatric patient and family by demonstrating your understanding of the child's feelings and displaying a kind and gentle manner. Include the child in the explanation of procedures on an age-appropriate level. Children who are helped to feel part of the examination frequently will be more cooperative.

Role of the Parents

Parents are a source of support and comfort to a child. Their presence minimizes stress in unfamiliar surroundings. Encourage parents to remain with the child

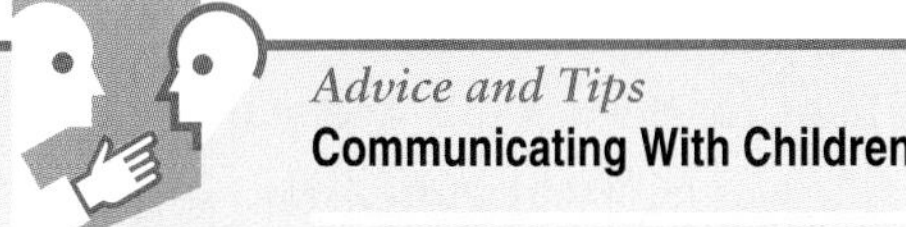

Advice and Tips
Communicating With Children

Pediatric patients require special communication techniques. Here are a few tips to help you speak more effectively with children:

- Ask the child how he or she feels, then speak to the parent. Make the child feel part of the communication.
- Use simple, easy-to-understand terms.
- Explain all procedures to both the parent and child, using age-appropriate explanations.
- Avoid using confusing medical terms.
- Avoid condescending language.
- Be honest. If a procedure is going to hurt, say so. Do not lie. Keep in mind that children may view pain as punishment. If a procedure is painful, explain that the procedure is necessary to promote the child's health.
- If you need to communicate with an adolescent about sexual history or other intimate circumstances, ask the parents if they feel comfortable leaving the room.

and to assist in care when appropriate. For instance, ask the parent to stand beside the child during the weight measurement as you adjust the scales. Many children are more compliant if much of the preliminary workup is performed while the parent holds the child. The child may be less anxious if the parent **restrains,** or holds, the head for ear examinations and is within the child's sight, rather than having the medical assistant in this position (Fig. 22-1).

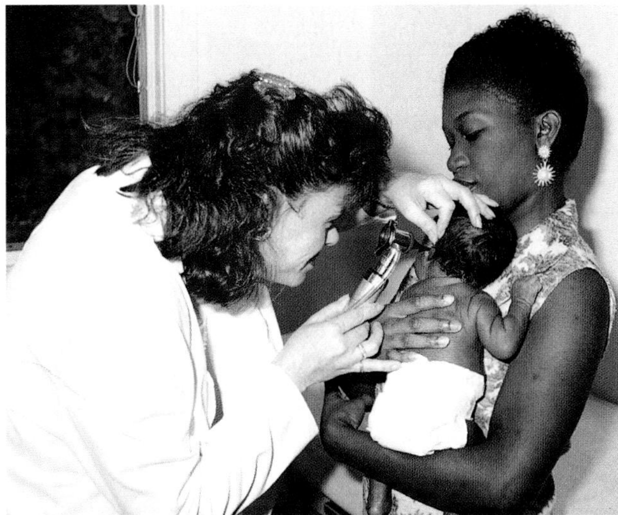

Figure 22-1 Much of the examination can be performed while the mother holds the baby.

As a child develops and becomes more **autonomous** (independent), a parent's immediate presence may be less meaningful as long as the child knows that the parent is close by. Many adolescent patients prefer to be alone with the physician to demonstrate their independence and to discuss matters that they may not be comfortable talking about with the parent present. Depending on the maturity of the adolescent, ask the patient, not the parent, if the parent is needed during the examination.

22

Checkpoint Question

2. *What kinds of feelings might a pediatric patient experience during an office visit?*

PHYSIOLOGIC ASPECTS OF CARE

Growth and Development

To anticipate age-appropriate behavior and to provide proper psychological support and physical care, the medical assistant must have a broad knowledge of child growth and development patterns. Never expect a child to react or respond beyond his or her developmental age. For example, a 2-year-old is naturally reluctant to be examined and may resist your advances. Many 4- or 5-year-olds are curious and willing to cooperate if you turn the examination into a game. Children older than 4 or 5 should have the reasoning capacity to understand the need to comply.

A normal child's growth and development follows an orderly progression involving mind, body, and personality. Table 22-1 describes the stages of growth and development and lists special considerations for the medical assistant.

One of the most popular tools for evaluating early childhood development is the Denver Development Screening Test (DDST) II. This tool is designed to assess fine motor, gross motor, language, and social development. The DDST II evaluates from the most basic reflexes to complex interpersonal reactions. The medical assistant who will perform the assessment should be educated in proper testing to evoke the most diagnostic response.

The indicators are registered in a vertical line drawn at the child's current age. Children should register within the normal range for age (Fig. 22-2).

Well-Child Visits

Well-child visits are scheduled at regular intervals, depending on the child's age. The goal of these visits is to maintain the child's optimum health, which is accomplished by a complete physical examination and an

22

Table 22-1 **Pediatric Growth and Developmental Stages, With Considerations for the Medical Assistant**

Age	*Growth*	*Development*	*Considerations for the Medical Assistant*
Infancy (0–1 y)	Triples birth weight Increases physical control of body Sits and stands May walk by first birthday	Trust versus mistrust	Involve the parent. Keep the parent in the child's view. Approach the child slowly. Use a soft, soothing voice. Verbalize reassurance.
Toddler (1–3 y)	Growth rate slows Body proportions change Language skills begin	Autonomy	Use all of the skills listed above. Explain procedures in terms the child can understand. Expect resistance. Use a firm, direct approach. Ignore negative behavior. Restrain to maintain the child's safety. Allow the child to hold a "security object."
Preschool (3–6 y)	Language and self-control develop Motor skills increase	Initiative	Use all of the skills listed above. Encourage the child to verbalize feelings. Explain why the procedure is being done. Have the child help as much as possible (eg, hold equipment).
School-age (6–12 y)	Social skills develop Peer group becomes important Self-concept develops	Industry	Involve the child in decision making. Involve the child in care, such as collecting specimens or choosing which procedure to do first. Encourage and support questions.
Adolescent (12–18 y)	Emotional changes Identity and place in the world defined	Biologic and identity	Discuss procedures in terms an adolescent can understand. Be aware that adolescents may resist authority figures. Be sure patient education includes information regarding smoking, alcohol, and, in some cases, birth control and sexually transmitted diseases. At the physician's discretion, this information may be discussed without the parent present.

evaluation of the child's neurologic and psychosocial development. During an infant's first few well-child visits, for example, the pediatrician will check reflexes. Responses are predictors of neurologic health and development (Table 22-2).

The physician discusses the examination results with the child's parents and prescribes treatment for any problems found. Guidance and answers are offered for any questions parents may have about their child's health and development. Parents also are counseled about what to expect as part of the child's upcoming stages of growth and maturation. A child who is old enough to understand also should be included in the discussion. As the child matures, these visits become less frequent (Table 22-3).

Immunizations

Immunizations are a scheduled, routine part of the well-child visit and have dramatically improved children's health over the past 50 years. Immunizations protect children from diseases that in the past caused early death or long-term health problems. Immunizations produce immunity by slowly introducing into the body an altered form of the disease-causing bacteria or virus, which in turn stimulates the body to produce antibodies to protect against the specific disease. Currently, immunizations are available for:

- Hepatitis B (HBV)
- Diphtheria, tetanus, and pertussis (DTP)
- Poliomyelitis (polio, both oral vaccine [OPV or TOPV] and injectable forms)
- Measles, mumps, and rubella (MMR)
- *Haemophilus influenzae* type B (Hib)
- **Varicella zoster** (VZV)—also known as chickenpox

Vaccine manufacturers have trade names for each product and have established protocols that must be followed to ensure full immunity to the specific dis-

Stage	Caution
The newborn can see, hear, smell, feel pain, and communicate. Protective mechanisms are in place, such as a blink reflex, pulling in for warmth, or pulling away from pain or restraint. Development is from cephalic to caudal. Head control comes first, then gradually evolves into full body control (eg, rolling over, crawling, walking) and, finally, fine motor development (eg, picking up small objects). The most phenomenal growth and development occurs during this time, from total dependence to walking and talking.	Advise the parents to call the physician if the child has a temperature over 100.5°F rectally; has breathing difficulties, diarrhea, or jaundice; is crying inconsolably or vomiting; is failing to nurse, or has low urine output.
Growth levels off, but exploration and social development continue. Negativism precedes autonomy. The child will begin to seek relationships and is acutely aware of strangers.	Advise parents to report any of the appropriate signs of illness as before, but also instruct them to be aware of the increased incidence of accidents with the need to explore. Children at this stage may indicate what hurts and how they feel, so you should not only talk with the parents, but also include the child when asking questions.
Socialization continues with fairly clearly marked stages of social development through the next 10 y. Many of the early-stage problems have resolved, and with the exception of the usual communicable diseases, this is generally a time of good health. Diseases such as leukemia, Hodgkin's, and various sarcomata may present in these next stages, but these years are usually spent establishing relationships with peers, exercising autonomy, and completing the growth process.	

eases. As a medical assistant, you are responsible for reading all package inserts to become familiar with the adverse effects and cautions for each vaccine and to alert parents to potential problems they might observe after routine immunizations. Manufacturers of vaccines require that parents read and sign a consent form regarding the possible side effects of routine immunizations (Box 22-1).

Immunization schedules, which are developed by the American Academy of Pediatrics (AAP), change periodically as new vaccines become available for current diseases or as information regarding vaccines requires an altered pattern. Immunization schedules should be posted prominently in the office and replaced as suggested by the AAP (Table 22-4).

For various reasons, some children may not be kept on the suggested immunization schedule. However, all children must be current with their immunizations before they are allowed to attend public school (Fig. 22-3).

Sick-Child Visits

Sick-child visits are made on an as-needed basis. The goal of these visits is the diagnosis and treatment of the child's immediate illness or injury. The pediatrician examines the child and prescribes treatment that may include x-rays, laboratory tests, medication, or simply the reassurance that the illness will run a predictable and manageable course. Table 22-5 lists three common childhood illnesses and their causes, symptoms, and treatments. (No immunizations for these illnesses are available at this time.)

Sick-child visits occur frequently during early childhood. Because children do not have well developed immune systems, they are more susceptible to viruses and bacterial infections. High fevers in young children may trigger seizures because of the child's immature nervous system. This does not mean that the child will be prone to seizures as he or she matures because the tendency to have seizures usually is out-

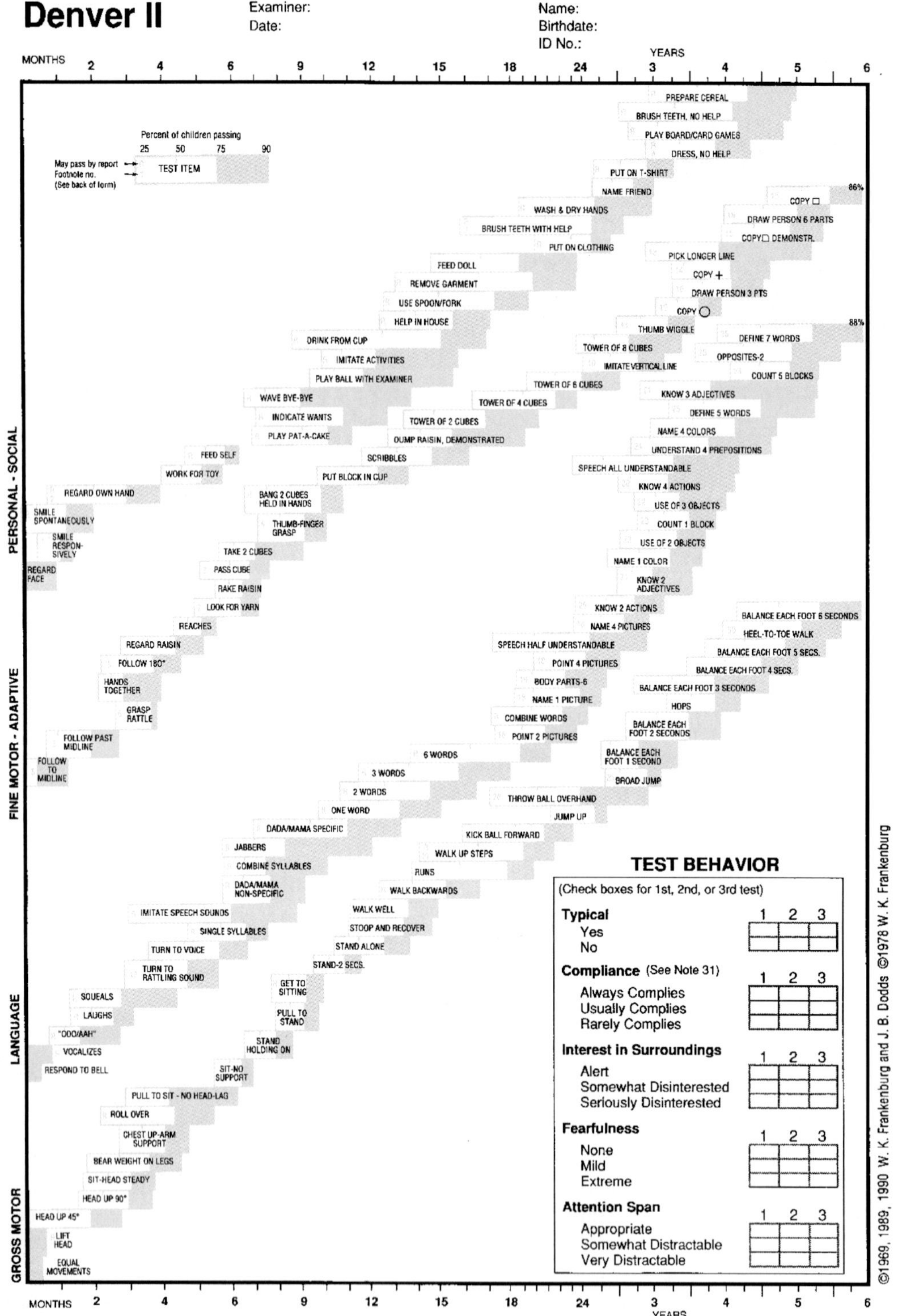
Denver II

Examiner:
Date:

Name:
Birthdate:
ID No.:

MONTHS 2 4 6 9 12 15 18 24 | YEARS 3 4 5 6

Percent of children passing
25 50 75 90
May pass by report
Footnote no.
(See back of form)
TEST ITEM

PERSONAL - SOCIAL
PREPARE CEREAL
BRUSH TEETH, NO HELP
PLAY BOARD/CARD GAMES
DRESS, NO HELP
PUT ON T-SHIRT
NAME FRIEND
WASH & DRY HANDS
BRUSH TEETH WITH HELP
PUT ON CLOTHING
FEED DOLL
REMOVE GARMENT
USE SPOON/FORK
HELP IN HOUSE
DRINK FROM CUP
IMITATE ACTIVITIES
PLAY BALL WITH EXAMINER
WAVE BYE-BYE
INDICATE WANTS
PLAY PAT-A-CAKE
FEED SELF
WORK FOR TOY
REGARD OWN HAND
SMILE SPONTANEOUSLY
SMILE RESPONSIVELY
REGARD FACE

FINE MOTOR - ADAPTIVE
COPY □ 86%
DRAW PERSON 6 PARTS
COPY □ DEMONSTR.
PICK LONGER LINE
COPY +
DRAW PERSON 3 PTS
COPY ○
THUMB WIGGLE
TOWER OF 8 CUBES
IMITATE VERTICAL LINE
TOWER OF 6 CUBES
TOWER OF 4 CUBES
TOWER OF 2 CUBES
DUMP RAISIN, DEMONSTRATED
SCRIBBLES
PUT BLOCK IN CUP
BANG 2 CUBES HELD IN HANDS
THUMB-FINGER GRASP
TAKE 2 CUBES
PASS CUBE
RAKE RAISIN
LOOK FOR YARN
REACHES
REGARD RAISIN
FOLLOW 180°
HANDS TOGETHER
GRASP RATTLE
FOLLOW PAST MIDLINE
FOLLOW TO MIDLINE

LANGUAGE
DEFINE 7 WORDS 88%
OPPOSITES-2
COUNT 5 BLOCKS
KNOW 3 ADJECTIVES
DEFINE 5 WORDS
NAME 4 COLORS
UNDERSTAND 4 PREPOSITIONS
SPEECH ALL UNDERSTANDABLE
KNOW 4 ACTIONS
USE OF 3 OBJECTS
COUNT 1 BLOCK
USE OF 2 OBJECTS
NAME 1 COLOR
KNOW 2 ADJECTIVES
KNOW 2 ACTIONS
NAME 4 PICTURES
SPEECH HALF UNDERSTANDABLE
POINT 4 PICTURES
BODY PARTS-6
NAME 1 PICTURE
COMBINE WORDS
POINT 2 PICTURES
6 WORDS
3 WORDS
2 WORDS
ONE WORD
DADA/MAMA SPECIFIC
JABBERS
COMBINE SYLLABLES
DADA/MAMA NON-SPECIFIC
IMITATE SPEECH SOUNDS
SINGLE SYLLABLES
TURN TO VOICE
TURN TO RATTLING SOUND
SQUEALS
LAUGHS
"OOO/AAH"
VOCALIZES
RESPOND TO BELL

GROSS MOTOR
BALANCE EACH FOOT 6 SECONDS
HEEL-TO-TOE WALK
BALANCE EACH FOOT 5 SECS.
BALANCE EACH FOOT 4 SECS.
BALANCE EACH FOOT 3 SECONDS
HOPS
BALANCE EACH FOOT 2 SECONDS
BALANCE EACH FOOT 1 SECOND
BROAD JUMP
THROW BALL OVERHAND
JUMP UP
KICK BALL FORWARD
WALK UP STEPS
RUNS
WALK BACKWARDS
WALK WELL
STOOP AND RECOVER
STAND ALONE
STAND-2 SECS.
GET TO SITTING
PULL TO STAND
STAND HOLDING ON
SIT-NO SUPPORT
PULL TO SIT - NO HEAD-LAG
ROLL OVER
CHEST UP-ARM SUPPORT
BEAR WEIGHT ON LEGS
SIT-HEAD STEADY
HEAD UP 90°
HEAD UP 45°
LIFT HEAD
EQUAL MOVEMENTS

TEST BEHAVIOR
(Check boxes for 1st, 2nd, or 3rd test)

	1	2	3
Typical			
Yes			
No			
Compliance (See Note 31)			
Always Complies			
Usually Complies			
Rarely Complies			
Interest in Surroundings			
Alert			
Somewhat Disinterested			
Seriously Disinterested			
Fearfulness			
None			
Mild			
Extreme			
Attention Span			
Appropriate			
Somewhat Distractable			
Very Distractable			

MONTHS 2 4 6 9 12 15 18 24 3 4 5 6 YEARS

Figure 22-2 Denver Developmental Screening Test II. © 1969, 1989, 1990 W. K. Frankenburg and J. B. Dodds © 1978 W. K. Frankenburg.

DIRECTIONS FOR ADMINISTRATION

1. Try to get child to smile by smiling, talking or waving. Do not touch him/her.
2. Child must stare at hand several seconds.
3. Parent may help guide toothbrush and put toothpaste on brush.
4. Child does not have to be able to tie shoes or button/zip in the back.
5. Move yarn slowly in an arc from one side to the other, about 8" above child's face.
6. Pass if child grasps rattle when it is touched to the backs or tips of fingers.
7. Pass if child tries to see where yarn went. Yarn should be dropped quickly from sight from tester's hand without arm movement.
8. Child must transfer cube from hand to hand without help of body, mouth, or table.
9. Pass if child picks up raisin with any part of thumb and finger.
10. Line can vary only 30 degrees or less from tester's line.
11. Make a fist with thumb pointing upward and wiggle only the thumb. Pass if child imitates and does not move any fingers other than the thumb.

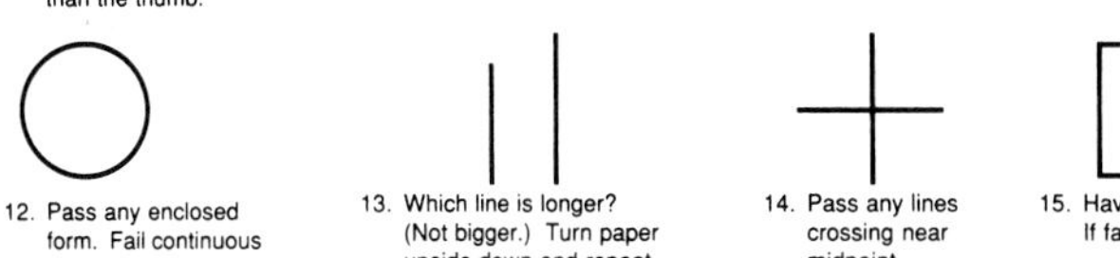

12. Pass any enclosed form. Fail continuous round motions.
13. Which line is longer? (Not bigger.) Turn paper upside down and repeat. (pass 3 of 3 or 5 of 6)
14. Pass any lines crossing near midpoint.
15. Have child copy first. If failed, demonstrate.

When giving items 12, 14, and 15, do not name the forms. Do not demonstrate 12 and 14.

16. When scoring, each pair (2 arms, 2 legs, etc.) counts as one part.
17. Place one cube in cup and shake gently near child's ear, but out of sight. Repeat for other ear.
18. Point to picture and have child name it. (No credit is given for sounds only.) If less than 4 pictures are named correctly, have child point to picture as each is named by tester.

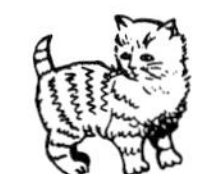
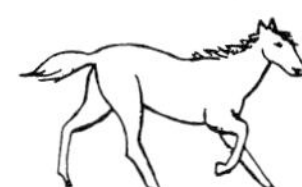
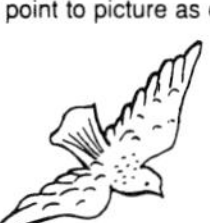
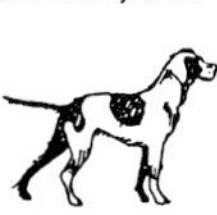
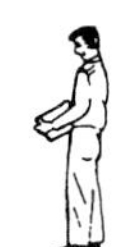

19. Using doll, tell child: Show me the nose, eyes, ears, mouth, hands, feet, tummy, hair. Pass 6 of 8.
20. Using pictures, ask child: Which one flies?... says meow?... talks?... barks?... gallops? Pass 2 of 5, 4 of 5.
21. Ask child: What do you do when you are cold?... tired?... hungry? Pass 2 of 3, 3 of 3.
22. Ask child: What do you do with a cup? What is a chair used for? What is a pencil used for? Action words must be included in answers.
23. Pass if child correctly places and says how many blocks are on paper. (1, 5).
24. Tell child: Put block **on** table; **under** table; **in front of** me, **behind** me. Pass 4 of 4. (Do not help child by pointing, moving head or eyes.)
25. Ask child: What is a ball?... lake?... desk?... house?... banana?... curtain?... fence?... ceiling? Pass if defined in terms of use, shape, what it is made of, or general category (such as banana is fruit, not just yellow). Pass 5 of 8, 7 of 8.
26. Ask child: If a horse is big, a mouse is __? If fire is hot, ice is __? If the sun shines during the day, the moon shines during the __? Pass 2 of 3.
27. Child may use wall or rail only, not person. May not crawl.
28. Child must throw ball overhand 3 feet to within arm's reach of tester.
29. Child must perform standing broad jump over width of test sheet (8 1/2 inches).
30. Tell child to walk forward, → heel within 1 inch of toe. Tester may demonstrate. Child must walk 4 consecutive steps.
31. In the second year, half of normal children are non-compliant.

OBSERVATIONS:

Figure 22-2 *(continued)*

grown fairly early. The physician determines the course to follow in the event of childhood febrile seizures.

Never give aspirin to young children with viral fevers. Aspirin has been associated with Reye's syndrome after cases of varicella zoster (chickenpox) and viral illnesses. Reye's syndrome, a condition of acute encephalopathy and fatty infiltration of the internal organs, may be fatal.

As children grow older and receive the full schedule of immunizations, and as parents become more

Table 22-2 **Infant Reflexes and Responses**

Reflex	*Response*
Suckling or rooting	Stroking the cheek causes the infant to turn toward the stroke with its mouth open to suck. This reflex subsides by 3–6 mo.
Moro or startle	A loud noise or sudden change in position causes the infant to look startled; the back arches, the arms and legs fly out and then are quickly brought back close to the body, and the infant cries. The Moro reflex results in the thumbs and forefingers forming a "C" while the other fingers spread open. (In the startle reflex, the fingers remain clenched.) Both reflexes disappear by 6 mo.
Grasp	Stroking the infant's palm causes the fingers to grasp; stroking the plantar surface causes the toes to flex to grasp. The palmar grasp disappears by 3 mo. The plantar grasp disappears by 9–12 mo.
Tonic neck or fencing	With the infant in a supine position, the physician turns the head to either side. The arm and leg on the side the infant is facing will flex and the limbs on the opposite side will extend. This reflex disappears by 3–4 mo.
Placing or stepping	The physician holds the infant at the edge of the examining table with the feet just below the edge. When the tops of the feet touch the table edge, the infant will place each foot up on the table and make walking movements. This reflex disappears by 6 wk.
Babinski	When the plantar surface is stroked, the toes flare outward. This reflex disappears by 12 mo.

Note: The absence of a response or a hyper-response may indicate a neurologic deficit.

Table 22-3 **Recommendations for Preventive Pediatric Health Care**

American Academy of Pediatrics

RECOMMENDATIONS FOR PREVENTIVE PEDIATRIC HEALTH CARE

Committee on Practice and Ambulatory Medicine (RE 9535)

Each child and family is unique; therefore, these **Recommendations for Preventive Pediatric Health Care** are designed for the care of children who are receiving competent parenting, have no manifestations of any important health problems, and are growing and developing in satisfactory fashion. **Additional visits may become necessary** if circumstances suggest variations from normal.

These guidelines represent a consensus by the Committee on Practice and Ambulatory Medicine in consultation with national committees and sections of the American Academy of Pediatrics. The Committee emphasizes the great importance of **continuity of care** in comprehensive health supervision and the need to avoid **fragmentation of care.**

A **prenatal visit** is recommended for parents who are at high risk, for first-time parents, and for those who request a conference. The prenatal visit should include anticipatory guidance and pertinent medical history. Every infant should have a newborn evaluation after birth.

	INFANCY[3]								EARLY CHILDHOOD[3]					MIDDLE CHILDHOOD[3]				ADOLESCENCE[3]										
AGE[4]	NEWBORN[1]	2-4d[2]	By 1mo	2mo	4mo	6mo	9mo	12mo	15mo	18mo	24mo	3y	4y	5y	6y	8y	10y	11y	12y	13y	14y	15y	16y	17y	18y	19y	20y	21y
HISTORY																												
Initial/Interval	•	•	•	•	•	•	•	•	•	•	•	•	•	•	•	•	•	•	•	•	•	•	•	•	•	•	•	•
MEASUREMENTS																												
Height and Weight	•	•	•	•	•	•	•	•	•	•	•	•	•	•	•	•	•	•	•	•	•	•	•	•	•	•	•	•
Head Circumference	•	•	•	•	•	•	•	•	•	•	•																	
Blood Pressure												•	•	•	•	•	•	•	•	•	•	•	•	•	•	•	•	•
SENSORY SCREENING																												
Vision	S	S	S	S	S	S	S	S	S	S	S	O[5]	O	O	S	S	O	S	O	S	S	O	S	S	O	S	S	S
Hearing[6]	S/O	S	S	S	S	S	S	S	S	S	S	O	O	O	S	S	O	S	O	S	S	O	S	S	O	S	S	S
DEVELOPMENTAL/ BEHAVIORAL ASSESSMENT[7]	•	•	•	•	•	•	•	•	•	•	•	•	•	•	•	•	•	•	•	•	•	•	•	•	•	•	•	•
PHYSICAL EXAMINATION[8]	•	•	•	•	•	•	•	•	•	•	•	•	•	•	•	•	•	•	•	•	•	•	•	•	•	•	•	•
PROCEDURES – GENERAL[9]																												
Hereditary/Metabolic Screening[10]	←—	—	•																									
Immunization[11]	•—	—	→	•	•	•		←	•	→			←	•	→			•—	—	—	—	—	→					
Lead Screening[12]							•—	→			•																	
Hematocrit or Hemoglobin			←	—	—	—	•											←	—	—	—	•[13]	—	—	—	—	—	→
Urinalysis														•				←	—	—	—	•[14]	—	—	—	—	—	→
PROCEDURES – PATIENTS AT RISK																												
Tuberculin Test[15]								*	*	*	*	*	*	*	*	*	*	*	*	*	*	*	*	*	*	*	*	*
Cholesterol Screening[16]											*	*	*	*	*	*	*	*	*	*	*	*	*	*	*	*	*	*
STD Screening[17]																		*	*	*	*	*	*	*	*	*	*	*
Pelvic Exam[18]																		*	*	*	*	*	*	←	*	•[18]	*	→*
ANTICIPATORY GUIDANCE[19]	•	•	•	•	•	•	•	•	•	•	•	•	•	•	•	•	•	•	•	•	•	•	•	•	•	•	•	•
Injury Prevention[20]	•	•	•	•	•	•	•	•	•	•	•	•	•	•	•	•	•	•	•	•	•	•	•	•	•	•	•	•
INITIAL DENTAL REFERRAL[21]								←	—	—	—	•																

1. Breastfeeding encouraged and instruction and support offered.
2. For newborns discharged in less than 48 hours after delivery.
3. Developmental, psychosocial, and chronic disease issues for children and adolescents may require frequent counseling and treatment visits separate from preventive care visits.
4. If a child comes under care for the first time at any point on the schedule, or if any items are not accomplished at the suggested age, the schedule should be brought up to date at the earliest possible time.
5. If the patient is uncooperative, rescreen within six months.
6. Some experts recommend objective appraisal of hearing in the newborn period. The Joint Committee on Infant Hearing has identified patients at significant risk for hearing loss. All children meeting these criteria should be objectively screened. See the Joint Committee on Infant Hearing 1994 Position Statement.
7. By history and appropriate physical examination: if suspicious, by specific objective developmental testing.
8. At each visit, a complete physical examination is essential, with infant totally unclothed, older child undressed and suitably draped.
9. These may be modified, depending upon entry point into schedule and individual need.
10. Metabolic screening (eg, thyroid, hemoglobinopathies, PKU, galactosemia) should be done according to state law.
11. Schedule(s) per the Committee on Infectious Diseases, published periodically in *Pediatrics*. Every visit should be an opportunity to update and complete a child's immunizations.
12. Blood lead screen per AAP statement "Lead Poisoning: From Screening to Primary Prevention" (1993).
13. All menstruating adolescents should be screened.
14. Conduct dipstick urinalysis for leukocytes for male and female adolescents.
15. TB testing per AAP statement "Screening for Tuberculosis in Infants and Children" (1994). Testing should be done upon recognition of high risk factors. If results are negative but high risk situation continues, testing should be repeated on an annual basis.
16. Cholesterol screening for high risk patients per AAP "Statement on Cholesterol" (1992). If family history cannot be ascertained and other risk factors are present, screening should be at the discretion of the physician.
17. All sexually active patients should be screened for sexually transmitted diseases (STDs).
18. All sexually active females should have a pelvic examination. A pelvic examination and routine pap smear should be offered as part of preventive health maintenance between the ages of 18 and 21 years.
19. Appropriate discussion and counseling should be an integral part of each visit for care.
20. From birth to age 12, refer to AAP's injury prevention program (TIPP®) as described in "A Guide to Safety Counseling in Office Practice" (1994).
21. Earlier initial dental evaluations may be appropriate for some children. Subsequent examinations as prescribed by dentist.

Key: • = to be performed * = to be performed for patients at risk S = subjective, by history O = objective, by a standard testing method ←—•—→ = the range during which a service may be provided, with the dot indicating the preferred age.
NB: Special chemical, immunologic, and endocrine testing is usually carried out upon specific indications. Testing other than newborn (eg, inborn errors of metabolism, sickle disease, etc.) is discretionary with the physician.
The recommendations in this publication do not indicate an exclusive course of treatment or serve as a standard of medical care. Variations, taking into account individual circumstances, may be appropriate.

Pediatrics Vol. 96 No. 2 August 1995

> *Box 22-1*
> **Educating Parents About Possible Side Effects of Childhood Immunizations**
>
> - **Diphtheria-pertussis-tetanus** (DPT) may produce discomfort, swelling and redness at the site of injection, slight fever, and **malaise** (a feeling of generalized weakness and discomfort) within 24–48 h. Parents can administer acetaminophen for discomfort and fever. The pertussis component may cause loss of consciousness, seizures, inconsolable crying, hyperpyrexia, and systemic allergic reactions. If these symptoms occur, parents should notify the physician immediately.
> - **Trivalent oral polio vaccine** (TOPV) usually causes no side effects, although vaccine-associated paralysis has been documented within 2 months of immunization. Be sure to question parents about the immune status of the family members and caregivers; immune suppression may lead to vaccine-induced polio.
> - **Measles-mumps-rubella** (MMR) may cause fever, rash, malaise, lymphadenopathy, and arthralgia. A delay in symptom onset may occur in some children. Antipyretics for discomfort may be ordered.
> - **Hemophilus B vaccine** (HiB) causes a low-grade fever with only a mild local reaction. Parents may give acetaminophen for discomfort.

knowledgeable about certain disorders, communicable diseases and common childhood illnesses occur less often.

Children are inquisitive, adventurous, and unaware of dangers that can lead to many of the accidents and injuries that account for a large percentage of visits to the pediatrician's office. As a child's reasoning abilities mature, accidents diminish as well. Closely supervising a child's diet, rest, and exercise as well as teaching stress reduction techniques helps to promote good health habits for a lifetime.

Checkpoint Question

3. *List the differences between well-child and sick-child visits.*

THE PHYSICAL EXAMINATION

Typically, the medical assistant prepares the pediatric patient for examination by the pediatrician and may also assist with the examination by restraining the child. The medical assistant usually is responsible for documenting much of the history and chief complaint information and for collecting appropriate specimens for diagnostic testing.

Pediatric Histories

A pediatric patient's medical history differs greatly from an adult patient's history. During the early years of a patient's life, it is important to know the history of the pregnancy, labor, and delivery. The length of the pregnancy, maternal illnesses or complications, neonatal complications, or risk factors must be recorded as predictors of infant health and development. Most newborn charts contain a copy of the delivery record or birth summary outlining the delivery with the Apgar score and progress notes from the newborn nursery (Box 22-2).

As the child grows, the information needed expands to include childhood illnesses, developmental milestones, immunizations, and nutritional status.

Figure 22-4 displays the kinds of forms used for documenting pediatric histories at various ages.

Preparing for the Physical Examination

You should approach the pediatric patient in a calm and cheerful manner and use a firm but gentle touch to increase the patient's feeling of security. Involve the parents as much as possible, and keep them in the patient's view to reduce anxiety for both the child and parents.

Prepare the pediatric patient for physical examination by obtaining some or all of the following measurements: height or length, head and chest circumference, weight, temperature, pulse and respiratory rate, and blood pressure. Many of the measurements needed depend on the child's age. The schedule preferred by the physician should be listed in the procedures manual.

Using Restraints

During the examination, the physician may need the medical assistant to help restrain the child. Restraining is sometimes necessary to protect the child from injury and to help the physician complete the examination in a timely manner. Children understandably resist the physician because they are frightened and do not want to be touched. Calm and gentle restraint is in the best interest of everyone involved.

In hospitals, many forms of restraints are used, including elbow, clove hitch, or abdominal. In the pediatrician's office, the medical assistant will most likely assist by using the papoose or mummy wrap or simply by holding the child in a position that the physician directs (Procedure 22-1).

text continues on page 500

Table 22-4 **Recommended Childhood Immunization Schedule**

Recommended Childhood Immunization Schedule
United States, January - December 1998

Vaccines[1] are listed under the routinely recommended ages. Bars indicate range of acceptable ages for immunization. Catch-up immunization should be done during any visit when feasible. Shaded ovals indicate vaccines to be assessed and given if necessary during the early adolescent visit.

Age ► Vaccine ▼	Birth	1 mo	2 mos	4 mos	6 mos	12 mos	15 mos	18 mos	4-6 yrs	11-12 yrs	14-16 yrs
Hepatitis B[2,3]	Hep B-1										
			Hep B-2		Hep B-3					Hep B[3]	
Diphtheria, Tetanus, Pertussis[4]			DTaP or DTP	DTaP or DTP	DTaP or DTP		DTaP or DTP[4]		DTaP or DTP	Td	
H influenzae type b[5]			Hib	Hib	Hib	Hib					
Polio[6]			Polio[6]	Polio		Polio[6]			Polio		
Measles, Mumps, Rubella[7]						MMR			MMR[7]	MMR[7]	
Varicella[8]							Var			Var[8]	

Approved by the Advisory Committee on Immunization Practices (ACIP), the American Academy of Pediatrics (AAP), and the American Academy of Family Physicians (AAFP).

IS 5081

(For **necessary footnotes** and important information, see reverse side.)

[1] This schedule indicates the recommended age for routine administration of currently licensed childhood vaccines. Some combination vaccines are available and may be used whenever administration of all components of the vaccine is indicated. Providers should consult the manufacturers' package inserts for detailed recommendations.

[2] **Infants born to HBsAg-negative mothers** should receive 2.5 μg of Merck vaccine (Recombivax HB) or 10 μg of SmithKline Beecham (SB) vaccine (Engerix-B). The 2nd dose should be administered at least 1 mo after the 1st dose. The 3rd dose should be given at least 2 mos after the second, but not before 6 mos of age.
Infants born to HBsAg-positive mothers should receive 0.5 mL of hepatitis B immune globulin (HBIG) within 12 hrs of birth, and either 5 μg of Merck vaccine (Recombivax HB) or 10 μg of SB vaccine (Engerix-B) at a separate site. The 2nd dose is recommended at 1-2 mos of age and the 3rd dose at 6 mos of age.
Infants born to mothers whose HBsAg status is unknown should receive either 5 μg of Merck vaccine (Recombivax HB) or 10 μg of SB vaccine (Engerix-B) within 12 hrs of birth. The 2nd dose of vaccine is recommended at 1 mo of age and the 3rd dose at 6 mos of age. Blood should be drawn at the time of delivery to determine the mother's HBsAg status; if it is positive, the infant should receive HBIG as soon as possible (no later than 1 wk of age). The dosage and timing of subsequent vaccine doses should be based upon the mother's HBsAg status.

[3] Children and adolescents who have not been vaccinated against hepatitis B in infancy may begin the series during any visit. Those who have not previously received 3 doses of hepatitis B vaccine should initiate or complete the series during the 11- to 12-year-old visit, and unvaccinated older adolescents should be vaccinated whenever possible. The 2nd dose should be administered at least 1 mo after the 1st dose, and the 3rd dose should be administered at least 4 mos after the 1st dose and at least 2 mos after the 2nd dose.

[4] DTaP (diphtheria and tetanus toxoids and acellular pertussis vaccine) is the preferred vaccine for all doses in the vaccination series, including completion of the series in children who have received 1 or more doses of whole-cell DTP vaccine. Whole-cell DTP is an acceptable alternative to DTaP. The 4th dose (DTP or DTaP) may be administered as early as 12 months of age, provided 6 months have elapsed since the 3rd dose, and if the child is unlikely to return at 15-18 mos. Td (tetanus and diphtheria toxoids) is recommended at 11-12 years of age if at least 5 years have elapsed since the last dose of DTP, DTaP or DT. Subsequent routine Td boosters are recommended every 10 years.

[5] Three *H influenzae* type b (Hib) conjugate vaccines are licensed for infant use. If PRP-OMP (PedvaxHIB [Merck]) is administered at 2 and 4 mos of age, a dose at 6 mos is not required.

[6] Two poliovirus vaccines are currently licensed in the US: inactivated poliovirus vaccine (IPV) and oral poliovirus vaccine (OPV). The following schedules are all acceptable to the ACIP, the AAP, and the AAFP. Parents and providers may choose among these options:
1) 2 doses of IPV followed by 2 doses of OPV.
2) 4 doses of IPV.
3) 4 doses of OPV.
The ACIP recommends 2 doses of IPV at 2 and 4 mos of age followed by 2 doses of OPV at 12-18 mos and 4-6 years of age. IPV is the only poliovirus vaccine recommended for immunocompromised persons and their household contacts.

[7] The 2nd dose of MMR is recommended routinely at 4-6 yrs of age but may be administered during any visit, provided at least 1 mo has elapsed since receipt of the 1st dose and that both doses are administered beginning at or after 12 mos of age. Those who have not previously received the second dose should complete the schedule no later than the 11- to 12-year visit.

[8] Susceptible children may receive varicella vaccine (Var) at any visit after the first birthday, and those who lack a reliable history of chickenpox should be immunized during the 11- to 12-year-old visit. Susceptible children 13 years of age or older should receive 2 doses, at least 1 month apart.

Immunization Protects Children

Regular checkups at your pediatrician's office or local health clinic are an important way to keep children healthy.

By making sure that your child gets immunized on time, you can provide the best available defense against many dangerous childhood diseases. Immunizations protect children against: hepatitis B, polio, measles, mumps, rubella (German measles), pertussis (whooping cough), diphtheria, tetanus (lockjaw), *Haemophilus influenzae* type b, and chickenpox. All of these immunizations need to be given before children are 2 years old in order for them to be protected during their most vulnerable period. Are your child's immunizations up-to-date?

The chart on the other side of this fact sheet includes immunization recommendations from the American Academy of Pediatrics. Remember to keep track of your child's immunizations—it's the only way you can be sure your child is up-to-date. Also, check with your pediatrician or health clinic at each visit to find out if your child needs any booster shots or if any new vaccines have been recommended since this schedule was prepared.

If you don't have a pediatrician, call your local health department. Public health clinics usually have supplies of vaccine and may give shots free.

American Academy of Pediatrics

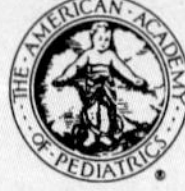

The information contained in this publication should not be used as a substitute for the medical care and advice of your pediatrician. There may be variations in treatment that your pediatrician may recommend based on individual facts and circumstances.

Patient's Name ______ Sex ______ D.O.B. ______

VACCINE			DATE GIVEN Mo.	Day	Yr.	Name of Physician and/or Local H.D. Stamp	DATE NEXT DOSE DUE
	DTP	DT					
DTP DT[1] (Diphtheria, Tetanus, Pertussis) 1							
2							
3							
4							
5[2]							
HEMOPHILUS INFLUENZA b (Hib) 1							
2							
3							
4							
	OPV	IPV					
Polio, Oral Trivalent Polio,[1] Inactivated 1							
2							
3							
4[2]							
5							
Hepatitis B 1							
2							
3							
MMR #1							
MMR #2							
MEASLES							
RUBELLA							
MUMPS							
Td Tetanus, Diphtheria BOOSTER EVERY 10 YEARS							

[1]Check the appropriate box for the specific vaccine administered.

[2]Administered on or after the fourth birthday and before enrolling in school (K-1).

VACCINE	Date Given	Administered By	Date Given	Administered By	Date Given	Administered By
INFLUENZA						

VACCINE	DATE GIVEN	ADMINISTERED BY	DATE NEXT DOSE DUE
PNEUMOCOCCAL (one dose only)			
HEPATITIS B: Recommended for persons at risk 1			
2			
3			

Medical Notes:

NORTH CAROLINA
DEPARTMENT OF ENVIRONMENT, HEALTH, AND NATURAL RESOURCES

LIFETIME IMMUNIZATION RECORD

Patient's Full Name ______ First ______ Middle ______ Last

Birthdate ______ Month/Day/Year Sex ______ SS# ______

Name of Parent/Guardian ______

Address ______

If properly completed this record can be used to comply with Immunization Laws for day care, primary school entry, and entry into N.C. colleges and universities. This card can also be used to comply with immunization requirements of various employers.

Present this record at each visit to your doctor or clinic. The date each dose was given and the name of the physician and/or local health department stamp are required as proof of immunization.

DEHNR 1065 (Revised 6/93)
Immunization (Review 6/95)

Figure 22-3 A standard form for recording immunizations.

Table 22-5 **Common Childhood Illnesses**

Illness	*Symptoms*	*Cause*	*Treatment*
Common cold	Congestion Cough Malaise Sore throat Fever	Virus	Increased fluids Rest Cold steam humidifier Antihistamines Decongestants
Gastroenteritis	Vomiting or diarrhea Fever	Virus or bacteria	Increased fluids (especially electrolyte-replacement fluids) Medication may be ordered to relieve symptoms
Otitis media (middle ear infection)	Earache (may accompany or follow a cold) Reduced hearing in affected ear Fever	Virus or bacteria	Increased fluids Antihistamines Decongestants Antibiotics

22

Box 22-2
The Apgar Score

Named for pediatrician Dr. Virginia Apgar, the Apgar score is a method for describing the general health of the newborn at 1 minute and 5 minutes after delivery. Signs assessed include:

- Heart rate
- Respiratory effort
- Muscle tone
- Response to a suction catheter in the nostril
- Color

A perfect score for each sign is 2; a total absence of any sign is 0. A perfect score of 10 indicates:

- Heart rate is greater than 100 beats/min.
- Respirations are eupneic, or the baby is crying.
- Muscle tone is good, and the baby is active.
- Cough or sneeze occurs in response to suction catheter.
- Skin is completely pink with no acrocyanosis.

Most babies have 1-minute scores of 7 to 9 because many have a bit of acrocyanosis until respirations are established. Babies with 1-minute scores below 4 usually require assistance, particularly respiratory interventions, such as oxygen.

The Apgar score is not considered an indicator of future intelligence or health problems. Rather, it is used by the obstetrician, pediatrician, and delivery room personnel to assess newborns who may require closer observation.

Obtaining Measurements

During a well-child visit, anthropometric measurements commonly obtained include height or length, head and chest circumference, and weight. These measurements show the child's growth and development patterns and are good indicators of the child's health status and of the parent–child bonding. For example, parents who are not bonding well may either overfeed or underfeed a child, resulting in either significantly above- or below-average measurements. Head versus chest measurements may alert the pediatrician to intracranial abnormalities.

Height is measured when the child is standing; length is measured when the child is lying down. Weight is the most frequently obtained measurement in pediatric practices. The way in which weight is measured depends on the child's ability to remain still. For instance, a young child can either sit or recline on an infant scale while an older child can stand on a larger scale (Procedures 22-2 through 22-5).

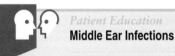

Patient Education
Middle Ear Infections

Explain to your pediatric patient's parents that children have short, narrow, straight eustachian tubes. Upper respiratory infections, particularly with coughing, may force microorganisms into the middle ear spaces. As the infection grows, the child's eustachian tubes swell and eventually close. Exudate from the mucous membrane continues to be produced, causing fluid to build with resulting pressure and pain.

Bacterial otitis media (middle ear infection) has been associated with, and may be caused by, putting the child to bed with a milk bottle. The milk and bacteria set up a medium for growth within the eustachian tube.

Checkpoint Question

4. *Why is it important to track a child's anthropometric measurements?*

Graphic Charts

Graphic charts are designed to show the child's growth patterns at a glance. The child's measurements commonly are plotted on percentile charts, then compared with those of children of the same age (Fig. 22-5).

Growth charts typically include the child's age, length or height, and weight. Notice that head circumference is not included on growth charts for children older than 36 months. Chest circumference usually is not graphed.

To use a growth chart, find the child's measurement (for length or height, in either inches or centimeters; for weight, in either pounds or kilograms), then move in that line across to the age column. Find the month or year opposite the measurement, and make a mark at the point where the two values intersect. Moving a straight edge across the page helps keep within the proper lines. If you make an error, mark through it with an X and initial it. Then make the correction in the proper lines.

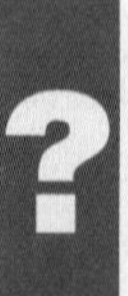

Checkpoint Question

5. *Using the chart in Figure 22-5B, find the mark for a 4-month-old girl whose head circumference is 43 cm. What is this child's percentile?*

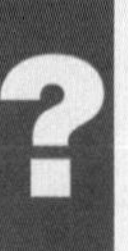

Checkpoint Question

6. *Using the chart in Figure 22-5A, find the mark for a 3-year-old girl who is 91 cm tall. What is this child's percentile?*

P.E. CODE:
Abnormalities described
✓ Normal
Ø Not done
Att: attempted

REVIEW OF SYSTEMS:
Recent illness: ____

☐ Crosses eyes
☐ Head tilt / Squints
☐ Problems with hearing
☐ Problems with vision
☐ Perceived developmental delay
☐ Problems with siblings
☐ Fails to have strong voiding stream
Favorite toy ____
Ipecac at home? ____

DEVELOPMENT:
☐ Sits well
☐ Crawls/creeps
☐ Pulls to stand
☐ Cruises
☐ Pincer grasp
☐ Finger feeds self
☐ 1-2 meaningful vocalization
☐ Peek-a-boo
☐ Pat-a-cake
☐ Reacts to stranger with anxiety
☐ Imitates gestures

✓ - pass / circle if failed

PERCENTILES:
Ht. ____
Wt. ____
H.C. ____
Daycare Y / N
Where? ____
Pleased? ____
Babysitters ____
Problems or changes at home? ____

3. PHYSICAL EXAMINATION/ASSESSMENT

	Normal for Age	Abnormal	Not Eval.
a. General Appearance			
b. Posture, Gait			
c. Speech			
d. Head			
e. Skin			
f. Eyes: (1) External Aspects ____			
(2) Optic Fundiscopic ____			
(3) Cover Test			
g. Ears: (1) External & Canals ____			
(2) Tympanic Membranes			
h. Nose, Mouth, Pharynx			
i. Teeth			
j. Heart			
k. Femoral Pulses			
l. Lungs			
m. Abdomen (include hernia)			
n. Genitalia			
o. Bones, Joints, Muscles			
p. Neurological/Social			
(1) Gross Motor ____			
(2) Fine Motor ____			
(3) Communication Skills ____			
(4) Cognitive			
q. Glands (Lymphatic/Thyroid)			
r. Hips - R.O.M. / Click			
s. Other Clavicles/Hernia			
Vision Screening			
Hearing Screening			
Other: Bonding:			

Concerns
Problems

Assessment/Plan:

☐ ViDaylin/F 0.25
☐ Hgb
☐ Hgb electrophoresis
☐ Nutrition/diet counseling
☐ Start using cup
☐ Change car seat at 20 pounds
☐ Accidents/safety discussed
☐ Teething
☐ Discipline/autonomy
☐ Sleep: anticipate night awakening

DATE:

9 Months

Figure 22-4 (**A**) Pediatric history form, age 9 months. (**B**) Pediatric history form, age preschool to 5 years.

22

P. E. CODE:
Abnormalities described
✓ Normal
⊘ Not done
Att: attempted

REVIEW OF SYSTEMS:
☐ Developmental concerns
☐ Behavioral problems
☐ Need for dental referral
☐ Vision/Hearing concerns

☐ Discuss parental activities/expectations.
☐ Promote interaction with other children.
☐ Encourage help with chores and tidy up of child's room.

DEVELOPMENT:
☐ Dresses without supervision
☐ Separates from mom easily
☐ Opposite analogies
☐ Defines 6-9 words
☐ Balances on one foot-10 seconds
☐ Catches bounced ball
☐ Interactive play
☐ Identify coins
☐ States age
☐ Tells simple story
☐ Right/wrong Fair/unfair
☐ Copies "☐"
☐ Imitates a demonstration of ☐
☐ Draws man - 3 parts
☐ Draws man - 6 parts
☐ Hops on one foot
☐ Backward heel/toe
☐ Cut/paste
☐ Reading
☐ Crossing of eyes?
☐ Voids w/good stream
☐ Daycare
☐ School
☐ TV
✓ - pass/circle if failed

PERCENTILES:

Ht. ____________

Wt. ____________

3. PHYSICAL EXAMINATION/ASSESSMENT

	Normal for Age	Abnormal	Not Eval.
BP /			
a. General Appearance			
b. Posture, Gait			
c. Speech			
d. Head			
e. Skin			
f. Eyes: (1) External Aspects ____			
(2) Optic Fundiscopic ____			
(3) Cover Test			
g. Ears: (1) External & Canals ____			
(2) Tympanic Membranes			
h. Nose, Mouth, Pharynx			
i. Teeth			
j. Heart			
k. Femorol Pulses			
l. Lungs			
m. Abdomen (include hemia)			
n. Genitalia			
o. Bones, Joints, Muscles			
p. Neurological/Social			
(1) Gross Motor ____			
(2) Fine Motor ____			
(3) Communication Skills ____			
(4) Cognitive			
q. Glands (Lymphatic/Thyroid)			
r. Spine			
s. Other Clavicles/Hernia			

Vision (R) (L) ☐ Snellen
Hearing Screening Audiometry ☐ Passed ☐ Failed
Color Vision ☐ Passed ☐ Failed

Concerns
Problems

Assessment/Plan:

☐ Vi Daylin/F 1.0 Chewable
☐ Hgb
☐ U/A ____________
☐ Urine culture - females
☐ Monovac
☐ DPT: Here / PHD
☐ OPV: Here / PHD
☐ Dental referral
☐ Safety-bicycle/water/fire
☐ Home telephone no. memorization
☐ T.V.
☐ Other

DATE:

Preschool/5 yr.

Figure 22-4 *(Continued)*

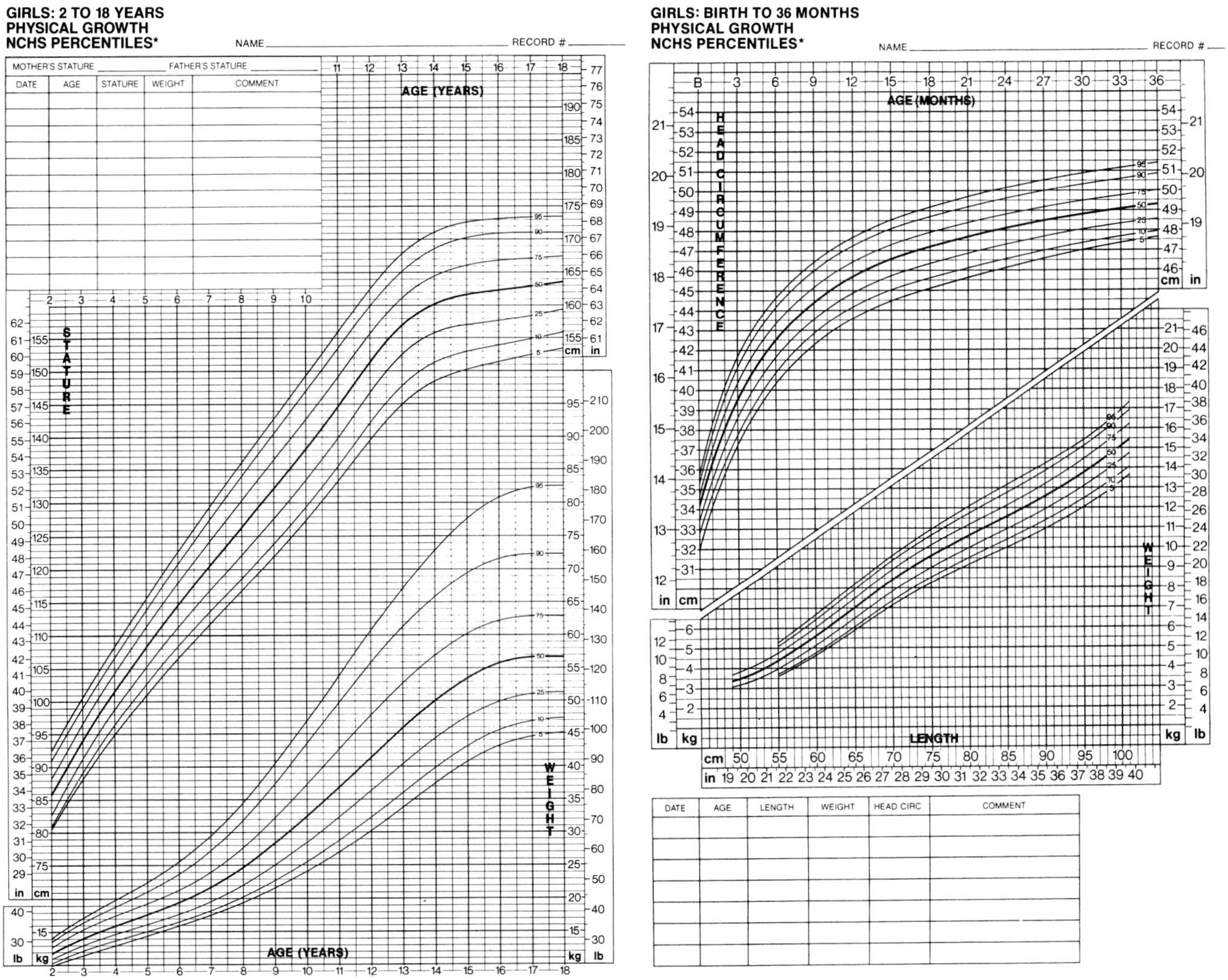

GIRLS: 2 TO 18 YEARS
PHYSICAL GROWTH
NCHS PERCENTILES*

NAME ________ RECORD # ________

MOTHER'S STATURE ________ FATHER'S STATURE ________

DATE	AGE	STATURE	WEIGHT	COMMENT

GIRLS: BIRTH TO 36 MONTHS
PHYSICAL GROWTH
NCHS PERCENTILES*

NAME ________ RECORD # ________

DATE	AGE	LENGTH	WEIGHT	HEAD CIRC	COMMENT

Figure 22-5 Pediatric growth charts (**A**) for girls 2–18 years—height and weight and (**B**) for girls birth to 36 months—length, weight, and head circumference. (Adapted from Hamill, P. V. V., Drizd, T. A., Johnson, C. L., Reed, R. B., Roche, A. F., Moore, W. M. [1979]. Physical growth: National Center for Health Statistics percentiles. *Am J Clin Nutr 32;* 607–629. Data from the National Center for Health Statistics [NCHS], Hyattsville, Maryland [Part A]. Data from the Fels Longitudinal Study, Wright State University School of Medicine, Yellow Springs, Ohio [Part B]. Used with permission of Ross Products Division, Abbott Laboratories, Inc. Columbus, OH 43216. © 1993 Ross Products Division, Abbott Laboratories, Inc.)

Checkpoint Question

7. *Using the chart in Figure 22-5B, find the weight/length percentile for a 7-month-old baby girl who weighs 16½ lb. What is this baby's percentile?*

Pediatric Vital Signs

Temperature

Infants and children have immature heat-regulating mechanisms, resulting in more temperature fluctuations than in adults. Factors that can influence a child's temperature include:

- Illness
- Infection
- Activity
- Dehydration
- Environmental temperature
- State of dress

Temperatures may be measured by the axillary, oral, rectal, or tympanic methods. If the child is compliant, the axillary route is a viable choice and is more acceptable to most children than rectal (Fig. 22-6). The oral route may be used for a child over 5 to 6 years of age if the child is not seriously ill or septic and is cooperative. Oral measurement should not be used if the child is congested, coughing, vomiting, or uncoopera-

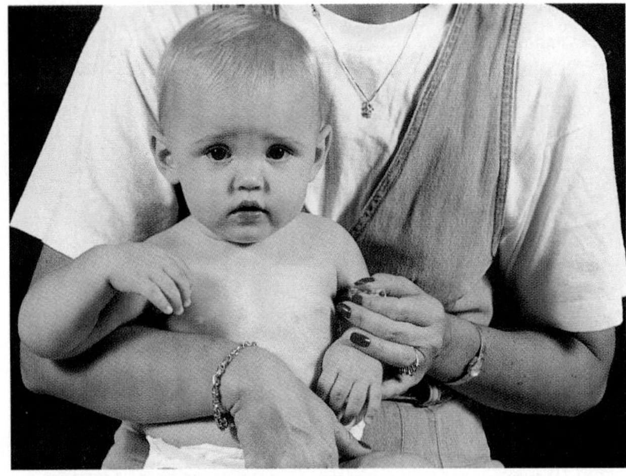

Figure 22-6 The axillary temperature is readily acceptable to most children and is considered accurate if the child is compliant.

tive. The rectal route should not be used if the child has diarrhea or objects strenuously to the procedure or is under the age of 2 months. The tympanic method is gaining popularity because it is rapid, reliable, and most readily accepted by all ages. (See Chap. 3, Anthropometric Measurements and Vital Signs, for more information about temperature.)

Checkpoint Question

8. *Besides illness and infection, what other factors can affect a child's temperature?*

Pulse

The pulse rate reflects the heart rate and is usually easily measured. Pulse rate can be affected by activity, temperature, emotions, and illness. For children under 2 years of age, measure the pulse apically. To do this, place the stethoscope on the chest between the sternum and left nipple. Count the heart rate for 1 full minute. For children older than 2 years, obtain the heart rate using the radial pulse site. (See Chap. 3, Anthropometric Measurements and Vital Signs.)

Expect a child's pulse to be considerably higher than an adult's. A newborn may have a pulse rate of 100 to 180 beats/min; with fever, a rate of 200 beats/min or more is not unusual. As the child matures, the rate will slow. By age 2, a child's rate may range from 70 to 110 beats/min; with fever or exercise, it may possibly reach 200 beats/min. By puberty, the rate is comparable to an adult's rate (Table 22-6).

Table 22-6 **Normal Pulse Rates for Children**

Age	*Rate/Minute*
Newborn	100–180 (may be over 200 with illness or crying)
3 mo–2 y	80–150 (may be up to 200 with illness or crying)
2–10 y	65–130
10 y and older	60–100

Respiration

Measure respiratory rate by observing the rise and fall of the child's chest. It is not necessary to disguise the fact that you are counting respirations, as you would with an adult patient. Because infants breathe by using the abdominal muscles more than the chest, observe abdominal movements and count 1 full minute. For children over age 2, use the same method as for adults. Count the respiration rate for 30 seconds and multiply by two.

Expect a newborn's respiratory rate to be as high as 35 per minute (Table 22-7). As with the pulse, the respiratory rate will slow as the child matures. At age 2, it will be about 25; by puberty, it will be comparable to an adult's.

Checkpoint Question

9. *How does a child's pulse and respiratory rate differ from an adult's?*

Blood Pressure

Blood pressure measurements are not required for most pediatric examinations but may be appropriate at times (Procedure 22-6). Blood pressure is the most difficult measurement to obtain in an infant or child because it is so difficult to prevent movement. Infants and children have smaller extremities than adults and require a smaller cuff. Select a cuff by the same method recommended in Chap. 3, Anthropometric Measurements and Vital Signs.

Because of their soft, nonresistant vessels and smaller bodies, children have lower blood pressures than adults. You may have problems determining a diastolic pressure in some children using standard sphygmomanometers. In children less than 1 year of age,

text continues on page 510

Table 22-7 **Normal Respiratory Rates for Children**

Age	*Rate/Minute*
Newborn	30–35
1–2 y	25–30
4–6 y	23–25
8 y and older	16–20

Procedure 22-1 Restraining a Child

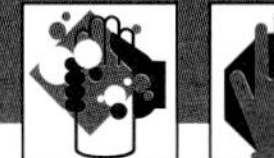
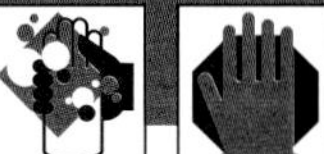

(as needed)

PURPOSE

To facilitate the pediatric examination or treatment while ensuring the patient's safety and comfort

EQUIPMENT/SUPPLIES

- receiving blanket (if using mummy restraint)

STEPS

1. Wash your hands.

2. Identify the patient.

3. Explain the purpose of the restraint to the child's parents.

Parents may become concerned that their child may be injured by the restraint. Explaining the need for the restraint and how it increases treatment safety will ease parents' fears.

4. Approach the child in a calm and purposeful manner. Speak softly close to the child's ear.

This reassures the child and decreases anxiety.

5. Restrain the child using one of these methods:

a. If only physical restraint is required, stabilize the child's joints.

This eliminates leverage that might allow the child to break from the proper restraint position. Holding the closest joint stabilizes the limb. For instance, to restrain the thigh for an injection, hold the child's knee rather than the lower leg.

b. If a mummy restraint is required, follow these steps:

(1) Place the child on a small receiving blanket.

(2) Wrap the left corner across the torso, covering the right arm and shoulder. Pull it snugly under the child's left arm and tuck it under the child's body.

(3) Pull the right corner across the child's left arm and shoulder and tuck it snugly under the torso at the back so that the child's weight secures the end.

(4) Tuck the bottom of the blanket around the child.

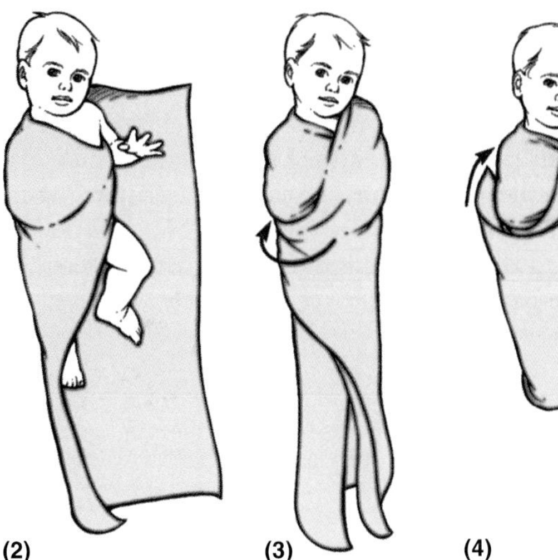

6. Guard against excessive pressure on the area of the child's body that is being restrained.

This avoids injury. In many instances, the restraint may be more frustrating for the child than the actual procedure.

7. Observe the child for any signs of respiratory distress or pain. Adjust the restraint or the holding position as necessary.

This provides for the child's physical comfort.

8. Wash your hands.

DOCUMENTATION GUIDELINES

- Date and time
- Reason for restraint
- Procedure requiring restraints
- Type of restraints and length of time the child was restrained
- Patient complaints/concerns
- Caregiver education/instructions
- Your signature

Charting Example

DATE	TIME 10 m/o/ presents with fever 102°F
	(R) × 2 days. Pulling on ears, fussy.
	Mother states she feels baby has ear
	infection. Today T - 102.4°F (R). Unable to
	hold baby still for Dr. Carson's exam.
	Mummy restraint applied for duration of
	exam (<5 mins). Baby tolerated procedure
	well. Mother instructed on fever control
	and antibiotic administration.
	—Your signature

22

Procedure 22-2 Measuring Height

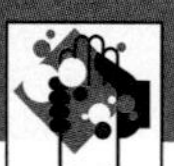

PURPOSE

To determine the proper growth pattern for the child's age

EQUIPMENT/SUPPLIES

- wall-mounted measuring unit
- growth chart

STEPS

1. Wash your hands.
2. Greet and identify the child.
3. Explain the procedure to the parent or to the child in an age-appropriate manner.
   This helps ensure cooperation.
4. Measure the child's height:
   a. Have the child stand as tall as possible against a wall-mounted measuring unit.
      Full extension to the child's tallest stature ensures a correct measurement.
   b. Make sure the child's heels are together and that the heels, buttocks, and shoulders are against the wall unit.
   c. Have the child look straight ahead.
   d. Place a horizontal bar against the crown of the child's head to determine the measurement.
5. Praise the child for cooperating.
   This may increase the child's positive response to the health care experience.
6. Record the child's height on the growth chart and in the patient chart.
7. Wash your hands.

DOCUMENTATION GUIDELINES

- Date and time
- Measurement reading
- Your signature
- (See Procedure 22-5, Weighing an Infant, for charting example.)

Procedure 22-3 Measuring Length

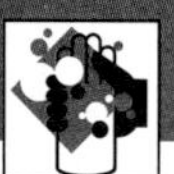

PURPOSE

To determine the proper growth pattern for the child's age

EQUIPMENT/SUPPLIES

- examining table with clean paper
- tape measure or measuring board
- growth chart
- pencil

STEPS

1. Wash your hands.
2. Identify the patient.
3. Place the child on a firm examining table covered with clean paper. If using a measuring board, cover with clean paper.
   Measurements may not be correct if the surface is not firm. Clean paper prevents cross-infection.
4. Measure the child's length:
   a. Fully extend the child's body by holding the head in the midline.
   b. Grasp the knees and gently press flat onto the table.
   c. Mark the top of the head and the heel of the feet on the paper.
   d. Have the parent pick up the child or move the child away from the section of the paper used for measuring.
   e. Measure between the marks in either inches or centimeters, or read the measurement indicated on the measuring board if this is the method used.
5. Record the child's length on the growth chart and in the patient chart.
6. Wash your hands.

DOCUMENTATION GUIDELINES

- Date and time
- Measurement reading
- Your signature
- (See Procedure 22-5, Weighing an Infant, for charting example.)

Procedure 22-4 Measuring Chest and Head Circumference

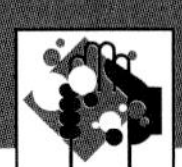

PURPOSE

To determine the proper growth patterns for the child's age

EQUIPMENT/SUPPLIES

- paper or cloth measuring tape
- growth chart

STEPS

1. Wash your hands.
2. Identify the patient.
3. Place the child supine on the examining table, or ask the parent to hold the child.
4. Measure around the chest at the nipple line, keeping the measuring tape at the same level anteriorly and posteriorly.
   Keeping the tape at the same level ensures an accurate measurement.

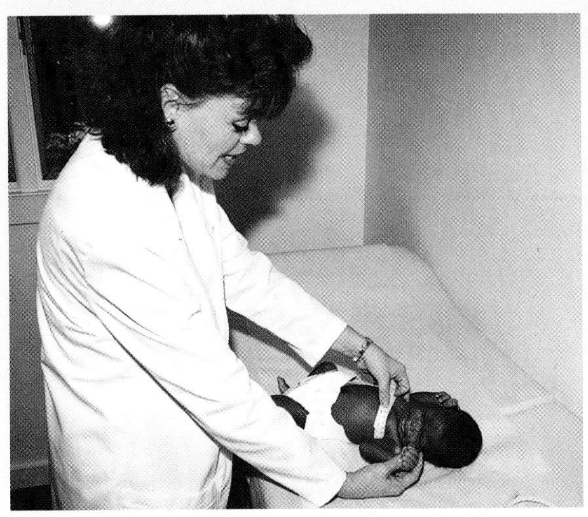

5. Measure around the head above the eyebrow and posteriorly at the largest part of the occiput.
   Measuring the largest circumference ensures an accurate measurement.

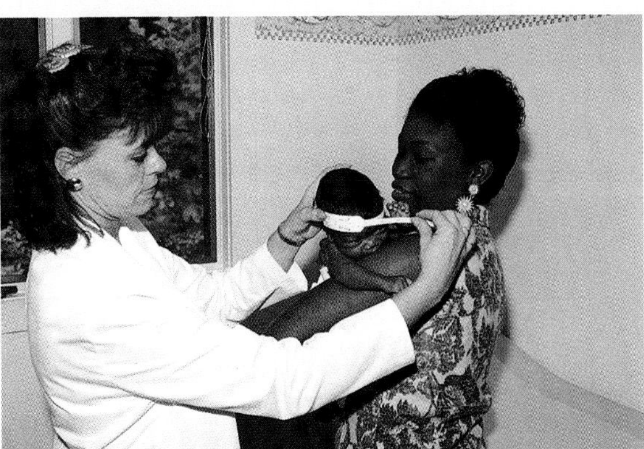

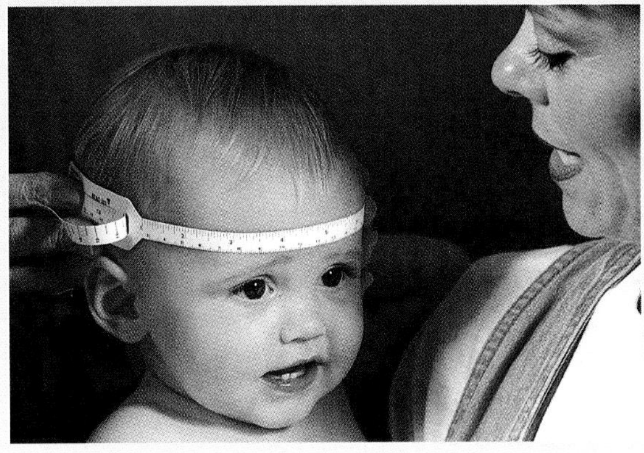

6. Record the child's chest and head circumference on the growth chart and in the patient chart.
7. Wash your hands.
   Note: If chest and head growth are within normal limits, these measurements usually are not required after 12 months.

DOCUMENTATION GUIDELINES

- Date and time
- Chest and head measurements (CC, HC)
- Your signature

Charting Example

DATE	TIME Mother arrived with 6 mo/o WF
	for recheck head and chest circumference
	to assess appropriate growth. CC—40.5
	cm, HC—41 cm (10% for 6 m/o).
	Percentiles unchanged from previous
	measurement. Dr. Boyce in to talk with
	mother. —Your signature

22

Procedure 22-5 Weighing an Infant

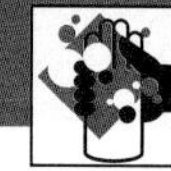
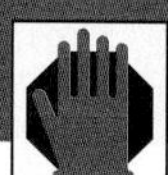

PURPOSE

To determine the proper growth pattern for the child's age

EQUIPMENT/SUPPLIES

- infant scale
- protective paper for the scale
- growth chart

STEPS

1. Wash your hands.
2. Identify the child.
3. Explain the procedure to the parent or to the child in an age-appropriate manner.
   This helps gain cooperation.
4. Place a protective paper on the scale.
   Protective paper prevents transmission of microorganisms.
5. Balance the scale.
   The balance beam must be centered before each use.
6. Follow these steps to weigh an infant:
   a. Place the infant gently on the scale, or have the parent place the infant.
   b. Infants are weighed lying down.

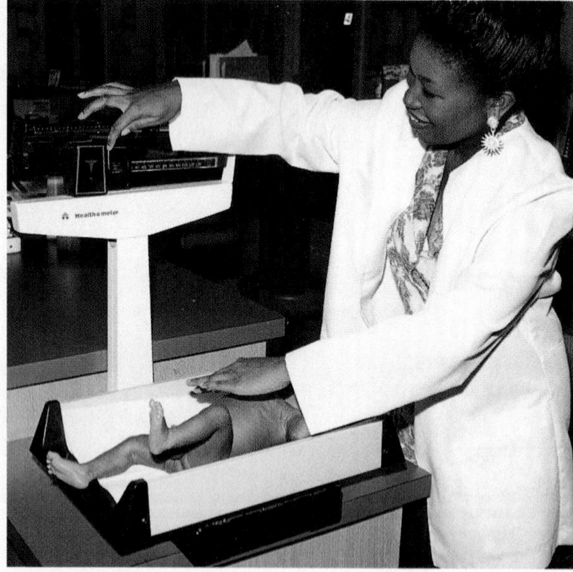

   c. Keep in mind that children who can sit may be weighed in a sitting position if this is less frightening for them.

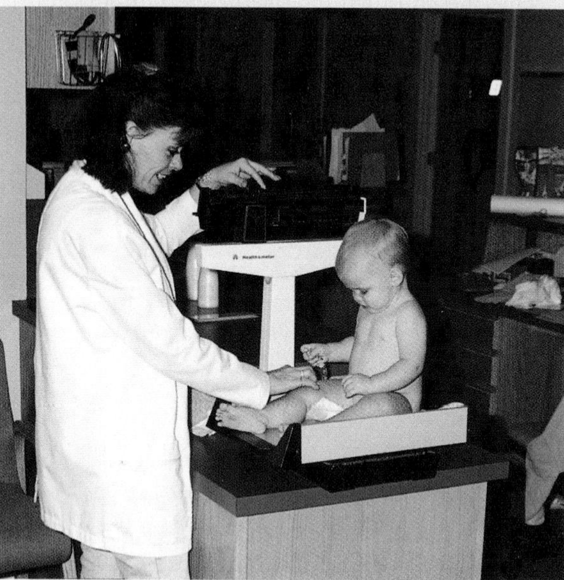

   d. Have the parent stand in the child's view.
   The child may feel insecure on the scale, and seeing a parent is reassuring.
   e. Keep one of your hands near the child at all times.
   Having a hand near the child reduces the risk of falling.
   f. Just before balancing the scale, remove an infant's diaper. *Note:* Wear gloves to handle diapers, as feces have been implicated in the transmission of disease. (Children may leave on undergarments while being weighed.)
   For the most accurate measurement, infants should be weighed without any clothing. Note that cool air against the infant's skin often causes voiding.
   g. Balance the scale quickly but carefully, moving the counterbalances to the proper places on the weight bar to balance the apparatus exactly.
   This ensures an accurate measurement.
   h. Have the parent pick up and soothe the child.
7. Record the child's weight on the growth chart and in the patient chart.
8. Wash your hands.

continued

Procedure 22-5 *Continued* Weighing an Infant

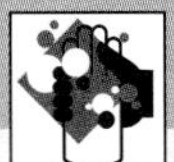
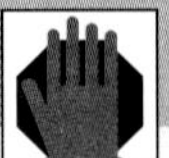

22

DOCUMENTATION GUIDELINES

- Date and time
- Measurement reading
- Your signature

Charting Example

DATE	TIME
	S: "My baby is doing great. He is now
	10 months old."
	O: 10-month-old infant. Ht—79.5 cm
	Wt—26 lb HC—46 cm T—98.4°F
	P—100 R—22. Child very alert,
	babbling various sounds, able to crawl,
	and able to pull self up. Child appears
	well nourished.
	A: Healthy 10-month-old. 95 percentile in
	growth chart.
	P: Educate parent on preventing ear
	infections and household safety tips.
	Physician in to see pt.
	—Your signature

Procedure 22-6 Measuring Pediatric Blood Pressure

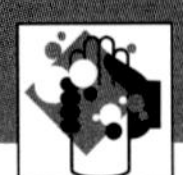

PURPOSE

To determine the hemodynamic status of the pediatric patient
To identify and monitor changes resulting from disease processes in the cardiovascular system

EQUIPMENT/SUPPLIES

- stethoscope
- sphygmomanometer

STEPS

1. Wash your hands.
2. Select the appropriate size cuff.

   Infants and children require a smaller cuff than adults. Choose the proper size cuff to accurately assess the child's blood pressure. (See Chap. 3, Anthropometric Measurements and Vital Signs, for an explanation of choosing cuff size.)
3. Identify the patient.
4. Explain the procedure to the child's parent or to the child in an age-appropriate manner. For instance, you might say, "This may squeeze your arm a little bit."

   This helps gain cooperation.

continued

22

Procedure 22-6 Continued Measuring Pediatric Blood Pressure

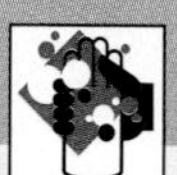

5. Expose the child's arm and determine the systolic pulse as described for adults. (See Chap. 3, Anthropometric Measurements and Vital Signs.)
   Doing this helps identify the proper site. Determining the systolic pulse avoids pumping the cuff too high and causing discomfort, or not pumping it high enough and missing the first systolic sounds.
6. Wrap the cuff around the arm 1/2 to 1 inch above the antecubitus.
   To avoid environmental noises, the cuff must not be against the area covered by the stethoscope.
7. Place the chestpiece of the stethoscope at the antecubital area. Pump the cuff about 30 mmHg above the last pulse felt.
   Pumping higher than necessary causes discomfort; not pumping high enough may cause the systolic to be missed.
8. Release the pressure 2–4 mmHg per second and note the first return of the pulse. This will be the systolic measurement. Note the last sound heard; this will be the diastolic pressure.
   Releasing more slowly interferes with circulation; releasing more quickly may cause the systolic to be measured too low.
9. Thank the child for cooperating.
   By providing praise and reassurance, you will help the child to develop a positive attitude about the pediatrician's office.
10. Care for the equipment as appropriate.
11. Wash your hands.

DOCUMENTATION GUIDELINES

- Date and time
- Patient complaints/concerns
- Blood pressure measurements and other vital signs as needed
- Patient/caregiver instructions and education
- Your signature

Charting Example

DATE	TIME 9/y/o for camp physical. Pt and
	mother state no complaints. Urine
	dipstick within normal limits. Hbg—14,
	Hct—40%. Immunizations current.
	Ht—4′11″ Wt—95 lbs T—98.2°F P—84
	R—22 BP—102/58. Dr. Hollowell to
	examine pt. —Your signature

expect a blood pressure of about 90/50. The blood pressure will gradually rise as the child matures. By age 10, a child's blood pressure will be in the low normal range of 110/60 (Table 22-8). Blood pressure checks become routine when children are about school age; they are done earlier if the patient history suggests the need.

Table 22-8 **Normal Blood Pressure for Children**

Age	*Systolic (mmHg)*	*Diastolic (mmHg)*
Newborn	<90	<70
1–5 y	<110	<70
10 y and older	<120	<84

ADMINISTERING MEDICATIONS

Administering medications to children presents a challenge to the medical assistant and to the parents, who are responsible for home administration. Medication dosage in children is calculated by weight or by body surface area. However, because children vary in weight, age, and fat/muscle ratio, they metabolize and absorb medication at varying rates. TO AVOID ERRORS, ALWAYS CHECK DRUG DOSAGE CALCULATIONS FOR A CHILD WITH ANOTHER STAFF MEMBER. Formulas for calculating pediatric dosages are discussed in Chapter 8, Preparing and Administering Medications.

You should be knowledgeable about the safe dosage amount, action, side effects, and signs of toxicity of any medication you administer. In most pediatric practices, the physician limits the choices to 50 or so medications that are suitable for children, making it relatively easy for you to learn all that is necessary about each medication. As for any medication, the seven "rights" of drug administration remain the same: *right patient, right drug, right dose, right route, right time, right method, and right documentation.*

Oral Medications

Use caution when administering oral medications to a child to prevent **aspiration** (inhaling the medication). Hold infants in a semi-reclining position, not lying. Place the medication in the mouth on either side of the tongue. Depending on the child's age, use a medication spoon, syringe, dropper, or medicine cup. Many children will suck medication from a syringe easily and safely. Administer small amounts of medication, allowing the child time to swallow. Older children who resist may need to be strongly encouraged to take medications. Always explain to children who are old enough to understand why medications are important, then proceed in a swift and safe manner to give the medication.

Injections

Medications are given to infants and children by injection when there is no other choice. Children commonly fear injections more than any other medical procedure. You should approach the child in a calm and firm manner. Never lie to the child or say that it will not hurt. For example, you might say, "You'll feel a prick, but it will hurt for only a few seconds. You can say 'ouch' but don't move."

Although it is important for the child to know that an injection is about to be given, some anxiety may be alleviated if the child does not see the syringe. Offer the child an age-appropriate explanation, then quickly give the medication. After administering any medication, praise and comfort the child. Childhood injections are more commonly given in the vastus lateralis, at least until age 2 (Fig. 22-7). The ventrogluteal site may be used if you are familiar with the landmarks. The dorsogluteal site is not used for children under age 2 because the muscles have not developed well.

The specific steps for administering an intramuscular injection are discussed in Chapter 8, Preparing and Administering Medications.

Checkpoint Question

10. *How is medication dosage calculated for children?*

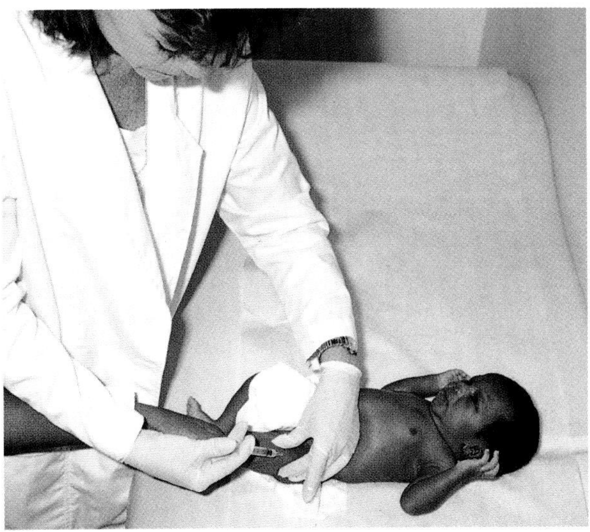

Figure 22-7 The vastus lateralis is the site of choice for infant injections.

COLLECTING A URINE SPECIMEN

You may need to obtain a urine specimen from an infant or young child for urinalysis. Because infants and young children cannot void on command into a specimen container, you will need to apply a pediatric urine collection device (Procedure 22-7). Ask parents to entertain or distract the child while waiting for the child to void.

UNDERSTANDING CHILD ABUSE

A child's social and physical well-being may be compromised by physical, emotional, or sexual abuse or by neglect. Abuse is thought to be the second most common cause of death in children under the age of 5. More die by the hands of their parents and caregivers than by accidents, fires, falls, or drowning. Many are permanently disabled or seriously injured; many more carry emotional scars that will never heal.

According to the National Center on Child Abuse and Neglect (NCCAAN), the following 1993 statistics represent the incidence of child abuse in the United States:

Emotional neglect	3.2/1000
Emotional abuse	3.0/1000
Physical neglect	8.1/1000
Physical abuse	4.9/1000
Sexual abuse	2.1/1000

The best available statistics only partially reflect the true incidence of child abuse and neglect.

22

Procedure 22-7 Applying a Pediatric Urine Collection Device

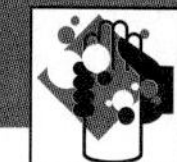 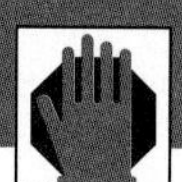

PURPOSE

To screen for abnormal components of the urinary output

EQUIPMENT/SUPPLIES

- personal antiseptic wipes or cotton balls and antiseptic solution
- pediatric urine collection bag
- completed laboratory request slip
- transport container

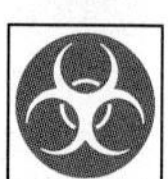

STEPS

1. Wash your hands.
2. Assemble the equipment and supplies.
3. Identify the patient.
4. Explain the procedure to the child's parents.
   This helps gain cooperation. Children who are old enough to understand the procedure will probably be able to provide a specimen without the use of a collection device.
5. Place the child in a supine position and ask for help from the parent, as needed.
   The urine collection bag must be properly attached to obtain the specimen. The child may be more cooperative if a parent is available to help.
6. Put on gloves.
   Standard Precautions must be followed when handling body fluids.
7. Clean the genitalia with the wipes or solution.
   a. For females: Cleanse front to back with separate wipes for each downward stroke on the outer labia. The last clean wipe should be between the inner labia (or labia minora).
      Cleansing front to back removes debris from the area and avoids introducing microorganisms into the urethra.
   b. For males: Retract the foreskin if the baby has not been circumcised, if possible. Cleanse the meatus in an ever-widening circle. Discard the wipe and repeat. Return the foreskin to position.
      Cleansing outward avoids introducing microorganisms into the urethra. Returning the foreskin to position prevents constriction of the penis.
8. Holding the collection device, remove the upper portion of the paper backing and press it around the mons pubis. Remove the second section and press it against the perineum. Loosely attach the diaper.
   The collection device must be securely attached to ensure collection of the next voiding. Reattaching the diaper avoids soiling if the child has a stool.

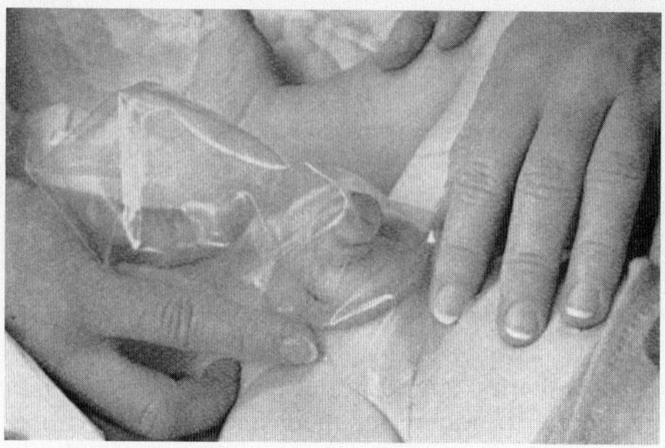

9. Give the baby fluids unless contraindicated, and check the diaper frequently for the specimen.
10. When the child has voided, remove the device, clean the skin of residual adhesive, and rediaper.
    Adhesive may be irritating to the skin.
11. Perform a routine urinalysis (see Chap. 28, Urinalysis), or route the specimen as required.
12. Remove gloves and wash your hands.

DOCUMENTATION GUIDELINES

- Date and time
- Application of urine collection device
- Description of urine (eg, cloudy, bloody, clear)
- Parent/caregiver education and instructions
- Your signature

Charting Example

DATE	TIME 5 m/o arrived for urine specimen
	as ordered by Dr. Perkins. Urine collection
	device applied after perineal prep, fluids
	offered. Pt voided qs cloudy urine for
	specimen to lab. Dr. Perkins to be notified
	stat of results to determine treatment
	plan. —Your signature

The Federal Child Abuse Prevention and Treatment Act mandates that threats to a child's physical and mental welfare must be reported. Some states require that all professionals report suspected child abuse or neglect to the proper authorities. Health care workers, teachers, and social workers who report in good faith will not be identified to the parents and will be protected against liability.

Medical assistants should be aware of the signs of abuse—either obvious indications or subtle warnings—that must be pursued for the child's safety.

Obvious Indications

- Reports of physical or sexual abuse by the child
- Previous reports of abuse in the family with current indicators
- Conflicting stories about the "accident" or injury from the parents and the child
- Injuries inconsistent with the history
- Injury blamed on siblings or someone other than the parent
- Repeated emergency room visits for injuries
- Fractures, burns, or skeletal injuries of a suspicious nature

Hidden Indicators

- Dislocations
- Nervous system trauma, particularly "shaken baby syndrome"
- Internal injuries, particularly to the abdominal area

Behavioral Indicators

- Overly compliant, too eager to please
- Passive avoidance, such as refusing to make eye contact, shrinking from contact
- Extremely aggressive, demanding, rage-filled behavior
- Role reversal, "parenting" the parent

What If?

What if you notice bruises and burn marks on the chest and back of the 3-year-old girl you are assessing?

If you suspect a child is being abused, approach the child and the parent in a calm and supportive manner. Any suspicions about the cause of a child's injuries should be discussed privately with the pediatrician right away. State laws vary regarding the procedure for reporting abuse; local regulations should be outlined in the policies and procedures manual. As a medical assistant, you have an ethical and moral responsibility to report suspected cases of abuse or neglect.

- Developmental delays (the child may be using energy needed for maturation to protect himself from abuse)

Warning Signs

- Malnutrition
- Poor growth pattern
- Poor hygiene
- Gross dental disorders
- Unattended medical needs

Answers to Checkpoint Questions

1. *Safety precautions that should be used in a pediatric practice include:*
   Keeping all medical equipment out of a child's reach
   Never leaving a child alone in the examining room
   Placing infant scales on a sturdy table and never leaving a child alone on a scale
   Storing disinfection solutions away from patient care areas
   Disposing of all sharps in proper containers
   Practicing stringent handwashing and Standard Precautions with every patient
2. *A pediatric patient might experience fear, anxiety, guilt, powerlessness, or curiosity during an office visit.*
3. *Well-child visits are scheduled at regular intervals, depending on the child's age, and are designed to maintain the child's optimum health. During a well-child visit, the pediatrician conducts a physical examination of the child and evaluates neurologic and psychosocial development. Sick-child visits are scheduled as needed. The goal of these visits is diagnosis and treatment of the child's immediate illness or injury.*
4. *A child's anthropometric measurements show growth and development and are good indicators of the child's health status and parent–child bonding.*
5. *75%*
6. *25%*
7. *10%*
8. *A child's temperature can be affected by activity, dehydration, environmental temperature, and state of dress.*
9. *In a child, both the pulse and respiratory rate are higher than in an adult.*
10. *Medication dosage in children is calculated by weight or by body surface area.*

Critical Thinking Challenges

During years of practice, Dr. Hernandez has found that many new parents are unfamiliar with basic child care needs. He decides to publish a short booklet for his new patients describing various aspects of child care. The booklet should be informative, professional, and show genuine concern for children. Topics to be covered include:

22

- General safety tips
- Types of office visits
- Immunizations (what they are, why they are important, at what ages they are given)
- What a parent can expect during an office visit
- Brief explanation of child development
- Tips for administering oral medications

Using your creativity and your knowledge of child care, write a sample booklet for Dr. Hernandez's patients.

Suggestions for Further Reading

Brown, J. L. (1994). *Pediatric Telephone Medicine: Principles, Triage, and Advice,* 2nd ed. Philadelphia: J.B. Lippincott.

Castiglia, P. T., & Harbin, R. E. (1992). *Child Health Care: Process and Practice.* Philadelphia: J.B. Lippincott.

Kozier, B., & Erb, G. (1993). *Techniques in Clinical Nursing,* 4th ed. California: Addison Wesley.

Marks, M. G. (1994). *Broadribb's Introductory Pediatric Nursing,* 4th ed. Philadelphia: J.B. Lippincott.

Pilliteri, A. (1995). *Maternal and Child Health Nursing: Care of the Childbearing and Childraising Family,* 4th ed. Philadelphia: J.B. Lippincott.

Schuster, C. S., & Ashburn, S. S. (1992). *The Process of Human Development. A Holistic Life-span Approach,* 3rd ed. Philadelphia: J.B. Lippincott.

Whaley, L. F., & Wong, D. L. (1991). *Nursing Care of Infants and Children,* 4th ed. St. Louis: C.V. Mosby.

23 Geriatric Patients

Chapter Outline

Role Delineation

GENERAL

Professionalism

- Project a professional manner and image.

Communication Skills

- Treat all patients with compassion and empathy.
- Adapt communications to individual's ability to understand.

Legal Concepts

- Practice within the scope of education, training, and personal capabilities.

Instruction

- Instruct individuals according to their needs.

Chapter Competencies

Learning Objectives

Upon successfully completing this chapter, you will be able to:

1. Spell and define the Key Terms.
2. Describe the changing concepts of the aging process.
3. Describe how aging affects the ability to remember and reason and how these changes affect thought processes.
4. List ways to ensure compliance with health maintenance programs among the elderly, and give reasons for noncompliance.
5. Outline steps to maintain open communication with the elderly patient.
6. Describe the coping mechanisms used by the elderly to deal with multiple losses and ways to recognize and alleviate the stressors.
7. List risk factors and signs of elder abuse, and give the responsibility of the medical office in suspected abuse.
8. Define the types of long-term care facilities available and the responses expected of the elderly at confinement.
9. Describe the affects aging will have on medication as it is processed in the body and the medical assistant's responsibility in patient education.
10. List and describe physical changes and diseases common to the aging process and how the medical assistant may alleviate the symptoms.

Key Terms

(See Glossary for definitions.)

activities of daily living (ADLs)
biotransforming
bradykinesia
cataracts
cerebrovascular accident (CVA)
degenerative joint disease (DJD)
dementia
dowager's hump (kyphosis)
dysphagia
glaucoma
keratoses
lentigines
osteoporosis
positron emission tomography (PET)
potentiation
presbycusis
presbyopia
syncope
transient ischemic attacks (TIAs)
vertigo

The elderly are the fastest growing segment of our population. They bring to the medical profession needs and concerns not generally faced by younger patients. Caring for these patients will test your skills in communication and will require the greatest degree of caring, compassion, and patience. The challenge of caring for the elderly may be one of the most rewarding aspects of the profession.

CONCEPTS OF AGING

As our older population has increased, established concepts of the aging process have changed. It is no longer expected that older relatives will be dependent on family members or that they will become incompetent by a specific age. Many are healthy enough to maintain homes well into their eighties and nineties. With many years spent in retirement, some are starting second careers at an age that their parents were either no longer alive or were incapacitated by ill health. College degrees are sought and earned, volunteering becomes a way of life, and hobbies become businesses. The greeting card image of the cozy, gray-haired grandmother in her rocking chair is more likely in reality to be a trim, active woman rushing out the door with a briefcase or tennis racket under her arm.

Compare these myths and stereotypes to the reality of the aging population (Box 23-1). How many of these are true? How many are far from typical of this age group?

Stereotyping the elderly, based on fear of aging, is a subtle and usually unconscious way to dissociate ourselves from the prospect of growing old. If these people are seen as somehow different, we may feel we can never be as they are now. This is striking when we compare the way children without preconceptions of aging respond to the elderly as opposed to the pulling away and separation adults may adopt when faced with someone who is not very many years older than they are themselves.

Although other cultures revere their elderly for their wealth of wisdom and experience, the American media perpetuate the myths and stereotypical reactions to the elderly by implying that graying hair and character lines are repulsive and should be avoided at all costs. Those "costs" range in the billions of dollars spent on delaying the physical signs of aging.

Consider how the following situations take on new meaning when applied through prejudice to different age groups.

- You are running late again. Dashing out of the door, locking it behind you, you remember that you left the keys to the house and car on the kitchen table . . . again.
- You stride purposefully from the bedroom into the kitchen with a specific goal in mind, only to reach the kitchen without any idea why you were in such a hurry to get there.

23

Box 23-1
Myths and Stereotypes About the Elderly

Myths
Old people are weak and sick.
Old people can no longer learn.
Old people have no more contributions to make.
Old people are boring.
Old people are a drag on the economy.
Old people are always lonely.
Old people cannot live alone.
Old people cannot be trusted to make rational decisions.
Old people have lost all interest in life.

Stereotypes
Old people have sensory losses.
Old people have erratic sleep patterns and nap a lot.
Old people do everything slower.
Old people have lost stature and slump a lot.
Old people cannot remember what happened this morning but can recall everything that happened 40 years ago.

We have all done these things and will no doubt do them again. However, if these things are done by an elderly person, they are considered to be a sign of approaching senility simply because the elderly are perceived as more forgetful than younger adults.

MEMORY ENHANCEMENT TO REINFORCE MEDICAL COMPLIANCE

Considering the differing functions of the aging mind and the interference of disease processes and medications with thought processes, it will be a challenge to help the patient work through methods of memory reinforcement. You might try these approaches:

1. Write out instructions in easy-to-understand terms. Use large print if the patient is vision impaired.
2. Have the patient repeat instructions to you for reinforcement.
3. Have the patient show you before leaving the office how he or she will perform a procedure.
4. Give the patient a large calendar or photocopy pages of a large appointment calendar and list times and days for treatments and medications to be crossed off as completed.

If a good rapport exists between the patient and the office staff, the patient is more likely to be truthful regarding the need for memory aids. If the importance of prescribed treatments and medications is explained in terms the patient can understand, compliance is more likely.

Many of the illnesses presented are long-term chronic situations that require medication for the remainder of the patient's life. In these situations, little improvement, if any, will be noticed by the patient, making compliance over a long period of time less probable. It may be explained in some circumstances that there is little chance for a return to former health but that the prescribed treatment will maintain health at a manageable level. This is especially important for patients with disorders such as diabetes or chronic heart disease. These patients will never be free of these diseases, but treatment will maintain a reasonable standard of health and independence. The patient may be helped to understand this with assistance from counselors and support groups.

Ask each time the patient visits the office for a complete account of all medications, prescribed and over-the-counter, and all current treatments. Ask the patient to list them. If you ask, "Mrs. Jones, are you still taking your heart medicine?", she may answer "Yes" whether or not she is actually taking this medication. A better question would be, "How do you take your medicine?" Many patients pick and choose what adjustments they make in their lives to comply with health restrictions, some grow tired of the constraints that illness and medications impose on their lives, some must choose between medication and food on the table, some forget, and some simply rebel. A stronger effort at remembering and adhering to treatment plans may depend on reinforcement of the patient's self-esteem and the will to be in control of one's own health status.

Assisting the patient to find ways to fit health requirements into a fairly normal life-style will help to ensure that treatment plans are followed and that the best level of health possible is achieved.

Checkpoint Question

1. *List memory enhancement techniques you might use to reinforce compliance.*

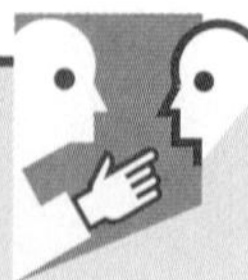

Advice and Tips
Communicating With the Hearing Impaired

When giving instructions to an elderly patient who is hearing impaired, do not shout. Instead, decrease the distance between you and the patient, face the patient directly, and speak slowly and distinctly. Call the patient the day after the office visit to assess compliance with and understanding of the instructions and to provide additional information if needed.

REINFORCING MENTAL HEALTH

With the recognized correlation between physical and mental health, we must be acutely aware of the patient's mental status. Elderly patients are adapting to new roles of dependency after a lifetime of social interaction, career objectives, and family development. Some have been relieved of social responsibility whether this is welcomed or not, and if they are ill, they must take on a dependent role. The presenting disease may be socially isolating, as in oxygen-assisted chronic obstructive pulmonary disease, a laryngostomy, or **dysphagia** (difficulty swallowing) requiring tube feedings.

Adjusting to pain or disability is often easier than adjusting to loss of social interaction. As we are better able to assist patients back to a semblance of health with advanced technology, more patients have to adjust to diseases that are not conducive to socialization. These patients experience all of the stages of grief as they lose their previous identities and lash out at the very people who are trying to help them. Their family members deal with stress, anger, frustration, and fear at the same time the patient is testing the patience of all caregivers.

Paradoxically, if you open yourself to the patient and are accessible and caring, you are more likely to be the object of anger and verbal abuse simply because you are seen as safe. A suffering patient is less likely to release pent up rage at someone who may respond with hostility or corresponding anger; consequently, the rage is held in, and the problem is compounded. Making yourself available to field these emotions can be as therapeutic as any treatment that might be administered to this patient. To do this effectively:

1. Maintain open communication, freely discussing hopes and fears realistically with the patient.
2. Help the patient to cope with and express feelings of guilt for being ill, anger at self and all nearby, and the loss of health and independence.
3. Work toward maintaining the patient's positive self-image.
4. Assist family members to maintain positive support.
5. Prepare the patient for the possibility that a return to the previous state of health may not be possible.
6. Direct the patient and family to support groups, such as the American Heart Association, the American Cancer Society, or other groups specific to the patient's problem.

Checkpoint Question

2. *How can you help promote good mental health in your elderly patients?*

COPING WITH AGING

Although the majority of the elderly are generally healthy and satisfied with their lives, those who are consigned to long-term care facilities or whose health and economic situations are precarious have every right to feel overwhelming stress and grief. Stress compromises the immune system, raises the blood pressure and blood sugar level, and strains the heart and lungs—all at a time when the patient needs all available resources to fight debilitating disease processes. Help patients to cope with stress by listening to their fears and concerns, respecting their rights to have these feelings, and helping them to reduce the stressors in their lives.

The coping mechanisms used to protect ourselves from stress become more pronounced with age. Young adults who handle stress by retreating into themselves will become withdrawn and stoical as older adults; young adults who handle stress by aggressive release will continue to be outspoken and vocal as older adults.

The ability of patients to cope with the losses that confront them is in direct relation to the importance of the losses. For instance, an artist with severe arthritis mourns the loss of artistic ability and may scarcely notice sags and wrinkles. Conversely, an actor who loses physical beauty minds that loss and may not notice fingers stiff with arthritis.

Be aware of the loss of specifics, such as sight, hearing, movement, perception, health, employment, home, and spouse. Also be alert to the loss of nonspecifics—life purpose, goals, a sense of achievement, self-worth, recognition, security.

Some patients have such difficulty adjusting to the multitude of losses that they might disengage emotionally and submit to decision making by family members that compounds the grieving process and leads to hopelessness and resignation. To avoid this reaction, the elderly must be involved in the personal decision making and have some voice in what becomes of them. The elderly who are encouraged to make decisions and take responsibility for themselves are happier, more sociable, and live longer.

Alcoholism

If coping fails, some elderly turn to alcohol as an escape. Alcohol slows brain activity and impairs mental processes, coordination, and judgment at a time when every available resource is needed. Alcohol may mask pain until the source of the pain becomes a danger. Alcohol abuse may be mistaken for **dementia** (mental deterioration), **transient ischemic attacks (TIAs)** (acute episodes of cerebrovascular insufficiency), or central nervous system impairment, and so may either be left

23

untreated or be treated incorrectly. Many of the medications used to treat the central nervous system react badly with alcohol and compound the problem. Alcohol increases the effect of narcotics, barbiturates, and depressants of all types, and the reason for the **potentiation** may go unrecognized.

The alcoholic patient is manipulative and convincing. The presenting symptoms may be explained away with no indication that alcohol is the problem. Such cases require the entire office staff to work with the patient's family or caregiver to uncover the cause of the symptoms. A situation like this also demands that the patient and those involved in the case work toward resolving the addiction.

Suicide

When ill health, multiple losses, and deep depression become too much for the patient to bear, suicide may seem preferable to life. Unlike suicide among younger people, suicide among the elderly is more likely to be well planned and successful. Approximately one-fifth of all suicides are persons over the age of 60. Most of those suicides are white men over the age of 65 who have recently lost a spouse. These suicides are not usually a cry for help, but a genuine effort to end life. Watch for these signs of intent:

- Deepening confusion and scattered attention span
- Increasing anger, hostility, or isolation
- Increase in alcoholism or requests for narcotics or sedatives
- Marked loss of interest in matters of health
- Secretive behavior
- Sharp mood swings from deep depression to euphoria
- Giving away favored objects

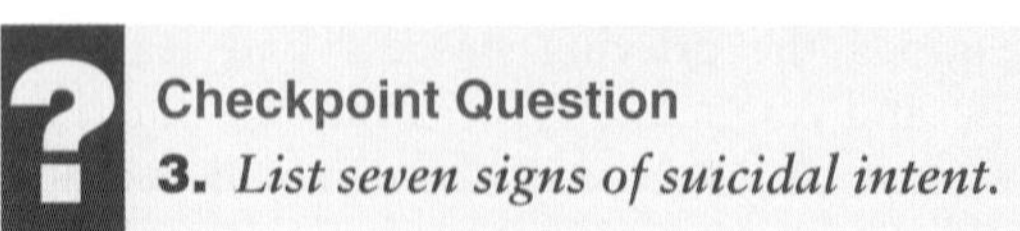

Checkpoint Question

3. *List seven signs of suicidal intent.*

Believe the patient who expresses an intent to commit suicide, and communicate this to the physician. Work with the health care team to restore mental health as aggressively as restoring physical health.

LONG-TERM CARE

More than 90% of the elderly live within the community, as many as 75% in their own homes. A small minority find that long-term care is the only option available if a return to health and independence is not possible.

Long-term care is divided into three main categories:

- *Group homes or assisted living homes* for the elderly who are able to tend to their own **activities of daily living (ADL)** (eg, bathing, dressing, self-feeding), but who need companionship and mild supervision for safety purposes. Bed and board are usually provided, along with a variety of other options.
- *Long-term care facilities* for those who need help with most areas of personal care as well as moderate medical supervision. Many are ambulatory but suffer from chronic diseases and disabilities that make living at home alone impossible.
- *Skilled nursing facilities* for those who are gravely or terminally ill and need constant supervision. If the illness is acute and short term, the patient may return to an intermediate stage of care after recovery.

Expect the elderly patient's move to long-term care to be met with sorrow and a deep sense of loss. The patient will probably show symptoms of bereavement: poor appetite, headaches, insomnia, deep depression, and vague aches and pains. All of these must be referred to the physician.

Many physicians continue to care for long-time patients who may be residing in long-term care facilities. As the medical assistant, you may be responsible to block time in the daily schedule for visits to patients in such facilities. You must direct calls from the facility to the physician regarding the patient's status and offer assistance to the family as they call with concerns about the care and physical condition of the patient.

Selecting a Long-Term Care Facility

A patient's relatives may turn to you for suggestions about facilities for elderly family members. It is generally not considered to be ethical to recommend a specific facility, but you may suggest several local sites. Urge the family to consider the following questions as they tour potential sites.

- Who owns and oversees the facility? How difficult would it be to contact the owner with questions and concerns?
- Ask to see the most recent inspection report. What deficiencies were noted, and were they corrected?
- Is there a large turnover of employees and supervisory staff? Do they seem open and friendly?
- Are rooms and common areas clean and odor free, bright and cheerful, barrier free, warm or cool enough?
- What is the ratio of assistants to residents? Do the assistants have time to assist with bathing and feeding?

- Glance through the rooms—Are many residents in their beds? Find out if residents are regularly assisted out of bed and given opportunities for exercise.
- Check the food service. Is the food service director a trained dietician? Can residents socialize in a central dining area for meals? Are the meals attractive, appetizing, and appropriate for the age group?
- Does the staff include a recreation director? Are residents' crafts and hobbies displayed and encouraged? Are group activities outside of the home planned and supervised?
- Is there a secure, shady place outside for pretty days? Is the area safe for short walks?
- Ask family members of other patients about the facility. Are they satisfied with the care provided?

Remind family members who ask you for referral advice to make sure that the facility director knows that they will be involved in their relative's care. They should not hesitate to make known any needs or concerns.

Checkpoint Question

4. *What is the difference between long-term care facilities and skilled nursing facilities?*

What If?

What if a patient's relative asks you about options for home care for an elderly parent?

You can explain that many options are available that allow patients to remain in the home. One option is the use of home health aides. Some insurance plans will pay for this service. The home health aides do light housecleaning, cooking, and will promote patient safety. A second option is community resource centers. Some communities have senior citizen programs that provide transportation for shopping, doctor appointments, or entertainment. These programs get the older patient out of the house, preventing boredom and enhancing self-esteem. A third option is placing the patient in a day-care program for the elderly. These programs keep the patient safe, entertained, and cared for during daytime hours. The advantage of day care is that it relieves the caregiver of the need to place a parent in a long-term care facility, yet provides for patient safety during the day and allows the relative the freedom to continue employment or attend to personal needs. Community programs for senior citizens are good sources of information for caregivers or for relatives searching for respite or permanent care.

ELDER ABUSE

Although elder abuse is not as well researched or as widely publicized as child abuse, it is thought to be almost as prevalent.

Risk Factors for Abuse

The following are common risk factors for elder abuse:

- Multiple chronic illnesses that stress the family's physical, emotional, and financial resources
- Senile dementia that precludes reasoning or interaction
- Bladder or bowel incontinence
- Age-related sleep disturbances that interfere with the caretaker's rest patterns
- Dependence on the caretaker for ADLs

Elder abuse may take several different forms, depending on the caretaker's need to exact punishment on the victim and the victim's access to resources.

Passive neglect may simply be ignorance on the part of the caretaker regarding the physiologic and psychological needs of the patient. The caretaker may be ill or elderly also and unable to supply the needs to the patient.

Active neglect may take many forms, including overmedicating (to render the patient passive and easier to care for) or purposely depriving the victim of adequate nutrition (to decrease physical resources).

Psychological abuse may include threatening imprisonment or physical abuse, withholding food or medication, or physical isolation.

Financial abuse may involve only small amounts of money or entire substantial estates. Financial resources may be embezzled, squandered, or frankly stolen, leaving the victim destitute.

Physical abuse may be as simple as pinches and slaps or may be life threatening, may be sexual in nature, and may be so well concealed as to be missed even by perceptive health care providers.

Checkpoint Question

5. *Name the different types of elder abuse. Describe each one.*

Signs of Elder Abuse

Be aware of these signs of elder abuse:

- Wounds of suspicious origins in various stages of healing
- Signs of restraint (wrist or ankle abrasions or bruising)
- Large, deep, neglected decubital ulcers
- Large amounts of physical debris and poor hygiene

- Poor nutrition with no efforts at correction
- Dehydration without related disease process
- Untreated injuries or medical conditions
- Excessive and unwarranted agitation or apathetic resignation

23

If you suspect abuse, you are responsible for bringing it to the attention of the physician, who should then assess the situation. If abuse is confirmed, referral should be made to the proper authorities. Most states now require that all suspected cases be reported to the Department of Social Services just as required for child abuse. Regulations for elder abuse are contained in statutes that address the concerns of the disabled adult. The entire medical staff may be held responsible if the abuse is not reported immediately.

The elderly fear reprisal or abandonment by their caregivers just as children do and are reluctant to complain of any improprieties. Separate the caregiver from the patient for the examination, if possible, and treat the patient with the utmost care and compassion. Document all findings with full descriptions. It may be necessary to photograph the suspected injuries to present with the documentation.

MEDICATIONS AND THE ELDERLY

Educating the elderly in self-medication is a challenge that will become increasingly common as the population ages. At a time when more medications are needed, the body is coping with the stress of illness or injury and a slowing down of all functions. The gastrointestinal system is no longer moving medications along as efficiently now that peristalsis has slowed. The circulatory system is not absorbing the dissolved medication from the intestines or the injection site and delivering it to the target tissue as quickly. The liver is not **biotransforming** (converting) the medication, causing it to remain in effect longer than might be desirable and possibly adding to a cumulative effect. Lastly, the kidneys are receiving less blood, thus less medication is being filtered, making the kidneys less effective at removing the medications from the system, with possible toxic effects.

The fact that the patient is ill adds to the problems of providing an education that will contribute to a return to an acceptable health status. Patients frequently have trouble understanding what is being explained to them because of their age-related barriers to understanding (poor hearing, slow response); these barriers are compounded by illness.

Your responsibility as a medical assistant is to elicit information regarding any and all of the prescribed and over-the-counter substances the patient is taking. Emphasize that the physician must be made aware of any change, addition, or deletion to the current list of substances. If the concept of interaction is understood, most patients will choose to adhere to suggestions made for their benefit.

Follow these guidelines to help ensure that your elderly patient adheres to the prescribed medication regimen:

1. Explain all side effects, precautions, interactions, and expected action in a manner that is appropriate for the patient's level of understanding.
2. Explain the proper dosage and how to measure. Mark plastic measuring cups with indelible ink at the appropriate level to be more easily read by patients with failing eyesight.
3. Write out a schedule and suggest methods for adherence. Suggestions may include daily dose packs available at pharmacies, egg cartons with hours of medication marked on the cups and filled with the proper medications each morning or evening, or calendars marked with the medications and hours to be checked off when the medication is taken.
4. Tell the patient to take the most important medication first. If it is not possible to take the other medications at this time, it may be acceptable to skip a dose of the less vital medications.
5. Help the patient understand not to rush taking the medication. The patient should be sitting or standing, not reclining. One pill should be taken at a time with lots of water. If the medication is difficult to swallow, have the patient try putting the pill on the back of the tongue and drinking with a straw.
6. Have the patient ask the pharmacist for large print on the label so that medication errors are less likely. Child-proof containers may not be necessary if there are no children in the home and the patient finds these hard to open.
7. Explain that the medication must be taken until it is gone (if this is the case) and must not be passed through the family or saved for another illness just like this one.
8. Encourage patients to take an active role in their therapy. Teach them to apply ointments or transdermal patches, even to give injections. A patient who feels in charge will more likely make the decision to complete a course of medication or to remain on the medication if its use is to be long term.

As a medical assistant, you are in control of the medication administration that occurs in the office, but responsibility to patients does not end there. To ensure that medications are used to their best benefit, emphasize to patients the importance of proper medication administration in their return to health.

Checkpoint Question

6. *Describe eight things you can do to make sure your elderly patient follows the prescribed medication regimen.*

SYSTEMIC CHANGES IN THE ELDERLY

Although longevity is considered largely hereditary, environmental factors play a considerable part in how long and how well we will live. The obese, physically inactive smoker is less likely to maintain a state of optimum health than the nonsmoker whose diet is well balanced and who is actively involved in an exercise program. In addition, certain occupational hazards, such as black lung disease or radiation exposure, may shorten a life that should have lasted for decades longer.

The aging changes are thought to be programmed into our cells along with our DNA. Theories now suggest that when cells have reached their allotted reproduction level, they either will not replace themselves or will replicate more slowly or ineffectively. These changes manifest themselves at varying rates for all persons but follow a recognized order as outlined in Table 23-1.

DISEASES OF THE ELDERLY

The degenerative conditions noted in Table 23-1 are part of the aging process. Many of the changes present problems that must be managed by the health care team; others are only inconveniences for the patient. Diseases specific for aging are covered in the chapters presenting each system. Below are two others commonly associated with aging, but they may present in the middle years as well.

Parkinson's Disease

Parkinson's disease is a slow, progressive neurologic disorder. It may take 10 years or more for complete debilitation or death. The initial presenting symptoms will frequently be muscle rigidity, involuntary tremors, and difficulty walking. It affects men more than women and is estimated to be present in some form in approximately 1 in 100 persons over the age of 60.

The cause is unknown but is thought to be a loss of dopamine in the brain cells. Normally dopamine and acetylcholine are in balance to inhibit involuntary movements of muscles. With the loss of normal levels of dopamine, acetylcholine has no counterbalance. This imbalance can be precipitated by cerebral injury or by cerebrotoxic medications in addition to idiopathic disease.

Signs and symptoms of Parkinson's disease include:

- Muscle rigidity
- **Bradykinesia** (abnormally slow voluntary movements)
- Difficulty walking, with a shuffling, mincing gait
- Forward-bending posture with no normal arm swing
- Laryngeal rigidity with a resulting monotone voice
- Pharyngeal rigidity with resulting dysphagia and drooling
- Facial muscle rigidity with resulting masklike, expressionless face and infrequent blinking reflex, causing eye infections.
- Small tremors in the fingers in a characteristic "pill-rolling" action. These start unilaterally and stop with purposeful action in the affected hand. Tremors are greater during times of stress and anxiety and are diminished at sleep or at rest. Muscles will resist passive stretching and will become rigid with passive manipulation (Fig. 23-1).

Diagnosis is usually made by excluding other possible causes. Testing may show decreased levels of dopamine in the urine. Symptomatic history remains the primary method of diagnosis after all other possibilities have been ruled out.

Parkinson's disease has no cure. Treatment is symptomatic, supportive, and palliative. Medications include:

- Levodopa (L-dopa). Dopamine replacement crosses the blood–brain barrier to restore the balance with acetylcholine. Individualized doses are gradually increased as the disease symptoms progress. Levodopa is fairly effective for a period of time but will gradually lose its effectiveness. Unfortunately, levodopa has serious side effects that include nausea and vomiting, tachycardia, and arrhythmias. It has severe adverse reactions with alcohol.
- Anticholinergics. By decreasing the levels of acetylcholine, depleted levels of dopamine are not so out of balance. This method works best in mild, early stages.
- Antihistamines with anticholinergic actions. In the early, mild stages, this method of lowering acetylcholine to balance with low levels of dopamine will alleviate symptoms.

text continues on page 525

23

Table 23-1 **Effects of Aging on Body Systems**

	Systemic Changes	*Manifestations*	*How the Medical Assistant Can Help*
Integumentary System	Loss of subcutaneous fat	Wrinkling, sagging, decreased ability to maintain hydration, less protection against temperature changes	Encourage the patient to drink plenty of fluids and dress appropriately for climate changes.
	Loss of pigment	Less protection against sun damage, paler skin, graying hair	Encourage the use of sunscreens with appropriate UV protection.
	Loss of elasticity	Increased incidence of trauma	Suggest using good lubricating lotions and bathing less often. Caution the patient to guard against injuries.
	Receding capillaries	Sallow skin, thicker nails	
	Slower reproduction of hair and skin cells	Balding; thin, fine hair; slower healing	Suggest ways to guard against injuries.
	Diminished oil and sweat production	Dry, fragile skin; intolerance to heat	Encourage the patient to use good lubricating lotions and bathe less often. Suggest ways to avoid becoming overheated.
	Erratic pigment and cell production	Senile **lentigines** (liver spots) and **keratoses** (skin thickening)	Show the patient how to conduct skin checks and consult a dermatologist with any concerns.
Musculoskeletal System	Loss of muscle strength and size	Loss of strength, flexibility, and endurance	Suggest frequent exercise appropriate to the patient's age and ability.
	Loss of bone density	Vertebral compression with diminished height and a **dowager's hump** (abnormal spinal curvature); **osteoporosis** (abnormal bone porosity) with frequent fractures	Educate the patient regarding weight-bearing exercises. Encourage the patient to conduct a home safety check to avoid falls. The physician may recommend calcium supplements, dietary consultations, or estrogen replacement.

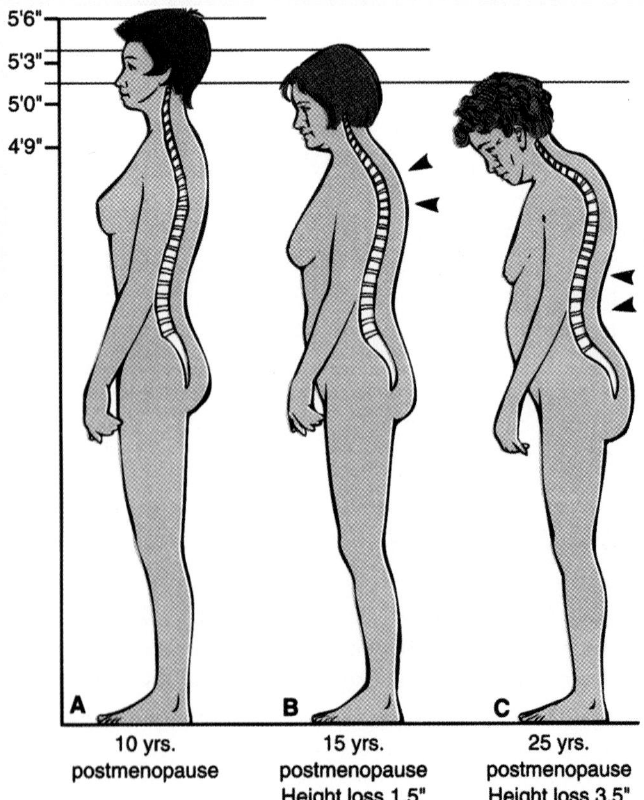

Typical loss of height associated with osteoporosis and aging. (Courtesy of Wilson Research Foundation.)

(continued)

Table 23-1 **Effects of Aging on Body Systems** *(Continued)*

	Systemic Changes	*Manifestations*	*How the Medical Assistant Can Help*
	Degenerative joint cartilage	Less clear margins with spurs of bone that restrict movement, **degenerative joint disease (DJD)**, arthritis	The physician may limit phosphorus intake.
Nervous System	Slower nerve conduction	Slower reaction time, slower learning, slower perception of pain with resulting increase in injuries	Allow extra time as needed, and educate the patient about possible hazards of delayed reaction times. Aim teaching at comprehension level. Encourage the patient to conduct home safety checks.
	Reduced cerebral circulation	Loss of balance and **vertigo** (whirling sensation), frequent falls	Have the patient install bath rails, remove throw rugs, conduct a home safety check. Encourage the patient to use ambulatory aids.
	Referred circulatory problems	Increase in cardiovascular diseases (atherosclerosis, arteriosclerosis) reflected as **cerebrovascular accidents (CVA)** (brain ischemia due to vessel occlusion), cerebral hypoxia, and transient ischemia attacks	Educate the patient and family about the danger signs for CVAs and transient ischemic attacks.
	Less time spent in deep sleep	Less restful sleep, more frequent naps	Allow the patient rest periods as needed.
Eyes	Diminished adjustment of lens to accommodation	**Presbyopia** (farsightedness)	Obtain a referral to an ophthalmologist. Provide adequate lighting, and use large print books.
	Lens cloud	**Cataracts** (lens opacity) that dim vision as less light reaches the retina	Obtain a referral to an ophthalmologist. Provide adequate lighting.
	Loss of ciliary function	**Glaucoma** (increased intraocular pressure as the pupils press on the canal of Schlemm), intolerance to light or glare, poor night vision	Obtain a referral to an ophthalmologist. Provide adequate lighting, and have the patient avoid night driving.
Ears	Loss of auditory hair cells (organ of Corti)	Hearing loss in upper frequencies, problems distinguishing Ch, S, Sh, and Z	Obtain a referral to an otologist. Speak clearly, facing the patient, in an area with few distractions.
	Ossicle becomes fixed	**Presbycusis** (hearing loss), strains to hear, misses cues, inappropriate responses	Obtain a referral to an otologist. Speak clearly, facing the patient, in an area with few distractions.
Other Senses	Diminished sense of smell	Loss of appetite, poor nutrition	Suggest dietary consultation.
	Diminished sense of taste	Loss of appetite, poor nutrition, may increase use of salt or spices	Suggest dietary consultation. Encourage use of spices rather than salt.
Cardiovascular System	Atherosclerosis and arteriosclerosis, narrowing of vessels	Loss of peripheral circulation, fatty plaques with resulting myocardial infarctions and CVAs, cold extremities, slower healing time, hypertension	Encourage the patient to exercise and to eat a balanced, low-fat, low-salt diet. Have the patient dress appropriately for temperature changes and conduct a home safety check.
	Slower response time to demands for increased output	Complaints of fatigue on exertion	Help the patient pace exercise and exertion.
	Diminished function	Pulmonary involvement with edema, dyspnea	Educate the patient regarding low-salt diets and orthopneic position.

(continued)

23

Table 23-1 **Effects of Aging on Body Systems** *(Continued)*

	Systemic Changes	*Manifestations*	*How the Medical Assistant Can Help*
Respiratory System	Stiffening costal cartilage	Decreased expansion and contraction, barrel chest, decreased lung capacity	Educate the patient about smoking hazards and emphysema. Encourage moderate exercise.
	Decreased gas exchange	Fatigue and breathlessness on exertion, impaired healing due to insufficient oxygen, **syncope** (sudden drop in blood pressure)	Encourage the patient to exercise, as appropriate, and to use ambulatory aids. Caution the patient to guard against upper respiratory infections and to conduct a home safety check.
	General loss of muscle mass	Difficulty coughing deeply (may lead to pneumonia)	Encourage the patient to drink adequate fluids to liquefy respiratory secretions.
Gastrointestinal System	Drying of secretions, including saliva	Dry mouth, dysphagia (difficulty swallowing)	Educate the patient regarding oral hygiene and adequate fluid intake.
	Decreased enzyme activity	Incomplete digestion, poor conversion of nutrients with malnourishment	Encourage the patient to eat small, frequent, well balanced meals.
	Slower peristalsis	Constipation, flatulence, indigestion	Suggest the patient increase fluid and fiber intake. Have the patient avoid laxative dependency.
	Loss of teeth	Poor chewing function, choking on large pieces, loss of appetite, poor nutrition	Refer the patient to dentist, and provide instruction regarding good oral hygiene. Suggest dietary counseling.
Urinary System	Decreased bladder capacity	Urinary frequency	Encourage the patient to respond to the initial urge to void.
	Decreased bladder muscle tone	Urinary retention with resulting urinary tract infections or incontinence	Suggest exercises for strengthening the pelvic floor. Urge the patient to completely empty the bladder with each voiding.
	Fewer functioning nephrons	Less blood flowing through the kidneys to be cleaned of wastes, creating possible lethal levels of medications or normal body wastes	Have the patient increase fluid intake to maintain hydration.
Endocrine System	Decreased hormonal activity	Menopause, glucose intolerance with non–insulin-dependent diabetes mellitus, slower metabolism	The physician will supplement as needed.
Immune System	Diminished production and function of T and B cells	Less resistance to illness	Encourage the patient to obtain immunizations as age appropriate.
	Diminished ability to distinguish "self" from "other"	Increase in autoimmune diseases	Educate the patient regarding symptoms of autoimmunity.
	Diminished defenses elsewhere (eg, gastrointestinal enzymes)	Overload on compromised immune system and more frequent serious illnesses	Encourage the patient to obtain immunizations as age appropriate and to guard against communicable diseases.
Female Reproductive System	Decreased egg production	Menopause or climacteric	The physician may prescribe supplemental estrogen.
	Decreased estrogen production	"Hot flashes"; thinner, drier vaginal walls with vaginal itching and painful intercourse; osteoporosis	The physician may prescribe supplemental estrogen.
	Poor perineal muscle tone	Rectocele, cystocele, stress incontinence	Suggest exercises for strengthening the pelvic floor.
Male Reproductive System	Decreased penile and testicle size	Loss of libido	The physician may refer the patient for counseling.
	Atherosclerosis and arteriosclerosis	Impotence	The physician may refer the patient for counseling. Educate the patient regarding good nutrition to avoid atherosclerosis.
	Benign prostatic hypertrophy (BPH)	Urgency, frequency, nocturia, retention	Encourage the patient to have yearly checks for BPH and provide instruction regarding testicular self-examination.

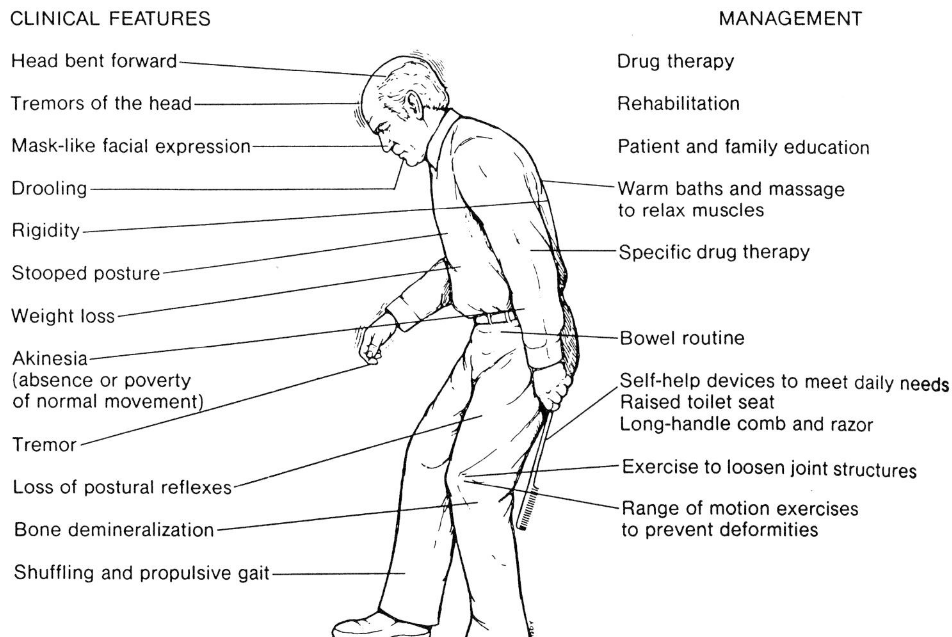

Figure 23-1 The patient with Parkinson's disease.

Neurosurgery exactly pinpointing the appropriate area of the thalamus involved will help to prevent involuntary movement. This method of treatment is rarely used except in young, otherwise healthy patients. As with all other methods, this is palliative and not curative.

Passive and active range-of-motion exercises will help to maintain a level of muscle tone and flexibility. Regular walking schedules, heat, and massage will help to keep muscle tissue supple. Parkinson's patients tire easily and must rest often but will ultimately benefit from regular schedules of moderately challenging exercise.

Parkinson's patients will retain their former level of intelligence unless an organic brain disturbance is also present. They are aware of the outward signs of the disease and are embarrassed and depressed. They will require great psychological support from the medical staff, family, and support groups. As a medical assistant, you can:

1. Encourage the patient to participate in all ADLs.
2. Encourage independence; do not infantilize the patient.
3. Be aware that rigidity extends to the gastrointestinal tract, so expect dysphagia and constipation. Suggest that the patient increase fluids, watch nutrition, and increase fiber intake.
4. Warn the patient that a decreased cough reflex can lead to choking.
5. Encourage the patient to use aids for safety and assistance in eating, such as no-spill cups, plates with high sides, and special utensils. Raised toilet seats and handrails in the bath will increase independence and safety.
6. Listen and talk to the patient. Intelligence is still intact and needs to be stimulated.
7. Educate the patient about safety factors; the forward-bending posture and altered gait frequently lead to falls.
8. Enlist the help of support groups. Include the caregiver, and urge respite care when exhaustion and stress become overwhelming.

Death is usually the result of aspiration pneumonia, falls, accidents, or opportunistic diseases secondary to the effects of long-term stress.

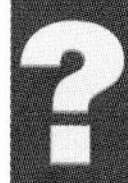

Checkpoint Question

7. *How can you assist a patient with Parkinson's disease?*

Alzheimer's Disease

Roughly half of the dementia seen in the elderly can be traced to Alzheimer's disease. Alzheimer's may masquerade as TIAs, cerebral tumors, and dementias other than Alzheimer's. There is no clearly defined cause or cure for this disease at this time. Research continues, and promising new therapies are available to slow the progression of the disease.

Symptoms may begin as early as age 40 with gradual loss of memory function and slight personality changes. The changes may cover a period as long as 15 years and are frequently so gradual that diagnosis is difficult and may only be made on the basis of symptoms. If swift and early diagnosis is necessary, **positron emission tomography (PET)** has been used with varied success. (PET is computerized radiography using radioactive substances to assess metabolic or physiologic functions within the body.)

Later diagnosis may sometimes be made by electroencephalography or computed tomography. However, diagnosis is generally made by excluding or ruling out all other possibilities. No reliable treatment is available at this time. On autopsy, organic brain changes are seen with loss of neurons and neurotransmitters. Plaques or deposits may be present as a residue of the neural cell deterioration.

Alzheimer's disease has seven recognized stages. The progression from one stage to the next may be gradual. Some stages may last for years, and some stages may be passed through so quickly that the progression may go unnoticed. Expect varying levels of response from patients as they present at each of these levels (Table 23-2).

As a medical assistant, your responsibility will be to remember that anger and hostility are symptoms of this disease and should not be taken personally. When caring for patients with Alzheimer's disease, be sure to:

- Respond with the utmost patience and compassion.
- Speak calmly and without condescension.
- Never argue with the patient, even if you are blamed unfairly for the patient's memory lapses.
- Reintroduce yourself. Do not expect the patient to remember the staff from previous visits.
- Explain even common procedures as if the patient has never had them explained.
- Approach quietly and professionally in a nonthreatening manner, and remind the patient of who you are and what you must do.
- Use short, simple, direct statements, and explain only one action at the time rather than a sequence of directions.
- Keep a list of support contacts for family members to call.

Home care agencies usually offer the respite care that is vital to the caregiver if mental and physical health are to be maintained. Remember that an exhausted, distraught family member may not be thinking clearly. The most therapeutic action may be for you to assist the family with the proper contacts to make the diagnosis of this devastating disease less traumatic.

MAINTAINING OPTIMUM HEALTH

No one realistically expects to maintain at age 70 the same strength and agility that is taken for granted at age 20. It is possible, however, to achieve a level of fit-

Table 23-2 **Levels of Alzheimer's Disease**

Level	*Description*
I and II	Presenile dementia may end here with no further progression. Brain changes are not significant, and the only remarkable symptom may be forgetfulness. Patients at this level still perform all activities of daily living (ADLs) with reasonable ease.
III	At this level, there will be an increased inability to remember facts, faces, and names. The patient will still have enough awareness to recognize the problem and will become increasingly frustrated and angry. Most ADLs are still performed reasonably well.
IV	Late confusional or mild Alzheimer's. The patient at this level will begin to misplace things, has increasing difficulty remembering, and will neglect ADLs. Most patients will be aware that a problem exists but will deny that it is a concern.
V	Early dementia or moderate Alzheimer's. By this level, the patient must have custodial care. There will be severe lapses in memory, disorientation, anger, and great frustration.
VI	Middle dementia or moderately severe Alzheimer's. The patient now has severe memory loss, is incapable of self-care at any level, and is disoriented most of the time. There is immense anger, hostility, and combativeness. At this level, a fear of water is present.
VII	Late dementia. The patient requires full-time care and will rarely be seen in the office setting. Unless home care is an option, the physician will probably make calls to the long-term care facility. The patient at this stage rarely speaks and almost never speaks intelligibly. There will be incontinence, and the patient may require tube feedings.

ness that adds a dimension to life not possible if proper nutrition and exercise are neglected.

Exercise

Exercise plays a vital role in maintaining overall physical and mental health (Table 23-3). Patients beginning an exercise program should only do so after a thorough physical examination and should proceed at the physician's recommendation.

Provide the following guidelines for elderly patients who are starting an exercise program:

1. Always warm up cold muscles for at least 10 minutes. Slow and rhythmic movements, such as walking, raise the heart rate and increase metabolism before beginning slow, easy stretching to lengthen sluggish muscles.
2. Begin by exercising for brief time periods. Expect to exercise 5 to 10 minutes a day the first week, then progress to 10 or 15 minutes a day the next week, and gradually work up to about 30 to 45 minutes of pleasantly challenging strength and cardiovascular/endurance activity after about a month. This routine will reduce the chance of injury and is more likely to be an attainable goal.
3. Stop if you feel pain, shortness of breath, or dizziness. Never try to work through pain.
4. Breathe deeply and evenly. If you cannot carry on a conversation, slow down. Never hold your breath while you exercise.
5. Rest when you get tired. Do not try to work to the point of exhaustion.
6. Keep a record of your progress. It helps to see how much your performance has improved.
7. Exercise with a friend, with a group, or to music that you enjoy.
8. Make exercise a part of your daily routine, do not make it a chore. Do something vigorous every day and take pride in it.

Table 23-3 **Benefits of Exercise**

System Targeted	*Benefits*
Cardiovascular	Increases endurance Lowers cholesterol to avoid atherosclerosis Maintains vascular elasticity to delay arteriosclerosis
Musculoskeletal	Increases bone mass to reduce osteoporosis Decreases fat/muscle ratio to maintain metabolism Retains strength and flexibility to ensure mobility and improve posture
Nervous	Improves mental health by reducing stress, fatigue, tension, and boredom Maintains or restores balance to reduce falls

Diet

The elderly have several factors that interfere with good nutrition. A decrease in activity will mean a corresponding decrease in hunger. Decaying teeth or poorly fitting dentures cause pain, making it hard to chew. Saliva production decreases, making it harder to swallow. The sense of smell diminishes, interfering with the cephalic phase of digestion. Taste perception does not work well, so nothing tastes good. Many eat alone or cannot enjoy the socialization that adds immeasurably to the joy of eating.

A balanced diet is vital to good health at any age. Although activity levels are lower among the elderly, decreasing the need for a certain amount of calories, vitamin and mineral requirements are not lowered with age. Efforts must be made to increase the nutritional level of the elderly. The food should be easy to chew but offer texture and variety. There should be a decrease in sugar, salt, and fat intake and an increase in vitamins, protein, and fiber consumption. Smaller, more frequent meals may be easier to digest than infrequent large meals. Water should be offered frequently to maintain hydration and to aid digestion and elimination. Constipation is a frequent complaint, but a diet high in fiber, water, and a regimen of exercise will help alleviate the problem.

Talk to patients or their families about valuable services, such as Meals on Wheels. Nutritious meals are delivered to the home either daily or 5 days a week (some do not operate on weekends). This ensures that at least one well balanced meal a day is available. Most prepare meals to meet special dietary needs, such as low sodium, low fat, and so on. In addition to the meals, contact with a caring volunteer is a daily occurrence. The volunteer will be alert to the needs of the patient and will report to a coordinator if the patient does not answer the door or seems ill or confused. This resource is reassuring to the patient and the family that nutritional and socialization needs are being met.

Safety

Alert the patient and caregivers to areas of concern for safety, and offer the following suggestions:

- Avoid scatter rugs, especially on highly polished floors.
- Never allow electrical cords across passageways.
- Increase lighting for better illumination.
- Remove or reduce clutter as much as possible.

- Strengthen handrails on stairs, and install them in tubs and near the commode.
- Install a telephone by the bedside and near a favorite chair. Consider having a telephone in the bathroom also.
- Install and frequently maintain smoke alarms and carbon monoxide detectors throughout the house.
- Establish a system for calling and checking every day. Many communities have available systems in which volunteers call the sick or elderly daily to check on needs and to offer a few minutes of conversation. If the patient fails to answer, someone is sent to the home to check on the patient. This service ensures that the patient will never be without contact for long periods of time. Lifeline, an emergency service contact worn by the patient, is also an option that increases the feeling of safety for patients who live alone.

Answers to Checkpoint Questions

1. *To reinforce compliance, you could write out instructions in easy-to-understand terms (using large print if the patient is vision impaired); have the patient verbalize instructions and demonstrate a procedure; or list times and days for treatments on a large calendar.*
2. *You can help your elderly patients maintain good mental health by encouraging open communication, helping them deal with their feelings, promoting a positive self-image, helping family members to be supportive, preparing the patient for the future, and suggesting support groups as needed.*
3. *The seven signs of suicidal intent are deepening confusion, increasing anger, increased alcohol or narcotic use, lack of interest in health, secretive behavior, sharp mood swings, and giving away personal possessions.*
4. *Long-term care facilities are for individuals who need help with personal care and some medical supervision. Skilled nursing facilities are for gravely or terminally ill individuals who need constant supervision.*
5. *Elder abuse can take the form of passive or active neglect or it can be psychological, financial, or physical in nature. Passive neglect refers to the caregiver's inability to identify the patient's needs; active neglect involves the caregiver's refusal to supply the patient's needs. Psychological abuse includes threats, withholding food or medication, or forced isolation. Financial abuse involves depriving the patient of material resources. Physical abuse includes varying degrees of physical injury.*
6. *To help your elderly patient follow the prescribed medication regimen: provide a full explanation of the medication in a way that the patient understands; explain the proper dosage and techniques for measuring; develop a written schedule for taking the medication; instruct the patient to take the most important medication first; tell the patient not to rush when taking the medication; have the patient ask the pharmacist for large print on the label; explain the appropriate use of the medication (eg, do not give it to others or save it); encourage patients to take an active role in their therapy.*
7. *To assist a patient with Parkinson's disease, encourage activity and independence, promote good nutrition and hydration, caution the patient about the potential for choking, educate the patient about safety, use therapeutic communication skills, and enlist the help of support groups.*

Critical Thinking Challenges

1. Mrs. Moss, age 78, lives with her son and daughter-in-law and their two school-age children. She has dysphagia and requires tube feedings, so she misses family mealtimes. Identify ways in which Mrs. Moss could participate in a family meal.
2. Mr. Brown is 90 and his wife is 86. They live alone, and Mrs. Brown is the primary caregiver. During the physical examination, Mr. Brown is found to have several large, deep decubital ulcers. Summarize the various types of elder abuse or neglect. What is likely the problem in this case?

Suggestions for Further Reading

Birchenall, J, M., & Streight, M. E. (1992). *Care of the Older Adult,* 3rd ed. Philadelphia: J.B. Lippincott.

Craven, R. F., & Hirnle, C. J. (1996). *Fundamentals of Nursing: Human Health and Function,* 2nd ed. Philadelphia: Lippincott-Raven.

Memmler, R. L., Cohen, B. J., & Wood, D. L. (1996). *The Human Body in Health and Disease,* 8th ed. Philadelphia: Lippincott-Raven.

Miller, C. A. (1995). *Nursing Care of Older Adults,* 2nd ed. Philadelphia: J.B. Lippincott.

Professional Guide to Diseases, 4th ed. (1992). Springhouse, PA: Springhouse.

Staab, A. S., & Hodges, L. C. (1995). *Essentials of Geriatric Nursing.* Philadelphia: J.B. Lippincott.

Unit 4

Assisting With Special Procedures

24 Diagnostic Imaging

Chapter Outline

X-rays and X-ray Machines
- Outpatient X-rays

Principles of Radiography
Patient Positioning
Examination Sequencing
Radiation Safety
Diagnostic Procedures
- Contrast Media Examinations
- Fluoroscopy
- Computed Tomography
- Sonography (Ultrasound)
- Magnetic Resonance Imaging
- Nuclear Medicine
- Mammography

Teleradiology
Interventional Radiologic Techniques
Radiation Therapy
The Medical Assistant's Role in Radiologic Procedures
- Patient Education
- Assisting With Examinations
- Handling and Storing Radiographic Films

Transferring Radiographic Information

Role Delineation

CLINICAL

Patient Care

- Prepare patients for examinations, procedures, and treatments.
- Assist with examinations, procedures, and treatments.

GENERAL

Professionalism

- Project a professional manner and image.
- Work as a team member.

Communication Skills

- Treat all patients with compassion and empathy.
- Serve as liaison.

Legal Concepts

- Practice within the scope of education, training, and personal capabilities.

Instruction

- Instruct individuals according to their needs.

Chapter Competencies

Learning Objectives

Upon successfully completing this chapter, you will be able to:

1. Spell and define the Key Terms.
2. Explain the theory and function of x-rays and x-ray machines.
3. State the basic principles of radiography.
4. Describe routine and contrast media, computed tomography, sonography, magnetic resonance imaging, nuclear medicine, and mammographic examinations.
5. Explain the basic concepts of therapeutic techniques.
6. Describe the basic concepts of radiation therapy.
7. Explain the principles of radiology in a manner that can be used in patient education.
8. State the legal and ethical considerations involved in radiology.
9. Explain the role of the medical assistant in radiologic procedures.

Key Terms

(See Glossary for definitions.)

cassettes
film
radiograph
radiographer
radiography
radiologist
radiology
radiolucent
radionuclides
radiopaque
tomography
x-rays

The discovery of x-rays in the late 19th century forever changed the practice of medicine. Today, **radiology** with its use of x-rays, radioactive isotopes and radiation, encompasses some of the most rapidly expanding diagnostic and therapeutic methodologies. Routine x-ray imaging, computed tomography (CT) scans, sonography, magnetic resonance imaging (MRI), and nuclear medicine are commonly used diagnostic procedures in the fight against disease. Advances in radiation therapy continue to be at the forefront of the treatment for cancer.

Radiology continues to evolve through technologic changes that provide ever-increasing diagnostic information to physicians. As the technology advances, the need to educate patients adequately becomes even more important. As part of interacting with patients, medical assistants are often in the ideal position to assist in the educational process.

X-RAYS AND X-RAY MACHINES

X-rays are high-energy electromagnetic radiation with several unique characteristics. They cannot be seen, heard, felt, tasted, or smelled. The rays travel at the speed of light and have the ability to penetrate fairly dense objects, such as the human body. This penetrating ability is what allows x-rays to be the diagnostic tools they are, creating two-dimensional shadow-like images on **film** that is similar to photographic film. The processed film containing a visible image is called a **radiograph** (Fig. 24-1). The process by which these films are produced is called **radiography.**

The production of x-rays occurs within the part of the machine called the x-ray tube. Electricity of extremely high voltage is applied to the tube, ultimately resulting in the production of x-rays. The x-rays exit the tube in one primary direction as a beam, through a collimator, the device used to control the size of the beam. The light seen by the patient is not part of the beam but is a positioning aid that demonstrates the area covered by the beam. A patient may hear noises coming from the tube area during an exposure, but these are made by the equipment, not the x-rays.

Today, x-ray machines are sophisticated and technologically advanced. Many are designed to work with computers to produce "digital" images of the body. Fluoroscopic images are capable of visualizing motion within the body. Most of the permanently installed radiographic units include a special table, some of which may be electronically rotated from the horizontal to the vertical position (Fig. 24-2).

Mobile radiographic units are designed to be moved to different areas of a hospital or clinic, to go to the patient's bedside or examination room when it is not advisable to transport the patient to the radiology area. This allows patients to have their studies done wherever they are being treated at that time: the emergency room, surgery, recovery room, in their bed in a hospital unit, or in an examining room. Mobile radiography is an essential part of critical care (Fig. 24-3).

Outpatient X-rays

Currently, the medical community is making a conscious effort to have as much patient treatment as possible done on an outpatient basis. In radiology, this has resulted in some medical offices (particularly specialties) having on-site x-ray equipment. Outpatient diagnostic imaging centers, separate from or a part of hospitals, have been created to offer these services. Many

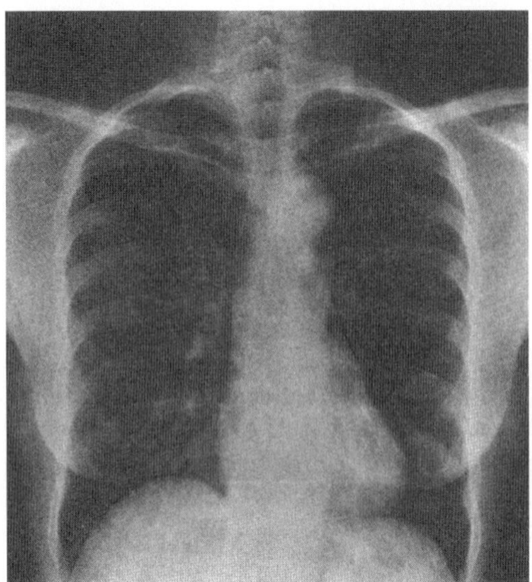

Figure 24-1 A radiograph of the chest.

patients may have their radiographic examinations or procedures done in one of these settings.

Inpatients have their examinations done in the hospital or other resident care facility. Some companies specialize in providing minimal x-ray services to patients in nursing homes and other long-term care facilities so that these patients do not have to be transported to hospitals.

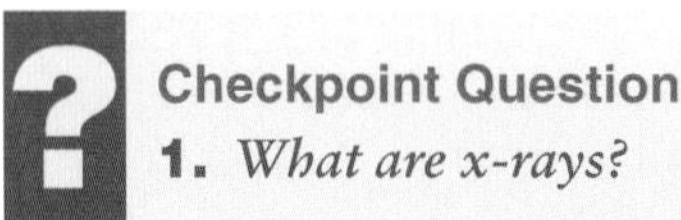

Checkpoint Question

1. *What are x-rays?*

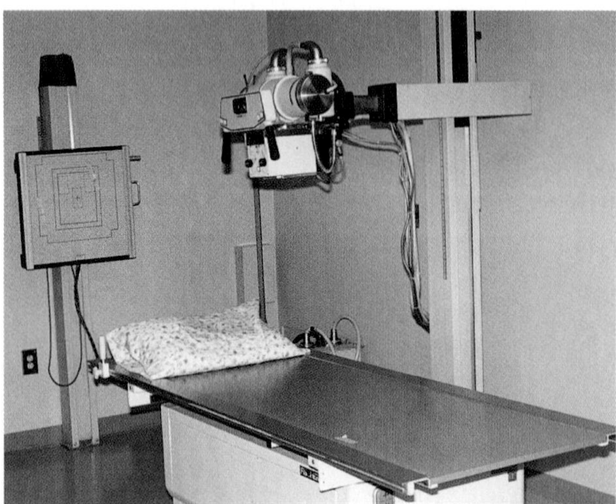

Figure 24-2 Permanently installed radiographic unit.

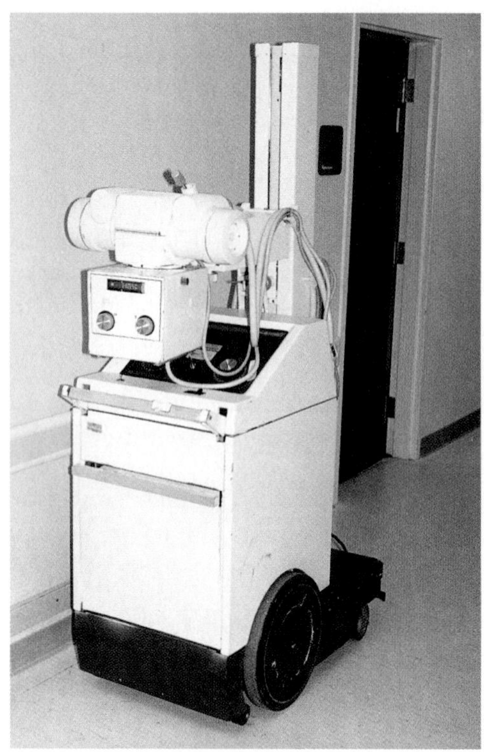

Figure 24-3 A mobile radiographic unit.

PRINCIPLES OF RADIOGRAPHY

The routine procedure for any radiographic examination generally includes:

1. Verifying the patient's identity and the examination to be performed.
2. Preparing the patient. This may involve undressing as necessary to remove objects (snaps, buttons, hooks) that could show up on the radiograph, obscuring vital parts of the image.
3. Preparing the room by setting up the equipment and readying supplies.
4. Performing the procedure, including positioning the patient and making exposures.
5. Processing the images.
6. Interpreting the images (performed by a physician).
7. Filing the images.

Paperwork is a critical part of this procedure. Before an examination can be performed, a requisition must be completed by a physician or his or her authorized agent. Radiographic procedures should only be performed by or on the order of a licensed physician. After the images have been interpreted, a written report becomes part of the patient's medical record.

PATIENT POSITIONING

The x-ray exposure on film is only a two-dimensional image. Because the human body is a three-dimensional structure, x-ray examinations usually require a minimum of two exposures taken at 90° to each other. For instance, a chest x-ray will require one exposure from the back and another from the side. Other examinations primarily interested in demonstrating joints will frequently involve the use of three or more exposures at different angles. These different angles of exposure are the basis for standard positioning for x-ray examinations (Box 24-1, Fig. 24-4).

Box 24-1
Standard Terminology and Illustrations for Positioning and Projection

Radiographic View
Describes the body part as seen by an x-ray film or other recording media, such as a fluoroscopic screen. Restricted to the discussion of a *radiograph* or *image.*

Radiographic Position
Refers to a specific body position, such as supine, prone, recumbent, erect, or Trendelenburg. Restricted to the discussion of the patient's *physical position.*

Radiographic Projection
Restricted to the discussion of the *path of the central ray.*

Positioning Terminology

A. Lying down
   1. *Supine*—lying on the back
   2. *Prone*—lying face downward
   3. *Decubitus*—lying down with a horizontal x-ray beam
   4. *Recumbent*—lying down in any position
B. Erect or upright
   1. *Anterior position*—facing the film
   2. *Posterior position*—facing the radiographic tube
   3. *Oblique positions*—(erect or lying down)
      a. Anterior—facing the film
         i. *Left anterior oblique*—body rotated with the left anterior portion closest to the film
         ii. *Right anterior oblique*—body rotated with the right anterior portion closest to the film
      b. Posterior—facing the radiographic tube
         i. *Left posterior oblique*—body rotated with the left posterior portion closest to the film
         ii. *Right posterior oblique*—body rotated with the right posterior portion closest to the film

EXAMINATION SEQUENCING

Most radiographic procedures can be performed in any order of convenience. However, certain sequences are followed in specific situations. For example, patients who present with gallbladder symptoms may go through a series of procedures, progressing from the simple, noninvasive oral cholecystogram to the more complex operative cholangiogram.

Another example involves "barium studies," the name given to examinations that involve the administration of barium sulfate as a part of the procedure. A patient with gastrointestinal (GI) symptoms may undergo a series of barium-based studies to assist in a diagnosis. Because of the nature of the barium studies and the length of time required to eliminate the barium from the digestive tract, barium enemas are usually scheduled before upper GI examinations. If fiberoptic studies are ordered, it is imperative that these be scheduled before any procedure involving barium.

Because barium enemas involve filling only the large intestine with barium and because the large intestine is the last part of the GI tract, this barium can be eliminated more quickly so that other examinations can be attempted. It an upper GI examination is performed first, it may be days later before all the barium is out of the system, allowing other examinations to be performed. Any residual barium could obscure vital structures, preventing other examinations from contributing diagnostic information. The proper sequencing of barium enema first and upper GI last will usually provide diagnostic information in a shorter period of time.

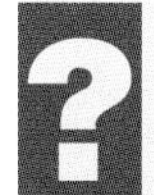

Checkpoint Question
2. *Why is a barium enema performed before upper GI studies?*

RADIATION SAFETY

Of primary concern to all radiation workers is the proper and safe use of radiant energy. The potential hazards of radiation have been known for many years, and warnings about x-ray radiation are usually posted in appropriate areas (Fig. 24-5). X-rays have the potential to cause cellular damage to the body, which may not manifest itself for years. The potential adverse effects are most critical for rapidly reproducing cells. Pregnant women, children, and adults of reproductive age are at the highest risk because of the rapid reproduction of the cells in these populations.

Radiation safety procedures generally directed toward patients include:

24

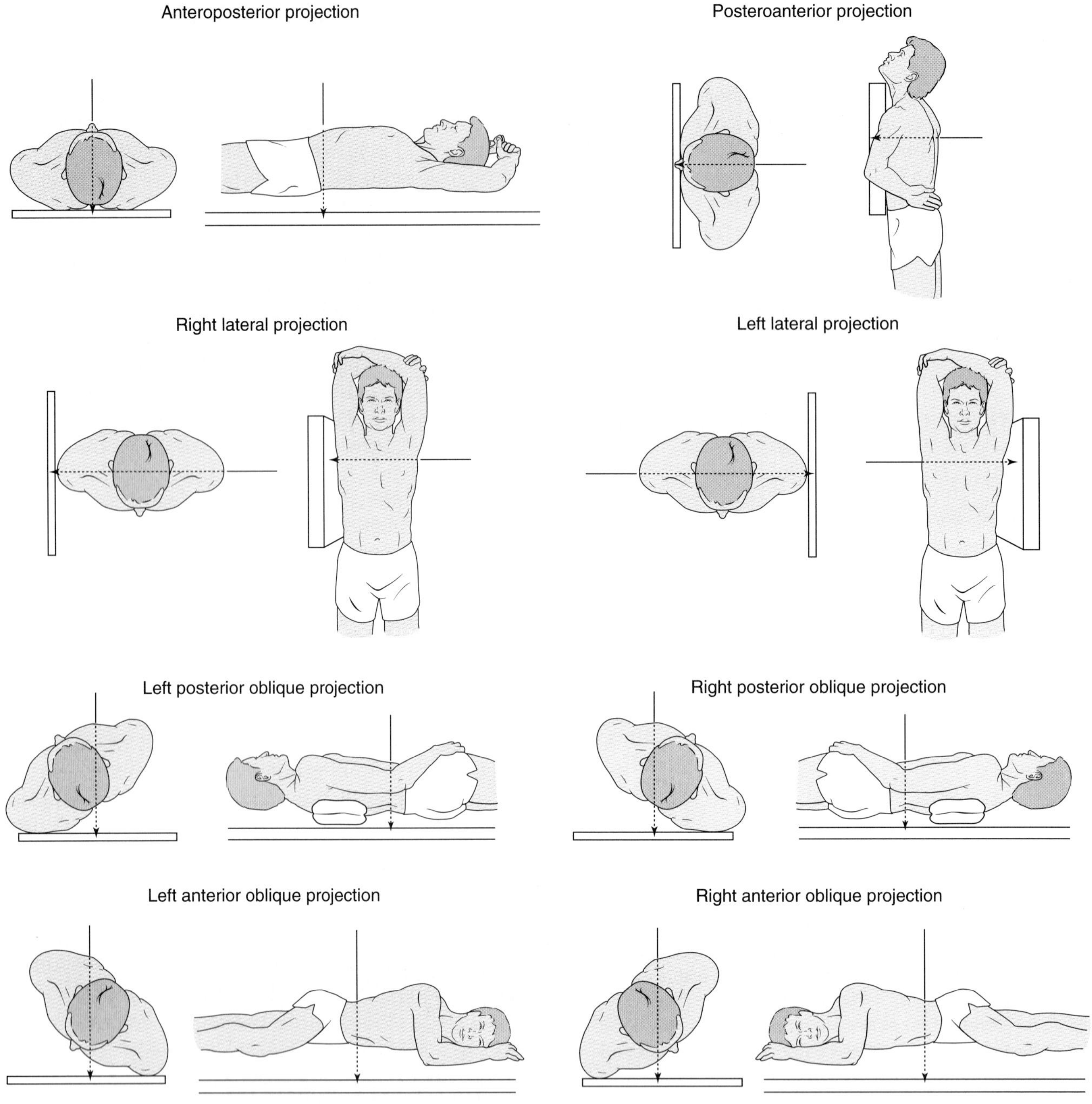

Figure 24-4 Standard positions for x-ray examinations. (© 1999, The American Registry of Radiologic Technologists, used with permission. The ARRT does not review, evaluate, or endorse publications. Permission to reproduce ARRT copyrighted materials within this publication should not be construed as an endorsement of the publication by the ARRT.)

1. Reducing exposure amounts as much as possible.
2. Avoiding unnecessary examinations.
3. Limiting the area of the body exposed.
4. Shielding sensitive body parts from the radiation.
5. Evaluating the potential pregnancy status of female patients before performing examinations.

Safety procedures for radiation workers include:

1. Limiting the amount of time exposed to x-rays.
2. Staying as far away from the x-rays as possible, preferably behind a barrier.
3. Using all available shielding for protection, such as lead aprons, gloves, and barrier walls.
4. Not holding patients during exposures. Sometimes small children need to be held to keep them still during an examination. A parent wearing a lead apron may be recruited for this procedure.
5. Wearing individual dosimeters, devices that record the amount of radiation to which the worker has

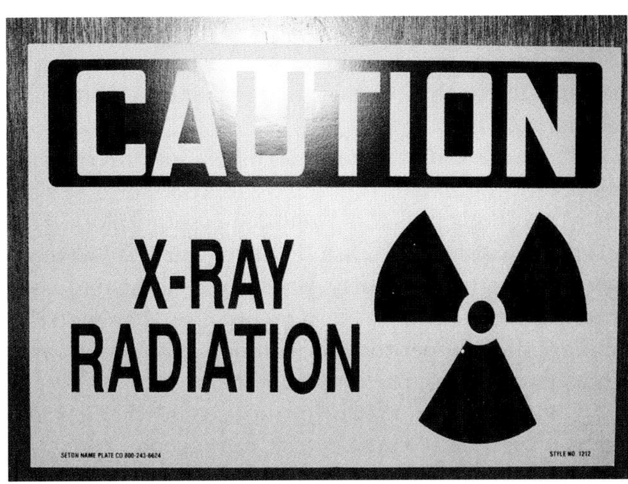

Figure 24-5 A posted x-ray warning sign.

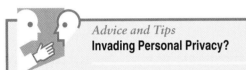

Advice and Tips

Invading Personal Privacy?

When a **radiographer** (the technician who produces routine x-ray images) asks a female patient if she may be pregnant, or when signs in x-ray facilities instruct patients to inform someone if they may be pregnant, is personal privacy being invaded? No; these measures are not intended to invade privacy but to ensure the safety of the unborn. The embryo is most sensitive to radiation damage during the first 3 months of formation. This is also a time when a woman may be pregnant and not be aware of it. (The patient is not asked if she knows she is pregnant, only if there is a possibility that she might be.) To save the patient any embarrassment, proper precautions are usually taken, regardless of the answer. If the examination includes the abdominopelvic area, the precaution may be to delay the procedure until pregnancy status is determined medically.

If You Suspect You Are Pregnant, Please Notify the Technician

This is not an invasion of privacy, but an effort to provide protection for patients.

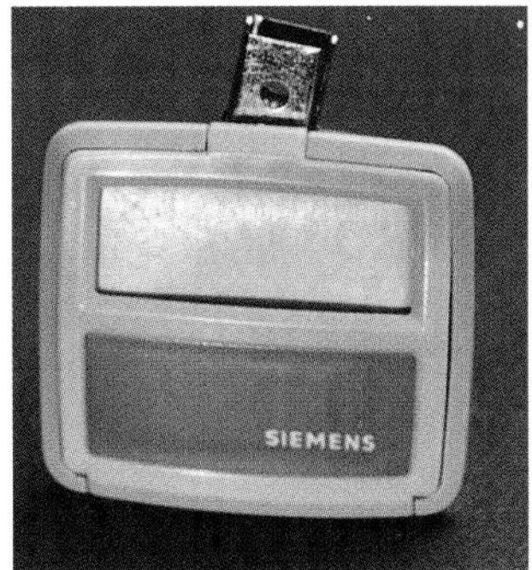

Figure 24-6 The dosimeter records the amount of radiation to which a worker has been exposed.

been exposed (Fig. 24-6), and protective equipment (Fig. 24-7).

6. Ensuring proper working condition of the equipment to avoid having to repeat examinations.

For both patients and radiation personnel, these concerns can be summed up in what is called the ALARA concept: doing whatever is necessary to keep radiation exposure As Low As Reasonably Achievable.

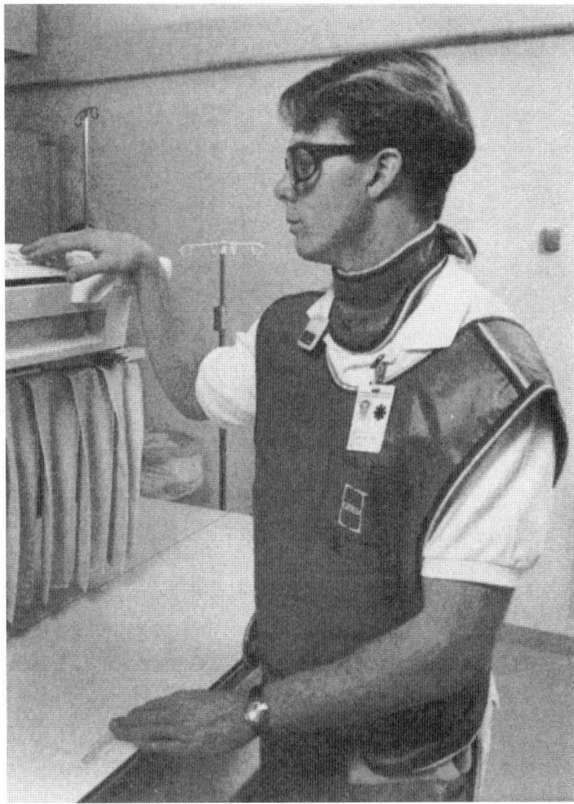

Figure 24-7 A radiographer wearing a dosimeter on the right collar, as well as protective glasses, an apron, and thyroid shield.

DIAGNOSTIC PROCEDURES

Routine examinations are those that require no patient preparation other than putting on a patient gown after removing only as much clothing as may be necessary to eliminate objects that might show up on the radiographs (eg, buttons, snaps, hooks). These are the most commonly performed examinations and are the most readily accepted by the patient. Routine radiographic examinations are named for the part of the body involved (Table 24-1).

24

Contrast Media Examinations

Images are formed on the x-ray film as the rays either pass through or are absorbed by the tissues of the body. **Radiolucent** tissues permit the passage of x-rays; **radiopaque** tissues do not. Bone is dense, absorbs much of the radiation beam, and shows white on a radiograph. Air is not dense, does not absorb much radiation, and therefore shows dark on a radiograph. Other body tissues (such as muscle, fat, and fluid) show as varying shades of gray because of the way each tissue absorbs x-rays.

Within the abdomen, many structures having similar radiation absorption rates are superimposed on each other. This makes it difficult to differentiate between structures, such as the components of the intestinal system. The use of radiopaque contrast media helps differentiate between body structures by artificially changing the absorption rate of a particular structure so that it may be distinctly visualized instead of blending in with adjacent structures. For example, barium sulfate absorbs radiation and shows white on a radiograph (Fig. 24-8).

There are different contrast media for different applications. Iodinated compounds are used for many areas of the body, including the kidneys and blood vessels and for some CT scans. Patients who may have an intestinal perforation may be given an iodinated contrast media instead of barium because that material spilling into the peritoneum is much less troublesome to the patient than barium would be.

Contrast media may be introduced in several ways, such as by swallowing, by the intravenous route, or through a catheter. A barium sulfate mixture is swallowed for an upper GI series. Other contrast media are introduced intravenously or by means of a catheter for studies of the vascular system. Examinations using contrast media often are used not only to evaluate a structure, but also to evaluate its function. The excretory urogram evaluates kidney structures as well as the organ's excretory functions.

Checkpoint Question

3. *How do contrast media help in differentiating between body structures?*

Of particular concern to patients is the preparation they must undergo before some contrast media examinations, especially barium studies. For contrast media to fill the intestinal tract properly, the intestine

Table 24-1 **Routine Radiographic Examinations by Body Region**

Region	*Patient Preparation*
Trunk	Patient preparation includes disrobing of the appropriate area: chest, ribs, sternum, shoulder, scapula, clavicle, abdomen, hip, pelvis, sternoclavicular, acromioclavicular, sacroiliac joints
Extremities	Patient preparation includes removing jewelry or clothing that might obscure parts of interest: finger(s), thumb, hand, wrist, forearm, elbow, humerus, toe(s), foot, os calcis, ankle, lower leg, knee, patella, femur
Spine	Patient preparation includes disrobing of the appropriate area: cervical, thoracic, or lumbar spine; sacrum; coccyx
Head	Patient preparation includes removing eyewear, false eyes, false teeth, earrings, hairpins, hairpieces from appropriate area: skull, sinuses, nasal bones, facial bones/orbits, optic foramen, mandible, temporomandibular joints, mastoid/petrous portion, zygomatic arch

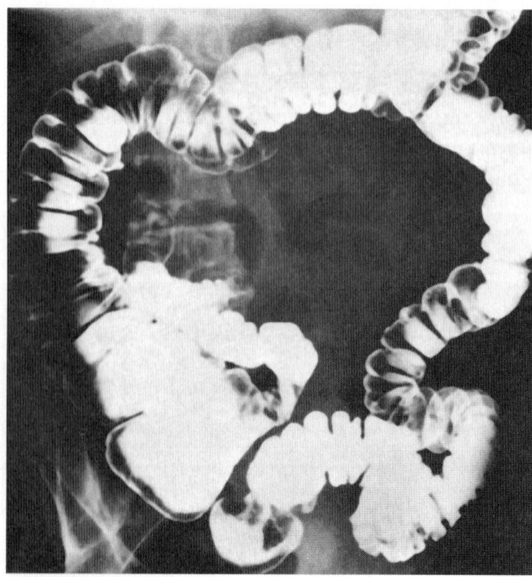

Figure 24-8 An x-ray of the large intestine with barium. The barium makes the large intestine show up as white on the radiograph.

must be completely empty. For example, patient preparation for a barium study might include:

- Liquid diet only for the evening meal on the day before the examination
- Laxatives to help clean the intestinal tract
- Nothing by mouth (NPO) after midnight. This usually includes no gum chewing or cigarette smoking because both activities increase gastric secretions that may interfere with the contrast media's ability to coat the wall of the intestine.

This general preparation could apply to any contrast media examination involving abdominal structures. Each facility may vary this to some extent. You should learn the specific preparations required for each procedure by each facility. It is to the advantage of the facility to provide its employees with this information to facilitate efficient and effective performance of x-ray procedures.

Examinations requiring that patients remain NPO past midnight should be scheduled as early in the morning as possible. If patients must remain NPO until late morning, they will be understandably upset.

If patients are not properly prepared for contrast studies, they may have to be rescheduled for another day and time and must go through the whole process again, sometimes adding cleansing enemas to the preparation. Explaining the importance of the preparation can be one of the most vital contributions a medical assistant can make to the patient's care in contrast examinations.

What If?

A patient who is scheduled to have a barium study has been kept waiting for over an hour. What if she asks you for a sip of water?

As a medical assistant, you must understand the reason for fasting and not give the patient anything by mouth just because it seems a benign request. Doing so could compromise the results and cause the patient to have to go through the whole process again. Give this explanation if you need to deny a patient's request for something to drink.

24

Table 24-2 **Common Radiographic Procedures**

Examination	*Contrast Media*	*Provides a Demonstration of:*
Angiogram	Iodinated	Blood vessels; named for those studied (eg, femoral, carotid, aorta)
Arthrogram	Iodinated	Joint capsule and related structures, often with stress applied to joint
Barium enema	Barium/air	Large intestine, sometimes using air for additional contrast
Barium swallow	Barium	Esophagus as patient swallows barium
Bronchogram	Iodinated	Bronchial tree by instilling contrast medium through a tube
Cardiac	Iodinated	Heart; may include angiography
Cystogram	Iodinated	Urinary bladder after contrast medium introduced through catheter
Endoscopic retrograde cholangiopancreatogram (ERCP)	Iodinated	Biliary and pancreatic duct structures after introducing contrast medium through endoscopy
Excretory urogram	Iodinated	Kidney structures, ureters, and urinary bladder after intravenous (IV) injection of contrast medium
Hysterosalpingogram	Iodinated	Patency of oviducts by filling uterus and ducts with contrast medium
IV cholangiogram	Iodinated	Gallbladder and biliary ducts after administration of IV drip of contrast medium
Lymphogram	Iodinated	Lymphatic structures after contrast medium injection into vessels in feet
Myelogram	Iodinated	Subarachnoid space around spinal cord after injection of contrast medium via lumbar puncture
Operative cholangiogram	Iodinated	Gallbladder and biliary ducts with direct injection of contrast medium during surgery
Oral cholecystogram	Iodinated	Gallbladder and biliary ducts after patient ingests contrast pills
Percutaneous transhepatic cholangiogram	Iodinated	Biliary system after percutaneous introduction of needle through the liver to the bile duct
Retrograde pyelogram	Iodinated	Kidney structures by filling with contrast medium from catheter in distal ureter
Sialogram	Iodinated	Salivary glands after injection into ducts
Small bowel series	Barium	Small bowel by following contrast medium through from stomach to beginning of large intestine
T-tube cholangiogram	Iodinated	Biliary ducts through tube left in place after cholecystectomy
Upper GI series	Barium	Upper GI tract through the duodenum
Voiding cystourethrogram	Iodinated	Urinary bladder and urethra and voiding function

Table 24-2 lists common radiographic procedures that use contrast media. Some examinations included here are being replaced by other techniques such as CT, MRI, and ultrasound in many institutions. Because they may still be performed, or may be referred to in a patient's medical record, they are included in this table.

Fluoroscopy

Fluoroscopy, or fluoro studies, use x-rays to observe movement within the body. The movement may be of barium sulfate through the digestive tract, the beating of the heart, or the movement of contrast media through blood vessels or even through the heart itself. Fluoroscopy is also used as an aid to other types of patient treatments, such as reducing fractures or implanting pacemakers.

Computed Tomography

Tomography is a procedure in which the x-ray tube and film move in relation to one another during the exposure, blurring out all structures except those in the focal plane. CT uses a combination of x-rays and computers to create cross-sectional images of the body. Some examinations are performed with contrast media, some without. Some units have the ability to create three-dimensional images (Fig. 24-9).

Sonography (Ultrasound)

Sonography uses high-frequency sound waves to create cross-sectional still or real-time (motion) images of the body, usually with the help of computers. This application is commonly used to demonstrate heart function or abdominal or pelvic structures. It is commonly used in prenatal testing to visualize the developing fetus. Some obstetricians routinely schedule at least one sonogram before the fourth month of pregnancy although this practice is being reconsidered for an "as-needed" basis (Fig. 24-10).

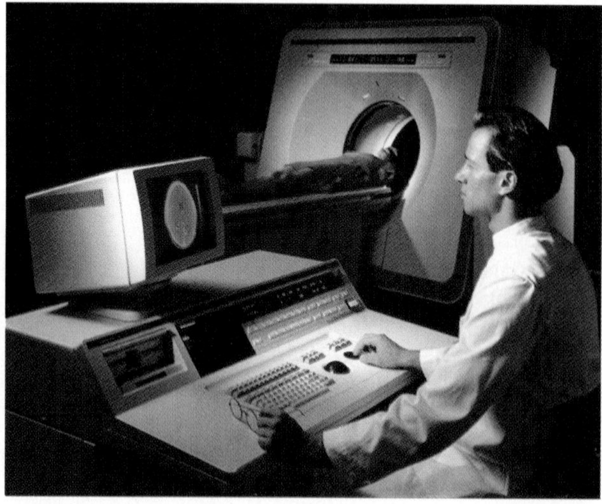

Figure 24-9 Computed tomography (CT) scanner. (Photograph courtesy of Philips Medical Systems.)

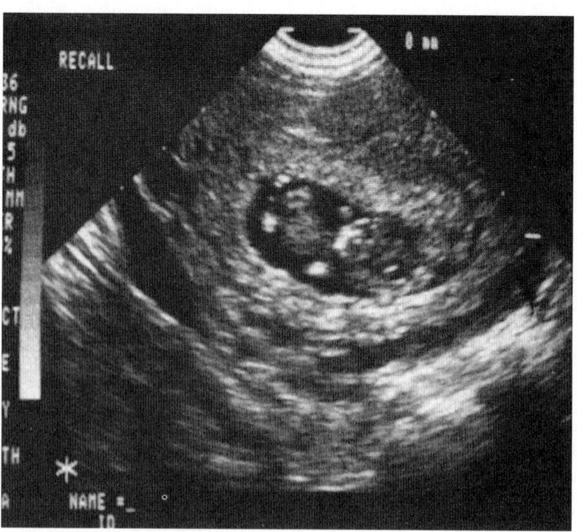

Figure 24-10 A sonogram showing an embryo 9 weeks after patient's last monthly period.

Magnetic Resonance Imaging

Magnetic resonance imaging uses a combination of high-intensity magnetic fields, radio waves, and computers to create cross-sectional images of the body. Some studies are performed with contrast media. Because MRI does not produce images using x-ray principles, but instead creates images based on the chemical makeup of the body, MRI studies provide information unavailable by other means. MRI is commonly used for a variety of studies, including the central nervous system and joint structure. The patient must be prepared for lengthy procedures while in a closely enclosed machine making knocking and whirring noises. It is not unusual for patients with a fear of enclosed places to require a mild sedative before this procedure. Newer machines are currently being designed that are less confining to reduce the patient's sense of enclosure.

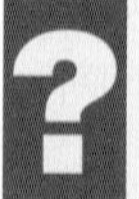

Checkpoint Question

4. *How does fluoroscopy differ from computed tomography and sonography?*

Nuclear Medicine

Small amounts of **radionuclides** are injected into the body and are designed to concentrate in specific areas. Radionuclides are radioactive materials with a short

Box 24-2
American Cancer Society Guidelines for Mammography Screening

- Mammography for women who do not have symptoms, such as palpable breast masses or masses found on prior radiologic examination:
  - If you are 40–49—every 1–2 years.
  - If you are 50 or over, every year
- Screening mammogram by age 40
- Discussion continues regarding the optimum frequency of mammographic studies. At this time it is suggested that women and their physicians assess the need within established guidelines but on an individual basis.

life span. Sophisticated computerized "cameras" detect the radiation and create an image. This technique is commonly used to study the thyroid, brain, lungs, liver, spleen, kidney, bone, and breast. These examinations are called scans.

Positron emission tomography (PET) is a sophisticated nuclear medicine study using specialized equipment to produce detailed sectional images of the body to measure blood flow volume, O_2 availability, and metabolism to an area.

Single photon emission computed tomography (SPECT) is a nuclear medicine technology that produces sectional images of the body as detectors move around the patient.

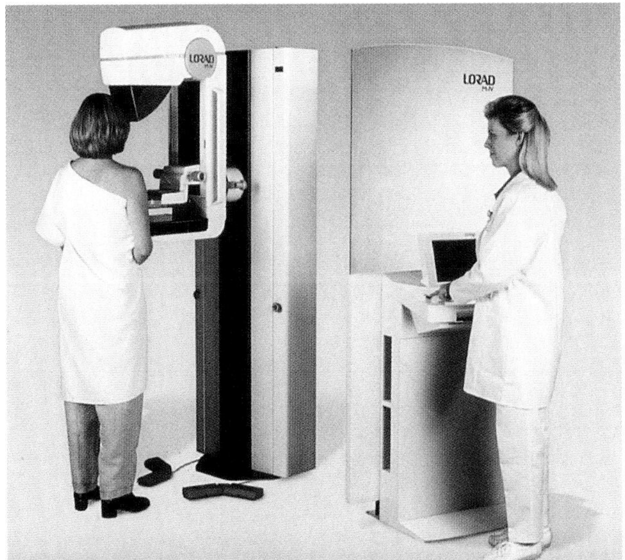

Figure 24-11 A patient being positioned for mammography. (LORAD M-IV mammography machine.)

Mammography

Mammography involves specialized x-rays of the breast and is used as a screening tool for breast cancer (Box 24-2). Compression of the breast is used to even the thickness, allowing a better diagnostic image. Needle localization studies using the information gained from the mammogram allow the physician to withdraw minute amounts of cells from suspicious areas in a minimally invasive procedure. Mammography has become a vital adjunct to biopsy procedures (Fig. 24-11).

24

TELERADIOLOGY

The use of computed imaging and information systems can be mutually beneficial in medicine. Many institutions today have a picture archiving and communication system (PACS) that uses computers to store and transmit images. Digital images from a CT scan, for instance, can be transmitted via telephone lines to distant locations. This allows consultation with experts on a difficult case within a matter of minutes. Previously unavailable expertise can be brought to rural areas for greatly improved patient care. The result is improved patient care over large geographic areas, not just in specific locations. The name teleradiology has been coined to describe this "radiology over a great distance."

INTERVENTIONAL RADIOLOGIC TECHNIQUES

Interventional radiologic techniques are designed to intervene in the normal process of specific disease conditions. For some patients, these therapeutic techniques can be so effective that the need for surgery will be eliminated. These interventional procedures, described below, may even be life saving.

Percutaneous transluminal coronary angioplasty (PTCA), also known as balloon angioplasty, is used to increase the size of the lumen of a coronary artery through the use of a balloon-tipped catheter. Under fluoroscopic guidance, the catheter is placed at a point of stenosis (narrowing). The balloon is inflated for a short time, usually resulting in an increase in the lumen of the vessel. After deflation, the catheter is removed. Balloon angioplasties may be performed in almost any vessel.

Laser angioplasties use laser beams to remove deposits in vessels.

A *vascular stent* (a plastic tube or wire) placed in the stenosed area of the vessel is used to maintain the patency of the lumen of a vessel. Fluoroscopy is used to guide the stent.

Embolizations artificially embolize a blood vessel to stop active bleeding or to reduce or stop blood flow to diseased areas.

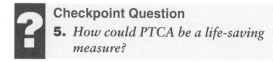

Checkpoint Question

5. *How could PTCA be a life-saving measure?*

RADIATION THERAPY

A major force in the fight against cancer for many years has been radiation therapy. The use of high-energy radiation to destroy cancer cells can not only prolong the lives of many patients, it may even save lives. Used in conjunction with surgery, chemotherapy, or both, radiation is possibly the best known treatment for cancer. With an intensity sufficient to destroy cancer cells, the potential damage to some adjacent normal cells does exist. Therefore, treatments must be planned carefully and precisely.

Treatment planning involves the establishment of a precise regimen of therapy, dictating the frequency and amount of radiation to be used as well as the number of exposures during a given period. The exact area of the body to be exposed must be defined precisely so that each treatment is identical.

The therapy consists of placing the patient in the exact position described by the treatment plan and administering the exact amount of radiation. The patient usually has little to do but lie still.

Each patient's prognosis varies according to the specific situation. Most patients have some side effects, which may include hair loss, weight loss, loss of appetite, skin changes, and digestive system disturbances. Once the treatment plan is completed, most of the side effects disappear.

THE MEDICAL ASSISTANT'S ROLE IN RADIOLOGIC PROCEDURES

Because medical assistants hold such a varied range of jobs related to patient care, they often are in ideal positions to help alleviate the anxiety that patients feel. This may be done by giving patients information about examinations they do not understand, by making the patients feel comfortable enough to ask questions, and by providing answers to those questions in terms the patients can understand.

Patient Education

Patients who have had prior experience with the medical system have sometimes learned to overcome their anxieties and to find answers to their questions. No matter how much they have been through before, there is always something new, something they do not understand that can make them feel they have lost control of their situation. Being sensitive to the feelings of patients is one of the greatest talents anyone in medicine can possess and is a prime component of the medical assistant's training and personality.

Unfortunately, many patients are confronted with procedures they do not understand and do not know enough about to ask questions. Many undergo procedures as a spectator rather than a participant in their own health care. As a medical assistant, you can have an impact on a patient's emotional response to radiologic procedures by explaining what to expect, not in technical terms, but in simple, everyday language (Fig. 24-12). The technical aspects of radiology make it one of medicine's most difficult areas for patients to understand. The key to success in explaining these procedures to patients is simplicity, leaving the details to the experts.

Explaining the preparations for examinations and their importance is vital to the success of many procedures. Equally important may be an explanation of what to do after the procedure. The barium enema, for instance, can lead to constipation if the patient does not increase fluid intake after the examination. This simple direction can save the patient much postexamination distress.

Assisting With Examinations

As a medical assistant, you may assist with examinations by:

- Giving the patient instructions for appropriate undressing and assisting with clothing as needed
- Assisting in positioning of the patient for the procedure, emphasizing to the patient the importance

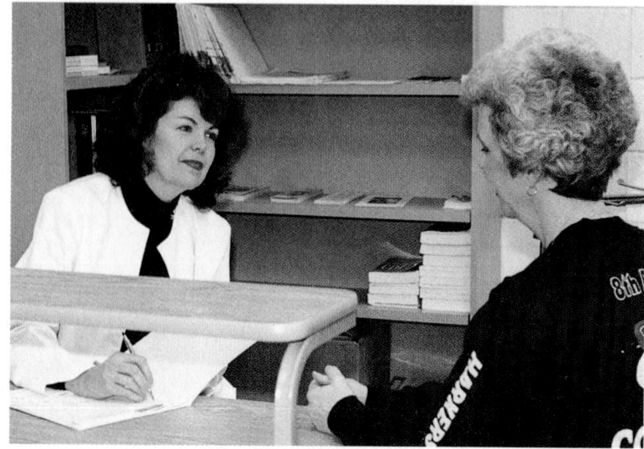

Figure 24-12 The medical assistant provides explanations of radiologic procedures that are easy to understand.

of remaining still and following breathing directions
- Processing film in a darkroom, removing film from **cassettes** (lightproof film holders), placing film into an automatic processor, reloading new film into the cassette
- Distributing or filing radiographs and reports

Handling and Storing Radiographic Films

Advancing technology and the need for quality control has led to automated film processing and developing to eliminate the human error factor. Automated processing machines produce a film usually in less than 2 minutes. Processors vary by manufacturer, requiring that the medical assistant be proficient in the operation of the particular facility's equipment.

Unexposed film must be protected from moisture, heat, and light by storage in a cool, dry place, preferably in a lead-lined box. Film packets, exposed or unexposed, must be opened in a darkroom with only the darkroom light for illumination. The film is placed in a cassette for use in any area outside the darkroom. Intensifying screens in the cassette are used to reduce the amount of exposure required.

Special sleeves or envelopes of varying sizes are available for storing the properly labeled film. Film must be protected in a cool, dry area.

Checkpoint Question

6. *How can medical assistants help with radiologic examinations?*

TRANSFERRING RADIOGRAPHIC INFORMATION

Radiography performed on site for use by the resident physician will remain as part of the patient's permanent record. In many cases, however, radiographic studies are performed at one site for consultation or referral to another site. X-ray films belong to the site where the study was performed, but the **radiologist** (physician who interprets the radiographs) or examining physician generally is required to return a written summary of the examination results to the referring physician. If the patient is a short-term referral, the examining physician will usually return the films to the referring physician. Patients with ongoing concerns who move from the area or who change physicians may request the information contained on their records and may obtain copies of the original radiographs.

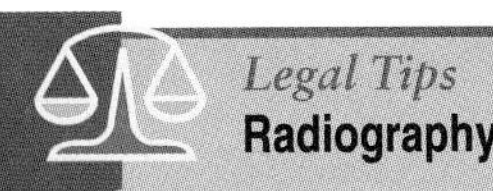

Legal Tips

Radiography

Follow these tips to help safeguard your patient and yourself:

- Be sure radiographic images are properly identified.
- Keep in mind that interventional procedures require a consent form, similar to those used for surgical procedures, to be signed by the patient.
- Remember that only physicians are legally permitted to make a diagnosis or interpret the radiographic images. If a patient asks you for the results of a radiographic study, you should not give any information unless directed to do so by a physician. The patient should be told in a calm, compassionate manner that only the physician is qualified to interpret the radiographs and that the physician will explain the results.
- Know your state laws regarding licensing for x-ray procedures. Many states now require the licensing of all personnel who perform x-ray procedures, which may exclude medical assistants from taking x-rays.

Answers to Checkpoint Questions

1. *X-rays are high-energy electromagnetic radiation that travel at the speed of light. X-rays can penetrate fairly dense objects, such as the human body. They cannot be seen, heard, felt, tasted, or smelled.*
2. *Barium enemas involve filling only the large intestine with barium. Because the large intestine is the last part of the GI tract, this barium can be eliminated more quickly. If an upper GI examination is performed first, it may be days later before barium can be eliminated—thus delaying other examinations.*
3. *Contrast media help differentiate between body structures by artificially changing the absorption rate of a particular structure so that it can be seen clearly instead of blending in with adjacent structures. For example, barium sulfate absorbs radiation and shows white on a radiograph.*
4. *Fluoroscopy uses x-rays to observe movement within the body. CT uses a combination of x-rays and computers to create cross-sectional images of the body. Sonography uses high-frequency sound waves to create cross-sectional still or real-time (motion) images of the body.*
5. *PTCA could save a patient's life by reopening the lumen of a coronary artery to allow sufficient blood flow to keep the heart muscle alive.*
6. *Medical assistants can help with radiologic examinations by providing instructions to patients, positioning patients, handling x-ray film, and distributing or filing radiographs and reports.*

24

Critical Thinking Challenges

1. A mother of a 6-year-old child voices concerns to you about the dangers of x-rays. How would you address her fears?
2. Summarize the key points of radiation safety, then write a policy booklet for new employees. Create a poster highlighting the most important points of radiation safety to hang in the staff lounge.
3. Constipation is a common problem among patients who have barium enemas. How could patient education diminish this problem? Develop a brief instruction sheet to give to these patients.

Suggestions for Further Reading

Andolina, V. F., Lille, S. L., & Willison, K. M. (1992). *Mammographic Imaging: A Practical Guide.* Philadelphia: Lippincott-Raven.

Bontrager, K.(1993). *Textbook of Radiographic Positioning and Related Anatomy,* 3rd ed. Mosby–Year Book.

Carlton, R., & Adler, A. (1992). *Principles of Radiographic Imaging—An Art and a Science.* Albany, NY: Delmar.

Cullinan, A. M. (1994). *Producing Quality Radiographs,* 2nd ed. Philadelphia: J.B. Lippincott.

Cullinan, A. M. (1992). *Optimizing Radiographic Positioning.* Philadelphia: J.B. Lippincott.

Torres, L. S. (1993). *Basic Medical Techniques and Patient Care for Radiologic Technologists,* 4th ed. Philadelphia: J.B. Lippincott.

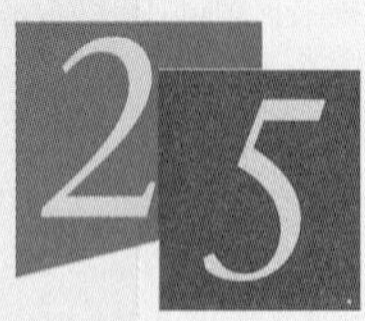

Medical Office Emergencies

Chapter Outline

Emergency Medical Services System
Medical Office Emergency Procedures
- Emergency Action Plan
- Emergency Medical Kit
- Who Do I Call for Emergency Help?
- What Should Be Done Before the Ambulance Arrives?
- What Should Be Done When the Ambulance Arrives?

Patient Assessment
- Scene Survey
- Personal Protective Equipment
- Initial Approach to the Patient
- Primary Survey
- Secondary Survey

Types of Emergencies
- Shock
- Bleeding and Soft-Tissue Injuries
- Burn Injuries
- Musculoskeletal Injuries
- Cardiovascular Emergencies
- Neurologic Emergencies
- Allergic and Anaphylactic Reactions
- Poisoning
- Heat- and Cold-Related Emergencies
- Behavioral and Psychiatric Emergencies

Role Delineation

CLINICAL

Patient Care
- Adhere to established triage procedures.
- Recognize and respond to emergencies.

GENERAL

Professionalism
- Work as a team member.
- Demonstrate initiative and responsibility.

Communication Skills
- Treat all patients with compassion and empathy.

Legal Concepts
- Practice within the scope of education, training, and personal capabilities.

Chapter Competencies

Learning Objectives

Upon successfully completing this chapter, you will be able to:

1. Spell and define the Key Terms.
2. Describe the role of the medical assistant in an emergency.
3. Explain the purpose of the primary survey.
4. Identify the five types of shock and the management of each.
5. Describe how burns are classified.
6. Discuss the management of allergic reactions.
7. Discuss the role of the poison control center.
8. List the three types of hyperthermic emergencies and the treatment for each type.
9. Discuss the treatment of hypothermia.
10. Discuss the role of the medical assistant in managing psychiatric emergencies.
11. Explain the technique for managing an adult patient with a foreign body airway obstruction.
12. Explain the technique for performing cardiopulmonary resuscitation on an adult.

Chapter Competencies *(continued)*

Performance Objectives

Upon successfully completing this chapter, you will be able to:

1. Manage an adult with a foreign body airway obstruction (Procedure 25-1).
2. Perform one-rescuer adult cardiopulmonary resuscitation (Procedure 25-2).

Key Terms

(See Glossary for definitions.)

anaphylactic shock
anaphylaxis
cardiogenic shock
contusion
ecchymosis
frostbite
full-thickness burn
heat cramps
heat exhaustion
heat stroke
hematoma
hyperthermia
hypothermia
hypovolemic shock
neurogenic shock
partial-thickness burn
primary survey
rule of nines
seizure
shock
secondary survey
septic shock
superficial burn

Emergency medical care is the immediate care given to the sick or injured person. When properly applied, it can mean the difference between life or death, rapid recovery or long hospitalization, temporary disability or permanent injury. Emergency medical care in the medical office consists of furnishing temporary assistance until a basic or advanced life support ambulance or rescue squad, if needed, is obtained.

An emergency situation can occur anywhere and to anyone. For example, a patient who is being seen for a routine examination may collapse from a heart attack and require immediate cardiopulmonary resuscitation (CPR); a coworker may forget to take her insulin and lapse into a diabetic coma; or an elderly person may fall down a flight of stairs. If first on the scene, the well prepared medical assistant can obtain important information and perform immediate lifesaving procedures before the ambulance or rescue squad arrives.

This chapter is not meant to provide a comprehensive study on all aspects of emergency care. Other chapters in this text should be read for details of various medical conditions. In addition, contact your local American Heart Association or American Red Cross chapter to obtain information about in-depth courses in first aid and CPR training. You should know what to do in an emergency *before* an emergency occurs.

EMERGENCY MEDICAL SERVICES SYSTEM

The initial element of any emergency medical services (EMS) system is citizen access. Speedy access for emergency help has been developed through the use of 911 as a nationally recognized emergency telephone number. The EMS system at its most visible level is the arrival of the ambulance or rescue squad at the scene of the call.

In most instances, the EMS system should be summoned as part of the initial response to any emergency. The need for rapid, systematic intervention by medically trained personnel to care for the sick and injured patient is an integral part of the EMS system.

MEDICAL OFFICE EMERGENCY PROCEDURES

Emergency Action Plan

Every medical office should have an emergency action plan. It should include:

- Appropriate emergency rescue service telephone number (usually 911)
- Location of the nearest hospital emergency department that provides 24-hour emergency care

- Telephone number of the local or regional poison control center in your area
- List of procedures outlining what to do in an emergency situation
- List of all personnel who are trained in CPR (this should include all office and medical staff)
- Location and list of contents of the emergency medical kit
- A protocol of responsibilities for each health care worker in the office

Emergency Medical Kit

Along with the emergency action plan, proper equipment and supplies should be available to use in a medical emergency. General equipment and supplies used for routine procedures may vary depending on the medical office specialty. Equipment used for emergency situations, however, is fairly standard with some exceptions, such as pediatric equipment in a pediatrician's office or precipitous delivery equipment for an obstetrician. This equipment should be made available for use and placed in a designated location that is accessible to all office staff. It should be the responsibility of at least one designated worker to inventory the kit at scheduled intervals to ensure that all items are present and within their expiration dates. Standard supplies in an emergency medical kit are listed in Box 25-1.

Box 25-1

Emergency Medical Kit and Equipment

These are standard supplies that can be used to stock an emergency medical kit:

Activated charcoal (used in cases of caustic poisoning)
Adhesive strip bandages, assorted sizes
Adhesive tape, 1- and 2-inch rolls
Alcohol (70%)
Alcohol wipes
Antimicrobial skin ointment
Chemical ice pack
Cotton balls
Cotton swabs
Disposable gloves, latex—sterile and nonsterile
Elastic bandages, 2- and 3-inch widths
Gauze pads, 2 × 2 and 4 × 4 inches—sterile in packs
Hemostats, various sizes, such as Kelly and mosquito—sterile
Roller, self-adhering gauze, 2- to 4-inch widths
Safety pins, various sizes
Scissors
Syrup of ipecac (an emetic, sometimes used in noncaustic poisoning)
Thermometer—1 oral, 1 rectal or fully charged tympanic thermometer
Triangular bandages, 2 or 3
Tweezers or thumb forceps

In addition to the kit contents listed above, the following equipment should be available:

Blood pressure cuff (pediatric and adult)
Stethoscope
Bag-valve-mask device with assorted size masks
Penlight
Portable oxygen tank with regulator
Oxygen masks—several sizes
Oxygen unit

Additional equipment, if available:

Defibrillator
Intravenous equipment (tourniquet, tubing, butterfly setups, angiocaths, IV solutions of various types)
Emergency drugs

Who Do I Call for Emergency Help?

Most communities have a 911 system for telephone access to report emergencies. The communications operator at a local EMS provider will answer the call, take the information, and alert the EMS, fire, or police departments as needed. In localities without the 911 system, emergency calls are usually made directly to the local ambulance, fire, or police department. The information is then routed to the appropriate agency. You should know which emergency system your community uses. The telephone numbers should be prominently displayed by all telephones in the medical office.

Some communities have what is called an enhanced 911 system. This system automatically identifies the caller's telephone number and location. If the telephone is disconnected or the patient loses consciousness, the communications operator still will be able to send emergency personnel to the scene.

Be sure to describe the emergency situation to the communications operator when you make the initial call. The operator will then know what level of emergency personnel and rescue equipment to send. Most of your emergency calls probably will be medical in nature. Ambulances are staffed by trained personnel who have met specific training and certification standards required by individual states.

What Should Be Done Before the Ambulance Arrives?

Whether confronted with a cardiac emergency or a traumatic injury, the medical assistant must be able to coordinate a multitude of ongoing events while rendering patient care. Contributing to the complexity of decisions are such distractions as hysterical family members, arrival of emergency personnel, police directives, and language barriers.

Documentation is an important responsibility in patient care. The information given to emergency medical personnel should be as complete as possible. Information should include but not be limited to:

1. Basic identification information of the patient (eg, name, age, address, or location of patient contact)
2. Patient's chief complaint
3. Times of events (eg, when it happened, how long ago)
4. Vital signs (blood pressure, pulse, and respiration)
5. Specific emergency management techniques rendered by the medical assistant (eg, cardiopulmonary resuscitation, bandaging, splinting)
6. Observations (not subjective conclusions) of the patient's condition (eg, patient's speech was slurred, rather than patient appears drunk; patient unresponsive to loud verbal stimuli, rather than lethargic)
7. Any past medical history, medication, or allergies.

Offer emotional support to the frightened patient, and explain everything that you are doing at each procedural step.

What Should Be Done When the Ambulance Arrives?

When emergency medical personnel arrive, escort the ambulance technician to the patient care area. Assist the technician as directed. Remove any obstacles, such as chairs or surgery stands, to allow room for stretchers and emergency personnel. Keep family members in the reception area or physician's private office. Calm other patients as needed.

Checkpoint Question

1. *What six items should you attempt to document before the ambulance arrives?*

PATIENT ASSESSMENT

The two primary objectives in patient assessment are to identify and correct any life-threatening problems and to identify and care for any associated problems. As a result of information gained from the patient assessment, each step must be managed effectively before proceeding to the next. For example, the scene must be free from life-threatening hazards before proceeding to the primary survey. Airway, breathing, and circulation must be intact before taking a patient history, and the patient's history guides the secondary survey. This section provides a general review of the components of patient assessment.

Scene Survey

The scene survey is the quick, yet observant, evaluation of potential hazards to you and other caregivers, the mechanism of injury, and clues to medical illness that are provided by the patient's environment. For example, in an elderly person found at the bottom of a flight of stairs outside your office suite, a head or neck injury may be probable. Coffee ground–like emesis found near a person may be a clue to the presence of peptic ulcer disease and gastrointestinal hemorrhage.

Personal Protective Equipment

25

For each situation you encounter, it is important to use the appropriate precautions to protect yourself. Because it is impossible to identify patients who carry infectious diseases just by looking at them, all body fluids must be considered infectious and appropriate precautions taken at all times. (See Chap. 1, Asepsis and Infection Control.) Protective equipment should be accessible and available for easy access in every medical office.

What If?
What if you encounter a person bleeding on the street and you do not have protective equipment with you?

If the person is conscious, instruct him or her to cover the wound with a hand or piece of cloth and to apply pressure. You can also make a large bulky dressing with a piece of clothing and hold it on the bleeding area; of course, try to keep your hands from contacting blood. In many cases, it is up to you to decide whether or not to participate in a street emergency. However, some states have specific laws that require health care professionals to render emergency care. You should be aware of your state's law regarding emergency care and acting as a Good Samaritan.

Initial Approach to the Patient

In providing emergency care in an injury situation, do not assume that the obvious injuries are the only ones present because less noticeable injuries may also have occurred. Look for the causes of the injury, which may provide a clue as to the extent of physical damage. The medical assistant should be especially careful not to move the victim any more than necessary during the primary and secondary survey. Any unnecessary movement or rough handling should be avoided because it might aggravate undetected fractures or spinal injuries. EMS personnel are trained in methods of movement that limit the potential for further injury to the patient.

Primary Survey

The **primary survey** is always the first step once the medical assistant is at the patient's side. The primary survey is a rapid evaluation, less than 45 seconds, to determine the patient's status in the following areas:

- Responsiveness
- Airway
- Breathing
- Circulation

The purpose of the primary survey is to identify and correct any life-threatening problems. Although several procedures are shown in this chapter, it is not the purpose of this text to teach CPR. Such instruction should be acquired by taking a complete CPR course designed for health care providers from a certified instructor associated with an organization such as the American Red Cross or the American Heart Association.

Responsiveness

The performance of the primary survey begins with attempts to awaken the patient by verbal and physical stimulation. Checking the patient's responsiveness should not be confused with assessing the more specific level of consciousness, which is part of the more thorough secondary survey. State of responsiveness is quickly noting whether the patient is conscious or unconscious.

Airway

Depending on the circumstances, the airway should be opened by using the head-tilt/chin-lift or jaw-thrust method as described below and shown in Figs. 25-1 and 25-2. The jaw-thrust method is recommended if cervical injury is a possibility. Excessive movement, such as the head-tilt/chin-lift maneuver, could cause neurologic damage to an already injured spine.

The mouth should be quickly inspected for any obvious obstruction; prompt removal of any obstructing foreign body is essential before continuing the patient survey. The tongue falling back into the oropharynx is the most common cause of airway obstruction.

HEAD TILT/CHIN LIFT. The head-tilt/chin-lift method of opening the airway should be used for a patient who is not suspected of having a cervical spine injury. The patient's head should first be tilted back by placing one hand on the forehead and applying firm backward pressure. The other hand should be placed with the fingers under the bony part of the patient's lower jaw, near the chin, thus lifting the mandible and helping to tilt the head back (see Fig. 25-1).

JAW THRUST. The jaw-thrust method requires forward displacement of the jaw without tilting the head. This is the safest method of opening the airway and should always be used on a patient suspected of having cervical spine injury. The angles of the patient's jaw should be grasped with both hands, one on each side, displacing the mandible forward (see Fig. 25-2). The head should be supported without tilting it backward or turning it from side to side.

OBSTRUCTION BY THE TONGUE. An unconscious patient who is in a supine position frequently has a partial or total airway obstruction caused by the tongue falling back into the oropharynx. The epiglottis occludes the airway by falling back over the laryngeal opening when its muscular attachments become weak. (See Chap. 17, Assisting With Diagnostic and Therapeutic Procedures Associated With the Respiratory System.) Patients with central nervous system depression from drugs, alcohol, or disease processes are more prone to this disorder because of poor tone in the facial muscles. Clinical signs include snoring respiration or total airway obstruction.

FOREIGN BODY ASPIRATION. Aspiration of foreign bodies has two effects on the airways. First, aspiration of any foreign material, including fluid, initiates a protective response that consists of sudden coughing and spasm of the airways. This spasm frequently causes labored or difficult breathing and may cause wheezing in

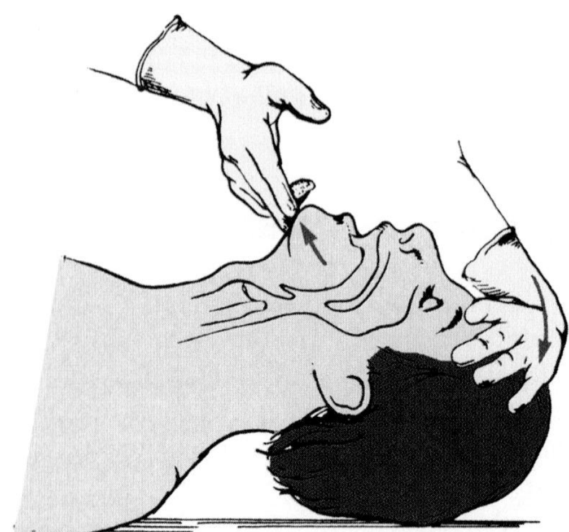

Figure 25-1 The head-tilt/chin-lift technique. The head is tilted backward with one hand (*down arrow*), while the fingers of the other hand lift the chin forward (*up arrow*).

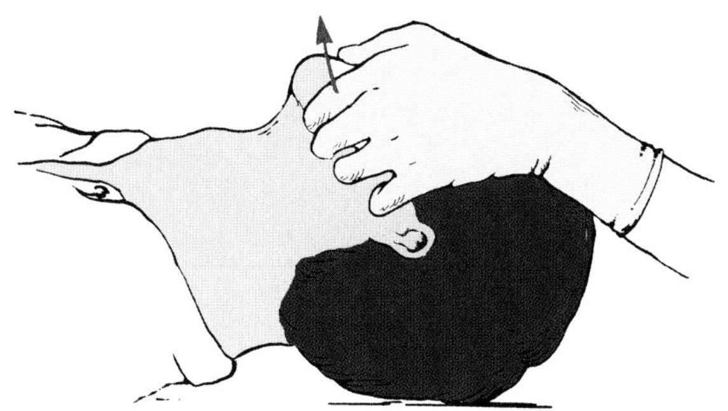

Figure 25-2 The jaw-thrust technique. The hands are placed on either side of the head. The fingers of both hands grasp behind the angle of the jaw, bringing it upward, as shown by the arrow.

severe cases. It can produce partial or total airway obstruction. In addition, if the aspirated material is large enough, it will cause a foreign body obstruction. Frequently, the object lodges in the larynx at the vocal cords because the airway is narrowest at this point.

As with obstruction by the tongue, foreign body aspiration in adults is associated most frequently with drug and alcohol ingestion or altered mental states, such as retardation or Alzheimer's disease. Often these patients have a decreased ability to feed themselves and a diminished gag reflex.

Management of Airway Disorders

After rapid assessment of the patient with airway compromise, immediate management must be started to establish and maintain an open airway. Various devices are available to assist in airway maintenance. Oropharyngeal and nasopharyngeal airways are used to open the upper airway and prevent the tongue from being an obstruction. Suction may be required to remove blood, mucus, or vomitus from the oropharynx.

Management techniques for airway obstruction are shown in Procedure 25-1. Medical assistants are not trained in the use of airway devices in the normal scope of practice.

Breathing

Once the airway is clear and secure, the patient's breathing is evaluated. You should watch the patient's chest while listening and feeling over the mouth and nose for adequate ventilation. If the patient is not breathing, artificial ventilatory support is given immediately. Any labored breathing is evaluated for the degree of distress involved.

Ventilation that is too slow, too fast, or irregular requires immediate intervention. The quality and pattern of breathing also are evaluated. Any obvious noises, such as stridor (a high-pitched, musical sound caused by airway obstruction) or wheezes, should be noted.

If the patient is breathing on his or her own, no intervention should be initiated by the medical assistant rescuer. EMS personnel are trained to respond to these emergencies.

Circulation

Circulation is evaluated in either the adult or child by checking the carotid pulse. The brachial pulse is used to evaluate circulation in the infant. (See Chap. 3, Anthropometric Measurements and Vital Signs.) If the patient has no pulse, external chest compressions should be initiated until the EMS arrives to relieve you. Any hemorrhage (profuse bleeding) should be observed and controlled.

If the pulse is present, the rate and quality are quickly noted. Perfusion (flow of blood through the tissues) is evaluated by skin temperature and moisture. Findings that indicate the presence of shock affect the steps of the secondary survey and ultimate patient management.

Management of Cardiopulmonary Resuscitation (CPR)

Although it is not the purpose of this text to teach CPR, it is important to describe some management techniques. The medical assistant is advised to use a face mask with a one-way valve or preferably a bag-valve-mask device when performing any rescue breathing (Fig. 25-3). These devices should be in the emergency medical kit. The technique for performing CPR on an adult patient is described in Procedure 25-2.

In the event of a cardiopulmonary crisis, you will need to respond quickly. Box 25-2 provides a flow chart of steps to follow during such an emergency.

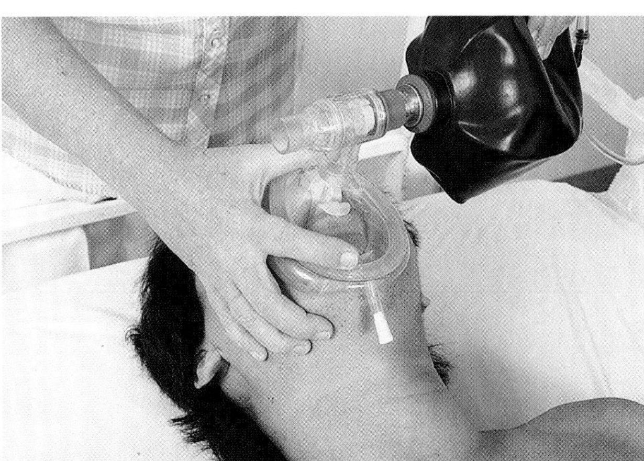

Figure 25-3 Bag and mask equipment for ventilating a patient during CPR. Note the oropharyngeal airway in the victim's mouth to maintain airway patency.

Box 25-2
Rescuer Decision Tree

In an emergency situation, you must make decisions quickly and accurately to prevent further damage to the patient and to reverse life-threatening conditions. Use the following set of decision prompts to help direct you through a cardiopulmonary crisis.

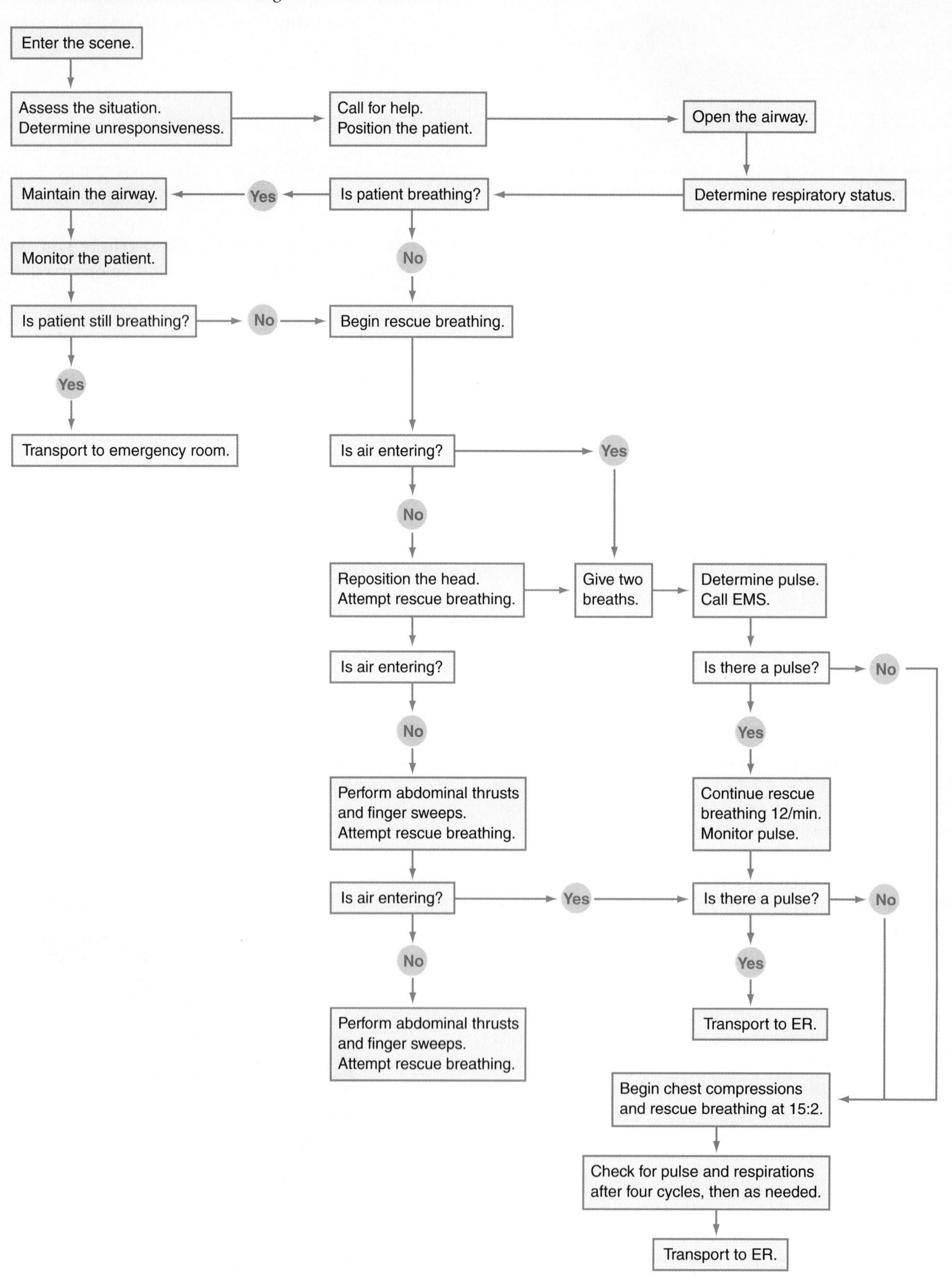

25

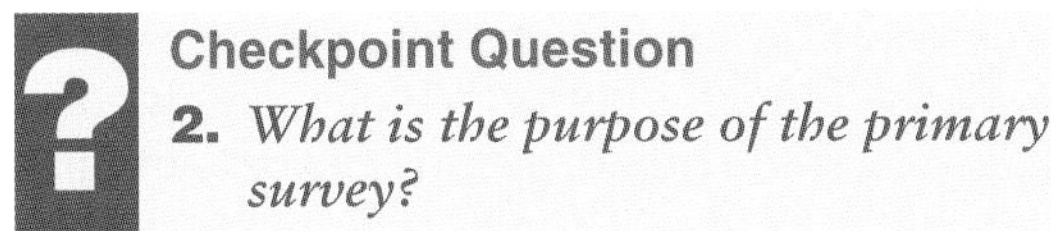

Checkpoint Question

2. *What is the purpose of the primary survey?*

Secondary Survey

The **secondary survey** is an assessment tool for making correct decisions regarding patient care. It is presumed that the patient is not in immediate danger of cardiopulmonary arrest at this point. The secondary survey includes a patient interview and a more thorough physical evaluation. Its aim is to find less obvious and less acute problems than those evaluated in the primary survey. Ideally, management follows as a logical extension of the examination.

Diagnostic Signs

Five diagnostic signs are necessary to gain an accurate impression during the secondary survey. They are:

1. General appearance. The patient's skin color and moisture, facial expression, posture, motor activity, speech, and state of awareness provide important clues about the patient's condition. Medic-Alert bracelets or medicine bottles in pockets can be helpful. The continuation of the secondary survey may confirm or deny initial suspicions seen by the patient's general appearance.
2. Level of consciousness. By the time you have completed the primary survey and noted the patient's general appearance, the level of consciousness may be apparent. The AVPU system is one example that uses a common language to describe the patient's level of consciousness. AVPU is an acronym that represents:
   A = Awake and alert
   V = Responds to voice
   P = Responds only to pain
   U = Unresponsive or unconscious
3. Vital signs. The next step in the secondary survey is assessment of vital signs. Vital signs should be determined before further assessment in most patients. Each vital sign should include a proper measurement technique and appropriate interpretation of the readings. This interpretation should be based on both the initial reading and on serial measurements of each vital sign. The proper techniques and interpretation of the respiration, pulse, and blood pressure are described in Chap. 3, Anthropometric Measurements and Vital Signs.
4. Temperature. Temperature determination is important for patients with altered skin temperature or patients who have been exposed to environmental temperature extremes. Patients with a history of infection, chills, or fever and children with seizures should have their temperatures taken. Taking a temperature is discussed in Chap. 3, Anthropometric Measurements and Vital Signs.
5. Skin. An initial evaluation of the skin that included both temperature and moisture should have been noted during the primary survey. A more thorough assessment should be made. Skin is normally dry and somewhat warm. Moist, cool skin may indicate poor blood flow to the tissues and possible shock. The color of the skin should also be noted as an indication of the circulation near the surface of the body and available oxygen levels. Table 25-1 summarizes abnormal skin colors.

Table 25-1 **Abnormal Skin Colors and Causes**

Color	*Possible Cause*	*Possible Conditions*
Pink	Vasodilation	Heat illness Hot environment
	Increased blood flow	Exertion Fever Alcohol consumption
White, pale	Decreased blood flow	Shock Fainting
	Decreased red blood cells	Anemia
	Vasoconstriction	Cold exposure
Blue	Inadequate oxygenation	Airway obstruction Congestive heart failure Chronic bronchitis
Yellow	Increased bilirubin	Liver disease
	Retention of urinary elements	Renal disease

From Jones S. A., Weigel, A., White, R. D., McSwain, N. E., & Breiter, M. (1992). *Advanced Emergency Care for Paramedic Practice,* p. 116. Philadelphia: J.B. Lippincott.

25

Physical Examination

If the patient appears to be in no immediate danger, make a quick assessment of the body while waiting for the EMS. Report the information you gather to the EMS personnel so they can use it to help determine the best course of action. The survey is organized as follows: head and neck, chest and back, abdomen, and extremities.

HEAD AND NECK. The head should be inspected and palpated. If a cervical spine injury is suspected, the spine should be immobilized immediately, and the neck should not be manipulated while the head is being evaluated. The face should be examined for edema, bruising, bleeding, or fluid from the nose or ears. The mouth should be examined for loose teeth or dentures. In infants, the condition of the anterior fontanel should be noted.

25

The pupils can provide important clues in certain patients. All trauma patients and every patient with an altered level of consciousness or a neurogenic complaint or finding should have the pupils checked. The pupils should be examined for several items:

- Equal size
- Dilation of both pupils when shielded from light
- Constriction of both pupils when exposed to light
- Constriction that occurs rapidly
- Reaction to light that is equal in both pupils

To evaluate these items, both eyes should be shaded from the light. Quickly shine a flashlight at each eye from an angle about 6 to 8 inches from the eye. The patient should not look directly into the light. Both pupils should quickly constrict.

CHEST AND BACK. The chest is evaluated to some degree when the patient's respirations are evaluated. A further inspection of the chest is necessary, especially in the trauma patient or in any patient with abnormal vital signs. The patient with a cardiac or respiratory complaint, finding, or history is also a candidate for a more thorough chest evaluation. Palpation of the chest and back may reveal tender areas that possibly indicate rib fractures.

ABDOMEN. The abdomen should be evaluated on all patients but particularly those with gastrointestinal symptoms or suspicion of blood or fluid loss as seen in vaginal bleeding, vomiting, or melena (blood in the stool). A distended abdomen may indicate hemorrhage within the abdomen.

ARMS AND LEGS. The examination of the arms and legs is the last step of the head-to-toe survey. The arms and legs are inspected and palpated for swelling, deformity, or tenderness. Tremors in the hands should be noted. Comparing one side to another is necessary.

The neurologic status of the arms and legs is determined and tested for strength, movement, range of motion, and sensation. Muscle strength is checked by having the patient squeeze both of your hands. Leg strength may be determined by having the patient push the feet against your hand. The ability to move each arm or leg is simultaneously evaluated. Sensation is assessed by using a safety pin or other tool to determine the patient's response to pain. Throughout the examination, a comparison of both sides is essential.

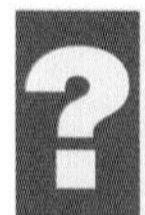

Checkpoint Question

3. *What are the five diagnostic signs that are evaluated in the secondary survey?*

TYPES OF EMERGENCIES

Shock

Shock is a lack of oxygen to the individual cells of the body. All of the body's tissues require oxygen for proper functioning, though the heart and brain have the most immediate response to lack of oxygen.

The body initially adjusts for shock by increasing the strength of contractions of the heart, increasing the heart rate, and constricting the peripheral blood vessels. These acts all help to pump blood throughout the body more efficiently. As shock progresses, the body has difficulty trying to adjust, and eventually tissues and body organs will have such severe damage that the shock becomes irreversible. Box 25-3 lists the signs and symptoms of shock.

Types of Shock

Hypovolemic shock is caused by the loss of blood or other body fluids. If hypovolemic shock occurs due to blood loss, it can also be called hemorrhagic shock. Dehydration caused by diarrhea, vomiting, or heavy sweating can also lead to hypovolemic shock.

Cardiogenic shock is the most extreme form of heart failure, occurring when the function of the left ventricle is so compromised that the heart can no longer adequately pump blood to body tissues.

Neurogenic shock is caused by a dysfunction of the nervous system (as seen in spinal cord injury). The diameter of the blood vessels in the body can no longer be controlled. This leads to a dilation of the blood vessels. Once the blood vessels are dilated, there is not enough blood in the circulation to fill the body's need, causing shock.

Anaphylactic shock is an acute generalized allergic reaction that occurs within minutes to hours after the body has been exposed to a foreign substance to which it is oversensitive.

Septic shock is caused by a generalized infection of the bloodstream in which the patient appears seriously

text continues on page 559

Procedure 25-1 Managing an Adult Patient With a Foreign Body Airway Obstruction (FBAO)

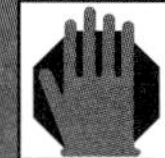
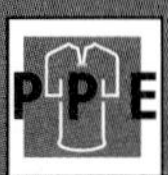

PURPOSE

To restore airway patency by removing foreign body obstruction

EQUIPMENT/SUPPLIES

- barrier respiratory devices
- gloves

Note: If time permits in an out-of-office emergency, secure barrier devices, such as gloves and a respiratory device, for your protection. In an office emergency, these items will be available on the crash cart or tray.

STEPS

1. Ask the patient, "Are you choking?" If the patient is able to speak or cough, the obstruction is not complete. Observe the patient for increased distress and assist the patient as needed, but do not perform thrusts.

This prevents injury to a patient who is not in need of assistance.

2. If the patient is unable to speak or cough and is displaying the universal sign for distress (grasping the throat), follow these steps to perform abdominal thrusts:

a. Stand behind the patient and wrap your arms around his or her waist.

b. Make a fist with your nondominant hand, thumb side against the patient's abdomen at midline between navel and xiphoid.

c. Grasp the fist with your dominant hand and give quick upward abdominal thrusts. Completely relax your arms between each thrust and make each thrust forceful enough to relieve the obstruction.

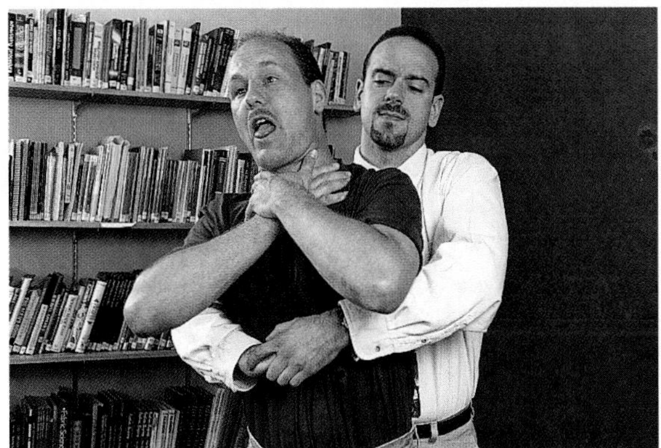

3. Repeat thrusts until effective or the victim becomes unconscious.

Several thrusts may be necessary to expel the object.

4. If the victim is unconscious, or becomes unconscious, activate the EMS system.

This will summon emergency personnel while you continue to provide assistance to the patient.

5. Glove now. Perform a tongue-jaw lift followed by a finger sweep to remove the object.

The object may become visible with the loss of consciousness and may be removed.

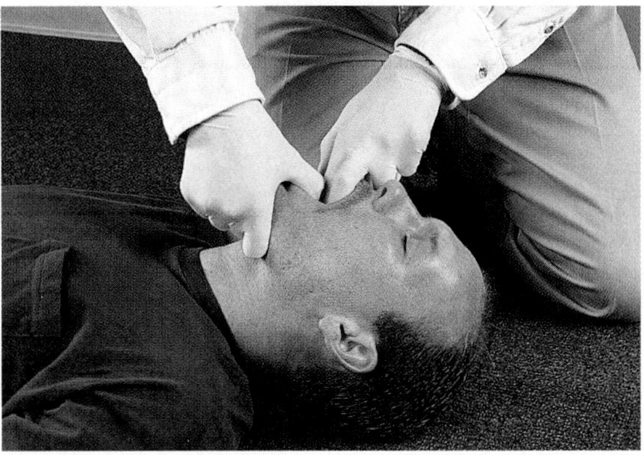

6. Open the airway and try to ventilate. If the airway is still obstructed, reposition the patient's head and try to ventilate again. Use a barrier respiratory device if available.

Repositioning the patient's head ensures that the airway obstruction is not caused by improper head position.

continued

Procedure 25-1 Continued Managing an Adult Patient With a Foreign Body Airway Obstruction (FBAO)

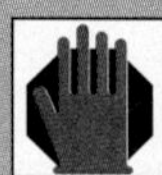
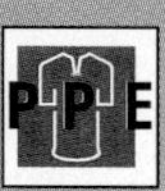

7. Begin abdominal thrusts:
   a. Straddle the patient's hips.
   b. Place the long axis of your nondominant palm between the patient's navel and xiphoid process.
   c. Lace your fingers with the dominant hand against the back of the properly positioned nondominant hand.
   d. Give up to five upward abdominal thrusts.
      This force may expel the object.

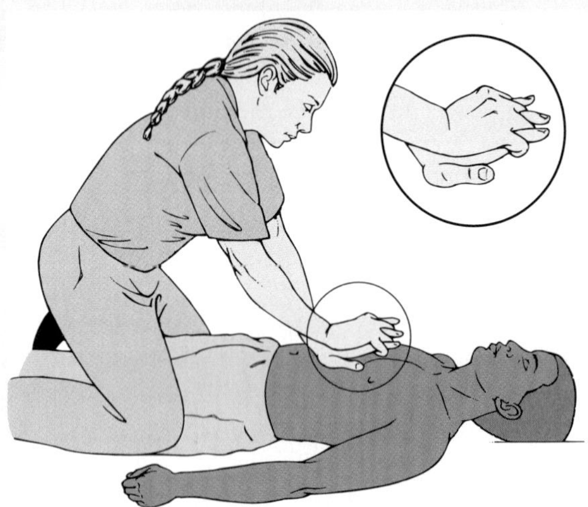

8. Repeat steps 5 through 7 until effective.
   Notes:
   - For detailed coverage of FBAO management and assessment of proficiency, apply for certification through your local American Heart Association or Red Cross.
   - If gloves are available in an emergency encountered outside of the medical office, put them on before doing a finger sweep to avoid exposure to oral secretions. Use your judgment in this situation if PPE and barrier respiratory devices are not available.
   - If the patient is significantly taller than you, you may need to have the patient sit or to raise yourself to a higher position (eg, step on a stool or other object). Achieving the proper effective upward angle for abdominal thrusts is difficult from a position that is lower than the patient's.
   - Obese or pregnant patients require chest thrusts rather than abdominal thrusts.
   - Children over 8 years of age are considered to be adults for the purposes of FBAO management.

DOCUMENTATION GUIDELINES

- Date and time
- Description of the incident that led to FBAO
- Number of thrusts required to dislodge the object
- Any signs or symptoms of respiratory distress
- Notification of physician
- Patient education, if appropriate
- Action taken at completion of emergency
- Your signature

Charting Example

DATE	TIME Pt choked while swallowing Keflex
	stat med. Universal sign of distress;
	obstruction complete. Abdominal thrusts
	administered × 6, object ejected.
	Dr. Kramer notified and checked pt.
	BP-160/98, P-104, R-26. Pt rested in
	room for 20 minutes. BP-118/76, P-76,
	R-16. Pt cautioned to drink full glass of
	water with meds. Dr. Kramer d/c pt to
	home. —Your signature

Procedure 25-2 Performing Cardiopulmonary Resuscitation (One Rescuer)

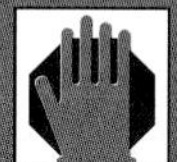

25

PURPOSE

To maintain or restore cardiopulmonary function after arrest until emergency services are available

EQUIPMENT/SUPPLIES

- barrier respiratory devices
- gloves

Note: If time permits in an out-of-office emergency, secure barrier devices, such as gloves and a respiratory device, for your protection. In an office emergency, these items will be available on the crash cart or tray.

STEPS

1. Establish patient unresponsiveness by shaking the patient and shouting "Are you okay?"

Establishing unresponsiveness prevents performance of rescue measures for a patient who does not need them.

2. Activate the EMS system if there is no response.

Quick access to EMS increases the patient's chance for survival.

3. Place the patient in the supine position with head level with the body. Kneel by his shoulders.

This position helps restore blood flow to the brain and makes chest compressions more effective.

4. Open the airway with the head-tilt/chin-lift maneuver.

If the obstruction is positional, this maneuver helps determine the patient's respiratory status.

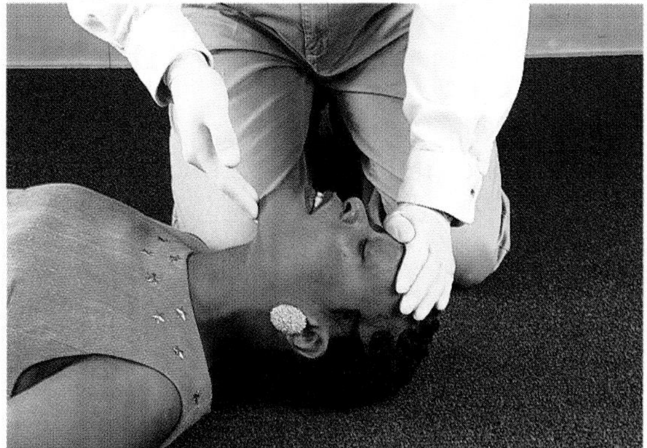

5. Determine breathlessness by looking, listening, and feeling for breaths.

Determining breathlessness avoids giving respirations to a patient who is breathing.

6. If the patient is breathing and his or her condition allows, place the patient in the recovery position (refer to Fig. 25-7) until consciousness returns or help arrives.

The recovery position (side-lying) facilitates respirations and helps prevent aspiration of vomitus.

7. If the patient is not breathing, maintain head-tilt/chin-lift and give two slow breaths just until the chest rises.

Slow breaths provide oxygen to the patient without overfilling the lung fields and causing gastric distention or vomiting.

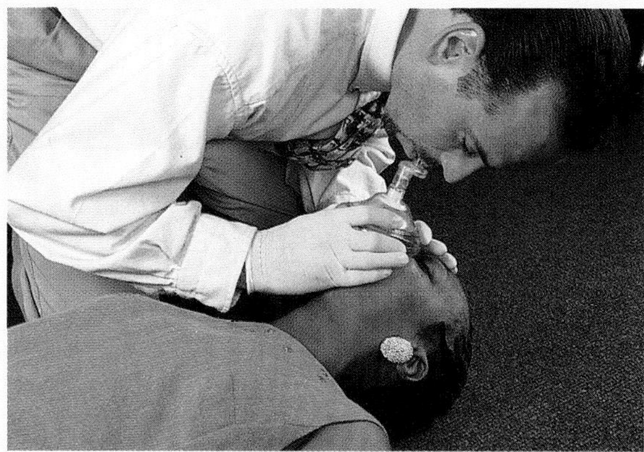

9. Check the carotid pulse.

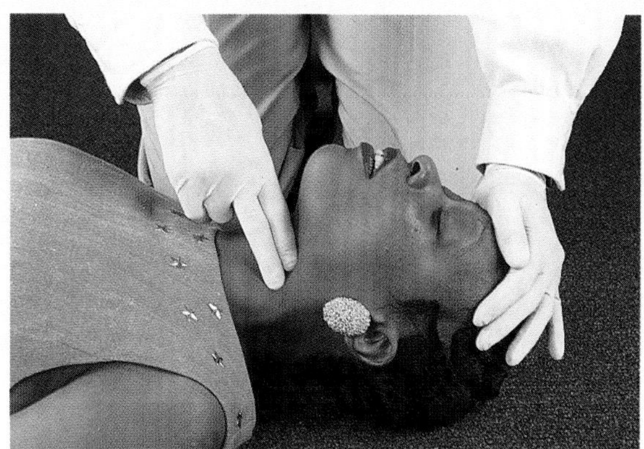

10. If no pulse is present, follow these steps to perform chest compression:

a. Locate the costal-xiphoid (xiphocostal) notch.

continued

Procedure 25-2 Continued Performing Cardiopulmonary Resuscitation (One Rescuer)

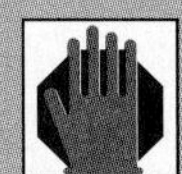
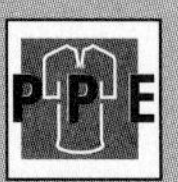

b. Place the long axis of the nondominant palm on the sternum two fingers above the costal-xiphoid notch.

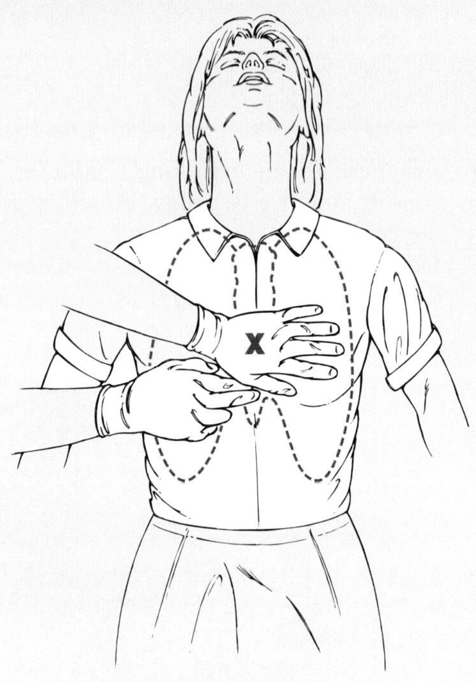

c. Lace the fingers with the dominant hand pressing against the back of the nondominant hand at the proper position.

d. With your upper body perpendicular to the patient's chest, rock from the hips with the force of the upper body and stiffened arms, compressing the sternum 1½ to 2 inches.

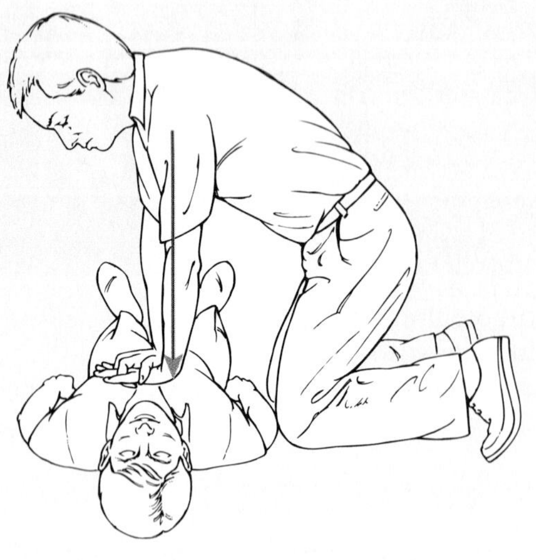

e. Keep your hands in position during the upstroke, but allow the patient's chest to expand completely before the next compression. Give cycles of 15 chest compressions and two breaths at a rate of 80 to 100 per minute.

11. After giving four cycles of 15 chest compressions and 2 breaths (about 1 minute), check the patient's carotid pulse. If no pulse is present, continue the 15:2 cycle beginning with chest compressions. Continue until help arrives or until a pulse is present at the pulse check. If the pulse returns but respirations do not, continue giving breaths at 14 to 16 per minute until help arrives. Transport the patient to an emergency facility.

WARNING! The physician or other trained personnel may use a defibrillation machine to convert the patient's heart rhythm. Stand clear of the patient when the rescuer activates the machine, and follow all of the rescuer's instructions. If a defibrillation machine is available in your office, ask for inservice instructions in its use to assist in future emergencies.

Notes:

- In the clinical situation, respiratory barrier devices and gloves will be available to protect you from the patient's oral secretions. In an out-of-office situation, these devices may not be at hand.
- All health care professionals should receive organized training for proficiency in CPR through an approved training program. The procedure described above is not intended to substitute for proficiency training performed with a mannequin and a structured educational protocol.

continued

Procedure 25-2 Continued **Performing Cardiopulmonary Resuscitation (One Rescuer)**

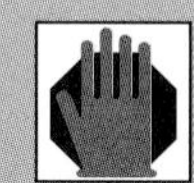
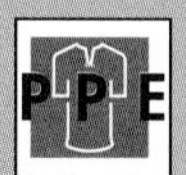

DOCUMENTATION GUIDELINES

- Date and time
- Description of incident
- Time CPR was initiated
- Time EMS arrived
- Hospital destination
- Notification of physician
- Your signature

Charting Example

DATE	TIME Pt scheduled for exercise stress
	test at 9:45 AM. Pt c/o chest pain
	3 minutes into testing. Testing stopped
	stat and Dr. Baker notified. Pt helped to
	examining table. Apparent cardiac arrest
	at 9:55 AM. EMS notified; CPR begun by
	Dr. Baker, assisted by Debra Mendez,
	RMA. EMS arrived at 10:12 AM. AED by
	EMS. Heart rhythm restored. Pt trans-
	ported to Metropolitan General Hospital.
	—Your signature

ill. It may be associated with an infection, such as pneumonia or meningitis, or it may occur without an apparent source of infection, especially in infants and children. History reveals that the patient may have become ill suddenly, or the illness may have developed over several days. Fever is present initially; however, hypothermia develops and is a clinical sign suggestive of sepsis.

Box 25-3
Signs and Symptoms of Shock

- Restlessness or signs of fear
- Thirst
- Nausea
- Cool, clammy skin
- Pale skin with cyanosis (bluish color) at the lips, earlobes, fingers, and toes
- Rapid and weak pulse
- Low blood pressure

Management of the Patient in Shock

Remember: Shock can be the result of many types of medical and trauma emergencies. The following should serve as a general guideline for managing a patient in shock.

1. Ensure an open airway and breathing.
2. Control bleeding.
3. Administer oxygen.
4. Immobilize for possible spinal injuries.
5. Splint fractures.
6. Prevent loss of body heat (use a blanket).
7. Transport to the closest hospital as soon as possible.

Checkpoint Question

4. *What does the term shock mean?*

Bleeding and Soft-Tissue Injuries

Soft-tissue injuries involve the skin and underlying musculature. An injury to these tissues is commonly referred to as a wound. Box 25-4 describes common soft-tissue injuries.

When a blunt object strikes the body, it may crush the tissue beneath the skin. Although the skin does not break, severe damage to tissue and blood vessels may cause bleeding within a confined area. This is called a closed wound.

Types of closed wounds include contusions, hematomas, and crush injuries. A **contusion** is a bruise. Blood collects under the skin or in damaged tissue. Swelling at the site may occur immediately or 24 to 48 hours later. As blood accumulates in the area, a characteristic black and blue mark, called **ecchymosis,** is seen. A blood clot that forms at the injury site is called a **hematoma.** Hematomas are generally caused when large areas of tissue are damaged. When a large bone such as the femur or pelvis is fractured, as much as a liter of blood can be lost in a confined space within the soft tissue. Crush injuries are usually caused by extreme external forces that crush both tissue and bone. Even though the skin remains intact, severe damage may occur to underlying organs.

In an open wound, the skin is broken, and the patient is susceptible to external hemorrhage and wound contamination. An open wound may be the only surface evidence of a more serious injury, such as a fracture. Open wounds include abrasions, lacerations, puncture wounds, impaled objects, avulsions, and amputations. When managing any patient with open wounds, follow Standard Precautions to protect yourself against disease transmission and to protect the patient from further contamination.

25

Box 25-4
Types of Soft-Tissue Injuries

- **Abrasion** is the scraping away of the top layers of skin. If large areas are involved, loss of tissue fluid is a concern. Because of the size of the areas usually involved and the debris that may be imbedded, infection is a serious risk. All abrasions, regardless of size, are extremely painful because of the nerve endings involved.
- **Laceration** results from snagging or tearing tissues that leaves a jagged wound that bleeds freely. Skin tissues may be partly or completely torn away, and the laceration may contain foreign matter that can lead to infection. An example of a laceration would be a wound caused by a broken bottle or a jagged piece of metal.
- **Major arterial laceration** can cause significant bleeding if the sharp or jagged instrument also cuts the wall of a blood vessel, especially an artery. If uncontrolled, major arterial bleeding can result in shock and death.
- **Puncture wound** can result from a number of causes, such as from sharp, narrow objects like knives, nails, and ice picks. Punctures also can be caused by high-velocity penetrating objects, such as bullets. A special case of the puncture wound is the *impaled object wound,* in which the instrument that causes the injury remains impacted in the wound. The object could be anything—a stick, piece of glass, a knife, a steel rod—that penetrates any part of the body.
- **Avulsion** is the tearing loose of a flap of skin, which may either remain hanging or tear off altogether. Avulsions usually bleed profusely. Most often, the patient who presents with an avulsion works with machinery. Home accidents that involve lawn mowers and power tools are common.
- **Amputation** is caused by the ripping, tearing, or cutting force of industrial and automobile accidents, which is often great enough to tear away or crush limbs from the body.

Management of Bleeding and Soft-Tissue Injuries

Management of open soft-tissue injuries includes controlling bleeding by direct pressure and elevation. Sterile gauze should be used to cover the wound. Elevation of the affected part above the level of the heart is effective in the control of both pain and bleeding.

Management of amputations includes controlling bleeding but also preserving the severed part. The severed part should be put in a plastic bag. Place the first bag in a second plastic bag and seal it closed. The second bag provides added protection against moisture loss. Place the sealed bags in a container of ice or ice water; never use dry ice.

An impaled object requires careful immobilization of the patient and the injured part. Any motion of the impaled object can cause additional damage to the surface wound and, particularly, the underlying tissues. Never attempt to remove an impaled object. This must be done by a trauma surgeon.

Burn Injuries

The four major sources of burn injury are thermal, electrical, chemical, and radiation. *Thermal burns,* also called heat burns, are a result of heat conducted by hot liquids, solids, and superheated gases, as well as flame burns from fire. *Electrical burns* are caused from contact with electricity. Lightning injuries are also considered electrical burns. *Chemical burns* result when corrosive substances come in contact with the skin. The amount of injury with a chemical burn depends on the concentration and quantity of the chemical agent. *Radiation burns* are similar to thermal burns and can occur from overexposure to ultraviolet light (sunburn) or from the heat of an atomic explosion.

Classification of Burn Injuries

Classification of burn injuries depends on the depth or tissue layers of the skin involved. Factors that determine the depth of the burn include the agent of burn, temperature, and length of time exposed. Burns are classified as **superficial** (first-degree), **partial-thickness** (second-degree), and **full-thickness** (third-degree). Table 25-2 describes the characteristics of burns according to depth.

Calculation of Body Surface Area

The extent of body surface area (BSA) burned is most commonly estimated by a method called the rule of nines. This method calculates the percentage of body surface occupied by individual sections of the body. To determine fully the extent of BSA burned, the percentage of superficial, partial-thickness, and full-thickness burns should be recorded. This process, however, is not practical in the out-of-hospital setting.

RULE OF NINES. The **rule of nines** is the most common method of determining the extent of burn injury (Fig. 25-4). With this technique, in the adult, 9% of the skin is estimated to cover the head and each upper extremity, including front and back surfaces. Twice as much, or 18%, of the total skin area covers the front and back of the trunk and each lower extremity, including front and back surfaces. The area around the genitals, called the perineum, represents the additional 1% of BSA. In the infant or child, the percentages remain the same with the exception of the head, which is 18%, and each lower extremity, which is 13.5% of total BSA. The rule of nines works well in adults but does not reflect the various anatomic differences seen in children of varying ages.

Management of the Burn Victim

The following should be used as management guidelines for burn victims. In the event of an electrical burn, protect yourself from the electrical source before attempting to rescue the patient.

1. Eliminate the source of the burn.
2. Assess the patient's airway, breathing, and circulation.
3. Remove all jewelry and clothing necessary to evaluate the burn.

25

Table 25-2 **Characteristics of Burns According to Depth**

Depth of Burn and Causes	*Skin Involvement*	*Symptoms*	*Wound Appearance*	*Recuperative Course*
Superficial (First-Degree)				
Sunburn Low-intensity flash	Epidermis	Tingling Hyperesthesia (supersensitivity) Pain that is soothed by cooling	Reddened; blanches with pressure Minimal or no edema	Complete recovery within a week Peeling
Partial-Thickness (Second-Degree)				
Scalds Flash flame	Epidermis and part of dermis	Pain Hyperesthesia Sensitive to cold air	Blistered, mottled red base; broken epidermis; weeping surface Edema	Recovery in 2–3 wk Some scarring and depigmentation Infection may convert it to third-degree
Full-Thickness (Third-Degree)				
Flame Prolonged exposure to hot liquids Electric current	Epidermis, entire dermis, and sometimes subcutaneous tissue	Possibly pain free Shock Hematuria (blood in the urine) and possibly hemolysis (blood cell destruction) Possible entrance and exit wounds (electrical burn)	Dry; pale white, leathery, or charred Broken skin with fat exposed Edema	Eschar (scab or dry crust) sloughs Grafting necessary Scarring and loss of contour and function Loss of digits or extremity possible

From Smeltzer, S. C., & Bare, B. G. (1996). *Brunner and Suddarth's Textbook of Medical-Surgical Nursing,* 8th ed., p. 1550. Philadelphia: Lippincott-Raven.

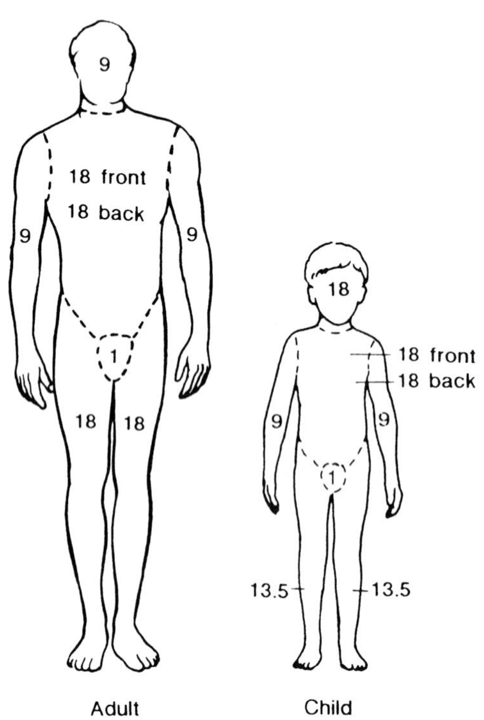

Figure 25-4 The rule of nines.

4. Wrap the patient in a clean, dry sheet.
5. Administer oxygen.
6. Keep the patient warm.
7. Treat the patient for shock.
8. Transport the patient to the hospital.

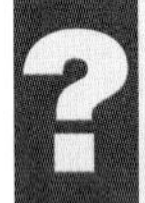

Checkpoint Question

5. *What are the four major sources of burn injuries?*

Musculoskeletal Injuries

Injuries to muscles, bones, and joints are some of the most common problems encountered in providing emergency care. The seriousness of these injuries varies widely from simple injuries, such as a fractured finger, to major life-threatening conditions, such as an open femur fracture or compromising spinal injuries. Injuries to muscle, tendons, and ligaments occur when a joint or muscle is either torn or stretched beyond its normal limits. Fractures and dislocations are usually associated with external forces, although some may occur through disease, such as bone degeneration.

Caring for patients with strains, sprains, fractures, and dislocations is described in Chapter 11, Assisting With Diagnostic and Therapeutic Procedures Associated With the Musculoskeletal System.

Management of Musculoskeletal Injuries

It is often difficult to distinguish between strains, sprains, fractures, and dislocations in an emergency situation. Therefore, in most cases, assume that the area is fractured and immobilize it accordingly. Proper splinting technique involves immobilizing above and below the fracture site. Splinting helps prevent further injury to soft tissues, blood vessels, or nerves from sharp bone fragments and relieves pain by stopping motion at the fracture site.

Never attempt to reduce (put back in place) a dislocated area. You may, however, gently realign a severely deformed limb before splinting it. This may be required when an angulated injury to the arm or leg cannot be fit into a rigid splint or if a pulse is absent distal to (below) the fracture site. Realignment is nothing more than pulling gently in line with the normal bone position. If there is pain or resistance to this procedure, splint the fracture as it is.

TYPES OF SPLINTS. Any device used to immobilize a fracture or dislocation is a splint. A splint may be soft or rigid. It can be improvised from almost any object that can provide stability. There are several kinds of commercially available splints, such as a traction splint, air splint, wire ladder splint, and padded board splint (Fig. 25-5).

Cardiovascular Emergencies

Cardiovascular disease accounts for nearly one million deaths each year in the United States. The most common problem is coronary artery disease, which usually leads to angina (chest pain due to ischemic heart disease) and eventually to heart attack (myocardial infarction) if left untreated. Approximately two thirds of sudden deaths due to coronary artery disease occur out of the hospital, and most occur within 2 hours of the onset of cardiovascular symptoms. Many of these deaths can be prevented by prompt basic or advanced life support, including rapid access to the EMS system, bystander CPR, and early defibrillation (an electrical shock to restore a normal heart rhythm).

If CPR is initiated promptly and the patient is successfully and rapidly defibrillated, survival chances are good. Defibrillation can be performed with manual, automatic, or semiautomatic external defibrillators. Manual defibrillation requires interpretation of a monitor or rhythm strip. Defibrillation using automatic or semiautomatic devices will analyze the rhythm and either automatically defibrillate or advise the operator to defibrillate (Fig. 25-6). Your responsibility during defibrillation is to assist the physician or skilled provider as needed and to stand clear of the patient as the machine is activated. If a defibrillator is used in your office, ask for an inservice in its use.

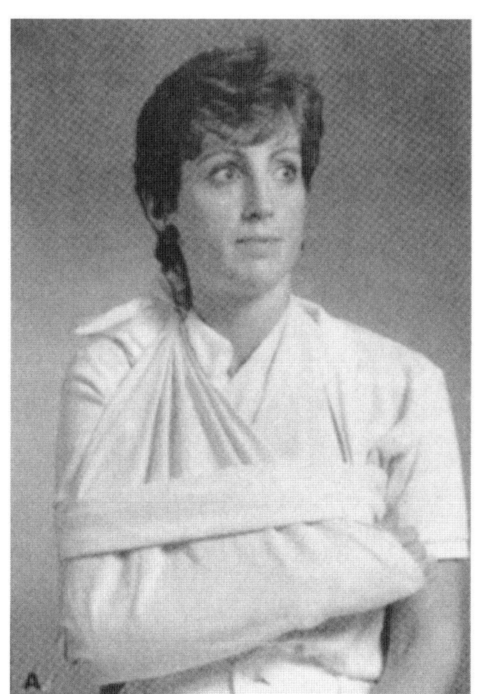

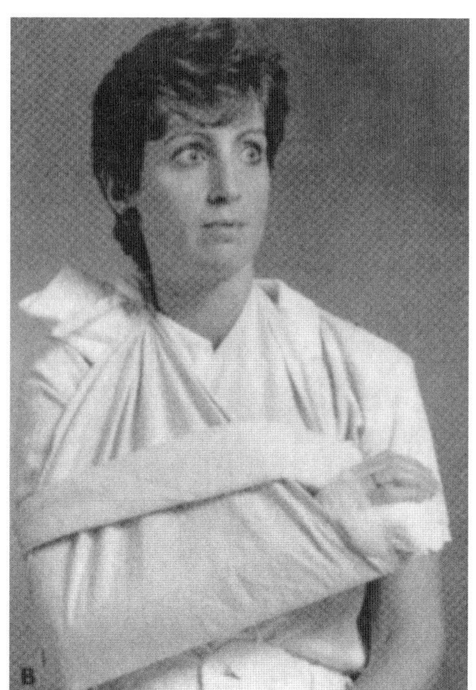

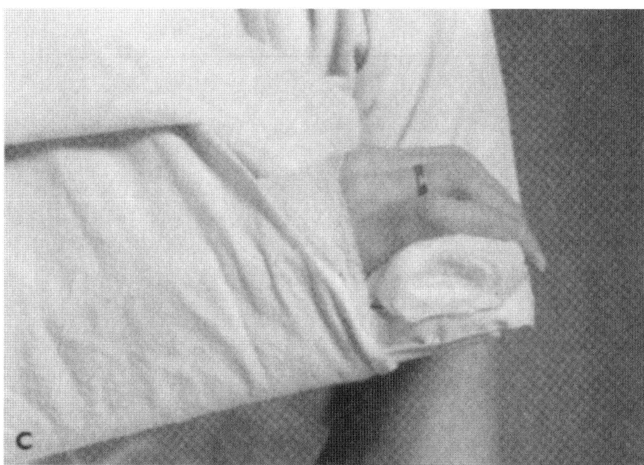

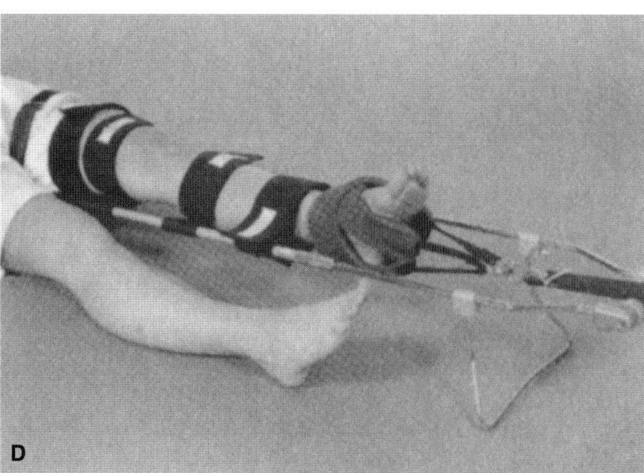

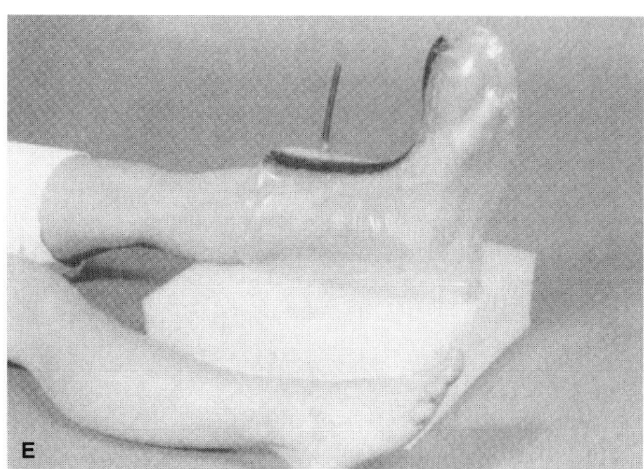

Figure 25-5 Types of splints. (**A**) Sling and swath. (**B**) Sling and swath with padded board on the anterior aspect of the forearm. (**C**) Roller bandage placed in the palm of the hand to splint the hand in a functional position. (**D**) Traction splint. (**E**) Air splint.

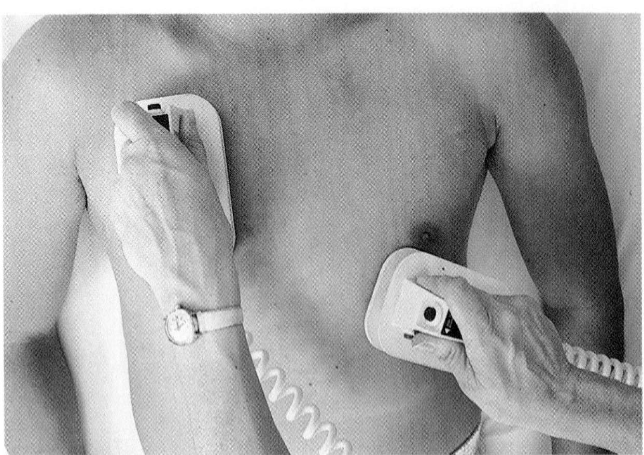

Figure 25-6 Paddles are placed on the chest exactly on locations indicated on the instruction panel of the attached defibrillation machine. Instructions are graphically displayed for the responder, either the physician or an EMT or paramedic.

Neurologic Emergencies

A seizure is caused by an abnormal discharge of electrical activity in the brain. During a seizure attack, bizarre muscle movements, strange sensations, and a complete loss of consciousness can occur. A seizure is not a disease but a manifestation or symptom of an underlying disorder.

When assessing the patient having a seizure, priority must be given to responsiveness, airway, breathing, and circulation. In certain types of seizure, the patient experiences a period of unconsciousness and, therefore, is unable to protect the airway. Frequently, these patients vomit during the seizure. Also, they have a tendency to bite their tongue. Particular attention and care should be given to clearing and maintaining the airway. Patient history is an important factor in the assessment of these patients. It should include information about past seizure disorders, frequency of the attacks, prescribed medications, and regularity in taking medications. Further, history of head trauma is a significant finding. Other important aspects to explore include alcohol and drug abuse, recent fever, stiff neck (as seen in meningitis), and a history of heart disease, diabetes, or stroke.

Care of the patient should always begin with opening and securing an airway. When maintaining the airway of the patient having a seizure, objects should never be forced between the patient's teeth. Padded tongue blades or bite sticks may cause further complications, such as broken teeth, vomiting, aspiration, and laryngeal spasm.

After maintaining patency of the airway, perhaps the most important thing you can do for a patient who is having a seizure is to protect the patient from injury. The patient will rarely need to be restrained. Placing the patient on the side in the recovery position (Fig. 25-7) will help secretions drain from the mouth and is an easier position to suction the patient, if necessary.

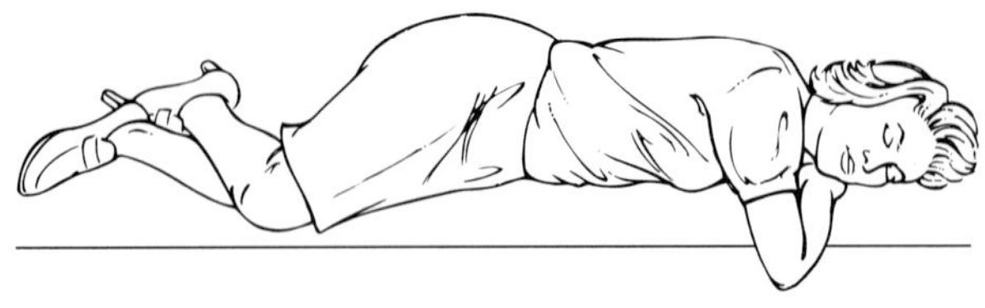

Figure 25-7 Patient in the recovery position.

Allergic and Anaphylactic Reactions

This section addresses allergic reactions, including the severe form, **anaphylaxis.** Anaphylaxis (or anaphylactic reaction) causes the most emergency department visits related to allergies. It is an acute generalized allergic reaction that occurs within minutes to hours after the body has been exposed to a foreign substance to which it is oversensitive. This anaphylactic reaction has systemic signs and symptoms that are exaggerated from a simple allergic reaction.

The exact incidence of anaphylactic reactions is difficult to pinpoint. Estimates in a study in the United States determined that 1% to 2% of all patients who receive penicillin have some form of allergy to the drug and that 1 in 50,000 injections of penicillin results in death. Estimates of anaphylactic death from insect stings number at least 50 per year.

As explained in Chap. 16, Assisting With Diagnostic and Therapeutic Procedures Associated With the Immunologic System, the immune response is a positive adaptive response. It is designed to guard the body against dangerous foreign substances, such as infections and antigens. In this normal immune response, the protective cells of the body recognize dangerous intruders, fight them, and destroy them. The allergic reaction, on the other hand, is an oversensitive and harmful response against foreign substances that may actually be harmless. The protective cells overestimate the danger of the harmless intruder and may produce needless damage to body tissue.

Common Allergens

An allergen is a substance that gives rise to hypersensitivity or allergy. Allergen groups include drugs, insect venom, food, and pollen. Other allergens include cigarette smoke, dust mites, and cats and dogs. The causative agent may be injected, ingested, absorbed through the skin or mucous membranes, or even inhaled. A patient may experience symptoms within seconds after exposure to an allergen, or the reaction may be delayed for several hours.

Signs and Symptoms

The initial signs and symptoms typically occur with severe itching, a feeling of warmth, tightness in the throat or chest, or a rash. Cardiovascular collapse and shock can occur if the situation becomes worse. The primary rule for any exposure is that the earlier the onset of symptoms after exposure, the more severe the reaction is likely to be.

Management of Allergic and Anaphylactic Reactions

Because the primary cause of death in anaphylaxis is airway obstruction, the medical assistant must observe closely for signs of airway involvement. Choking or tightness in the neck and throat may signal this danger. In addition to the upper airway, the entire respiratory system frequently is involved. The patient may exhibit wheezing, shortness of breath, coughing, spitting up blood (hemoptysis), or pulmonary edema. A fast heart rate (tachycardia), low blood pressure (hypotension), pale skin, dryness of the mouth, sweating, and other classic signs of shock may be seen. The patient is likely to be anxious, and reassurance is an important part of the immediate intervention.

MedicAlert tags can be life saving, particularly for patients who have severe anaphylactic reactions. The tags are available as a bracelet or necklace and have engraved medical information.

Some allergic reactions are mild, without respiratory problems or signs of shock. These simple reactions can be managed with giving the patient oxygen (2–4 L/min) by nasal cannula or simple face mask. If respiratory involvement occurs without shock, the physician may order that epinephrine (1:1,000) be given subcutaneously to enhance bronchodilation. In the patient with a severe anaphylactic reaction who is in shock, more aggressive therapy is indicated. Along with administering oxygen, the physician may order intravenous epinephrine (1:10,000). Monitoring the cardiac rhythm and additional drug therapy may be required. The primary goal of therapy in the patient with a severe anaphylactic reaction is to restore respiratory and circulatory function.

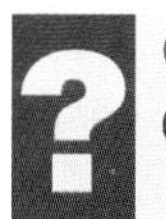

Checkpoint Question

6. *What is the primary cause of death in anaphylaxis?*

Poisoning

The likelihood that one will be exposed to toxins in the home or workplace is increasing. Over-the-counter and prescription medications are common in the home. Household chemicals are a hazard, many times designed to have a pleasant odor and color. Industrial chemicals offer another dimension of potential toxic exposures. These chemicals may involve a single victim or may create a triage problem in a widespread hazardous materials incident requiring the sorting of a large number of patients to concentrate on those most in need.

Overall, most toxic exposures occur in the home. Almost 50% of exposures reported occur in children between the ages of 1 and 3 years. About 90% of all reported poisonings are accidental. In adolescents and adults, intentional toxic exposures can occur. Although deaths from poisoning and drug overdose are not frequent, intentional toxic exposures tend to have a higher death rate and result in more serious symptoms than accidental exposures or adverse drug actions.

Poison Control Center

When information about a poisoning or drug overdose is not readily available, the poison control center is a valuable resource. Poison control centers are designed to answer questions from health care professionals and the public. Many times, they can evaluate a nontoxic or mildly toxic exposure by telephone, instruct the caller in the use of syrup of ipecac to induce vomiting, and check on the progress by follow-up telephone calls. In questionable or more potentially serious toxic exposures, the poison control center can be consulted from the emergency scene (ie, physician's office).

The American Association of Poison Control Centers has established standards and recognizes regional poison control centers throughout the country. These centers are staffed by physicians, nurses, and pharmacists who are specifically trained or experienced in collecting information from a caller and retrieving information from many sources. Exactly how and when a poison control center is consulted should be part of the medical office's protocol.

Management of Poisoning Emergencies

Few toxic substances have specific antidotes. As a result, management of the poisoning emergency is aimed at the signs and symptoms present and organ systems involved. Decontamination and prevention of further absorption are done once the patient is relatively stable and initial priorities have been addressed.

INHALED POISON. Protect yourself from the fumes, and remove the victim from the area as quickly as possible. Fresh air is imperative, and oxygen should be administered if available while waiting for the EMS. Assess respiratory function, and begin CPR or rescue breathing if necessary.

CONTACT POISON. Wear gloves to protect yourself from the substance, and strip contaminated clothing away from the victim. Rinse the skin with large amounts of room temperature water. Avoid soap if unsure of the poisonous substance to prevent an additional chemical reaction.

INGESTED POISON. Remove any remaining poison in the victim's mouth if possible. Contact the Poison Control Center in your area with the name of the poison before attempting to administer an antidote. Transport the container with the victim to the nearest emergency center by EMS. Do not induce vomiting unless told to do so by the Poison Control Center.

Heat- and Cold-Related Emergencies

25

Temperature is one of the many variables to which the body adjusts in the process of maintaining equilibrium. As warm-blooded animals, human beings depend on the ability to limit core body temperature within a range of several degrees. This range centers around a normal core temperature of 37.6°C or 99.6°F, measured rectally. Peripheral temperature is usually lower, as seen by a normal value of 37°C (98.6°F) for oral readings. The definition of normal thus varies with location. Temperature also fluctuates over a range of several degrees under entirely healthy circumstances. To take advantage of the body's temperature as an assessment tool, both rectal and oral thermometers should be available. If neither is available or advisable, tympanic measurement is an excellent alternative.

Several conditions disrupt the normal heat-regulating mechanisms of the body. They are divided into two main categories, hyperthermia and hypothermia.

Hyperthermia

Hyperthermia refers to the general condition of excess body heat. Correct management depends on assessment of underlying causes.

Heat cramps result from profuse sweating. Most often, the cramping follows a period of physical exertion in a hot environment. Heavy sweating leads to high sodium losses, and at some point, the sodium deficit compromises muscle function. The cramps are a consequence of sweating, a healthy compensatory mechanism, and usually present without evidence of more severe problems.

The patient complains of cramps most commonly in the calves of the legs and in the abdomen. Cramps may occur in the hands, arms, and feet. The patient's skin is cool and usually wet. Mental status and blood pressure should be normal, although an increased pulse rate is common.

Heat cramps signal the need for cooling and rest. In uncomplicated cases, the patient is often able to take fluid by mouth, but nausea may make intravenous infusion of 0.9% sodium chloride the desired management. If the patient is able to take fluid by mouth, add ½ to 1 teaspoon of salt per pint of water or fruit juice or give one of the commercial electrolyte solutions, such as Gatorade. Cramps can sometimes be prevented entirely with similar oral intake before physical exertion. Salt tablets are not recommended because they may cause nausea or upset the body's sodium balance.

Heat exhaustion results most often from physical exertion in the heat without adequate fluid replacement. Body temperature usually remains normal or only slightly above normal. Patients often present with central nervous system symptoms, such as headache, fatigue, dizziness, or syncope (fainting). Skin is typically moist, and the pulse rate is high. Skin color, blood pressure, and respiratory rate are all variable depending on the degree to which the body is able to hold off the distress. Patients with later stages of heat exhaustion have pale skin, low blood pressure, and increased respiratory rate.

Management used for heat cramps may be sufficient in the early stages of heat exhaustion, but any hint of decreased mental status or unstable vital signs demands closer attention. Aggressive cooling measures must be used, as described for heat stroke, if rectal temperature is above 39°C (102°F).

Heat stroke is a true emergency. The body is no longer able to compensate for the rise in body temperature. Core body temperature threatens brain damage as it rises rapidly past 41°C (105°F). Heat stroke victims can deteriorate quickly to coma. They often have

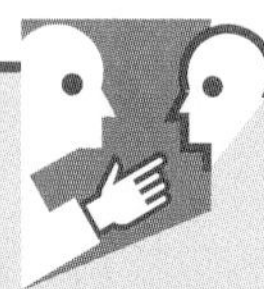

Advice and Tips

Recognizing Groups at High Risk for Hypothermia

Heat loss can be more serious in groups at high risk for hypothermia.

Children, particularly newborns and infants, have heat-regulating systems that are not completely developed, and their ratio of skin surface to body mass is higher than that of adults. Both of these factors predispose them to rapid heat loss.

The elderly tend to lose heat gradually. Their heat-balancing mechanisms and other defense systems that would otherwise protect them from excessive heat loss lose sensitivity with age. Additional risks for the elderly may include poor circulation, physical immobility, the tendency of friends and family to dismiss early mental changes as senility, and other factors, such as malnutrition and poorly heated homes. Hypothermia in the elderly can develop over a period of days in indoor surroundings that feel comfortable to the young healthy adult.

Hypothermia can be prevented in both age groups through patient education.

seizures, and the skin is classically hot, flushed, and dry, although gradual onset, age, and other factors can alter this sign. Vital signs rise initially, then drop later, resulting in cardiopulmonary arrest.

Heat stroke demands rapid cooling. The patient should be moved quickly to a cool area, clothing removed, and cold water or wet sheets placed on the patient's body. Concentrate on the core surface areas where the ability to cool central blood is greatest: the scalp, neck, axillae, and groin. The patient should be given oxygen and placed on a cardiac monitor. Transport to the hospital with continued cooling en route is required.

Hypothermia

The body's core temperature can drop several degrees in the normal course of body function. Even when the heat loss is not routine, the body usually tolerates a 3° to 4° drop without symptoms. **Hypothermia** is an abnormally low body temperature, with rectal readings below 35°C (95°F). Internal metabolic factors and heat loss to the external environment can lead to hypothermia. The rate of onset of hypothermia is variable. Very cold air and immersion in cold water can cause rapid drops in core temperature.

Basic management of hypothermia includes handling the patient gently, removing wet clothing, and covering the patient to prevent further cooling. Give warm oral fluids only if evidence of active rewarming is seen. The patient should be alert and able to swallow easily before taking fluids. The patient must be able to control shivering to achieve active rewarming. Avoid drinks that contain caffeine (coffee and tea), which constricts peripheral blood vessels, and alcohol, which dilates them. Warm beverages with sugar, such as hot chocolate, can be given to begin replacement of the fuel the body needs to restore normal heat production. No oral fluids should be given to patients with changing levels of consciousness.

Frostbite

Windy, subfreezing weather creates the greatest risk for frostbite. **Frostbite** occurs when small body parts with a high ratio of surface area to tissue mass (fingers, toes, ears, and nose) are exposed to extreme cold. Larger areas of the extremities are vulnerable in more profound cooling. This cold exposure causes tissues to freeze, and cells will eventually die.

The type and duration of contact are the two most important factors in determining the extent of frostbite injury. Touching cold fabric is not nearly as dangerous as coming into direct contact with cold metal, particularly if the hands are wet or even damp. In the latter case, the skin usually is cemented instantly to the cold metal and is torn off when the hand is removed. The combination of wind and cold is a dangerous factor in freezing.

Superficial frostbite appears as firm and waxy gray or yellow skin in an area that loses sensation after hurting or tingling. Prolonged exposure can lead to blistering and eventually *deep frostbite,* which most often afflicts hands and feet. No warning symptoms appear after the initial loss of feeling. Freezing progresses painlessly once the nerve endings are numb. Skin becomes inelastic, and the entire area feels hard to the touch.

Superficial frostbite can be managed by warming the affected part with another body surface, for example, placing an ungloved hand over a cold spot on the cheek. Management for more than superficial frostbite is rapid rewarming after any system-wide hypothermia has been corrected. Deep frostbite should only be managed in the hospital to prevent further damage. Immerse the frozen tissue in lukewarm water (41°C [105°F]) until the tissue becomes pliable, and color and sensation return. Because this effect may take at least 20 minutes in most cases, transport to the hospital should not be delayed. Dry heat, cold therapy, massaging, and any handling that breaks blisters are harmful actions.

Apply dry sterile dressings, and handle gently after thawing. If rewarming is not attempted, the frostbitten part should be bandaged with dry sterile dressings and the patient transported to the hospital. Frostbitten flesh also shares burned tissue's vulnerability to infection, so care should be taken to keep the affected part as clean as possible.

All frostbite victims should be assessed for signs of hypothermia as well. Clothing offers good protection against weather only if it is loose enough to avoid restricting circulation. Tight gloves, cuffs, boots, and straps add to the danger.

Behavioral and Psychiatric Emergencies

It is important to remember that psychological distress may be mild, moderate, or severe. The degree of intensity determines the type and amount of intervention necessary. When working with a behavioral problem in a patient, the medical assistant should know what constitutes a psychiatric emergency and what is better classified as an emotional crisis. A psychiatric emergency is any situation in which patients' moods, thoughts, or actions are so disordered or disturbed that they have the potential to produce danger, harm, or death to themselves or to others if the situation is not quickly controlled.

An emotional crisis, on the other hand, is a situation with much less intensity. It is distressing but in most cases is not likely to end in danger, harm, or death if not responded to immediately. However, if neglected entirely, an emotional crisis may escalate to a full psychiatric emergency.

A true behavioral emergency, like a medical emergency, has an element of serious threat to it. Without immediate intervention, true behavioral emergencies can end in injury or death to the patient or to someone else near the patient. Urgent behavioral situations usually require some form of professional intervention; the patient should be transported to a hospital for evaluation. The nonemergency cases have a far less degree of urgency attached to them. Nonemergency situations are less likely to result in potentially dangerous behaviors. Kindness, reassurance, and general support are usually sufficient until specialized services are available.

Answers to Checkpoint Questions

1. *Before the ambulance arrives, you should document basic identification information, chief complaint, times of events, vital signs, techniques used to treat the patient, and any observations.*
2. *The purpose of the primary survey is to identify and correct any life-threatening problems.*
3. *The five diagnostic signs of the secondary survey are general appearance, level of consciousness, vital signs, temperature, and skin appearance.*
4. *Shock is defined as the lack of oxygen to the individual cells.*
5. *The four major sources of burn injuries are thermal, electrical, chemical, and radiation.*
6. *The primary cause of death from anaphylaxis is airway obstruction.*

Critical Thinking Challenges

1. When an emergency occurs, the patient's family members may become anxious and, in some cases, emotionally distraught. How would you help to calm an anxious family member?
2. Reread the "What If?" question in this chapter. Analyze how you would respond to such a situation.

Suggestions for Further Reading

Grant, H. D., Murray, R. H., & Bergeron, D. J. (1990). *Brady Emergency Care,* 5th ed. Englewood Cliffs, NJ: Brady Division of Prentice Hall.

Harwood-Nuss, A. L., & Luten, R. C. (1995). *Handbook of Emergency Medicine.* Philadelphia: Lippincott-Raven.

Jones, S. A., et al. (1992). *Advanced Emergency Care for Paramedic Practice.* Philadelphia: Lippincott-Raven.

Unit 5

Performing Laboratory Procedures

26

Introduction to the Clinical Laboratory

Chapter Outline

Role Delineation

GENERAL

Professionalism

- Adhere to ethical principles.
- Demonstrate initiative and responsibility.

Legal Concepts

- Comply with established risk management and safety procedures.

Operational Functions

- Evaluate and recommend equipment and supplies.

Chapter Competencies

Learning Objectives

Upon successfully completing this chapter, you will be able to:

1. Spell and define the Key Terms.
2. List reasons for laboratory testing.
3. Outline the medical assistant's responsibility in the clinical laboratory.
4. Name the kinds of laboratories available to the medical assistant and the functions of each.
5. List the types of personnel found in laboratories and describe their jobs.
6. Name the types of departments found in most large laboratories and give their purposes.
7. Explain how to use a package insert to determine the procedure for a laboratory test.
8. List the equipment found in most small laboratories and give the purpose of each.

Chapter Competencies *(continued)*

9. List and describe the parts of a microscope.
10. List the safety rules for laboratories.
11. Explain the significance of the Clinical Laboratory Improvement Amendments (CLIA) and how to follow CLIA regulations to ensure quality control.

Performance Objective

Upon successfully completing this chapter, you will be able to:

1. Care for the microscope (Procedure 26-1).

Key Terms

(See Glossary for definitions.)

aerosol
anticoagulant
calibrations
capillary action
centrifugal force
Clinical Laboratory Improvement Amendments (CLIA)
material safety data sheet (MSDS)
National Committee for Clinical Laboratory Standards (NCCLS)
normal values
quality assurance (QA)
quality control (QC)
reagents
reference values
specimens

The medical laboratory provides the physician with one of medicine's most powerful diagnostic tools. It can aid the physician in evaluating the patient's response to medications and in following the progress of a disease process. Laboratory personnel analyze blood, urine, and other body samples to identify diseases and disorders. Results of laboratory testing are compared with **normal** or **reference values** (acceptable ranges for a healthy population) to determine the relative health of body systems or organs. Blood levels of various medications are determined to adjust dosages to therapeutic levels. Bacteria, viruses, parasites, and other microorganisms are identified to begin the treatment process. (See Appendix VI for a list of commonly performed laboratory tests and their normal values.)

Laboratory testing is most commonly used for:

- Diagnosing a disease
- Following the progress of a disease
- Meeting legal requirements (eg, drug testing, a marriage license)
- Monitoring a patient's medication levels
- Determining the levels of essential substances produced by the body
- Identifying the cause of an infection
- Determining a baseline value

As a medical assistant, you will play an important role in laboratory analysis—even in instances in which testing is performed at sites other than the medical office. In general, you may be responsible for:

- Educating patients before obtaining laboratory **specimens** (small samples of substances, such as blood or urine, used to evaluate a patient's condition)
- Obtaining a quality specimen
- Arranging for appropriate transport if the specimen is to be analyzed at another site
- Performing common laboratory tests in the physician's office and clinics
- Maintaining **quality assurance** (QA), a program designed to ensure a high level of patient care, and **quality control** (QC), protocol designed to monitor and evaluate testing procedures, supplies, and equipment to ensure accuracy in laboratory performance.
- Maintaining laboratory instruments and equipment

Medical assistants also may control purchasing of laboratory supplies and selection of **reagents,** substances used to produce a reaction in testing situations. In addition, they may be in charge of biohazard safety and waste disposal for their workplace. This chapter outlines the basic information you will need to ensure the quality of the laboratory testing in your facility.

TYPES OF LABORATORIES

There are many kinds of laboratories, but three of the most common types you may encounter include reference, hospital, and physician's office laboratories (POLs). Hospital and reference laboratories may perform hundreds of different specialized tests and may process thousands of patient samples per day. In contrast, POLs perform only a few types of tests on a limited number of patients.

Reference Laboratory

A reference laboratory is a large facility, similar to a factory, in which thousands of tests of different types are performed each day. A reference laboratory seldom has contact with patients. Instead, it receives specimens from physicians' offices, hospitals, and clinics across the region it serves. The specimens are delivered by special courier, U.S. mail, or other ground or air transportation delivery services. Specimens sent to reference laboratories must be packaged to withstand rough handling, pressure changes, and temperature extremes during shipment. Packaging includes placement in special leak-proof secondary transport containers (Fig. 26-1) that meet federal regulations for transportation of biohazardous materials.

Tests are performed in large batches, and results and reports are managed by large computer systems. Reference laboratories usually are not responsible for reporting test results to patients. Test results generally are returned to the referring physician, who then relays the results to the patient.

Most employees of reference laboratories have specific job descriptions. *Specimen processors* accept (receive) the specimens and log patient data and specimen information into the computer, which assigns each specimen an *accession* (testing) number. Processors also centrifuge, separate, and aliquot (prepare a portion of a specimen for testing) specimens if indicated and send them to the correct departments for testing.

Testing is performed by *laboratory assistants, medical technicians,* or *medical technologists,* depending on the complexity of the testing procedures. Most testing is performed in large batches on automated instruments. Testing personnel are responsible for performing QC procedures, such as checking instruments, performing daily maintenance, and running control specimens. Testing duties include loading specimens and reagents into the instruments, running the tests, and accepting or rejecting, recording, and reporting results of quality control and test specimens.

Customer (or client) services personnel answer questions, track specimens, report results, add or delete tests requested by physicians, and trouble-

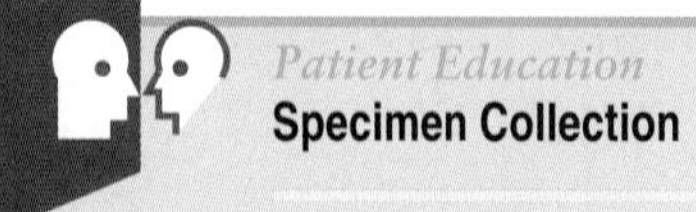

Patient Education

Specimen Collection

Before collecting a quality specimen, instruct the patient on the proper preparation for testing. For instance, does the test require that the patient fast for a period of time or follow a specific dietary regimen? Is the timing of collection imperative, or will a random sample be sufficient? Failure to educate the patient properly before testing may result in erroneous (invalid) test results, which could cause a delay in treatment or incorrect diagnosis.

At the time of specimen collection, educate the patient about:

- The name of the test (eg, blood cell count)
- The type of specimen required (eg, blood, stool, urine)
- Why the test is being performed

Be sure to tell the patient approximately how long it will take for the results to be available and how and by whom the patient will be contacted regarding the results.

Patient education requirements for drawing a human immunodeficiency virus (HIV) test vary from state to state, although most require pretest and post-test counseling. Additionally, most states do not allow HIV test results to be given over the telephone.

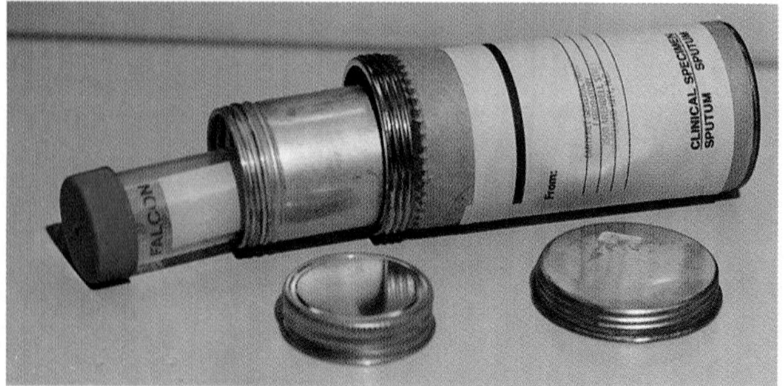

Figure 26-1 Transport containers are constructed to maintain the integrity of the transported specimen and to protect those who are responsible for the care and handling of potentially hazardous body fluids and substances.

shoot problems primarily by phone. Medical assistants often find employment in specimen processing or client services. They also may find employment in testing, provided that they meet the Clinical Laboratory Improvements Amendments of 1988 (CLIA '88) federal requirements, which include documented testing experience and supervision by a CLIA qualified person.

Hospital Laboratory

The hospital laboratory primarily serves inpatients (patients who stay overnight or longer). However, due to an increase in hospital ambulatory care facilities, including clinics and day surgery services, laboratories are serving increasing numbers of outpatients (patients who come for services and go home the same day).

Hospital laboratory workers include *phlebotomists,* who collect and sometimes process blood specimens; *laboratory assistants,* who collect and process specimens and perform limited testing; and *medical technicians* and *medical technologists,* who perform the majority of the testing. Laboratories also have *receptionists* or *secretaries,* who check in outpatients and manage the large volume of requisitions, test results, and other information and paperwork generated daily. Medical assistants often find employment as laboratory secretaries or receptionists or receive additional training to become phlebotomists or laboratory assistants.

A hospital laboratory performs many different types of tests on blood and other body fluids to aid physicians in assessing patient health and detecting, diagnosing, treating, and monitoring the disease process. Most testing is performed using large automated and computerized machines capable of sequentially testing many samples from different patients in one batch or run. Many machines are capable of performing a number of different tests on the same specimen at the same time. At times, STAT testing is required when there is a need to respond to life-threatening situations. Most often it is ordered for patients in the emergency room, surgery, or intensive care units. Because STAT testing requires immediate testing and results, regular test runs may be interrupted, or separate machines may be used to perform these tests.

Because maintaining equipment, reagents, and personnel for testing is expensive, hospital laboratories do not perform every possible type of test. The test menu is restricted to tests that are most commonly requested and STAT tests for which results are needed immediately. Less commonly ordered tests and those that require sophisticated testing usually are sent to reference laboratories. Whether performed on site or sent to a reference laboratory, results of most tests generally are available within a day or two. Results for some of the less common or more sophisticated tests may take up to a week or longer.

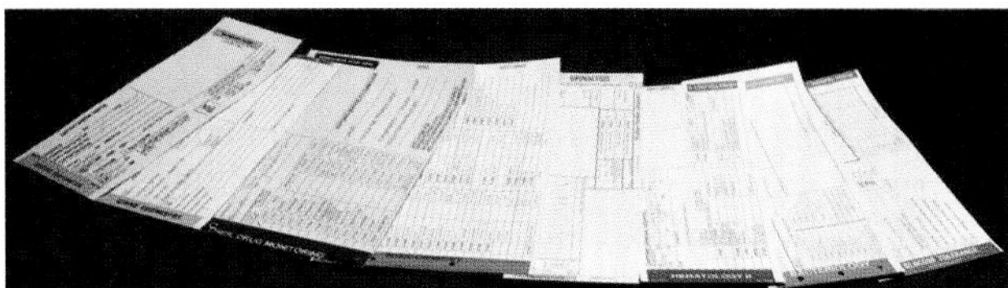

Figure 26-2 Laboratory request forms commonly used in a hospital setting.

Laboratory Request Forms

Hospital and reference laboratories design test request forms to suit their individual operations (Fig. 26-2). All forms should be convenient to use, with clear instructions for complete patient and physician identification to avoid errors. Most request forms cover a variety of tests so that a single form can be used for tests in hema-

Box 26-1

Laboratory Request Forms: Commonly Required Information

- Patient data base. This includes name, address, Social Security number, and the medical office identification number to avoid errors with identical names. Other identifying information may be included.
- Patient birth date and gender. Some test results will vary with age and sex.
- Date and time of collection. Many types of test results will be altered or affected by the passage of time or the time of day the specimen was collected.
- Physician's name and address or identification number (if a contract exists with the office and laboratory). Results may need to be reported immediately; having this information also avoids errors in reporting.
- Checklist of the test(s) to be performed. These may be grouped under one heading as a "profile" (such as a thyroid profile or a liver profile), which will include more than one test to determine the state of health of one organ, or a general health profile, such as a complete blood count.

Other information that may be required might include the source of the specimen (such as culture swabs for microbiology tests), a list of medications the patient is taking that may alter certain test results (eg, anticoagulants affect prothrombin time), directions for reporting (eg, an immediate need should be marked STAT), and total volume of a 24-hour urine specimen.

tology, chemistry, serology, and so on. Some forms serve as both a request and a report form. These forms often list test normal values as an instant alert. Many requisitions now contain barcodes that allow fast, accurate processing and reduce specimen identification errors. Most hospitals use computer-generated forms that also contain specimen labels. Box 26-1 lists the information required on all laboratory request forms.

Physician's Office Laboratory

The third common type of laboratory is the POL. There are more of these laboratories than any other type, and they vary greatly in size and quality. POLs generally perform a limited number of waived (or low complexity) to moderate-complexity tests (see section "Levels of Testing," below). Samples for less common or high-complexity tests may be obtained here but are sent to hospital or reference laboratories for testing.

The most common tests in this type of laboratory are urinalysis, blood cell counts, hemoglobin and hematocrit, and blood glucose or cholesterol levels. In some small laboratories, pregnancy tests and quick screening tests for diseases such as mononucleosis and strep throat are available. Like hospital and reference laboratories, some POLs use forms that list normal adult ranges for various tests (Fig. 26-3).

A small office laboratory may have only one or two employees who perform all of the duties: collecting samples, performing tests, managing quality control, maintaining instruments, keeping accurate records, and reporting results. In many of these laboratories, medical assistants perform all of these tasks, with a physician monitoring quality control and abnormal results. The chapters in this unit will introduce you to the skills and knowledge necessary to operate a small POL.

Checkpoint Question

1. *What is a reference laboratory, and how does it differ from a physician's office laboratory? Name and describe the kinds of positions that a medical assistant may hold in a reference laboratory.*

LABORATORY DATA SHEET

(Patient Identification)

LAB TEST	ADULT NORMAL RANGE	DATES AND RESULTS
WBC x 10^3	4.8-10.8	
RBC x 10^6	M.4.4-6.0 F.4.2-5.4	
Hgb gm	M.13.0-17.0 F.12.0-16.0	
Hct %	M.41-51 F.37-47	
MCV m3	80-96	
MCH mmg	27-31	
MCHC %	32-36	
Polys %	25-62	
Band %	0-22	
Lymph %	20-53	
Mono %	2-12	
Eos %	0-2	
Sed Rate (West)	M.0-10 mm/hr. F.0-20 mm/hr.	
Color	amber	
Sp. G	1.001-1.035	
pH	4.6-8.0	
Protein	0	
Sugar	0	
Ketones	0	
Bilirubin	0	
Blood	0	
WBC	0-5/HPF	
RBC	0-3/HPF	
Bacteria	0	
Vag. Saline	0 trich.	
KOH	0 monilia	
Uricult	0	
Throat	0 Gp. A Strep	
G.C.	0	

LABORATORY DATA SHEET

(Patient Identification)

LAB TEST	ADULT NORMAL RANGE	DATES AND RESULTS
Gluc. (Random)		
Gluc. (Fasting)	65-110 mg/dl	
Gluc. 2 hr. pc.	Less than 120	
BUN	10-25 mg/dl	
Creatinine	0.7-1.4 mg/dl	
Na	135-145 meg/L	
K	3.5-5.0 meg/L	
Cl	95-105 meg/L	
Co_2	24-32 meg/L	
Uric A.	2.5-8.0 mg/dl	
T. Protein	6.0-8.0 g/dl	
Albumin	3.5-5.0 g/dl	
Globulin	2.5-3.2 g/dl	
A/G	0.9-1.9	
Calcium	8.5-11.0 mg/dl	
Phos.	2.5-4.5 mg/dl	
Chol.	150-300 mg/dl	
Trig.	30-200 mg/dl	
Alk. Phos.	30-115 U/L	
SGOT	7-40 U/L	
SGPT	7-40 U/L	
LDH	100-225 U/L	
T. Bili.	0.2-1.5 mg/dl	
D. Bili.	0.2-0.5 mg/dl	
Ind. Bili.	0.2-1.0 mg/dl	
T_4 RIA	3.8-11.4 meg %	
T_3 Uptake	25-35 %	
T_7 Index	0.9-3.9 units	
TSH	2-10 microunits/ml	

Figure 26-3 Laboratory data sheet. Note that normal values are provided for the various tests.

LABORATORY DEPARTMENTS

Most large laboratories are divided into departments. This makes it easier to divide the workload and to group similar kinds of tests together. Small laboratories, such as POLs, may have only one department in which all tests are done. Even so, it may be easier to understand the nature of the tests and the information they provide if the basic divisions of laboratory testing are understood.

Below is a list of common laboratory departments, their possible subdivisions, and the kinds of testing performed in each. (See the appropriate chapters in Unit 5 for more specific information about the testing mentioned here.)

Hematology

The hematology department performs tests that detect abnormalities of the blood and blood-forming tissues. The various types of cells in the blood and the amount or number of each type of cell are determined in this department. Common tests include complete blood count (CBC), white blood cell count (WBC), red blood cell count (RBC), platelet count, hemoglobin (Hgb or Hb), hematocrit (Hct), differential (diff), erythrocyte sedimentation rate (ESR), and reticulocyte (retic) count.

Coagulation

Often a part of the hematology department, coagulation testing involves evaluating how well the body reacts when blood vessels are injured. The most common tests are prothrombin times (PT), partial prothrombin times (PTT), fibrinogens, and bleeding times. These tests also are used to monitor levels of anticoagulant drugs, such as heparin and Coumadin, during medication therapy. An **anticoagulant** is anything that prevents or delays blood clotting.

Clinical Chemistry

In the clinical chemistry department, chemical substances in blood or serum are measured. These substances may include hormones, enzymes, electrolytes, gases, medicines and drugs, sugars, proteins, fats, and waste products. In large laboratories, chemistry profiles often contain as many as 20 or more different chemical analyses. The most common tests in small laboratories are glucose, cholesterol, blood urea nitrogen (BUN), and electrolytes.

Toxicology

Toxicology is often a separate department in the chemistry laboratory. Toxicology testing involves measuring blood levels of both therapeutic drugs and drugs of abuse.

Urinalysis

This department often is housed within the chemistry, hematology, or microbiology departments. The most common urinalysis test is the complete urinalysis (UA), which is an evaluation of the physical, chemical, and microscopic properties of urine. UA tests can be performed manually or by automated instruments. Urine pregnancy tests also may be performed in this department.

Blood Bank or Immunohematology

This department generally is found only in hospitals and special blood donor centers. This department performs blood typing and compatibility testing of patient's blood with blood products for transfusion purposes. Blood products prepared, stored, and dispensed include whole blood, packed red cells, platelets, fresh-frozen plasma, cryoprecipitate, and Rh immune globulin (RhIg), such as RhoGam. Other services may include autologous donation (donation of blood by prospective patients for their own use), tissue typing for transplant purposes, and paternity testing.

Serology/Immunology

Testing in the serology or immunology department is based on the reactions of antibodies formed against certain diseases in the presence of proteins called antigens. Recent advances in serology testing have produced quick and accurate tests for diagnosing many diseases, including syphilis, human immunodeficiency virus (HIV), mononucleosis, and streptococcus A and B.

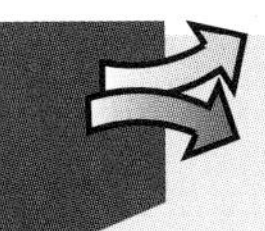

Ethical Tips

Test Results

While working in a laboratory setting, you will have access to the results of many confidential blood and urine tests, such as tests for human immunodeficiency virus, drugs, pregnancy, and sexually transmitted diseases. You have an ethical responsibility not to communicate any results to unauthorized persons. Only patients and their physicians are entitled to the results. The only exception is the provision in state laws requiring the reporting of certain test results for public safety; however, reporting this information is not the responsibility of the medical assistant.

Microbiology

The microbiology department identifies the various microorganisms that cause disease. Through sensitivity testing, microbiology identifies which antibiotics will successfully treat infections grown from patient specimens. Microbiology may include one or more of the following:

- Bacteriology—study of bacteria
- Virology—study of viruses
- Mycology—study of fungi and yeasts
- Parasitology—study of parasitic protozoa and worms

Anatomic and Surgical Pathology

The anatomic and surgical pathology department studies tissue and body fluid specimens from aspirations, autopsies, biopsies, organ removal, and other procedures to identify the presence or evaluate the effects of cancer and other diseases. The following are common subdivisions of pathology, which may be individual departments in larger institutions.

Histology

Histology is the study of the microscopic structure of tissue. In histology, samples of tissue are prepared, stained, and evaluated under a microscope to determine the presence of disease. Types of specimens examined include tissue obtained through biopsy, and surgical frozen sections that must be evaluated immediately to determine if further surgery is needed.

Cytology and Cytogenetics

Cytology involves the study of the microscopic structure of cells. In cytology, the individual cells in body fluids and other specimens are evaluated microscopically for the presence of disease, such as cancer. The most common cytology test is the PAP smear in which vaginal secretions containing cells brushed or scraped from the cervix are evaluated.

Cytogenetics is a type of cytology in which the genetic structure of the cells obtained from tissue, blood, or body fluids, such as amniotic fluid, are examined or tested for the presence of chromosome deficiencies related to genetic disease.

Checkpoint Question

2. *What departments may be found in a large laboratory? Summarize the testing done in each one.*

LABORATORY PERSONNEL

Within the various departments of reference and hospital laboratories, specially trained professionals oversee laboratory operations or perform the diagnostic tests

Box 26-2
Laboratory Personnel

- **Pathologist:** A physician who studies disease processes. Commonly, a pathologist oversees the technical aspects of a laboratory, a histology department, or a blood bank.
- **Chief technologist or laboratory manager:** A supervisor who manages the day-to-day operations of a laboratory, including staffing, test menu and pricing, purchasing, and quality control.
- **Medical technologist (MT)/Clinical laboratory scientist (CLS):** A graduate of a bachelor's (4-year) degree program (or equivalent) in medical laboratory science, who has been certified by a national certification agency. Laboratory technologists perform all levels of testing and often supervise laboratory departments.
- **Medical laboratory technician (MLT)/Clinical laboratory technician (CLT):** A graduate of an associate's (2-year) degree program (or equivalent) in medical laboratory science, who is nationally certified. Laboratory technicians perform waived, moderate-complexity, and certain high-complexity testing.
- **Laboratory assistant:** A person with a high school diploma or GED who is a graduate of a vocational or on-the-job laboratory assistant training program. Laboratory assistants collect and process specimens and can perform waived and certain moderate-complexity testing if CLIA qualified.
- **Phlebotomist:** A professional trained to draw blood and to process blood and other samples. Phlebotomists may be laboratory assistants, medical assistants, or persons trained specifically in phlebotomy. A nationally certified phlebotomist has a high school diploma or GED and either is a graduate of an approved training program or has a minimum of 1 year full-time work experience in phlebotomy.
- **Histologist:** A technician trained to process and evaluate tissue samples, such as biopsy or surgical samples.
- **Cytologist:** A professional trained to examine cells under the microscope and to look for abnormal changes; Pap smears are generally examined by cytologists.
- **Specimen processor or accessioner:** A professional trained to accept specimens that are received by the laboratory and to centrifuge, separate, or otherwise process the samples to prepare them for testing. In addition, this position usually involves numbering and labeling the specimens and entering specimen information into a computer.

required by physicians. Each professional position requires a particular level of education and training and has specific responsibilities (Box 26-2).

PHYSICIAN'S OFFICE LABORATORY TESTING

Many tests can be performed in an office laboratory that meet the standards set forth by Congress in the 1988 **Clinical Laboratory Improvement Amendments (CLIA)** (see section "Clinical Laboratory Improvement Amendments," below). Most tests performed in the POL fall into one of two general categories: tests performed on a semiautomated machine or tests conducted using a self-contained kit. Tests in either of these categories will vary slightly among manufacturers.

The best source of information for safe and accurate testing is the package insert that is issued with the testing kit or the instrument reagents and quality control instructions specific for various office testing instruments. Box 26-3 outlines the type of information contained in test package inserts. For many kit tests, the package insert is the only information provided to guide the performance of the test and to evaluate the results.

Determining the key or basic information needed for test performance and quality control will make using package inserts a simple and integral part of office laboratory testing. Ask your laboratory procedures instructor for examples of package inserts from pregnancy test kits or serology test kits for practice in obtaining this information.

Box 26-3

Understanding Test Package Inserts

Test package inserts will provide the following basic pieces of information.

- Procedure: Explains the test method in numbered steps, usually with illustrations.
- Test principles: Outlines the method required for the test.
- Specimen required: Tells whether the test is done on blood, urine, or other body fluids and what collection method is acceptable.
- Reagents needed (or included): Lists the reagents included in the kit and any other reagents or materials that are necessary to perform the test.
- Quality control: States recommendations for testing procedures to ensure that test results are accurate.
- Expected values: Lists normal values for comparison to results obtained.
- Interferences: Explains any factors that may alter test results or compromise test accuracy.

Checkpoint Question

3. *Why are package inserts crucial for safe and accurate testing?*

LABORATORY EQUIPMENT

Laboratory equipment and supplies for performing physician's office tests come in hundreds of different types and sizes. It is not necessary to become familiar with every possible type of laboratory equipment. However, a few basic pieces are common to most small laboratories. These include:

- Automated cell counter
- Microscope
- Chemistry analyzer
- Centrifuge
- Urine refractometer
- Incubator
- Refrigerator or freezer
- Glassware

Cell Counter

A cell counter is an automated machine used to perform hematology testing on blood specimens. The simplest cell counter is limited to counting red and white blood cells and performing hemoglobin and hematocrit testing. Specimens are inserted one at a time by the technician operating the machine, and results may be printed or may be read from a screen. (See Chap. 30, Hematology, for information on performing a cell count in the medical office.)

Cell counters increase from the basic level of complexity needed for a medical office to large machines that accept hundreds of specimens and perform 12 to 15 tests and calculations on each specimen, recording results directly into a computer. Medical assistants can test specimens using a cell counter if the cell counter is categorized as a moderate-complexity machine and if they have received documented training in its use from a CLIA-qualified person.

Microscope

The microscope is used to identify and count cells and microorganisms in blood and various other body specimens. Learning how to use a microscope properly requires time and patience. Microscopes vary somewhat, but the type most commonly used in the medical office is the compound microscope. This kind of microscope uses a two-lens system in which one system increases the magnification of the other. A light source in combination with the lenses illuminates the objects as they are magnified. Figure 26-4 shows a microscope and its various parts.

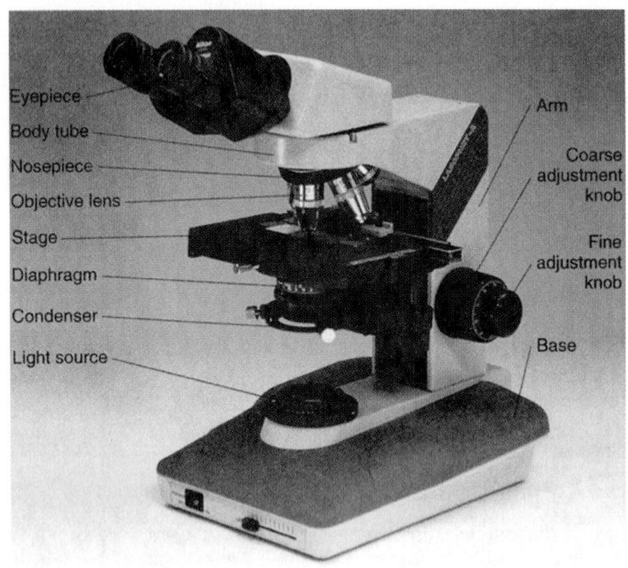

Figure 26-4 Basic components of the standard light microscope (Courtesy of Nikon Inc., Melville, NY.)

The *frame,* which consists of the arm and base, is the basic nonworking structural component of the microscope. The *eyepiece* is located at the top of the instrument for the user's eye. It is marked with its magnification, usually 10×. Many microscopes are binocular (two eyepieces) to reduce eyestrain; these also have adjustments to allow for the individual differences in widths between eyes. For most people, binocular instruments are easier to use than the monocular (one eyepiece) microscope.

The eyepiece is connected by the *body tube,* which directs the visual path from the light source. To bring the object to be viewed into focus, the body tube is raised and lowered by the coarse and fine adjustment knobs. The *coarse adjustment knob* is usually used with the lower powered objective to focus on the object; the *fine adjustment knob* is used with the higher powered objective or the oil immersion lens for the greatest definition.

The *nosepiece* houses the three objective lenses and revolves to bring down the lens required for a specific test. The magnification power of the objectives is referred to as the numerical aperture. The shorter objective, or low power objective, magnifies 10 times for scanning. The higher power magnifies 40 times for closer observation. With the use of oil, the third objective, called the oil immersion lens, magnifies 100 times. If the manufacturer has not identified the lenses, the shorter is the low power and the longest is the oil immersion. In conjunction with the lens in the eyepiece, each total magnification is multiplied by 10; therefore:

- Low power equals 10 × 10 = 100 magnification
- High power equals 10 × 40 = 400 magnification
- Oil immersion equals 10 × 100 = 1,000 magnification

The *stage* is the flat surface that holds the slide for viewing. An opening in the solid surface allows illumination of the slide from the power source below. Many stages have clips to hold the slide in place and to move manually as needed. Some stages mechanically adjust the position vertically or horizontally by moving adjustment knobs.

The *condenser* or *substage condenser* concentrates the light rays to focus on the slide. The condenser is adjustable. In the lower position, the light focus is reduced; in the higher position, it is increased.

The *diaphragm* is located in the condenser. It consists of interlocking plates that adjust into a variable-sized opening, or iris, to regulate the amount of light from the source in conjunction with the condenser. The more highly magnified the slide must be, the greater the need for light. To visualize all structures on a slide, it is usually necessary to adjust the light source and illumination level by opening and closing the diaphragm during the entire inspection to avoid missing objects visible at variable light levels.

The *light source* is housed within the base and provides the necessary illumination.

Microscopes are delicate and expensive instruments. To ensure that the microscope used in your clinical laboratory is kept in good working order, you must handle it properly and maintain it according to the manufacturer's standards (Procedure 26-1).

Checkpoint Question

4. *How do the three objective lenses of the microscope differ?*

Chemistry Analyzers

Like cell counters, traditional chemistry analyzers vary from simple instruments that perform one or at most a few different tests and require manual operation to large complex machines that perform 20 or more tests per sample and are operated by computer.

Advances in laboratory instrumentation have led to the development of small, portable, and often hand-held testing devices designed for point-of-care-testing (POCT). These devices are especially suited to POL testing because they are simple to operate, require only small amounts of sample for testing, and provide results in minutes. A variety of glucose analyzers originally designed for home use but equally suited to POL testing require only a single drop of blood, which is placed on a reagent strip that has been inserted into the machine. The machine computes the result and displays it on a screen. Other analyzers use a cartridge or test pack system to perform panels of tests, such as blood gases and electrolytes, or individual tests, such as glucose and BUN. Tests are performed by inserting the appropriate cartridge or test pack into the machine and injecting a few drops of the patient's blood into it. These machines often provide a paper printout of results as well as displaying them on a screen. Examples of POCT chemistry instruments are the i-STAT (i-STAT Corp., Princeton, NJ), the IRMA (Diametrics Medical, Inc., St. Paul, MN), and the AVL OPTI (AVL Scientific, Roswell, GA).

For higher volume testing and to perform a larger variety of tests, there are a number of bench top chemistry analyzers suitable for POL testing. Several use dry reagent technology in which all the reagents are impregnated into a special strip or card. The strip or card is inserted into the machine, and a drop of whole blood or serum is applied to the strip using an automated pipette. Other analyzers use wet reagent systems with special reagent packs required for each type of test. These machines can usually be interfaced with an office computer system to allow for storage and retrieval of results.

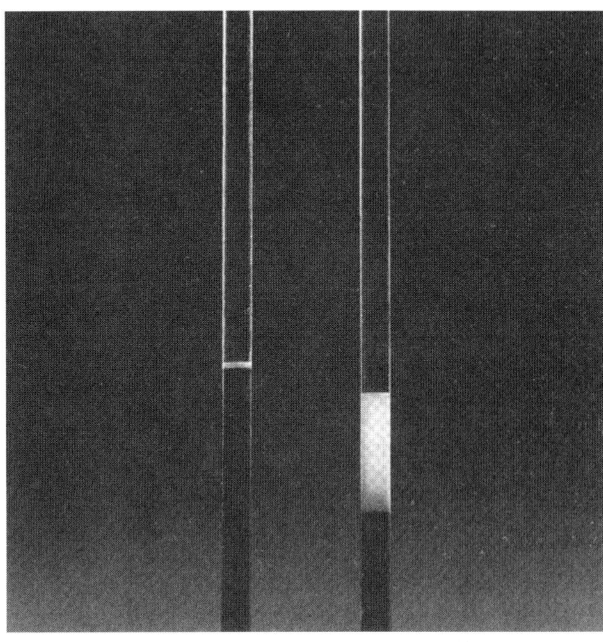

Figure 26-5 Comparison of a small (*left*) and large (*right*) buffy coat in hematocrit samples from two patients. Large buffy coat results from increased WBC and platelet counts.

Centrifuges

Many kinds of centrifuges are used in laboratories. A centrifuge uses **centrifugal force**, a spinning motion that exerts force outward, to separate liquids into their component parts. For instance, a whole blood specimen can be placed into a centrifuge and separated into a bottom layer of heavy red blood cells, a tiny middle layer of platelets and white blood cells called the buffy coat (Fig. 26-5), and a top liquid layer that is the lightest of the components. The top layer is serum if the specimen was allowed to clot before centrifuging or plasma if the specimen was anticoagulated and not allowed to clot.

Tubes must always be balanced in the centrifuge. If an uneven number of tubes are to be spun, a tube with water must balance the tube without a counterbalance. Try to place tubes with approximately the same level of liquid in opposing spaces. All tubes must be securely capped. Never start the machine until the lid is locked (many will not start until the lid is securely locked). NEVER open the centrifuge until all motion has stopped, and NEVER stop the spin with your hand. Follow the manufacturer's recommendations for cleaning, oiling, and maintaining the machine. As with all equipment, read the instructions before operating the machine.

A special type of centrifuge called a microhematocrit centrifuge is used to perform an hematocrit (Hct) test. A special capillary tube filled with blood is spun in the centrifuge. The percentage of packed red blood cells compared to the total volume of specimen is determined, and the result is the hematocrit.

Urine Refractometer

A urine refractometer is used to determine the specific gravity of urine if the chemical reagent strip is not diagnostic. It requires a drop of urine and uses a light scale to compare particulate matter to arrive at a value for the specimen. See Chap. 28, Urinalysis, for the specific procedure for using a urine refractometer.

Incubator

Microbiologic specimens require a suitable environment to simulate the conditions they need to thrive and reproduce. Culture media are stored in an incubator for a specified time to determine the presence or type of microbes in patient specimens. The incubator is set at about body temperature (99°F or 37°C), and a log is maintained daily to record the incubator setting.

Refrigerators and Freezers

Laboratory refrigerators and freezers are similar to those used in the home, but their uses are very different. They are used to store reagents, kits, and patient specimens. The temperature is critical and must be measured and recorded daily. Food should never be stored in these refrigerators because of the possibility of biohazard contamination.

Glassware

For general purposes, the term glassware also includes the disposable plastic supplies used in many medical offices. As with all other medical supplies, sizes and shapes vary with the purpose. Many forms are named for their inventor or for their use. The term glassware includes the following items:

- Beakers. Containers with wide mouths and straight sides for mixing, holding, or heating liquids. They may be marked with **calibrations** (measurements for size or volume) and are supplied in various sizes.
- Flasks. Containers with narrow necks and a rounded base used for holding or transporting liquids in a laboratory. Most are marked with calibrations. Names include Florence, volumetric, and Erlenmeyer.
- Glass slides and coverslips. Used with the microscope for holding the specimen to be viewed and are usually disposable.
- Graduated cylinders. Used for measuring quantities of substances or solutions.
- Petri dishes or plates. Shallow, covered dishes filled with a solidified medium to support the growth of microorganisms for diagnosis.
- Pipettes (pipets). Narrow tubes (glass or plastic) sometimes graduated, open at both ends, used to transport or measure small amounts of liquid. Some pull liquid in by **capillary action,** others by mechanical suction (Fig. 26-6*A*). Pipettes marked TC (To Contain) are designed to hold a certain volume; those marked TD (To Deliver) are designed to dispense a certain volume. Names include Pasteur, serologic, volumetric, and Mohr (Fig. 26-6*B*). Box 26-4 describes how to use a pipette.
- Test tubes. Cylindrical containers open at one end and rounded or pointed on the other, used for holding laboratory specimens.

Figure 26-7 displays various kinds of glassware.

LABORATORY SAFETY

Technicians must always be safety conscious when using laboratory equipment. All specimens studied in the laboratory should be considered potentially hazardous and must be treated as such. (See Chap. 1, Asepsis and

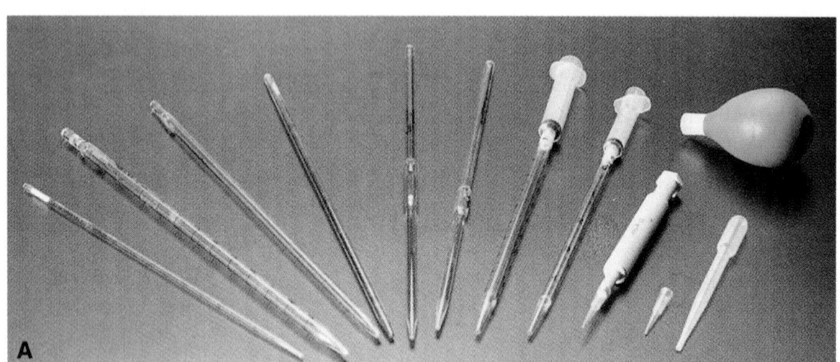

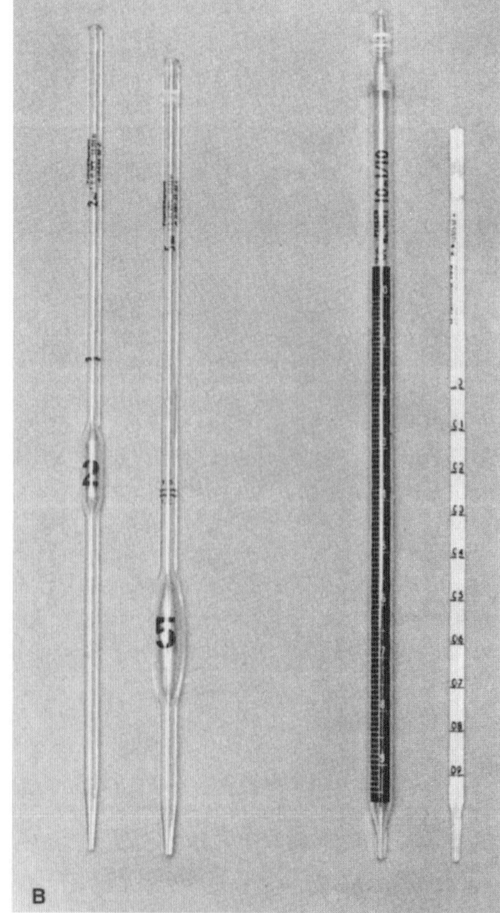

Figure 26-6 Assorted pipettes. (A) Pipettes on the right have attached or integrated suction. The bulb at top is used for suction with standard pipettes. (B) *From left to right:* volumetric pipette, Ostwald-Folin pipette, serologic pipette (10 mL), serologic pipette (1 mL), Mohr pipette.

Box 26-4

How to Use a Pipette

Hold the pipette upright, not at an angle, with the tip slightly under the surface of the liquid. Use a slight suction on the suction apparatus until the meniscus is slightly above the desired level. Maintain the level by holding the finger over the top of the tube or maintaining constant pressure on the mechanical apparatus. Raise the pipette from the liquid, and wipe the tip with a tissue. Allow the lowest meniscus curve to reach the desired calibration by releasing a small amount of the liquid into a waste receptacle. With the pipette in a vertical position, place the side of the pipette against the receiving vessel and allow the contents to drain.

Some pipettes, such as the Unopette, are available with premeasured amounts of reagents supplied. The whole unit is discarded in a biohazard receptacle after use. Reusable glass pipettes or the mechanical components of automated pipettes should be cleaned by the manufacturer's instructions. Some may be autoclaved after soaking and rinsing, whereas some require special chemical disinfectants or sterilization.

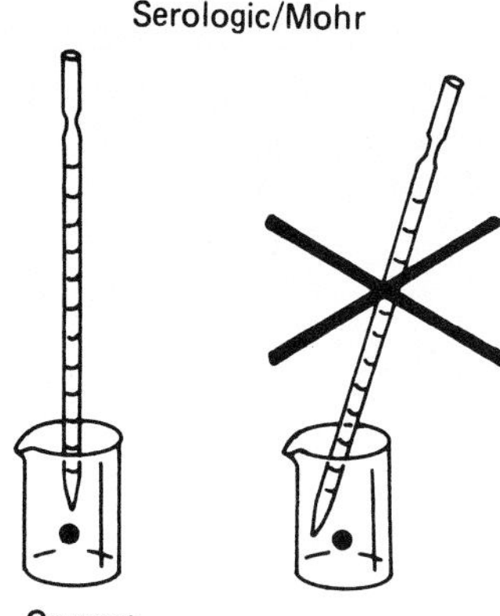

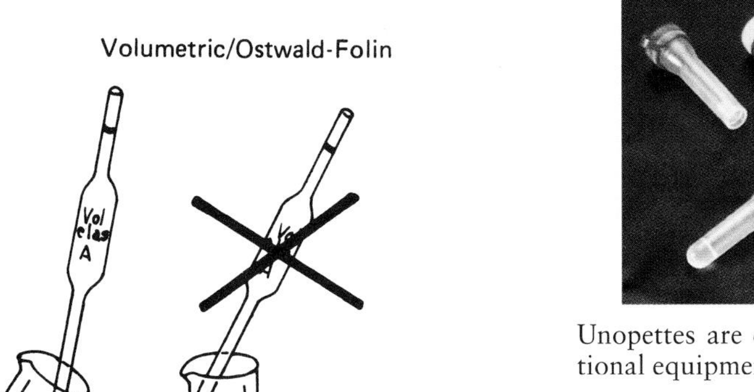

Correct and incorrect pipette positions.

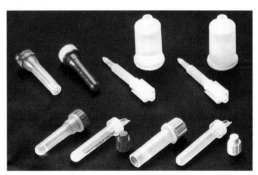

Unopettes are complete units and do not require additional equipment or supplies.

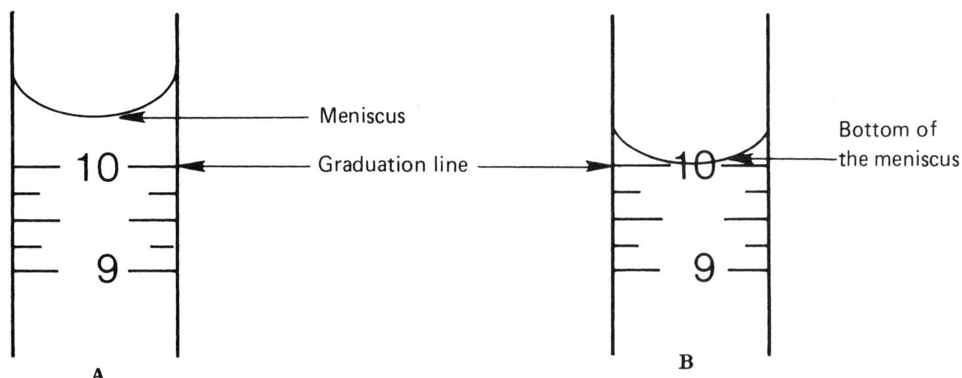

Pipetting technique. (**A**) Meniscus is brought above the desired graduation line. (**B**) Liquid is allowed to drain until the bottom of the meniscus touches the desired calibration mark.

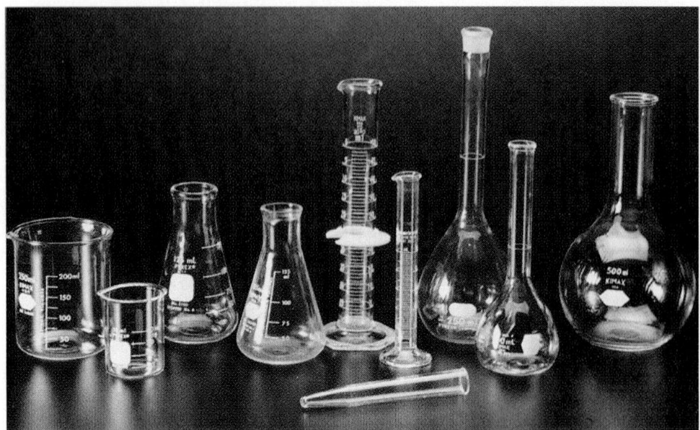

Figure 26-7 Glassware. *From left to right:* beakers, Erlenmyer flasks, graduated cylinders, volumetric flasks. *Front:* test tube.

Infection Control.) A technician who is aware of the types of hazards presented by the clinical laboratory is much more likely to work safely and avoid injury (Fig. 26-8).

There are three basic types of hazards in the laboratory:

- Physical hazards (fire, broken glass, liquid spills)
- Chemical hazards (acids, alkalis, chemical fumes)
- Biologic hazards (diseases such as HIV, hepatitis, and tuberculosis)

Methods for handling each of these hazards must be outlined in detail in your facility's policies and procedures manual. Each member of the staff must be familiar with safety protocol to ensure that risks are kept to a minimum.

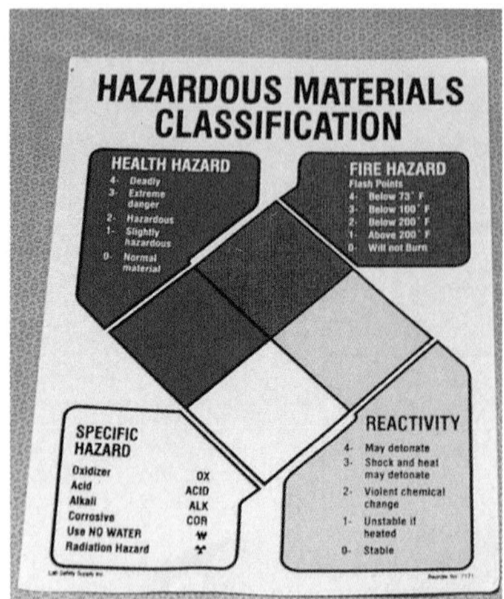

Figure 26-8 Hazardous materials classification posters should be prominently displayed in all laboratory areas.

Occupational Safety and Health Administration (OSHA)

The Occupational Safety and Health Administration (OSHA) is a federal agency within the U.S. Department of Labor charged with the responsibility of monitoring and protecting the health and safety of workers. OSHA standards are federal laws that are designed to protect workers by eliminating or minimizing chemical, physical, and biologic hazards and preventing accidents. OSHA standards supersede all other regulatory agency requirements. Two OSHA standards of particular importance to medical laboratories are the Occupational Exposure to Bloodborne Pathogens Standard and the Hazardous Communication (HazCom) Standard, also referred to as the "right to know law."

Prevention of disease transmission in a medical facility is often referred to as infection control or biohazard risk management. The OSHA Bloodborne Pathogens Standard requires all medical employers to provide training for their employees in techniques that will protect them from occupational exposure to infectious agents, including bloodborne pathogens. Safety manuals must be available or incorporated into the policies and procedures manual to guide employees in correct procedures and emergency protocols.

In addition, OSHA standards require that all workers who are at risk for exposure to potentially hazardous material wear personal protective equipment (PPE) supplied by the employer and readily available for use. PPE includes:

- Gloves
- Gowns
- Aprons
- Face shields
- Goggles
- Glasses with side shields
- Masks
- Lab coats

Workers who are sensitive to allergens such as latex must be supplied with hypoallergenic gloves.

All PPE must be appropriate to the level of exposure. (Review the use of Standard Precautions in Chap. 1, Asepsis and Infection Control.) A medical assistant performing phlebotomy or assisting with the collection of most tissue samples should be considered safe with glove protection. Situations that may result in splashes, splatters, or aerosolization, however, require full coverage, including footwear, such as shoe covers. (**Aerosol** refers to suspended particles in gas or air.)

According to OSHA requirements, employers are required to provide free immunization against hepatitis B Virus (HBV) (and other bloodborne pathogens if vaccines are available) to employees within 10 days of being assigned to duties with possible exposure to

Procedure 26-1 Caring for a Microscope

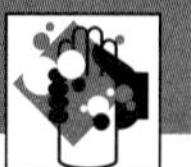

PURPOSE

To protect the integrity and function of laboratory equipment

EQUIPMENT/SUPPLIES

- lens paper
- lens cleaner
- gauze
- mild soap solution
- microscope

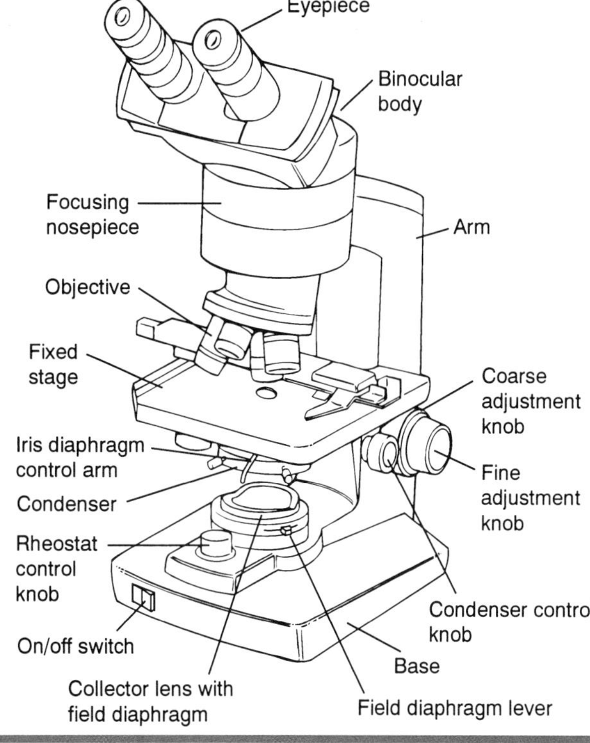

STEPS

1. Wash your hands.
2. Assemble the equipment.
3. If you need to move the microscope, carry it using two hands—one to hold the base and the other to hold the arm.
4. Clean the ocular areas, following these steps:
   a. Place a drop or two of lens cleaner on a piece of lens paper. Never use tissue or gauze because these may scratch the ocular areas.
   b. Wipe each eyepiece thoroughly with the lens paper. To prevent the transfer of oils from your skin, avoid touching the ocular areas with your fingers.
   c. Wipe each objective lens, starting with the lowest power first and continuing to the highest power (usually an oil immersion lens). If the lens paper appears to have dirt or oil on it, use a clean section of the lens paper, or use a new piece of lens paper with cleaner.
      Wiping in this manner ensures that you progress from the cleanest area (eyepieces) to the least clean area (oil immersion lens).
   d. Using a new piece of lens paper, wipe each eyepiece and objective lens so that no cleaner remains.
      Removing the cleaner completely prevents distortion that can be caused by residue.
5. Clean the nonocular areas, following these steps:
   a. Moisten gauze with mild soap and wipe down all nonocular areas, including the stage, base, and adjustment knobs.
   b. Moisten another gauze with water and rinse the washed areas.
      This removes oil and dirt from mechanical and structural surfaces.
6. To store the cleaned microscope, ensure that the light source is turned off. Rotate the nosepiece so that the low-power objective is pointed down toward the stage. Cover the microscope if appropriate.
   This protects the mechanism and surfaces between uses.

Note: Follow the manufacturer's recommendations for changing the light bulb and servicing the microscope.

bloodborne pathogens. Medical assistant patient care and laboratory testing duties involve possible exposure to bloodborne pathogens. Exposure can occur when the skin is pierced by a needle or other contaminated sharp object or when blood or other body fluid splashes into the eyes, nose, or mouth or comes in contact with a cut, scratch, or other skin abrasion.

The OSHA HazCom Standard requires all hazardous materials to be labeled by their manufacturers. Hazardous chemicals must be labeled with a warning, such as "danger"; a statement of the hazard, such as "flammable"; precautions to avoid exposure; and first aid measures for exposure incidents. In addition, manufacturers must supply **material safety data sheets (MSDS)** for their products. Employers are responsible for obtaining or developing a protocol for each hazardous agent used on site. This protocol should include MSDS supplied by the manufacturer for each substance used in the medical office. The information on the MSDS is extensive and includes items such as storage guidelines, flammability, and exposure precautions. These sheets should be maintained in an office binder near the site of use and should be reviewed routinely by all office staff (Box 26-5).

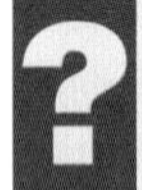

Checkpoint Question

5. *What are three types of hazards found in the laboratory? Give examples of each.*

Box 26-5

Material Safety Data Sheet (MSDS)

An MSDS is required for all of the hazardous materials at a particular site. In the laboratory, these can include disinfectants, cleaning compounds, laboratory chemicals, and some office supplies (eg, toners, printing compounds). All of these must be labeled as hazardous, with the contents listed on the label. Protocols for each hazardous agent used on site must be listed on the MSDS and should include the following information:

- Product name and identification. Include all names (trade and generic) by which it may be known.
- Hazardous components. List all hazardous components if the agent contains more than one hazardous ingredient.
- Health hazard data. Note the potential danger that exists for those using the agent.
- Fire and explosive data. If this is a volatile agent, note what precautions are necessary to prevent an accident.
- Spill and disposal procedures. Note how to handle spills and disposal to avoid danger.
- Recommendations for personal protection equipment. Note whether gloves, gown, face shield, or other equipment should be worn during use of this agent.
- Handling, storage, and transportation precautions. List any special precautions that must be observed.

Any other pertinent information for the protection of the worker should also be included. All of the information necessary to complete the MSDS is available on package inserts, instrument manuals, from the Occupational Safety and Health Administration, or from the manufacturer of the chemical.

Safety Guidelines

The guidelines outlined below are some of the most important safety factors required in all laboratories. Follow these guidelines carefully to protect yourself, your coworkers, and your patients.

1. Never eat, drink, or smoke in the laboratory area.
2. Do not apply makeup or lipstick or insert contact lens in the laboratory.
3. Wear gloves and appropriate protective barriers whenever contact with blood, body fluids, secretions, excretions, nonintact skin, or mucous membranes is possible. If splatters, splashes, spills, or aerosolization are possible, wear appropriate PPE.
4. Label all specimen containers with biohazard labels.
5. Store all chemicals according to the manufacturer's recommendations. Discard any container with an illegible label. Never store chemicals in unlabeled containers.
6. Wash hands frequently for infection control. Hands must always be washed before and after gloving and before and after leaving the laboratory work site.
7. Never touch your face, mouth, or eyes with your gloves or with items such as pens or pencils used in the laboratory.
8. Clean reusable glassware and other containers with soap and water or recommended solutions, and dry thoroughly before reuse. Wear gloves to prevent cuts.
9. Avoid inhaling the fumes of any chemicals found in the laboratory.
10. Know the location and operation of all safety equipment, such as fire extinguishers, eye washes (Fig. 26-9), and safety showers. Keep fire extinguishers close at hand because many chemicals are flammable.
11. Use safe practices when operating laboratory equipment. Read the manuals and know how to operate the equipment. Avoid contact with damaged electrical equipment.
12. Disinfect all laboratory surfaces concurrently and at the end of the day with a 10% bleach solution or appropriate disinfectant. Never allow clutter to accumulate.
13. Dispose of needles and broken glass in sharps con-

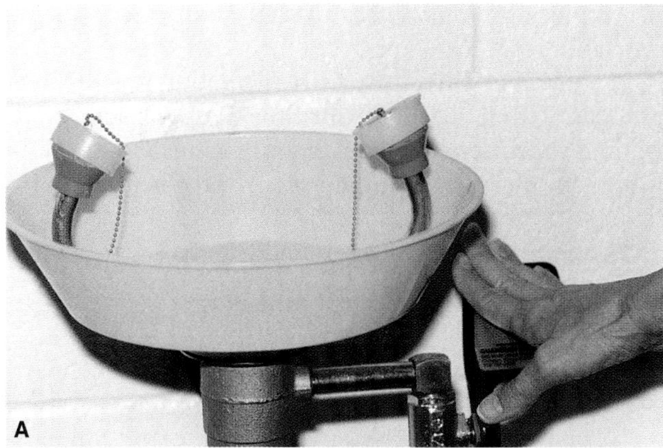

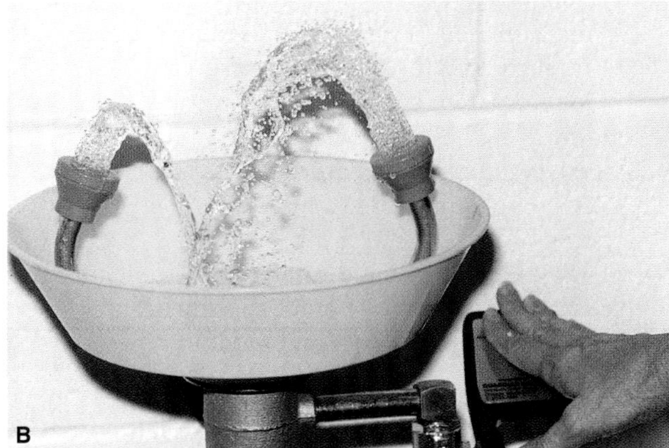

Figure 26-9 Eye wash basin. (**A**): Press the lever at the right of the basin. (**B**) The caps are forced from the water source by the stream. Lower your face and eyes into the stream, and continue to wash the area until the eyes are clear.

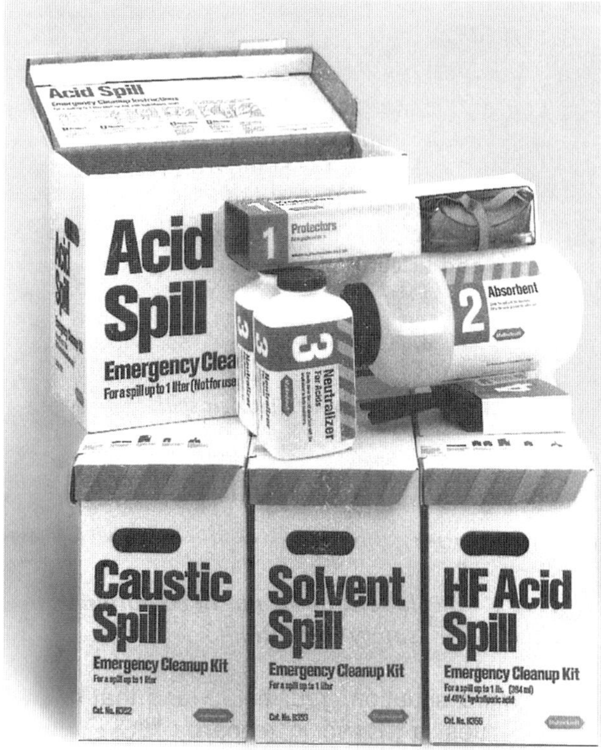

Figure 26-10 Spill cleanup kits for safely caring for clinical spills. (Photo courtesy of Scientific Products Division, Baxter Healthcare Corporation.)

tainers. Use biohazard containers for any other contaminated articles.

14. Never mouth pipette; use mechanical pipetters.
15. Use the proper procedure for removing chemical or biologic spills. If the spill is chemical, follow the manufacturer's directions; commercial kits are available for such cleanups (Fig. 26-10). If the spill is biologic:
    - Put on gloves.
    - Cover the area with disposable material, such as paper towels; discard in a biohazard container.
    - Flood the area with disinfecting solution, allowing it to sit for 10 to 15 minutes.
    - Wipe up the spill.
    - Dispose of all waste in a biohazard container.
16. Avoid spills by:
    - Pouring carefully (palm the label)
    - Pouring at eye level if possible or practical; never pour close to the face
    - Tightly capping all containers immediately after use
17. Use splatter guards or splash shields in any instance of possible splatter or aerosolization. Spills, splatters, and aerosolization commonly occur when:
    - Unstoppering blood collection tubes
    - Transferring blood from a collection syringe to a specimen receptacle
    - Conducting centrifugation
    - Preparing smears
    - Flaming the inoculation loop
18. When removing stoppers, hold the opening away, use gauze around the cap, and twist gently. Avoid glove contact with the specimen.
19. Report all work-related injuries or biohazard exposure to your supervisor immediately.
20. Follow all guidelines for Standard Precautions and the requirements of the various types of transmission-based precautions as described in Chapter 1, Asepsis and Infection Control.

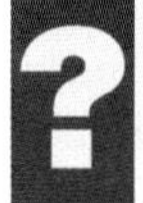

Checkpoint Question

6. *How would you clean up a biologic spill?*

26

What If?
What if your laboratory is not in compliance with OSHA's safety regulations?

In such a situation, your health and that of your colleagues is placed in jeopardy. OSHA developed the guidelines to protect you from serious injury or death. OSHA can impose significant fines for noncompliance. Continued noncompliance may result in loss of laboratory privileges. In some situations, the physician may not be allowed to file for Medicare compensation. To bring the laboratory back into compliance, any citations issued must be addressed and corrected. OSHA inspectors will then revisit the site and reconsider licensure.

CLINICAL LABORATORY IMPROVEMENT AMENDMENTS

In an effort to standardize and improve the quality of laboratory testing, Congress passed the Clinical Laboratory Improvement Amendments (CLIA) in 1988 to address the issue of regulations governing any facility that performs testing for the diagnosis, prevention, or treatment of human disease or for assessment of patients' health status. Standards were developed to cover all laboratory areas from the most complex regional laboratory to the smallest POL. The Health Care Financing Administration (HCFA) is responsible for implementing and enforcing CLIA regulations.

Before the passage of CLIA, POLs, private clinics, and long-term care facilities were not covered by regulations that govern larger, established laboratories. CLIA regulations were developed by the Department of Health and Human Services (DHHS) and set standards for:

- Laboratory operations
- Application and user fees
- Procedures for enforcement of the amendment
- Approval of programs for accreditation

Levels of Testing

CLIA regulations established the following three levels of testing based on the complexity of the testing method:

Waived Tests

Waived tests are low-complexity tests that require minimal judgment or interpretation and include many tests simple enough for the patient to perform at home (eg, dipstick urinalysis and glucose monitoring). If these are the only types of tests performed on site, the laboratory can apply for a certificate of waiver (CLIA HCFA Waiver Registration), but it still must practice within the guidelines for proper procedures. All manufacturers' recommendations must be followed for each piece of equipment or product used for testing.

The following are considered waived tests:

- Urine dipstick or reagent tablets
- Fecal occult blood packets
- Ovulation testing in packets with color comparison charts
- Urine pregnancy testing kits using color comparison charts
- Nonautomated erythrocyte sedimentation rate tests, such as Wintrobe or Westergren
- Nonautomated copper sulfate testing for hemoglobin
- Centrifuged microhematocrits
- Low-complexity blood glucose determination testing
- Hemoglobin by single analyte instruments with self-contained reagent and specimen interaction and direct measurement and readout

Moderate-Complexity Tests

Most of the testing performed in large, established laboratories falls under the moderate-complexity heading. The following are some of the moderate-complexity tests commonly performed in POLs that have been granted a moderate-complexity testing registration certificate:

- Urine and throat cultures
- Packaged rapid strep tests
- Automated testing for cholesterol, high-density lipoproteins, and triglycerides
- Gram's staining
- Helminth testing
- Microscopic urinalysis
- Automated hematology procedures with or without a differential requiring no operator intervention during the analytic process and no interpretation of a histogram
- Manual WBC differentials without identification of atypical cells
- Automated coagulation procedures that do not require operator intervention during the analytic process
- Automated chemistry procedures that do not require operator intervention during the analytic process
- Automated urinalysis procedures that do not require operator intervention during the testing process

A subcategory of moderate-complexity testing called provider-performed microscopy (PPM) requires a special registration certificate if POLs perform this type of testing. PPM procedures can be performed only by a physician or dentist or a nurse midwife, nurse practitioner, or physician assistant under the direct supervision of a physician. PPM tests include the following:

- All direct wet mount preparations for the presence or absence of bacteria, fungi, parasites, and human cellular elements
- All potassium hydroxide (KOH) preparations
- Pinworm examinations
- Fern tests
- Postcoital direct, qualitative examinations of vaginal or cervical mucus
- Urine sediment examinations
- Nasal smear examinations for granulocytes
- Fecal leukocyte examinations
- Qualitative semen analysis (limited to the presence or absence of sperm and detection of motility)

High-Complexity Tests

These kinds of tests, which are rarely performed in medical offices, include:

- Advanced cell studies (cytogenetics)
- Cytology (Pap smears)
- Histocompatibility
- Histopathology
- Manual cell counts

If the level of testing to be performed is in question, it must be considered high complexity until its level can be designated by the HCFA. HCFA publishes a list of all tests in the moderate-complexity category. States may establish local rules that are more strict than those set by the governing body, but they may not adopt less strict rules.

Laboratory Standards

Laboratories that perform moderate- or high-complexity testing may be inspected in an unannounced visit every year by representatives from HCFA or the Centers for Disease Control and Prevention (CDC) under the direction of the DHHS. As discussed below, they must meet all standards set by CLIA.

Patient Test Management

It must be proven that a system is in place to ensure that the specimens are properly maintained and identified and that the results are accurately recorded and reported. Policies must be written for standards of patient care and employee conduct. Each test performed

Quality Control Log

Test: ______________________ Control Lot Number: ______________________

Date	Control Value	Performed By	Accept	Reject	Corrective Action Taken

Figure 26-11 Quality control log. (From *Physician's Office Laboratory Guidelines and Procedure Manual,* 3rd ed.; Tentative Guideline. Wayne, PA: NCCLS, 1995, with permission.)

will be evaluated for safety, reliability, and diagnostic indication for its performance.

Policies and procedures manuals will clearly outline patient preparation, specimen handling, how tests are to be performed, alternatives to the usual testing methods for specific situations, and what to do in the event of questionable testing results.

Quality Control

The policy and procedure manual must include written directives for each division to ensure that all QC for monitoring the accuracy and quality of each test are in place. The protocols established by the manual must include a control sample, management of reagents, and instrument calibration, as explained below.

CONTROL SAMPLE. Manufacturers provide a specimen that is comparable to a human specimen with a known reference range. Testing the control sample at the same time the patient specimen is tested or when a new kit or batch of reagents is received ensures that all testing components are performing as required. Sam-

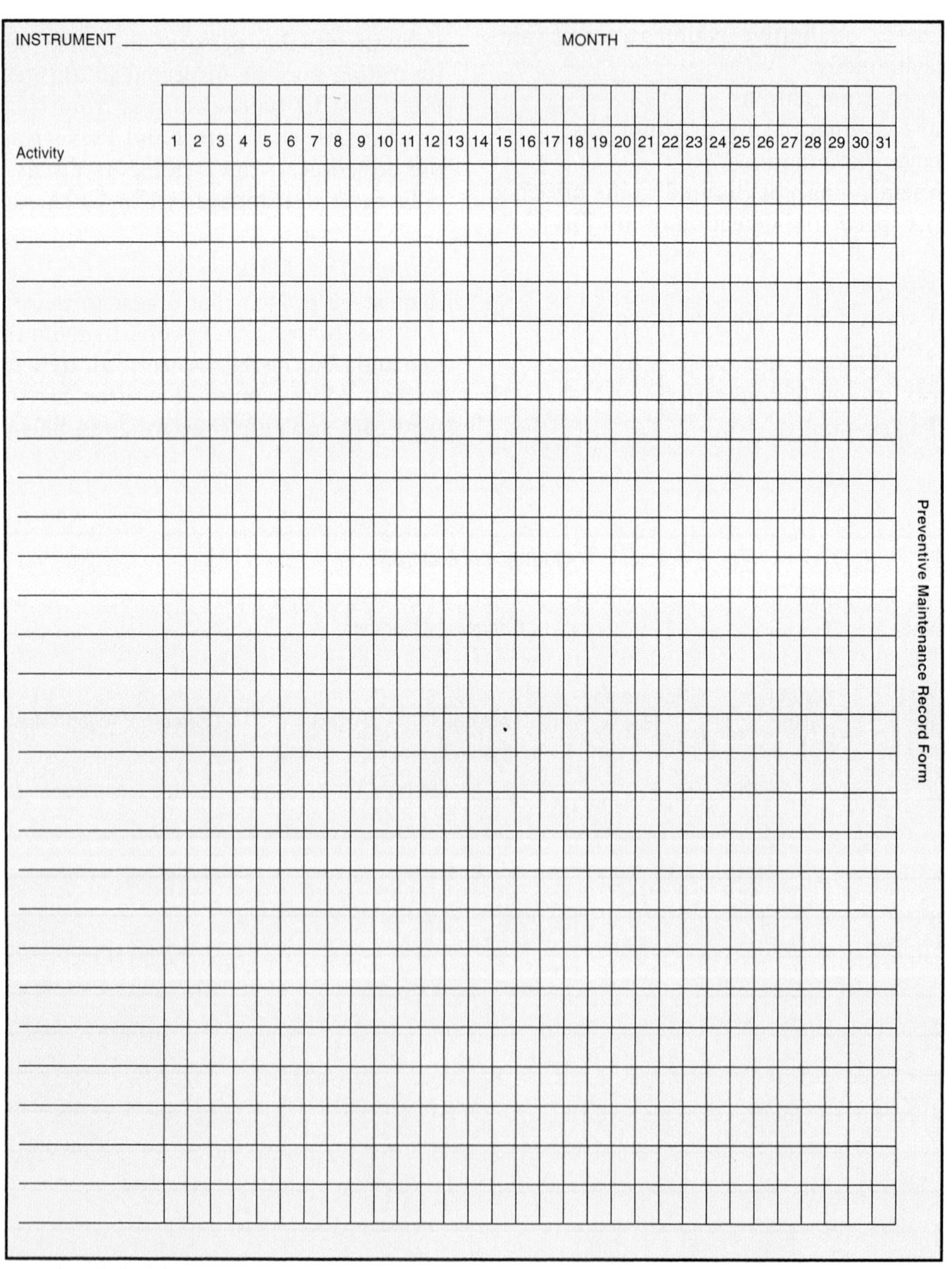
INSTRUMENT ____________ MONTH ____________

Activity	1	2	3	4	5	6	7	8	9	10	11	12	13	14	15	16	17	18	19	20	21	22	23	24	25	26	27	28	29	30	31

Preventive Maintenance Record Form

Figure 26-12 Preventive maintenance record form. (From *Physician's Office Laboratory Guidelines and Procedure Manual,* 3rd ed., Tentative Guideline. Wayne, PA: NCCLS, 1995, with permission.)

ples should also be performed at the start of each day before testing begins. The performance of these controls must be recorded in the quality control log book.

The **National Committee for Clinical Laboratory Standards (NCCLS)** establishes rules to ensure the safety, standards, and integrity of all testing performed on human specimens. Fig. 26-11 is an example of an NCCLS form on which control sample testing can be recorded.

MANAGEMENT OF REAGENTS. Reagents are chemicals used to produce a reaction in a testing situation. All reagents are given a manufacturer's lot number and expiration date. These must be recorded in a quality control log book with the date received, the date opened, and the initials of the person who opened the package. If the reagent consistently performs inappropriately, the lot number will help the manufacturer identify defects. All supplies and equipment, reagents, and testing components must be labeled with identification, storage requirements, date of preparation or when opened, and expiration date.

INSTRUMENT CALIBRATION. Highly complex laboratory equipment is very sensitive and requires strict operation and maintenance standards. Manufacturers provide maintenance schedules and methods of evaluating performance. Maintenance on equipment and supplies must be documented in the quality control log book; this includes maintenance either by an employee or by a manufacturer's representative. Any corrective action required for equipment or supply malfunction must be documented. Figures 26-12 and 26-13 show sample NCCLS forms on which this information can be recorded.

Instruments are designed to register within a set of standard calibrations. If the specimen test results are not within a normal range, the instrument's calibration should be checked by the manufacturer's instructions, and the specimen should be retested. If the calibration is correct and the specimen is still outside the normal value, the results are probably correct for this patient. A control specimen tested at the same time and in the same manner as the patient specimen will ensure that proper testing procedures were followed. The flow chart in Figure 26-14 shows how you can evaluate test results for errors.

The manual must state the manufacturer's recommendation for the performance of calibration proce-

Instrument History Record

	Instrument: ______
Model No.: ______	Serial No.: ______
Date Purchased: ______	Cost: ______
Manufacturer: ______	
______	State: ______ Zip: ______
Telephone: ______	Contact Person: ______
Dealer: ______	
______	State: ______ Zip: ______
Telephone: ______	Contact Person: ______
Warranty: ______	Expiration Date: ______
______	

Technical Service Representative: ______

Telephone: ______

Service Record

Date	Comments Who was contacted, action taken

Figure 26-13 Instrument history record. (From *Physician's Office Laboratory Guidelines and Procedure Manual,* 3rd ed., Tentative Guideline. Wayne, PA: NCCLS, 1995, with permission.)

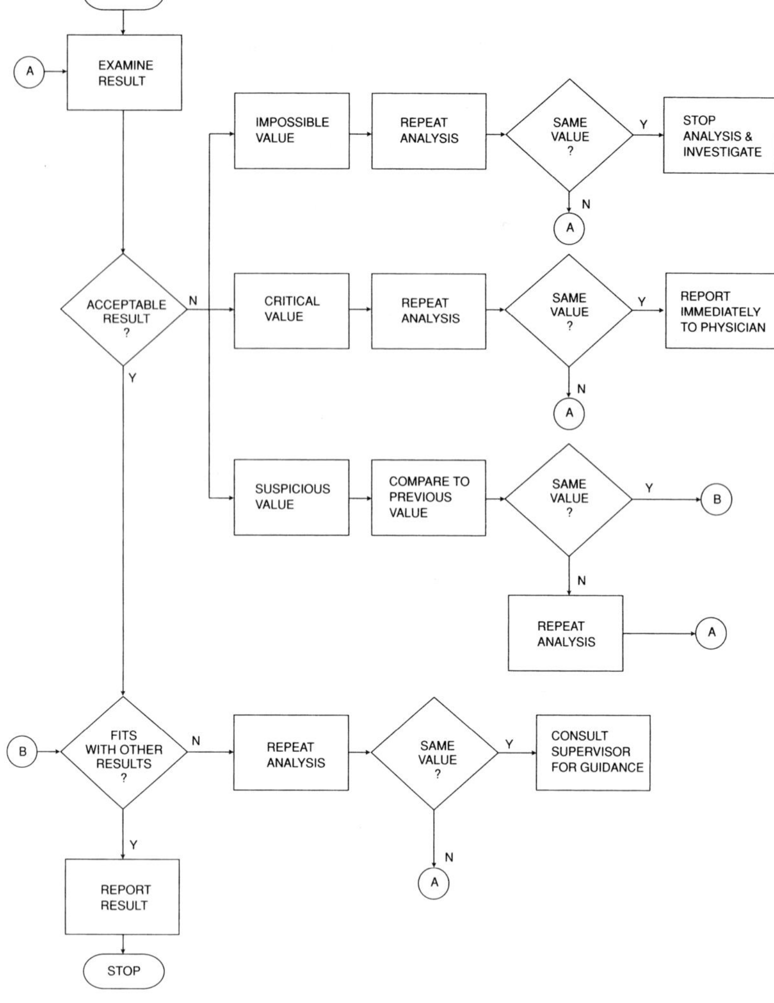

Figure 26-14 Flow chart for evaluation of test result for random error: A simple strategy for determining whether individual test result is reasonable and correlates with other results. *Y*, yes; *N*, no. Symbols *A* and *B* show interconnection between results of evaluation of repeat testing and where decision-making strategy should resume (*far left*). For example, if an impossible value is obtained, and repeat analysis does not show same value, uppermost horizontal line of chart says that testing procedure should return to symbol *A*, where the steps are begun again with EXAMINE RESULT. (Adapted from Cembrowski, GS: Use of patient data for quality control. *Clin Lab Med*, 6:715 [1986].)

dures, and supporting documentation must show that controls are performed as directed. Some procedures may require that controls be performed at each testing. Documentation must show the action taken to verify results, what was done when a problem arose, what the solution to the problem was, when the testing equipment was serviced and by whom, and what was done.

Quality Assurance

The policy and procedure manual should cover recommendations for continuing education for the laboratory personnel and evaluation methods for ensuring worker competence. The qualifications and responsibilities of all laboratory workers are specified by CLIA, giving education and training requirements for all levels of personnel. Employers are responsible for ensuring the educational background of employees, providing opportunities for continuing education, and conducting or providing for proficiency testing. This information must be documented and available for inspection by CLIA representatives.

Proficiency Testing

This requirement allows external evaluation of the laboratory. All laboratories, even those conducting only waived tests, must participate in three proficiency tests a year and must be available for at least one on-site inspection to continue testing and maintain Medicare eligibility. Three times a year, the laboratory will be shipped specimens prepared by an approved agency. These specimens must be tested by the same procedures used for patient evaluation and the results mailed to the proficiency testing agency.

Quality Control Log Book

To record compliance with CLIA measures, a record must be kept of each control sample and standard test. The log must reflect the date and time of the test, the control or standard results expected, what results were obtained, and the action taken for correction, if any. Documentation must be consistent, and a policy must exist for retaining the records for at least 2 years.

Answers to Checkpoint Questions

1. *A reference laboratory is a large facility that serves a particular region, performing thousands of different specialized tests daily. In contrast, the POL performs only a few kinds of common tests; some specimens may actually be sent to a reference laboratory for testing. Medical assistants working in reference laboratories may be employed as specimen processors, sorting specimens and entering data into computers. They may also work as customer service personnel, answering telephones, tracking specimens, and reporting results to the centers from which the specimens were collected.*
2. *A large laboratory may have the following departments:*
   - *Hematology—performs tests that detect abnormalities of blood and blood-forming tissues*
   - *Coagulation—measures clotting time*
   - *Clinical Chemistry—measures chemicals in blood*
   - *Toxicology—measures drug levels in blood*
   - *Urinalysis—evaluates physical, chemical, and microscopic properties of urine*
   - *Blood Bank or Immunohematology—performs blood typing and compatibility testing for transfusion purposes*
   - *Serology/Immunology—evaluates antibody reaction*
   - *Microbiology—identifies pathogens*
   - *Anatomic and Surgical Pathology—studies tissue and body fluid specimens to identify the presence or evaluate the effects of disease*
3. *Because tests may vary among manufacturers, the package insert is the best source of information on performing the test and evaluating the results.*
4. *The low-power objective lens magnifies objects 10 times and is used for scanning. The high power objective lens magnifies objects 40 times and is used for close observation. The oil immersion lens magnifies objects 100 times for greater visualization.*
5. *The three basic types of hazards are physical (eg, fire, broken glass, and liquid spills), chemical (eg, acids, alkalis, and chemical fumes), and biologic (eg, diseases such as HIV, hepatitis, and tuberculosis).*
6. *To clean up a biologic spill, first put on gloves. Cover the area with disposable material, such as paper towels; discard these in an appropriate container. Next, flood the area with disinfecting solution, allowing it to sit for 10 to 15 minutes. Wipe up the spill. Dispose of all waste in a biohazard container.*

Critical Thinking Challenges

1. Review the laboratory safety rules, then create a poster summarizing these rules for display in the laboratory.
2. Develop a list of all the items that must be documented in the laboratory setting. Design a form that can be used to meet these documentation requirements. Who should complete the form? Where should it be kept? Explain your responses.

Suggestions for Further Reading

Bishop, M. L., Duben-Englekirk, J. L., & Fody, E. P. (1996). *Clinical Chemistry, Principles, Procedures, Correlations,* 3rd ed. Philadelphia: Lippincott-Raven.

Linn, J. J., & Ringsrud, K. M. (1992). *Basic Techniques in Clinical Laboratory Science,* 3rd ed. St. Louis: C.V. Mosby.

McCall, R. E., & Tankersley, C. M. (1998). *Phlebotomy Essentials,* 2nd ed. Philadelphia: Lippincott-Raven.

Walters, N. J., Estridge, B. H., & Reynolds, A. P. (1990). *Basic Medical Laboratory Techniques.* Albany, NY: Delmar Publishers.

27 Microbiology

Chapter Outline

Role Delineation

CLINICAL

Fundamental Principles

- Apply principles of aseptic technique and infection control.

Diagnostic Orders

- Collect and process specimens.
- Perform diagnostic tests.

GENERAL

Legal Concepts

- Practice within the scope of education, training, and personal capabilities.
- Document accurately.
- Comply with established risk management and safety procedures.

Chapter Competencies

Learning Objectives

Upon successfully completing this chapter, you will be able to:

1. Spell and define the Key Terms.
2. List and describe primary bacteria.
3. Identify various bacterial illustrations.
4. Describe the purpose for the formation of spores.
5. Describe the classifications of fungi, Rickettsia, chlamydia, protozoa, and metazoa.
6. State the factors necessary for microbial growth.
7. Describe the medical assistant's responsibilities in microbiologic testing.

Performance Objectives

Upon successfully completing this chapter, you will be able to:

1. Properly label and identify specimen for transportation and handling (Procedure 27-1).
2. Prepare a wet mount slide.
3. Prepare a hanging drop slide.
4. Prepare a dry specimen smear (Procedure 27-2).
5. Prepare a specimen with Gram's stain (Procedure 27-3).
6. Inoculate a tube of broth medium.
7. Inoculate a culture and conduct sensitivity testing (Procedure 27-4).

Key Terms

(See Glossary for definitions.)

aerobic
anaerobic
agar
bacteriology
bacilli (sing. bacillus)
bibulous
binary fission
centesis
Chlamydia
diplococci
flagella
mordant
morphology
mycology
nosocomial infections
obligate
parasitology
Petri plate
Rickettsia
spirochetes
spores
staphylococci
streptococci
swab
virology

Microbiology is the study of microorganisms too small to be seen without a microscope. Microorganisms exist in the polar ice caps and in the steaming water in hot springs, but the ones most likely to present problems in the health care field are those that thrive at temperatures between 96°F and 101°F in a basically neutral environment. Of course, many normal flora live and thrive on the human body without causing disease. As a medical assistant, you need to be aware of the organisms present around us and their potential for causing disease to protect yourself, the physician, patients, and all coworkers from **nosocomial infections** (infections acquired in a medical setting).

Medical microbiology is performed using cultures and smears of the specimens referred to the laboratory. The specimens may be taken from wounds or other areas, such as the throat, vagina, urethra, or skin, by using a **swab,** a stick topped with cotton or other absorbent manmade fiber. Specimens may be drawn from the body by **centesis** (surgical puncture) or by venipuncture. Specimens are also excreted from the body as sputum, stool, or urine.

The medical assistant frequently collects specimens or assists the physician with the collection. Medical assistants may collect specimens from wounds or from the throat, but the physician usually collects specimens from the eye, ear, rectum, or reproductive organs. In all instances, aseptic technique must be practiced to ensure the integrity of the specimen. In addition, Standard Precautions must be observed to protect all health care workers and patients.

MICROBIOLOGIC LIFE FORMS

Bacteria

Bacteriology is the science and study of bacteria. Several groups of bacteria are significant in medical microbiology, including the spore-forming bacteria. Bacteria are unicellular (one-celled) simple organisms, each with its own specific characteristics. Bacteria reproduce by **binary fission** (direct division of the cell into two equal parts) and do not require a host for their life stages as long as all other requirements for replication are met. (See Chapter 1, Asepsis and Infection Control, for information on requirements for replication.) Bacteria can be identified by their distinct shapes, or **morphology** (Table 27-1).

Cocci are responsible for many of the diseases transmitted through the population. **Staphylococci** are found on all surfaces of the skin and many mucous membranes. They are generally nonpathogenic unless they reach areas that are usually sterile, where they may cause abscess formation or other forms of infection. **Streptococci** cause sore throats, scarlet fever, rheumatic fever, many pneumonias, and various skin infections. **Diplococci** cause bacterial meningitis, gonorrhea, and some of the pneumonias.

Bacilli are usually **aerobic** (requiring oxygen to live), may be gram-positive or -negative, and some are spore forming. Diseases caused by bacilli include tetanus, botulism, gas gangrene, tuberculosis, pertussis, salmonellosis, certain pneumonias, and otitis media.

Spirochetes are long, spiral, flexible organisms classified as spirilla if they are rigid rather than flexible. Spirochetes are responsible for syphilis and Lyme disease; spirilla cause rat bite fever.

27

Table 27-1 **Categorizing Bacteria**

Morphology	*Types*
Round (spherical)	Cocci
Grapelike clusters	Staphylococci
Chain formations	Streptococci
Paired	Diplococci
Single	Micrococci
Rod-shaped	Bacilli
Somewhat oval	Coccobacilli
End-to-end in chains	Streptobacilli
Spiral-shaped	
Flexible (usually with **flagella;** whiplike extremities that aid movement)	Spirochetes
Rigid	Spirilla
Curved rods (comma-shaped)	Vibrios

Vibrios are curved, comma-shaped bacteria. They are very motile and cause cholera. Figure 27-1 shows the various forms of bacteria.

Bacterial Spore Formation

Some of the microorganisms present in our environment produce **spores** to protect themselves under adverse conditions. The bacterium, usually a bacillus, forms a capsule around itself and enters a resting state that is resistant to most means of asepsis, such as heat or chemicals. When conditions are favorable for reproduction, the spore will revert to its active form and resume its life cycle. Examples include:

- *Clostridium botulinum* (food poisoning)
- *Clostridium tetani* (tetanus)
- *Clostridium perfringens* (gas gangrene)
- *Bacillus anthracis* (anthrax)

Spores are destroyed by autoclaving with the proper components of heat, steam, pressure, and time. (See Chap. 5, Instruments and Equipment, for the autoclave procedure.)

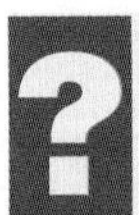

Checkpoint Question

1. *What are the four main categories of bacteria?*

Rickettsias and Chlamydias

Specialized forms of bacteria that fit in a category of their own are the ***Rickettsias*** and the ***Chlamydias.*** Both are smaller than bacteria but larger than viruses. Because they both require a living host for replication and survival, they are referred to as **obligate** intracellular parasites. *Rickettsias* cause Rocky Mountain spotted fever. The *Chlamydias* cause trachoma and lymphogranuloma venereum.

Fungi

Mycology is the science and study of fungi. Fungi are small organisms like bacteria, with the potential to produce disease processes in susceptible hosts. Some forms are microscopic, but many can be seen without the aid of a microscope. Fungi resemble plants, whereas bacteria appear to resemble one-celled animals. Fungi may be in the form of yeasts or molds in the human body. They are opportunistic, usually becoming pathogenic when the host's normal flora can no longer counterbalance the colony's growth.

Fungal diseases are referred to as mycoses or mycotic infections and include those listed below:

Molds

- Aspergillus—often affects the ear but may affect any organ or surface; may be fatal if widespread
- Blastomycosis—usually asymptomatic but may cause skin ulcers or bone lesions and may spread to the viscera
- Coccidiomycosis—may present with acute flulike respiratory symptoms or may become chronic and infect almost any body part
- Histoplasmosis—spreads through contaminated soil, usually asymptomatic but may lead to pneumonia
- Tinea—cutaneous mycoses (eg, tinea pedis [athlete's foot], tinea corporis [ringworm of the body], tinea capitis [ringworm of the scalp], and tinea unguinum [nail fungus])

Yeasts

- Candidiasis—causes thrush (skin and mouth), vaginitis, and endocarditis; may be spread by contact (Fig. 27-2).

What If?

What if your patient asks you how to prevent cutaneous mycoses, such as tinea pedis?

Explain to your patient that tinea pedis is a common fungal infection that affects many people. Then offer the following suggestions, which can aid prevention:

- Practice good basic hygiene.
- Thoroughly dry between the toes.
- Do not share footwear.
- Use antifungal powders between the toes and in shoes.
- Wear foot protection when using public showers.

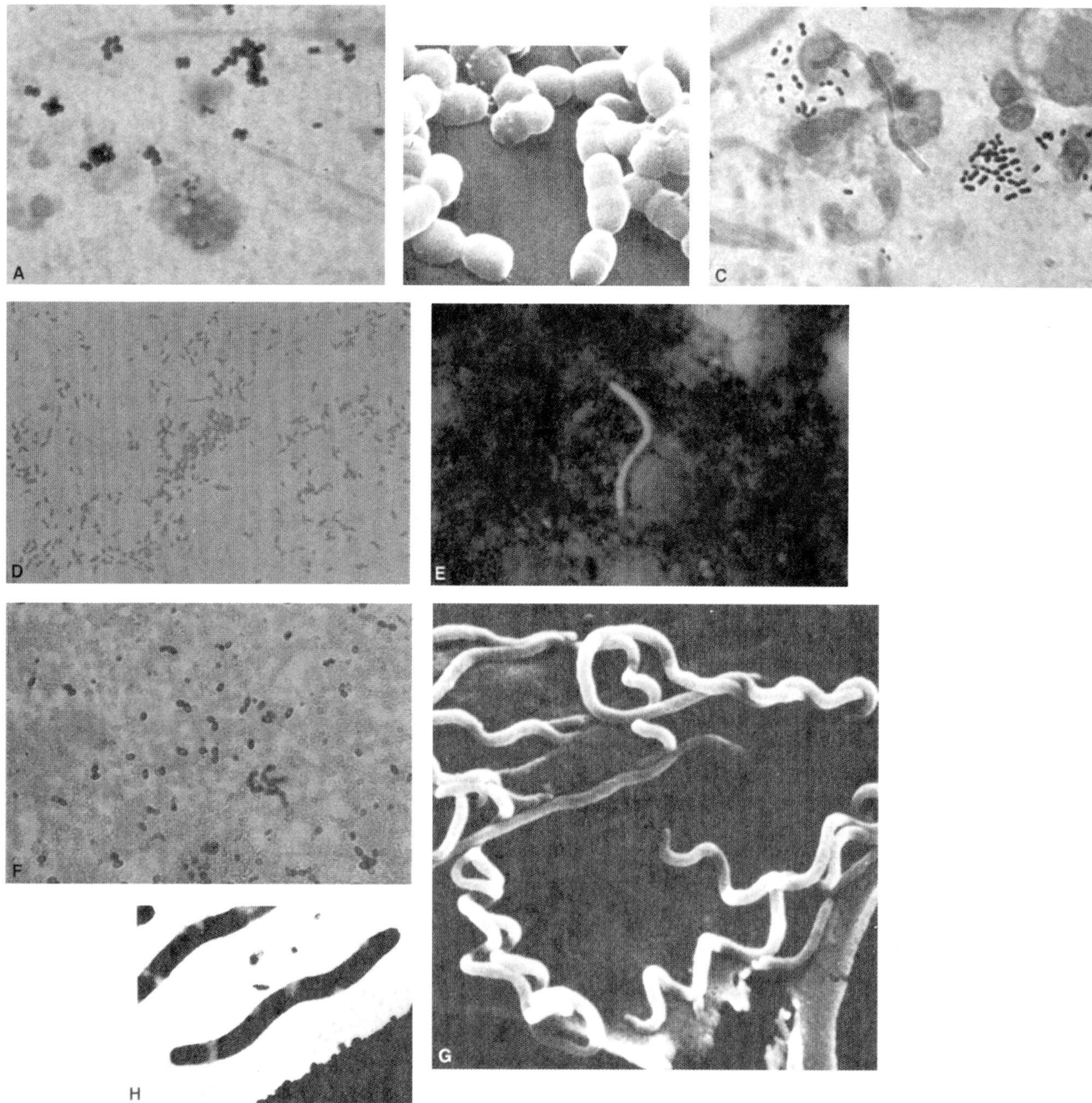

Figure 27-1 Forms of bacteria. (A) Gram-positive *Staphylococcus.* (B) *Streptococcus* in short chains (electron microscopic view). (C) Gram-positive diplococci. (D) Gram-negative bacilli. (E) A long, rod-shaped bacterium. (F) Gram-positive, spore-forming bacilli. (G) The spirochete *Treponema pallidum* responsible for syphilis. (H) *Vibrio.*

Viruses

Virology is the science and study of viruses, the smallest form of microorganisms. Viruses cause influenza, infectious hepatitis, rabies, polio, and acquired immunodeficiency syndrome (AIDS). They are so small that they can be seen only with a special electron microscope, not the usual microscope found in the medical office. They require a living host for survival and replication and are referred to as obligate intracellular parasites. Because viruses are not susceptible to antibiotics, they are extremely difficult to treat at this time. Antiviral therapy is in various stages of development and shows great promise.

Protozoa

Single-celled parasitic animals that may be diagnosed in the **parasitology** laboratory are the protozoa. These

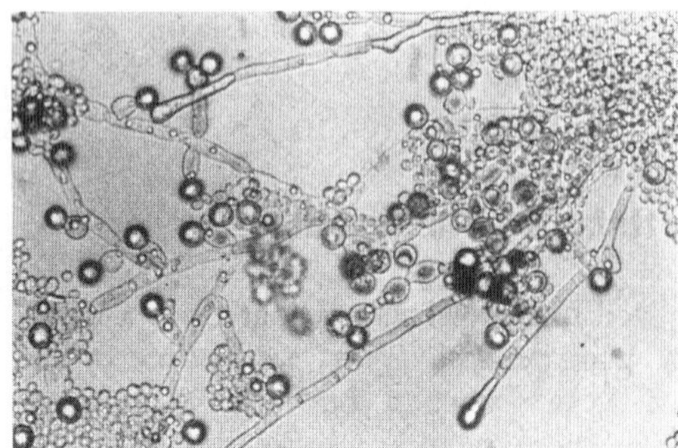

Figure 27-2 Fungus—*Candida albicans.*

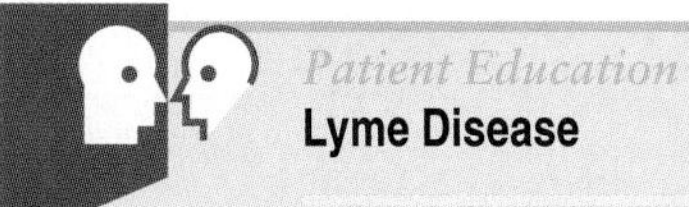

Patient Education

Lyme Disease

Deer ticks are a type of arthropod capable of transmitting the spirochete responsible for Lyme disease. The spirochete is called *Borrelia burgdorferi.* When the infected deer tick bites a human, the spirochete enters the body and can produce mild to severe symptoms, including a rash, joint aches, fever, general body aches, and alterations in neurologic and cardiac functioning.

Lyme disease, which has been documented in 47 states, can be prevented with proper education. Instruct patients to avoid tick habitats, to apply insect repellant, and to wear shoes and light-colored clothing when working outside in wooded areas. Clothing should be checked for the presence of ticks and washed in hot water with strong soap. Stress the importance of observing for ticks and removing them properly when they are found.

microorganisms and conditions they cause include the following:

- Entamoeba—diarrhea, dysentery, and liver and lung disorders
- Giardia—giardiasis, diarrhea, and malabsorption of nutrients
- Trichomonas—trichomoniasis, vaginitis, and urinary tract infection
- Plasmodium—malaria
- Toxoplasma—toxoplasmosis and fetal abnormalities

Metazoa

Metazoa include helminths, nematodes, and arthropods.

The helminth family includes round worms, flat worms, and flukes. Most will survive almost anywhere in the human body or may migrate through the body until they find a place to settle. Helminths can cause schistosomiasis, liver fluke infestations, and beef or pork tapeworm infestation.

The nematodes cause roundworm infestations, gastrointestinal obstruction, bronchial damage, pinworm infestation, and trichinosis.

Arthropods include mites, lice, ticks, and fleas. Also included are bees, spiders, wasps, mosquitoes, and scorpions. All may cause injury by their bites or stings, but several are also capable of transmitting disease by their bite or sting.

MICROBIOLOGIC TESTING: THE MEDICAL ASSISTANT'S ROLE

The medical assistant's role in microbiologic testing is extensive. Although it varies from office to office and sometimes from state to state, it will include both administrative and clinical responsibilities.

Administrative duties in microbiologic testing include:

- Routing specimens
- Handling and filing reports
- Ensuring patient safety and education
- Billing and insurance filing

Clinical skills require the medical assistant to:

- Collect and process many of the specimens obtained
- Assist the physician and patient as needed
- Maintain Standard Precautions and safety
- Perform terminal cleaning procedures after testing is complete

SPECIMEN COLLECTION AND HANDLING

Laboratory tests are most often performed on specimens that are easily obtained from the body, such as blood, urine, feces, sputum, and other body secretions and fluids. The specimen gives the physician a view of the condition of the system from which the specimen was obtained. For instance, a urine culture will indicate the infectious process at work within the urinary system; a sputum culture will grow the organism responsible for the patient's presenting respiratory symptoms.

As a medical assistant, you may be responsible for collecting most of the specimens obtained in the medical office. To ensure that the laboratory receives a sample that represents the disease process for which the specimen was collected, you must collect the specimen from the appropriate site using the proper method. You also must handle the specimen appropriately so that it will yield accurate diagnostic test results (Box 27-1).

Types of Specimens

Microbiology laboratories work extensively with cultures of the referred biologic specimen. Cultures are colonies of microorganisms that are encouraged to replicate under controlled conditions for the purpose of diagnosing disease. These may be *mixed cultures,* which are used to investigate any or all of the microorganisms found at a site, or *secondary cultures,* which remove from the mixed cultures only those organisms that need to be encouraged to grow for more extensive study. *Pure cultures* contain only one organism and may be a primary or secondary culture.

Blood is frequently examined in the microbiology laboratory and may be collected by the medical assistant. Care must be taken in any instance of venipuncture, of course, but for the purpose of culture, the specimen must remain uncontaminated for a diagnostic result. (See Chap. 29, Phlebotomy.) The yellow-stopper tube should be anticoagulated with sodium polyethanol sulfonate unless the pathogen is suspected to be *Neisseria gonorrhoea.* In adults, usually 10 to 20 mL is collected; in children, from 1 to 5 mL is collected.

Box 27-1
Guidelines for Specimen Collection and Handling

- Follow Standard Precautions for specimen collection as outlined by the Centers for Disease Control and Prevention (CDC).
- Review the requirements for collecting and handling the specimen, including the equipment needed, the type of specimen to be collected (exudate, blood, mucus, and so on), the amount required for proper laboratory analysis, and the procedure to be followed for handling and storage.
- Assemble the equipment and supplies. Use only the appropriate specimen container for the sample to be submitted as specified by the medical office or laboratory.
- Ensure the specimen container is sterile to prevent contamination of the specimen by organisms not present at the collection site.
- Examine each container before use to make sure that it is not damaged, the medium is intact and moist, and it is well within the expiration date.
- Label each tube or specimen container with the patient's name and/or identification number, the date, the name or initials of the person collecting the specimen, the source or site of the specimen, and any other information required by the laboratory. Use an indelible pen or permanent marker. Make sure you print legibly, document accurately, and include all pertinent information.

Sputum is often tested for the diagnosis of respiratory diseases. It should be the first morning specimen collected by deep coughing with care that saliva is not also expectorated into the container. You may be responsible for educating the patient regarding the proper procedure for sputum collection. (See Chap. 17, Assisting With Diagnostic and Therapeutic Procedures Associated With the Respiratory System.)

Wound specimens may be collected by the medical assistant or the physician. It may be necessary to collect wound specimens from several sites within the wound area. (See Chap. 10, Assisting With Diagnostic and Therapeutic Procedures Associated With the Integumentary System.)

Other commonly obtained specimens include throat cultures (see Chap. 17, Assisting With Diagnostic and Therapeutic Procedures Associated With the Respiratory System), urine cultures (See Chap. 28, Urinalysis), and stool specimens (see Chap. 18, Assisting With Diagnostic and Therapeutic Procedures Associated With the Gastrointestinal System).

Checkpoint Question

2. *What are the differences between mixed cultures, secondary cultures, and pure cultures?*

Types of Culture Media

Media support the growth of microorganisms for easier identification. The microorganism will proliferate for easier diagnosis of disease when it has been provided an environment for optimal growth.

Various types of media are prepared with a mixture of substances that nourish pathogens. All of the requirements for replication must exist for the suspected microorganism. Nutrients, moisture, and the proper pH are provided by the medium. The temperature and darkness will be maintained by an incubator, and the presence or absence of oxygen will be provided as needed. Some media are solid, some are semisolid, and some are in the form of a liquid or broth.

Media may contain additives to support the growth of specific organisms and inhibit the growth of others; these are referred to as selective media. Nonselective media will grow almost any microorganism introduced to its surface.

Media designed for **anaerobic** bacteria (bacteria that live without oxygen) may contain a tablet that generates carbon dioxide and eliminates oxygen in the closed environment of the medium. Many laboratories use special sealed jars containing a pouch of chemicals that maintain an anaerobic environment. In some instances, the plate may be placed in a jar with a lighted candle. The jar is tightly sealed and the candle will consume the available oxygen and gradually burn itself out. Figure 27-3 displays one type of anaerobic culture set.

Specimens submitted for laboratory study are most frequently cultured on blood **agar.** Blood agar is a solid medium that is prepared by adding 5% sheep's blood to agar, a transparent and colorless substance made from seaweed. The agar congeals the blood and forms a firm surface to support the growth of microorganisms. The firm surface makes it easier to read the culture growth. The blood adds the nourishment required for replication of the microorganisms.

A **Petri plate** is a glass or plastic dish used to hold a solid culture medium such as blood agar. The plate is fitted with a cover to maintain the integrity of the specimen. Petri plates are clear and allow visual examination of a culture as it grows.

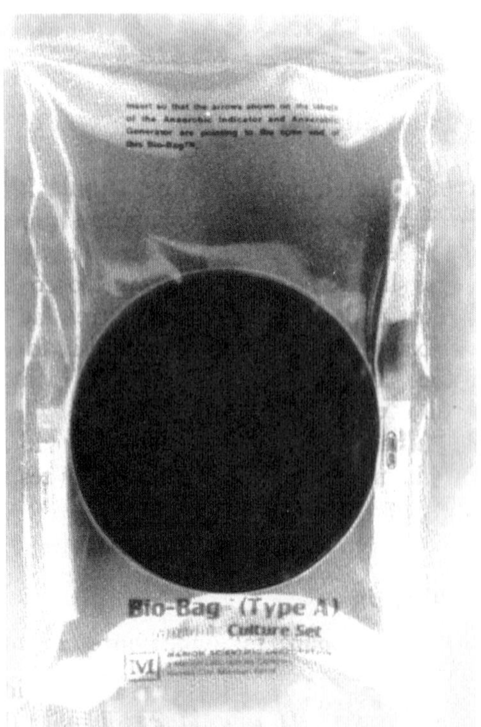

Figure 27-3 The Bio-Bag anaerobic culture set (Becton Dickinson Microbiology Systems, Cockeysville, MD). This culture set includes a plate of CDC-anaerobic blood agar contained within an oxygen-impermeable bag. The system contains its own gas-generating kit and cold catalyst.

A liquid or broth medium is usually provided in a small jar or tube. Many special broth media are supplied with swabs to be used for specimen collection and are enclosed in special envelopes for transporting the specimen.

Caring for the Media

Commercially prepared culture media contained in disposable plastic Petri plates are available for use in medical offices. The plates are supplied in a plastic sleeve and must be stored in the refrigerator with the side containing the medium uppermost (Fig. 27-4). The plates should be stored in the plastic wrapper to keep the media moist. Petri plates stored with the medium downward may form condensation on the lids that will drip onto the surface, making it too moist for an accurate culture. Check the expiration date and the condition of the medium surface before using the plates. Discard any plates that are past the expiration date or any medium that has dried or cracked.

Culture media may also be prepared in the medical office from a commercially available dehydrated form. A culture medium is effective for 72 hours once it has been inoculated with a specimen. Transportation or on-site testing within that time frame is essential.

Agar medium must be refrigerated until needed, then warmed to room temperature before use. A cold plate or tube will kill many of the microorganisms that require a warmer temperature for growth. Most physician's offices will be equipped with an incubator set at about 99°F (37°C) or just about body temperature. Check and record the incubator temperature daily.

Checkpoint Question

3. *Why is it important to store the Petri plates with the media side uppermost?*

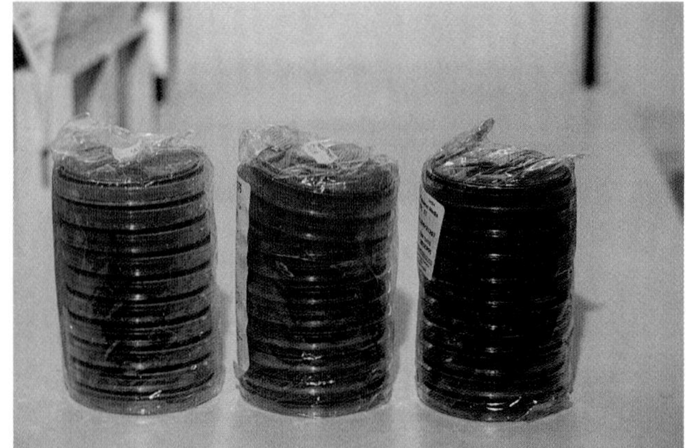

Figure 27-4 Solid media are supplied on petri plates wrapped in a plastic sleeve. Petri plates are always stored media side up.

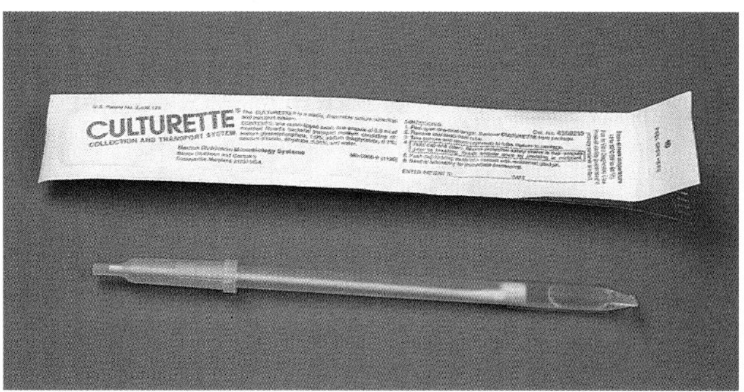

Figure 27-5 Transport media.

Transporting the Specimen

Many pathogens are not particularly fragile, but care must be taken to transport or process the specimen as soon as possible to avoid the death of any of the organisms present. The quicker the specimen is processed, the sooner the pathogen can be identified and treatment can begin. Some microorganisms, such as *N. gonorrhoea,* are very fragile and must be cultured under controlled conditions as quickly as possible.

Specimens to be processed in outside or regional laboratories must be placed in transport media, such as the Culturette (Marion Scientific Corporation) (Fig. 27-5) or Precision Culture CATS (Precision Dynamics Corporation). All directions appropriate to the specimen will be specified by the manufacturer on the packaging. Most of the transport systems are designed to be self-contained and include a plastic tube with a sterile swab and transport medium appropriate for the type of specimen usually collected by this particular system (Fig.

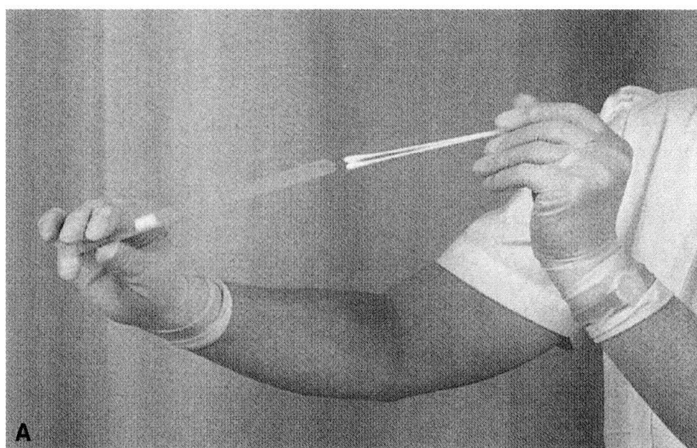

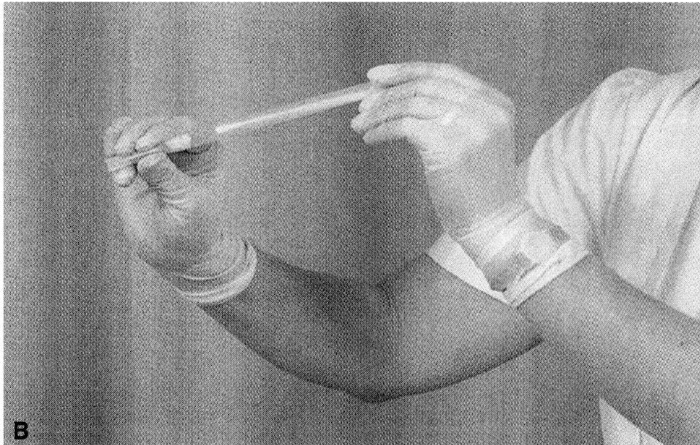

Figure 27-6 (**A**) Place the swab in a Culterette tube. (**B**) Crush the ampule of medium at the bottom of the tube.

Table 27-2 **Handling and Storing Commonly Collected Specimens**

Handling	*Storage*
Urine	
The specimen should be clean-catch midstream with care to avoid contaminating the inside of the container. Do not let the specimen stand for more than 1 h after collection.	If the urine specimen cannot be tested within 1 h after collection, it must be refrigerated. An appropriate preservative may be added at the direction of the laboratory; however, preservatives are not usually added to specimens for urine culture.
Blood	
Handle the specimen carefully; hemolysis may destroy the microorganisms necessary for diagnosis. Collect the specimen in an anticoagulant tube that is at room temperature. The specimen must remain free of contaminants. Refer to the reference laboratory manual for the proper anticoagulant.	For most blood specimens, refrigerate at 4°C (39°F) to slow changes in the physical and chemical composition of the specimen.
Stool	
Collect the specimen in a clean container. To test for ova and parasites, keep the stool warm.	Deliver the specimen to the laboratory immediately. If there is a delay in transporting, mix the stool with preservatives provided or recommended by the laboratory, or place it in a transport medium.
Microbiologic specimens	
Do not contaminate the swab or the inside of the specimen container by touching either to surfaces other than the site of collection. Protect anaerobic specimens from exposure to air.	Transport the specimen as soon as possible. If transport is not possible, refrigerate the specimen at 4°C (39°F) to maintain its integrity.

Note: Observe Standard Precautions while handling any of these specimens.

27

27-6). Most are stored at room temperature. Because transported specimens will be handled by a large laboratory, special care must be taken in filling out all identification slips and information. Procedure 27-1 describes the steps for preparing a specimen for transport.

Properly prepared transport media may be mailed or routed by a courier. The outside laboratory may provide specific mailing or shipping containers, either cardboard or styrofoam, to protect the specimen during transport. A label indicating the presence of a biohazardous biologic specimen is attached to the outside of the container. In many instances, specimens are only collected and transported on days that ensure their arrival during the business week to avoid having them remain in transit until the start of a new week. Delays in testing may cause some of the microorganisms to die or to overproliferate, possibly compromising the results of the test.

For the most reliable results, laboratory tests should be performed on fresh specimens within 1 hour after collection. When this is not possible, the speci-

Procedure 27-1 Preparing a Specimen for Transport

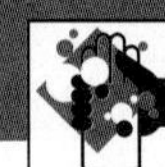
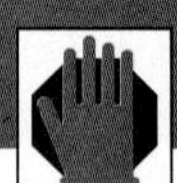
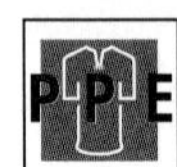

PURPOSE

To maintain and ensure the viability of a specimen for testing purposes

EQUIPMENT/SUPPLIES

- appropriate laboratory requisition
- specimen container/mailing container

STEPS

1. Assemble the equipment.
2. Complete the laboratory request form.
   All information must be filled into the appropriate blanks. If information is not applicable or is not available, indicate this on the slip. Do not leave any questions unanswered.
3. Wash hands and put on gloves.
4. Check the expiration date and the condition of the transport medium.
   Out-of-date media must not be used. If the medium appears to be dried, or looks different than it normally does, do not use it.
5. Peel the envelope away from the transport tube about one-third of the way and remove the tube.
   Many of the envelopes are used for repackaging the specimen. This will be indicated on the package.
6. Label the tube with the date, the patient's name, the source of the specimen, and initials of the person processing the specimen.
   The specimen container must be identified to accompany the laboratory slip.
7. Obtain the specimen as directed by the physician or receive the specimen as the collection procedure is performed by the physician.
   The specimen may be obtained by various methods and from many different sites.
8. Return the swab to the tube and follow the manufacturer's recommendation for immersion into the medium.
   Instructions vary and are specific to the manufacturer. All instructions must be followed to ensure accurate test results.
9. Remove and dispose of gloves and wash hands.
10. Package for transport as directed by the manufacturer's recommendations on the packaging. Some specify returning the tube to the peel-apart envelope.
    The laboratory slip and all components of the transport system must be packaged together to avoid misidentification.
11. Route the specimen.
    The specimen may be mailed, or a courier may be contacted.

DOCUMENTATION GUIDELINES

- Date and time
- Site of collection
- Type of specimen
- Destination of specimen
- Your signature

Charting Example

DATE	TIME Wound swab taken from left lower
	leg wound. Yellow-green drainage noted.
	Culture of wound sent by courier to
	Wakefield lab. —Your signature

men must be stored properly to preserve the physical and chemical properties necessary for accurate diagnosis. Specimens should never be subjected to extreme temperature changes. Table 27-2 lists general guidelines for handling and storing specimens commonly collected in the medical office.

27

MICROSCOPIC EXAMINATION OF MICROORGANISMS

Smears and Slides

Specimens collected by a swab or spatula from the site of a disease process or by inoculation loop from a pri-

text continues on page 609

Box 27-2
Preparing a Wet Mount Slide

To prepare a wet mount, follow these steps:

1. Place a drop of the specimen on a glass slide with sterile saline or 10% potassium hydroxide (KOH).
2. Place a coverslip over the specimen to reduce evaporation.
3. To decrease further evaporation, place petrolatum around the rim of the coverslip.
4. Inspect the slide by microscope using the high power objective with diminished light.

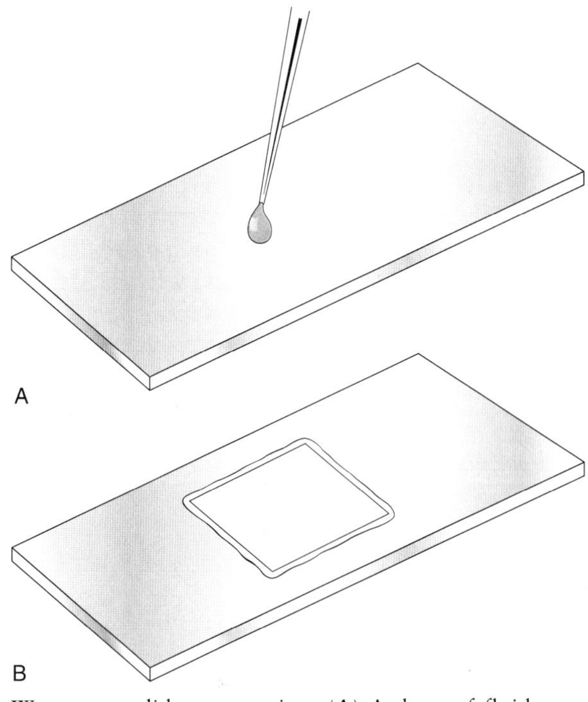

Wet mount slide preparation. (**A**) A drop of fluid containing the organism is placed on a glass slide. (**B**) The specimen is covered with a coverslip ringed with petroleum jelly.

Box 27-3
Preparing a Hanging Drop Slide

This method requires a special slide with a depression in the center. A coverslip edged with petrolatum keeps the specimen from drying out.

1. Place a drop of the specimen in the center of the coverslip with the petrolatum around the edges.
2. Place the depression in the slide over the coverslip with the specimen in the center.
3. Lightly press the slide against the coverslip to seal the edges; this will hold the slide tightly to the coverslip.
4. Invert the slide so that the specimen on the coverslip hangs into the depression on the slide.
5. Inspect the slide arrangement by microscope with the high power objective and diminished light.

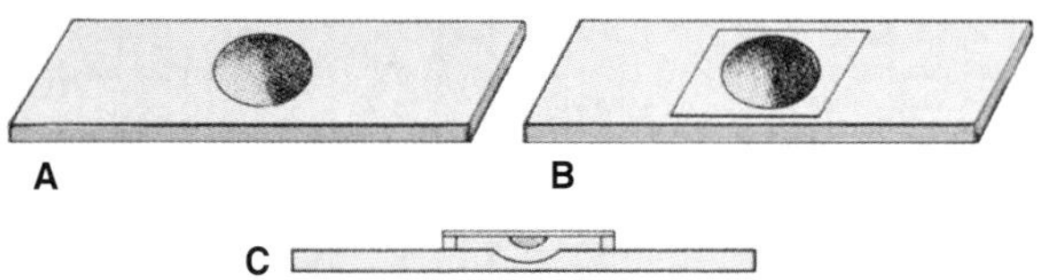

Hanging drop preparation for study of living bacteria. (**A**) Depression slide. (**B**) Depression slide with coverglass over the depression area. (**C**) Side view of hanging drop preparation, showing the drop of culture hanging from the center of the coverglass above the depression. (Volk, W.A., Wheeler, M.F. [1984]. *Basic Microbiology*, 5th ed. Philadelphia: JB Lippincott.)

Box 27-4
Gram's Staining: A Diagnostic Tool

Gram's staining provides important diagnostic information. Even before a culture can be incubated, a physician may tentatively diagnose a patient's disease and begin treatment based on the results of Gram's staining, the organism's morphology, and the patient's reported symptoms.

Below are some common diseases and their Gram's staining results:

Gram-Positive	*Gram-Negative*
Strep throat	Whooping cough (pertussis)
Scarlet fever	*Escherichia coli* (present in some forms of cystitis)
Diphtheria	*Haemophilus influenzae*
Meningitis	Certain pneumonias
Tetanus	Gonococcus
Botulism	Salmonella
Certain pneumonias	Shigella
Gardnerella vaginitis	Cholera
Staphylococcal skin lesions	
Toxic shock syndrome	

27

Procedure 27-2 Preparing a Dry Smear

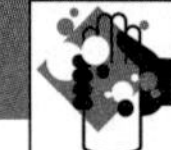
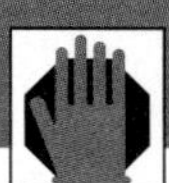
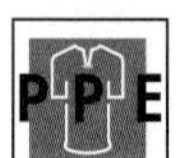

PURPOSE

To aid in the identification of microorganisms in a specimen

EQUIPMENT/SUPPLIES

- specimen
- slide forceps
- sterile swab or inoculating loop
- Bunsen burner
- slide
- pencil or diamond-tipped pen

STEPS

1. Wash your hands.

2. Assemble the equipment.

3. Label the slide with the patient's name and the date on the frosted edge.

Labeling will ensure proper patient identification.

4. Put on gloves and face shield. Hold the edges of the slide between the thumb and index finger. Starting at the right side of the slide and using a rolling motion of the swab or a sweeping motion of the inoculating loop, gently and evenly spread the material from the specimen over the slide. The material should thinly fill the center of the slide within ½ inch of each end.

The face shield should be worn to avoid splatters from the inoculating loop. The material should be spread thinly to avoid obscuring the slide with too much material. Rolling ensures that as much of the specimen as possible is deposited on the slide. Sweeping the loop accomplishes the same purpose. Confining the specimen to the area within ½ inch of the edges avoids contaminating the gloves.

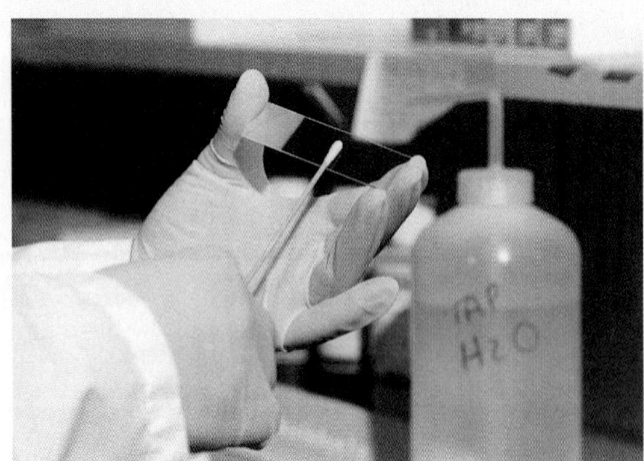

5. Do not rub the material vigorously over the slide.

Doing so may destroy fragile microorganisms.

6. Dispose of the contaminated swab or inoculating loop in a biohazard container. If you are not using a disposable loop, sterilize it as follows:

The swab and the loop contain body fluid and are considered biohazardous.

a. Hold the loop in the colorless part of the flame of the Bunsen burner for 10 seconds.

b. Raise the loop slowly (to avoid splattering the bacteria) to the blue part of the flame until the loop and its connecting wire glow red.

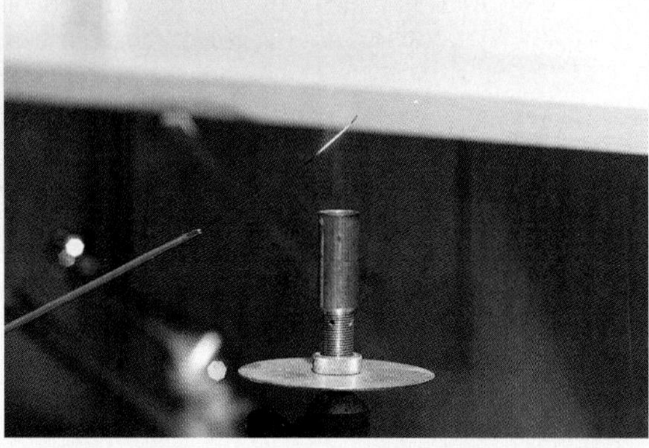

c. If reusing the loop, cool the loop so the heat will not kill the bacteria that must be allowed to grow. Do not wave the loop in the air because doing so may expose it to contamination. Do not stab the medium with a hot loop to cool; this creates an aerosol.

7. Allow the smear to air dry in a flat position for at least ½ hour. Do not wave it about in the air. Heat should not be applied until the specimen has been allowed to dry. Some specimens require a fixative spray (eg, Pap smears).

The cells will dry slowly if allowed to dry at room temperature. Fixatives may be sprayed from a distance of 4 to 6 inches to protect the cells from contaminants or to keep them from becoming dislodged. Heat at this point may destroy the microorganisms.

continued

27

Procedure 27-2 *Continued* Preparing a Dry Smear

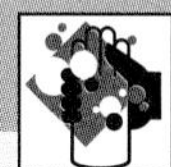 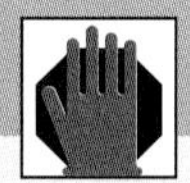 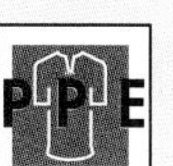 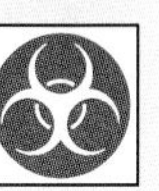

8. Hold the dried smear slide with the slide forceps. Pass the slide quickly through the flame of a Bunsen burner three or four times. The slide has been fixed properly when the back of the slide feels slightly uncomfortably warm to the back of the gloved hand. It should not feel hot.
   Passing the slide through the heat kills the microorganisms and attaches them firmly to the slide so they do not wash off during the staining process or are not dislodged during the viewing process if they are not to be stained. Excessive heat may distort the specimen cells.

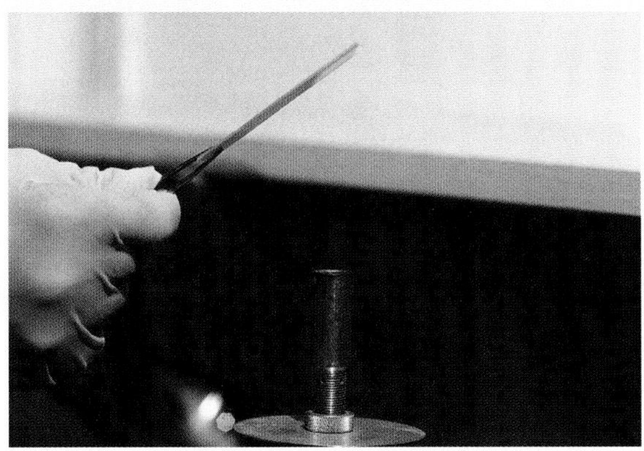

9. Examine the smear under the microscope, or stain it according to office policy. In most instances, the physician examines the slide for identification.
10. Dispose of equipment and supplies in appropriate containers. Remove and dispose of gloves and wash your hands.

DOCUMENTATION GUIDELINES

- Date and time
- Site of collection
- Type of specimen
- Results of testing, if applicable
- Action taken, if any
- Patient education/instructions
- Your signature

Charting Example

DATE	TIME Specimen taken from nasal cavity
	and prepared as a dry smear. Gram's
	stain positive. Dr. York read the slide.
	—Your signature

Procedure 27-3 Gram's Staining a Smear Slide

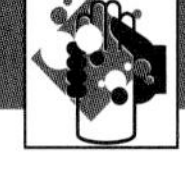 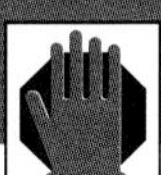

PPE

PURPOSE

To aid in the identification of pathogens in a specimen

EQUIPMENT/SUPPLIES

- crystal violet stain
- Gram's iodine solution
- alcohol-acetone solution
- counterstain (eg, Safranin)
- specimen on a glass slide labeled using a diamond-tipped pen
- Bunsen burner
- slide forceps
- staining rack
- wash bottle with distilled water
- absorbent (**bibulous**) paper pad
- immersion oil
- microscope
- stop watch or timer

STEPS

1. Wash your hands.
2. Assemble the equipment.
3. Make sure that the specimen is heat fixed to the labeled slide and that the slide is room temperature before beginning. (See Procedure 27-2: Preparing a Dry Smear.)
   Labeling the slide with a diamond-tipped pen ensures that the identification will not wash off during the repeated staining and washing steps of the procedure.
4. Put on gloves.

continued

Procedure 27-3 Continued **Gram's Staining a Smear Slide**

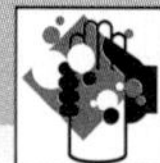
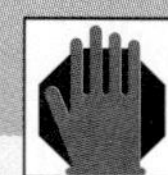

5. Place the slide on the staining rack with the smear side upward.

The staining rack collects the dye as it runs off the slide for disposal.

6. Flood the smear with crystal violet. Time with the stop watch or timer for 30 to 60 seconds.

To stain the bacteria purple.

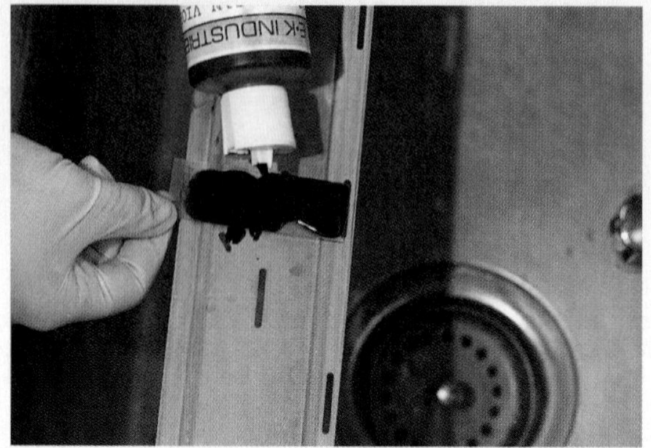

7. Hold the slide with slide forceps.

a. Tilt the slide to an angle of about 45 degrees to drain the excess dye.

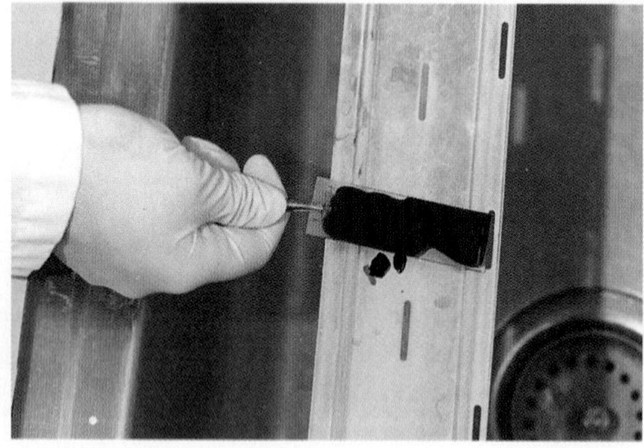

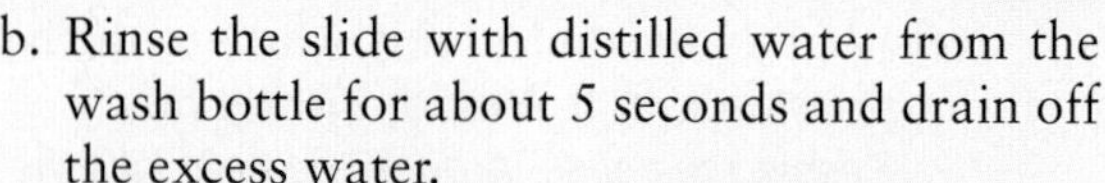

b. Rinse the slide with distilled water from the wash bottle for about 5 seconds and drain off the excess water.

Washing off the stain stops the coloring process.

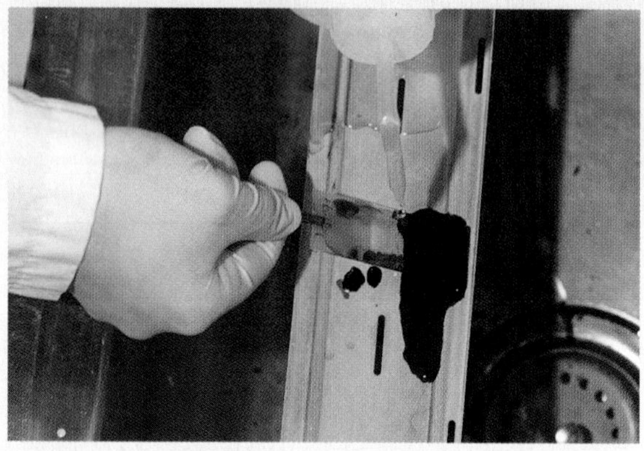

8. Replace the slide on the slide rack. Flood the slide with Gram's iodine solution and time for 30 to 60 seconds.

The iodine acts as a ***mordant*** *and fixes, or binds, the crystal violet to the gram-positive bacteria. The stain will be permanent in the receptive gram-positive cells after being fixed with the iodine solution.*

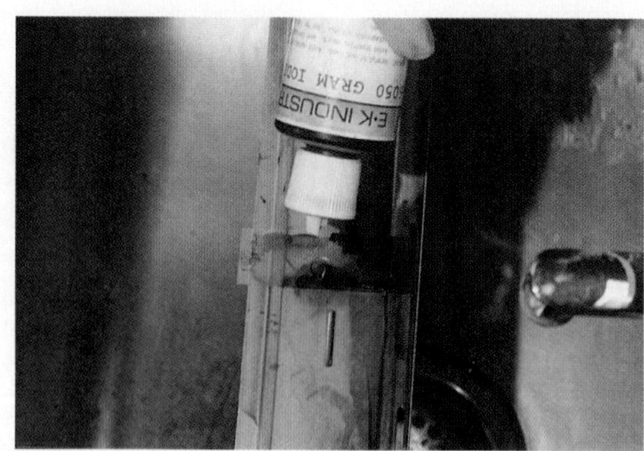

continued

Procedure 27-3 Continued **Gram's Staining a Smear Slide**

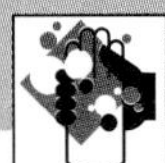
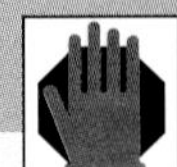

9. Using the forceps, tilt the slide at a 45-degree angle to drain iodine solution. With the slide tilted, rinse the slide with distilled water from the wash bottle for about 5 to 10 seconds. Slowly and gently wash with the alcohol-acetone solution until no more purple stain runs off.

The alcohol-acetone removes the crystal violet stain from the gram-negative bacteria. The gram-positive bacteria retain the purple dye. If the process is carried on too long or too vigorously, dye may leech out of the gram-positive bacteria and lead to incorrect test results.

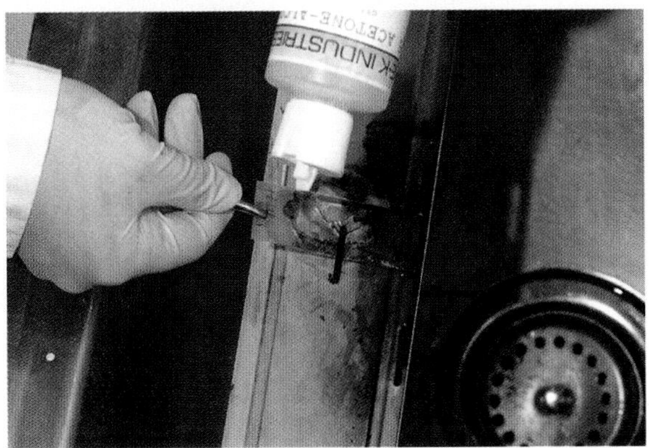

10. Immediately rinse the slide with distilled water for 5 seconds and return the slide to the rack.

Rinsing with the wash bottle stops the decolorizing process.

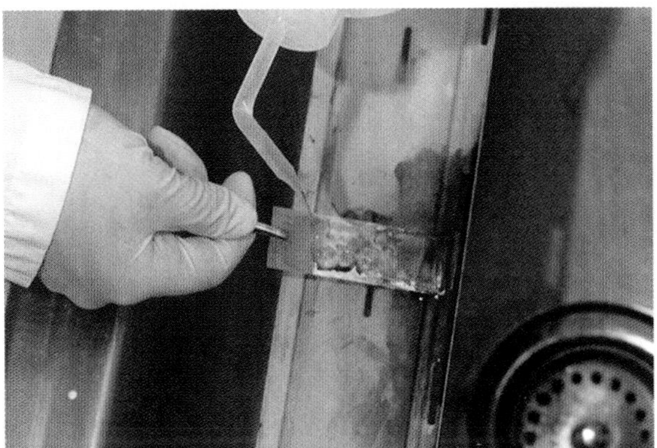

11. Flood with the Safranin or suitable counterstain. Time process for 30 to 60 seconds.

The gram-negative bacteria stain pink or red with the counterstain.

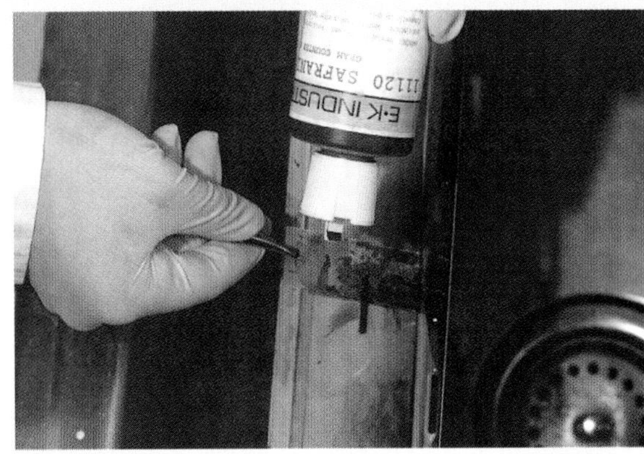

12. Drain the excess counterstain from the slide by tilting it at a 45-degree angle.

Moisture or excess solution may obscure the slide and hinder identification.

a. Rinse the slide with the distilled water for 5 seconds to remove the counterstain.

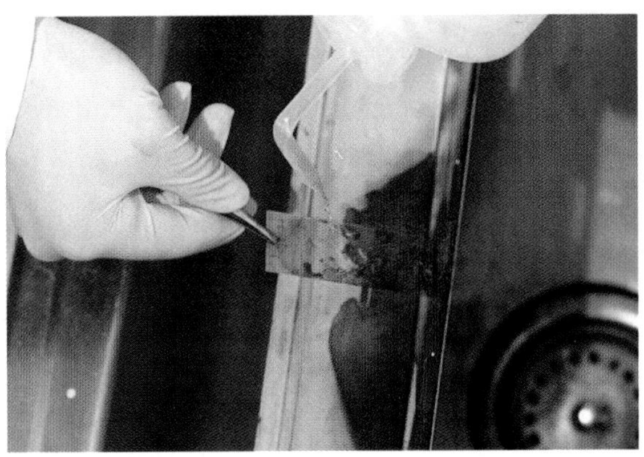

continued

Procedure 27-3 *Continued* Gram's Staining a Smear Slide

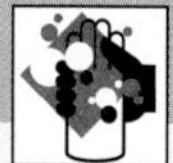
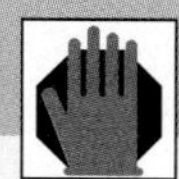
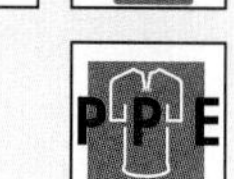

b. Gently blot the smear dry using absorbent bibulous paper. Take care not to disturb the smeared specimen. Wipe the back of the slide clear of any solution. It may be placed between the pages of a bibulous paper pad and gently pressed to remove excess moisture.

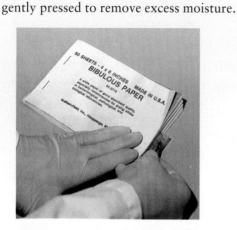

13. Inspect the slide using oil immersion objective lens for greatest magnification. The physician interprets the slide.
14. Properly care for or dispose of equipment and supplies. Clean the work area. Remove gloves and wash your hands.

Special Precautions: Results may be misinterpreted if the reagents are defective or near expiration or if the timing factors in the staining process are not as directed. The bacteria may overstain or may have color leeched from the cells if care is not taken to observe the time limits. The results will not be accurate if the specimen was not heated properly (causing the bacteria to die) or was not incubated long enough or if the general technique was not performed correctly. Premade smears of known gram-positive and gram-negative organisms are processed with the patient's specimen for quality control. See Procedure 27-2 for documentation guidelines and charting example.

Procedure 27-4 Inoculating a Culture

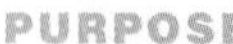
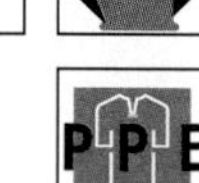

PURPOSE

To introduce a portion of a specimen into the culture medium for growth and replication of microorganisms present in a sample

EQUIPMENT/SUPPLIES

- specimen on a swab or loops
- Bunsen burner
- china marker or permanent lab markers
- labeled Petri dish (The patient's name should be on the side of the plate containing the medium, because it is always placed upward to prevent condensation from dripping onto the culture.)

STEPS

1. Assemble the equipment.
2. Put on gloves and the face shield.
   The face shield should be worn to avoid splatters from the inoculating loop.
3. Label the plate with the patient's name, identification number, source of specimen, time collected, time inoculated, your initials, and date.
   Because culture incubation may take 24–72 hours, dating ensures that the plate is read at the proper time.
4. Remove the Petri plate from the cover (the Petri plate is always stored inverted with the cover downward), and place the cover with the opening upward on the work surface. Do not open the cover unnecessarily.
   Each time the cover is removed, there is the chance of contamination. Placing the cover with the opening upward avoids contamination from the work surface.

continued

Procedure 27-4 Continued Inoculating a Culture

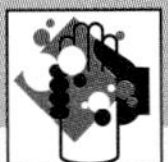
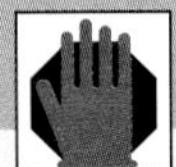

PPE

27

5. Using a rolling and sliding motion, streak the specimen swab completely across ½ of the plate starting from the top and working to a midpoint or at the diameter of the plate. Dispose of the swab in a biohazard container. If the inoculating loop is used for lifting a secondary culture, streak in the same manner.

   The specimen will be spread in gradually thinning colonies of bacteria.

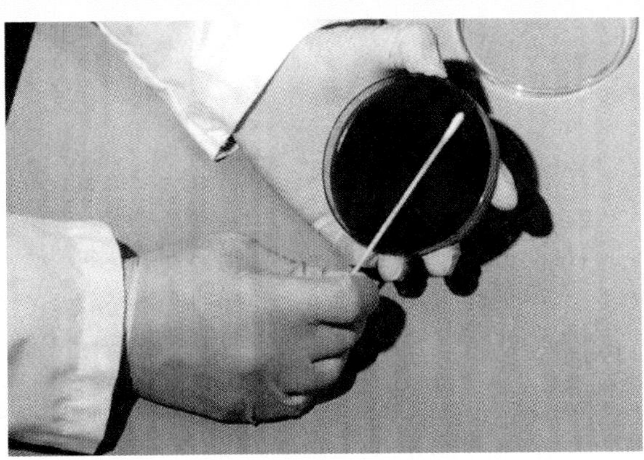

6. Dispose of this loop. If your office does not use disposable inoculating loops, sterilize the loop as described in step 6 of Procedure 27-2.
7. Turn the plate ¼ turn from its previous position. Pass the loop a few times in the original inoculum then downward into the media approximately ¼ of the surface of the plate. Do not enter the originally streaked area after the first few sweeps.

   The loop draws into the clean surface a bit of the specimen that was streaked in the first part of the procedure.

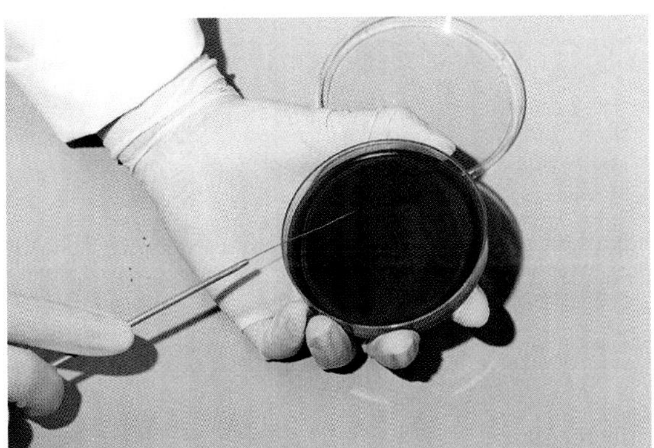

8. Dispose of this loop. If you are not using a disposable loop, flame loop and allow it to cool again.

   The loop must be flamed again to avoid contamination from the previous pass.
9. Turn the plate another ¼ turn so that now it is 180 degrees to the original smear. Working in the previous manner, draw the loop at right angles through the most recently streaked area. Again, do not enter the originally streaked area after the first few sweeps. (The accompanying photograph shows *Staphylococcus aureus* on a properly streaked plate.)

   The loop pulls out gradually thinning bits of the specimen to isolate colonies. Large groups of colonies close together are more difficult to identify than isolated colonies.

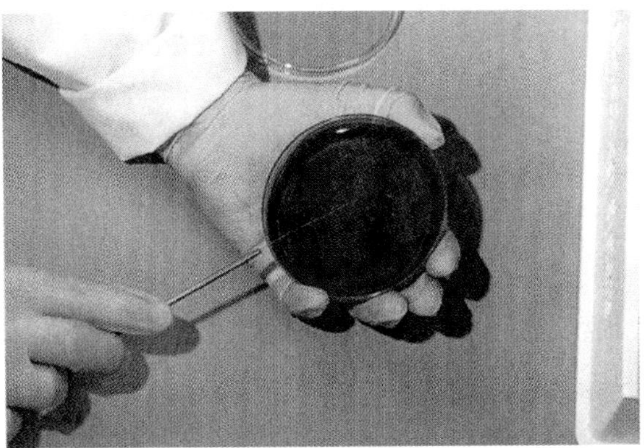

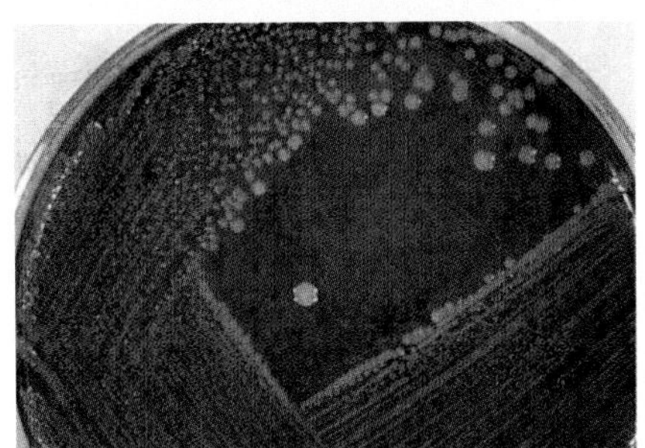

continued

27

Procedure 27-4 Continued Inoculating a Culture

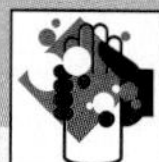
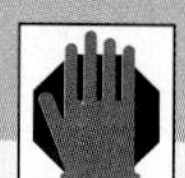

10. If the plate is to be used for sensitivity, follow these steps:
    a. Using sterile forceps or an automatic dispenser, place the specified disks on areas of the plate equidistant from each other.

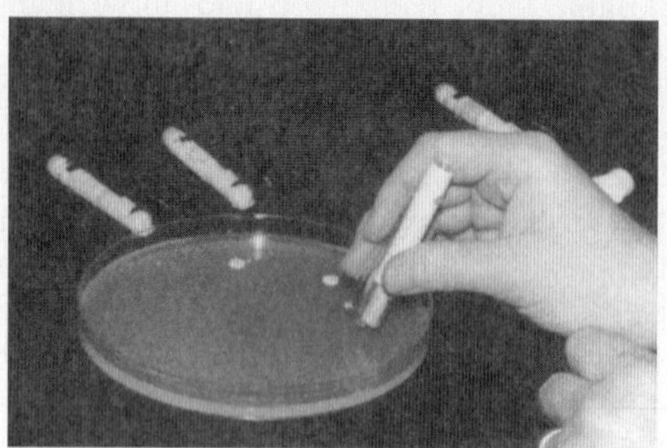

    b. Press them gently with the sterilized loop or forceps until good contact is made with the surface of the agar. (The accompanying photograph shows a sensitivity culture with areas of resistance and susceptibility.)

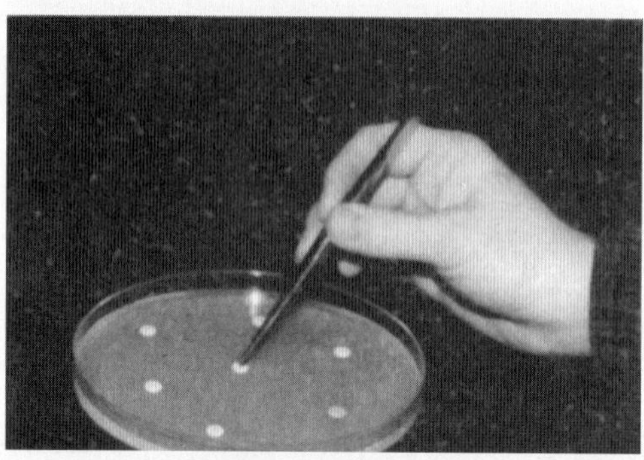

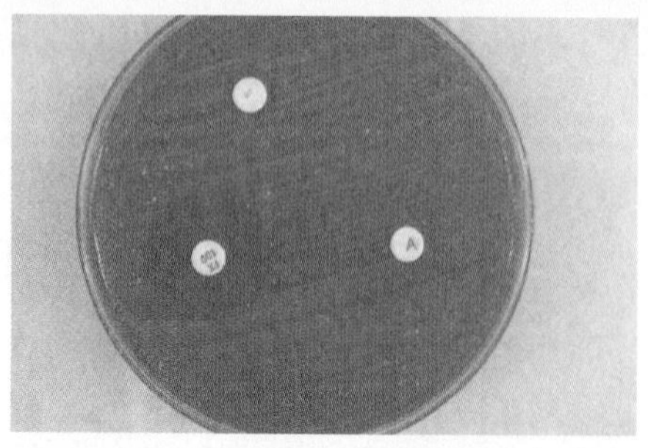

PPE

11. Properly care for or dispose of equipment and supplies. Remove gloves and wash your hands.
12. Incubate for the specified period of time. Read the results and record as directed by office policy.

DOCUMENTATION GUIDELINES

- Date and time
- Site of specimen
- Performance of test
- Results of test at appropriate time
- Action taken, if any
- Patient education/instructions
- Your signature

Charting Example

7/14/99	9:15 am Swab specimen taken of (L) heel
	wound, transferred to culture medium for
	incubation. To be read 7/16/99.
	Pt instructed on wound care and infection
	control; verbalized understanding of
	instructions. —Your signature
7/16/99	8:30 am Specimen checked by
	Dr. Persons. Pt instructed to RTC today
	for wound débridement and further
	treatment. —Your signature

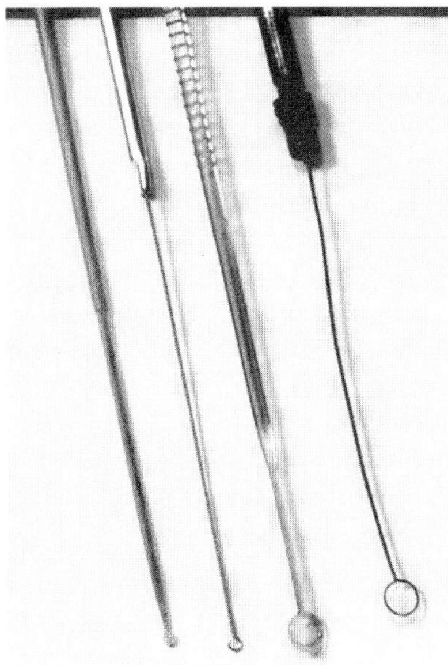

Figure 27-7 Bacteriology loops for inoculation and transfer of bacterial cultures. The two loops to the left (plastic and wire construction, respectively) are calibrated to deliver 0.001 mL of fluid for performing semiquantitative colony counts. The plastic and the wire loops to the right are calibrated to deliver 0.01 mL of fluid.

mary or secondary culture are frequently spread onto a glass slide to be inspected by microscope in the clinical setting. Sometimes a special treatment with stains or fixatives will be applied to aid in identification. Some pathogens are more easily identified if they are allowed to move freely in what is called a wet mount (Box 27-2) or a hanging drop slide (Box 27-3). These should always be viewed immediately or within 30 minutes of collection.

If multiple smears are to be made from one culture, the colonies to be observed should be numbered on the back of the Petri plate(s). Number the slides with corresponding numbers with a diamond-tipped pen on the frosted edge of the slide for proper identification of the culture sites (see Procedure 27-2: Preparing a Dry Smear).

27

Identification by Staining

Staining the microorganisms may help the physician narrow the field of possible pathogens and initiate treatment before a culture has been incubated (see Box

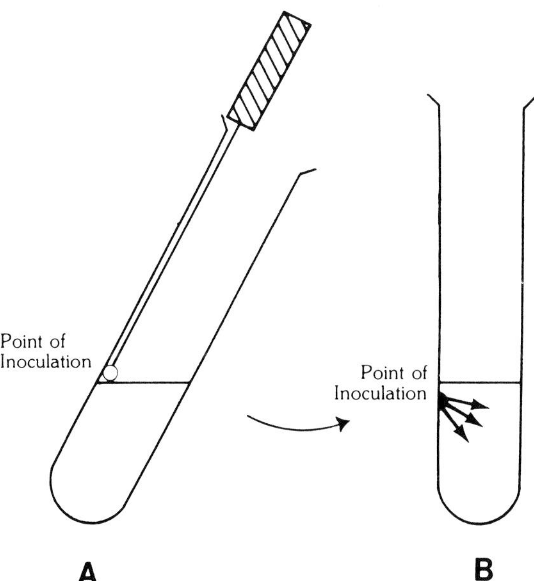

Figure 27-8 Technique for inoculating a tube of broth medium. (**A**) Slant and inoculate the side of the tube as shown. (**B**) Replace the tube upright. This submerges the inoculation site under the surface.

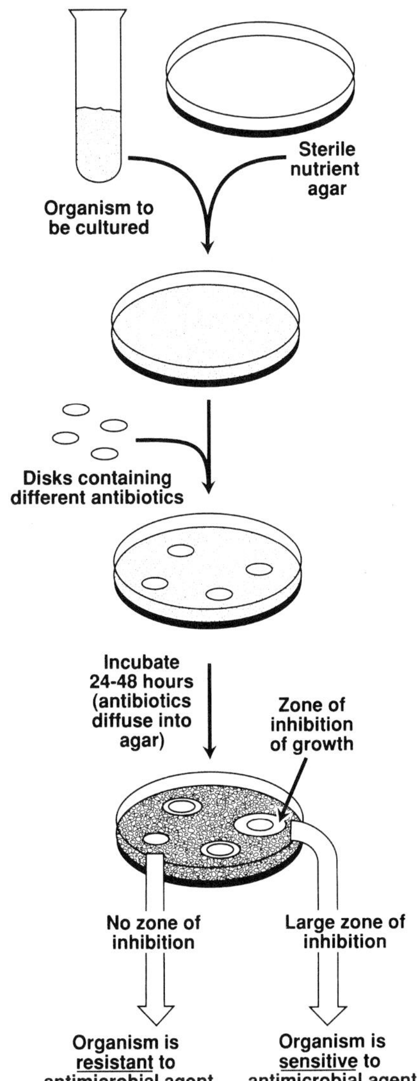

Figure 27-9 Disk diffusion method for determining the sensitivity of bacteria to antimicrobial agents.

27

27-4). Most bacteria are colorless and hard to see or to identify without special treatment such as staining.

The Gram's stain process was developed by Dr. Hans Gram, a Dutch physician who discovered that certain bacteria (cocci and bacilli) retain crystal violet dye through a process to decolorize the specimen. Those bacteria that retain the purple color are gram-positive. Those that do not are gram-negative and must be counterstained to be seen under a microscope. The gram-negative bacteria will retain a pink or red color from the counterstain. Procedure 27-3 details the steps for Gram's staining a smear slide.

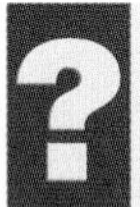

Checkpoint Question

4. *Why are bacteria stained?*

Microbiologic Inoculation

Microbiologic inoculation refers to the practice of introducing a microorganism into a hospitable environment. To ensure that the specimen is placed on or in the culture medium in the proper manner to encourage maximal growth, the medical assistant will *streak* it with a swab or with an inoculating loop (Fig. 27-7). Broth is considered to be inoculated when the swab is inserted below its surface (Fig. 27-8).

Generally, a swab is used when the specimen is lifted directly from the site to the medium. An inoculating loop is used when lifting a specimen from a culture to inoculate a secondary culture. The specific colonies will be lifted from the primary plate and streaked onto the second plate to be re-incubated for further study. Procedure 27-4 describes the steps for culture inoculation.

Sensitivity Testing

Once an organism has been identified, its susceptibility to medication must be established. In many cases, pure or secondary cultures are used to avoid confusion of the results. Filter paper disks impregnated with various antimicrobial agents are placed on the inoculated agar plate just before the plate is incubated. After the plate has been incubated for the prescribed length of time (usually 18–24 hours), it will be inspected for a zone of nongrowth around each disk. Those that exhibit a margin with no bacterial growth indicate that the pathogen is sensitive or susceptible to this medication (Fig. 27-9).

Streptococcal Testing

Streptococcal pharyngitis in children and young adults is one of the most common presenting infections in the medical office. Because of the need for rapid diagnosis to begin appropriate treatment, many kits are available to test quickly for the pathogen group A beta hemolytic *streptococcus* or *Streptococcus pyogenes*. The results are read in a few minutes while the patient waits. Treatment can begin at once.

The theory behind the rapid tests for *Streptococcus* relies on the antigen–antibody reaction that causes a change to occur on the testing material. Quick, easy-to-follow instructions are provided by the manufacturer of the testing equipment chosen by the physician. Quality control measures are included with the testing packages. See Chap. 31, Serology and Immunohematology, for further discussion of strep testing.

Checkpoint Question

5. *What is the purpose of sensitivity testing?*

Answers to Checkpoint Questions

1. *The four main categories of bacteria are cocci, bacilli, spirochetes, and vibrios.*
2. *Mixed cultures are used to investigate any or all of the microorganisms found at a site. Secondary cultures remove from the mixed cultures only those organisms that need to be encouraged to grow for more extensive study. Pure cultures contain only one organism and may be either a primary or a secondary culture.*
3. *If Petri plates are stored with the medium downward, condensation may form on the lids and drip onto the surface, making it too moist for an accurate culture.*
4. *Staining bacteria helps the physician narrow the field of possible pathogens and begin treatment before a culture has been incubated. Most bacteria are colorless and hard to see or identify without special treatment such as staining.*
5. *Sensitivity testing is done to determine which antibiotic affects the bacterial replication.*

Critical Thinking Challenges

1. You are asked to give a brief talk to a group of elementary school children on microbiologic life forms. Develop an age-appropriate discussion of this topic. How would you make it possible for the children to correlate the presence of microbacteria with the need to wash their hands?
2. Write a policy that explains how to care for media and how to transport specimens. Be sure to include who can participate in this process.
3. Create a patient education brochure for streptococcal pharyngitis infections. Include information about what it is, how it is transmitted, signs and symptoms, and the testing procedure.

Suggestions for Further Reading

Atkinson, L. J. (1992). *Berry and Kohn's Operating Room Technique,* 7th ed. St. Louis, MO: Mosby–Year Book.

Burton, G. R. W. (1992). *Microbiology for the Health Sciences,* 4th ed. Philadelphia: J.B. Lippincott.

Fischbach, F. (1998). *Quick Reference to Common Laboratory and Diagnostic Tests,* 2nd ed. Philadelphia: Lippincott-Raven.

Fischbach, F. (1992). *Microbiology for the Health Sciences,* 4th ed. Philadelphia: J.B. Lippincott.

Koneman, E. W., et al. (1994). *Introduction to Diagnostic Microbiology.* Philadelphia: J.B. Lippincott.

Koneman, E. W., et al. (1992). *Color Atlas and Textbook of Diagnostic Microbiology.* Philadelphia: J.B. Lippincott.

Hamann, B. (1992). *Disease: Identification, Prevention and Control.* St. Louis: C.V. Mosby.

Memmler, R. L., Cohen, B. J., & Wood, D. L. (1996). *The Human Body in Health and Disease,* 8th ed. Philadelphia: Lippincott-Raven.

Volk, W. A., et al. (1995). *Essentials of Medical Microbiology,* 5th ed. Philadelphia: J.B. Lippincott.

28 Urinalysis

Chapter Outline

- **Specimen Collection Methods**
  - Clean Catch Midstream Urine Specimen
  - Bladder Catheterization
  - Suprapubic Aspiration
  - 24-Hour Urine Collection
- **Physical Properties of Urine**
  - Color
  - Clarity
  - Specific Gravity
- **Chemical Properties of Urine**
  - pH
  - Glucose
  - Ketones
  - Proteins
  - Blood
  - Bilirubin
  - Urobilinogen
  - Nitrite
  - Leukocyte Esterase
- **Urine Sediment**
  - Structures Found in Urine Sediment
- **Urine Pregnancy Testing**

Role Delineation

CLINICAL

Fundamental Principles

- Apply principles of aseptic technique and infection control.
- Comply with quality assurance practices.

Diagnostic Orders

- Collect and process specimens.
- Perform diagnostic tests.

Patient Care

- Prepare patient for examinations, procedures, and treatments.

GENERAL

Legal Concepts

- Practice within the scope of education, training, and personal capabilities.
- Document accurately.

Instruction

- Instruct individuals according to their needs.

Chapter Competencies

Learning Objectives

Upon successfully completing this chapter, you will be able to:

1. Spell and define the Key Terms.
2. Describe the methods of urine collection.
3. List and explain the physical and chemical properties of urine.
4. State the conditions that can be detected by abnormal urinalysis findings.
5. List and describe the components that can be found in urine sediment.
6. Correlate chemical strip results with sediment findings.

Performance Objectives

Upon successfully completing this chapter, you will be able to:

1. Explain and/or assist a patient in obtaining a clean-catch midstream urine specimen (Procedure 28-1).
2. Explain the method of obtaining a 24-hour urine collection (Procedure 28-2).
3. Determine urine color and clarity (Procedure 28-3).
4. Determine specific gravity by urinometer (Procedure 28-4).

Chapter Competencies *(continued)*

5. Determine specific gravity by refractometer (Procedure 28-5).
6. Accurately interpret chemical reagent strip reactions (Procedure 28-6).
7. Perform copper reduction test (Procedure 28-7).
8. Perform a nitroprusside reaction (Acetest) for ketones (Procedure 28-8).
9. Perform acid precipitation test (Procedure 28-9).
10. Perform diazo tablet test (Ictotest) for bilirubin (Procedure 28-10).
11. Prepare a urine sediment (Procedure 28-11).
12. Prepare a urine sediment for microscopic examination (Procedure 28-12).

Key Terms

(See Glossary for definitions.)

ammonia
bilirubinuria
creatinine
culture
diazo
electrolytes
enumerate
Ehrlich units
esterase
flocculation
galactosuria
hemoglobinuria
hydrogen ions
lyse
nitroprusside
particulate matter
phosphates
precipitation
quantitative
sulfosalicylic acid
urates

A complete urinalysis (UA) involves a physical, chemical, and microscopic examination of urine to assess renal function. Insight into many systemic diseases or conditions can be gained from urinalysis. Diabetes mellitus, shock, malnutrition, preeclampsia, and blood transfusion reactions are several of the disorders that can be diagnosed or assessed by an examination of the urine.

SPECIMEN COLLECTION METHODS

Proper collection of a urine specimen varies depending on the test to be performed. For a routine UA, a freshly voided specimen is all that is necessary. This is called a "random urine." The patient voids the urine into a clean dry container. Often, however, a sterile specimen must be obtained to diagnose a urinary tract infection (UTI). Detecting the pathologic microorganism may require that a **culture** be performed. A culture is a laboratory process in which microorganisms are grown in a special medium, often for the purpose of identifying a causative agent in an infectious disease. All cultures require an uncontaminated specimen. Results of a urine culture and a microscopic analysis can be misleading if the specimen was contaminated with microorganisms from the perineal area.

Once the urine is collected, testing should be done within 1 hour. If testing cannot be performed within this time, the specimen requires refrigeration at 4°C–6°C until testing can be performed. If the specimen is not properly refrigerated, alteration of certain chemical and cellular components contained in the urine can occur, causing the specimen to deteriorate. The presence and multiplication of microorganisms in an unrefrigerated specimen change the pH from acidic to alkaline. Glucose present in the urine may be used as a nutrient by the microorganisms, resulting in a false-negative or lowered glucose result. Some preservatives can be used to prevent deterioration if refrigeration is not possible.

The timing of collection may be an important consideration as well. First-morning urine specimens are the most concentrated and are useful for many tests that are more easily read with concentrated components (eg, pregnancy testing). Double-voided (two separate specimens collected at a timed interval) and 2-hour postprandial (after a meal) specimens are often used for glucose testing. Random UA is the most common of the specimens required for office testing.

Clean Catch Midstream Urine Specimen

A clean catch midstream (CCMS) urine is the most commonly ordered random specimen. It is useful when the physician suspects an infection because any microorganisms present after a correctly collected CCMS will be from the urinary tract and not from contamination such as the perineal area. This specimen can then be used for a culture if nothing has been allowed to contaminate the urine, such as a pipette or chemical strip. Collection is done after the urinary meatus and surrounding skin have been cleansed. The urine is voided into a sterile container. Be aware that the procedure for obtaining a CCMS urine specimen for males differs from the procedure for females (Procedure 28-1).

28

Bladder Catheterization

Another method for aseptic urine collection is catheterization. A thin sterile tube (catheter) is placed into the bladder through the urethra. This procedure usually is performed by a physician or a nurse. In some

Procedure 28-1 Obtaining a Clean Catch Midstream (CCMS) Urine Specimen

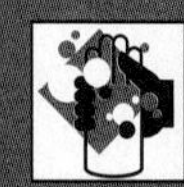
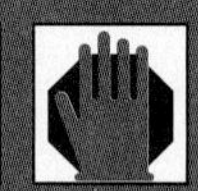

PURPOSE

To minimize contamination of a voided urine specimen

EQUIPMENT/SUPPLIES

- sterile cotton balls or appropriate antiseptic wipes
- antiseptic (if using cotton balls)
- sterile water
- sterile urine container labeled with patient's name
- bedpan or urinal (if necessary)

STEPS

1. Wash your hands. If you are to assist the patient, put on gloves.
2. Assemble the equipment.
3. Identify the patient and explain the procedure. Ask for and answer any questions.
4. If the patient is to perform the procedure, provide the necessary supplies.
5. Have the patient perform the procedure.
   a. *Instruct the male patient to:*
      (1) Expose the glans penis by retracting the foreskin, then clean the meatus with a cotton ball or wipe soaked in a mild antiseptic or a towelette. The glans should be cleaned in a circular motion away from the meatus. A new wipe should be used for each cleaning sweep.
      Antiseptic solutions remove bacteria from the urinary meatus and the surrounding skin. Wiping away from the meatus will remove bacteria from the area; wiping toward the meatus or returning to the area with a used wipe would reintroduce bacteria to the site.
      (2) Keeping the foreskin retracted, void the first 30 mL into the toilet or urinal.
      Organisms in the lower urethra and at the meatus will be washed away. Collecting the middle of the stream ensures the least contamination with skin bacteria.
      (3) Bring the sterile container into the urine stream and collect a sufficient amount (about 30–100 mL). Instruct the patient to avoid touching the inside of the container with the penis.
      Touching the inside with the penis may contaminate the specimen.
      (4) Finish voiding into the toilet or urinal.
      Prostatic fluid may be expressed at the end of the stream and may contaminate the specimen.
   b. *Instruct the female patient to:*
      (1) Kneel or squat over a bedpan or toilet bowl. Spread the labia minora widely to expose the meatus. Using cotton balls soaked in a mild antiseptic or wipe, cleanse on either side of the meatus then the meatus itself. Use a wipe or cotton ball only once in a sweep from the anterior to the posterior surfaces, then discard it. Rinse with cotton balls soaked in sterile water in the same manner.
      Antiseptic solutions remove bacteria from the urinary meatus. Bringing a cotton ball or wipe back to the surface already cleaned will recontaminate the area. The antiseptic solution must be washed away before the specimen is collected.

continued

Procedure 28-1 Continued **Obtaining a Clean Catch Midstream (CCMS) Urine Specimen**

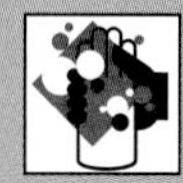
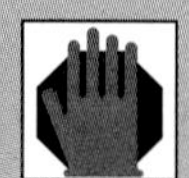

(2) Keeping the labia separated, void the first 30 mL into the toilet.
Organisms remaining in the meatus will be washed away.
(3) Bring the sterile container into the urine stream and collect a sufficient amount (about 30–100 mL).
(4) Finish voiding into the toilet or bedpan.

6. Recap the filled container and drop it into the outside carry container or place it in a designated area.
The specimen should be transported in a biohazard container for testing.
7. Properly care for or dispose of equipment and supplies. Clean the work area. Remove gloves and wash your hands.

DOCUMENTATION GUIDELINES

- Date and time
- Performance of procedure
- Physical observations
- Chemical testing results
- Action taken (if any)
- Patient education/instructions
- Your signature

Charting Example

DATE	TIME Pt instructed in midstream
	collection of urine with Zephiran wipe.
	U/A: Color—straw;
	clarity—clear; specific gravity by
	urinometer—1.020; dipstick negative;
	pH 7.0. —Your signature

Warning! Some antiseptic wipes may interfere with protein testing. Note the type of antiseptic used on the patient's chart.

instances, medical assistants may be trained by their physicians to perform uncomplicated catheterizations. Bladder catheterization is recommended when the patient is unable to give a urine specimen in a sterile manner using the clean catch method. (See Chap. 19, Assisting With Diagnostic and Therapeutic Procedures Associated With the Urinary System, for more information about catheterization.)

Suprapubic Aspiration

Suprapubic aspiration is the least common method of urine collection. A needle is inserted into the bladder through the skin of the abdominal wall above the symphysis pubis, and urine is withdrawn (aspirated). This method is used in rare situations and is performed by a physician.

24-Hour Urine Collection

Because substances such as proteins, **creatinine**, and **electrolytes** are variably excreted during a 24-hour period, a 24-hour collection is a better indicator of values than a random specimen. (Creatinine is a substance formed from creatine metabolism. Electrolytes are chemical substances dissolved in the blood that have numerous basic functions, such as conducting electrical currents.) To obtain this kind of specimen, the patient collects all voided urine within a 24-hour period (Procedure 28-2).

Checkpoint Question

1. *What is the time frame for testing unrefrigerated urine? Why is this important?*

PHYSICAL PROPERTIES OF URINE

The physical properties include the urine's color, appearance (such as clarity or turbidity), specific gravity, and odor (for instance, a diabetic patient's urine may smell sweet and bacteria may give urine a strong odor). Color and clarity are assessed visually and are subjective, meaning the individual performing the testing will determine whether these properties can be considered within the normal range.

Color

Urine color can be affected by many things: diet, drugs, diseases, and the concentration of the urine. The normal color of urine is a pale straw color to dark yellow. The yellow color is due to a urine pigment called urochrome. A pale urine is typically very dilute and is seen after high fluid intake and after diuretic therapy.

text continues on page 617

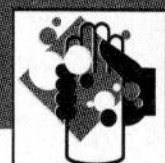
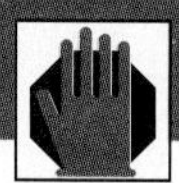

Procedure 28-2 Obtaining a 24-Hour Urine Specimen

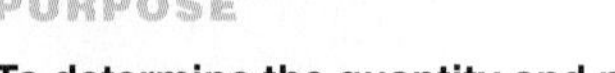

28

PURPOSE

To determine the quantity and proportion of substances in the urine within a 24-hour period

EQUIPMENT/SUPPLIES

- patient's labeled 24-hour urine container (some patients may require more than one container)
- preservatives required for the specific test
- hazard labels
- volumetric cylinder (holds at least 1 L)
- serologic or volumetric pipettes
- clean random urine container
- fresh 10% bleach solution
- patient log form

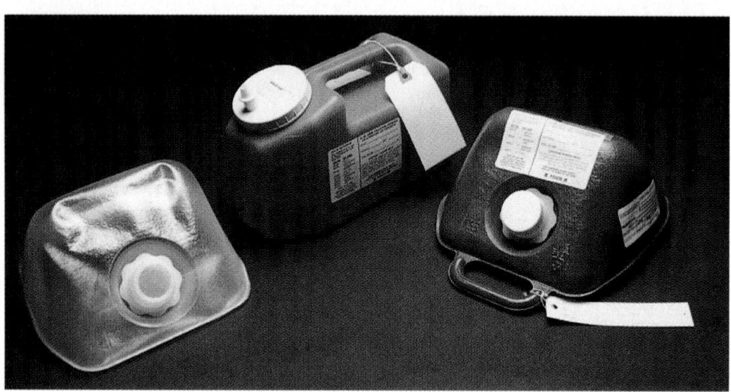

24-hour specimen containers. Each type pictured is used for specific testing procedures.

STEPS

1. Wash your hands.
2. Assemble the equipment.
3. Identify the type of 24-hour urine collection requested and check for any special requirements, such as any acid or preservative that should be added. Label the container appropriately.
   Proper identification avoids errors. Special additives protect the integrity of the specimen.
4. Put on gloves and PPE.
5. Add the correct amount of acid or preservative, if needed, using a serologic or volumetric pipette to the 24-hour urine container.
   This prevents altered testing results due to incorrect preparation.
6. Use a label provided or write on the 24-hour urine container "Beginning Time ____ and Date ____" and "Ending Time ____ and Date ____" so that the patient can fill in the appropriate information.
   This ensures that the patient documents the correct testing times.
7. Instruct the patient to collect a 24-hour urine sample as follows:
   a. Void into the toilet, and note this time and date as "beginning."
   b. After the first voiding, collect each voiding and add it to the urine container for the next 24 hours.
   c. Precisely 24 hours after beginning collection, empty the bladder even if there is no urge to void.
   d. Note on the label the "ending" time and date.
8. Explain to the patient that, depending on the test requested, the 24-hour urine may need to be refrigerated the entire time. Instruct the patient to return the specimen to you as soon as possible after collection is complete.

continued

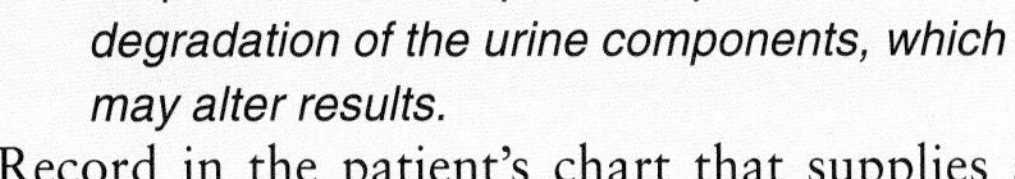

Procedure 28-2 Continued **Obtaining a 24-Hour Urine Specimen**

Proper care of the specimen prevents degradation of the urine components, which may alter results.

9. Record in the patient's chart that supplies and instructions were given to collect a 24-hour urine specimen and the test that was requested.
   This documents patient education and instructions.
10. After receiving the 24-hour urine specimen from the patient, verify beginning and ending times and dates before the patient leaves. Check for required acids or preservatives that need to be added before routing the specimen to the laboratory, if applicable.
   The addition of needed preservatives protects the integrity of the specimen.
11. Pour the urine into a cylinder to record the total volume collected during the 24-hour period. Pour a small representative sample (aliquot) of the urine into a clean container to be sent to the laboratory. (Label the specimen with a biohazard label if this is not prominently displayed on the container.) Record the volume of the urine collection and the amount of acid or preservative added (if needed) on the sample container and on the laboratory requisition. If permissible, you may dispose of the remainder of the urine.
12. Record the volume on the patient log form.
13. Clean the cylinder with fresh 10% bleach solution, then rinse with water. Let it air dry.
14. Clean the work area and dispose of waste properly. Remove PPE and wash your hands.

DOCUMENTATION GUIDELINES

- Date and time
- Performance of procedure
- Testing results
- Action taken
- Patient education/instructions
- Your signature

Charting Example

3/8/99	9:30 AM Pt instructed to
	collect urine for 24 hours and verbalized
	understanding. Pt was given container
	and written instructions. To begin
	collecting at 8:00 AM on 3/9 and to end
	on 3/10 at 8:00 AM. Will bring specimen
	in on 3/10.
3/10/99	10:10 AM Pt returned with completed
	24-hour specimen collection. Total
	volume = 1,850 mL. Labeled 50 mL
	aliquot to Control Path Lab.
	—Your signature

Warning! Use caution when handling acids or other types of hazardous materials. Be familiar with the MSDS for each chemical in your site.

Note: Depending on the type of office and laboratory in which you work, you may not need to aliquot a portion of the 24-hour urine collection.

Likewise a deep, dark yellow can signify a highly concentrated urine, such as when fluids are withheld or the patient is dehydrated. It also may mean that the patient recently took a multiple vitamin pill.

Clarity

Normal, freshly voided urine is usually clear (transparent). Haziness or turbidity (cloudiness) indicates the presence of **particulate matter** (material composed of particles). Some alkaline urine may appear turbid because of the presence of certain chemicals, such as **phosphates,** a compound containing phosphorus and oxygen. Some acidic urine may become turbid on standing as a result of **precipitation** (settling out) of **urates** (nitrogenous compounds derived from protein use and excreted in the urine). Turbidity caused by either of the above is considered normal. The presence of cells, such as red and white blood cells, bacteria, and other particulate matter, such as mucus, can also cause a urine specimen to become turbid.

Laboratories may vary in terminology used to express clarity or turbidity of urine. However, most agree that when a small amount of turbidity is present so that black lines drawn on white paper can still be seen through the specimen, it is termed hazy. As turbidity increases and these black lines can no longer be seen, it is called cloudy (Procedure 28-3). The three terms most commonly used to describe clarity are clear, hazy,

text continues on page 619

28

Procedure 28-3 Determining Color and Clarity of Urine

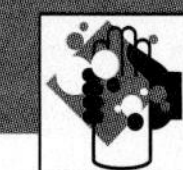
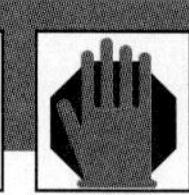
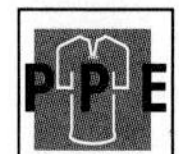

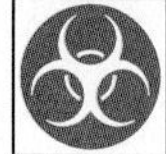

PURPOSE

To determine by visual inspection the presence of particulate and soluble matter in a urine specimen

EQUIPMENT/SUPPLIES

- patient's labeled urine specimen
- clear glass tube, usually a centrifuge
- white paper scored with black lines

28

STEPS

1. Wash your hands.
2. Assemble the equipment.
3. Put on gloves, gown, and face shield.
4. Verify that the names on the specimen container and the laboratory form are the same.
5. Pour 10–15 mL of urine into the tube.

   This provides an adequate quantity for testing and allows for visual assessment of the urine.
6. In bright light, examine the urine for color. The most common colors are straw (very pale yellow), yellow, dark yellow, and amber (brown-yellow). Other colors include blue, green, red, orange, brown, and black.

   The yellow color is due to urochrome and can range in intensity depending on urine concentration. (Refer to Table 28-1 for information about other urine colors.)
7. Determine urine clarity. Hold the urine tube in front of the white paper scored with black lines. If the lines are seen clearly (not obscured), record as clear. If the lines are seen but are not well delineated, record as hazy. If the lines cannot be seen at all, record as cloudy.

   The lines help discern urine clarity by providing contrast.
8. Properly care for or dispose of equipment and supplies. Clean the work area. Remove gloves, gown, and face shield. Wash your hands.

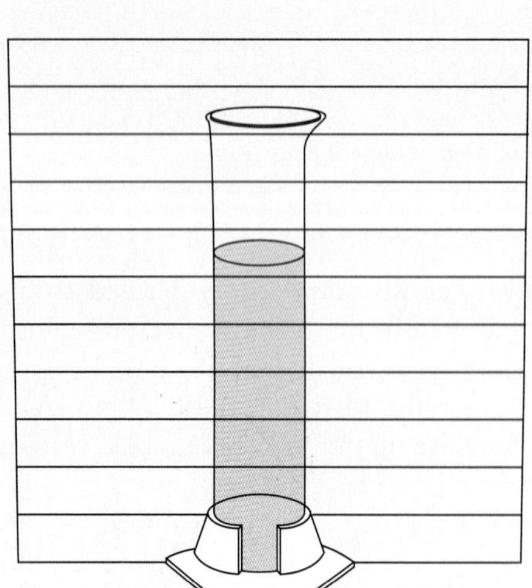

DOCUMENTATION GUIDELINES

- Date and time
- Performance of procedure
- Testing results
- Action taken (if any)
- Your signature

Charting Example

DATE	TIME Random urine collected. Yellow/clear.
	—Your signature

Notes:

- *Rapid determination of color and clarity is necessary because some urine turns cloudy if left standing.*
- *Bilirubin, which may be found in urine in certain conditions, breaks down when exposed to light. Protect the specimen from light if UA is ordered but testing is delayed.*
- *If further testing is to be done but is delayed, refrigerate the specimen to avoid alteration of urine chemistries.*

Table 28-1 **Common Causes for Variations in the Color and Clarity of Urine**

Color/Clarity	*Possible Causes*
Yellow-brown or green-brown	Bile in urine (as in jaundice), phenol poisoning (AKA carbolic acid, used as an antimicrobial agent)
Dark yellow or orange	Concentrated urine, low fluid intake, dehydration, inability of kidney to dilute urine, fluorescein (an intravenous dye), excessive carotene (carotenemia)
Bright orange-red	Pyridium (a urinary tract analgesic)
Red or reddish-brown	Fresh blood (indicating bleeding in the lower urinary tract), porphyrin menstrual contamination (porphyrin binds with iron to form heme), pyrvinium pamoate (Povan) for intestinal worms, sulfonamides (sulfa-based antibiotics)
Brownish-black	Methylene blue medication (commonly used as an antiseptic or in the treatment of a form of anemia)
Black	Melanin (the pigmenting cell)
Grayish or smokey	Hemoglobin or remnants of old red blood cells (indicating bleeding in the upper urinary tract), chyle, prostatic fluid, yeasts
Cloudy	Phosphate precipitation (normal after sitting for a prolonged time), urates (a compound of uric acid), leukocytes, pus, blood, epithelial cells, fat droplets, strict vegetarian diet

Note: In addition to the causes noted above, foods such as blackberries, rhubarb, beets, and those with red dye are common causes of dark or reddish urine that might resemble hematuria.

and cloudy. Table 28-1 summarizes the common causes for variations in the color and clarity of urine.

Specific Gravity

The specific gravity reflects the relative concentration of a urine specimen. The weight of the urine is compared with the weight of water. Urine is heavier than water by a small amount. If you were to compare the weight of distilled water to itself, the specific gravity of the water would be 1.000. If salt water were compared with fresh water, its specific gravity would be higher, approximately 1.040, because there are salt particles present that give it more weight. In the same manner, urine (which has particles such as sodium, potassium, chloride, and cells) will be heavier than water. The range of specific gravity for a normal urine specimen is 1.003 to 1.035.

Low specific gravity urines (less than 1.003) are very dilute. As stated previously, this may result from a high fluid intake. Abnormal conditions that produce a dilute urine are diabetes insipidus and kidney infections or inflammations.

High specific gravity urines (those greater than 1.030) are very concentrated. A patient who is dehydrated, perhaps from sweating, vomiting, or diarrhea, may have a more concentrated urine specimen because the body is trying to conserve water. High specific gravities can occur with congestive heart failure and hepatic disease.

28

Specific gravity can be determined by a variety of methods. The oldest is the urinometer, which requires a relatively large amount of urine (Procedure 28-4). The refractometer requires a drop of urine and is read using a scale (Procedure 28-5). This method uses the principle that light travels slower in liquids with dissolved particles when compared with pure water. The refractometer measures this difference in light velocities. The specific gravity chemical strip also needs a drop of urine, and the color change is compared to a chart to determine the value.

Checkpoint Question

2. *What are the three physical properties of urine, and which two are assessed visually?*

CHEMICAL PROPERTIES OF URINE

Urine contains a number of chemicals, many of which are measured in the UA test. If more **quantitative** (measurement of a specific amount or quantity) information is needed (eg, creatinine), the tests are performed in the chemistry laboratory. (See Chap. 32, Clinical Chemistry.) Detecting and measuring urine chemical properties can indicate many conditions. Included in the discussion of each urine chemistry are the disease processes that might be indicated by abnormal readings.

Many biotechnology companies offer chemical strips that can be dipped into urine (hence the name "dipsticks"). These strips have chemicals imbedded on pads that react with the chemicals in the urine. Each pad will turn certain colors as reactions take place. These colors are then compared with a color chart that is used to interpret the reactions (Procedure 28-6).

Prior to the invention and general use of chemical strips, other methods existed to determine urine chemistries. Some of these are still used as backup methods, or confirmation, for quality control and assurance to check the accuracy of the reagent strips, or

text continues on page 624

Procedure 28-4 Determining Specific Gravity of Urine Using a Urinometer

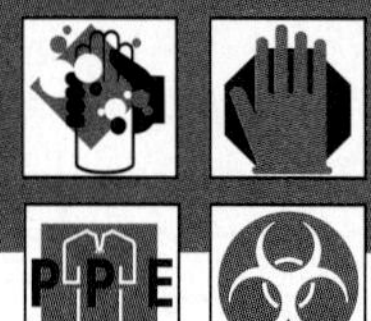

28

PURPOSE

To determine by a weighted float the concentration of solutes in the urine
To aid in determining the concentrating or diluting ability of the kidneys

EQUIPMENT/SUPPLIES

- patient's labeled urine specimen
- urinometer with cylinder (Note: Urinometers also are known as hydrometers.)
- patient report form
- Kemwipe or clean paper towel

STEPS

1. Wash your hands.
2. Assemble the equipment.
3. Put on impervious gown, gloves, and face shield.
4. Verify that the names on the specimen container and the laboratory form are the same.
5. Make sure the urinometer is clean before beginning. Use distilled water and a Kemwipe or paper towel to wipe the inside of the cylinder and urinometer free of lint and moisture.
   A clean urinometer reduces errors in testing.
6. Add the patient's well-mixed, room-temperature urine specimen to the cylinder until it is two-thirds full.
   Urine must be at room temperature for accurate test results. Very warm urine will test falsely low; cold urine will test falsely high.
7. Add the urinometer to the cylinder with a spinning motion.
   This motion frees the urinometer to reflect an accurate reading.
8. Read the specific gravity of the urine specimen from the urinometer scale. Observe the value from the bottom of the meniscus.

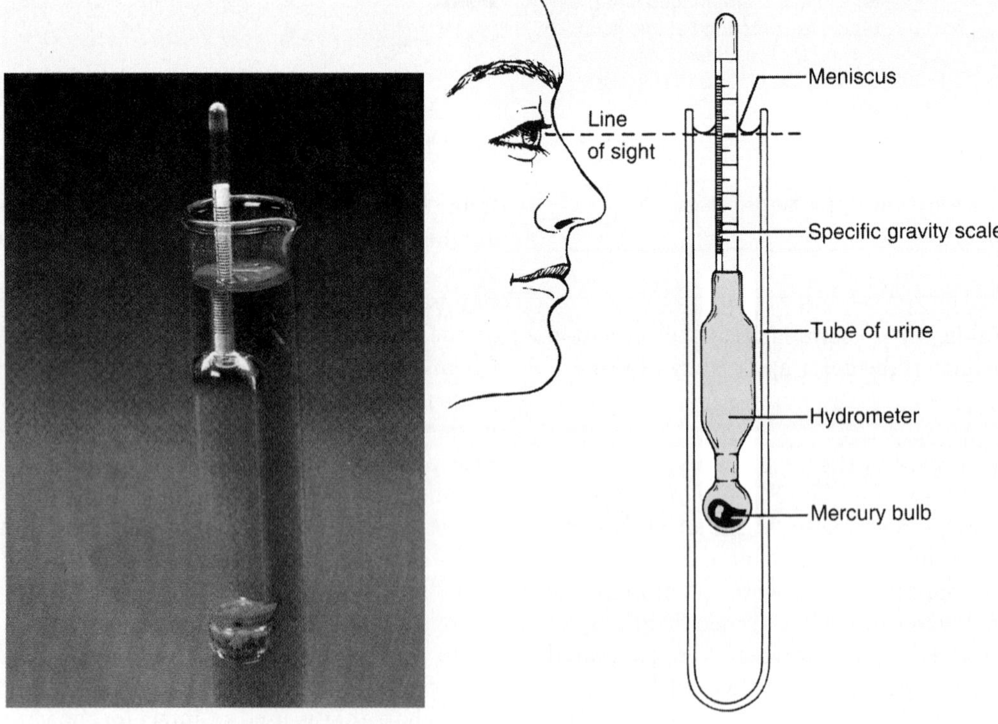

continued

Procedure 28-4 Continued — Determining Specific Gravity of Urine Using a Urinometer

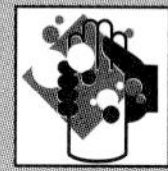
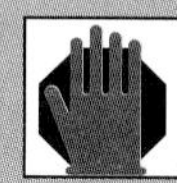
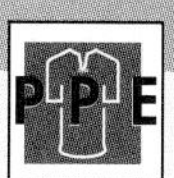
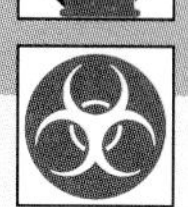

9. Record the value on the patient's report form and in the patient's chart.
10. With a Kemwipe or paper towel, wipe the urinometer dry after the testing procedure.
11. Clean the work area, and dispose of waste properly. Remove gown, gloves, and face shield. Wash your hands.

DOCUMENTATION GUIDELINES

- Date and time
- Performance of procedure
- Testing results
- Action taken (if any)
- Your signature
- (See Procedure 28-1: Obtaining a Clean Catch Midstream [CCMS] Urine Specimen for charting example.)

28

Notes:

- *Quality controls (QC) must be performed daily and recorded in the appropriate QC record. Use distilled water for the negative control and NaCl for the positive control. Follow office policies and procedure for assuring accurate calibration.*
- *A sufficient amount of specimen is needed for the urinometer to float accurately. If not enough urine is provided, report quantity not sufficient (QNS), and notify the physician. To avoid a QNS sample, check the quantity of urine before the patient leaves the area.*
- *Urinometers vary. Read the manufacturer's instructions before beginning the test.*

Procedure 28-5 Determining Specific Gravity of Urine Using a Refractometer

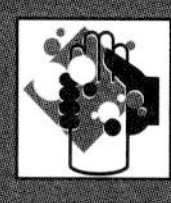
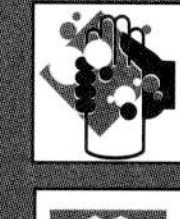
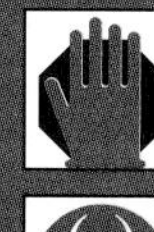
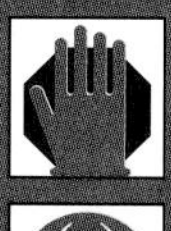
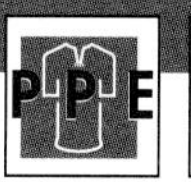
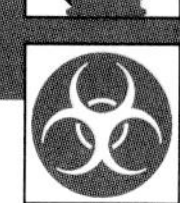

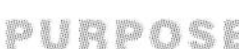

PURPOSE

To determine the concentration of solutes in a specimen using a lighted meter
To aid in determining the concentrating or diluting ability of the kidneys

EQUIPMENT/SUPPLIES

- patient's labeled urine specimen
- transfer pipettes
- refractometer
- Kemwipe or clean gauze
- light source

STEPS

1. Wash your hands.
2. Assemble the equipment.
3. Verify that the names on the specimen container and the laboratory form are the same.
4. Put on impervious gown, gloves, and face shield.
5. Make sure the refractometer is clean before beginning. Use distilled water and a Kemwipe or gauze to wipe the cover and the prism clean and free of moisture.
   A clean refractometer reduces the risk of errors.
6. Using a clean pipette, place a drop of the patient's well-mixed, room-temperature urine onto the notch of the cover. (If the urine has been refrigerated, allow it to reach room temperature because cold affects specific gravity readings.) The urine should flow over the prism.
   This delivers the urine specimen for reading.
7. Point the refractometer toward a light source, and observe the level where the dark and the light portions meet. Record the patient's specific gravity on the worksheet and in the patient's chart.
8. Wipe the refractometer clean with distilled water and dry with a gauze or Kemwipe.
   This prepares the instrument for the next use.

continued

Procedure 28-5 Continued Determining Specific Gravity of Urine Using a Refractometer

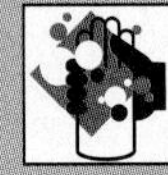
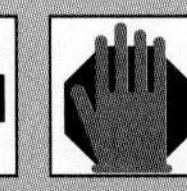
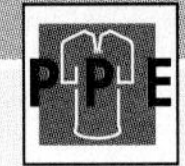
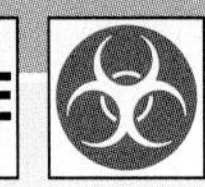

9. Clean the work area and dispose of waste properly. Remove PPE and wash your hands.

DOCUMENTATION GUIDELINES

- Date and time
- Performance of procedure
- Testing results
- Action taken (if any)
- Your signature

Charting Example

DATE	TIME Urine specimen collected and tested
	for specific gravity using refractometer—
	results 1.005. —Your signature

Notes:

- *Quality controls must be performed daily and recorded in the appropriate QC record. Use distilled water for the negative control and a manufactured control or NaCl for the positive control. Follow office policies and procedure for assuring accurate calibration.*
- *The prism is delicate; avoid scratching the surface as you clean it.*
- *Refractometers vary. Read the manufacturer's instructions before beginning the test.*
- *If the specific gravity for the test is greater than the highest marking on the refractometer (usually 1.035), dilute the specimen with distilled water (10 drops of water to 10 drops of urine) in a glass tube. Mix and read the results and multiply by 2.*

Procedure 28-6 Performing Chemical Reagent Strip Analysis

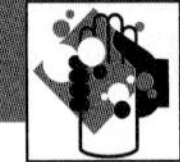
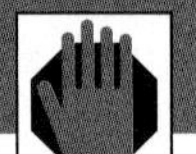
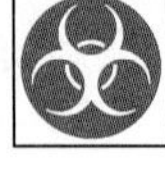

PURPOSE

To determine the level of urine constituents in a patient's sample
To aid in the diagnosis and treatment of urinary or metabolic disorders

EQUIPMENT/SUPPLIES

- patient's labeled urine specimen
- chemical strip (such as Multistix or Chemstrip)
- manufacturer's color comparison chart
- stopwatch or timer

STEPS

1. Wash your hands.

2. Assemble the equipment.

3. Put on gloves, impervious gown, and face shield.

4. Verify that the names on the specimen container and the laboratory form are the same.

5. Mix the patient's urine by gently swirling the covered container.

6. Remove the reagent strip from its container, and replace the lid to prevent deterioration of strips by humidity.

7. Immerse the reagent strip in the urine completely, then immediately remove it, sliding the side edge of the strip along the lip of the urine container to remove excess urine from the pads.

Immersing the reagent strip resuspends particulate matter into urine. Immediate removal of the strip prevents leaching colors from prolonged exposure to urine.

8. Start your stopwatch or timer immediately.

Reactions must be read at specific intervals as directed on the package insert and on the color comparison chart.

continued

Procedure 28-6 Continued Performing Chemical Reagent Strip Analysis

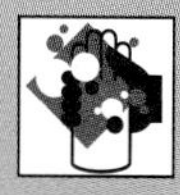
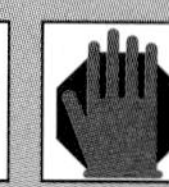
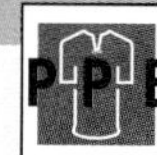

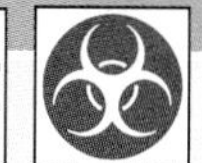

28

9. Compare the reagent pad areas to the color chart, determining results at the intervals stated by the manufacturer. Example: Glucose is read at 30 seconds. To determine results, examine that pad at 30 seconds post-dipping, and compare with color chart for glucose.

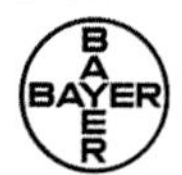

2161

Multistix® 10 SG

COLOR CHART

Reagent Strips for Urinalysis

For In Vitro Diagnostic Use

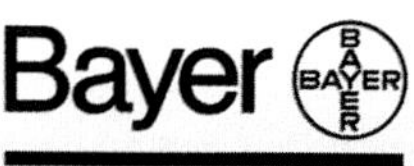

READ PRODUCT INSERT BEFORE USE.
IMPORTANT: Do not expose to direct sunlight.
Do not use after 12/99.

TESTS AND READING TIME

Test							
LEUKOCYTES 2 minutes	NEGATIVE		TRACE	SMALL +	MODERATE ++	LARGE +++	
NITRITE 60 seconds	NEGATIVE		POSITIVE	POSITIVE	(Any degree of uniform pink color is positive)		
UROBILINOGEN 60 seconds	NORMAL 0.2	NORMAL 1	mg/dL 2	4	8	(1 mg = approx. 1EU)	
PROTEIN 60 seconds	NEGATIVE	TRACE	mg/dL 30 +	100 ++	300 +++	2000 or more ++++	
pH 60 seconds	5.0	6.0	6.5	7.0	7.5	8.0	8.5
BLOOD 60 seconds	NEGATIVE	NON-HEMOLYZED TRACE	NON-HEMOLYZED MODERATE	HEMOLYZED TRACE	SMALL +	MODERATE ++	LARGE +++
SPECIFIC GRAVITY 45 seconds	1.000	1.005	1.010	1.015	1.020	1.025	1.030
KETONE 40 seconds	NEGATIVE	mg/dL	TRACE 5	SMALL 15	MODERATE 40	LARGE 80	LARGE 160
BILIRUBIN 30 seconds	NEGATIVE		SMALL +	MODERATE ++	LARGE +++		
GLUCOSE 30 seconds	NEGATIVE	g/dL (%) mg/dL	1/10 (tr.) 100	1/4 250	1/2 500	1 1000	2 or more 2000 or more

 5 Rev. 12/97 0401123

Multistix package insert. (Courtesy of Bayer Corporation, Elkhart, IN.)

10. Read all reactions at the times indicated and record results.

This adheres to strict time-sensitive testing protocol.

11. Discard the reagent strips in the proper receptacle. Discard urine unless more testing is required.

continued

Procedure 28-6 Continued Performing Chemical Reagent Strip Analysis

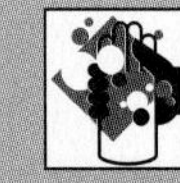
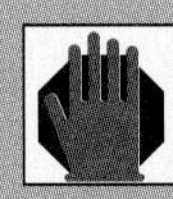
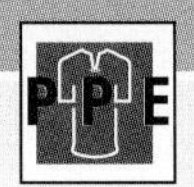

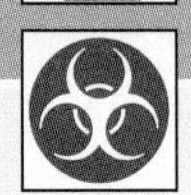

12. Clean the work area. Remove gown, gloves, and face shield. Wash your hands.

DOCUMENTATION GUIDELINES

- Date and time
- Performance of procedure
- Testing results
- Action taken (if any)
- Your signature
- (See Procedure 28-1: Obtaining a Clean-Catch Midstream [CCMS] Urine Specimen for charting example.)

WARNING: Do not remove the desiccant packet in the strip container because it ensures that minimal moisture affects the strips. Be aware that the desiccant is toxic and should be discarded appropriately after all the strips have been used.

Notes:

- *The manufacturer's color comparison chart is assigned a lot number that must match the lot number of the strips used for testing. Record this in the quality assurance (QA/QC) log.*
- *False-positive and false-negative results are possible. Review the manufacturer's package insert accompanying the strips to learn about factors that may give false results and how to avoid them.*
- *Aspirin may cause false-positive ketones. Document if the patient is taking aspirin or other medications. If the patient is taking pyridium, do not use a chemical strip for testing.*
- *Outdated materials give inaccurate results. If the expiration date has passed, discard the materials.*

28

they may be used in place of some of the more expensive chemical strips. Confirmation of positive chemical strip reactions (eg, bilirubin, protein) are sometimes part of laboratory protocol as outlined in the Clinical Laboratory Improvement Amendments (CLIA). (See Chap. 26, Introduction to the Clinical Laboratory, for more information on CLIA.)

pH

The kidneys excrete acids produced during normal metabolic processes. **Hydrogen ions** and **ammonia** are excreted as well. (A hydrogen ion is hydrogen that is missing an electron and therefore readily binds with substances having extra electrons; it is an important constituent of acids. Ammonia is a substance produced by decomposition of organic matter containing nitrogen.) In this manner, the kidneys regulate the acid–base balance of the body. Because the body produces more acids than bases, the pH of urine reflects this by being more acidic also.

Expected values for urine pH can range from 5.0 (acidic) to 8.0 (slightly basic). The typical value for a freshly voided urine is 6.0. Neutral is 7.0. Although considered normal, acidic urine is also seen with high-protein diets and uncontrolled diabetes. Alkaline urine (above 7.0) can occur after meals, with vegetarian diets, certain renal diseases, and urinary tract infections. Usually, pH is tested by using the chemical strip reagents described for this purpose.

Glucose

Glucose is filtered and resorbed in the kidneys. If plasma renal threshold levels exceed approximately 175 to 190 g/dL, not all of the glucose will be reabsorbed, and detectable amounts of it will be present in the urine. However, this can vary greatly and will require more specific testing for a diagnostic assessment. The amount of glucose in urine corresponds to plasma levels; normal urine will not contain glucose. This corresponds to a plasma level of less than 175 mg/dL. In hyperglycemic states, such as diabetes mellitus, glycosuria (glucose in urine) can occur if plasma levels are greater than 175 mg/dL (Box 28-1). A urine glucose test can be performed as a quick check for a diabetic patient experiencing symptoms.

> *Box 28-1*
> **Renal Threshold and Glycosuria**
>
> Glucose is resorbed in the proximal convoluted tubule. When blood glucose levels exceed a certain level (175–190 mg/dL or higher, depending on the individual), not all of the glucose can be reabsorbed into the bloodstream.
>
> Rarely will a healthy person's blood glucose level exceed this threshold value. Diabetics, however, will pass some glucose in their urine due to high levels in their blood. A frequently used term, "spilling sugar," means that not all of the sugar is reabsorbed and is excreted in the urine.

The copper reduction method (trade name, Clinitest, by Miles Inc.) has been used for many years to detect reducing sugars in urine (Procedure 28-7). This test is used to detect any of the substances that reduce copper (eg, glucose, galactose, and other sugars). It is used also for pediatric patients, aged 2 years or less, to screen for **galactosuria.** (Galactosuria, or increased levels of galactose in the blood and urine, is a condition in newborns lacking an enzyme that metabolizes galactose.) The results of this test may be inaccurate because other sugars and ascorbic acid (vitamin C) can react with the reagent. The chemical strips are specific for glucose and are preferred for their accuracy; how-

Procedure 28-7 Performing a Copper Reduction Test (Clinitest) for Glucose

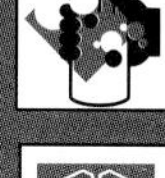
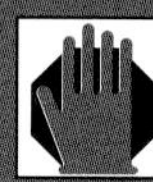
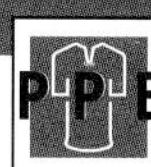

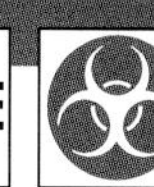

PURPOSE

To determine the presence of reducing sugars when testing by reagent strip is not appropriate

EQUIPMENT/SUPPLIES

- patient's labeled urine specimen
- positive and negative controls
- Clinitest tablets (tightly sealed or new bottle)
- 16 3 125 mm glass test tubes
- test tube rack
- transfer pipettes
- distilled water
- stopwatch or timer
- five-drop Clinitest color comparison chart
- daily sample log
- patient report form or data form

STEPS

1. Wash your hands.
2. Assemble the equipment.
3. Put on impervious gown, gloves, and face shield.
4. Identify the patient's specimen to be tested, and record patient and sample information on the daily log.
5. Record the patient's name or identification information, catalog and lot numbers for all test and control materials, and expiration dates on report or data form.
   This complies with QA/QC requirements.
6. Label test tubes with patient sample identification or as controls, and place them in the test tube rack.
   Proper labeling avoids misidentification.
7. Using a transfer pipette, add 10 drops of distilled water to each labeled test tube in the rack. Add drops by holding the dropper vertically to ensure proper delivery.
8. Add 5 drops of the patient's urine or control sample to the appropriately labeled tube, using a different transfer pipette for each.
   This prevents diluting the urine with water or contaminating the water with urine.
9. Open the Clinitest bottle, and shake a Clinitest tablet into the lid without touching it. Then drop the tablet from the lid into the sample in the test tube rack. Repeat for all patient and control samples being tested. Close the Clinitest bottle.
   Touching the tablet may result in a false test result. The Clinitest bottle must be tightly capped at all times because moisture causes the tablets to deteriorate, thus affecting test results.
10. Observe reactions in the test tubes as the mixture boils. After the reaction stops, wait 15 seconds, then gently shake the test tubes.
    This mixes the contents so you can read the results.
11. Compare results for the patient specimen and controls with the 5-drop method color chart immediately after shaking. (If positive or negative controls do not give expected results, the test is invalid and must be repeated.)
    This ensures testing accuracy.

continued

28

Procedure 28-7 Continued Performing a Copper Reduction Test (Clinitest) for Glucose

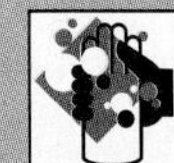
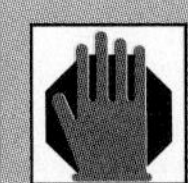
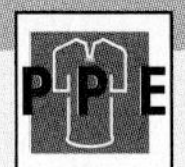
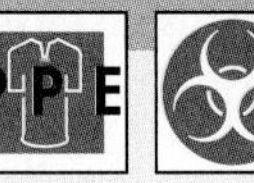

5-Drop Method Standard Procedure

DIRECTIONS FOR TESTING:

1. Collect urine in clean container. With dropper in upright position, place **5 drops** of urine in test tube. Rinse dropper with water and add 10 drops of water to test tube.

2. Drop one tablet into test tube. Watch while complete boiling reaction takes place. Do not shake test tube during boiling, or for the following 15 seconds after boiling has stopped.

3. At the end of this 15-second waiting period, shake test tube gently to mix contents. Compare color of liquid to Color Chart below. Ignore sediment that may form in the bottom of the test tube. Ignore changes after the 15-second waiting period.

4. Write down the percent (%) result which appears on the color block that most closely matches the color of the liquid.

NEGATIVE **1/4%** **1/2%** **3/4%** **1%** **2% or more**

Clinitest package insert. (Courtesy of Bayer Corporation, Elkhart, IN.)

12. Clean and disinfect the work area, and dispose of all waste properly. Remove gown, gloves, and face shield. Wash your hands.

DOCUMENTATION GUIDELINES

- Date and time
- Performance of procedure
- Testing results
- Action taken (if any)
- Your signature

Charting Example

DATE	TIME Pt diagnosed IDDM on last visit.
	Random urine tested for glucose.
	Clinitest, results ¾%. —Your signature

WARNING! Always use glass test tubes—never plastic. Do not touch the test tube bottoms because they become very hot during the test reaction.

Notes:

- *Watch carefully during the boiling reaction to see if the tube contents pass through all the colors on the five-drop color chart, resulting in a final color that reflects a lower score than one seen during the reaction. This is known as "pass-through phenomenon" and should be reported as "exceeds 2%." If your office requires a precise quantitative result on samples that exhibit the pass-through phenomenon, perform the two-drop method. (Refer to the Clinitest package insert, and use the 2-drop color chart for interpretation.)*
- *Clinitest test may be used as a confirmatory test:*
  —When dipstick urine tests for glucose result in a trace value or greater or cannot be interpreted
  —On children under age 2 who are having urine tested for problems with glucose metabolism (regardless of dipstick result)
- *Certain medications (ascorbic acid) and reducing substances other than glucose (galactose and lactose) may give false-positive results. If this occurs, further testing is necessary.*

ever, the Clinitest tablets may be used as confirmation for chemical reagent strips.

Ketones

Ketones are a group of chemicals that result from fat metabolism. In normal circumstances, energy is derived primarily from carbohydrate metabolism. In the absence of sufficient carbohydrates, as in starvation, fats are then used and ketones are produced.

In normal urine, ketones are typically too low to be measurable. A positive ketone test indicates that the body is burning more fat than normal. Conditions that can cause an increase in ketones (ketonuria) include starvation and inadequately managed diabetes.

Nitroprusside reactions are used to detect ketones (Procedure 28-8). (Nitroprusside is a nitrogen cyanic compound that reacts with ketones.) This method is used with chemical strips and tablet tests. Many laboratories choose to confirm results with the nitroprusside tablet (brand name: Acetest, Ames Co.).

Checkpoint Question

3. *What does a positive ketone test indicate?*

Proteins

Small quantities of proteins are found in normal urine. Proteinuria (increased amounts of protein in the urine) is an important indicator of renal disease. Chemical strips are usually used to determine the presence of proteins in urine. Other conditions that can cause proteins to appear in urine are strenuous physical exercise, pregnancy, infections, hematuria (blood in urine), pyuria (white cells in urine), and multiple myeloma. Microscopic examination of the urine can help determine what is causing the proteinuria.

Turbidity or precipitation tests are often used to confirm a positive chemical strip reaction (Procedure 28-9). The simplest and most common test involves observing the amount of cloudiness that occurs when equal amounts of urine and **sulfosalicylic acid** (an acid used to test for protein) are added together. The urine used must be centrifuged to remove all particulate matter before adding the acid.

If the amount of protein is negligible and produces a negative reaction with the chemical strip, there should be no cloudiness when the sulfosalicylic acid is added to the urine. When the concentration of urine protein reaches approximately 20 mg/dL, there will be perceptive turbidity. As protein levels increase, so will the degree of turbidity during the reaction with the acid.

Blood

Small numbers of red blood cells occasionally occur in urine. Intact capillaries in the glomerulus usually will not allow the passage of cells into the Bowman's capsule. Hematuria (not due to contamination from menstrual flow) indicates bleeding in the urinary tract that may result from renal disorders, certain neoplasms, UTI, or trauma to the urinary tract. Chemical reaction strips are usually used to test for blood in the urine, and confirmation is made by microscopic examination.

The chemical strip reacts to hemoglobin, which is the primary constituent of red cells. Free hemoglobin also gives a positive reaction. **Hemoglobinuria** can be seen with transfusion reactions, chemical toxicity, and burns. The strip also reacts to myoglobin, a protein found in muscles. Myoglobin may be released into the bloodstream in crushing injuries and other traumas and then excreted in the urine.

Bilirubin

Bilirubin is formed from the breakdown of hemoglobin. It is processed in the liver before being excreted into the intestines as bile. Urine contains very low levels of bilirubin, reflecting the usual low serum levels. **Bilirubinuria** (bilirubin in the urine) can be seen with certain liver diseases (eg, hepatitis), biliary tract obstruction, and hemolytic states, such as transfusion reactions.

The chemical strip for bilirubin is specifically designed to react to its presence. However, a dark yellow urine can make it difficult to read the reaction because bilirubin is also a yellow pigment. Many laboratories confirm a positive strip by a **diazo** tablet method (brand name: Ictotest, by Miles, Inc.). Diazo is a double nitrogen compound that reacts with bilirubin (Procedure 28-10).

IMPORTANT NOTE: Bilirubin is a highly unstable substance and will break down with prolonged light exposure. Specimens must be shielded from light and processed as soon as possible to avoid deterioration of the specimen.

Urobilinogen

When bilirubin is secreted into the intestines in the bile, bacterial action converts it into urobilinogen. Some of this is reabsorbed into the bloodstream and is excreted by the kidneys. The remaining urobilinogen leaves the body in the feces.

Small amounts of urobilinogen are normally found in urine, usually 0.1 to 1.0 **Ehrlich units**/dL (mg/dL). (An Ehrlich unit is a unit of measurement for

text continues on page 631

28

Procedure 28-8 Performing Nitroprusside Reaction (Acetest) for Ketones

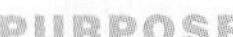

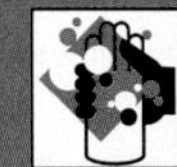
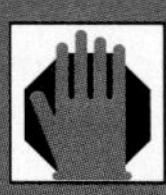
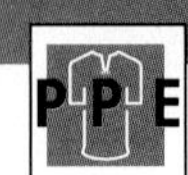

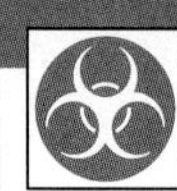

PURPOSE

To determine the level of ketones in the urine
To aid in the diagnosis and treatment of diseases and disorders of fat metabolism

EQUIPMENT/SUPPLIES

- patient's labeled urine specimen
- white filter paper
- plastic transfer pipette
- Acetest tablet
- manufacturer's color comparison chart

STEPS

1. Wash your hands.
2. Assemble the equipment.
3. Put on gloves, impervious gown, and face shield.
4. Place an Acetest tablet on the filter paper by shaking one into the cap and dispensing it onto the paper. Replace the cap.
   Dispensing the tablet in this manner prevents contamination of the tablet or bottle contents. The white background of the filter paper allows for contrast.
5. Using a transfer pipette, place 1 drop of well-mixed urine on top of the tablet.
   When the urine and the tablet meet, the reaction begins.
6. Wait 30 seconds for the complete reaction.
   Nitroprusside reaction occurs if ketones are present.
7. Compare the color of the tablet to the color chart, and record the results as negative, trace, small amount, moderate amount, or large amount.
   Nitroprusside reaction gives a color change of varying degrees of purple if ketones are present. The color correlates to the amount of ketones in the urine.
8. Properly care for or dispose of equipment and supplies. Clean the work area. Remove gloves, gown, and face shield, and wash hands.

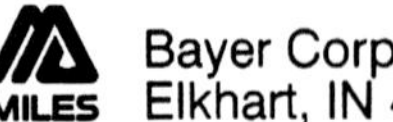

Bayer Corporation
Elkhart, IN 46515 USA

Colors shown below are for use with ACETEST Reagent Tablets only.

NEGATIVE

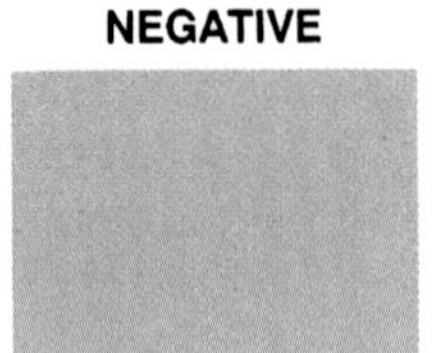

SMALL

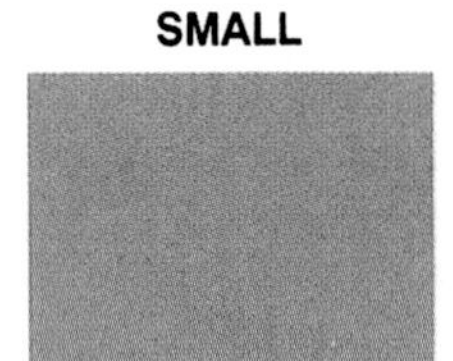

MODERATE

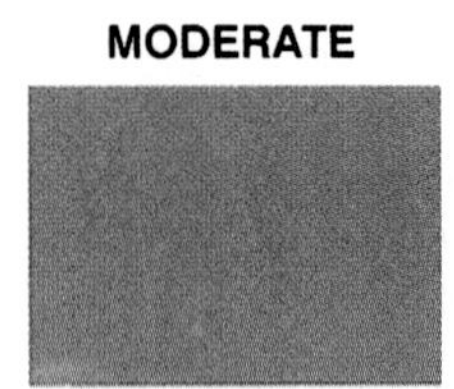

LARGE

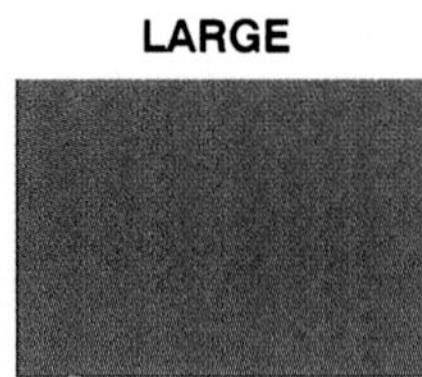

Acetest package insert. (Courtesy of Bayer Corporation, Elkhart, IN.)

DOCUMENTATION GUIDELINES

- Date and time
- Performance of procedure
- Testing results
- Action taken (if any)
- Your signature

Charting Example

DATE	TIME Urine specimen collected and tested
	for ketones—results showed large
	amount. Dr. Wendt notified.
	—Your signature

Procedure 28-9 Performing an Acid Precipitation Test for Protein

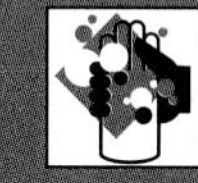
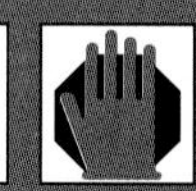
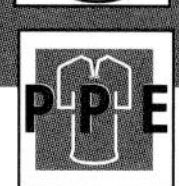

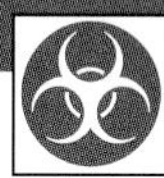

PURPOSE

To determine the presence of increased levels of protein in the urine

To aid in the diagnosis and treatment of diseases and disorders resulting in increased protein metabolism

EQUIPMENT/SUPPLIES

- patient's labeled and centrifuged urine specimen
- positive and negative controls
- 3% sulfosalicylic acid (SSA) solution
- clear glass test tubes
- test tube rack
- transfer pipettes
- stopwatch or timer
- daily sample log
- patient report form or data form

STEPS

1. Wash your hands.
2. Assemble the equipment.
3. Put on impervious gown, gloves, and face shield.
4. Identify the patient's specimen to be tested, and record patient and sample information on the daily log.

   Proper identification and recording avoids errors and complies with QA/QC requirements.
5. Record the patient's name or identification information, catalog and lot numbers for all test and control materials, and expiration dates on report or data form.

   This complies with QA/QC requirements.
6. Label the test tubes with patient sample identification or as controls, and place in test tube rack.

   Proper labeling avoids misidentification.
7. Centrifuge at 1,500 RPM for 5 minutes.
8. Add 1 to 3 mL of supernatant urine (top portion of spun urine) or control sample to appropriately labeled tube in rack. Repeat for all samples and controls, using a clean transfer pipette for each. (*Note:* If supernatant from centrifuged urine is not used or the specimen is not mixed after centrifugation, a false-positive result may occur.)

   Using a clean pipette avoids contamination of test results.
9. Add an equal amount of 3% SSA solution to sample quantity in each tube. Use a clean transfer pipette for each addition if your 3% SSA solution does not have a repeating dispenser.

   Adding equal amounts of 3% SSA solution reduces errors in testing.
10. Mix the contents of the tubes, and let stand for a minimum of 2 minutes but no longer than 10 minutes. Use a stopwatch or timer to make sure you perform the next step within the appropriate time frame.

    The reactants must be mixed together. Adherence to timing guidelines provides for accuracy in testing.
11. Mix the contents of tubes again, then observe the degree of turbidity seen in each test tube and score as follows:

    NEG: No turbidity or cloudiness; urine remains clear

    TRACE: Slight turbidity

    11: Turbidity with no precipitation (print on a page held behind tube is visible)

    21: Heavy turbidity with fine granulation

    31: Heavy turbidity with granulation and flakes

    41: Clumps of precipitated protein

    The specimen may be matched against a McFarland standard to decrease the degree of subjective interpretation.
12. Clean work area, and dispose of all waste properly. Remove gown, gloves, and face shield. Wash your hands.

DOCUMENTATION GUIDELINES

- Date and time
- Performance of procedure
- Testing results
- Action taken (if any)
- Your signature

Charting Example

DATE	TIME Urine specimen collected and tested
	for protein—results 31 using acid
	precipitation test. —Your signature

Notes:

- *This is a confirmatory test used for specimens with dipstick urine test results greater than TRACE value for protein.*
- *If positive and negative controls do not give expected results, the test is invalid and must be repeated.*

28

Procedure 28-10 Performing a Diazo Tablet Test (Ictotest) for Bilirubin

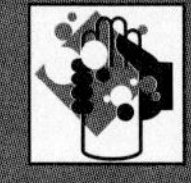
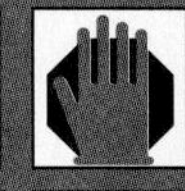
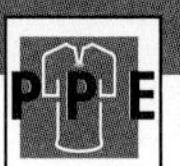

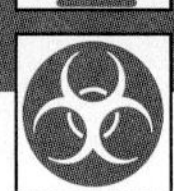

PURPOSE

To determine the presence and level of bilirubin excreted by the kidneys

To aid in the diagnosis of liver, gallbladder, or hemolytic diseases

EQUIPMENT/SUPPLIES

- patient's labeled urine specimen
- Ictotest (diazo) tablets
- Ictotest white mats
- clean paper towel
- transfer pipette
- stopwatch or timer

STEPS

1. Wash your hands.
2. Assemble the equipment.
3. Put on impervious gown, gloves, and face shield.
4. Verify that the names on the specimen container and the laboratory form are the same.
5. Place an Ictotest white mat on a clean, dry paper towel.

   The mat provides a testing surface. The paper towel must be dry because moisture may cause a false result.
6. Using a clean transfer pipette, add 10 drops of the patient's urine to the center of the mat. (If the urine is red, it may be difficult to read the reaction properly. Pour a representative sample [aliquot] of the urine into a urine tube or test tube, and centrifuge as you would for preparing urine sediment. Use 10 drops of supernatant in this step.)
7. Shake a tablet into the bottle cap, and dispense onto the center of the mat. Do not touch the tablet with your hands.

   Touching the tablet contaminates it and may cause a false-positive result.
8. Recap the bottle immediately.

   The bottle must be recapped to prevent deterioration of the contents.
9. Using a clean transfer pipette, place 1 drop of water on the tablet and wait 5 seconds.
10. Add another drop of water to the tablet so that the solution formed by the first drop runs onto the mat.

    This allows the diazo chemical to react with the urine.
11. Within 60 seconds, observe for either a blue or purple color on the mat around the tablet. Either color indicates a positive result. Pink or red indicates a negative result.

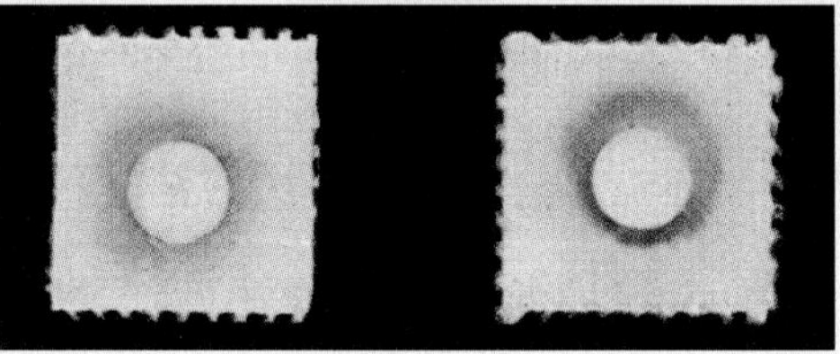

Ictotest package insert. (Courtesy of Bayer Corporation, Elkhart, IN.)

12. Clean the work area, and dispose of waste properly. Remove gown, gloves, and face shield. Wash your hands.

DOCUMENTATION GUIDELINES

- Date and time
- Performance of procedure
- Testing results
- Action taken (if any)
- Your signature

Charting Example

DATE	TIME Urine specimen collected and tested
	for bilirubin using diazo test. Results 1.
	—Your signature

Notes:

- *Quality controls must be performed daily and recorded appropriately. Follow office policies and procedures for assuring compliance with QA/QC requirements.*
- *The specimen should be free of pyridium, chlorpromazine, or other drugs that interfere with color interpretation.*
- *The tablets must be protected from exposure to light, heat, and moisture to prevent deterioration.*

urobilinogen.) As with bilirubin, increased levels of urobilinogen can be found with conditions that have a high rate of red cell destruction. Also, bowel obstructions cause the feces to remain in the intestines for longer periods, resulting in greater reabsorption of urobilinogen along with the rest of the fluid portion. Urobilinogen levels will rise both in urine and in serum when this occurs. Liver impairment can also lead to increased levels of urobilinogen because some of the urobilinogen that is reabsorbed from the intestinal tract is processed by the liver and re-excreted in the feces. Urobilinogen is tested by chemical reagent strips.

Nitrite

Most types of bacteria that infect the urinary tract have an enzyme that can reduce nitrate to nitrite. This factor is used to assess the presence of bacteria in urine. In the nitrite test, urine is applied to a pad impregnated with nitrates. If bacteria are present, nitrates will be changed into nitrites, and the resulting color development can be observed. A positive nitrite test result indicates bacteriuria, which occurs with urinary tract infections.

Leukocyte Esterase

Leukocytes in the urine indicate a urinary tract infection. Phagocytic white cells, such as neutrophils, are called to the kidney to fight the infection. These leukocytes contain an enzyme called **esterase.** This is detected with the leukocyte esterase reaction on the chemical strip. Normal urine may contain a few white cells but not in sufficient numbers to produce a positive leukocyte esterase test.

Checkpoint Question

4. *Which two indicators on a dipstick would suggest a urinary tract infection?*

URINE SEDIMENT

The microscopic examination of urine can corroborate the findings of the UA and may produce new data of diagnostic value. Cells and other structures are noted and **enumerated** (counted) during a microscopic examination. Microscopic examination of urine is generally considered to be an advanced procedure and is not usually performed by medical assistants.

Urine sediment is prepared by centrifuging urine and saving the button of cells and other particulate matter that collects in the bottom of the tube. This button is resuspended, and a drop of this suspension is placed on a slide and viewed with a microscope. Making a sediment concentrates all the structures present in the urine so that it is unlikely that any urine components will be missed (Procedures 28-11 and 28-12).

Many manufacturers have a slide system that is used in conjunction with a centrifuge tube, also made by that company, to examine urine sediments. This provides some standardization of the procedure so that when quantifying the structures seen microscopically, the numbers have meaning with regard to abnormal results. Although glass slides and coverslips may still be used by some laboratories, this technique is rarely used and is not recommended.

28

Structures Found in Urine Sediment

The following structures may appear in the urine: red blood cells, white blood cells, bacteria, epithelial cells, crystals, casts, and others (Fig. 28-1). Correlations with chemical properties of the urine are given when appropriate.

Red Blood Cells

The presence of red cells in urine, as stated previously, can indicate a number of conditions, including renal damage. A few red cells in every high power field (HPF) is considered normal. Greater than 3 per HPF is abnormal.

When greater than normal numbers of red cells are present in urine sediment, the chemical strip reaction for blood should be positive. Protein may be positive if hemolysis is occurring. A positive chemical strip test for blood with no red cells seen microscopically correlates with various kinds of hemolysis, such as with transfusion reactions and sickle cell crisis. (See Chap. 30, Hematology, for an explanation of sickling.) As stated earlier, myoglobin will cause a positive reaction.

White Blood Cells

Leukocytes in the sediment indicate a UTI. A finding of 0 to 5 white blood cells per HPF is normal; greater than 5 per HPF is considered abnormal.

The leukocyte esterase test on the chemical strip will be positive when white cells are present in increased numbers. Protein may be positive if some of the white blood cells have **lysed** (broken apart) or if the infection is damaging the renal tubules, as in glomerulonephritis.

Bacteria

Bacteria are always present on the surface of the skin but are not usually present in the bladder. Urine normally will not contain bacteria if a clean-catch urine specimen is collected properly. The presence of

text continues on page 636

Procedure 28-11 Preparing a Urine Sediment

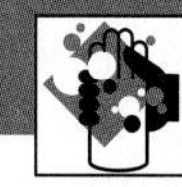 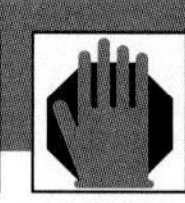
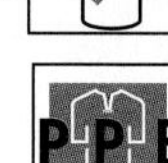 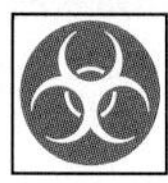

PURPOSE

To aid in the determination and identification of formed elements and solid particles in a urine specimen

EQUIPMENT/SUPPLIES

- patient's labeled urine specimen
- urine centrifuge tubes
- transfer pipette
- centrifuge (1,500–2,000 rotations per minute [RPM])

28

STEPS

1. Wash your hands.
2. Assemble the equipment.
3. Put on impervious gown, gloves, and face shield.
4. Verify that the names on the specimen container and the laboratory form are the same.
5. Pour 10 to 15 mL of the patient's well-mixed urine into a labeled centrifuge tube (or a standardized system tube). Cap the tube with a plastic cap or parafilm.
6. Place the labeled urine tube in the centrifuge, and balance it with another tube (filled to the same level with water or another patient's urine).
   This prevents damage to the centrifuge due to imbalance of the rotator wheel.
7. Close the centrifuge cover and set it to spin at 1,500 RPMs for 5 minutes.
   Centrifugation ensures that cellular and particulate matter is pulled to the bottom of the tube.
8. When the centrifuge has stopped, remove the tubes. Make sure no tests are to be performed first on the supernatant. Remove the caps and pour off the supernatant, leaving a small portion of it (0.5–1.0 mL). Resuspend the sediment by flicking the tube with your finger or aspirating up and down with a transfer pipette, or follow manufacturer's directions for standardized system.
   The concentrated urine is now prepared for microscopic examination.
9. Properly care for and dispose of equipment and supplies. Clean the work area. Remove gown, gloves, and shield. Wash your hands.

Notes:

- *If the urine is to be tested by chemical reagent strip, perform the dip test before spinning the urine.*
- *Preparing a urine for sediment with less than 3 mL is not recommended because that is not enough urine to create a true sediment. However, some patients are unable to provide a large amount of urine. In such cases, document the volume on the chart under sediment to ensure proper interpretation of results.*
- *Check the centrifuge periodically to ensure the speed and timing are correct. Document this information on the maintenance log.*

Procedure 28-12 Performing a Microscopic Examination of Urine

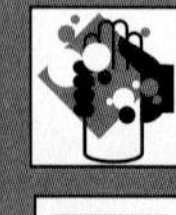 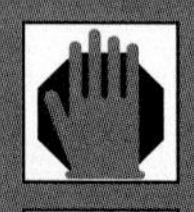

PURPOSE

To aid in determining the presence and identity of formed elements and solid particles in a urine specimen

EQUIPMENT/SUPPLIES

- patient's labeled urine tube
- transfer pipette
- microscope
- lens cleaner
- lens paper
- glass slide
- coverslip
- standardized sediment slide (if applicable)

STEPS

1. Wash your hands.
2. Assemble the equipment.
3. Put on impervious gown, gloves, and face shield.
4. Verify that the names on the specimen container and the laboratory form are the same.

continued

Procedure 28-12 Continued Performing a Microscopic Examination of Urine

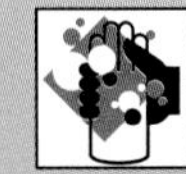
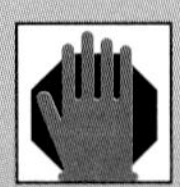

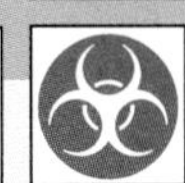

5. Using a spun urine specimen, make sure the sediment is well mixed with the remaining 1 mL of urine.
   Proper mixing ensures accurate results.
6. Using the transfer pipette, place 1 drop of the urine mixture onto a clean glass slide or into the chamber of the standardized slide.
   This distributes the sediment for examination.
7. Place a coverslip on the drop of urine if using the glass slide.
   The coverslip secures the specimen to the slide for viewing.
8. Place the slide on the microscopic stage between the holding clips. Using the 103 objective, focus until the sediment structures (eg, cells) become clear.
   Proper focusing ensures that no components are overlooked.
9. Scan the edges of the slide for casts, about 10 to 15 fields. If a cast is present, use the 403 objective to identify the type (waxy, granular, hyaline, white blood cells [WBC], red blood cells [RBC]). To report the amount of casts present, take the average seen on *low power,* 103 objective. Example: 0-1 hyaline casts/LPF. Record on the worksheet and lab form any casts observed.
   Greater magnification is required to identify the type of casts. Accuracy in reporting is essential.
10. Scan the slide using the 403 objective for about 10 to 15 fields. Average the number of RBC, WBC, and epithelial cells observed. Record on the worksheet and lab form.
11. Observe the presence of bacteria, mucus, crystals, sperm, yeast, and trichamotis using 403 objective for 10 fields. Use references located in the laboratory area to identify structures as needed. Average the number or amount observed, and record on the worksheet and lab form.
12. Report your observations as follows:
    Epithelial: Rare, few, moderate, many
    Casts: Number per LPF
    Mucus: Trace, 11, 21, 31, 41
    WBCs: Lowest number and highest number seen in 10 fields per HPF (*Example: 0–5 WBC/HPF*)
    RBCs: Lowest number and highest number seen in 10 fields per HPF (*Example: 2–10 RBC/HPF*)
    Bacteria: Trace, 11, 21, 31, 41
    Crystals, yeast, sperm, trichamotis: Few, moderate, many
    (Note: 11 5 few in some fields; 21 5 few in all fields; 31 5 many in all fields; 41 5 too numerous to count [TNTC].)
13. Clean the work area and dispose of waste properly. Remove gown, gloves, and shield. Wash your hands.

DOCUMENTATION GUIDELINES

- Date and time
- Performance of procedure
- Testing results
- Action taken (if any)
- Your signature

Charting Example

DATE	TIME Microscopic examination of urine.
	Results: WBC 8/HPF and RBC casts
	1/LPF. —Your signature

Notes:

- *According to CLIA regulations, medical assistants may perform the microscopic examination to step 8 to have the slide in focus for the physician and to point out types of sediment. Medical assistants who have been trained to complete the procedure may continue with the remaining steps.*
- *The 103 objective is used to focus and scan; the 40/453 objective is used to identify components.*

ATLAS OF URINE SEDIMENT

CELLS IN URINE

Epithelial Cells Three types of epithelial cells may appear in urine sediment: renal tubular, transitional and/or squamous. Other types of cells may appear in urine but are difficult to identify due to morphologic changes caused by urine. Tubular cells are approximately ⅓ larger than white blood cells. Transitional epithelial cells may arise from the renal pelvis, ureters, bladder or urethra. They tend to be pear-shaped. Squamous cells are large and flat with a prominent nucleus. They originate in the urethra.

RENAL TUBULAR

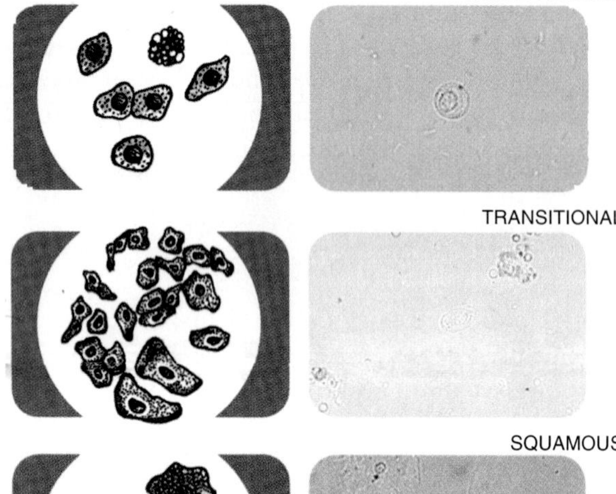

TRANSITIONAL

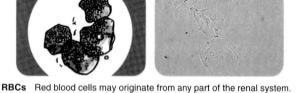

SQUAMOUS

RBCs Red blood cells may originate from any part of the renal system. The presence of large numbers of RBCs in the urine suggests infection, trauma, tumors, renal calculi, etc. However, the presence of 1 or 2 RBC/(HPF) in the urine sediment, or blood in the urine from menstrual contamination, should not be considered abnormal.

RBCs

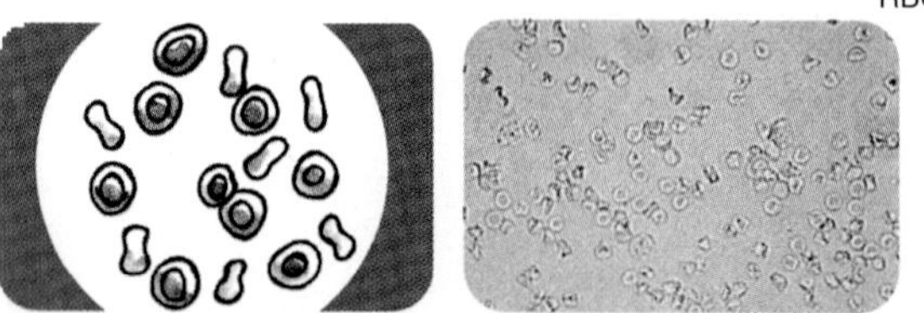

WBCs White blood cells in the urine (pyuria) may originate from any part of the renal system. The presence of more than 5 WBCs per HPF may suggest infection, cystitis, or pyelonephritis.

RENAL TUBULAR & WBC (SEDI-STAIN*)

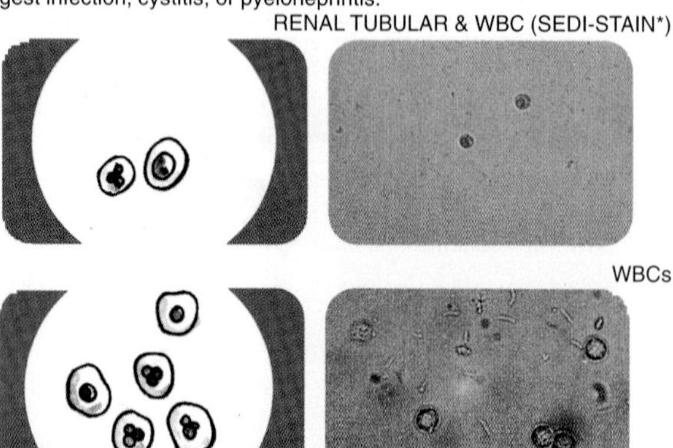

WBCs

CASTS IN URINE

Hyaline Casts Hyaline casts are formed from a protein gel in the renal tubule. Hyaline casts may contain cellular inclusions. Hyaline casts will dissolve very rapidly in alkaline urine. Normal urine sediment may contain 1 to 2 hyaline casts per low power field (LPF).

HYALINE

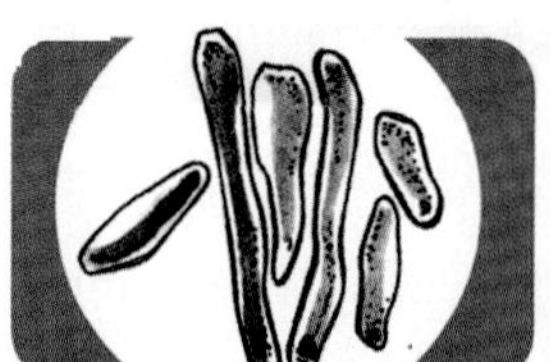

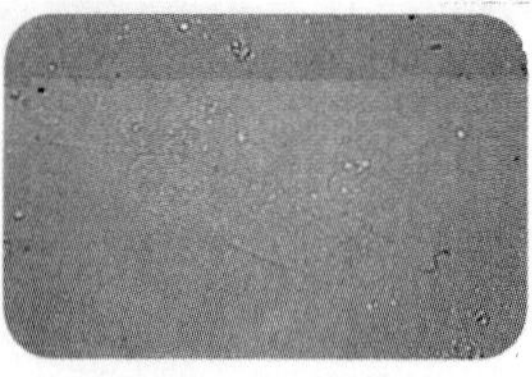

Granular Casts Granular casts are casts with granules present throughout the cast matrix. They are quite refractile. If the granules are small, the cast is defined as a finely granular cast. If granules are large, it is termed a coarsely granular cast. Granular casts can appear in urine in normal or abnormal states.

GRANULAR

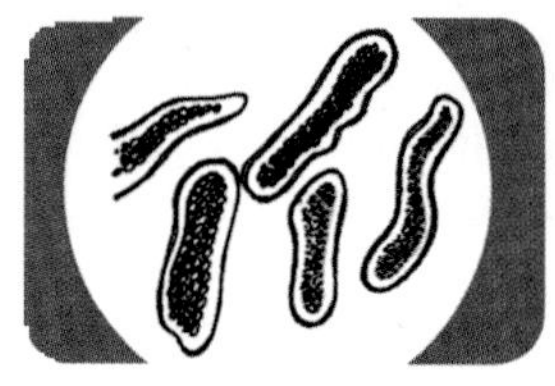

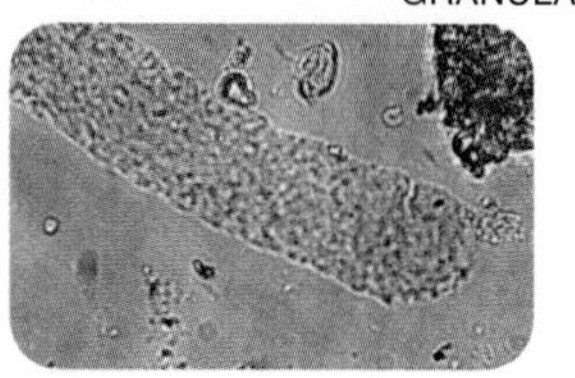

RBC Casts RBC casts are pathologic and their presence is usually indicative of severe injury to the glomerulus. Rarely, transtubular bleeding may occur, forming RBC casts. RBC casts are found in acute glomerulonephritis, lupus, bacterial endocarditis and septicemias. "Blood" casts are granular and contain hemoglobin from degenerated RBCs.

RBC CASTS

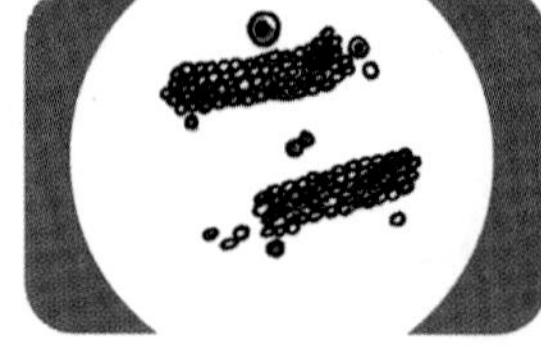

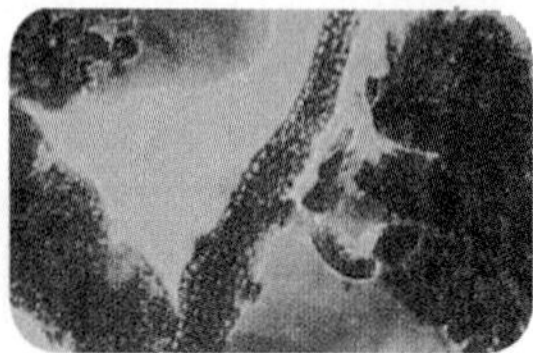

WBC Casts WBC casts occur when leukocytes are incorporated within the cast matrix. WBC casts will usually indicate an infection, most commonly pyelonephritis. They may also be seen in glomerular diseases. WBC casts may be the only clue to pyelonephritis.

WBC CASTS

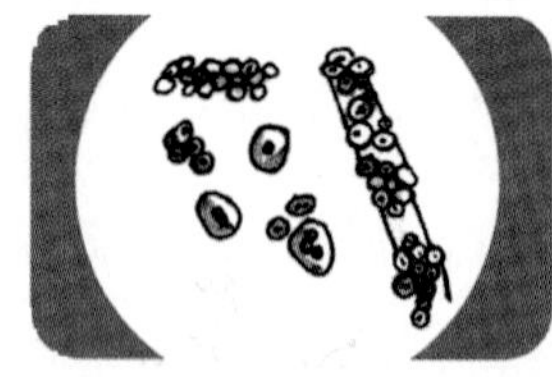

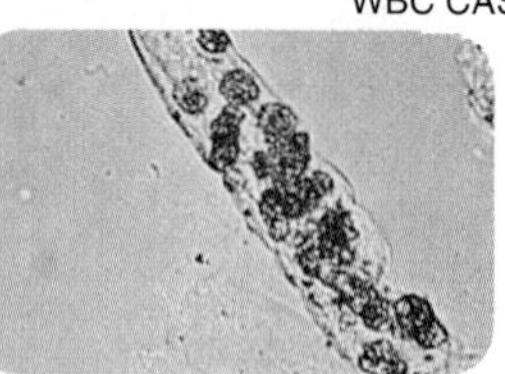

CRYSTALS FOUND IN ACID URINE

Uric Acid Crystals Uric acid has birefringent characteristics; therefore, it polarizes light, giving multi-colors. Uric acid crystals are found in acid urine. Uric acid may assume various forms, e.g., rhombic, plates, rosettes, small crystals. The color may be red-brown, yellow or colorless. Although increased in 16% of patients with gout, and in patients with malignant lymphoma or leukemia, their presence does not usually indicate pathology or increased uric acid concentrations.

URIC ACID (BRIGHTFIELD)

Figure 28-1 Atlas of urine sediment.

CRYSTALS FOUND IN ACID URINE

URIC ACID (POLARIZED)

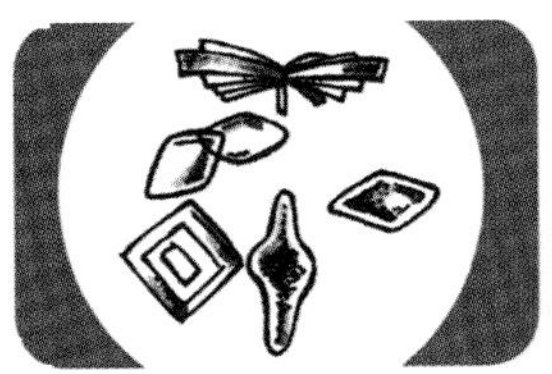

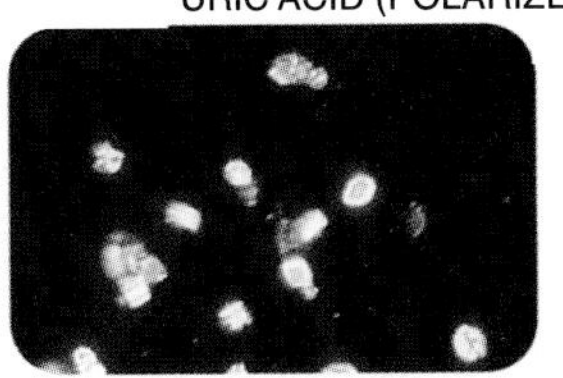

Leucine/Tyrosine Crystals Leucine and tyrosine are amino acids which crystallize and often appear together in the urine of patients with severe liver disease. Tyrosine usually appears as fine needles arranged as sheaves or rosettes and appear yellow. Leucine is usually yellow, oily-appearing spheres with radial and concentric striations.

TYROSINE (BRIGHTFIELD)

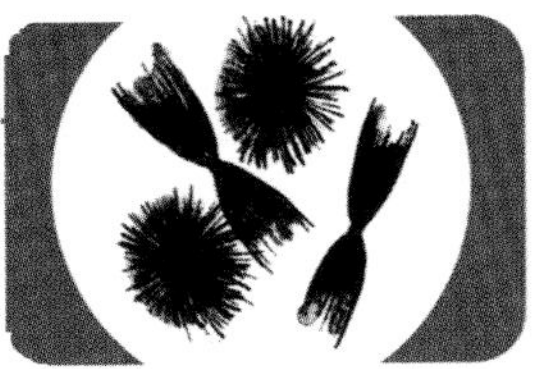

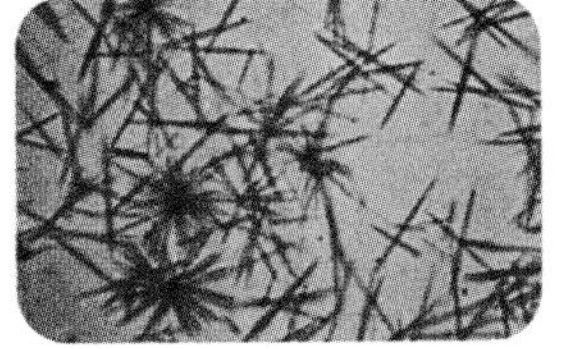

LEUCINE (BRIGHTFIELD)

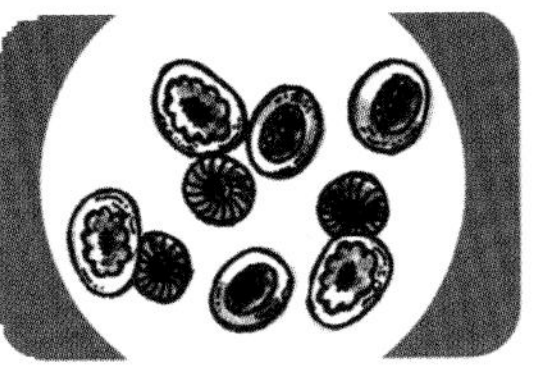

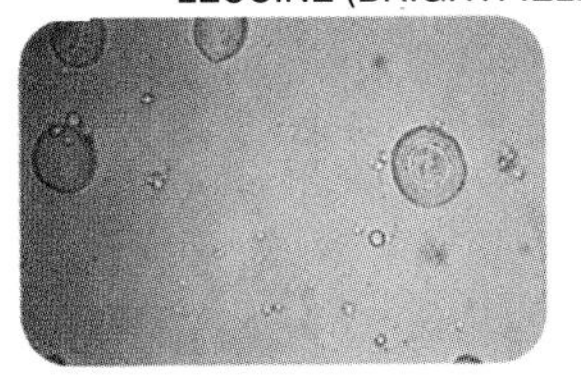

Cystine Crystals Cystine crystals are thin, hexagonal-shaped (6-sided) structures. They appear in the urine as a result of a genetic defect. Cystine crystals and stones will appear in the urine in cystinuria and homocystinuria. Cystine crystals are frequently confused with uric acid crystals. Cystine crystals do not polarize light.

CYSTINE (BRIGHTFIELD)

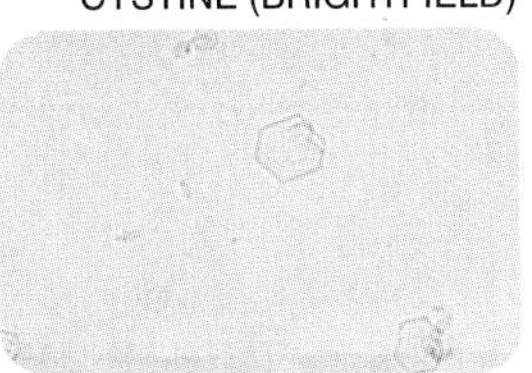

CYSTINE (POLARIZED)

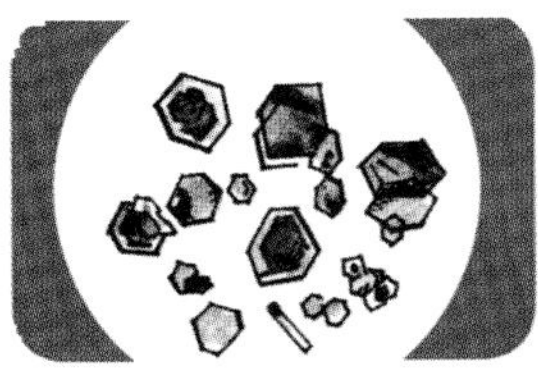

CRYSTALS FOUND IN ACID, NEUTRAL AND ALKALINE URINE

Calcium Oxalate Calcium oxalate crystals most frequently have an "envelope" shape and appear in acid, neutral or slightly alkaline urine. They appear in the urine after the ingestion of certain foods, i.e., cabbage, asparagus.

CALCIUM OXALATE (BRIGHTFIELD)

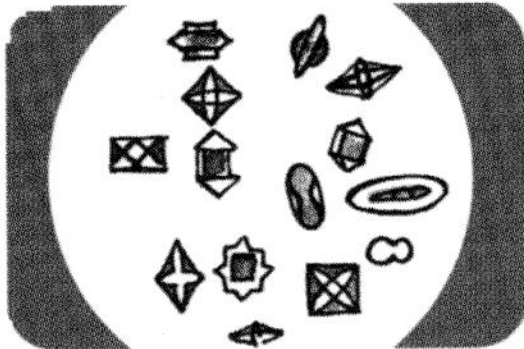

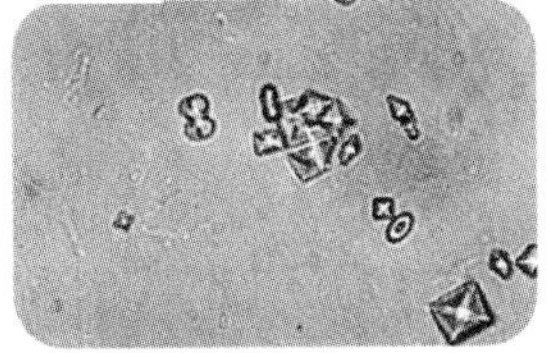

Hippuric Acid Hippuric acid crystals are colorless or pale yellow. They occur as needles, six-sided prisms, or star-shaped clusters. They appear in urine after the ingestion of certain vegetables and fruits with benzoic acid content. They have little clinical significance.

HIPPURIC ACID (BRIGHTFIELD)

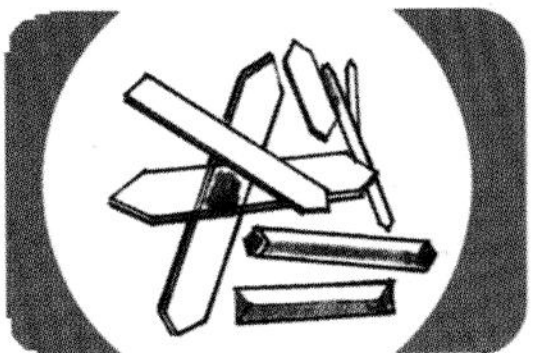

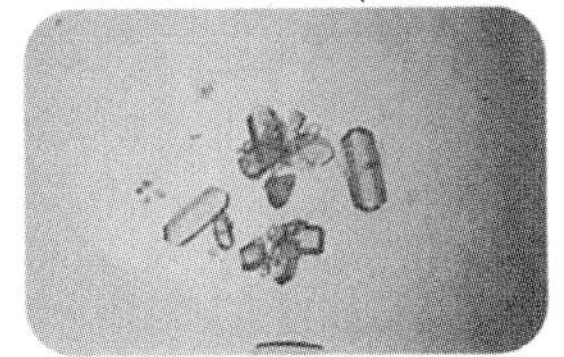

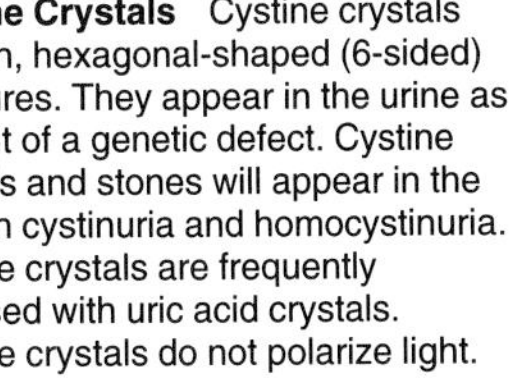

CRYSTALS FOUND IN ALKALINE URINE

Ammonium Biurate or Ammonium Urates Ammonium urates are yellow-brown in appearance and occur in urine as spheres or spheres with spicules ("thorny apples"). Both forms are frequently seen together. They appear in urine when there is ammonia formation in the urine present in the bladder. They are considered to have little clinical significance.

AMMONIUM URATES (BRIGHTFIELD)

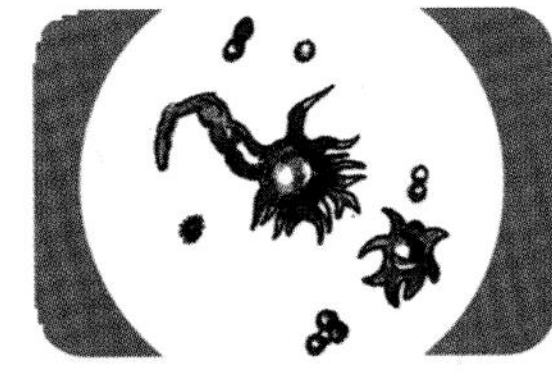

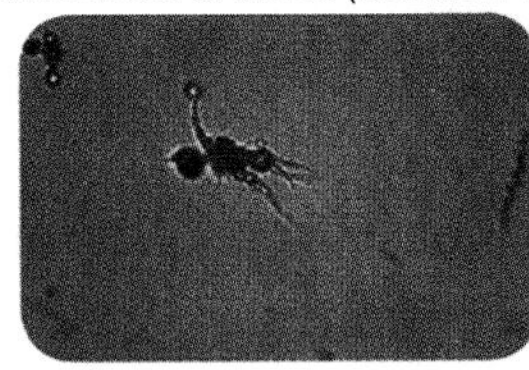

Triple Phosphate Triple phosphate crystals are common in urine sediment. They have a "coffin-lid" shape, are colorless and appear in alkaline urine. The ingestion of fruit may cause triple phosphate to appear in urine.

TRIPLE PHOSPHATE (BRIGHTFIELD)

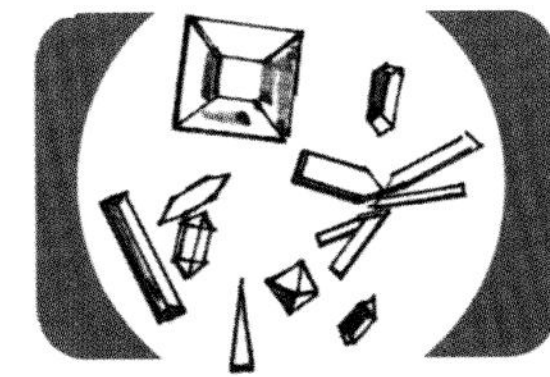

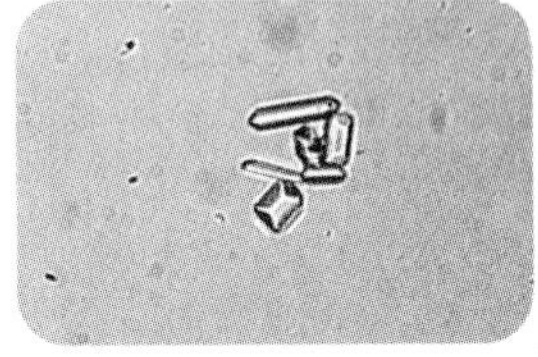

BACTERIA, FUNGI, PARASITES IN URINE

Bacteria Bacteria in the urine (bacteriuria) can result from contaminants in collection vessels, from periurethral tissues, the urethra, or from fecal or vaginal contamination as well as from true urinary infection.

BACTERIA

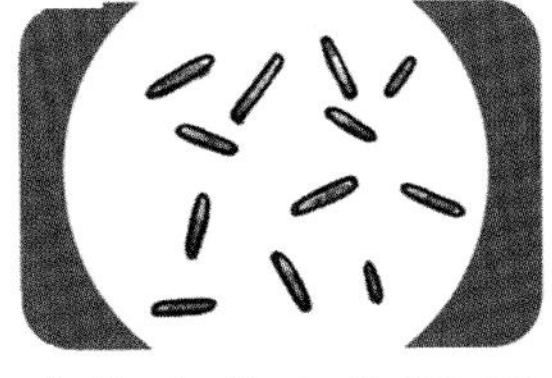

Yeast Yeast cells vary in size, are colorless, ovoid, and are often budding. They are often confused with RBCs. *Candida albicans* is often seen in diabetes, pregnancy, obesity and other debilitating conditions.

YEAST

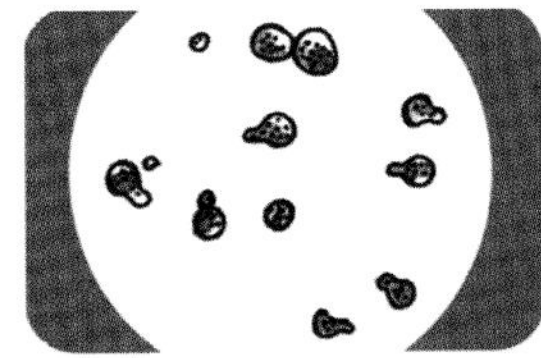

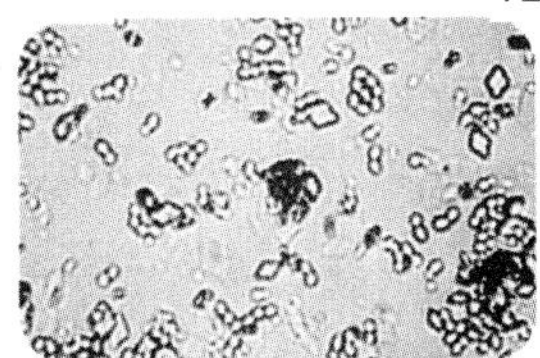

Trichomonas Vaginalis Trichomonas vaginalis is a flagellate protozoan which affects both males (urethritis) and females (vaginitis).

TRICHOMONAS VAGINALIS

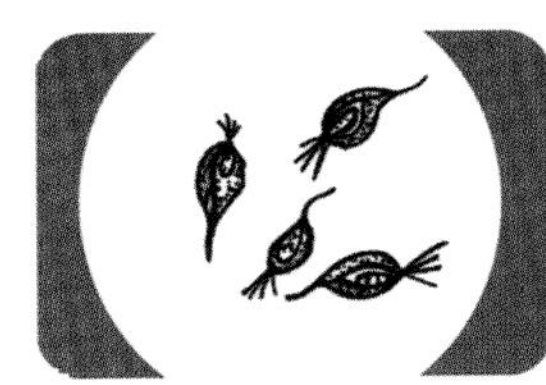

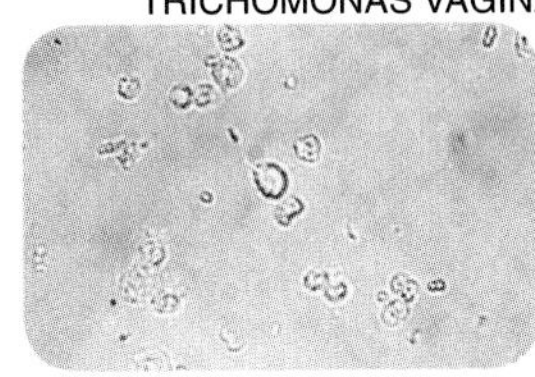

Figure 28-1 (continued)

significant amounts (more than a trace) of bacteria in a urine specimen is considered an indication of a urinary tract infection (UTI).

A positive nitrite test on the chemical strip will correlate with bacteria seen in the sediment. The only bacterium that will not give a nitrite-positive report is *Streptococcus faecalis*. However, *S. faecalis* causes only 1% of UTIs.

Epithelial Cells

Epithelial cells cover the skin and organs and line pathways, such as the digestive or urinary tracts. Their shapes vary according to location. Epithelial cells will normally slough off and are found in the urine, but increased amounts can indicate an irritation, such as inflammation somewhere in the urinary system. Three different types of epithelial cells may be found in the urine: squamous, transitional, and renal. Squamous epithelial cells cover external surfaces and are considered a normal finding. Transitional epithelial cells line the bladder and are seen with infections of the lower urinary tract, such as cystitis. Renal epithelial cells line the nephrons and are seen with infections and inflammations of the upper urinary tract.

No chemical test exists for epithelial cells. However, if renal epithelial cells are seen in urinary sediment, damage to the renal tubules is likely, and the protein test may be positive.

Crystals

Crystals are made up of a chemical substance present in the urine in sufficient quantities to form a solid three-dimensional structure that can be seen microscopically. The three most common crystals found in urine sediment—calcium oxalate, uric acid (both of which occur in acidic urine with a pH below 7.0), and triple phosphate (found in alkaline urine, above 7.0)—are not pathologic. Uric acid crystals can, however, be seen with fevers, leukemia, or gout.

Crystals can also contribute to the formation of stones in the urinary tract. Box 28-2 describes urinary tract stone formation and specimen collection.

Casts

Cast formation occurs in the tubules of the nephron. When protein is present in sufficient quantities, it will cement together whatever solutes or cells are in the tubule as well; this is a cast. Most casts eventually break free and flow into the urine. The type of cast can indicate certain pathologies. For instance, in pyelonephritis, white cells that are present to combat the infection become trapped in the protein network and form white cell casts. Casts are counted on low

Box 28-2

Urinary Tract Stone Formation

Stones are formed in the urinary system by crystals of normally occurring substances, such as calcium oxalate, calcium phosphate, and uric acid. Uroliths range in size from minute particles as fine as sand to huge staghorn calculi that fill the renal pelvis and cystoliths that fill the bladder.

Many disorders contribute to the formation of renal calculi. These disorders include hypercalcemia, excessive dietary vitamin D, and certain bone disorders, such as leukemia or polycythemia vera. Stones also may form as a sequela to an ileostomy or a bowel resection.

Patients may present with symptoms ranging from mild discomfort to severe and debilitating pain. Symptoms may include pyelonephritis, cystitis, generalized signs of infection, dysuria, flank pain, hematuria, and pyuria. As stones pass into the ureter, pain may become excruciating.

Diagnosis is confirmed by radiography and blood chemistries. Patient history is important to determining patient predisposition to stone formation.

Patients are instructed to collect a 24-hour urine specimen for measurement of calcium, uric acid, creatinine, sodium, and pH. In many cases, the medical assistant will assist with instructions for collection. Patients with uroliths are usually required to strain the urine before adding it to the collection. Urine may be collected in a bedpan or toilet collection receptacle ("nun's cap" or "Mexican hat"), or it may be voided into a small collection bottle before adding to the 24-hour receptacle. In acute onset situations, the patient may bring to the office a specimen collected at home that must be strained at the office. Retain all evidence of solids for analysis.

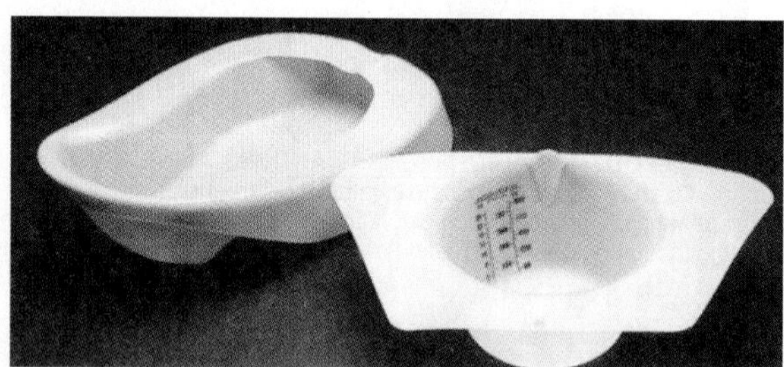

Bedpan (*left*) and toilet collection receptacle ("nun's cap" or "Mexican hat").

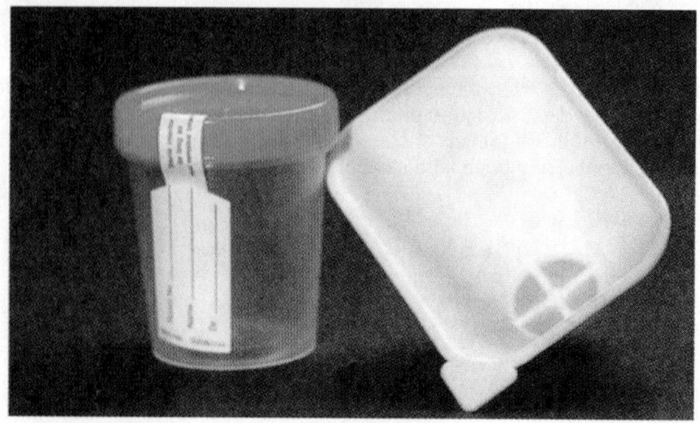

Urine specimen container (*left*) and urine strainer for stone collection.

power with reduced light and are reported as a number per low power field (LPF).

Checkpoint Question

5. *What are three of the most common crystals found in urine?*

Other Structures

Many other structures can be found in the urine sediment. Yeast found in the urine can result from a vaginal contamination of the specimen or may be the causative agent of a UTI, especially in a diabetic patient. The parasite *Trichomonas vaginalis* is a frequent contaminant from the genital tract of an infected person. Mucus may be present if there is an inflammation in the urinary tract. Mucous threads are usually reported in quantities, such as few, moderate, or many. Spermatozoa may be found when there has been a recent emission.

What If?

What if a patient asks you what drugs can be detected in the urine? What would you say?

Many employers are requiring routine drug testing for their employees using urine specimens. Urine tests are preferred to blood tests because they are less expensive and are noninvasive. The following drugs can be detected in the urine: amphetamines, barbiturates, benzodiazepines, cocaine, marijuana, opiates, PCP, and methadone. If you are involved in obtaining urine specimens for drug testing, it is essential that you ensure security of the urine and confidentiality of the results.

URINE PREGNANCY TESTING

Human chorionic gonadotropin (HCG) is a hormone secreted by the developing placenta shortly after conception. Its appearance and rapid rise in concentration in the mother's serum and urine make it an excellent marker for confirming a pregnancy. Many test kits are available that can detect levels as low as 25 mIU/mL. These levels are typically seen within 10 to 12 days after fertilization, often before the first missed period. Most test kits simply require the addition of urine to test and are very easy to use. First-morning urine specimens are the specimen of choice because the urine is most concentrated at that time. Many laboratories will test the specific gravity and will not report a negative pregnancy result if it is below 1.005 because the urine may be too dilute to detect low HCG serum levels.

Answers to Checkpoint Questions

1. *Urine should be tested within 1 hour of collection. (If testing cannot be performed within 1 hour, refrigerate the specimen at 4°C–6°C until testing can be performed.) If the urine is not properly refrigerated, the specimen can deteriorate.*
2. *The three physical properties of urine are color, clarity, and specific gravity. Color and clarity are assessed visually.*
3. *A positive ketone test indicates that the body is burning more fat than normal.*
4. *Positive nitrates and leukocytes on a dipstick would suggest a urinary tract infection.*
5. *Three of the most common crystals found in urine are calcium oxalate, uric acid, and triple phosphate.*

Critical Thinking Challenges

1. Most laboratories pour off a portion of a urine specimen to test rather than dipping the chemical reagent strip directly into the urine container. Why?
2. Why would burn and trauma patients need a urinalysis? What results would you expect to see and why?

Suggestions for Further Reading

Bullock, B. L. (1996). *Pathophysiology: Adaptations and Alterations in Function,* 4th ed. Philadelphia: Lippincott-Raven.

Fishbach, F. (1996). *A Manual of Laboratory and Diagnostic Tests,* 5th ed. Philadelphia: Lippincott-Raven.

Graff, S. L. (1983). *A Handbook of Routine Urinalysis.* Philadelphia: J.B. Lippincott.

Memmler, R. L., Cohen, B. J., & Wood, D. L. (1996). *The Human Body in Health and Disease,* 8th ed. Philadelphia: Lippincott-Raven.

Rubin, E., & Farber, J. L. (1994). *Pathology,* 2nd ed. Philadelphia: J.B. Lippincott.

29 Phlebotomy

Chapter Outline

Blood Collection Sites
- Capillary Blood
- Venous Blood
- Arterial Blood

General Blood Drawing Equipment
- Blood Drawing Station
- Gloves
- Disinfectants and Antiseptics
- Sterile Gauze Pads
- Bandages
- Needle and Sharps Disposal Containers
- Slides

Venipuncture Equipment
- Tourniquets
- Needles

Blood Collection Systems
- Evacuated Tube System
- Syringe System
- Wing Infusion Set

Order of Draw
- Evacuated Tube System
- Syringe System

Skin Puncture (Microcollection) Equipment
- Lancets
- Microcollection Tubes
- Microcollection Containers
- Micropipet Dilution Systems
- Filter Paper Devices
- Warming Devices

Patient Preparation

Performing a Venipuncture
- Complications of Venipuncture

Performing a Skin Puncture
- Complications of Skin Puncture

Role Delineation

CLINICAL

Fundamental Principles
- Apply principles of aseptic technique and infection control.

Diagnostic Orders
- Collect and process specimens.
- Perform diagnostic tests.

Patient Care
- Prepare and maintain examination and treatment areas.
- Prepare patient for examinations, procedures, and treatments.

GENERAL

Professionalism
- Project a professional manner and image.

Legal Concepts
- Practice within the scope of education, training, and personal capabilities.
- Document accurately.
- Comply with established risk management and safety procedures.

Chapter Competencies

Learning Objectives

Upon successfully completing this chapter, you will be able to:

1. Define and spell the Key Terms.
2. Identify equipment and supplies used to obtain a routine venous specimen and a routine capillary skin puncture.
3. List the anticoagulants used, the order of draw, and color coding recognized with each type for the collection of blood specimens.
4. Discuss the location and selection of the blood collection sites for capillaries and veins.

Chapter Competencies *(continued)*

5. Explain the importance of correct patient identification and complete specimen and requisition labeling.
6. Describe the steps in preparation of the puncture site for venipuncture and skin puncture.
7. Describe care for a puncture site after blood has been drawn.
8. List precautions to be observed when drawing blood.

Performance Objectives

Upon successfully completing this chapter, you will be able to:

1. Obtain a blood specimen from a patient by venipuncture (Procedure 29-1).
2. Obtain a blood specimen from a patient by skin puncture (Procedure 29-2).
3. Use a butterfly collection system.
4. Use a Unopette system for diluting blood specimens.

Key Terms

(See Glossary for definitions.)

antecubital area	**edema**	**palmar**
antiseptic	**gel separator**	**thromboplastin**
arteriole	**hemolysis**	**venule**
cyanotic	**Luer adapter**	**whorls**

The literal translation of the word phlebotomy means incision into a vein. Phlebotomy is performed today by one of two procedures:

1. *Venipuncture*—collecting blood by penetrating a vein with a needle and syringe or other collection apparatus
2. *Skin puncture*—collecting blood after puncturing the skin with a lancet or similar puncture device

Most blood collection procedures are performed by the medical assistant or phlebotomist. You will need to study and practice to obtain blood specimens successfully. You also will need to ensure that blood collection is performed in the safest manner possible. Blood is recognized as a hazardous material, so it should be handled with the use of Standard Precautions and appropriate barrier devices.

BLOOD COLLECTION SITES

The three main types of blood vessels are capillaries, veins, and arteries. Blood can be obtained from all three types of vessels. You will routinely use capillaries and veins for collecting blood specimens. Arterial blood is not drawn by medical assistants.

Capillary Blood

Capillaries are the smallest vessels that carry blood, and they form the link between arterioles (small arteries) and venules (small veins). Blood from a capillary puncture (skin puncture) may be taken when:

- Small amounts of blood are needed
- The patient is a child under age 2
- The patient's veins are inaccessible or damaged
- Veins must be preserved for parenteral therapy

The puncture sites most often used to obtain capillary blood are the finger, heel, and big toe. The earlobe is rarely used as a collection site but may be chosen under certain circumstances. In adults and older children, the usual puncture site is the **palmar** surface (palm of the hand) of the end segment of the second or third finger (middle or ring finger) of the nondominant hand.

The puncture should be made in the central, fleshy portion of the finger, slightly to the side of center and perpendicular to the **whorls** (spirals and ridges) of the fingerprint. This procedure will allow the blood to form a bead or drop that is easily collected. Infants 3 months of age or younger have capillary blood drawn from a prewarmed heel; older infants may have blood taken from their big toes. Skin puncture sites should be warm, pink, and free of scars, cuts, bruises, **edema** (fluid accumulation), calluses, and rashes.

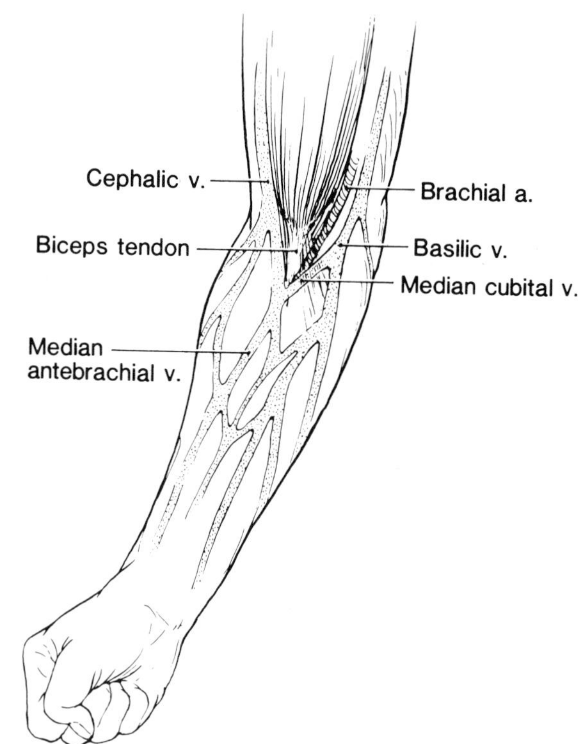

Figure 29-1 The venous structure. (a = artery; v = vein.) (Redrawn from Valaske, M.D. [ed] [1982]. *So You're Going to Collect a Blood Specimen*, College of American Pathologists, rev ed, p 16. Skokie, IL.)

Venous Blood

Systemic veins carry blood toward the heart after oxygen and nutrients from the blood have been delivered to the cells of the body. **Venules** are very small veins that are connected to capillaries. Venules widen as they travel toward the heart and become veins that gradually increase in size until they reach the vena cavae. Most laboratory testing is done on blood drawn from veins because they are easily accessible and can yield large amounts of blood.

The forearm veins located in the **antecubital area** (the inner surface of the bend of the elbow) are commonly used for venipuncture. The three main veins in this area are the cephalic, median cubital, and the basilic (Fig. 29-1). The primary vein for venipuncture is the median cubital vein. The fingertips are used to palpate (feel) or press on the vein gently to determine its direction and to estimate its size and depth. Veins will feel spongy, like an elastic tube. Alternative sites may be indicated if the area is **cyanotic** (bluish skin discoloration caused by lack of oxygen), scarred, bruised, edematous, or burned. Veins on the lower forearm, the back of the hand, or wrist may also be used. Use foot or ankle veins only if the patient has good circulation to the legs and permission is received from the patient's physician.

Arterial Blood

Arteries in the systemic circulation are vessels that carry oxygenated blood away from the heart. Arteries branch into smaller vessels called **arterioles,** which then connect with capillaries. Physicians order arterial punctures to assess how well the lungs are functioning. Medical assistants do not normally draw arterial blood specimens but should be aware of artery locations so the arteries will not be entered when performing a venipuncture. Arteries can be distinguished from veins because they have a pulse, and veins do not.

Inadvertent arterial puncture can be suspected if the blood spurts or pulses into the tube and the color of the blood is bright red compared with the darker red color of venous blood. If an artery is entered by mistake, maintain pressure on the site for 5 to 10 minutes or until all bleeding has stopped. If the specimen has already been collected, it may be used for testing. However, the tube, the request, and the laboratory report must be labeled as arterial blood.

Checkpoint Question

1. *Name four situations that may require capillary puncture?*

GENERAL BLOOD DRAWING EQUIPMENT

Blood Drawing Station

A blood drawing station is equipped for performing phlebotomy procedures on outpatients or patients in medical offices (Fig. 29-2). This station includes a

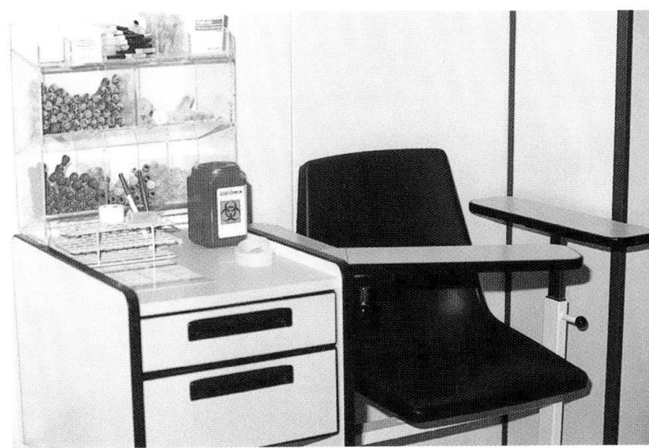

Figure 29-2 A well-stocked blood drawing station.

table for supplies close at hand and a chair or bed for the patient. The table should be a convenient height for working with enough space to hold numerous supplies. The chair should be comfortable and have an adjustable armrest with a safety device to lock the armrest in place to prevent the patient from falling if fainting occurs. A bed or reclining chair should be available for patients with a history of fainting and to perform heel sticks or other procedures on infants and small children.

Gloves

Guidelines from the Centers for Disease Control and Prevention (CDC) and the Occupational Safety and Health Administration (OSHA) require that gloves be worn when performing phlebotomy procedures. A new pair of gloves must be used for each patient and removed when the procedure is finished. Latex, vinyl, or polyethylene nonsterile, disposable gloves are acceptable.

Disinfectants and Antiseptics

Disinfectants kill bacteria. They are used on inanimate objects, such as instruments and surfaces. They are not to be used on human skin. Household bleach in a 1:10 solution is commonly used to wipe surfaces and clean up blood spills in the phlebotomy station. This disinfectant will kill viruses that cause acquired immunodeficiency syndrome (AIDS) and hepatitis.

Antiseptics prevent or inhibit the growth of bacteria. They are safe for use on human skin and are used to clean the skin before skin puncture or venipuncture. The most commonly used antiseptic for routine blood collection is 70% isopropyl alcohol. Another antiseptic frequently used for blood culture collection is povidone-iodine.

What If?

What if you or your patient is allergic to latex products?

If you are allergic to latex, OSHA requires your employer to provide other appropriate gloves and supplies for you. If your patient is allergic to latex, you must use products such as gloves and tourniquets made from substances other than latex. Latex is also found in catheters, some elastic bandages, wheelchair tires, disposable diapers, and disposable underpads. Latex is made from the sap of the *Hevea brasiliensis* tree. Latex allergies were first identified in 1989 and have resulted in many deaths when used in surgical procedures involving extended exposure to the inner surfaces of the body. The signs of allergic reactions can be minor (redness, rash, itching at the site) or more severe (hives, wheezing, angioedema, and bronchospasm). The signs and symptoms are treated with epinephrine and bronchodilators. Tests are available to determine latex allergies.

Sterile Gauze Pads

Sterile 2 × 2 gauze pads are used to hold pressure over the site after skin puncture or venipuncture. Cotton or rayon balls may be used, but these have a tendency to stick to the site and may cause bleeding to start again when pulled from the site.

Bandages

Adhesive bandages are used to cover the site once the bleeding has stopped. If a patient is allergic to adhesive bandages, use paper cloth, or knitted tape over a folded gauze square. Do not use bandages on infants under 2 years of age because of the danger of aspiration and suffocation.

Needle and Sharps Disposal Containers

Immediately dispose of used needles, lancets, and other sharp objects in puncture-resistant, leakproof, disposable containers referred to as "sharps" containers. These containers are usually marked as "biohazard" and are red or bright orange for easy identification. Needles should not be cut, bent, or broken before disposal. If the needle must be recapped, use the single-handed scoop technique.

Slides

Slides are available either plain or with a frosted end where the patient's name and other information can be written in pencil. Precleaned 1 × 3-inch glass microscope slides are used to make blood films for hematology studies.

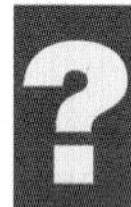

Checkpoint Question

2. *Explain when disinfectants are used, and when antiseptics are used.*

VENIPUNCTURE EQUIPMENT

Venipuncture procedures require the use of the following special equipment.

Tourniquets

The tourniquet constricts the venous flow of blood in the arm and makes the veins more prominent, making them easier to find and penetrate with a needle. The most common type of tourniquet is a soft, pliable rubber strip, usually 1 inch wide by 15 to 18 inches long. It can be released easily with one hand, does not cut into the patient's arm, can be wiped with a disinfectant to prevent the spread of infection, and is inexpensive enough to be replaced often. Some offices require a fresh tourniquet for each patient.

The tourniquet should be placed 3 to 4 inches above the proposed venipuncture site and secured by using the half-bow. The half-bow makes it easy to remove the tourniquet with just one hand. Velcro-closure, rubber tubing, or a blood pressure cuff may also be used as a tourniquet.

Needles

Sterile, disposable, single-use-only needles are used for venipuncture. They are silicon-coated, which enables them to penetrate the skin smoothly. The end of the needle is cut on a slant or bevel. The bevel allows the needle to penetrate the vein easily and prevents "coring," or the removal of a portion of skin or vein. The long, cylindrical portion of the needle is called the shaft, and the end that connects to the blood-drawing apparatus is called the hub.

The gauge of a needle indicates the size of the needle and refers to the lumen or "bore" of the needle. The larger the gauge number, the smaller the actual diameter of the needle (eg, 20 gauge is larger than 25 gauge). Gauge selection depends on the size and condition of the vein.

Figure 29-3 shows the special equipment and supplies used for phlebotomy.

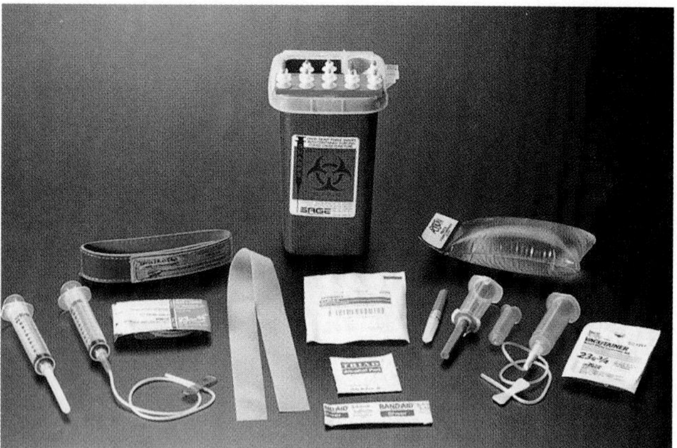

Figure 29-3 Equipment and supplies used for phlebotomy.

BLOOD COLLECTION SYSTEMS

Two blood collection systems are commonly used for venipuncture. One is the vacuum or evacuated tube system, and the other is the syringe system (Fig. 29-4).

Evacuated Tube System

The evacuated tube system consists of a special double-pointed multisample needle, a tube holder (or adapter), and vacuum tubes. The needle screws into

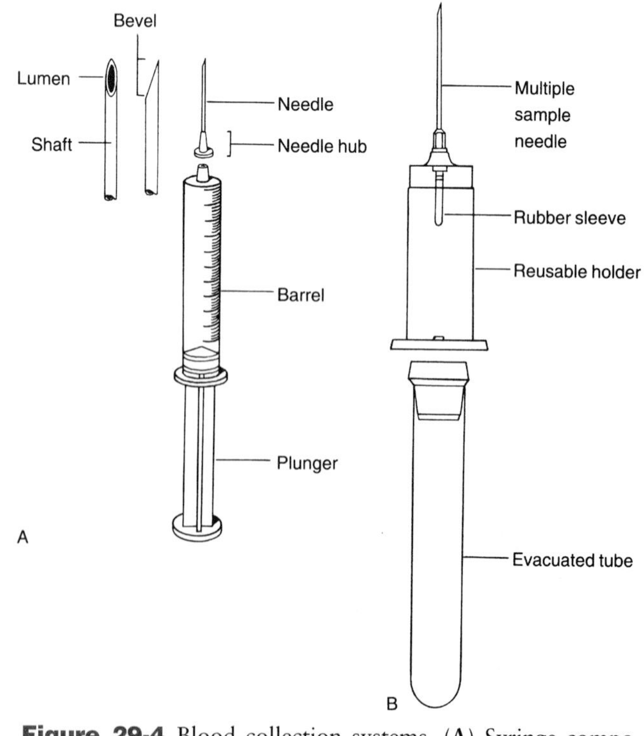

Figure 29-4 Blood collection systems. (**A**) Syringe components. (**B**) Components of the evacuated tube collection system.

Table 29-1 **Tube Guide**

Tube Guide

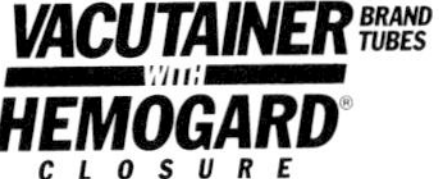

VACUTAINER® Tubes with HEMOGARD Closure	VACUTAINER Tubes	Additive	Number of Inversions at Blood Collection (Invert gently, do not shake)	Laboratory Use
Gold		• Clot activator and gel for serum separation	5	SST Brand Tube for serum determinations in chemistry. Tube inversions ensure mixing of clot activator with blood and clotting within 30 minutes.
Light Green		• Lithium heparin and gel for plasma separation	8	PST Brand Tube for plasma determinations in chemistry. Tube inversions prevent clotting.
Red		• None	0	For serum determinations in chemistry, serology and blood banking.
Orange		• Thrombin	8	For stat serum determinations in chemistry. Tube inversions ensure complete clotting, usually in less than 5 minutes.
Royal Blue		• Sodium heparin • Na_2EDTA • None	8 8 0	For trace element, toxicology and nutrient determinations. Special stopper formulation offers low levels of trace elements (see package insert).
Green		• Sodium heparin • Lithium heparin	8 8	For plasma determinations in chemistry. Tube inversions prevent clotting.
Gray		• Potassium oxalate/ sodium fluoride • Sodium fluoride • Lithium iodoacetate • Lithium iodoacetate/ lithium heparin	8 8 8 8	For glucose determinations. Tube inversions ensure proper mixing of additive and blood. Oxalate and heparin, anticoagulants, will give plasma samples. Without them, samples are serum.
Brown		• Sodium heparin	8	For lead determinations. This tube is certified to contain less than .01 µg/mL (ppm) lead. Tube inversions prevent clotting.
Yellow		• Sodium polyanetholesulfonate (SPS) OR • ACD - Acid Citrate Dextrose Additives: Solution A - 22.0g/L trisodium citrate, 8.0g/L citric acid, 24.5g/L dextrose Solution B - 13.2g/L trisodium citrate, 4.8g/L citric acid, 14.7g/L dextrose	8 8 8	For blood culture specimen collections in microbiology. Tube inversions prevent clotting. For use in blood bank studies, HLA phenotyping, DNA and Paternity testing.

(continued)

29

Table 29-1 **Tube Guide** *(Continued)*

VACUTAINER® Tubes with HEMOGARD Closure	VACUTAINER Tubes	Additive	Number of Inversions at Blood Collection (Invert gently, do not shake)	Laboratory Use
Lavender		• Liquid K_3EDTA • Spray-dried K_2EDTA	8 8	For whole blood hematology determinations. Tube inversions prevent clotting.
Light Blue		• .105M sodium citrate (3.2%) • .129M sodium citrate (3.8%)	8 8	For coagulation determinations on plasma specimens. Tube inversions prevent clotting. NOTE: Certain tests require chilled specimens. Follow recommended procedures for collection and transport of specimen.

For technical information, call **1-800-631-0174**

BECTON DICKINSON

Becton Dickinson VACUTAINER Systems, Franklin Lakes, New Jersey 07417
VACUTAINER, HEMOGARD, SST and PST are trademarks of Becton Dickinson and Company.

© 1990 Printed in USA 4/96 U.S. Pat No. 4,741,446 and foreign

VACUTAINER BRAND QUALITY MAKES THE DIFFERENCE

Becton Dickinson VACUTAINER Systems, Franklin Lakes, New Jersey 07417
VACUTAINER, HEMOGARD, SST and PST are trademarks of Becton Dickinson and Company. © 1990

(Courtesy of Becton Dickinson. Used with permission.)

threads on one end of the tube holder, and tubes are inserted into the wide-mouthed opposite end of the holder. The needle and tube holder function as a unit; neither is able to function without the other.

The evacuated tube system needle is threaded in the middle with a beveled tip on each end. One end of the needle is used to enter the patient's vein; the other end attaches to the tube holder. The needle is enclosed in a sterile twist-apart shield. Twisting apart the shield uncovers the end of the needle that threads into the tube holder. The other end of the needle remains covered by a removable cap until it is time to insert the needle into a vein. The end of the needle that attaches to the tube holder is covered by a rubber sleeve that retracts when inserted into an evacuated tube, allowing the tube to fill with blood. The needle is called a multisample needle because the sleeve recovers the needle as the tube is removed, preventing blood from leaking into the tube holder when changing tubes during a multiple tube draw and when the tube is removed before withdrawing the needle from the vein. Needles are available in two lengths, 1 inch and 1½ inches, and in 20 to 22 gauge, with 21-gauge being the one most commonly used for routine venipuncture.

The holder, sometimes called an adapter, makes the task of collecting the blood sample easier. It has an indentation about ½ inch from the hub. This indentation marks the point where the short, sleeved end of the needle starts to enter the rubber stopper of the tube. If the tube is inserted past this point before entering the vein, the tube will fill with air, and it will not be possible to draw a blood sample. There are flanges (extensions) on the sides of the rim of the holder to aid in tube placement and removal.

Evacuated collection tubes contain a vacuum with a rubber stopper sealing the tube. These tubes range in size from 2 to 15 mL. The tubes are sterile to prevent contamination of the specimen and the patient. Evacuated tubes may or may not contain an additive. Blood collected in tubes without additives will clot and separate into serum and cells on centrifugation.

Tube Additives

An additive is any substance (other than the tube coating) that is placed in a tube. Additives have specific functions. Below is a list of the most common types of additives and their functions:

- Anticoagulant—prevents the blood from coagulating or clotting
- Clot activator—enhances coagulation
- Thixotropic **gel separator**—a special inert substance that forms a physical barrier between the cells and the serum or plasma portion of a specimen after the specimen is centrifuged

The evacuated tube system uses color-coded stoppers as a means of identifying the additive content of each type of tube (Table 29-1).

Syringe System

Syringes are made of either glass or disposable plastic, varying in volume from 1 to 50 mL. Both types must be sterile for use. The barrel of the syringe is graduated in milliliters. Pulling on the plunger of the syringe creates a vacuum within the barrel. The plunger often sticks and is hard to pull. A technique called "breathing the syringe" makes the plunger easier to move. To do this, before beginning the procedure, pull back the plunger to about halfway the length the barrel, then push the plunger back. This makes the plunger move more smoothly and reduces the tendency to jerk when first pulled after insertion into the vein.

The vacuum created by pulling on the plunger while a needle is in a patient's vein fills the syringe with blood. Pulling the plunger slowly and resting between pulls allows the vein time to refill with blood. Blood specimens collected by syringe must be transferred to evacuated tubes following proper order of draw (see the section "Order of Draw," below).

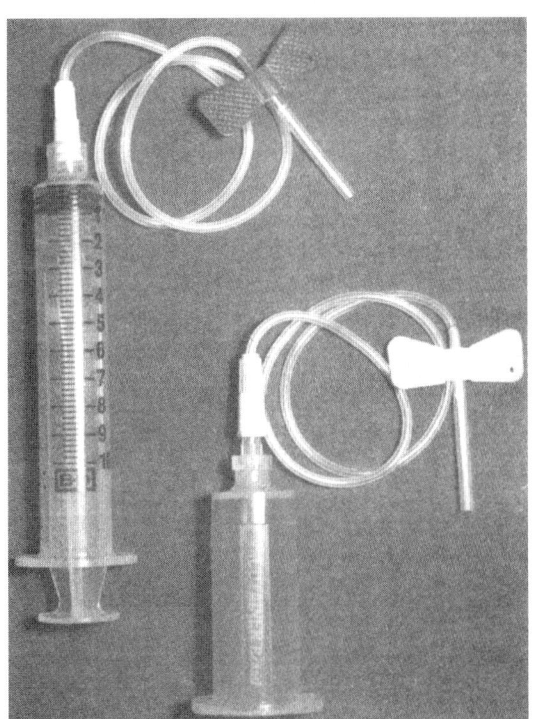

Figure 29-5 Wing infusion sets: (*left*) attached to a syringe; (*right*) attached to evacuated tube holder by means of a Luer adapter.

Wing Infusion Set

The butterfly collection system or wing infusion set has a stainless steel beveled needle with attached wing-shaped plastic extensions connected to a 6- to 12-inch length of tubing. The most common butterfly needle sizes are 21 to 23 gauge with ½- to ¾-inch lengths. Butterflies come with attachments to be used with syringes and a special multisample **Luer adapter** (a device for connecting a syringe or evacuated holder to the needle) that allows them to be used in an evacuated tube system (Fig. 29-5). The set is routinely used to collect blood from patients who have difficult or small veins and from pediatric patients. Figure 29-6 shows how to use the butterfly system.

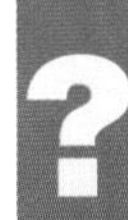

Checkpoint Question

3. *What three chemical substances may be added to collection tubes? Explain the function of each.*

➤ ORDER OF DRAW

Evacuated Tube System

When multiple tubes are to be drawn in the evacuated tube system, the following "order of draw" is recommended to avoid contamination of nonadditive tubes by additive tubes as well as cross-contamination between different types of additive tubes:

1. Blood culture tubes (and other tests requiring sterile specimens)
2. Red stopper or red/gray stopper (nonadditive and gel separator)
3. Light blue stopper (If a light blue-stoppered tube is the first and only tube to be drawn, draw a 5-mL red-stoppered tube first and discard it to eliminate contamination from tissue **thromboplastin,** a substance that aids clotting, picked up during needle penetration.)
4. Green stopper
5. Lavender stopper
6. Gray stopper

29

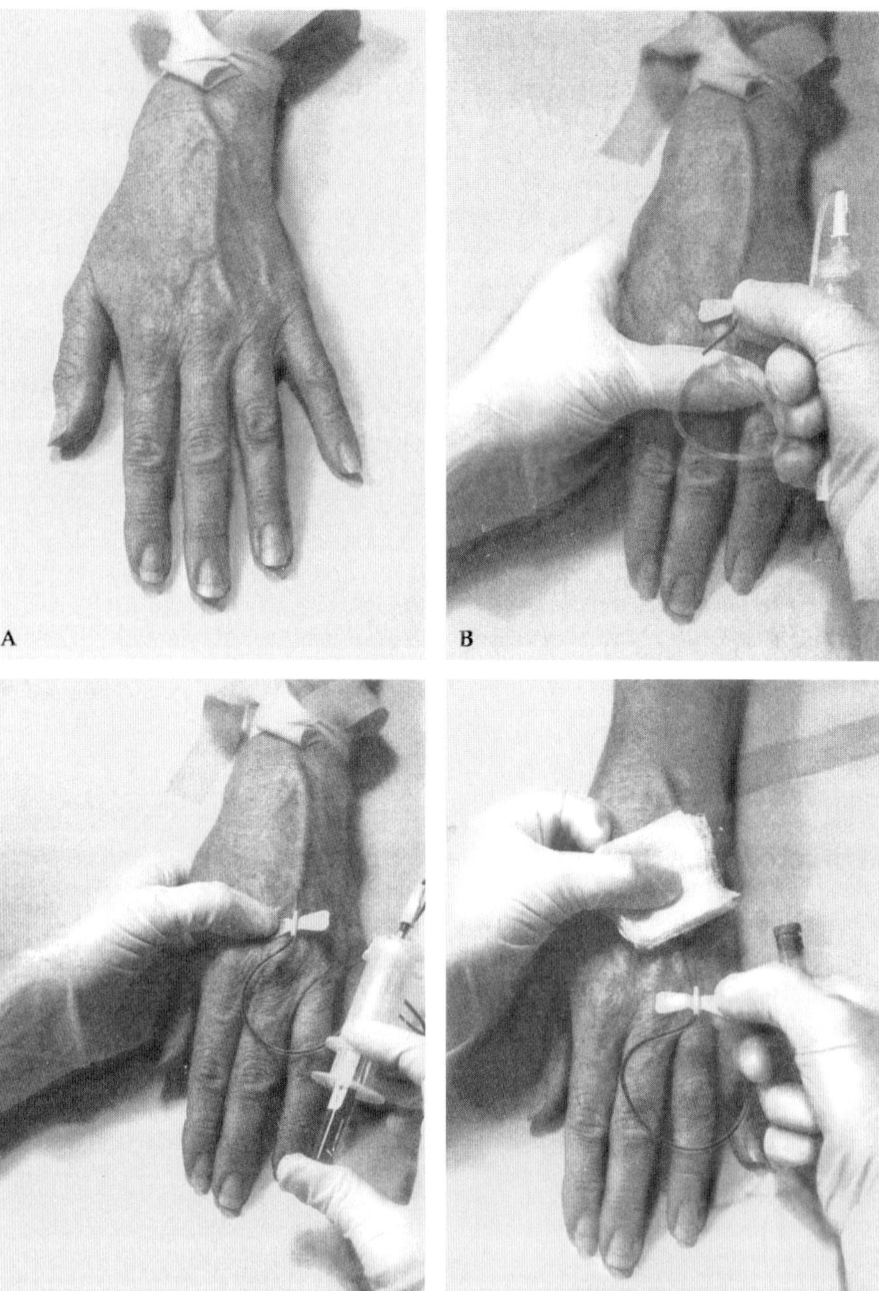

Figure 29-6 Procedure for using butterfly in a hand vein. (**A**) Hand with tourniquet in place reveals prominent vein. (**B**) With the skin pulled taught over the knuckles, the needle is inserted into the vein until there is a "flash" of blood in the tubing. (**C**) Using the nondominant hand, a wing of the butterfly is held against the patient's hand to steady the needle while the blood collecting tube is pushed onto the blood collecting needle. (**D**) Once the proper tubes have been drawn, release the tourniquet, then release the needle. Gauze is placed over the vein, and the needle is removed.

Syringe System

The order of draw for this system differs from the evacuated tube system's order of draw. The blood that enters the syringe last is the freshest and will be the first blood out of the syringe in the transfer process. The clotting process begins the second the blood enters the syringe; therefore, it is important to transfer the blood quickly and fill anticoagulant tubes before serum tubes. The suggested order of draw for syringes is:

1. Blood culture
2. Light blue
3. Lavender
4. Green
5. Gray
6. Red

> **Checkpoint Question**
>
> **4.** *What is the proper order of draw when using the evacuated tube system? Why is this important?*

SKIN PUNCTURE (MICROCOLLECTION) EQUIPMENT

In some instances, a blood specimen cannot be obtained by a venipuncture. Microcollection of a sample through a skin puncture can produce a quality specimen. The equipment used to collect the specimen depends on the test being performed.

Lancets

Different sterile disposable lancets are available to pierce the skin for an adequate blood flow. Lancets are now designed to control depth of puncture. You may insert the lancet into a spring-loaded device, or you may hold the blade in your hand and push it into the skin to a selected depth. Automatic puncturing devices are popular. Most consist of a platform and a spring-loaded lancet; the platform controls the tissue penetration depth. Three color-coded platforms are available for use with the automatic lancet device: white (1.8 mm), yellow (2.4 mm), and orange (3.0 mm). The platform and lancet are both disposable. Some devices feature a safety mechanism that inhibits the use of the device unless first reloaded with a new platform and lancet. Figure 29-7 shows lancets and other supplies used for microcollection.

These devices should be regularly sanitized and disinfected according to the manufacturer's recommendation. The blades must be sterile; follow the directions for loading the replacement blades and platforms.

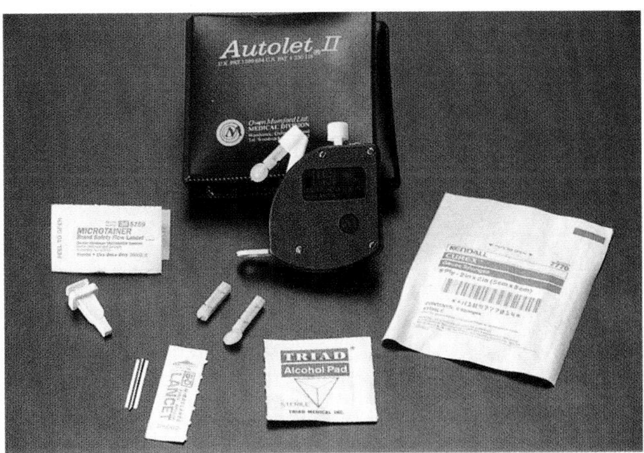

Figure 29-7 Microcollection supplies.

Microcollection Tubes

These tubes are narrow-bore glass or plastic disposable capillary tubes used for hematocrit determinations on 50 to 75 μL of blood. Microcollection tubes for collecting serum specimens are plain; those used for hematocrit or other tests requiring plasma may be coated with ammonium heparin. Plain tubes have a blue band on one end of the capillary tube, and ammonium heparin-coated tubes have a red band. Clay sealants are used to seal one end of the tubes used in microhematocrit and chemistry determinations (Fig. 29-8).

Microcollection Containers

These microtainers consist of nonsterile, small, round-bottomed plastic tubes and color-coded stoppers that indicate the presence or absence of an additive. The color-coding is identical to blood collection tubes used in venipuncture. Microtainers are used for filling, measuring, stoppering, centrifuging, and storing all in one container. Samples collected for bilirubin are collected in an amber-colored plastic tube that protects the blood from light.

Micropipet Dilution Systems

The brand name for this type of system is the Unopette, manufactured by Becton Dickinson. Components of this system include a sealed plastic reservoir containing a premeasured amount of reagent or diluent, a disposable self-filling diluting pipette, and a pipette shield for puncturing the reservoir covering before adding the sample. Figure 29-9 shows how to use the Unopette system.

Filter Paper Devices

Another microcollection device is blood collection on filter paper, which is used for lead screening or to test newborns for genetic defects such as hypothyroidism

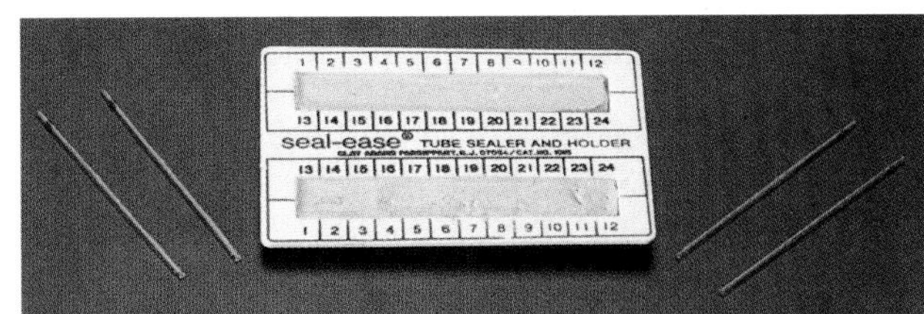

Figure 29-8 Microcollection tubes and clay sealant.

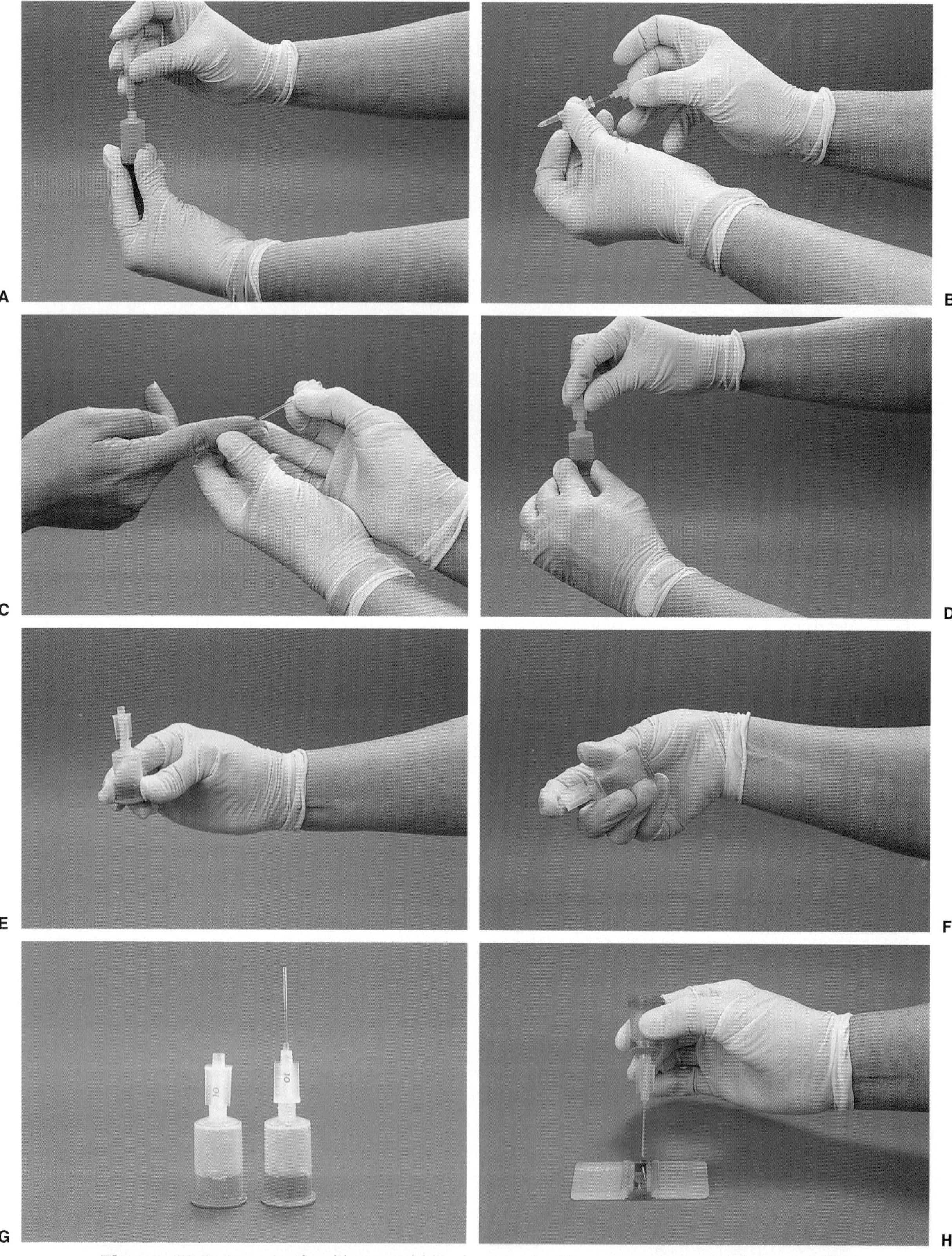

Figure 29-9 Steps in the dilution of blood using the Unopette system. (**A**) Puncture diaphragm. (**B**) Remove shield from pipet assembly with a twist. (**C**) Draw sample into pipet from free-flowing skin puncture or tube. Remove excess blood on outside of pipet carefully with a gauze. (**D**) Squeeze reservoir slightly to force out some air. Do not expel liquid. Cover opening of pipet overflow chamber with finger and seat pipet securely in reservoir neck. (**E**) Squeeze reservoir gently two or three times to rinse capillary bore, forcing diluent into, but not out of, overflow chamber. (**F**) Cover opening with finger and gently invert to mix. (**G**) Convert to dropper assembly. Mix well, invert, and expel first few drops of mixture on waste cloth. Maintain pressure on reservoir to avoid air bubbles. (**H**) Charge hemocytometer. (Courtesy Becton Dickinson Vacutainer Systems, Franklin Lakes, NJ.)

or phenylketonuria. The lateral surface of the newborn's heel is punctured, and the blood droplet is absorbed into individual circles on a filter paper card.

Warming Devices

These units can increase blood flow before the skin is punctured. Several heel-warming devices are available; these commercial devices provide a temperature not exceeding 42°C. A diaper or towel may be wet with warm tap water and used to wrap the hand or foot before skin puncture. Do not use water so hot that it might burn the patient.

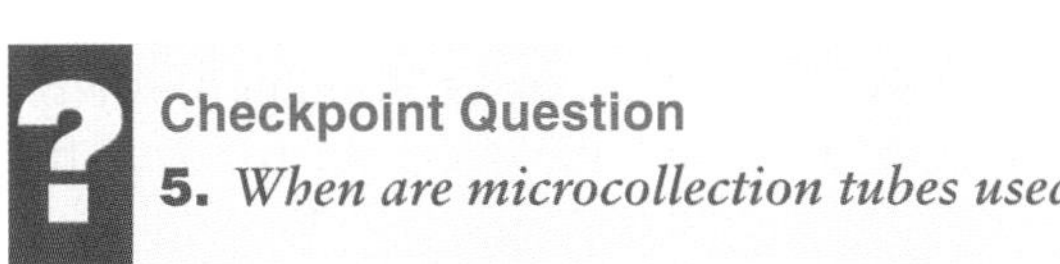

Checkpoint Question
5. *When are microcollection tubes used?*

PATIENT PREPARATION

Gaining the patient's trust and confidence and putting the patient at ease help minimize anxiety and divert attention from any discomfort associated with the procedure. To do this, display a cheerful, confident, and pleasant manner; introduce yourself; explain the procedure in simple terms; and communicate effectively with the patient. Ask the patient for preference of sites. Many patients know from experience where it is easiest to find an accessible vein. In conjunction with your knowledge and skill, knowing the best site will make the procedure less traumatic. Talk quietly with the patient, and progress through the procedure with confidence.

Always believe patients who say they faint during venipuncture. Have these patients lie down during the procedure. This reduces the chance of syncope (fainting), and if fainting does occur, the patient will already be lying down. If the patient is sitting and feels faint, have him or her lower the head between the knees. Never draw blood from a patient who is likely to faint unless the physician is in the office.

One of the most important steps in specimen collection is patient identification. When identifying a patient, ask the patient to state his or her name, date of birth, or any other information to verify identity. After the blood specimen has been collected, the sample must be labeled with the patient's first and last names, an assigned identification number if available, the date and time, and the medical assistant's initials to verify who drew the sample.

PERFORMING A VENIPUNCTURE

The steps for performing a venipuncture (Procedure 29-1) are organized according to the guidelines established by the National Committee for Clinical Laboratory Standards. There may be variations in some methods performed at various clinical settings because of individual technique and specific circumstances.

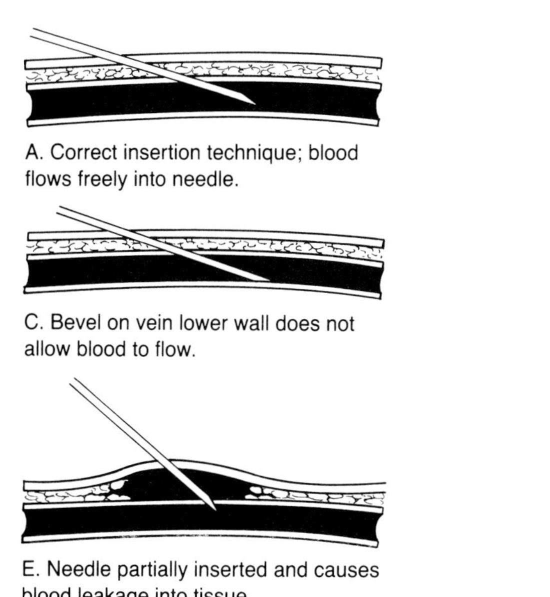

A. Correct insertion technique; blood flows freely into needle.
C. Bevel on vein lower wall does not allow blood to flow.
E. Needle partially inserted and causes blood leakage into tissue.

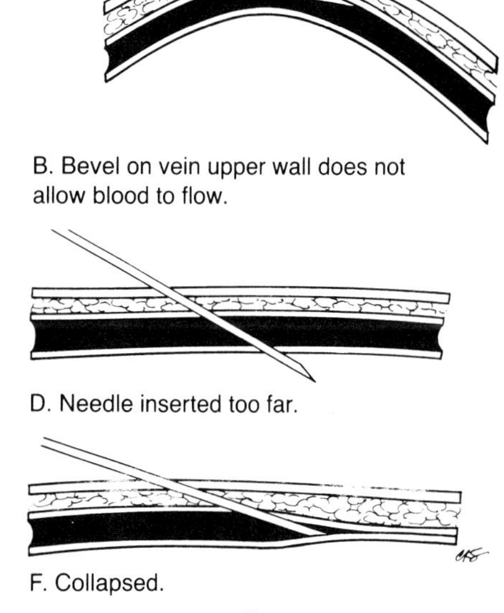

B. Bevel on vein upper wall does not allow blood to flow.
D. Needle inserted too far.
F. Collapsed.

Figure 29-10 Proper and improper needle positioning. (**A**) Proper needle position. (**B**) Needle bevel against the upper wall of a vein. (**C**) Needle bevel against or embedded in opposite wall of vein. (**D**) Needle inserted all the way through a vein. (**E**) Needle partially inserted into a vein. (**F**) Needle in collapsed vein.

Complications of Venipuncture

When a blood sample cannot be obtained, you may need to change the position of the needle. Figure 29-10 shows proper and improper needle positions. Rotate the needle half a turn; the bevel of the needle may be against the wall of the vein. If the needle has not penetrated the vein, slowly advance it further into the vein. If the needle has penetrated too far into the vein, pull back a little. The tube being used may not have sufficient vacuum; try another tube before withdrawing. If the vein feels very thick and hard, try for one with more elasticity; this one may roll away. If the patient has a history of collapsing veins during evacuated tube draws, try a syringe; you will have a more controlled withdrawal. Never attempt a venipuncture more than twice. If a blood specimen cannot be obtained in two tries, do a microcollection (skin puncture) if possible, or have another person attempt the draw. Table 29-2 lists some common sources of errors in venipuncture that you need to guard against.

Table 29-2 **Sources of Error in Venipuncture**

Errors in Venipuncture Preparation
Improper patient identification
Failure to check patient adherence to dietary restrictions
Failure to calm patient prior to blood collection
Use of improper equipment and supplies
Inappropriate method of blood collection
Errors in Venipuncture Procedure
Failure to dry the site completely after cleansing with alcohol
Inserting needle bevel side down
Use of needle that is too small, causing hemolysis of specimen
Venipuncture in an unacceptable area
Prolonged tourniquet application
Wrong order of tube draw
Failure to mix blood collected in additive-containing tubes immediately
Pulling back on syringe plunger too forcefully
Failure to release tourniquet prior to needle withdrawal
Errors After Venipuncture Completion
Failure to apply pressure immediately to venipuncture site
Vigorous shaking of anticoagulated blood specimens
Forcing blood through a syringe needle into tube
Mislabeling of tubes
Failure to label appropriate specimens with infectious disease precaution
Failure to put date, time, and initials on requisition
Slow transport of specimens to laboratory

(From Lotspeich-Steininger, C. A., Stiene-Martin, E. A., & Koepke, J. A. [1992]. *Clinical Hematology,* p. 17. Philadelphia: J.B. Lippincott.)

PERFORMING A SKIN PUNCTURE

Some veins will not endure a venipuncture. Microcollection of a sample through a skin puncture can provide a medical assistant with a quality specimen with less trauma to the patient (Procedure 29-2).

Complications of Skin Puncture

Several precautions should be observed to produce the most accurate specimen. The greatest concern with microcollection specimens is **hemolysis,** the rupture of erythrocytes with the release of hemoglobin. Do not squeeze or milk the heel or finger to produce a greater blood flow. Never scrape the microcollection device on the skin surface; only allow the container to touch the drop of blood. You should also be careful to avoid additional sources of errors, which are listed in Table 29-3.

Obtaining a specimen without clots is also a challenge in microcollection. The body's clotting system is activated to stop the bleeding as soon as the skin is punctured. If an ethylenediaminetetraacetic acid (EDTA) specimen is required, this specimen should be drawn first to get an adequate volume of blood before the blood begins to clot. Any other additive specimens are collected next, and clotted specimens are collected last. If the blood has begun to produce microscopic clots while filling the last tube, this is not a problem because clotting is required in this tube.

Checkpoint Question

6. *How should you label the patient's blood sample?*

text continues on page 658

Table 29-3 **Sources of Error in Skin Puncture**

1. Misidentification of patient
2. Puncturing wrong area of infant heel
3. Puncturing bone in infant heel
4. Puncturing fingers of infants
5. Puncturing wrong area of adult finger
6. Contaminating specimen with alcohol or Betadine
7. Failure to discard first blood drop
8. Excessive massaging of puncture site
9. Collecting air bubbles in pH or blood gas specimen
10. Hemolyzing specimen
11. Failure to seal specimens adequately
12. Failure to chill specimens requiring refrigeration
13. Erroneous specimen labeling
14. Failure to note skin puncture collection
15. Failure to warm site
16. Delaying specimen transport
17. Bruising site as a result of excessive squeezing

(From Bishop, M. L., ed. [1996]. *Clinical Chemistry,* 3rd ed. Philadelphia: Lippincott-Raven.)

Procedure 29-1 Obtaining a Blood Specimen by Venipuncture

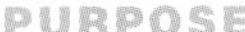

PPE

PURPOSE

To secure a sample of venous blood safely for diagnostic purposes with minimal patient discomfort

EQUIPMENT/SUPPLIES

- needle, syringe, and tube(s) or evacuated tubes
- tourniquet
- sterile gauze pads
- bandages
- needle and adaptor
- sharps container
- 70% alcohol pad or alternative antiseptic
- permanent marker or pen

STEPS

1. Check the requisition slip to determine the tests ordered and specimen requirements.

This ensures proper specimen collection.

2. Wash your hands.

3. Assemble the equipment. Check the expiration date on the tubes.

Expired tubes may no longer have a vacuum; additives may no longer be functional.

4. Greet and identify the patient. Explain the procedure. Ask for and answer any questions.

5. If a fasting specimen is required, ask the patient the last time food was eaten.

For fasting specimens, food should not have been eaten within at least 12 hours.

6. Put on nonsterile latex or vinyl gloves.

7. Break the seal of the needle cover, and thread the sleeved needle into the adaptor, using the needle cover as a wrench. Tap the tubes that contain additives to ensure that the additive is dislodged from the stopper and wall of the tube. Insert the tube into the adaptor until the needle slightly enters the stopper. Do not push the top of the tube stopper beyond the indentation mark. If the tube retracts slightly, leave it in the retracted position. If using a syringe, tighten the needle on the hub and "breathe" the syringe.

This ensures proper needle placement, tube positioning, and prevents loss of vacuum in the evacuated tubes or sticking of the plunger in the barrel of the syringe.

8. Instruct the patient to sit with the arm well supported in a downward extended position if possible.

Veins in the antecubital fossa are more easily located when the elbow is straight. The tourniquet makes the veins more prominent.

a. Apply the tourniquet around the patient's arm 3 to 4 inches above the elbow.

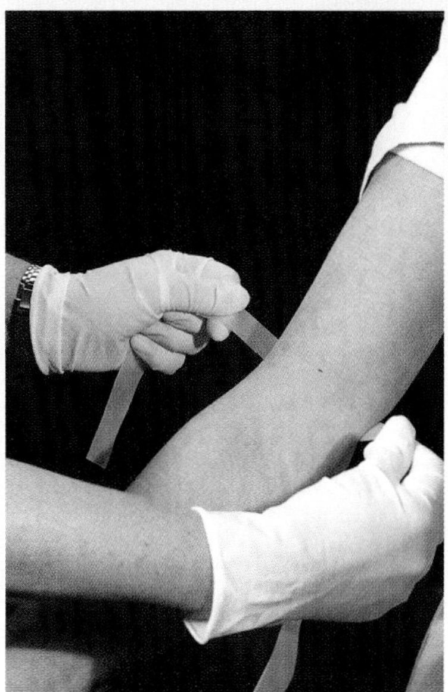

b. Apply the tourniquet snugly, but not too tightly.

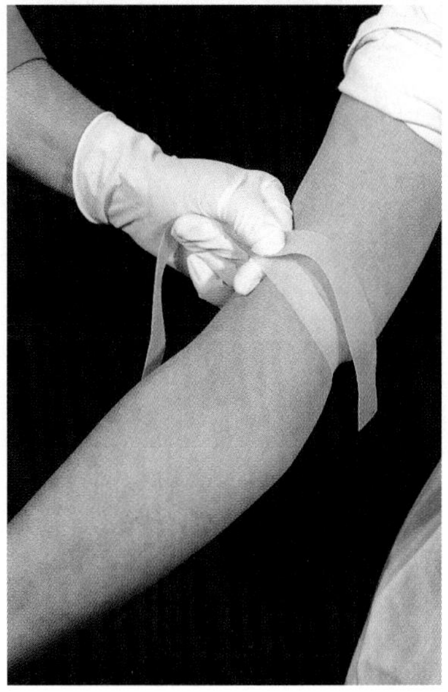

continued

Procedure 29-1 Continued Obtaining a Blood Specimen by Venipuncture

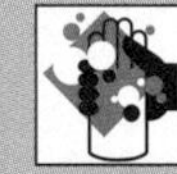
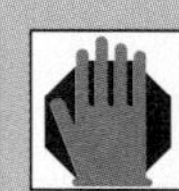
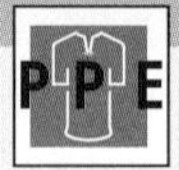

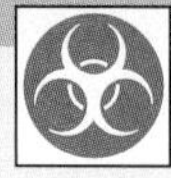

c. Secure the tourniquet by using the half-bow.

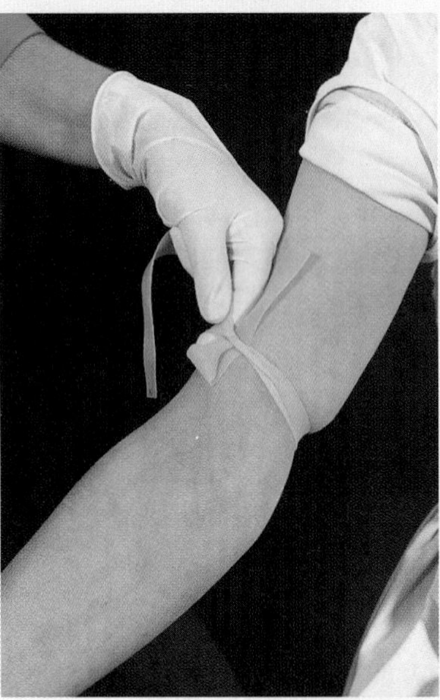

d. Make sure the tails of the tourniquet extend upward to avoid contaminating the venipuncture site.

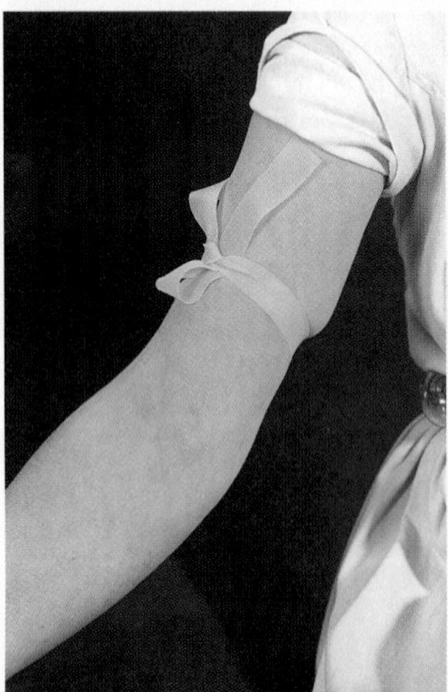

e. Ask the patient to close his or her hand into a fist, but not to pump the fist.
Making a fist raises the vessels out of the underlying tissues and muscles.

9. Select a vein by palpating. Use your gloved index finger to trace the path of the vein and judge its depth.
The index finger is most sensitive for palpating.

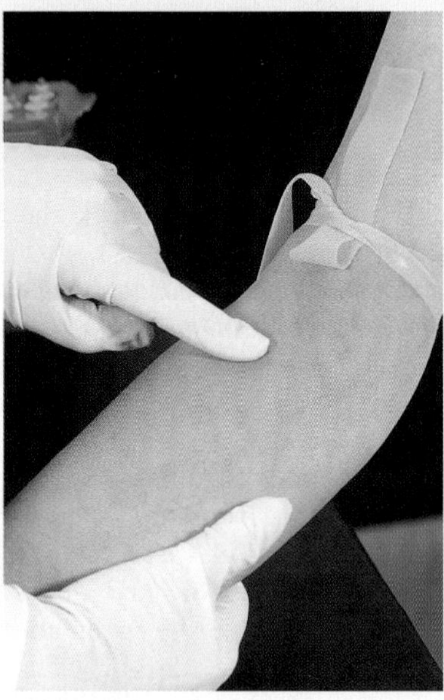

10. Release the tourniquet after palpating the vein if it has been left on for more than 1 minute.
The tourniquet should not be left on for more than 1 minute at a time during the procedure.

11. Cleanse the venipuncture site with an alcohol pad starting in the center of puncture site and working outward in a circular motion. Allow the site to dry or dry the site with sterile gauze. Do not touch the area after cleansing.
The circular motion helps avoid contamination of the area. Puncturing a wet area stings and can cause hemolysis of the sample.

12. If blood being drawn for culture will be used in diagnosing septic conditions, make sure the specimen is sterile. To do this, apply alcohol to the area for 2 full minutes. Then apply a 2% iodine solution in ever-widening circles. Never move the wipes back over areas that have been cleaned; use a new wipe for each sweep across the area. Allow the iodine to dry completely.
Ensuring sterility of the specimen will aid accurate diagnosis. Iodine contamination of the specimen can inhibit the growth of microorganisms and cause a false-negative result.

continued

29

Procedure 29-1 Continued Obtaining a Blood Specimen by Venipuncture

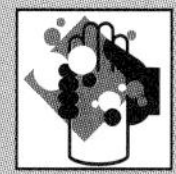
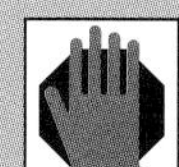
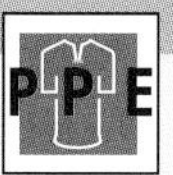

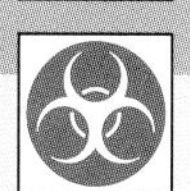

13. Reapply the tourniquet if it was removed after palpation.

If tourniquet time is greater than 1 minute, test results could be altered.

14. Remove the needle cover. Hold the syringe or evacuated assembly in your dominant hand. Your thumb should be on top of the adaptor and your fingers underneath. Grasp the patient's arm with the nondominant hand while using your thumb to draw the skin taut over the site and anchor the vein about 1 to 2 inches below the puncture site.

Anchoring the vein allows for easier needle penetration and less pain.

15. With the bevel up, line up the needle with the vein at approximately ¼ to ½ inch below the site where the vein is to be entered. At a 15 to 30-degree angle, rapidly and smoothly insert the needle through the skin.

The sharpest point of the needle is inserted first.

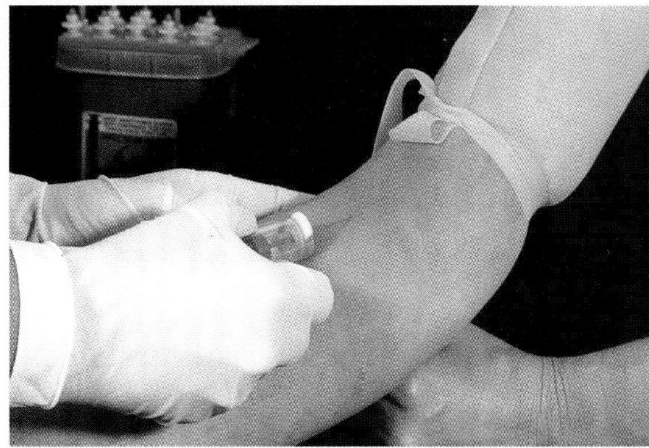

16. Remove your nondominant hand, and slowly pull back the plunger of the syringe. Instead, you may place two fingers on the flanges of the adapter, and with the thumb, push the tube onto the needle inside the adapter. When blood flow begins in the tube or syringe, release the tourniquet and allow the patient to release the fist. Allow the syringe or tube(s) to fill to capacity. When blood flow ceases, remove the tube from the adapter by gripping the tube with your nondominant hand, and place your thumb against the flange during removal.

Proper tube filling ensures correct ratio of blood to additive. Removal of the tourniquet releases pressure on the vein and helps prevent blood from seeping into adjacent tissues and causing a hematoma.

17. Gently pull out the tube. If the tube contains an additive, immediately invert it 5 to 10 times.

This allows for mixing additives and blood.

18. Steady the needle in the vein. To prevent discomfort, try not to pull up or press down on the needle while it is in the vein. Insert any other necessary tubes into adapter and allow to fill to capacity.

19. Remove the tube from the adapter before removing the needle from the arm. If the tourniquet has not been previously released, do so now.

Removing the last tube from the adapter before removing the needle from the vein prevents any excess blood from dripping from the tip of the needle onto the patient.

a. Place a sterile gauze pad over the puncture site at the time of needle withdrawal. Do not apply any pressure to the site until the needle is completely removed.

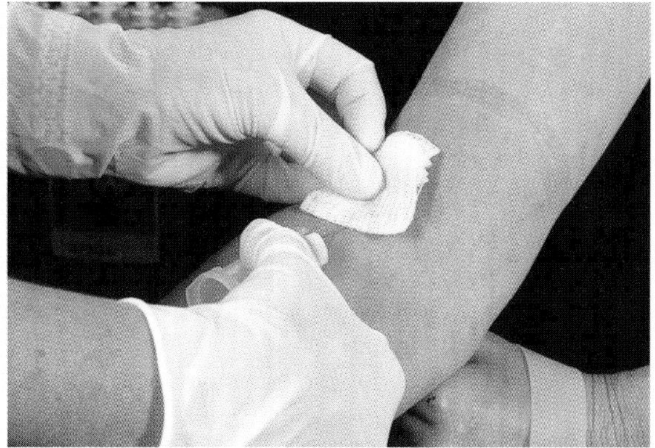

continued

Procedure 29-1 Continued Obtaining a Blood Specimen by Venipuncture

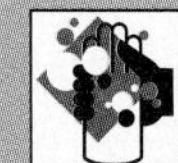
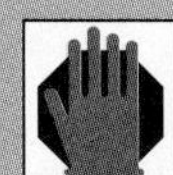
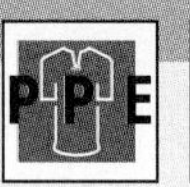

b. After the needle is removed, apply pressure or have the patient apply direct pressure for 3 to 5 minutes. Do not bend the arm at the elbow.
Pressure decreases the amount of blood escaping into the tissues. Bending the arm increases the chance of blood seeping into the subcutaneous tissues.

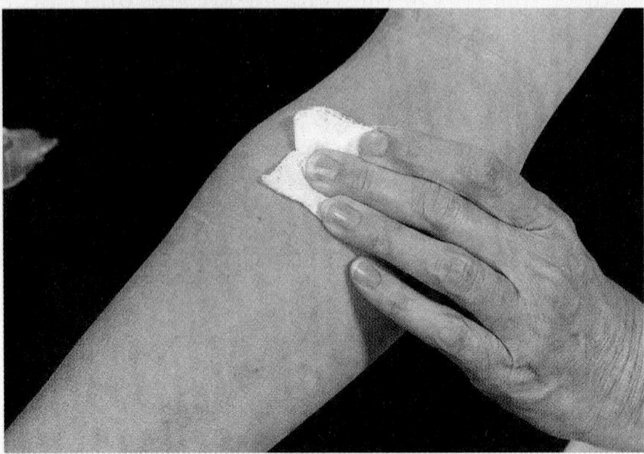

20. Transfer the blood from a syringe into the proper order of draw tubes by inserting the needle through the stopper and allowing the vacuum to fill the tubes. Do not hold the tube when puncturing the stopper and filling the tube; place it in a tube rack and carefully insert the needle through the stopper. If the vacuum tubes contain an anticoagulant, they must be mixed immediately by gently inverting the tube 8 to 10 times. Do not shake the tube. Label the tubes with the proper information.
Mixing anticoagulated tubes prevents clotting of blood. Holding the tube increases the chance of accidental stick. Proper labeling of blood specimens avoids mix-up of samples.

21. Check the puncture site for bleeding. Apply a bandage.

22. Properly care for or dispose of all equipment and supplies. Clean the work area. Remove gloves and wash your hands.

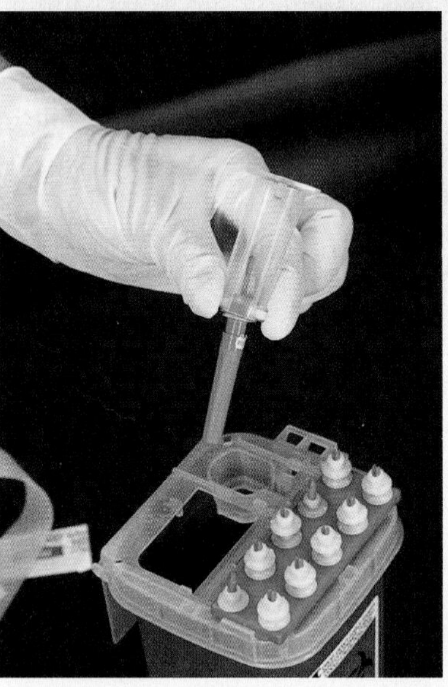

23. Test, transfer, or store the blood specimen according to the medical office policy.

DOCUMENTATION GUIDELINES

- Date and time
- Site of venipuncture
- Performance of procedure
- Patient observations
- Routing of specimen or on-site testing results
- Patient education/instructions
- Your signature

Charting Example

DATE	TIME Venipuncture (left) anticubitus.
	Specimen routed for CBC to Med-Path lab.
	Pt tolerated procedure well.
	—Your signature

Procedure 29-2 Obtaining a Blood Specimen by Skin Puncture

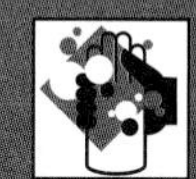
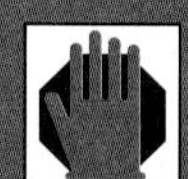
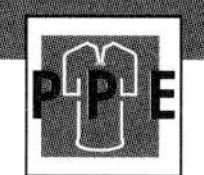

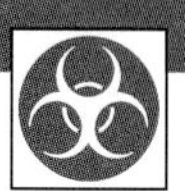

PURPOSE

To secure a small blood sample safely without venous access and with minimal patient discomfort

EQUIPMENT/SUPPLIES

- sterile disposable lancet or automated skin puncture device
- 70% alcohol or alternate antiseptic sterile gauze pads
- collection containers (Unopettes, capillary tubes)
- heel-warming device, if needed

STEPS

1. Check the requisition slip to determine the tests ordered and specimen requirements.
   This ensures proper specimen collection.
2. Wash your hands.
3. Assemble the equipment.
   Having the equipment ready will speed the collection process so the blood does not clot before the entire specimen has been collected.
4. Greet and identify the patient. Explain the procedure. Ask for and answer any questions.
5. Put on nonsterile latex or vinyl gloves.
6. Select the puncture site (the lateral portion of the tip of the middle or ring finger of the nondominant hand, lateral curved surface of the heel, or the great toe of an infant). The puncture should be made in the fleshy, central portion of the second or third finger, slightly to the side of center, and perpendicular to the grooves of the fingerprint. Perform heel puncture only on the plantar surface of the heel, medial to an imaginary line extending from the middle of the great toe to the heel, and lateral to an imaginary line drawn from between the fourth and fifth toes to the heel. Puncture should not exceed 2.4 mm in depth.
   The ring and middle fingers are less calloused. The lateral part of the tip is the least sensitive part of the finger. A puncture made across the fingerprints will produce a large, round drop of blood. In an infant skin puncture, the area and the depth designated reduces the risk of puncturing the bone.

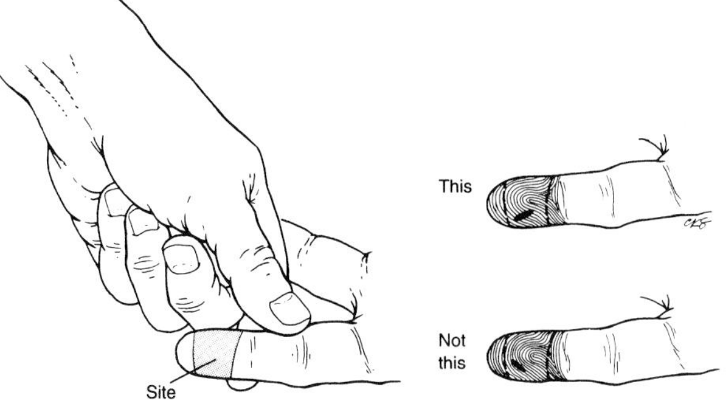

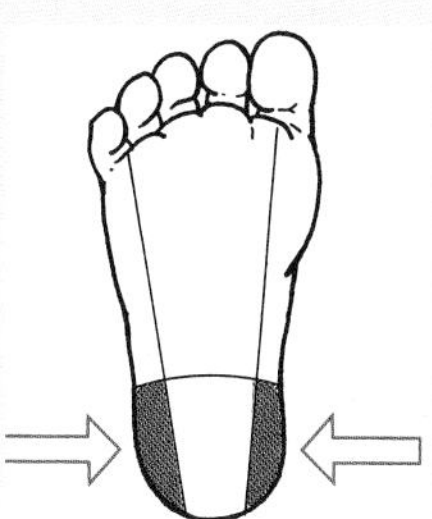

7. Make sure the site chosen is warm and not cyanotic or edematous. Gently massage the finger from the base to the tip or warm the site for 3 minutes with a warm washcloth or commercial heel warmer.
   Massaging and warming the area increases the blood flow. Good circulation at the chosen site yields a better blood sample for analysis.

continued

Procedure 29-2 Continued Obtaining a Blood Specimen by Skin Puncture

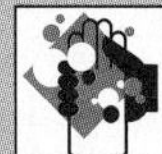
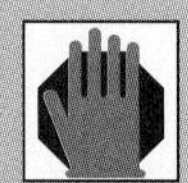
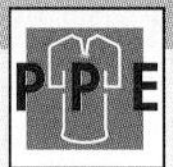

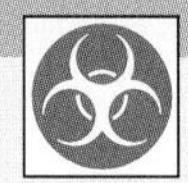

29

8. Grasp the finger firmly between your nondominant index finger and the thumb, or grasp the infant's heel firmly with the index finger wrapped around the foot and the thumb wrapped around the ankle. Cleanse the ball of the selected finger or heel with 70% isopropyl alcohol and wipe dry with a sterile gauze pad or allow to air dry.

The area must be dry to eliminate alcohol residue, which can cause the patient discomfort or interfere with test results. Securing the site prevents the patient from contaminating the cleansed puncture area and allows you to have control of the puncture site.

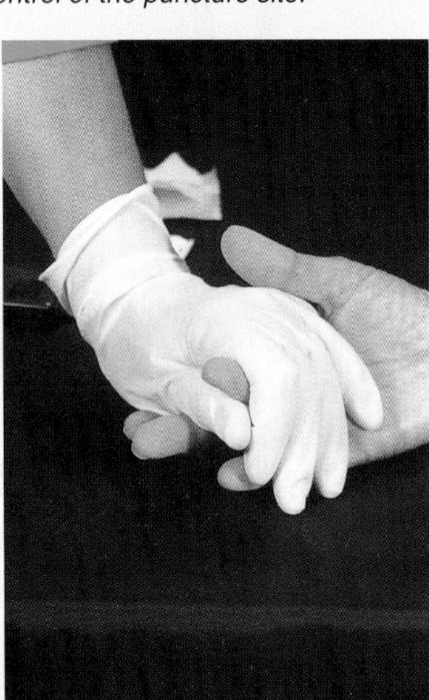

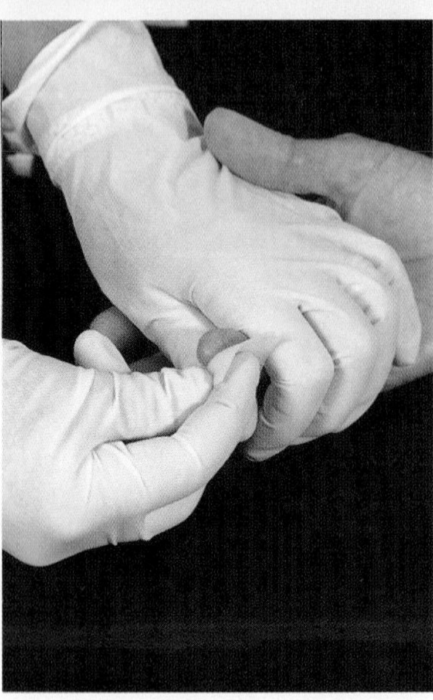

9. Hold the patient's finger or heel firmly, and make a swift, deep puncture. Perform the puncture perpendicular to the whorls of the fingerprint or footprint in a recommended safe area.

The proper puncture will allow the blood to form a rounded drop that can be easily collected. Puncturing in a recommended area avoids damage to underlying structures such as nerves, tendons, bone, or cartilage.

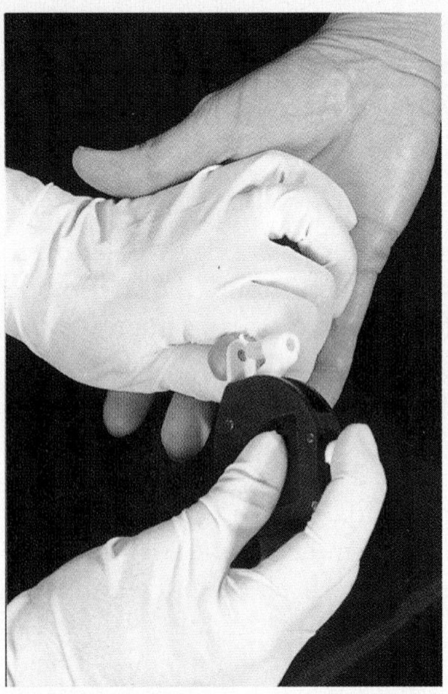

a. Wipe away the first drop of blood with a sterile dry gauze.

The first discarded drop may be contaminated with tissue fluid or alcohol residue.

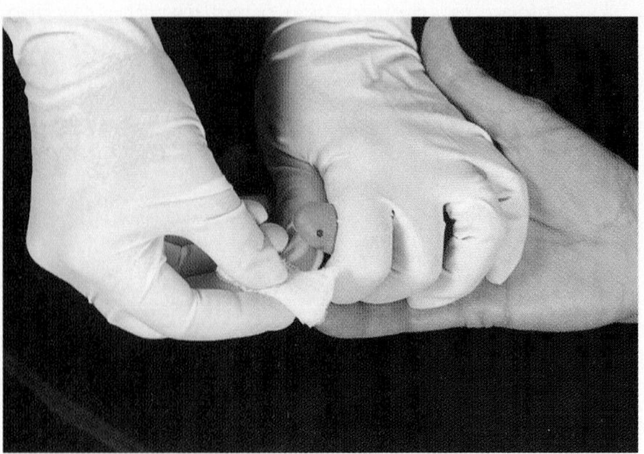

continued

Procedure 29-2 Continued **Obtaining a Blood Specimen by Skin Puncture**

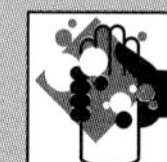
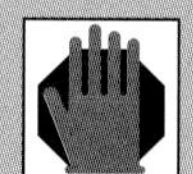
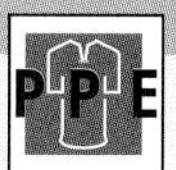

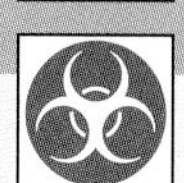

b. Apply pressure toward the site, but do not "milk" or squeeze the site.

Excessive manipulation of the collection site, such as squeezing or milking, will dilute the specimen with tissue fluid.

10. Collect the required specimen in the chosen containers or slides. Touch only the tip of the collection device to the drop of blood. Blood flow is encouraged if the puncture site is held in a downward, or dependent, angle and a gentle pressure is applied to the site. Cap microcollection tubes with the caps provided, and mix the additives by gently tilting or inverting the tubes 8 to 10 times.

Scraping the collection device on the skin activates platelets and may cause hemolysis. Mixing the specimens prevents clotting. Touching the tube to the site may cause contamination.

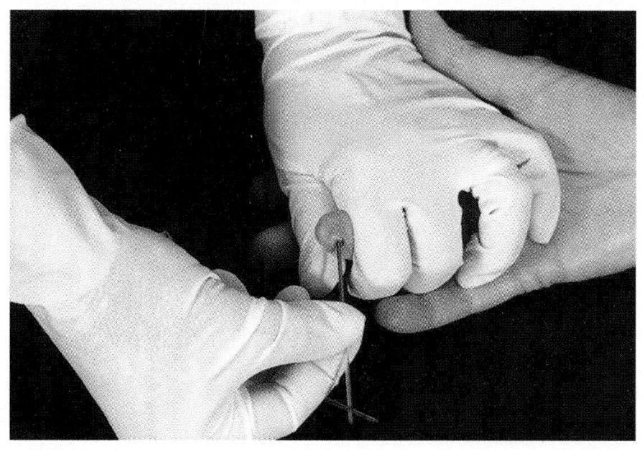

11. When collection is complete, apply pressure to the site with a clean gauze until bleeding stops. Label the containers with the proper information. Do not apply bandages to skin punctures of infants under 2 years of age. Never release a patient until the bleeding has stopped.

Proper labeling prevents a mix up of specimens. Newborns have delicate skin that may be injured when an adhesive bandage is removed. Younger children may develop a skin irritation from the adhesive bandage. Also, a young child might aspirate the bandage and choke.

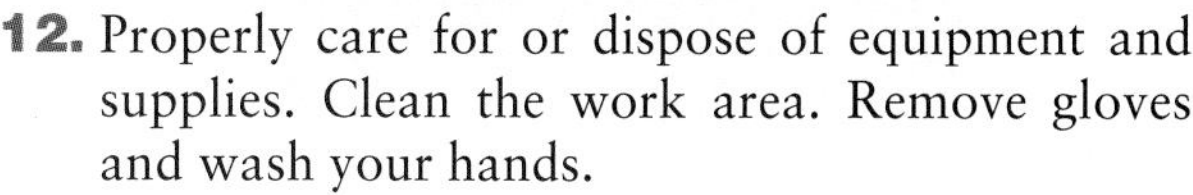

12. Properly care for or dispose of equipment and supplies. Clean the work area. Remove gloves and wash your hands.

13. Test, transfer, or store the blood specimen according to the medical office policy.

DOCUMENTATION GUIDELINES

- Date and time
- Site of puncture
- Performance of testing, if appropriate
- Action taken, if any
- Routing of specimen, if appropriate
- Patient education/instructions
- Your signature

Charting Example

DATE	TIME Capillary puncture to (R) ring finger.
	Hct 42%. —Your signature

Answers to Checkpoint Questions

1. *Capillary puncture may be required when small amounts of blood are needed, when the patient is under age 2, or when the veins either are inaccessible or must be preserved for parenteral therapy.*
2. *Disinfectants are used to kill bacteria on equipment and surfaces. Antiseptics are safe for people and are used to clean the skin before skin puncture or venipuncture.*
3. *Common additives include anticoagulants (prevent the blood from coagulating or clotting); clot activators (enhance coagulation); and thixotropic gel separator (forms a physical barrier between the cellular portion of a specimen and the serum or plasma portion after centrifugation).*
4. *When using the evacuated tube system, the proper order of draw is blood culture tubes, red or red/gray, light blue, green, lavender, gray. It is important to follow the correct order of draw to avoid contamination between additives.*
5. *Microcollection tubes are commonly used for hematocrit determinations.*
6. *You should label the blood sample with the patient's first and last names, an identification number, the date and time, and your initials to verify who drew the sample.*

Critical Thinking Challenges

1. How will you help ease patient anxiety about venipuncture? Explain exactly what steps you will take.
2. Review Chap. 22, Pediatric Patients. How would you draw blood on a child? How would you help the child and the parent?
3. Your patient asks you how long you have been drawing blood and if you are "good." How would you respond? Justify your response.

Suggestions for Further Reading

Bishop, M. L. (1996). *Clinical Chemistry,* 3rd ed. Philadelphia: Lippincott-Raven.

Marshall, J. (1993). *Fundamental Skills for the Clinical Laboratory Professional.* Albany, NY: Delmar Publishers.

McCall, R., & Tankersley, C. M. (1998). *Phlebotomy Essentials,* 2nd ed. Philadelphia: Lippincott-Raven.

30 Hematology

Chapter Outline

Formation of Blood Cells
Hematologic Testing
Complete Blood Count
- White Blood Cell Count and Differential
- Red Blood Cell (RBC) Count
- Hemoglobin
- Hematocrit
- Indices
- Platelet Count

Erythrocyte Sedimentation Rate
Coagulation Tests
- Prothrombin Time
- Partial Thromboplastin Time
- Bleeding Time

Role Delineation

CLINICAL

Fundamental Principles

- Apply principles of aseptic technique and infection control.

Diagnostic Orders

- Collect and process specimens.
- Perform diagnostic tests.

GENERAL

Legal Concepts

- Practice within the scope of education, training, and personal capabilities.
- Document accurately.
- Maintain and dispose of regulated substances in compliance with governmental guidelines.
- Comply with established risk management and safety procedures.

Instruction

- Instruct individuals according to their needs.
- Teach methods of health promotion and disease prevention.

Chapter Competencies

Learning Objectives

Upon successfully completing this chapter, you will be able to:

1. Spell and define the Key Terms.
2. List the indices measured in the complete blood count and their normal ranges.
3. Explain the principle of automated cell counters.
4. State the conditions associated with abnormal complete blood count findings.
5. Explain the functions of the three types of blood cells.
6. Describe the purpose of performing an erythrocyte sedimentation rate.
7. List the leukocytes seen in the blood and their functions.
8. Explain the hemostatic mechanism of the body.
9. List and describe the tests that measure the body's ability to form a fibrin clot.
10. Explain the methodology used to determine the prothrombin time and partial thromboplastin time.

Performance Objectives

Upon successfully completing this chapter, you will be able to:

1. Perform a manual white blood cell count (Procedure 30-1).
2. Make a peripheral blood smear (Procedure 30-2).
3. Stain a peripheral blood smear (Procedure 30-3).

Chapter Competencies *(continued)*

4. Perform a white blood cell differential (Procedure 30-4).
5. Perform a red blood cell count (Procedure 30-5).
6. Perform a hemoglobin determination (Procedure 30-6).
7. Perform a manual microhematocrit determination (Procedure 30-7).
8. Perform a Wintrobe erythrocyte sedimentation rate (Procedure 30-8).
9. Perform a Westergren erythrocyte sedimentation rate.
10. Determine a bleeding time (Procedure 30-9).

Key Terms

(See Glossary for definitions.)

agranulocytes
anisocytosis
Autolet
coumarin
elliptocytosis
enzymes
erythrocytes
erythropoietin
femtoliter
folate
granulocytes
hematocytometer (hemacytometer)
hematopoiesis
hemoglobin C disease
hemolytic anemia
heparin
hyperosmolarity
indices
intravascular coagulation
leukocytes
megaloblastic anemia
myelofibrosis
parameters
poikilocytosis
sickle cell anemia
spherocytosis
spicules
thalassemia
thrombocytes
thromboplastin
yolk sac

The hematology laboratory analyzes the blood cells, their quantities, and their characteristics for diagnosis and management of many conditions. Anemias, leukemias, and infections are some of the more common disorders detected by hematologic tests.

FORMATION OF BLOOD CELLS

Blood is made up of two parts: fluid (plasma) and formed elements (cells). There are three types of cells, **erythrocytes** (red blood cells), **leukocytes** (white blood cells), and **thrombocytes** (platelets) (Fig. 30-1).

Blood cells are formed in the bone marrow. The long bones, skull, pelvis, and sternum are the usual sites for the manufacture of these cells. Alternative sites include the liver and spleen. The **yolk sac** of the developing fetus also produces blood cells. (The yolk sac is the structure that nourishes the embryo until the seventh week, when the placenta takes over.)

Hematopoiesis (blood cell production) starts with very young, immature cells within the marrow that eventually divide and differentiate (acquire distinct or individual characteristics; to mature). These cells become erythrocytes, leukocytes, and thrombocytes according to the body's current needs. Each type of cell has a particular function that is discussed later in this chapter. Hematopoiesis is influenced by hormones and depends on adequate nutrients, such as iron, to produce functional cells. Once these cells have reached maturity, they are released from the bone marrow and travel into the bloodstream.

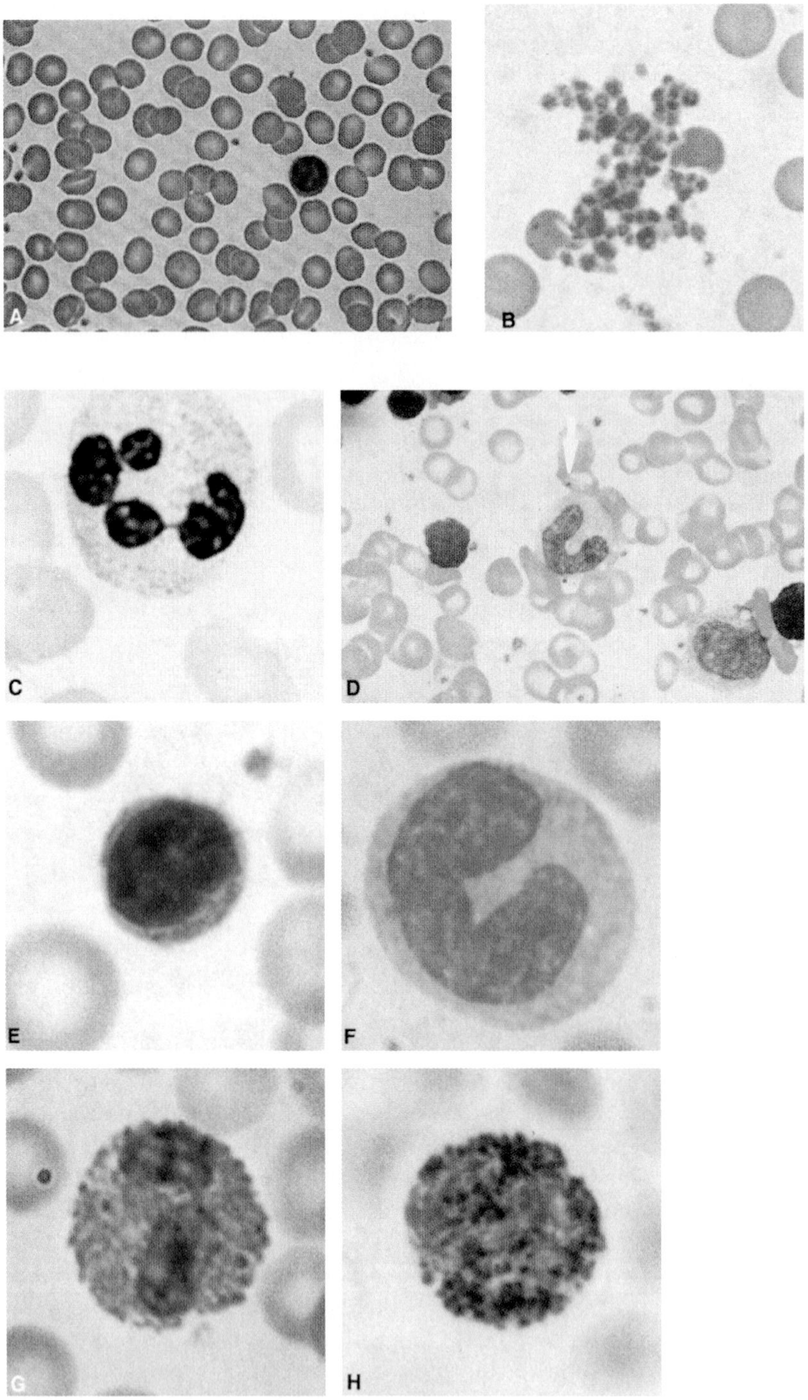

Figure 30-1 (A) A blood smear; (B) red blood cells (large, round cells) and platelets (stained purple); (C) segmented neutrophil; (D) neutrophil band; (E) lymphocyte; (F) monocyte; (G) eosinophil; (H) basophil.

Checkpoint Question

1. *What is hematopoiesis, and how is it influenced?*

HEMATOLOGIC TESTING

In the hematology laboratory, blood testing is done to detect disease-producing conditions. Common hematologic tests include the complete blood count (CBC), erythrocyte sedimentation rate (ERS or Sed rate), and coagulation tests.

COMPLETE BLOOD COUNT

The CBC is one of the most frequently ordered tests in the laboratory. It consists of a number of **parameters** (characteristics that are measured), including:

- White blood cell (WBC) count and differential
- Red blood cell (RBC) count

- Hemoglobin (Hgb) determination
- Hematocrit (Hct) determination
- Mean cell volume (MCV)
- Mean corpuscular hemoglobin (MCH) and mean corpuscular hemoglobin concentration (MCHC)
- Platelet count

Most laboratories use the term CBC; a few, however, may use the term hemogram. Each of the blood cells (white, red, and platelets) can be counted using a counting chamber called a **hematocytometer** or a **hemacytometer.** Historically, WBCs, RBCs, and platelets were counted manually. Since the introduction of automated cell counters, manual cell counts are rarely performed because of the subjectivity of the testing. Automated cell counters are fast, simple, and accurate. With training, the medical assistant usually is allowed to perform automated cell counts. Most laboratories use automated cell counters to determine the CBC parameter values (Box 30-1), virtually eliminating the subjectivity and human error factors present in manual cell counts.

Box 30-1
Automated Blood Cell Counters

A number of biotechnology companies have instruments that can count and size the blood cells. Coulter and Technicon are two of these companies. Although each has its own specific method, the main operating principle is similar.

A portion of whole blood (anticoagulated with ethylenediaminetetraacetic acid [EDTA]) is fed into the machine and automatically diluted. The diluted specimens are moved into counting chambers where they are drawn through tiny holes (apertures). As the cells pass through the holes, either an electrical current, a light beam, or a laser beam is interrupted. The instrument registers the interruption as a cell. It can tell the size of the cell by the length of time the beam is interrupted.

These instruments have become so sophisticated that even the complicated WBC differential can be reported accurately. RBC measurements and other parameters are calculated also, adding to the diagnostic value of the complete blood count.

30

White Blood Cell Count and Differential

White blood cells (leukocytes) provide the main line of defense against foreign invaders, such as bacteria and viruses. Some types circulate in the peripheral blood, and others migrate into tissues and cavities to perform their functions. The normal range for a *WBC count* is 4,300 to 10,800/mm^3. Test results may depend on the method used for testing, and normal references will vary in different regions and populations. A patient's WBC count can be determined by using the hematocytometer counting chamber (Procedure 30-1) or by an automated cell counter.

text continues on page 666

Procedure 30-1 Performing a Manual White Blood Cell Count

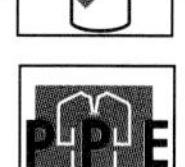
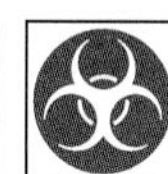

PURPOSE

To determine the number of leukocytes per cubic millimeter in a blood sample
To aid in the diagnosis and treatment of infectious processes or blood dyscrasias

EQUIPMENT/SUPPLIES

- Unopette system for WBC count
- Neubauer hemacytometer
- cover glass
- gauze
- moist filter paper or moist cotton ball
- Petri dish
- hand tally counter

STEPS

1. Wash your hands.
2. Assemble the equipment.
3. Using the shield on the capillary pipette, pierce the diaphragm in the neck of the reservoir, pushing the tip of the shield firmly through the diaphragm before removing it. Remove the shield from the capillary pipette using a twisting motion. Fill the pipette with free-flowing whole blood obtained through skin puncture or from a properly obtained, well-mixed EDTA (lavender top) tube specimen. (See Chap. 29, Phlebotomy, for the procedure for performing a skin puncture.)
4. If filling from a tube, place the tip of the Unopette just below the surface of the blood. Allow capillary action to fill the Unopette system completely.

   The tube must be filled completely to obtain the proper blood-to-diluent concentration.
5. Wipe off the pipette with gauze, being careful not to draw it across the tip.

   Wiping the assembly free of blood removes surface contaminants. The gauze may absorb some of the blood sample if it comes in contact with the pipette tip, causing erroneous results.

continued

Procedure 30-1 Continued Performing a Manual White Blood Cell Count

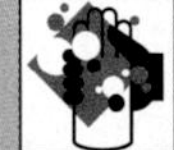
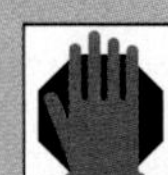
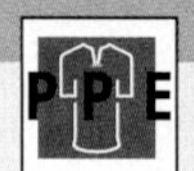

6. Squeeze the reservoir gently to press out the air without expelling any of the specimen. Place your finger over the opening of the overflow chamber of the pipette.
   Air in the reservoir will prevent the blood from entering the chamber; expressing the air creates a vacuum that assists in filling the unit. Covering the opening prevents loss of the specimen.
7. Maintain the pressure on the reservoir and your finger position on the pipette, and insert the pipette into the reservoir.
   Entry into the reservoir must be provided for the blood to combine with the diluent.
8. Release the reservoir pressure. Then remove your finger from the pipette.
   The vacuum created draws the blood into the reservoir to begin the reaction.
9. Gently press and release the reservoir several times, forcing the diluent into but not out of the overflow chamber.
   Gentle swishing action rinses blood from the pipette without destroying the fragile cells and ensures an accurate dilution. Solution escaping the overflow chamber adversely affects the dilution ratio and becomes a source of contamination.
10. Place your index finger over the opening of the overflow chamber, and gently invert or swirl the container several times. Remove your finger, and cover the opening with the pipette shield.
    The specimen must be well mixed to ensure proper results but must be done gently to maintain the integrity of the cells. Covering the unit prevents leakage and evaporation.
11. Label with the required patient information, and set the unit aside for 10 minutes.
    Labeling ensures proper patient identification. Standing time allows RBCs to lyse.
12. At the proper interval, mix the contents again by gently swirling the assembly.
13. Remove the pipette from the Unopette reservoir, and replace it as a dropper assembly.
    The dropper adaptor allows the diluted specimen to charge the hemacytometer.
14. Invert the reservoir and gently squeeze the sides, discarding the first 3 to 4 drops.
    The capillary lumen must be cleaned of blood that might not be adequately mixed.
15. Charge the hemacytometer by touching the tip of the assembly to the V-shaped loading area of the covered chamber. Control the flow gently, and do not overfill. Do not allow the specimen to flow into the H-shaped moats that surround the platform loading area.
    Forceful charging may cause bubble formation or may overfill the chamber, either will make counting and identifying the cells very difficult.

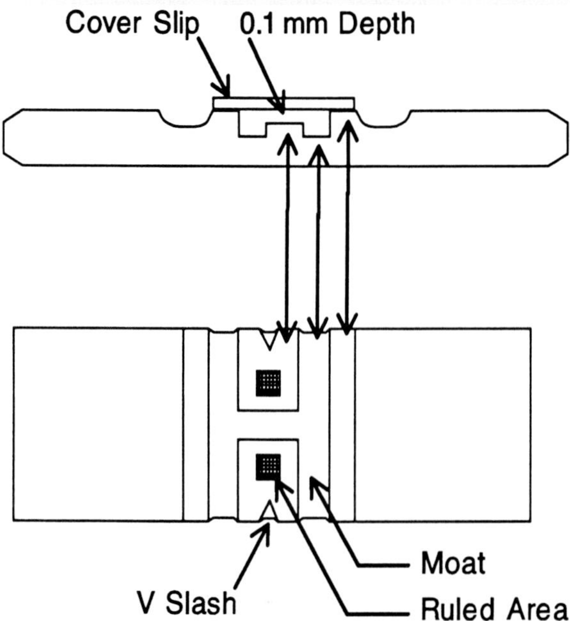

The Neubauer hemacytometer.

16. Place the hemacytometer and the moistened filter paper or cotton ball in the Petri dish, and cover the entire assembly for 5 to 10 minutes.
    The added moisture keeps the cells moist and allows the cells to settle for counting.
17. Place the prepared hemacytometer on the microscope stage, and turn to the 100 × magnification.
    The specimen is ready for the cell count.
18. Using a zigzag counting pattern; starting at the top far left, count the top row left to right. At the end of the top row, drop to the second row, and count from right to left.
    The traditional counting pattern avoids omitting or overcounting cells.

continued

Procedure 30-1 Continued Performing a Manual White Blood Cell Count

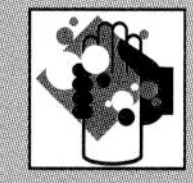
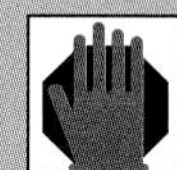
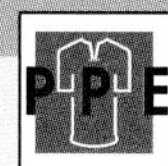
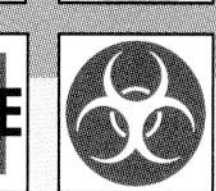

19. Using the tally counter, count all of the WBCs within the boundaries and those that touch the top and left borders. Do not count those that touch the bottom or right borders.

Using this protocol prevents an inaccurate estimation of cells.

20. Record the number. Return the tally counter to 0, and move to the next square until all nine squares have been counted. If the numbers do not match by within 10%, the hemacytometer was improperly charged, and the test must be repeated. Count the opposite side of the hemacytometer.

Comparing the results between squares as you go helps ensure accuracy of testing results.

30

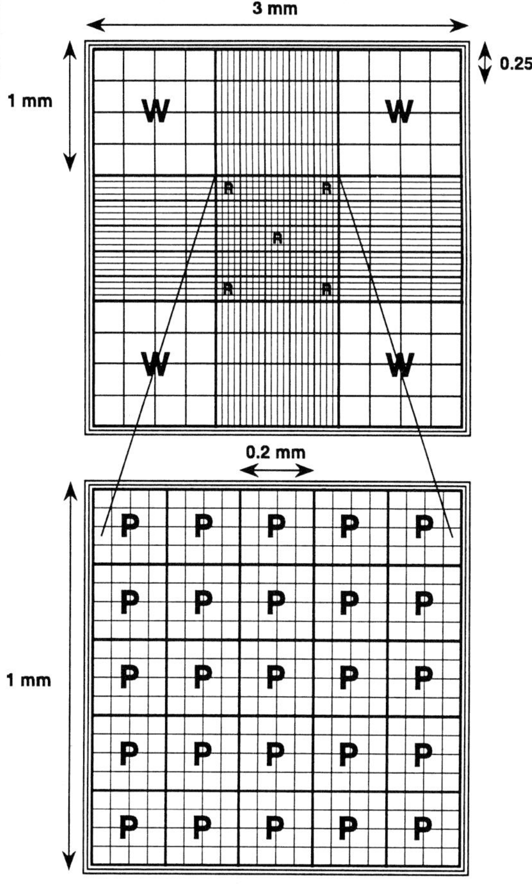

(**A**) The ruled area of the Neubauer hemacytometer. There are nine large (1 mm) squares. Each of the four corner 1-mm squares is subdivided into 16 smaller squares and is marked W to indicate use for counting leukocytes. The center 1-mm square is subdivided into 25 smaller squares, each 0.04 mm^2. The squares marked R were used for counting erythrocytes when they were historically counted manually. The higher magnification of this center square (*bottom*) illustrates all 25 0.04-mm^2 squares marked P where platelets are counted.

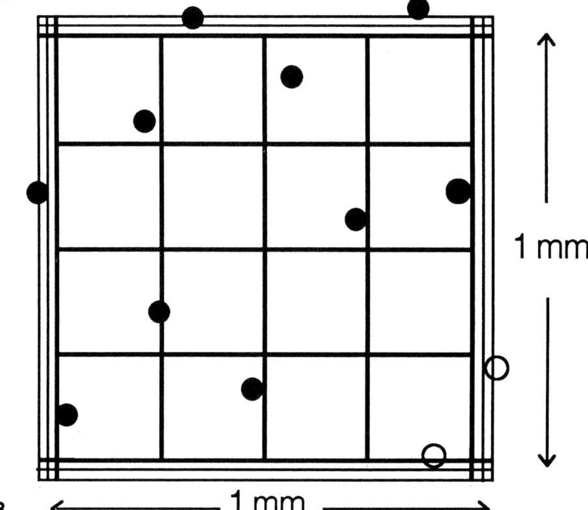

(**B**) Rules for microscopic counting of leukocytes on the Neubauer hemacytometer. One square millimeter is illustrated. Leukocytes are counted in 9 of these 1-mm squares. Leukocytes that touch the top or left triple boundary lines are counted; those that touch the bottom or right boundaries are not. (Solid circle, cells counted; open circle, cells not counted.)

continued

Procedure 30-1 Continued Performing a Manual White Blood Cell Count

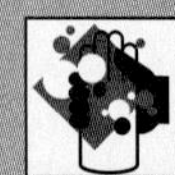
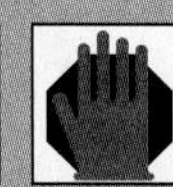
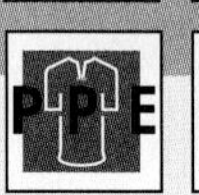
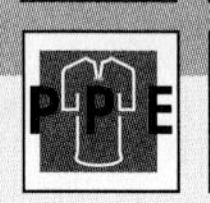

30

21. Add the total from both sides of the hemacytometer and divide by 2. Add 10% to the averaged total.
    The calculation will be simpler by allowing for a total of 10 squares rather than 9.
22. Multiply this figure by 100.
    The result calculates the total WBC by mm^3.
23. Clean the hemacytometer and cover glass with 10% bleach solution, and wipe dry with lens paper.
24. Clean the work area. Remove your PPE, and wash your hands.

DOCUMENTATION GUIDELINES

- Date and time
- Performance of procedure
- Site of venipuncture
- Results of testing
- Action taken, if any
- Patient education/instructions
- Your signature

Charting Example

DATE	TIME Venipuncture to left antecubitus.
	Hematology results as follows:
	WBC: 4880
	WBC diff:
	Neutrophils 60%
	Lymphocytes 25%
	Monocytes 5%
	Eosinophils 8%
	Basophils 2%
	RBC: 4.6
	Hgb 17
	Hct 50%
	MCV 88
	Platelets 250,000
	ESR 16
	PT 18
	Ptt 45
	—Your signature

Note: When performing a manual WBC count, always refer to the manufacturer's directions for counting and calculating results.

Conditions with diminished numbers of leukocytes (leukopenia or leukocytopenia) can result from several factors, including:

- Chemical toxicity
- Nutritional deficiencies
- Chronic or overwhelming infections
- Certain malignancies

The patient may be vulnerable to infections when the leukopenia is pronounced. Leukocytosis (increased amounts of WBCs) may indicate many factors, such as:

- Infections
- Inflammatory conditions
- Certain drugs

- Injuries to tissues
- Certain malignancies

The *WBC differential* is performed to determine the amounts of various WBC types present in the peripheral blood. These types include:

- Neutrophils (see Fig. 46-1*C* and *D*)
- Lymphocytes (see Fig. 46-1*E*)
- Monocytes (see Fig. 46-1*F*)
- Eosinophils (see Fig. 46-1*G*)
- Basophils (see Fig. 46-1*H*)

Because all of these types of leukocytes are colorless, a drop of blood is smeared on a glass slide and then stained so that leukocytes may be seen with a microscope. Once the peripheral blood is stained, 100 WBCs are counted, each tallied as to the type of cell seen, and then reported as percentages (Procedures 30-2, 30-3, and 30-4). These cell types are divided into two categories: the **granulocytes** (so called because of the granules in their cytoplasm that have distinctive staining characteristics) and the **agranulocytes** (meaning their cytoplasm does not contain visibly stained granules).

Checkpoint Question

2. *What is leukopenia, and what are four conditions that may cause it?*

Neutrophils

Neutrophils—also called polymorphonuclear neutrophils, PMNs, polys, segmented neutrophils, or segs—are the most abundant leukocyte and are the main granulocyte. Following release from the bone marrow, they circulate in the blood for about 7 hours. They then move into the tissues, where they perform their function. Neutrophils defend against foreign invaders by phagocytizing them. The invaders are then destroyed inside the cells with digestive **enzymes** contained within the granules. (Enzymes are substances that speed or initiate reactions.) These digestive enzymes eventually cause the neutrophil to die because

text continues on page 669

Procedure 30-2 Making a Peripheral Blood Smear

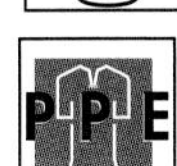

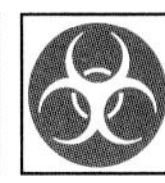

PURPOSE

To prepare a blood sample for microscopic examination

EQUIPMENT/SUPPLIES

- clean glass slides with frosted ends
- transfer pipette
- whole blood
- pencil
- well-mixed patient specimen

STEPS

1. Wash your hands.
2. Assemble the equipment.
3. Greet and identify the patient. Explain the procedure. Ask for and answer any questions.
4. Put on gloves, impervious gown, and face shield.
5. Obtain an EDTA (lavender-top tube) blood specimen from the patient, following the steps for venipuncture described in Chap. 29, Phlebotomy.
6. Label the slide on the frosted area.

   The slide must be labeled with the patient's name or identification number; the frosted end will retain the markings.

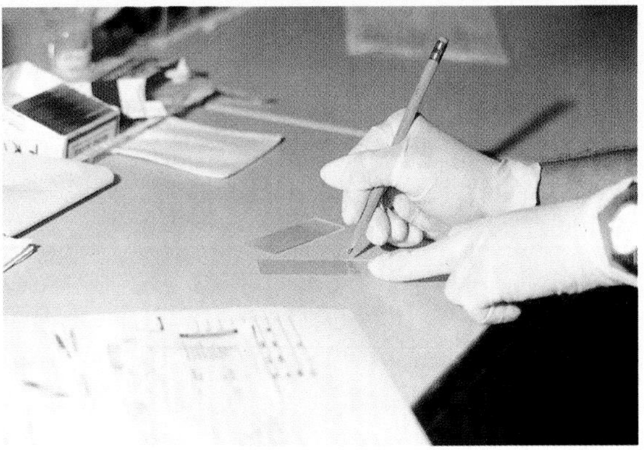

continued

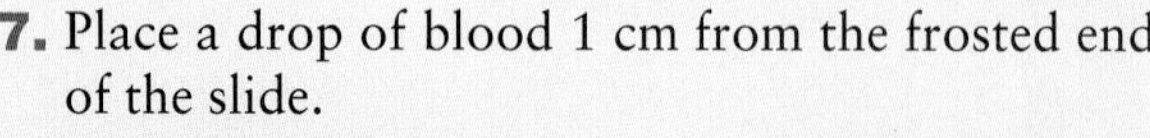

Procedure 30-2 Continued Making a Peripheral Blood Smear

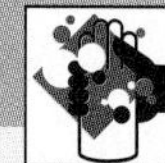
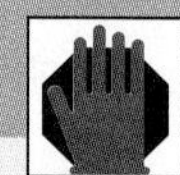

7. Place a drop of blood 1 cm from the frosted end of the slide.

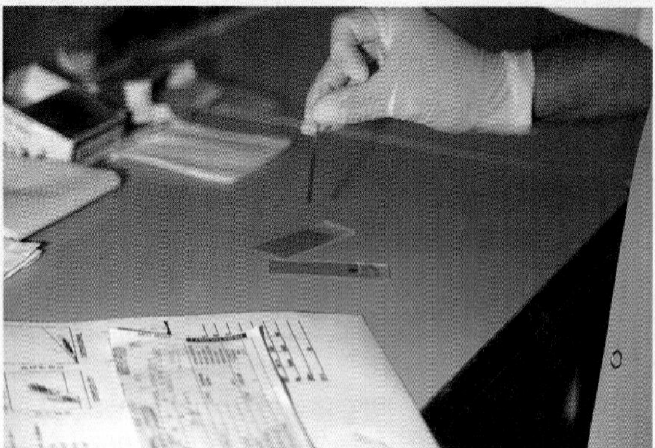

8. Place the slide on a flat surface. With the thumb and forefinger of the right hand, hold the second (spreader) slide against the surface of the first at a 30-degree angle. Draw the spreader slide back against the drop of blood until contact is established. (*Note:* The angle of the spreader slide may have to be greater than 30 degrees for larger or thinner drops of blood, and less than 30 degrees for smaller or thicker drops of blood.) Allow the blood to spread out under the edge, then push the spreader slide at a moderate speed toward the other end of the slide, keeping contact between the two slides at all times.

   A flat surface allows for smooth movements. A 30-degree angle allows the blood to be spread out in a thin film for viewing.

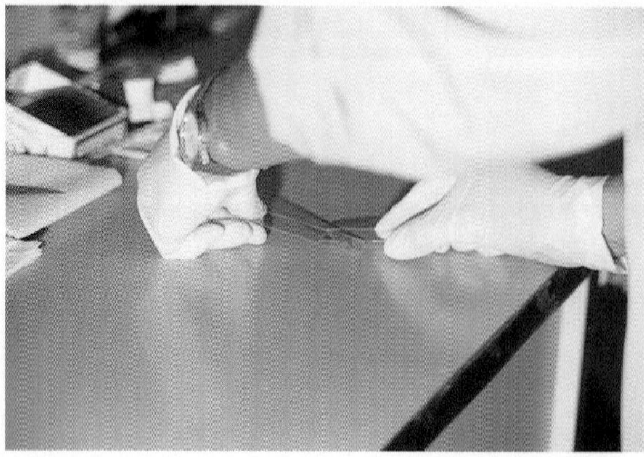

9. Allow the slide to air dry. (See the figures for examples of properly and improperly prepared smears.)

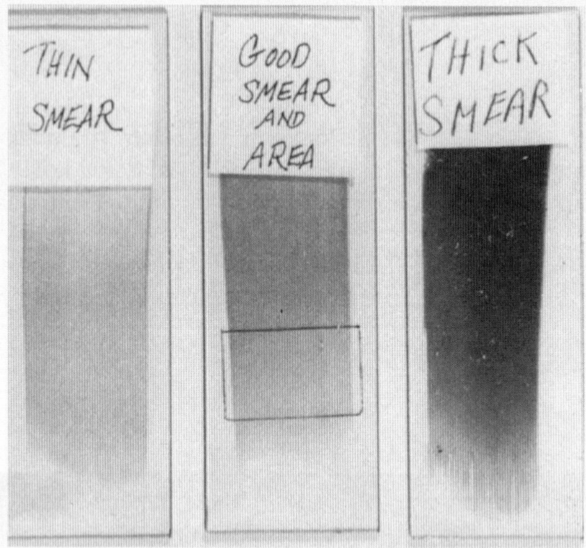

A properly prepared smear will yield a slide that is easy to read.

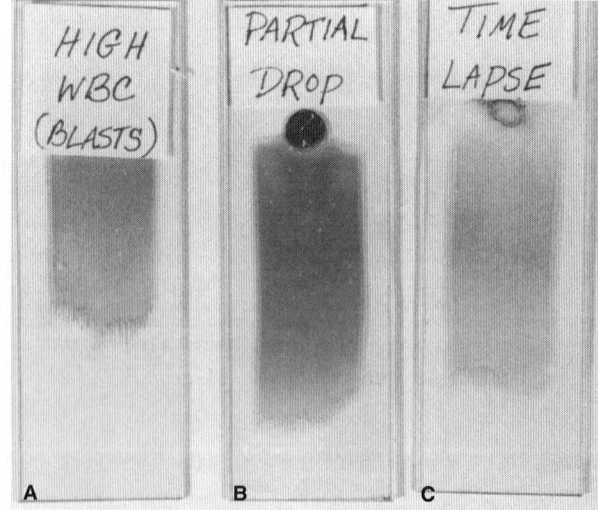

Improperly prepared smears will yield slides that are difficult to read. Slides B and C should be discarded and new slides prepared properly.

10. Properly care for or dispose of equipment and supplies. Clean the work area. Remove gloves, gown, and face shield, and wash your hands.

Note: Too much blood will make the smear invalid. (See Procedure 30-1 for documentation guidelines and charting example.)

Procedure 30-3 Staining a Peripheral Blood Smear

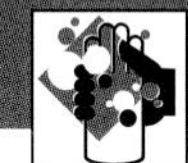
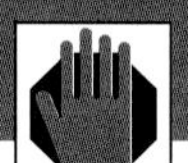

PPE

PURPOSE

To aid in identifying the types of blood cells in a patient sample
To aid in the diagnosis and treatment of infectious processes and blood dyscrasias

EQUIPMENT/SUPPLIES

- staining rack
- Wright's stain
- Giemsa stain
- prepared slide
- tweezers

STEPS

1. Wash your hands.
2. Assemble the equipment.
3. Put on gloves, impervious gown, and face shield.
4. Obtain a recently made, dried blood smear.
   A smear that is more than 2 hours old may deteriorate.
5. Place the slide on a stain rack blood side up.
   This provides a stable surface for staining.
6. Flood the slide with Wright's stain. Allow the stain to remain on the slide for 3 to 5 minutes or for the time specified by the manufacturer.
   Wright's stain contains alcohol to fix blood to the slide as well as to stain the blood cells according to their characteristics.
7. Using tweezers, tilt the slide so that the stain drains off. Apply equal amounts of Giemsa stain and water. A green sheen will appear on the surface. Allow the stain to remain on the slide for 5 minutes or the time specified by the manufacturer.
   This buffers the Wright's stain and enhances staining.
8. Holding the slide with tweezers, gently rinse the slide with water. Wipe off the back of the slide with gauze. Stand the slide upright and allow it to dry.
   This rinses and removes the excess stain for viewing under a microscope.
9. Properly care for or dispose of equipment and supplies. Clean the work area. Remove gloves, gown, and face shield, and wash your hands.

Note: Some manufacturers provide a simple one-step method that consists of dipping the smear in a staining solution, then rinsing. Directions are provided by the manufacturer for this procedure and will vary with the specific test. (See Procedure 30-1 for documentation guidelines and charting example.)

30

they are fatal to the cell and to all it ingests. The normal range for neutrophils is 50% to 70%; increased numbers are seen with bacterial infections.

When stained, the neutrophil has a light pink cytoplasm. This is due to the many small granules it contains. Its dark purple nucleus is segmented, and the typical number of lobes can range from 2 to 5. A hyperseg is one that has five or more lobes or segments. This can indicate a chronic infection or **folate** deficiency. (Folate, a salt of folic acid, is an essential nutrient.) A band (or stab) is a younger, less mature version of the neutrophil. The band's appearance is the same as the more mature counterpart, but its nucleus is not segmented. The normal range for bands is 0% to 5%. Increased amounts of bands (left shift or bandemia) can be an indicator of various acute situations that need more immediate attention than chronic conditions usually require.

Checkpoint Question

3. *What is the function of neutrophils?*

Lymphocytes

Lymphocytes (lymphs) are the second most numerous WBCs and the main agranulocyte. The main function of lymphocytes is to recognize that a particular cell or particle is foreign to the body and to make antibodies specific to its destruction. The antibodies then coat this foreign mass, resulting in one of two possible outcomes: The phagocytic system is activated to destroy the pathogen, or the complement system (a series of chemicals in the blood) is activated to destroy the cellular invaders by puncturing holes in their membranes. The normal range for lymphocytes is 20% to 35%. Increased numbers, especially atypical ones, can signal a viral infection. The life span of the lymphocyte is generally 3 to 4 days, which is longer than that of the neutrophil. However, some have much longer lives spanning into years or even decades.

In appearance, a normal lymphocyte is the smallest of the leukocytes. When stained, it has a small, round, dark purple nucleus. The surrounding cytoplasm is scant and sky blue. Atypical lymphs are larger with more cytoplasm that is either darker or lighter in color.

Procedure 30-4 Performing a White Blood Cell Differential

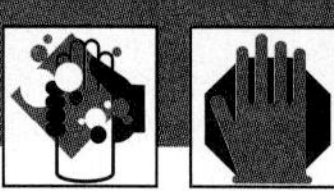

PURPOSE

To identify and quantify leukocytes present in a blood sample
To aid in the diagnosis and treatment of infectious processes and blood dyscrasias

EQUIPMENT/SUPPLIES

- stained peripheral blood smear
- microscope
- immersion oil
- paper
- recording tabulator

STEPS

1. Wash your hands.
2. Assemble the equipment.
3. Put on gloves.
4. Place the stained slide on the microscope. Focus on the feathered edge of the smear and scan to ensure an even distribution of cells and proper staining. (See the figure showing a properly prepared smear in Procedure 30-2, Step 9.) Use the low-power objective.
   Stage mounting sets up the slide to be read. Scanning the slide is a quality control assurance of staining performance.
5. Carefully turn the nosepiece to the high-power objective and bring the slide into focus using the fine adjustment.
6. Place a drop of oil on the slide, and rotate the oil immersion lens into place. Focus and begin to identify any leukocytes present.
   Oil is always used with the oil immersion lens. The oil immersion lens allows the greatest magnification and provides a path for the light source.
7. Record on a tally sheet or tabulator the types of white cells found.
   Tallying the types seen is necessary to record accurate percentages.
8. Move the stage so that the next field is in view. Identify any white cells in this field, and continue to the next field to identify all that are present until 100 white cells have been counted.
   Many fields must be viewed before 100 cells have been counted. The systematic movement of the stage so that another field comes into view ensures that this is accomplished correctly.
9. Calculate the number of each type of leukocyte as a percentage.
   Since 100 cells are counted, each represents one percentage point.
10. Properly care for or dispose of equipment and supplies. Clean the work are. Remove gloves, and wash your hands.

Note: A WBC differential is performed by a trained laboratory technologist. Abnormal cells can appear in the peripheral blood; recognizing them is an important diagnostic procedure that requires specific training. (See Procedure 30-1 for documentation guidelines and charting example.)

Monocytes

Monocytes (or monos) are the third most abundant leukocyte. They are agranulocytes. Like neutrophils, monocytes are capable of phagocytizing foreign material. They also aid the lymphocyte in providing the humoral response (destruction of foreign particles by antibodies). Monocytes stay in the bloodstream for about 3 days and then move into tissues.

The monocyte has a nucleus similar to the lymphocyte in that it is rounded and has no lobes. However, it is much larger than the lymph and closer in size to the neutrophil. When stained, the monocyte's cytoplasm is gray blue and has a ground-glass appearance. The normal range of monocytes is 3% to 8%. Monocytosis (increase in monos) is found in inflammatory responses and certain bacterial infections, such as syphilis and tuberculosis. Monocytopenia may occur after administration of certain drugs or an overwhelming infection.

Eosinophils

Eosinophils (or eos) are fourth in abundance. Their function is not completely understood. The normal range for eosinophils is 0% to 7%. They will, however, increase in allergic reactions and some infections (especially parasitic). The eosinophil has a bilobed nucleus with large distinctive red-orange granules in the cytoplasm.

Basophils

Basophils (or basos) are the least numerous, representing less than 1% of circulating WBCs. The nucleus is either bilobed or trilobed, and on staining, very large dark blue-purple granules are seen in the cytoplasm, making them granulocytes. Basophils appear to be involved in allergic asthma, contact allergies, and hypothyroidism and chronic myeloid leukemia.

Checkpoint Question

4. *Elevated eosinophils and basophils are both seen with what condition?*

Red Blood Cell Count

Red blood cells (erythrocytes) are designed to transport gases (mainly oxygen and carbon dioxide) between the lungs and the tissues. Their special structure as a biconcave disk containing hemoglobin enables them to exchange gases readily in the tissues and lung fields. As blood moves through the capillary bed of the lungs, RBCs release carbon dioxide that was picked up at the tissues and then binds oxygen. As the blood leaves the lungs and circulates to the periphery, oxygen is released from the RBCs into the tissues. At the same time, carbon dioxide (the by-product of metabolism) diffuses into the blood and is brought back to the lungs so that it can be removed from the body by exhalation.

Red blood cells are made in the bone marrow along with all other blood cells. Their production is influenced by the hormone **erythropoietin,** which is released mainly from the kidneys. When tissue hypoxia is detected, this hormone migrates to the marrow, which then steps up RBC production (erythropoiesis) and corrects the anemia by releasing more RBCs into the circulation. Other factors can also influence the quality and quantity of erythropoiesis. For example, vitamin B_{12} and folic acid are important substances for the cells to mature properly. Iron is needed for incorporation into the globin molecule to make functional hemoglobin. Initially, erythrocytes have a nucleus, but as they mature, the nucleus is pushed out, and the color of its cytoplasm changes from blue to red. The mature RBC is a pale red biconcave disk that can squeeze through very small capillaries. The average RBC lives about 120 days.

Measurement of RBCs and associated tests, such as hemoglobin, hematocrit, and **indices** provide a useful guide in detecting anemia, which can be caused by decreased erythrocyte production (as in iron deficiency), increased RBC destruction (as in **hemolytic anemia**), or blood loss. The normal range of RBCs for men is 4.6 to 6.2 million/mm^3 (per cubic millimeter) and for women, 4.2 to 5.4 million/mm^3 (Procedure 30-5).

When performing a differential on a peripheral blood smear, the laboratory technician also notices and comments on the variation in size (**anisocytosis**) and shape (**poikilocytosis**) of the RBCs. Findings such as target cells can indicate liver impairment. Table 30-1 describes some common erythrocyte abnormalities and their associated conditions.

Hemoglobin

Hemoglobin is the functioning unit of the RBC. Each hemoglobin molecule contains four protein chains called globins. There are different types of globin chains: A and B are the most common with some F (fetal) in newborns as well as abnormal hemoglobins such as S (sickle) found in persons having sickle cell disease or carrying the sickle trait. Located in the folds of each globin is a heme unit that contains one iron molecule each; the iron can reversibly bind gases, such as oxygen and carbon dioxide. The iron also gives RBCs their distinctive red color. There are millions of hemoglobin molecules in each RBC. The normal range for hemoglobins is 13 to 18 g/dL (or g/1,000 mL) for men and 12 to 16 g/dL for women. Anemia is detected with a hemoglobin measurement, which is a direct indicator of the body's ability to oxygenate itself (Procedure 30-6).

30

Hematocrit

The hematocrit is the percentage of RBCs contained in whole blood. It is expressed as a percentage. For example, a hematocrit of 40% indicates that of the total blood volume, 40% of it consists of RBCs. The remaining 60% is plasma, which includes the WBCs and platelets.

To measure the hematocrit, the blood is centrifuged to pack the RBCs. The percentage is then read. Automated instruments do not measure the hematocrit but rather calculate the hematocrit from the RBC count and MCV. The purpose for measuring the hematocrit is

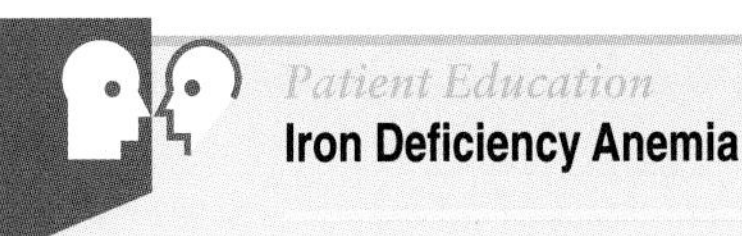

Patient Education

Iron Deficiency Anemia

Patients who have iron deficiency anemia should be educated regarding proper dietary management. They should be instructed to eat foods high in iron, such as liver, oysters, kidney beans, lean meats, turnips, egg yolks, whole wheat bread, carrots, raisins, and dark greens. Many vitamin supplements with iron are available and can be added to the diet. Patients should be alerted that iron supplements can cause constipation and dark stools.

Procedure 30-5 Performing a Manual Red Blood Cell Count

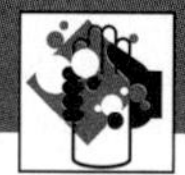
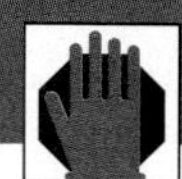
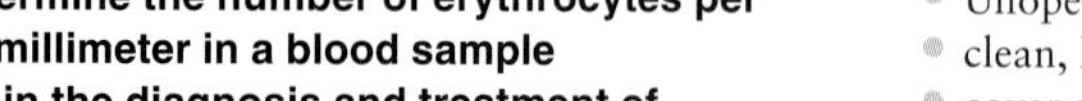
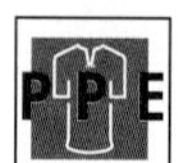

PURPOSE

To determine the number of erythrocytes per cubic millimeter in a blood sample
To aid in the diagnosis and treatment of anemias and blood dyscrasias

EQUIPMENT/SUPPLIES

- Unopette system for red cell count
- clean, lint-free hemacytometer
- cover glass
- gauze
- moist filter paper or moist cotton ball
- Petri dish
- microscope
- hand tally counter

STEPS

1.–16. Follow steps 1–16 listed in Procedure 30-1: Performing a Manual White Blood Cell Count.

17. Place the hemacytometer on the microscope stage so that the ruled area can be surveyed with the low-power objective. Focus the microscope, then progress to the 400× magnification to count the RBCs.

The slide is ready for evaluation.

18. Count the RBCs in the four corner squares and the center square following the zigzag pattern described in Procedure 30-1. Starting at the top far left, count the top row left to right. At the end of the top row, drop to the second row, and count from right to left. Continue this pattern until all of the rows are counted. Count cells touching the upper and left side, but do not count those on the lower and right side.

The traditional counting pattern avoids omitting or overcounting cells.

19. Tally the count and record the number. Return the counter to 0 and count the next grid. Count the opposite side of the hemacytometer.

20. The count within the squares should not vary by more than 20 cells. If the variance is greater, the test must be repeated.

Comparing results as you count helps ensure accuracy of testing.

21. Average the two sides, and multiply the result by 10,000.

This calculation gives the total number of RBCs per mm³.

22. Clean the hemacytometer and cover glass with 10% bleach, and wipe dry with lens paper. Dispose of or care for any other equipment and supplies appropriately. Clean the work area. Remove gloves and gown, and wash your hands.

Note: Always read and follow the manufacturer's instructions for performing this procedure. (See Procedure 30-1 for documentation guidelines and charting example.)

to detect anemia. The normal range is 45% to 52% for men and 37% to 48% for women (Procedure 30-7).

Checkpoint Question

5. *A patient has a hematocrit of 20%. What does this percentage represent?*

Indices

Indices are used in the differentiation of anemias. Indices give the physician an idea of the size and hemoglobin content of the RBCs. They also serve as a quality control check because of their relationship to the hemoglobin, hematocrit, RBC count, and the microscopic RBC evaluation. Indices are calculated automatically by many hematology analyzers. However, they can be calculated by hand using Hgb, Hct, and RBC results. The three main indices calculated are MCV, MCH, and MCHC.

Mean Cell Volume

Red blood cells can vary in size. The mean corpuscular (cell) volume or MCV computes the average size of RBCs. For example, a patient with an MCV of 85 cubic micrometers or **femtoliters** (one quadrillionth of a liter) may have RBCs that range in size from 75 to 95, but the average would be 85. The MCV can be used as an indicator for anemias caused by the nutritional deficiencies that affect RBC production. The normal range for MCV is 80 to 95 cubic micrometers (or femtoliters).

Microcytosis (MCV < 80) is most commonly caused by iron deficiency. This finding coupled with RBC parameters (RBC count, hemoglobin, and hematocrit) will indicate anemia and lead to a diagnosis of

text continues on page 674

Table 30-1 **Erythrocyte Abnormalities**

Abnormality	*Associated Conditions*
Hypochromasia—diminished hemoglobin in RBCs; appear paler with more area of central pallor.	Anemias (especially iron deficiency), **thalassemia** (a hemolytic anemia)
Hyperchromasia—increased hemoglobin in RBCs; appear to have less or no area of central pallor.	**Megaloblastic anemia** (characterized by large, dysfunctional RBCs), hereditary **spherocytosis** (condition in which nearly all the RBCs are spherocytes)
Polychromasia—some RBCs have a blue color.	Hemolysis, acute blood loss
Microcytosis—RBCs are smaller than usual.	Iron deficiency anemia, thalassemia
Macrocytosis—RBCs are larger than normal.	B_{12} and folate deficiencies, megaloblastic anemias
Elliptocytes/ovalocytes—RBCs are distinctly oval in shape.	Hereditary **elliptocytosis,** iron deficiency anemia, **myelofibrosis** (disorder in which bone marrow tissue develops in abnormal sites), **sickle cell anemia** (hereditary anemia characterized by the presence of sickle-shaped RBCs)
Target cells—RBCs resemble a target with light and dark rings.	Liver impairment, anemias (especially thalassemia), **hemoglobin C disease** (genetic blood disorder)
Schistocytes—RBCs are fragmented.	Hemolysis, burns, **intravascular coagulation** (clot formation within the vessels)
Spherocytes—RBCs show no area of central pallor.	Hereditary spherocytosis, hemolytic anemias, burns
Burr cells—RBCs have small, regular **spicules** (sharp points).	Artifact as blood dries, **hyperosmolarity** (a condition of increased numbers of dissolved substances in the plasma)

30

Procedure 30-6 Performing a Hemoglobin Determination

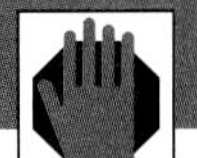

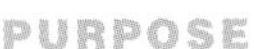

PURPOSE

To determine the oxygen-carrying capacity of the blood in a patient sample
To aid in the diagnosis and treatment of anemia

EQUIPMENT/SUPPLIES

- hemoglobinometer
- applicator sticks
- whole blood

PPE

STEPS

1. Wash your hands.
2. Assemble the necessary equipment.
3. Put on gloves, gown, and face shield.
4. Obtain an EDTA (lavender-top tube) blood specimen from the patient, following the steps for capillary puncture described in Chap. 29, Phlebotomy.
5. Place a drop of well-mixed whole blood (obtained by skin puncture) on the glass chamber of the hemoglobinometer. Place the coverslip into the holding clip over the chamber and slide it into the holding clip.
   This prepares the sample for the hemoglobin determination.
6. At one of the open edges, push the applicator stick into the chamber. Gently move the stick around until the specimen no longer appears cloudy.
   This lyses the red cells, thereby releasing the hemoglobin.
7. Slide the chamber into the hemoglobinometer. Remove the face shield.
   The chamber must be inserted into the receiving slot to perform the color comparison reading.

continued

Procedure 30-6 Continued Performing a Hemoglobin Determination

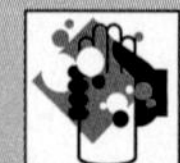
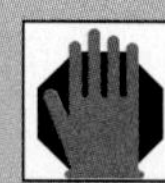
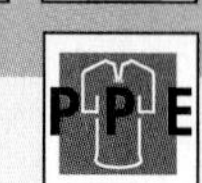

8. With your left hand, hold the meter and press the light button. View the field through the eyepiece. With your right hand, move the dial until both the right and left sides match each other in color intensity. Note the hemoglobin level indicated on the dial.

   The chamber must be illuminated to compare the colors. Matching fields indicate that the amount of hemoglobin in the sample matches the internal standard.

9. Clean the chamber and work area with 10% bleach solution. Dispose of equipment and supplies appropriately. Remove gloves and gown, and wash your hands.

30

DOCUMENTATION GUIDELINES

- Date and time
- Site of capillary puncture
- Performance of test
- Results of testing
- Action taken, if any
- Patient education/instructions
- Your signature

Charting Example

DATE	TIME Pt c/o no energy. Periods have been
	heavy, awaiting hysterectomy for
	dysfunctional bleeding. Cap puncture
	L ring finger. Hgb 9.5. Dr. Royal notified,
	Fe supplement ordered. —Your signature

Note: Regarding quality assurance, calibration chambers are included in the hemoglobinometer kit and are used to verify proper functioning of the meter. This procedure may vary according to the instrument used. Some manufacturers offer a digitally read hemoglobin device that is less subjective and is therefore considered more accurate and easier to use.

iron deficiency anemia. Likewise, macrocytosis (MCV > 95) may be caused by a deficiency of B_{12} or folic acid. These abnormalities can also result in anemia. Liver disorders may sometimes give increased MCVs.

Mean Cell Hemoglobin and Mean Cell Hemoglobin Concentration

As technology becomes increasingly sophisticated, more measurable parameters are added to the CBC. Among the most useful are MCH and MCHC. MCH and MCHC indicate relative hemoglobin concentration in the blood; when anemia is present, both measurements will be decreased. Other conditions may be indicated by these measurements as well.

Both the MCH and MCHC are calculated. The MCH is derived from the ratio of hemoglobin and the number of RBCs present in the specimen. The MCHC is derived from the ratio of hemoglobin and hematocrit.

Platelet Count

Platelets (thrombocytes), like other blood cells, are made in the bone marrow. However, they are not actually cells but cell fragments that adhere to damaged endothelium. Platelets are essential to hemostasis because they not only aid in sealing wounds until a clot can form, but they also help initiate the clotting factors to form the more stable fibrin clot.

The normal range for platelets is 150,000 to 200,000 to 400,000/mm³. Thrombocytopenia (decreased platelets) can be caused by a variety of conditions and is the most common cause of bleeding disorders. The bleeding usually occurs from many small capillaries. Treatment requires a specific diagnosis of the cause of the thrombocytopenia. Administration of drugs is usually stopped because almost any drug can cause its onset. Thrombocytosis (increased platelets) is typically benign. It can be seen after splenectomies or during inflammatory diseases.

Platelets are much smaller than RBCs. They stain a light purplish blue, have an irregular shape, and contain no nucleus.

ERYTHROCYTE SEDIMENTATION RATE

The ESR measures the rate at which RBCs settle out in a tube. Anticoagulated blood is placed into a calibrated glass column and then allowed to settle undisturbed for 1 hour. At the end of the hour, the distance the RBCs have fallen is measured. This is expressed in millimeters per hour (mm/h). Although there are several different methods for performing the ESR, such as the Wintrobe and the Westergren methods, the principle remains the same. Procedure 30-8 describes the

text continues on page 678

Procedure 30-7 Performing a Manual Microhematocrit Determination

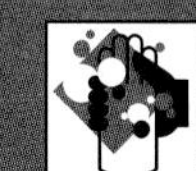
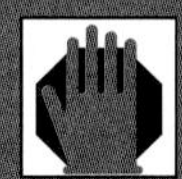
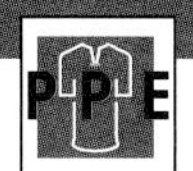

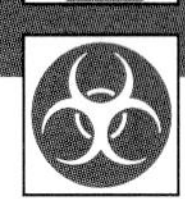

PURPOSE

To determine the quantity of erythrocytes in a centrifuged blood specimen
To aid in the diagnosis and treatment of anemia

EQUIPMENT/SUPPLIES

- microcollection tubes
- sealing clay
- microhematocrit centrifuge
- microhematocrit reading device

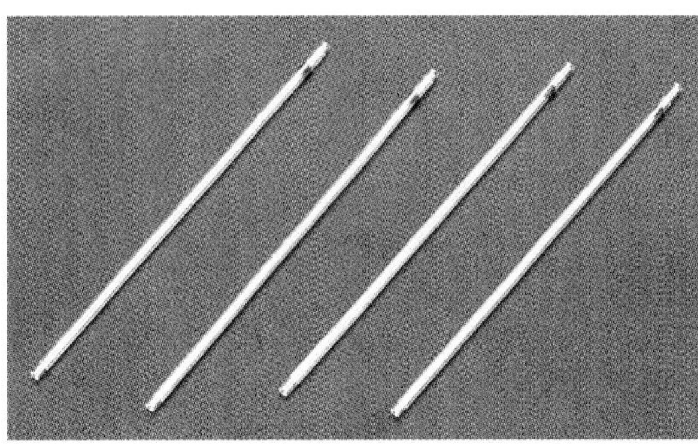

Microcollection tubes.

30

STEPS

1. Wash your hands.

2. Assemble the equipment.

3. Put on gloves, gown, and face shield.

4. Draw blood into the capillary tube by one of two methods: (1) directly from a capillary puncture where the tip of the capillary tube is touched to the blood at the wound and allowed to fill ¾ of the tube or to the indicated mark (see Chap. 29, Phlebotomy); or (2) from a well mixed anticoagulated (EDTA) tube of whole blood where, again, the tip is touched to the blood and allowed to fill ¾ of the tube. Place the forefinger over the top of the tube, wipe excess blood off the sides, and push the bottom into the sealing clay. Draw a second specimen in the same manner.

Whole blood from a capillary puncture has not clotted yet and is acceptable. If blood from a tube is not well mixed, the reading is likely to be inaccurate. Holding the finger over the tip stops blood from dripping out the bottom. The clay seals one end of the tube to contain it during centrifugation. A second tube is necessary for duplicate testing as a quality control measure.

5. Place the tubes in the radial grooves of the microhematocrit centrifuge opposite each other. Place the cover on top of the grooved area, and tighten by turning the knob clockwise. Close the lid. Spin for 5 minutes or as directed by the manufacturer.

Specimens should always be placed opposite each other to balance the centrifuge. Read the manufacturer's directions for the specific centrifuge used in your facility; 5 minutes is a normal time limit.

6. Remove the tubes from the centrifuge and read the results from the reading device available (instructions are printed on the device). (The accompanying figure shows two methods for determining microhematocrit values.) Results should match within 5% of each other. Take the average and report as a percentage. (*Note:* Some microhematocrit centrifuges have the scale printed within the machine at the radial grooves.)

Results greater than 5% variation have been found to offer unreliable results.

continued

Procedure 30-7 Continued Performing a Manual Microhematocrit Determination

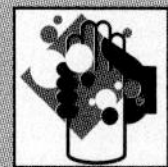
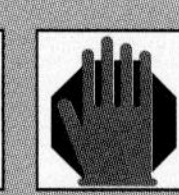
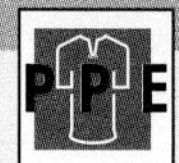

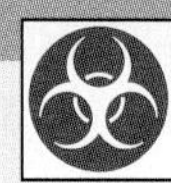

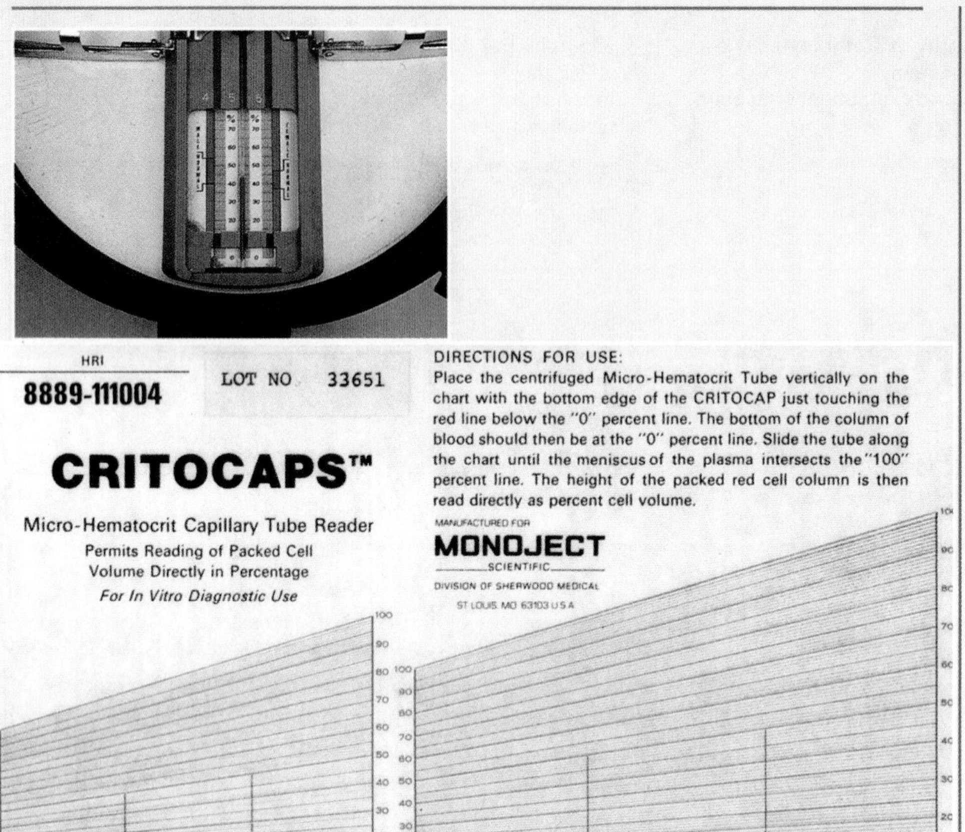

HRI
8889-111004
LOT NO 33651
CRITOCAPS™
Micro-Hematocrit Capillary Tube Reader
Permits Reading of Packed Cell Volume Directly in Percentage
For In Vitro Diagnostic Use
DIRECTIONS FOR USE:
Place the centrifuged Micro-Hematocrit Tube vertically on the chart with the bottom edge of the CRITOCAP just touching the red line below the "0" percent line. The bottom of the column of blood should then be at the "0" percent line. Slide the tube along the chart until the meniscus of the plasma intersects the "100" percent line. The height of the packed red cell column is then read directly as percent cell volume.
MANUFACTURED FOR
MONOJECT
SCIENTIFIC
DIVISION OF SHERWOOD MEDICAL
ST LOUIS MO 63103 USA

7. Dispose of the microhematocrit tubes in a biohazard container. Properly care for or dispose of other equipment and supplies. Clean the work area. Remove gloves, gown, and face shield, and wash your hands.

DOCUMENTATION GUIDELINES

- Date and time
- Site of capillary puncture
- Performance of test
- Results of testing
- Action taken, if any
- Patient education/instructions
- Your signature

Charting Example

DATE	TIME Capillary tube filled from skin
	puncture, left ring finger. Hct: 42%.
	Dr. Erikson notified. —Your signature

Procedure 30-8 Performing a Wintrobe Erythrocyte Sedimentation Rate

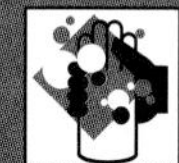
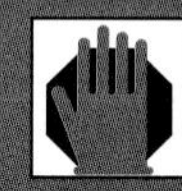
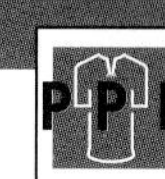

PURPOSE

To determine the rate at which erythrocytes separate from plasma and settle in a tube
To aid in the diagnosis of nonspecific inflammatory processes

EQUIPMENT/SUPPLIES

- anticoagulation tube
- Wintrobe tube
- transfer pipette
- timer

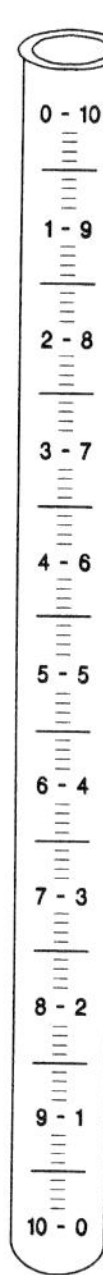

Wintrobe tube for erythrocyte sedimentation rate determination.

STEPS

1. Wash your hands.
2. Assemble the necessary equipment.
3. Put on gloves, impervious gown, and face shield.
4. Draw blood (see Chap. 29, Phlebotomy) into an EDTA lavender-stoppered anticoagulation tube.
   The blood must not be allowed to clot; it must be drawn in an anticoagulation tube.
5. Fill a graduated Wintrobe tube to the 0 mark with the well mixed whole (EDTA) blood using the provided transfer pipette. Be sure to eliminate any trapped bubbles and fill exactly to the 0 line.
   Bubbles and incorrect filling will alter the test results.
6. Place the tube in a holder that will allow the tube to remain in a vertical position.
7. Wait exactly 1 hour; use a timer for accuracy. Keep the tube straight upright and undisturbed during the hour.
   Never use a shorter time and multiply the reading; less time will give inaccurate results. Tilting or disturbing the tube also will alter the results.
8. Record the level of the top of the red blood cells after 1 hour. Normal results for men are 0–10 mL/h; for women, 0–15 mL/h.
9. Properly care for or dispose of equipment and supplies. Clean the work area. Remove gloves, gown, and face shield. Wash your hands.

DOCUMENTATION GUIDELINES

- Date and time
- Site of venipuncture
- Performance of test
- Results of testing
- Action taken, if any
- Patient education/instructions
- Your signature

Charting Example

DATE	TIME 45-year-old WF presented with
	vague aches. Specimen drawn L
	antecubitus in lavender-top tube per
	Dr. North's order. Wintrobe ESR test
	results 12 mL/h. Dr. North notified.
	—Your signature

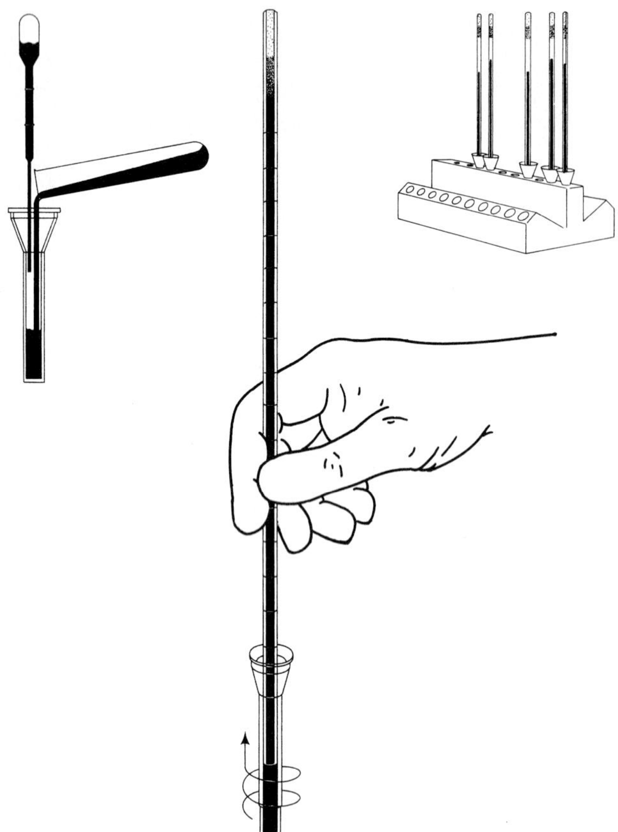

Figure 30-2 Westergren Dispette System for erythrocyte sedimentation rate (ESR) determination. (*Left*) After mixing four parts EDTA-anticoagulated whole blood with one part 0.85% saline, mixture is poured into a vial. (*Center*) Dispette is placed in vial using a twisting motion until blood reaches bottom of safety autozeroing plug. (*Right*) Vial and Dispette are placed vertically in a special rack for 60 minutes before reading the ESR. (Courtesy of Ulster Scientific, Inc., Highland, NY.)

steps for performing a Wintrobe ESR. Figure 30-2 outlines the steps for using the Westergren method.

The normal range for men is 0 to 10 mm/h and for women, 0 to 20 mm/h. Elevations in ESR values are not specific for any disorder; however, they do indicate the presence of either inflammation or any other condition that causes increased or altered proteins in the blood (eg, rheumatoid arthritis). The more rapidly the RBCs fall in the column, the greater the degree of inflammation. Physicians use this as a guideline when monitoring the course of inflammation in rheumatoid arthritis. ESRs can also be elevated with infections, pregnancy, and malignancy.

COAGULATION TESTS

Coagulation tests measure the ability of whole blood to form a clot. Thirteen factors (proteins) in the blood act in sequential order when stimulated by cell membrane disruptions (eg, cuts, tears, or other injuries) to form a clot. This clot is more stable than a platelet plug, which is the first in the chain of events that occur on injury. Both the platelet plug and the fibrin clot are needed for continued hemostasis. When vascular damage occurs, the following sequence of events occurs:

1. *Vasoconstriction.* The vein constricts to reduce blood loss.
2. *Platelet plug formation.* The platelets adhere to the wound and form a plug, temporarily slowing the blood flow.
3. *Fibrin clot formation.* When activated, the clotting factors form an insoluble clot at the wound site. (The two most common tests for determining how well a fibrin clot can form are prothrombin time and partial thromboplastin time; see below.)
4. *Clot lysis and vascular repair.* Another set of proteins slowly dissolves the fibrin clot as the surrounding endothelial tissue of the blood vessel wall replicates to repair the damage.

Prothrombin Time

The prothrombin time (PT) is a one-stage test in which calcium and **thromboplastin** (a complex substance that starts the clotting process) are added to the patient's plasma. The clotting time is then observed. The normal

What If?

What if your patient is receiving Coumadin (the brand name for warfarin) and does not return for scheduled prothrombin tests? What should you do?

Inform the physician, who will then determine whether or not to order a refill prescription for Coumadin for the patient. Be sure to document all phone conversations with the patient, including the date, time, and message given. Also document the patient's responses, using quotes whenever possible. Educate the patient regarding the dangers of self-medicating Coumadin, which can include excessive bleeding (with overmedicating) or clotting (with undermedicating). Make sure the patient understands the purpose of the medication and the importance of blood tests. Determine why the patient is refusing to come into the office for blood work; the reason may be as simple as lack of transportation. If this is the case, investigate your community's health care resources. For example, many communities have visiting nurse associations or hospital outreach programs staffed with health care professionals who will draw blood for patients in the home.

Procedure 30-9 Determining Bleeding Time

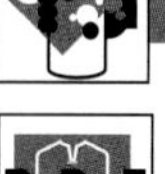
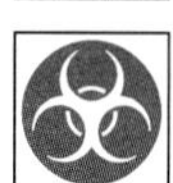

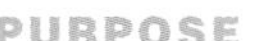

PURPOSE

To determine the time required for clot formation
To aid in the diagnosis and treatment of clotting disorders

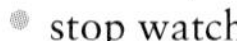

EQUIPMENT/SUPPLIES

- blood pressure cuff
- Autolet device
- alcohol or antiseptic wipe
- filter paper
- butterfly bandage
- stop watch

STEPS

1. Wash your hands.
2. Assemble the equipment.
3. Greet and identify the patient. Explain the procedure. Ask for and answer any questions.
   Some patients will be nervous before the incision is made; reassure them that the cut is very small and will barely be felt.
4. Put on gloves, impervious gown, and face shield.
5. Position the patient so that the arm is extended in a manner that is both comfortable and stable.
   The test requires a moderate length of time and requires that the patient remain still; a comfortable position will help ensure that the patient does not move until the procedure is complete.
6. Have the patient turn the palm upward so that the inner aspect of the arm is exposed. Select a site several inches below the antecubital area. The area should be free of lesions and with no visible veins. Clean the site with alcohol or antiseptic wipe.
   The inner aspect provides a surface relatively free of hair. (Rarely, the patient's arm may need to be shaved at the site.) There are no large surface vessels at this site.
7. Apply the pressure cuff and set it at 40 mmHg for the length of the test. Adjust it as needed throughout the test to maintain the pressure.
   Placing the pressure cuff on the arm stabilizes the pressure to the arm.
8. Twist the tear-away tab on the Autolet. Make an incision 1 mm in depth on the cleaned skin surface by placing the Autolet bleeding time device on the site and pressing the trigger button on the side. This will spring the blade to make the incision. At the same time, start the stop watch.
   A 1-mm incision is sufficiently deep to disrupt the surface capillaries but not the underlying veins.
9. At 30-second intervals, bring the filter paper near the edge of the wound to draw off some of the accumulating blood. Avoid touching the wound with the filter paper.
   Removing the blood from the wound site is essential for observing the slowing of the blood flow. The filter paper should not touch the wound because disruption of the platelet plug may occur, resulting in an inaccurate measurement of bleeding time.
10. The test is complete when the blood flow stops completely. Stop the watch when the blood no longer stains the filter paper; note the time to the nearest 30 seconds.
    When the blood flow stops, this indicates that the platelet plug has formed.
11. Apply a butterfly bandage across the wound to keep it sealed and cover the site with a waterproof bandage. Instruct the patient to keep the site dry and not to remove the bandage for a minimum of 24 hours.
    Butterfly bandages work best to reduce scarring.
12. Properly care for or dispose of all equipment and supplies. Clean the work area. Remove gloves, gown, and face shield, and wash your hands.

DOCUMENTATION GUIDELINES

- Date and time
- Site of puncture
- Performance of test
- Results of test
- Action taken, if any
- Patient education/instructions
- Your signature

Charting Example

DATE	TIME Skin puncture of L inner forearm,
	bleeding time test done, results 14 min.
	Dr. Lancaster notified. —Your signature

WARNING! Be sure you are away from superficial veins. Puncturing superficial veins will cause a prolonged bleeding time. If the patient is having clotting problems, excessive bleeding could occur.

Note: Low platelet counts and aspirin ingestion will prolong the bleeding time. Each laboratory has a set policy for stopping the test if the flow continues for too long. Most laboratories stop the bleeding test at 15 to 30 minutes. Any testing beyond this point is not needed because it is established that the bleeding time is not normal.

range is 12 to 15 seconds, but each laboratory establishes its own range. A patient's PT may be prolonged when a deficiency of certain factors exists, such as liver disease or vitamin K deficiency, or as a result of **coumarin** (anticoagulant) therapy. Current restrictions are in place that do not allow medical assistants to perform the PT test.

Partial Thromboplastin Time

The partial thromboplastin time (PTT) is a two-stage test in which partially activated thromboplastin is incubated with the patient's plasma followed by the addition of calcium. The clotting time is then determined. The normal range is 32 to 51 seconds, but again, each laboratory establishes its own range, so there may be a slight variation. A PTT may be prolonged in certain factor deficiencies, especially those that cause hemophilia. **Heparin** (anticoagulant) therapy also will prolong the PTT, so this test is used for monitoring and determining dosages.

30

Bleeding Time

The bleeding time test is performed to determine the time required for blood to stop flowing from a very small wound. An incision is made on the inside of the forearm with an automated cutting device, such as an **Autolet,** to a depth of 1 mm. Normal bleeding times range from 2 to 6 minutes (Procedure 30-9).

Although it is a rather nonspecific test, prolonged bleeding times can occur with decreased platelets or impaired platelet function. Ingestion of aspirin or other anti-inflammatory medications can also inhibit platelet function. A prolonged bleeding time may indicate the use of medications or such disease states as uremic syndrome. Bleeding times are often performed before surgeries to detect various bleeding problems that may interfere with surgical hemostasis.

Checkpoint Question

6. *What are the two most common tests used to determine how well a fibrin clot will form?*

Answers to Checkpoint Questions

1. *Hematopoiesis is the medical term for blood cell production. It is influenced by hormones and depends on adequate nutrients, such as iron.*
2. *Leukopenia is a diminished number of leukocytes. It can be caused by chemical toxicity, nutritional deficiencies, overwhelming or chronic infections, and certain malignancies.*
3. *Neutrophils defend against foreign invaders by phagocytosis.*
4. *Elevated eosinophils and basophils are both seen with allergic reactions.*
5. *A hematocrit of 20% indicates that of the total blood volume, 20% of it consists of red blood cells.*
6. *The two most common tests for determining how well a fibrin clot can form are prothrombin time and partial thromboplastin time.*

Critical Thinking Challenges

1. A patient was taking a medication that caused him to become neutropenic. To what might he be susceptible?
2. A patient lives at a very high elevation, where there is less oxygen than at sea level. Would you expect her hemoglobin to be greater, lesser, or the same in comparison to living at sea level?
3. A patient with rheumatoid arthritis has an erythrocyte sedimentation rate of 77 mm/h when she has her blood tested at the doctor's office. Two weeks later, she returns and now the rate is 31 mm/h. With her condition in mind, would you expect that she is improving or not?

Suggestions for Further Reading

Bullock, B. L. (1996). *Pathophysiology: Adaptations and Alterations in Function,* 4th ed. Philadelphia: Lippincott-Raven.

Fishbach, F. (1996). *A Manual of Laboratory and Diagnostic Tests,* 5th ed. Philadelphia: Lippincott-Raven.

Lotspeich-Steininger, C., Stein-Martin, E. A., & Koepke, J. A. (1992). *Clinical Hematology Principles, Procedures and Correlations.* Philadelphia: J.B. Lippincott.

Rubin, E., & Farber, J. L. (1998). *Pathology,* 3rd ed. Philadelphia: Lippincott-Raven.

Chapter Competencies (continued)

Performance Objectives

Upon successfully completing this chapter, you will be able to:

1. Perform an agglutination test.
2. Perform an enzyme immunoassay test.
3. Perform a chromatographic assay test.
4. Perform a mononucleosis test (Procedure 31-1).
5. Perform an HCG pregnancy test (Procedure 31-2).
6. Perform a group-A rapid strep test (Procedure 31-3).

Key Terms

(See Glossary for definitions.)

agglutination
conjugate
donor
hemolysis
immunohematology
sensitivity
serology
specificity
substrate

Serology is the study of antigens and antibodies. The term serology refers to the source of most of the samples, the liquid part of blood called serum, produced when whole blood is allowed to clot. Serologic methods are used to:

- Identify bacterial and viral infections (eg, streptococcus, hepatitis A, hepatitis B, human immunodeficiency virus, rubella, and Epstein-Barr virus)
- Diagnose *Chlamydia* infections, syphilis, and Rocky Mountain spotted fever
- Measure substances such as human chorionic gonadotropin (HCG) found in pregnant women, drugs found in the urine, and hormones found in serum

Immunohematology refers to the testing done in the blood bank on red blood cells (RBCs, erythrocytes) and serum to ensure that blood from a **donor** (one who contributes blood) is compatible with a recipient's blood. It involves testing for antigens on the surface of RBCs using reagents containing antibodies called antisera as well as testing for antibodies in the patient's serum using reagent RBCs. These tests are based on the attraction between antigens and antibodies.

All testing described requires the use of Standard Precautions.

ANTIGENS AND ANTIBODIES

As noted in Chapter 16, Assisting With Diagnostic and Therapeutic Procedures Associated With the Immune System, antigens are substances recognized as foreign to the body that cause the body to initiate a defense response, including the production of antibodies. Antibodies are proteins produced by the body in response to a specific antigen and that bind to that specific antigen to destroy it. Antibodies float freely in the bloodstream and are found in serum.

Each antibody produced by the body will combine with and destroy (in most instances) only one antigen; this is called **specificity**. It allows laboratory personnel to test the exact substance desired without interference from all the other substances found in serum.

Because an antibody has a particularly strong attraction for its antigen, little antigen need be present in a sample for the antibody to find it; this is referred to as **sensitivity**. A test is very sensitive if it can measure a substance even if only a small amount is present. Tests using antigen–antibody reactions as their bases are very specific and very sensitive. These tests can measure small amounts of a substance and pick it out of a solution such as serum that contains millions of other unrelated substances.

The body's immune system can recognize many different areas or sites on a single antigen and therefore will produce several antibodies that can combine with that one antigen. They will each, however, bind with only that one antigen at different areas or sites of that antigen. For example, the body's immune system produces at least three antibodies to the hepatitis B virus. One is against an antigen found on the surface of the virus; one is against an antigen found in the core or center of the virus; and one is against an antigen named E. These antibodies will combine with different parts of the hepatitis B virus but will not combine with the hepatitis A or the hepatitis C virus.

An antibody is named by using its specific antigen's name and adding the prefix "anti." If the antigen's name is A, the antibody's name is anti-A. If the antigen is B, the antibody is anti-B. The antibodies mentioned above for the hepatitis B virus are named anti-hepatitis B surface antigen (anti-HBs), anti-hepatitis B core antigen (anti-HBc), and anti-hepatitis B E antigen (anti-HBe).

Checkpoint Question

1. *How would you describe a test that is both specific and sensitive?*

SEROLOGY TEST METHODS AND PRINCIPLES

In serology, the substance to be tested is identified or the amount present (quantity) is measured using the binding of a specific antibody to its specific antigen. Either the antigen is measured by using a solution containing the antibody (antisera), or the antibody is measured by using a solution containing the antigen. Usually the binding of an antigen and antibody is not visible to the naked eye. The reaction has to be enhanced or enlarged. Methods commonly used to do this include:

- **Agglutination** (clumping) of visible particles, such as RBCs or latex particles
- Enzyme immunoassays (EIA) that produce a color change from colorless to a specific color, such as blue or red
- Chromatographic assays in which fluid migration through a membrane leaves a bar of color in a viewing "window"

Other methods include agglutination inhibition and competitive binding assays.

Agglutination Test

Agglutination is a term used to describe the clumping together of particles caused by the binding of antibodies and antigens. For agglutination testing, only two things are necessary:

1. A solution containing the particles (usually RBCs or latex particles)
2. The patient's sample

To perform an agglutination test, follow these steps:

1. Mix together the solution and the patient's sample on a paper card or glass plate.
2. Gently rock the solution and sample back and forth for a few seconds or a few minutes.
3. Observe for agglutination or clumping of particles. If agglutination does not occur, the test solution appears smooth and milky. If agglutination does occur, the test solution appears rough and granular with areas of clumped particles in a clear background.

Both the antigen and antibody will be present in the test mixture formulated for a specific disease. If the suspected disease-causing antigen, or antibodies against the disease, are present in the patient's sample, agglutination will occur. Agglutination is a positive test and indicates that the test substance is present. If no agglutination occurs, the test is negative, indicating that the test substance is absent. Some tests are designed so that agglutination must appear within a specified time period to indicate a positive reaction.

Agglutination tests can be used in two ways:

1. If the specific antigen is on the particle (RBCs or latex), the patient's serum can be tested for the presence of the specific antibody. This method is used to test for infectious mononucleosis, rheumatoid arthritis, syphilis, and rubella.
2. If the manufacturer produces a particle (usually latex) with the antibody attached, the patient's serum or other specimen can be tested for the presence of a specific antigen. This method is used in some tests for streptococci.

Agglutination tests are quick and easy to perform. They are also inexpensive and have a wide range of uses. The procedure for a test must be followed exactly for the results to be accurate (Box 31-1).

Enzyme Immunoassays

Enzyme immunoassays often have more steps and more reagents than agglutination tests, but the end point is an easy-to-read color change. Agglutination, particularly if the clumps are small, can be difficult to read. EIA tests usually come with all the necessary reagents packaged together in a kit that also contains any additional components needed for test completion, including:

Box 31-1
Tips for Performing Agglutination Testing

1. Start with a clean test slide, one that is free of fingerprints and dust.
2. Follow the times exactly.
3. View the test mixture under a direct light source.
4. Mix reagents before using.
5. Mix samples before using.
6. Do not touch reagent droppers to test area.
7. Do not smear one test mixture into another test area.

- A solid surface (plastic test pack, test tube, bead) coated with the first antibody to the antigen to be tested
- A solution containing a **conjugate,** which is a second antibody specific to the antigen to be tested. The conjugate has an enzyme attached (conjugated) to it that will help to initiate the reaction.
- A wash solution used to remove excess conjugate not bound to the antigen or antigen–antibody complex
- A color specimen (a **substrate,** or substance that is acted on) that turns from colorless to a specific color in the presence of the enzyme

All that needs to be added is the patient specimen. To perform the EIA test, follow these steps:

1. Remove the plastic test pack and other components from a protective pouch.
2. Add the patient's sample to a specially marked area of the test pack, then add conjugate to that same marked area.
3. Allow time for the first antibody to combine with the antigen and the second antibody (conjugate) to combine to the antigen–antibody complex. The antigen is "sandwiched" between the two antibodies.
4. Rinse the test pack or area one or more times using the wash solution. This removes the excess second antibody (conjugate) not attached to the antigen–antibody complex. The wash removes all the conjugate if no antigen is present in the patient sample.
5. After completing the wash step, add the color solution (substrate) to the test area. If the "sandwich" formed and the conjugate is attached, the color solution will produce a color. If no conjugate is attached, no color will be produced. Color is a positive test and indicates the presence of the antigen in the patient's sample. No color is a negative test and indicates the absence of the antigen in the patient's sample.

This test method is often referred to as the sandwich method. Some important tips for obtaining accurate results are listed in Box 31-2.

Chromatographic Assay

Chromatographic assay tests reduce the number of steps involved in an EIA test but retain the color change end point. These tests are usually more expensive than agglutination tests but are easy to read.

In these tests, fluid flows or migrates through a paper-like membrane combining with reagents embedded in the test pack. The parts of the test include:

- Test pack
- Patient's sample
- Diluting fluid

To perform the test, follow these steps:

1. Add the patient's sample to a special area of the test pack followed quickly by several drops of the diluting fluid.
2. Allow time for the fluid to flow through the paper membrane.
3. Observe the test pack for the presence of a colored line or bar.

As the fluid flows across a special area containing antibodies, the antigen in the patient's sample attaches to the antibody conjugated to a color substance. This complex continues to migrate across a line or bar containing stationary antibodies. A "sandwich" is formed of stationary antibody–antigen–antibody with color substance producing a line or bar of color. If a color bar develops, the test is positive, and the antigen is present in the patient sample. If no color bar develops, the test is negative, and the antigen is absent from the patient sample.

The test packs for some tests already have a horizontal line or bar. Fluid migration containing the antigen produces a vertical line or bar. A positive test is indicated by the presence of a plus or positive (+) sign

Box 31-2
Tips for Performing Enzyme Immunoassays

1. Follow the times exactly.
2. Add reagents in correct order.
3. Use reagents only with other reagents from the same kit.
4. Use exact amount of reagents stated in directions.
5. Ensure that reagents and samples are at room temperature.
6. Ensure that reagents have not expired.

31

produced by the two lines. A negative test is indicated by a minus or negative (−) sign produced by the initial single line. Tips to follow in performing these tests are the same as those for EIA tests (see Box 31-2).

Checkpoint Question

2. *What are three serology test methods, and how do they indicate the presence of the test substance?*

SPECIMEN COLLECTION AND HANDLING

Whether a patient's result is correct, false, or incorrect depends to a large extent on the quality of each step involved in testing the patient's sample. This starts with the collection of the sample (venipuncture if serum or blood) and ends with the reporting of the result. Mistakes can be made at any step. Each person involved in testing patients' samples must ensure that mistakes are not made and if they are made, that they are discovered and corrected. This whole process of checking and rechecking to be sure the correct result is reported is called quality assurance. Some of the key areas to address in the assurance of a correctly processed specimen include:

- Specimen collection and handling
- Reagent and kit storage and handling
- Adherence to test procedures
- Quality assurance and quality control

Serum

Many serology tests require a serum specimen. For some tests, plasma or whole blood may be substituted for serum. It is important to use the correct specimen type for a particular test because using the wrong type may result in an incorrect reading.

To obtain serum, collect a red top evacuated tube using standard venipuncture procedure (see Chap. 29, Phlebotomy). A serum-separation or a clot-activator evacuated tube is also acceptable. Immediately label the tube with the patient's name, the date and time, your initials, and any other required information. Because there is no premeasured anticoagulant in a red top tube to be matched by a certain amount of blood, the volume of blood drawn into the tube may vary without affecting the test results. It is not critical that the tube be completely full. There must be enough blood, however, to yield sufficient serum to perform the test and repeat it if necessary.

After obtaining the serum, follow these steps:

1. Allow blood to clot for at least 15 minutes.
2. Invert the tube to be sure the blood has solidified into a firm clot.
3. Allow to stand longer if not clotted.
4. Centrifuge at moderate speed for 10 minutes.

The serum must then be separated from the clot and cells. This can be done by one of three methods:

1. Transfer the serum into a clean test tube using a plastic or glass transfer pipette, label with patient's name and other required information and the word "serum," and cap the tube. Be careful not to stir up the cells and to transfer only clear serum.
2. Use a serum-separation tube. This tube contains gel that migrates between the cells and serum, separating them when the tube is centrifuged.
3. Insert a special plastic tube with a rubber bottom called a serum filter into the already centrifuged tube. The serum filter is pushed through the serum to a level just above the cells. This filter keeps cells from mixing with the serum.

The first method is the best for long-term storage and the only acceptable method if the serum must be frozen. The last two methods are for same-day use only.

If the serum is not tested shortly after separation from cells, it should be stored according to the directions for the test to be performed. For some tests, this will be room temperature. For other tests, this will be in the refrigerator at 2° to 8°C. For still others this will be in the freezer at −4°C or maybe even −18°C. The proper storage of a sample also depends on when the testing is to be performed. For example, a sample that may be left at room temperature if tested within 8 hours may need to be refrigerated if testing is to be performed in 24 to 48 hours or frozen if not to be tested until the next week or next month.

Checkpoint Question

3. *How can serum be separated from a clot?*

Urine

Urine for serology testing is usually collected by the clean-catch method. (See Chap. 28, Urinalysis, for a description of urine collection methods.) The first voided morning specimen is the most concentrated and so the most suitable sample for measuring an antigen. Mark the specimen container with the patient's name, date and time of collection, and your initials. In general, urine samples should be tested immediately or refrigerated at 2° to 8°C until testing. In some instances, it may be necessary to freeze the sample. If the urine is moderately cloudy or bloody, it should be centrifuged before testing.

Other Specimens

Sometimes an infected area of the body is swabbed to collect bacteria for testing in the laboratory. Swabs that have been collected from the throat, the vaginal area, and occasionally other areas of the body are sent to the laboratory for testing. If both a culture and a serology test are ordered, two swabs should be collected. The swab should be made of cotton or Dacron with a plastic or wooden shaft. Calcium alginate swabs should not be used. A transport medium (solution), such as found in Culturettes, is not needed as it is for growing the bacteria. If a medium is used, it should be liquid modified Stuart's medium. A medium that is semisolid or contains charcoal, agar, or gelatin will interfere with serologic tests.

Swab specimens should be tested as soon as possible after collection. Some tests allow for storage up to 8 hours at room temperature or 72 hours refrigerated. The test procedure should be checked for specific specimen storage.

REAGENT AND KIT STORAGE AND HANDLING

For most serology tests, reagents come packaged in kits from the manufacturer. These kits contain all the reagents and often include supplies, such as pipettes, tubes, and cups, needed to perform tests on a certain number of samples.

The kits must be stored at the temperature recommended on the kit box or package insert (the information sheet that comes inside the kit). Some kits are stored at room temperature and others in the refrigerator. Some kits need to be divided with some reagents stored at room temperature and others in the refrigerator. Still others are stored in the refrigerator until opened and then stored at room temperature. It is important to follow the manufacturer's directions. If the kits are stored improperly, the reagents may deteriorate, and false results may be obtained.

Each kit has a lot number and expiration date stamped on the box or package. All reagents with the same lot number were made at the same time in the same manufacturing facility. The expiration date is the day past which the reagents are no longer guaranteed to perform correctly. Reagents from kits with different lot numbers should not be used together. The manufacturer will not guarantee that they will work correctly when components from different lots are mixed.

Reagents should never be used past their expiration date. The date should be written on the kit box when it is received in the laboratory. The date and the initials of the worker who opened the kit should also be written on the box when the kit is opened and used for the first time. Some kits have a new expiration date starting from the day the kit is opened. The package insert that comes in the kit should always be read for details about storing and handling the reagents and supplies.

Checkpoint Question

4. *Why is it important to store reagent kits at specified temperatures?*

FOLLOWING TEST PROCEDURES

All tests performed in serology should have written procedures. These procedures must be followed each time a patient's sample is tested to ensure correct results. Test procedures typically cover:

- Test principle and clinical use of the test
- Reagents and materials needed to do the test
- Precautions
- Specimen collection and handling
- Controls to be run and how often
- Step-by-step procedure to follow
- Interpretation and reporting of results
- Normal or expected values
- Test limitations

QUALITY ASSURANCE AND QUALITY CONTROL

Reagents do not always function properly even though they are well within the expiration date. Sometimes a reagent is left at room temperature when it should be refrigerated. Sometimes serum or other solutions are accidentally added to a reagent, causing it to test or register incorrectly. Kits should be tested periodically for continued reactivity of all reagents. A check needs to be performed each time the reagents are used. Other forms of checks may be performed once a day or only when a new kit is opened. Solutions used to perform some of these checks are called controls.

External Controls

An external control is a solution similar to a patient sample that is tested in the same manner as a patient sample; however, its value or expected result is already known. These controls are often part of the serology

31

kit. In some instances, separate controls can be purchased from the manufacturer.

For most serology tests, positive and negative controls are needed. The positive control should give a positive reaction (agglutination, color, or colored bar). The negative control should give a negative reaction (no agglutination, no color, no colored bar or other specified result). If the controls do not give the expected result, patient results should not be reported and the test should be repeated. If a problem still exists, it should be further investigated (Box 31-3).

Internal Controls

Besides external control solutions, some serology tests also have internal controls that are built into the test packs themselves; such controls monitor that the test procedure is followed correctly and that the reagents are working properly. Sometimes positive and negative test zones exist on each test pack. Sometimes there is only a positive test zone or a test completed zone. These zones are separate from the patient test zone or area. The positive control zone must give a positive color reaction and the negative control zone must give a negative (usually no color) reaction for the test to be valid and patient results to be reported. Do not report patient results if controls do not give proper reactions.

The positive control zone ensures that the correct reagents have been added in the proper order. The negative control zone ensures there is not a nonspecific reaction of patient sample and test reagents. Problems with internal controls can be investigated in the same manner as used for external controls (see Box 31-3). Positive and negative internal controls do not completely take the place of external control solutions, which should be performed on a daily basis.

Box 31-3
Test Troubleshooting Tips

If a serology test using a control is not producing expected results, try:

1. Re-reading the procedure to be sure a step was not omitted.
2. Checking labels of reagents to be sure the correct reagents were added in the correct order.
3. Visually checking reagents for signs of contamination, such as cloudiness or color change.
4. Repeating testing with new bottles of control.
5. Repeating testing with new kit or reagents.
6. Calling the manufacturer for assistance.

SEROLOGY TESTS

Rheumatoid Factor/Rheumatoid Arthritis

Rheumatoid factor is an antibody found in the serum of 70% of people with rheumatoid arthritis. Rheumatoid arthritis is an autoimmune progressive inflammatory disease of the joints causing pain on motion, swelling, stiffness, and subcutaneous nodules near the joints involved. Rheumatoid arthritis can affect people of all ages. Initial occurrence in most cases is between the ages of 30 and 50. It is two to three times more common in women than in men.

Testing

The most common tests for rheumatoid factor are based on agglutination of latex particles. The rheumatoid factor in the serum of patients with rheumatoid arthritis causes agglutination of latex particles that are coated with the antigen (immunoglobulin G, IgG). The sample used is serum tested soon after separation from cells or stored at 2° to 8°C for up to 72 hours. External positive and negative controls are run with each batch of patient samples. If agglutination occurs with a patient's undiluted serum, the serum is diluted 1:20 with a diluting fluid and tested with another drop of latex particles. A 1:20 solution can be obtained by adding 0.1 mL (100 μL) of patient's sample to 1.9 mL of diluting fluid, such as saline or distilled water. If the diluted serum agglutinates with the latex particles, the test is positive for rheumatoid factor. If the serum does not agglutinate on the undiluted or on the diluted serum, the test is negative for rheumatoid factor.

The external controls must give appropriate reactions for the test to be valid and patient results to be reported. That is, the positive control must agglutinate and the negative control must not agglutinate for testing to be valid.

False-Negative and False-Positive Results

Even when the controls react appropriately, laboratory tests are not a perfect indicator of disease. Physicians use test results along with physical examination and patient history to make clinical decisions about disease. Sometimes a negative result occurs even when a patient has a disease. This is called a false-negative result. Because only 70% of patients with rheumatoid arthritis are positive for rheumatoid factor, 30% of patients with rheumatoid arthritis will have a false-negative result.

Sometimes a positive result occurs when the patient does not have the disease. This is called a false-positive result. False-positive results sometimes occur in the elderly and in patients with lupus erythematosus, syphilis, or hepatitis.

False-negative and false-positive results can occur because of biologic conditions of patients as the examples above show. They can also be due to technical difficulty with samples or with performing the test. Testing personnel cannot control the biologic conditions, but they can sometimes control the technical conditions. If testing personnel wait too long to read agglutination, a false-positive test result can occur. This can be avoided by following directions carefully. Hemolyzed and lipemic samples (samples with increased fat levels) can give a false-positive result. These samples must be recollected to ensure accurate testing.

Checkpoint Question

5. *What is the difference between a false-negative and a false-positive test result, and why do these sometimes occur?*

Infectious Mononucleosis

Infectious mononucleosis is caused by the Epstein-Barr virus. About 50% of exposures reported in medical offices occur before the age of 5, and most of the other 50% occur between the ages of 15 and 24. Children under the age of 5 rarely exhibit symptoms. Adults present with general symptoms, such as fatigue, malaise, sore throat, and enlarged lymph nodes. A patient may sometimes exhibit an enlarged spleen or hepatitis. The white blood cell count may be normal, slightly decreased, or slightly increased with atypical lymphocytes visible on blood smears. Infectious mononucleosis is usually self-limiting and most patients fully recover.

Testing

Tests for infectious mononucleosis include agglutination of RBCs or latex particles, EIAs, and chromatographic assays (Procedure 31-1). The substance tested for in each method is heterophil antibodies. These are antibodies produced by a person with infectious mononucleosis that combine with antigens found on the RBCs of other animals, such as horses, oxen, and sheep. For most tests, serum, plasma, or whole blood (purple top tube or capillary sample) may be used. Whole blood must be tested as soon as possible. Serum and plasma may be stored in the refrigerator for 2 to 3 days. External or internal controls must give appropriate reactions for testing to be valid and patient results to be reported.

False-Negative and False-Positive Results

False-negative results can occur early in the disease before heterophil antibodies are produced. Only 50% of children under the age of 4 produce heterophil antibodies. The other 50% will give a false-negative reaction. Only 85% to 90% of adults produce heterophil antibodies. False-positive results can be obtained by waiting too long to read agglutination tests.

C-Reactive Protein

The C-reactive protein (CRP) is a test used to detect inflammatory diseases, such as bacterial infections, malignant diseases, and autoimmune disorders. It is not a diagnostic test for a particular disease, but rather a test for monitoring the inflammatory process. It can be used to monitor the effect of therapy on disease.

Testing

C-reactive protein is an antigen found in serum. Most tests use latex particles coated with antibodies to CRP. Patient serum is tested undiluted and diluted 1:5 (0.1 mL serum and 0.4 mL diluting fluid). Agglutination with either or both the undiluted and diluted serum is considered positive for CRP. If no agglutination occurs in either sample, the test is negative. A positive and negative external control run with each batch of patient samples must give appropriate reactions for the test to be valid and results to be reported.

False-Negative and False-Positive Results

Too much CRP in the serum samples can cause a false-negative result. This is due to antigen excess. The 1:5 dilution of the serum helps avoid this problem. False-positive results can occur from using lipemic or hemolyzed samples.

Rubella

The rubella virus causes a disease also known as German or 3-day measles. Measles occurs most commonly in childhood. Today there is widespread immunization for rubella. Before immunization, epidemic outbreaks occurred every 6 to 9 years, resulting in stillbirths and birth defects from congenital rubella. In children and adults with measles, the symptoms are mild, low-grade fever and a rash on the face, neck, and trunk. For a fetus of less than 3 months, measles can cause death or birth defects, such as bone abnormalities, mental retardation, cataracts, and cardiovascular defects.

Testing

Tests available for rubella include agglutination of RBCs or latex particles, hemagglutination (RBCs) inhibition, and EIAs. In latex agglutination tests, particles are coated with rubella antigens. The presence of antibodies in the patient's serum will agglutinate the latex particles. Agglutination is a positive test indicating the patient has immunity to the rubella virus. If there is no agglutination, the serum should be diluted 1:10 with dilution fluid and the diluted serum tested. If both the undiluted and diluted samples show no agglutination, the test is negative for antibodies to the rubella virus. Controls must react appropriately for the tests to be valid.

Latex agglutination tests do not distinguish between present and past infections. EIAs are available that determine if the antibodies present belong to the IgG or to the IgM class of immunoglobulins. The IgM class is generally seen in current infections, and the IgG class indicates immunity from past infection or vaccination.

False-Negative and False-Positive Results

Very high levels of antibodies can give a false-negative result. Negative serums should be diluted 1 : 10 and retested. Allowing the test to sit too long before observing for agglutination can cause a false-positive result.

Rapid Plasma Reagin Test for Syphilis

Rapid plasma reagin (RPR) is a screening test for syphilis, a sexually transmitted disease caused by a spirochete bacteria, *Treponema pallidum.* Incidence of the disease declined after World War II, but it has been increasing in recent years. The highest incidence is seen in individuals between the ages of 20 and 24. It can be transmitted from mother to fetus, resulting in congenital syphilis causing notched teeth, nerve deafness, and other symptoms. Syphilis is treated with penicillin. Untreated syphilis is a chronic disease in which the patient demonstrates symptoms at times and is asymptomatic at other times. Untreated syphilis progresses in stages, including primary, secondary, latent, and tertiary.

Testing

T. pallidum does not grow in culture; the best test to demonstrate the organism is darkfield microscopy. More frequently the serum is tested for the presence of antibodies and antibody-like substances called reagins. Venereal Disease Research Laboratories (VDRL) and RPR are the most common screening tests for these nonspecific reagins. The microhemagglutination assay for *T. pallidum* (MHA-TP) and fluorescent treponemal antibody absorption test (FTA-ABS) are two confirmatory tests for the organism itself.

The RPR is an agglutination test. The antigen solution contains charcoal to increase the visibility of the clumping. Serum is the specimen of choice, even though the name implies that plasma is used. One drop of the patient's serum is added to the appropriate circle on a plastic-coated card. One drop of antigen is then added to each circle from a calibrated syringe with a special 18-gauge needle. The card is placed on a mechanical rotator, rotating at 95 to 110 rotations per minute for 8 minutes. The circles are observed for agglutination. Reactive (positive), weakly reactive, and nonreactive (negative) controls are run with each batch of patient samples. They must react appropriately for the test to be valid and patient results to be reported. The rotator is checked each day for the number of rotations per minute, which should average 100/min. The 18-gauge needle is checked periodically for the number of drops it delivers per milliliter of antigen solution, which should be 60 ± 2.

Agglutination of the antigen solution is considered reactive for the reagin (presumptive positive test for syphilis). Even a weakly reactive agglutination is considered positive or reactive. No agglutination of the antigen solution is considered nonreactive. Determination of titer is performed on any reactive serum. This involves performing a serial dilution to obtain dilutions of the serum of 1:2, 1:4, 1:8, 1:16, and so forth. The diluting of the serum is continued until a diluted specimen gives a nonreactive result (no agglutination). The titer reported is the last dilution showing agglutination. If the last diluted specimen showing agglutination was the 1:8 dilution, the titer would be reported as 1:8. If only the undiluted specimen showed agglutination, the titer would be reported as 1:1.

The patient's physician and the health department must be notified of all reactive results for syphilis. Serum should be sent to the state laboratory or reference laboratory for confirmation of a syphilis infection using the MHA-TP or FTA-ABS tests.

False-Negative and False-Positive Results

The RPR is reactive in 80% of cases of primary syphilis, 99% of secondary, and 1% of tertiary. The MHA-TP, in contrast, is reactive in 65% of cases of primary syphilis, 100% of secondary, and 95% of tertiary. A false-negative RPR will be obtained in 20% of primary syphilis cases. A false-negative MHA-TP will be obtained in 35% of primary syphilis cases. A false-positive RPR can be seen in patients with lupus erythematosus, infectious mononucleosis, hepatitis, rheumatoid arthritis, and in pregnancy and the elderly. Improper rotation of specimen can also cause a false-negative result.

Pregnancy Test

The test for pregnancy is based on the detection of the hormone HCG, which is produced by the developing placenta starting at about 10 days after the fertilization of the ovum by sperm. Modern pregnancy tests can determine pregnancy before the first missed menses. HCG increases during the first 3 months of pregnancy and then decreases to undetectable levels a few days after childbirth. A pregnancy test is frequently used to rule out pregnancy before performing medical procedures that might be harmful to the fetus (Procedure 31-2).

Testing

Tests of HCG include agglutination inhibition (the absence of agglutination), EIA, and chromatographic assay. Many popular test kits are based on the EIA "sandwich" method. Urine or serum is added to the test pack in the test area containing antibodies to HCG. If the kit uses either urine or serum, the serum usually has to be pretreated before testing. Next, the conjugate containing the second antibody attached to an enzyme is added. Time is allowed for the binding of antigen to antibodies. Unbound conjugate–antibody–enzyme is washed off, and the color reagent (substrate) is added. Development of color indicates a positive test. No color is a negative test (Fig. 31-1).

Internal positive and negative control areas must react appropriately for results to be valid. Not adding one of the reagents or adding reagents in the wrong order can result in all control and patient test areas appearing negative (no color). Some patients have antibodies to test reagents causing all test areas to appear positive. Either of these patterns indicates an invalid result.

False-Negative and False-Positive Results

A urine specimen that is too dilute can give a false-negative reaction. The first morning urine specimen is the most likely to contain HCG if the patient is pregnant. Certain tumors produce HCG and can cause a false-positive result.

Group A Streptococcus

Group A streptococcus (*Streptococcus pyogenes*) is one of the most common bacterial causes of sore throat and upper respiratory tract infections. Infections are usually found in school-aged children, especially in winter and spring. These infections can be treated with antibiotics. If not treated, the disease may lead to rheumatic fever and acute glomerulonephritis.

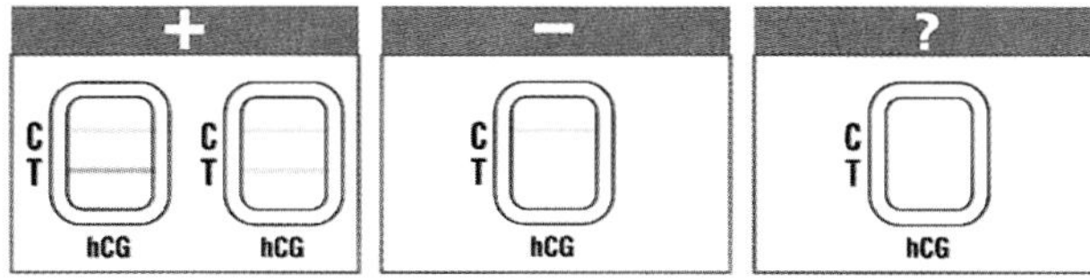

Figure 31-1 QuickVue One-Step hcg-urine test. (Courtesy of Quidel Corp.)

Testing

Group A strep infection can be diagnosed by bacterial culture or serologic tests for the antigenic presence of the bacteria (Procedure 31-3). Serologic tests include agglutination, EIA, and chromatographic assay. The bacteria do not need to be alive for serology tests as they do for culture. Serologic tests are easier and more rapid (5–15 minutes) than culture, which takes 18 to 24 hours; however, culture is considered more sensitive.

The specimen used is a swab of the patient's throat. (See Chap. 17, Assisting With Diagnostic and Therapeutic Procedures Associated With the Respiratory System, for a description of performing a throat culture.) The bacterial antigen is extracted from the swab using an acid solution and a nitrite solution. The mixture is then neutralized with a buffer solution. Color indicators are added to these solutions to monitor that correct extraction procedure has been followed. If the color changes described in the procedure do not occur, the extraction process should be repeated using a new specimen (throat swab). The extraction fluid is then filtered before addition to the test. The extracted specimen is tested using one of the methods listed in the section "Serology Test Methods and Principles," above. Internal or external controls must be performed with the patient sample and give appropriate reactions for the test to be valid (Fig. 31-2).

False-Negative and False-Positive Results

If improper technique is used in collecting the throat swab or an inadequate specimen is obtained, a false-negative result can occur. If the test is allowed to stand too long before results are read, a false-positive result can occur. High levels of *Staphylococcus aureus* in the specimen can interfere with the interpretation of results.

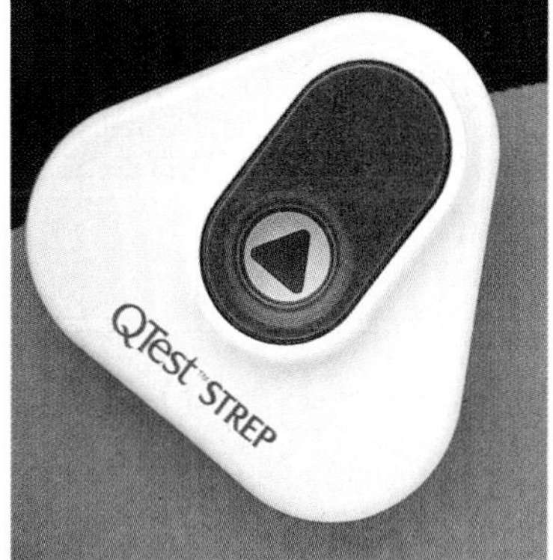

Figure 31-2 Qtest strep test for group A streptococcus. (Courtesy of Becton-Dickinson Primary Care Diagnostics, Sparks, Maryland.)

31

Checkpoint Question

6. *What are the benefits and drawbacks of using serology tests versus cultures for group A streptococcus?*

Other Serologic Tests

Antinuclear Antibody

Normal antibodies react against foreign cells, causing their destruction; autoantibodies react by destroying the body's own normal cells. Antinuclear antibodies react against the nucleus of the body's cells. Antinuclear antibodies are present in the sera of patients with rheumatoid arthritis, systemic lupus erythematosus, progressive systemic sclerosis, and other autoimmune diseases.

Antistreptolysin-O (ASO) Titer

Streptolysin-O is an exotoxin (a poison excreted by an organism) produced by most group A and some C and G streptococci. Streptolysin-O causes **hemolysis** (breakdown) of RBCs and the loss of hemoglobin. An ASO titer identifies and measures the antibodies produced by the body in response to the presence of the exotoxin (the streptolysin-O). Antistreptolysin antibodies oppose the action of the streptolysin. Streptolysin-O indicates that the exotoxin is inactivated by the presence of oxygen. The antistreptolysin antibodies' presence in serum is used to help diagnose rheumatic fever.

Cold Agglutinins

The sera of patients with atypical pneumonia and certain blood diseases, such as hemolytic anemia, may contain circulating antibodies that cause RBC agglutination and hemolysis at a less than normal body temperature. Their presence in the serum may indicate certain viral or mycoplasmic infections. Cold agglutinins are more common in women over the age of 50.

Radioallergosorbent Test

The radioallergosorbent test is a radiologic test of the serum capable of measuring and identifying small quantities of IgE. This test is capable of detecting the presence of as many as 45 allergens. Agglutination indicates that an allergic response is present.

IMMUNOHEMATOLOGY

Testing in the blood bank is directed at determining if a donor's blood is suitable for transfusion to a patient (recipient) who needs blood. If the donor's blood is compatible, the patient's immunosurveillance will not immediately recognize it as foreign, and the RBCs may circulate in the patient's body for a longer time after they are transfused. If the donor's blood is incompatible, the patient's body will immediately recognize the blood as foreign and begin destroying it as soon as it is transfused. This can rapidly lead to death.

Blood Group Antigens

ABO Group

Transfusion compatibility is determined by testing the antigens present on RBCs (patient's and donor's) and the antibodies present in the patient's serum. The main RBC antigens belong to the ABO system. Each person belongs to one of four blood groups: A, B, O, or AB. People, however, are not equally divided among the four groups. Approximately 45% are O, 40% are A, 11% are B, and 4% are AB. Consequently, some blood groups are easier to obtain, and some are more in demand than others. The ABO group of each donor and each patient who will need a transfusion is determined as described below under "Testing."

Almost every person's serum contains antibodies to the ABO antigens that he or she lacks. These antibodies occur naturally. Shortly after birth these antibodies are found in serum, even though the person has never received blood. A person in the A group has the A antigen. A person in the B group has the B antigen. A person in the O group lacks both antigens. A person in the AB group has both the A and B antigen. A person in the A group lacks the B antigen and has an antibody to B (anti-B) in serum. Someone who is B lacks the A antigen and has anti-A in serum. One who is O has both anti-A and anti-B in serum. A person who belongs to the AB group has neither antibody in serum.

These antibodies are crucial to safe transfusion of blood to a patient. They are the reason it is unsafe to give B blood to an A patient. An A patient has anti-B in the serum that would bind and destroy the B cells, causing breakdown products that are toxic and can lead to death. The lack of either A or B antigens on O cells makes it the universal donor. This means type O blood may be given to patients no matter what their ABO group. If B blood is unavailable for a patient, O blood can be given safely.

Rh Group

Another group of antigens important to the blood bank is the Rh group. This includes the antigens D, E, C, e, and c. However, D is the most important. The presence of the D antigen is termed Rh positive. The absence of the D antigen is termed Rh negative. Antibodies to D do not occur naturally. A person lacking the D antigen must be exposed to the D antigen of for-

Procedure 31-1 Performing a Mononucleosis Test

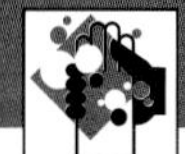

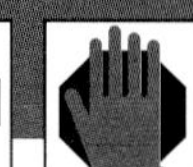

PURPOSE

To determine the presence of the Epstein-Barr virus

EQUIPMENT/SUPPLIES

- patient's labeled specimen (whole blood, plasma, or serum depending on the kit)
- mononucleosis kit (slide or card, controls, reagents, capillary tubes, bulb and stirrers)
- stopwatch or timer
- saline, test tubes, pipettes (if titration is required)

STEPS

1. Wash your hands.
2. Verify that the names on the specimen container and the laboratory form are the same.
3. Assemble the equipment, and ensure that the materials in the kit are at room temperature before beginning the procedure.
4. Label the slide or card (depending on the type of kit used) with the patient's name, positive control, and negative control. One circle or space is provided per patient and control.

   Doing this ensures accurate documentation.
5. Place the rubber bulb on the capillary tube, and aspirate the patient's specimen up to the marked line. Dispense the sample in the middle of the circle labeled with the patient's name. Avoid air bubbles to ensure accurate results.
6. Gently mix the positive control. Using the capillary tube, aspirate the positive control up to the marked line. Dispense the control in the middle of the circle labeled "negative control." Avoid air bubbles.

   These steps adhere to quality assurance and quality control requirements.
7. Mix the latex reagent, and add 1 drop to each circle or space (patient sample, positive control, negative control). Avoid splashing the reagents, which can result in cross-contamination and incorrect results.
8. Using a clean stirrer for each test, mix the reagent with the patient sample and controls. Mix only one circle at a time, keeping within each circle. Going outside of the circle may lead to cross-contamination and incorrect results.
9. Gently rock the slide for 2 minutes, and observe for agglutination (clumping). Testing time may vary if using a disposable card.
10. Verify the results of the controls before documenting the patient's results. Log controls and patient information on the worksheet.
11. Read the kit's instructions if titration is required.
12. Clean the work area and dispose of waste properly. Wash the slide thoroughly with bleach and rinse with water before using again. Remove gown, gloves and shield. Wash your hands.

DOCUMENTATION GUIDELINES

- Date and time
- Performance of procedure
- Testing results
- Action taken (if any)
- Your signature

Charting Example

DATE	TIME Mono spot = neg on serum.
	—Your signature

Note: Kits vary depending on the manufacturer; read instructions carefully before beginning the procedure. Controls for test kits are usually done once per day or kit. Follow office policies and procedures for ensuring testing accuracy and maintaining quality control. Be aware that controls are needed when performing a titration.

eign RBCs to produce antibodies. This can happen if an Rh-negative (D-negative) patient is transfused with Rh-positive (D-positive) blood. This can also happen if an Rh-negative mother is exposed to the Rh-positive cells of her baby before or during childbirth. Rh negative mothers can be prevented from producing antibodies to the Rh (D) antigen by injection of immune-D serum or RhoGAM. This injection prevents the production of antibodies that might cause hemolytic disease of the newborn by destroying the RBCs of children born after this birth.

Other Blood Groups

Although the ABO and Rh groups are of greatest importance to immunohematology, there are many more

text continues on page 696

31

Procedure 31-2 Performing an HCG Pregnancy Test

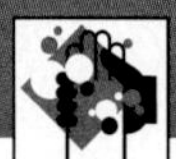
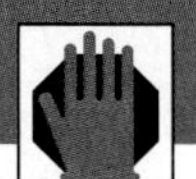
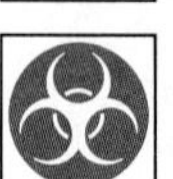
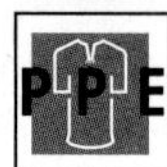

PURPOSE

To detect the production of HCG to determine pregnancy

EQUIPMENT/SUPPLIES

- patient's labeled specimen (plasma, serum, or urine depending on the kit)
- HCG pregnancy kit (test pack and transfer pipettes; kit contents will vary by manufacturer)
- HCG positive and negative control (different controls may be needed when testing urine)
- timer

STEPS

1. Wash your hands.
2. Assemble the equipment.
3. Verify that the names on the specimen container and the laboratory form are the same.
4. Label the test pack (depending on type of kit) with the patient's name, positive control, and negative control. Use one test pack per patient and control.
5. Note in the patient's information and in the control log if you are using urine, plasma, or serum for testing. Be sure that the kit and controls are at room temperature for accurate testing.
6. Aspirate the patient's specimen using the transfer pipette and place three drops (180 μL) on the sample well of the test pack labeled with the patient's name.
7. Aspirate the positive control using the transfer pipette and place three drops (180 μL) on the sample well of the test pack labeled "positive control." Avoid splashing to eliminate cross-contamination.

    This adheres to quality assurance and quality control standards.
8. Aspirate the negative control using the transfer pipette, and place three drops (180 μL) on the sample well of the test pack labeled "negative control." Avoid splashing to eliminate cross-contamination.

    This adheres to quality assurance and quality control standards.
9. Report the results when the "End of Assay Window" is red. This will take approximately 7 minutes for serum samples and 4 minutes for urine samples. Check to verify controls before reporting the results. Repeat the test if the "End of Assay Window" does not appear and if the controls do not work.

    Waiting the appropriate amount of time ensures that testing is complete.
10. Record controls and patient information on the worksheet and log form.
11. Clean the work area and dispose of waste properly. Remove gown, gloves, and shield. Wash your hands.

DOCUMENTATION GUIDELINES

- Date and time
- Performance of procedure
- Testing results
- Action taken (if any)
- Your signature

Charting Example

DATE	TIME Pt presented with c/o late period —
	LMP 11/22/99. C/o nausea in the am,
	breast tenderness. Urine sample positive
	for pregnancy. Dr. Wong in to examine pt.
	Pregnancy brochures explained to pt. RTC
	2/14/00. —Your signature

Note: Kits vary depending on the manufacturer; read instructions carefully before beginning the procedure. Controls for test kits are usually done once per day or kit. Follow office policies and procedures for ensuring testing accuracy and maintaining quality control.

Procedure 31-3 Performing Group A Rapid Strep Test

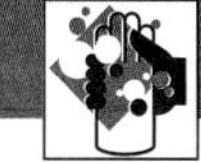
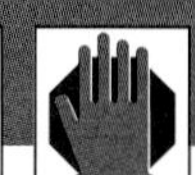
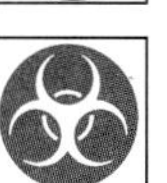
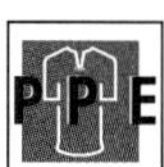

PURPOSE

To determine the presence of *Streptococcus pyogenes* in the specimen

EQUIPMENT/SUPPLIES

- patient's labeled throat culture (use a culturette with two swabs provided)
- group A strep kit (controls may be included, depending on the kit)
- timer
- beta strep agar
- bacitracin disks

Note: Beta strep agar and bacitracin need to come to room temperature before being used.

STEPS

1. Wash your hands.
2. Verify that the names on the specimen container and the laboratory form are the same.
3. Label one extraction tube with the patient's name, another with the positive control, and one with the negative control.
4. Follow the directions for the kit. Add the appropriate reagents and drops to each of the extraction tubes. Avoid splashing, and use the correct number of drops.

   Following the manufacturer's instructions exactly will ensure that you adhere to the appropriate testing guidelines.
5. Insert the patient's swab (one of the two swabs present) into the labeled extraction tube. If only one culture swab was submitted, first swab a beta strep agar plate, then use the swab for the rapid strep test.

   This begins the testing process without contaminating the culture specimen.
6. Add the appropriate controls to each of the labeled extraction tubes.

   This begins the chemical reaction for proper control results.
7. Set the timer for the appropriate time to ensure testing accuracy.
8. Add the appropriate reagent and drops to each of the extraction tubes.
9. Use the swab to mix the reagents. Then press out any excess fluid remaining on the swab by placing your fingers on the outside of the extraction tube while pinching the swab against the inside of the tube.

   This helps deposit the maximum amount of substance to be tested.
10. Add three drops from the well mixed extraction tube to the sample window of the strep A test unit labeled with the patient's name. Do the same for each control.
11. Set the timer for the appropriate time.
12. Be aware that a positive result appears as a line in the result window within 5 minutes. An internal control is present in the strep A test unit; if a line appears in the control window, the test is valid.
13. Read a negative result at exactly 5 minutes to avoid a false-negative.
14. Verify results of the controls before recording test results. Log the controls and the patient information on the worksheet.
15. Note that depending on laboratory protocol, you may need to culture all negative rapid strep screens onto beta strep agar. A bacitracin disk may be added to the first quadrant while setting up or after 24 hours if a beta hemolytic colony appears. A culture is more sensitive than a rapid immunoassay test.
16. Clean the work area and dispose of waste properly. Remove gown, gloves, and shield. Wash your hands.

DOCUMENTATION GUIDELINES

- Date and time
- Performance of procedure
- Testing results
- Action taken (if any)
- Your signature

Charting Example

DATE	TIME Pt C/o sore throat × 2 days. Group
	A rapid strep test positive. Dr. Harrison
	notified. —Your signature

Note: Kits vary depending on the manufacturer; read instructions carefully before beginning the procedure. Controls for test kits are usually done once per day or kit. Follow office policies and procedures for ensuring testing accuracy and maintaining quality control.

31

Patient Education
Expectant Mothers and RhoGAM

If you are employed in an obstetrician's office, you will have the opportunity to educate many expectant mothers who are Rh negative regarding the purpose of RhoGAM. Here are some educational pointers:

- Explain what it means to be Rh negative in terms appropriate to the patient's level of understanding.
- Point out that if the Rh factor of the baby's father is either positive or unknown, the baby could be born with Rh-positive blood. Also note that if the Rh factor of the baby's father is negative, there should be no problem.
- Explain that if the baby's Rh-positive blood comes in contact with the mother's Rh-negative blood, she will make antibodies against the baby's blood. In future pregnancies, her antibodies will fight with the fetal blood (if Rh positive), causing severe hemolytic anemia in the fetus.
- Tell the patient that RhoGAM is an immune globulin that prohibits the production of Rh-positive antibodies in the mother. It is given intrapartum and postpartum and will require that a patient consent form be signed.

It is important to note that after a miscarriage or abortion, the Rh-negative mother must receive RhoGAM, unless it is documented that the baby's father was Rh negative.

significant antigens and antibodies. Some other groups include Duffy, Lewis, MNS, Kidd, and Kell. These are all RBC antigens. White blood cells and platelets also have antigens. Most of these antigens belong to a system called human leukocyte antigens. Antibodies to these antigens can cause fever during transfusion of RBCs because of the presence of white blood cells (leukocytes). Antibodies to these antigens are also responsible for the rejection of an organ transplant, such as kidney, heart, or liver. Most of these antibodies do not occur naturally. A person must be exposed to blood or tissue that is foreign before producing antibodies.

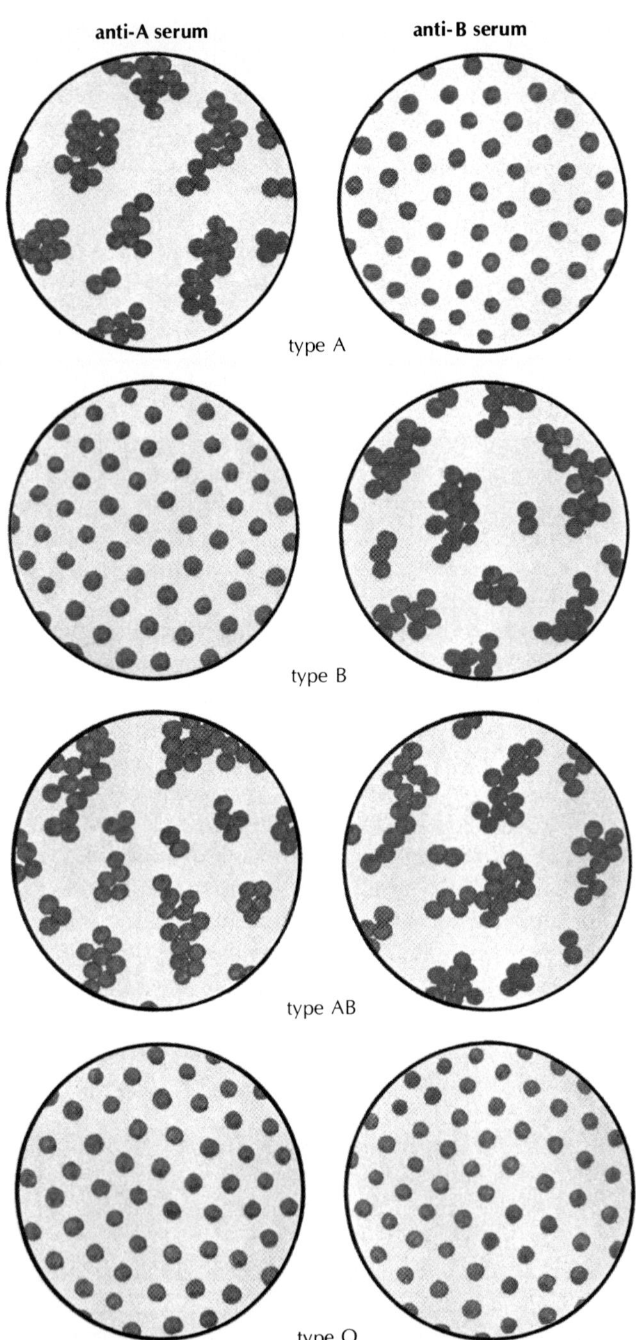

Figure 31-3 Blood typing. Red cells in type A blood are agglutinated (clumped) by anti-A serum; those in type B blood are agglutinated by anti-B serum. Type AB blood cells are agglutinated by both sera, and type O blood is not agglutinated by either serum.

Blood Group Testing

ABO Testing

To test for the ABO group of a patient or blood donor, two reagent antisera are used. One is anti-A. The other is anti-B. The RBCs to be tested are diluted with saline to approximately a 3% solution (3 drops of cells and about 100 drops of saline). One drop of 3% RBCs is mixed with one drop anti-A in a glass tube labeled "A." One drop of 3% RBCs is mixed with one drop anti-B in another tube labeled "B." The tubes are centrifuged for 15 seconds at low speed. The RBC button on the bottom of the tube is gently resuspended. The solution is examined for agglutination.

The antisera will agglutinate the RBCs if the antigen is present. No agglutination will be observed if the

Table 31-1 **ABO Group Testing Results**

RESULT	*Reagents*				*Group*
	anti-A	*anti-B*	*"a" Cells*	*"b" Cells*	
	+	−	−	+	**A**
	−	+	+	−	**B**
	−	−	+	+	**O**
	+	+	−	−	**AB**

antigen is not present. If a patient's RBCs agglutinate with anti-A but not anti-B, the patient belongs to the A group. If the RBCs agglutinate with anti-B and not with anti-A, the cells belong to the B group (Fig. 31-3). This procedure is called direct or forward typing (Table 31-1).

The serum can be used to verify the ABO group of a patient or blood donor. Reagent "a" group cells and "b" group cells are mixed with serum, centrifuged, and examined for agglutination. If a patient is A, serum will contain anti-B only. Agglutination will be observed with the "b" cells. This procedure using serum is called indirect or reverse typing (see Table 31-1).

Rh Testing

Anti-D reagent is used to determine the Rh of RBCs. Add one drop of 3% cell suspension and one drop anti-D reagent in a test tube labeled "D." Centrifuge for 15 seconds. Resuspend the RBC button, and observe for agglutination. If agglutination is present, RBCs are Rh positive. If no agglutination is present, RBCs are Rh negative.

Many anti-D reagents require a control. One drop of 3% cell suspension and one drop of control reagent are added to a test tube labeled "DC" ("D" control). It is then centrifuged for 15 seconds and resuspended RBCs examined for agglutination. The control should always be negative for the test to be valid. Often in the blood bank, agglutination is graded according to the strength of the clumping. A positive is graded 1+, 2+, 3+, or 4+.

Checkpoint Question

7. *What ABO blood group is the universal donor? What does this mean?*

BLOOD SUPPLY

Today one of the major problems facing the blood banks is obtaining sufficient amounts of safe blood and blood products to meet patient needs. There is a shortage of volunteer donors. The American Red Cross and other agencies collect blood from donors at blood mobiles or sometimes at fixed sites. One donor blood unit containing about 450 mL whole blood can be divided into three products:

1. Packed RBCs, which can be stored at 2° to 8°C for 42 days and used to treat anemia.
2. Plasma, which can be frozen for 1 year and used to treat bleeding caused by a lack of coagulation factors, such as fibrinogen
3. Platelet concentrates, which can be stored at room temperature for 5 days and used to treat bleeding due to low platelet count or dysfunctional platelets

The American Red Cross tests each donor blood unit for ABO group, Rh type, and unexpected antibodies to RBC antigens. It also tests each unit for infectious agents such as hepatitis, human immunodeficiency virus (HIV), and syphilis. The donors are also asked questions about their medical history to protect the safety of the blood supply.

A patient in an accident who needs blood quickly has few options except volunteer donor blood. Patients scheduled for elective surgery, however, have alterna-

What If?
What if a patient asks you about the criteria for donating blood?

The criteria for donating blood are determined by the American Red Cross based on recommendations from government agencies, the Centers for Disease Control and Prevention, and through various research projects. In addition, each state has its own laws regulating blood donors. Generally, blood donors must meet the following criteria:

- Age 18 years or older (individuals 17 years of age require a parent's permission; individuals 65 years of age or older require a physician's consent)
- Weight 110 lb or more
- Hemoglobin 12.5 g/dL (women) or 13.5 g/dL (men) or higher values
- Pulse 50 to 110 beats/min
- Blood pressure lower than 180 (systolic)/100 (diastolic)

The donor also will need to complete a brief patient history. The entire procedure will last approximately an hour; the actual blood donation time is about 10 minutes. Blood can be donated every 56 days. Only 1 U (pint) will be taken at a time. All blood will be tested by the American Red Cross for HIV, hepatitis, and syphilis.

31

tives. Patients who are not anemic may give blood in advance of surgery for themselves. Under the physician's care, they can give up to 6 U starting 6 weeks before surgery. This is called autologous donation. During surgery, blood can be saved and returned to the patient using blood salvage equipment. The patient can ask family and friends to give in the directed donor program. The units are marked for the patient and cannot be given to anyone else. Both the autologous blood units and directed donor blood units are more costly than volunteer donor units. Directed donor units are no safer than volunteer donor units. Patients need to know they have options. The choice is made with the assistance of the physician.

Checkpoint Question

8. *What are three products that can be obtained from 1 U whole blood and how are they used?*

Answers to Checkpoint Questions

1. *A test that is specific and sensitive can measure a substance even if only a tiny amount is present (specificity), and it can pick that substance out of a solution containing millions of other related substances (sensitivity).*

2. *Three serology test methods are agglutination, enzyme immunoassay, and chromatographic assays. Enzyme immunoassays produce a color change and chromatographic assays produce a color bar if the test substance is present. With agglutination tests, clumping of particles (agglutination) occurs if the test substance is present.*

3. *Serum can be separated from a clot by using a pipette, a serum separation tube, or a serum filter.*

4. *Improperly stored kits may result in deterioration of the reagents, which may lead to false test results.*

5. *A false-negative result occurs when a patient tests negative for a disease, even though the disease is present. A false-positive result occurs when a test indicates that a patient has a particular disease, even though the patient is disease free. These results can be caused by technical problems in performing the test or by the patient's biologic condition.*

6. *Serology tests are easier to perform and provide results more quickly, but cultures are considered to be more sensitive.*

7. *Type O is the universal donor because it lacks A or B antigens, making it safe to give patients—no matter what their ABO group.*

8. *A single unit of whole blood can be divided into packed RBCs (used to treat anemia); plasma (used to treat bleeding from a lack of coagulation factors); and platelet concentrates (used to treat bleeding caused by low platelet count or dysfunctional platelets).*

Critical Thinking Challenges

1. You are working for Dr. Mathers, a cardiothoracic surgeon. Dr. Mathers performs many surgeries during which patients experience substantial blood loss, requiring transfusions. Identify the available options for blood transfusions. How would you explain these to a patient facing elective surgery?
2. Your local chapter of the American Red Cross is in great need for volunteer donors. Formulate a plan for encouraging more community members to donate blood. How can you put your plan into action?

Suggestions for Further Reading

Barrett, J. T. (1991). *Medical Immunology: Tests and Review.* Philadelphia: F. A. Davis.

Bryant, N. J. (1992). *Laboratory Immunology and Serology,* 3rd ed. Philadelphia: W.B. Saunders.

Fischbach, F. (1996). *A Manual of Laboratory and Diagnostic Tests,* 5th ed. Philadelphia: Lippincott-Raven.

Fischbach, F. (1998). *Quick Reference for Common Laboratory and Diagnostic Tests,* 2nd ed. Philadelphia: Lippincott-Raven.

Miller, L. E. (1991). *Manual of Laboratory Immunology,* 2nd ed. Philadelphia: Lea & Febiger.

Quinley, E. D. (1998). *Immunohematology: Principles and Practice,* 2nd ed. Philadelphia: Lippincott-Raven.

Sheehan, C. (1997). *Clinical Immunology: Principles and Laboratory Diagnosis,* 2nd ed. Philadelphia: Lippincott-Raven.

Turgeon, M. L. (1990). *Immunology and Serology in Laboratory Medicine.* St Louis: Mosby–Year Book.

32 Clinical Chemistry

Chapter Outline

Role Delineation

CLINICAL

Fundamental Principles

- Apply principles of aseptic technique and infection control.

Diagnostic Orders

- Collect and process specimens.
- Perform diagnostic tests.

Patient Care

- Prepare patient for examinations, procedures, and treatments.

GENERAL

Legal Concepts

- Practice within the scope of education, training, and personal capabilities.
- Document accurately.

Instruction

- Instruct individuals according to their needs.

Chapter Competencies

Learning Objectives

Upon successfully completing this chapter, you will be able to:

1. Spell and define the Key Terms.
2. List the common electrolytes, explain the relationship of electrolytes with fluid and acid–base balance, and identify some conditions in which imbalances may occur.
3. Describe the nonprotein nitrogenous compounds and how they are formed, and name conditions with abnormal values.
4. Describe glucose utilization, regulation, and the purpose of the various glucose tests.
5. Describe the function of cholesterol and associated lipids in the body and their correlation to heart disease.
6. List and describe the substances commonly tested in liver function assessment.
7. Explain thyroid function assessment tests and hormones that regulate and are produced by the thyroid gland.
8. Describe how an assessment for a myocardial infarction is made with laboratory tests.

Chapter Competencies *(continued)*

9. Describe how pancreatitis is diagnosed with laboratory tests.
10. List the components of blood gas analysis and the purpose in determining their levels.

Performance Objectives

Upon successfully completing this chapter, you will be able to:

1. Determine blood glucose (Procedure 32-1).
2. Perform a glucose tolerance test (GTT) (Procedure 32-2).

Key Terms

(See Glossary for definitions.)

adenosine triphosphate (ATP)
artifactual
azotemia
basal metabolic rate
bicarbonate
bile
biliary obstructions
body fluids
catalyzes
challenge
cortisol
creatine
diuretics
extracellular
gestational diabetes
intracellular
iodine
ions
Krebs cycle
lipase
lipids
lipoproteins
metabolic acidosis
muscular dystrophies
nitrogenous
pancreatitis
quantification
screening

Clinical chemistry involves testing for many of the chemical components found in serum, plasma, whole blood, and other **body fluids** (fluids that accumulate in the body's compartments). The chemical components can be electrically charged atoms called **ions** (K^+, Na^+, Cl^-), *metabolic by-products* (urea, creatinine), *proteins* (albumin, globulin), or *hormones* (testosterone, thyroid-stimulating hormone [TSH]). Determining the amount of these chemicals, or **quantification,** can help the physician to:

- Assess organ function (eg, bilirubin level is an indicator of liver function)
- Gain a better understanding of the patient's overall health status (eg, glucose and cholesterol levels are two chemical tests that can aid in assessing a patient's current level of health)

INSTRUMENTATION AND METHODOLOGY

A spectrophotometer is one of the earliest chemistry instruments. It is still widely used today for quantifying (determining the concentrations) various substances in a patient's blood. Certain chemical substances, when reacted with other chemicals, will cause a color formation or a color change. The higher the concentration of the substance, the more intense the color reaction. When this solution is placed in the spectrophotometer, a light source is directed at the solution. The greater the intensity of the color, the more light is absorbed and the less light is allowed to pass through. A photodetector measures the amount of light that passes through the solution. This measurement is translated into an absorbance reading shown on a galvanometer. The absorbance is compared with a graph that contains the readings for all the concentrations, and the unknown quantity in the solution being analyzed can be determined in this manner (Fig. 32-1).

A large portion of chemistry analysis is performed on automated systems that mechanically sample, dilute, or add reagents (chemicals) to the patient's blood for quantifying components. Automation has allowed more rapid analyses, reduced the occurrence of operator error, and helped control the cost of testing by reducing human intervention.

32

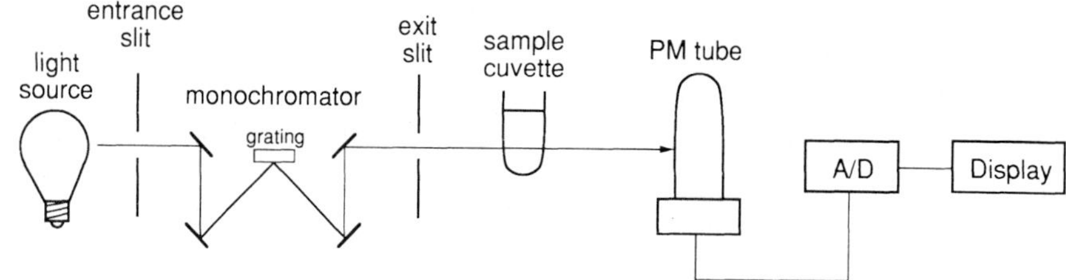

Figure 32-1 Single-beam spectrophotometer.

Many methods are used to detect and quantify chemical compounds in blood. For example, certain chemicals will produce colors when burned in an instrument called a flame photometer and can be measured during the process. Other compounds will fluoresce (produce visible radiation rays) under certain circumstances, and this method can be used for determining the level or presence of that compound. Substrate (a substance that is acted on by an enzyme) utilization for enzyme levels is another testing method. An example of substrate utilization involves introducing starch into the serum and measuring the length of time for all the starch to be broken down. This can determine the amount of amylase present.

Many office analyzers (also called bench-top analyzers) use the color change principle to determine chemistry levels. Kodak, Baxter, and Miles Diagnostic are a few companies that manufacture bench-top analyzers.

Normal (reference) ranges for all chemistry results will vary from laboratory to laboratory depending on the assay used. The normal ranges that follow in this text may be altered in laboratories because of the use of different substrates, temperatures, and instrumentation.

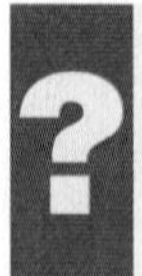

Checkpoint Question

1. *What types of chemical components are tested in the chemistry laboratory? Give examples of each.*

RENAL FUNCTION

The kidneys rid the body of waste products and help maintain *fluid balance* and *acid–base balance.* When the kidneys begin to fail, waste products, such as urea, ammonia, and creatinine, build up in the blood. The patient will become edematous, and the delicate acid–base balance will be upset. Abnormal increases or decreases in the substances that affect acid–base balance will seriously compromise health and may cause death. To assess renal function, the physician may order tests for serum measurements of electrolytes, blood urea nitrogen (BUN), creatinine, and other components. These tests, combined with information gained from urinalysis, can significantly aid in renal assessment.

Electrolytes

Electrolytes are ions (chemicals that carry a charge) found in blood and body fluids. They may be positively charged (cations) or negatively charged (anions). Electrolytes conduct electric impulses across cell membranes to maintain fluid and acid–base balance and aid in the functioning of nerve cells and muscle tissue.

Major body electrolytes include sodium, potassium, chloride, calcium, magnesium, phosphorus, and **bicarbonate** (dissolved form of carbon dioxide). The renal system helps regulate electrolytes and fluid and acid–base balance. In the presence of an electrolyte imbalance, electric impulses are not transmitted properly, resulting in fluid and acid–base imbalances and impaired functioning of nervous and muscle tissue. Table 32-1 summarizes common electrolyte imbalances, which are described below.

Sodium

Sodium (chemical symbol Na) is the major cation of the **extracellular** fluid (the fluid outside the cell). Normal serum levels range from 135 to 145 mEq/L. *Hyponatremia* (sodium level below 135 mEq/L) is one of the most common electrolyte imbalances and can result from many factors, including gastrointestinal losses (vomiting, diarrhea), burns, cardiac or renal failure, and hypothyroidism. Symptoms of hyponatremia

Table 32-1 **Terms Describing Electrolyte Imbalances**

Imbalance	*Definition*
Hypernatremia	An excess of sodium in the blood
Hyponatremia	A deficit of sodium in the blood
Hyperkalemia	An excess of potassium in the blood
Hypokalemia	A deficit of potassium in the blood
Hyperchloremia	An excess of chloride in the blood
Hypochloremia	A deficit of chloride in the blood
Hyperphosphatemia	An excess of phosphate in the blood
Hypophosphatemia	A deficit of phosphate in the blood
Hypercalcemia	An excess of calcium in the blood
Hypocalcemia	A deficit of calcium in the blood
Hypermagnesemia	An excess of magnesium in the blood
Hypomagnesemia	A deficit of magnesium in the blood

(From Timby, B. K., & Lewis, L. W., [1992]. *Fundamental Skills and Concepts in Patient Care,* 5th ed., p. 678. Philadelphia: J.B. Lippincott.)

range in severity, depending on how low the value is. These may be manifested as subtle changes in energy levels and mental activity or, in severe forms, as neurologic malfunctions, including seizures.

Hypernatremia (sodium level above 145 mEq/L) can be caused by drug therapies, Cushing's syndrome, diabetes insipidus, and other pathologies. Typically, the kidneys help the body adjust to this more saline (salty) environment by not excreting as much water. In this way, sodium is diluted back to an acceptable level. Because water is retained in hypernatremia, the patient may present with signs of edema.

Potassium

Potassium (chemical symbol K) is the major cation of the **intracellular** fluid (fluid within the cell). Only 2% of potassium is extracellular; therefore, serum levels are much lower than sodium: 3.5 to 5.0 mEq/L. *Hypokalemia* (potassium level below 3.5 mEq/L) is seen with insulin therapy, gastrointestinal losses, and renal disease. *Hyperkalemia* (potassium level above 5.0 mEq/L) can occur with cell injuries and renal failure. **Artifactual** (caused by outside interference) hyperkalemia can result from red blood cell lysis, as in a traumatic venipuncture, or if the tourniquet is left on the arm too long or is applied too tightly. Abnormal blood levels of potassium can have profound effects on the neuromuscular system, resulting in muscle weakness, paralysis, and cardiac arrhythmias.

Chloride

Chloride (chemical symbol Cl) is the major anion of the extracellular fluid. The normal range for chloride is 96 to 110 mEq/L. *Hypochloremia* is a condition in which the serum chloride level is below 96 mEq/L. In *hyperchloremia,* the serum chloride level is above 110 mEq/L. Chloride is closely associated with acid–base balance and is adversely affected in such conditions as diabetic ketoacidosis and **metabolic acidosis** (a condition of increased metabolic acids). Renal disease can alter chloride levels in either direction.

Calcium

Calcium (chemical symbol Ca) is a cation, with normal serum levels ranging from 8.5 to 10.5 mg/dL. *Hypocalcemia* (calcium level significantly below 8.5 mg/dL) is associated with acute or chronic renal failure or electrolyte imbalances due to hypoparathyroidism. *Hypercalcemia* (calcium level above 10.5 mg/dL) is associated with metabolic conditions, such as hyperparathyroidism or excessive calcium intake or absorption due to medications or alterations in gastrointestinal metabolism.

Magnesium

Magnesium (chemical symbol Mg) is a cation found in intracellular fluid. Normal magnesium levels range from 1.3 to 2.1 mEq/L. *Hypomagnesemia* (magnesium level below 1.3 mEq/L) may result from shifts in body fluids and other electrolytes. *Hypermagnesemia* (magnesium level above 2.1 mEq/L) may also result from fluid and electrolyte shifts as well as from impaired excretion caused by kidney failure. Symptoms of hypermagnesemia are similar to those for hyperkalemia (see above).

32

Phosphorus

Phosphorus (chemical symbol P) is the major anion in the intracellular fluid. Normal phosphorus levels range from 2.5 to 4.5 mg/dL. *Hypophosphatemia* (phosphorus level below 2.5 mg/dL) can result from a number of factors, including inadequate absorption, gastrointestinal losses, electrolyte shifts, and endocrine disorders. *Hyperphosphatemia* (phosphorus level above 4.5 mg/dL) is associated with hypocalcemia, hypoparathyroidism, and renal impairment or failure. In patients with renal failure, soft-tissue calcification is seen as a long-term effect of hyperphosphatemia.

Bicarbonate

Bicarbonate (chemical symbol HCO_3) is formed when carbon dioxide (CO_2) dissolves in the bloodstream, providing another negatively charged ion to the extracellular fluid. Bicarbonate is the major factor in acid–base balance; increased levels result in *alkalosis* (the body pH is too basic), and decreased levels may be due to *acidosis* (the body pH is too acidic).

The acid–base system is extremely sensitive and cannot tolerate large pH fluctuations. The body's normal pH range is 7.35 to 7.45, very slightly basic from the neutral 7.0. The renal and respiratory systems work to regulate acid–base balance. Bicarbonate is breathed out in the form of CO_2 and is also excreted through the kidneys. Measurement of CO_2 is considered more useful for pH balance assessment than for measuring renal functioning, but it also aids in the overall assessment of renal function.

Checkpoint Question

2. *What is hyponatremia? Name four possible causes.*

Nonprotein Nitrogenous Compounds

More than 15 different nonprotein **nitrogenous** (nitrogen-containing) compounds are recognized. Three that can be increased as a consequence of impaired renal function are urea, creatinine, and uric acid. However, other diseases can also affect the concentrations of these substances, making this a relatively nonspecific indicator.

Urea

Urea is the major end-product of protein and amino acid metabolism. Because urea is formed in the liver and excreted mainly by the kidneys, it can be an indicator for both liver and renal function. Typically, urea is measured as BUN and ranges from 10 to 20 mg/dL. Various other factors affect BUN levels besides renal and liver functions, such as dietary intake of protein and state of hydration.

Creatinine

Creatinine is a breakdown product of **creatine,** which aids in delivering energy to cells. Creatine is a chemical compound that adds phosphorus to adenosine diphosphate (ADP) to make **adenosine triphosphate (ATP),** the energy currency of the body. Normal range for creatinine is 0.8 to 1.7 mg/dL for men and 0.6 to 1.0 mg/dL for women depending on the muscle mass of the patient. Creatinine is more effective in assessing renal function than BUN. This is because only trace amounts of creatinine are reabsorbed in the renal tubules. Urinary excretion of this compound equals the amount produced in the body, whereas urea is reabsorbed to a certain extent. This is useful in determining the filtering ability of the kidneys.

A test called creatinine clearance is used for this purpose. A 24-hour urine sample is collected for a creatinine clearance because excretion of creatinine varies throughout the day. (See the procedure for 24-hour urine collection in Chap. 28, Urinalysis.)

The term used to describe elevated levels of urea and creatinine is **azotemia** (azo- means compounds containing nitrogen). A large increase in urea alone is called uremia. Liver and renal dysfunction can cause azotemia. Other conditions include dehydration, shock, trauma, congestive heart failure, skeletal muscle necrosis, starvation, and **muscular dystrophies** (diseases characterized by progressive atrophy of skeletal muscles). As levels of these toxins rise, systemic affects may include neurologic alterations (eg, memory loss, hallucinations, seizures, coma), cardiovascular alterations (eg, hypertension, congestive heart failure), and respiratory distress.

Uric Acid

Uric acid is a metabolic end-product of proteins containing purine. For men, the normal range is 4.0 to 8.5 mg/dL, and for women, it is 2.7 to 7.3 mg/dL. Like other nitrogen-containing compounds, uric acid is formed in the liver and excreted mostly by the kidneys; therefore, it can be an indicator of organ dysfunction. Clinically, increased amounts of uric acid are more significant than decreased amounts. *Hyperuricemia* is seen with renal failure, use of **diuretics** (substances that promote urine formation and excretion), obesity, and atherosclerosis. Diets high in proteins (meat, legumes, and yeast) can cause a mild case of hyperuricemia. The disease gout is characterized by a high uric acid accumulation in the joints; the joints become inflamed, producing significant discomfort. Typically, gout is due to an inborn error of metabolism (an inherited trait wherein an enzyme is missing or decreased so that a normal metabolic process is not fully functional). Gout can be treated with various drugs and diet therapy.

What If?
What if a patient is diagnosed with gout and asks you about dietary restrictions?

First and foremost, speak to the physician to determine if there are any other medical conditions that warrant a special diet. Patients with gout are usually placed on a low purine diet initially. Foods that are high in purine are liver, kidneys, sweetbreads, sardines, anchovies, and meat extracts. Diet and medications can often keep gout under control. Dietary retraining is usually done by the physician or a registered dietitian.

Checkpoint Question

3. *Name the nonprotein nitrogenous compounds important for assessing renal function.*

LIVER FUNCTION

The liver is the largest gland of the body and one of the most complex. More than 500 of its functions have been identified. Among the major functions are the production of **bile** (bitter yellow-green secretion of the liver), metabolism of many compounds used by the body (glucose, fats, proteins, and vitamins), processing of bilirubin, and detoxifying substances found in the blood that could prove dangerous to the body.

Liver malfunction is an extremely serious condition. It can be brought on by disease, acute or chronic toxicities, cancer, or inherited abnormalities. Discussed below are some of the commonly tested chemistries that help determine liver function. Many laboratories offer a panel of tests often called liver function tests. Typically included in this panel would be bilirubin, alkaline phosphatase (ALP or AP), alanine aminotransferase (ALT), aspartate aminotransferase (AST), total protein, and albumin. Table 32-2 shows how these tests are affected by abnormal liver conditions.

Bilirubin

When red blood cells break down, hemoglobin is released into the plasma. Hemoglobin, through a series of steps, is then converted into bilirubin. At this stage

32

Table 32-2 **Chemistry Tests Affected by Abnormal Liver Conditions**

Chemistry Test	*Normal Values*	*Acute Hepatitis*	*Cirrhosis*	*Obstructive Jaundice*	*Liver Cancer*
Albumin	3.5–5.0 g/dL	NL/↓	↑	NL/↓	↓
Bilirubin	Direct: 0.4 mg/dL Total: 1.0 mg/dL	↑↑	↑	↑	NL/↓
Alkaline phosphatase	30–115 IU/L	↑	NL/↑	↑	NL/↓
Aspartate aminotransferase	0–41 IU/L	NL/↑	NL/↑	NL/↑	NL/↑
Alanine aminotransferase	0–45 IU/L	↑↑	NL/↑	↑	NL/↑

NL, normal; ↑, increased; ↑↑, marked increase; ↓, decreased

it is unconjugated (not attached to another compound) and is insoluble in water. It travels through the bloodstream until it enters the liver. Here it is converted into conjugated bilirubin, which is water soluble and excreted into the bile. Testing for serum bilirubin provides valuable information for diagnosis and evaluation of liver disease, **biliary obstructions** (blockage of bile ducts), and hemolytic anemias. Bilirubin is yellow-orange; if excess amounts settle into the skin and sclera, its presence will make the patient appear yellow (jaundiced).

Note: Bilirubin is extremely sensitive to light and will break down readily when exposed to ultraviolet rays. A bilirubin specimen should be protected from light from the time it is collected until testing has been completed and results verified. Testing should be performed within 1 hour of collection.

Enzymes

An enzyme is a protein produced by living cells and **catalyzes** (speeds up) chemical reactions. The liver has many enzymes to speed up its various processes. Some of these can be found in the serum and in quantities sufficient for analysis.

Alkaline Phosphatase

Alkaline phosphatase is present in the bones, liver, intestines, kidneys, and placenta. Circulating ALP is primarily from the liver and bone. Levels of ALP will rise in disorders such as Paget's disease (bone) or hepatitis (liver).

Normal values vary with age. Increased levels of ALP are considered normal during periods of bone growth activity, such as childhood growth spurts and third-trimester pregnancy. These elevated levels are not indicators of a disease process.

Alanine Aminotransferase (ALT [SGPT]) and Aspartate Aminotransferase (AST [SGOT])

These enzymes are present in the liver. AST (SGOT), however, is present in many other organs as well. Increased levels of ALT (SGPT) and AST are seen with liver damage; AST also rises in myocardial infarctions.

Albumin

Albumin is the major protein in the blood. The liver is responsible for its manufacture. Albumin serves as a transport protein linking up with other chemical compounds that otherwise could not be processed. When liver function is impaired or in conditions of malnutrition, albumin values decrease. The normal range for albumin is 3.6 to 5.2 g/dL.

Other Tests

Other laboratory tests used to evaluate liver function are total protein (normal range, 6–8 g/dL), cholesterol (discussed in the section "Lipids and Lipoproteins," below), and the prothrombin time. (See Chap. 30, Hematology, for a discussion of prothrombin time.) Techniques such as imaging (eg, ultrasound) and biopsies also help in diagnosis.

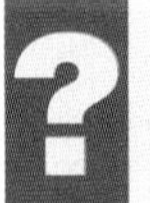

Checkpoint Question

4. *Name three diseases that can be diagnosed by testing bilirubin levels.*

THYROID FUNCTION

The thyroid gland regulates metabolism by secreting the hormones triiodothyronine (T_3) and thyroxine (T_4). Its primary function is to establish the **basal**

metabolic rate, which is the amount of energy used in a unit of time to maintain vital functions. The thyroid gland is controlled by another hormone, TSH, which is produced in the anterior pituitary gland.

Thyroid-Stimulating Hormone

In the absence of a disease process, when additional thyroid hormones are needed, more TSH is secreted to stimulate the thyroid gland. In the same manner, when lesser amounts of the hormones are required, less TSH is secreted so the thyroid gland will reduce its production. However, many situations can cause an imbalance in this delicate endocrine system. There may be a malfunction in the anterior pituitary gland so that it oversecretes or undersecretes TSH. If the thyroid gland is malfunctioning, it cannot be stimulated, regardless of the amount of TSH secreted. TSH levels may be quite high in cases such as this.

Triiodothyronine and Thyroxine

The thyroid hormones, T_3 and T_4, target many organs to control various processes (see above). For T_3 and T_4 to be present in sufficient quantities, a functional thyroid gland and adequate amounts of **iodine** (an essential micronutrient) are required. Elevations of one or both hormones along with TSH levels aid in the diagnosis of various conditions.

CARDIAC FUNCTION

Several enzymes can be analyzed for the diagnosis of a myocardial infarction (MI). When an MI occurs, these enzymes are released in large quantities by the damaged heart muscle into the bloodstream.

Lactate Dehydrogenase

Lactate dehydrogenase (LDH or LD) is widely distributed in body tissues but concentrated in the myocardium, liver, kidney, and muscle. LDH is markedly increased within 24 hours of an MI; elevations usually return to normal in 8 to 14 days. Elevations are also seen with certain leukemias, pulmonary infarctions, hemolytic anemias, and progressive muscular dystrophy. LDH has five isoenzymes, LDH-1 to LDH-5. Isoenzymes are similar but not identical structures that have the same function but originate in different organs. In a normal profile, LDH-2 is in greater quantity than LDH-1, but an MI causes LDH-1 to be much higher.

Creatine Kinase

Creatine kinase (CK) is found almost exclusively in skeletal muscle and myocardium. Within 2 to 8 hours of an MI, CK levels will increase. CK will also be increased in crushing injuries to muscles, such as those sustained in car accidents. CK has three isoenzymes, designated MM (muscle), MB (hybrid), and BB (brain). Most of the normal levels of CK consist of the MM fraction. The MB fraction rises with an MI.

Note: The AST level (see section on "Liver Function") will also rise after an MI but takes longer to detect (2–3 days). Other techniques, such as electrocardiograms, are also used for assessing cardiac function (Table 32-3).

Cardiac Troponin T

Cardiac troponin T (TnT) is a protein specific to heart muscle, making it a valuable tool in the diagnosis of acute myocardial infarction. Cardiac TnT blood levels begin to rise within 4 hours of the onset of myocardial damage and stay elevated for up to 14 days, which means levels can be measured to monitor the effectiveness of thrombolytic therapy in heart attack patients. A one-step, whole-blood test kit for TnT is available from Boehringer Mannheim Corp., Indianapolis, IN.

Table 32-3 **Enzymes Elevated After a Myocardial Infarction**

Enzyme	*Timing of Release*	*Special Notation*
Lactate dehydrogenase	• Begins rise at 24 h • Peaks at 3–6 d • Reaches baseline at approximately 2 wk	Isoenzyme LDH-1 is greater in relation to LDH-2.
Creatine kinase	• Begins rise at 2–8 h • Peak is variable • Reaches baseline at 4 d	Isoenzyme CK-MB is the increased fraction.
Aspartate amino transferase	• Begins rise at 8 h • Peaks at 18–36 h • Reaches baseline at 4 d	

Checkpoint Question

5. *Which enzyme will assist the physician in the diagnosis of an MI within 3 hours of onset? Why?*

LUNG FUNCTION

The lungs are the organs that bring oxygen into contact with the circulatory system and aid in the removal of the waste product carbon dioxide. The lungs, along with the kidneys, help regulate acid–base balance. There are many methods of assessing lung function using respiratory therapy; in the laboratory, assessment is accomplished with blood gases.

Blood Gases

Specimens for blood gases are usually drawn from an artery; therefore, they are typically termed arterial blood gases (ABGs). However, venous or capillary specimens are used on occasion. Blood gases consist of oxygen, carbon dioxide, and nitrogen. These gases are given as percentages and partial pressures. By comparing blood gas values to the normal ranges, the physician can assess a patient's ventilatory status (how well the patient is oxygenated). Also included in the determination is the patient's acid–base balance or pH (Tables 32-4 and 32-5). The blood gas determination is often used to aid in the evaluation of cardiac failure, hemorrhage, kidney failure, diabetes, shock, and drug overdose.

PANCREATIC FUNCTION

The pancreas functions in both the endocrine and exocrine systems and produces many secretions. Amylase and **lipase,** two of its exocrine system products, are released as excretory enzymes into the intestines to aid in digestion. Insulin and glucagon are hormonal products of its endocrine function and are released into the bloodstream to regulate carbohydrate metabolism.

Pancreatic Enzymes

Amylase

Amylase is markedly increased with pancreatitis (inflammation of the pancreas). The salivary glands also produce amylase, which accounts for the elevated levels found with sialoadenitis and other inflammatory diseases of the salivary glands such as mumps.

Lipase

Lipase levels also rise with pancreatitis. For a differential diagnosis of pancreatitis, it is recommended that both of the enzymes be quantitated.

Pancreatic Hormones

Glucose is one of the main energy sources for the body. When foods are broken down by the metabolic processes, many nutrients are released. These nutrients are absorbed from the intestines into the bloodstream, carried to the liver by the hepatic portal system, and designated for use immediately or for storage as needed. Sugars, mainly glucose, provide energy by entering a complex biochemical pathway called the **Krebs cycle,** also known as the citric acid cycle. As glucose works through this metabolic chain of events, one of the co-events in the breakdown of glucose into carbon dioxide (CO_2) and water is the generation of ATP, a compound that stores energy in muscles for release as needed—our body's energy currency.

For glucose to be used for stored energy in the form of glycogen, it must be brought into the cells where the Krebs cycle occurs. Two hormones regulate this process: insulin and glucagon. Blood glucose levels need to be maintained within narrow limits so that there are no adverse physical effects. By their actions, insulin and glucagon keep these levels within the approximate range.

Glucose-Regulating Hormones

Insulin brings the glucose used for energy into cells for immediate use or for storage. If there is sufficient energy available for cell use, the glucose is stored as either glycogen (long chains of glucose) in the liver and mus-

Table 32-4 **Blood Gases in Relation to Acid–Base Balance in the Body**

Condition in the Body	*pH*	*Oxygen Tension*	*Oxygen Saturation*	*Carbon Dioxide Tension*	*Bicarbonate*
Normal	7.35–7.45	75–100 mmHg	96%–100%	35–45 mmHg	22–26 mEq/L
Respiratory acidosis	<7.35			>45 mmHg	
Metabolic acidosis	<7.35				<22 mEq/L
Respiratory alkalosis	>7.45			<35 mmHg	
Metabolic alkalosis	>7.45				>26 mEq/L

32

Table 32-5 **Causes of Acid–Base Imbalance**

Condition	*Possible Causes*
Respiratory acidosis	Obstructive lung disease, respiratory depression due to drug toxicity or disease, other causes of hypoventilation
Metabolic acidosis	Diarrhea (bicarbonate loss), diabetic acidosis, renal failure, aspirin toxicity, ammonium chloride therapy, starvation, diabetes, heart failure, shock
Respiratory alkalosis	Hypoxia, anxiety, pulmonary embolus, pregnancy, other causes of hypoventilation
Metabolic alkalosis	Diuretic therapy, severe gastrointestinal losses, Cushing's syndrome, excessive ingestion of antacids

cles or as fat. Insulin is an important hormone; cells would starve if insulin were not available or if the cells were not able to bring glucose in for energy. By arranging for glucose storage, insulin keeps glucose levels down, thereby maintaining a stable normal range.

Glucagon is a hormone that causes glucose stored in the form of glycogen to be released into the bloodstream, thereby raising glucose levels. Whenever blood glucose levels drop, glucagon acts on glycogen to break it apart so molecules of glucose are available for cellular use.

Common Glucose Tests

The time during which a blood sample is taken for glucose testing can assist in the diagnostic or monitoring process. The tests described below are the most frequently ordered.

The glucose reflectance photometer (glucose meter) is often used as a quick, accurate, easy-to-perform in-office procedure to measure a patient's blood glucose level. Glucose meters are commercially available under different names: the Glucometer made by Ames, the Accu-Chek by Boeringer Mannheim, and the Glucosan by Lifescan. The basic testing principles involves the application of whole blood to a reagent strip, which is read optically by the instrument after a designated time (Procedure 32-1). The amount of color change (to blue) correlates with glucose concentration and a value is reported.

FASTING BLOOD GLUCOSE (SUGAR). A fasting blood sugar (FBS) can be obtained from the patient after a 12- to 14-hour fast (nothing but water is taken in during the fast). Procedure 32-1 describes the process for obtaining an FBS using a glucose meter. The normal range for an FBS is typically 50 to 110 mg/dL, but there may be a slight interlaboratory variation, depending on the population used to establish the normal range.

The main purpose of an FBS is to detect either diabetes mellitus or hypoglycemia. Fasting glucose levels of 125 to 140 mg/dL or greater are considered indicative of diabetes. Further testing by either another FBS, a 2-hour postprandial glucose test, or a glucose tolerance test (GTT) is used to corroborate the initial high result. Hypoglycemia is a syndrome characterized by FBS levels below 45 mg/dL and a variety of symptoms: sweating, weakness, dizziness, headache, trembling, lethargy, and other nervous manifestations.

RANDOM BLOOD GLUCOSE. Although a random glucose is not as diagnostically useful as a fasting test, it is a good **screening** tool (preliminary test) on otherwise healthy patients. A random glucose can be drawn anytime during the day and has a slightly broader range: 45 to 130 mg/dL.

2-HOUR POSTPRANDIAL GLUCOSE. A 2-hour postprandial glucose (2-hour PP) is used to screen for diabetes and to monitor insulin therapy of diabetic patients. The patient must eat a high carbohydrate meal after a 12-hour fast. Patients who may not be compliant are given a glucose solution to drink as a substitute for the meal for better control of the testing results. Two hours after the meal, a blood sample is drawn, and glucose is measured. Timing of the specimen collection is extremely important in this test result. "Good control" of diabetes has been defined as a 2-hour pp of less than 130 mg/dL.

GLUCOSE TOLERANCE TEST. The GTT is used for diagnosing diabetes and hypoglycemia. The patient is **challenged** (tested) with a large dose of glucose, then blood glucose levels are checked at intervals to see how the body is metabolizing the glucose. Many conditions can affect a GTT. Strict control should be maintained when possible to minimize extraneous factors. A diet of 150 g of carbohydrate per day is usually ordered for 3 days before the test. Other carbohydrate levels will be calibrated by body weight if the patient's weight is not what is expected for a normal adult. The patient should fast for 12 hours before the time of testing and should not smoke or exercise before the test. Also, the patient should have been free of illnesses during the previous 2 weeks. These precautions are taken because glucose utilization is affected by many factors and can interfere with an accurate picture of how the body would normally metabolize glucose.

Briefly, the GTT is performed by administering an amount of glucose calculated by the patient's weight. Blood is obtained ½, 1, 2, and 3 hours after the glucose has been administered. Blood sampling *must* occur at the precise times indicated for valid diagnosis. Urine specimens may also be collected during the timed intervals.

Blood may be drawn by venipuncture (see Chap. 29, Phlebotomy). A serum or plasma specimen can be collected, depending on laboratory preference. The specimen should be centrifuged and separated as soon as possible to prevent the metabolism or breakdown of glucose by the red blood cells. Specimens collected in gray stopper tubes containing sodium fluoride are stable for up to 3 days even without centrifugation.

Blood also may be drawn using capillary puncture (see Chap. 29, Phlebotomy). The number of samples required make capillary collection more acceptable to the patient and the accuracy of the glucose meter make this method a viable option. Procedure 32-2 describes the steps to follow when performing a GTT.

Interpretation of GTT Results. The medical assistant does not interpret the results of the GTT. However, knowledge of how patients with various conditions (diabetes, hypoglycemia) will respond to this testing can be useful.

Numerous methods can be used to interpret the values obtained from a GTT. The criteria proposed by the National Diabetes Data Group and the World Health Organization, and endorsed by the American Diabetes Association, recommend that a diagnosis of diabetes be established if the fasting glucose level is greater than 125 to 140 mg/dL, and the 2-hour measurement is equal to or above 200 mg/dL. Some sources recommend as well that another value between fasting and the 2-hour (ie, either the ½ or 1 hour) be above 200 mg/dL.

Hypoglycemia can also be diagnosed by the GTT. Symptoms of hypoglycemia include headaches, weakness, shakiness, fatigue, sweating, and light-headedness. Whenever any of these occur during a GTT, it is important to obtain a blood specimen from the patient even if it is not at an appointed time. Unfortunately, many times a lower-than-normal range glucose level does not correspond to the symptoms presented. Different authors noting this theorize that emotional states and anxieties may be causing the symptoms, not lowered glucose levels. Frequently, these same patients will improve when their food intake is divided so that they eat many small meals (thereby introducing smaller glucose loads) rather than several large ones. This leads to the consideration that an imbalance of glucose levels has some merit in explaining why these symptoms appear.

32

Checkpoint Question

6. *What is hypoglycemia? List the symptoms associated with this disorder.*

DIABETIC GLUCOSE TESTING. Although blood glucose levels are used to detect and monitor the diabetic patient, the test of choice is hemoglobin A_{IC}. This allows the physician to form a more accurate picture of the diabetic's physiologic state over long periods of time (weeks to several months).

Glucose converts the A portion of hemoglobin into A_{IC}, which is simply the glucose attached to a portion of hemoglobin A. As glucose levels increase over long periods of time, increasing amounts of hemoglobin A are converted to A_{IC}. A certain amount of conversion is considered to be in the "good control" range. A measurement above a certain level of hemoglobin A_{IC} indicates to the physician that the patient has "poor control" of the condition even if the fasting blood sugar at the time is acceptable.

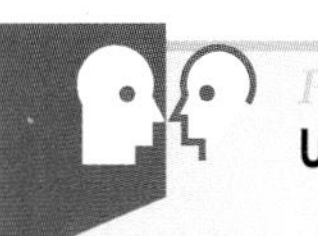

Patient Education

Using a Glucose Meter

Many diabetic patients are discharged from the hospital with instructions for using a glucose meter. As a medical assistant, you can help reinforce patient education regarding this procedure. Here are points to stress:

- Teach patients about the need to test and document glucose levels regularly.
- Offer instructions in the proper technique for obtaining a blood sample (eg, do not "milk" the finger, cleanse the area well before beginning).
- Caution patients against "self-regulating" insulin. Have patients call the physician for abnormal glucose levels.
- Alert patients to the signs and symptoms of high and low glucose levels and the treatments for each.

Most pharmacies and surgical supply stores that sell glucose meters will be able to educate patients in their use. The strips for glucose meters are expensive and may be covered by certain insurance companies if the physician clearly documents the need.

32

Procedure 32-1 Determining Blood Glucose

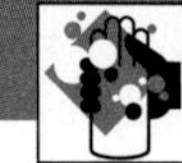
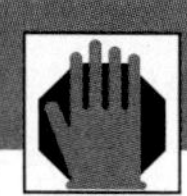

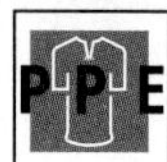

PURPOSE

To determine the level of glucose in the blood
To aid in the diagnosis and treatment of hypoglycemia and hyperglycemia

EQUIPMENT/SUPPLIES

- glucose meter of the physician's choice
- glucose reagent strips
- lancet
- alcohol pad
- sterile gauze
- paper towel

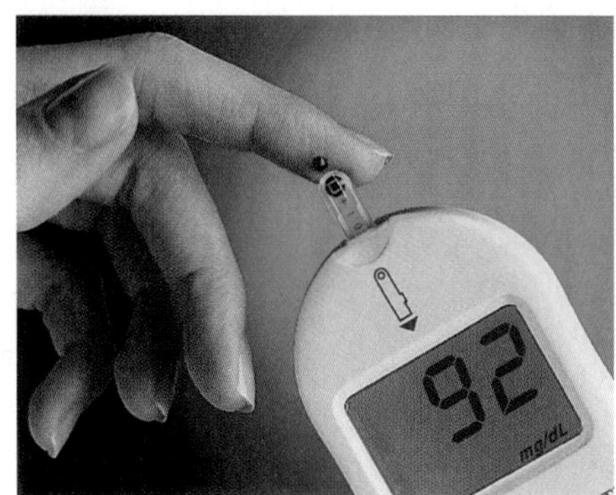

Glucometer Elite blood glucose monitoring device. (Courtesy of Bayer Corporation, Elkhart, Indiana.)

STEPS

1. Wash your hands.
2. Assemble the equipment and supplies.
3. Put on gloves before removing reagent strip.
   Sugar residues on hands can falsely elevate glucose results if the strip is contaminated by touching.
4. Turn on the instrument, and ensure that it is calibrated. The digits 888 appear on the display screen followed by the code of the strips being used.
   Calibration of the glucose meter is essential for accurate test results.
5. Remove one reagent strip, lay it on the paper towel, and recap the container.
   The strip is ready for testing. The paper towel will serve as a disposable work surface and will absorb excess blood added to the strip. The strips are sensitive to humidity and will deteriorate if allowed to absorb moisture.
6. Greet and identify the patient. Explain the procedure. Ask for and answer any questions.
7. Have the patient wash his or her hands.
   Washing removes sugar residues from the skin and the warm water stimulates blood flow.
8. Cleanse the selected puncture site (finger) with alcohol.
   Alcohol removes bacteria from the site.

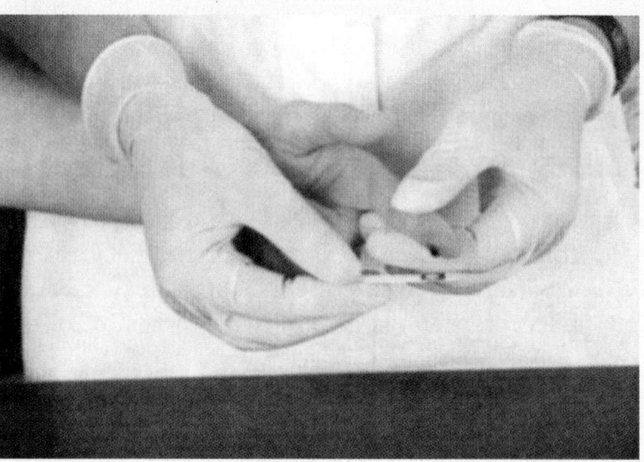

9. Puncture the site with a lancet, following the steps described in Chap. 29, Phlebotomy. Wipe away the first drop of blood.

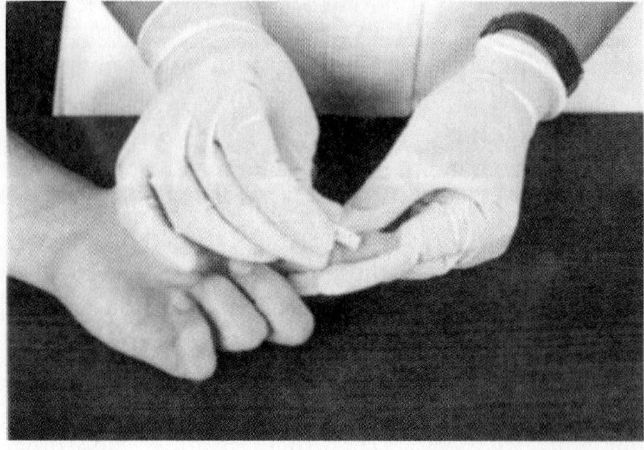

continued

Procedure 32-1 Continued **Determining Blood Glucose**

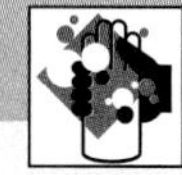
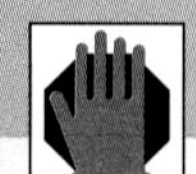
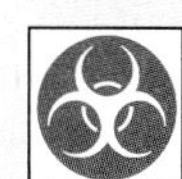

32

10. Turn the patient's hand palm down and gently squeeze the finger to form a large drop of blood.
Gentle squeezing obtains a blood specimen without diluting the sample with tissue fluid.

11. Bring the reagent strip up to the finger and touch the pad to the blood. Do not touch the finger. Completely cover the pad with blood.
The entire pad must be covered for accurate reading. There is no chance of contamination by oils or other residue remaining on the finger if this surface is not touched.

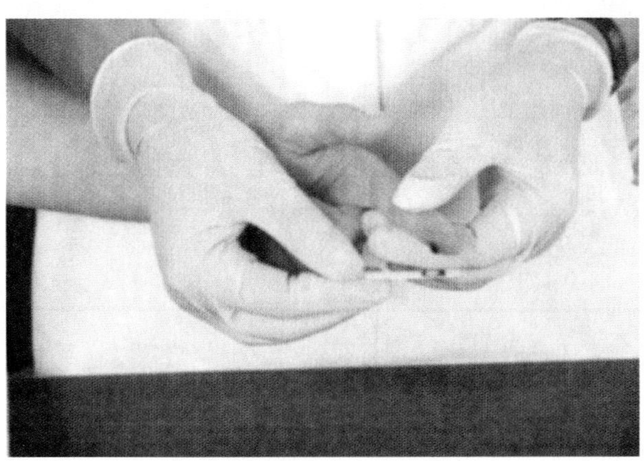

12. Immediately press the TIME button. Most meters count up to 60 seconds. (Meanwhile, apply pressure to the puncture wound with gauze.) At the end of 60 seconds, firmly wipe the blood off with a clean gauze. The meter will continue to count for another 60 seconds. During this time, insert the reagent strip into the chamber with the pad side down.
This time frame allows the reaction changes to occur.

13. Be aware that at 120 seconds, the instrument reads the reaction strip and displays the result on the screen in mg/dL. If the glucose level is higher or lower than expected, refer to the troubleshooting guide provided by the manufacturer.
The reaction is now complete. The color change is photo-optically measured and reported in mg/dL.

14. Properly care for or dispose of equipment and supplies. Clean the work area. Remove gloves, and wash your hands.

DOCUMENTATION GUIDELINES

- Date and time
- Testing site
- Test results
- Action taken (if any)
- Patient education
- Your signature

Charting Example

DATE	TIME Lancet skin puncture right index
	finger. Glucose tested with Glucometer.
	Results: 60 mg/dL. Dr. Peters notified.
	Pt was given a glass of orange juice.
	—Your signature

Quality assurance measure: Controls are available in the low, normal, and high range to ensure that the glucose meter is functioning properly. These controls should be run daily or every time a patient glucose test is performed if the meter is not used daily.

OBSTETRIC GLUCOSE TESTING. An increase of glucose intolerance has been noted among pregnant patients in the second and third trimesters. Because **gestational diabetes** can endanger the fetus, the pregnant patient's glucose level needs to be monitored. The widely accepted screening method used for this purpose is to administer a 50-g glucose load in drink form and draw blood samples 1 hour later. If the value exceeds 155 mg/dL, a GTT is indicated for a diagnosis of gestational diabetes. This screening method is usually done during the second trimester.

LIPIDS AND LIPOPROTEINS

Cholesterol and associated **lipids** (free fatty acids) and **lipoproteins** (substances composed of lipids and proteins) have long been implicated as the culprits in heart

32

Procedure 32-2 Glucose Tolerance Testing (GTT)

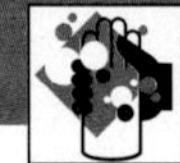
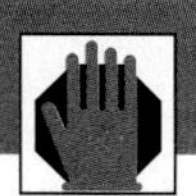
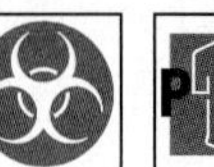

PURPOSE

To determine the body's ability to metabolize a premeasured quantity of glucose over a specified time

EQUIPMENT/SUPPLIES

- calibrated amount of glucose per the physician's order
- phlebotomy equipment
- glucose test strips
- glucose meter equipment
- alcohol wipes
- stopwatch

STEPS

1. Wash your hands.
2. Assemble the equipment and supplies.
   A stopwatch is necessary because the timing of the collections is important to the test results.
3. Greet and identify the patient. Explain the procedure. Ask for and answer any questions.
4. Obtain a fasting glucose (FBS) specimen (red top) from the patient using the steps as outlined in the venipuncture procedure (see Chap. 29, Phlebotomy). It is recommended that laboratories test the blood sample before the glucose drink is administered; if the FBS exceeds a certain reading (eg, greater than 140 mg/dL), do not perform the GTT. Notify the physician.
   Fasting glucose gives a baseline for further interpretation. Giving more glucose to a patient whose blood glucose level is already too high could cause serious harm.
5. Give the glucose drink to the patient to consume within a 5-minute period. Note the time the patient finishes the drink; this is the "START" of the test.
   The body begins to metabolize the glucose immediately, so rapid ingestion of the drink is necessary.
6. Exactly 30 minutes after the patient has finished the glucose drink, obtain another blood specimen. Label the specimen with the patient's name and time of collection.
   Precise timing of specimen collection is vital for accurate interpretation of results. Many specimens will be received from this patient, making proper notation of the sequence extremely important.
7. Exactly 1 hour after the glucose drink, repeat step 6.
8. Exactly 2 hours after the glucose drink, repeat step 6.
9. Exactly 3 hours after the glucose drink, repeat step 6. Unless a GTT of longer than 3 hours has been requested, the testing is complete at this time. (For a longer GTT, continue specimen collection in the same manner for as many additional hours as required.)
10. If the specimens are to be tested by an outside laboratory, package as required, and arrange for transportation.
    Careful handling and transport helps ensure accurate testing.
11. Properly care for or dispose of equipment and supplies. Clean the work area. Remove gloves and gown, and wash your hands.

DOCUMENTATION GUIDELINES

- Date and time
- Test results, if performed on site
- Patient observations
- Patient education
- Your signature

Charting Example

DATE	TIME 0800 GTT test
	0800 FBS: 100 mg/dL glucose
	0810 Glucose drink given to pt
	0815 Glucose drink finished
	0845 Glucose: 125 mg/dL
	0915 Glucose: 132 mg/dL
	1015 Glucose: 120 mg/dL
	1115 Glucose: 110 mg/dL Pt tolerated
	procedure well, discharged by Dr. Lynch.
	—Your signature

Note: Ensure that the patient remains fairly sedentary throughout this procedure (eg, no long walks between blood draws); exercising will alter the glucose levels by burning it for more energy. The patient also should avoid smoking because it may artificially increase the glucose level. Only water should be ingested. Encourage the patient to drink water to increase the blood volume and make it easier to draw blood from venipuncture. If the patient experiences any severe symptoms (eg, headache, dizziness, vomiting), end the test and notify the physician. These symptoms could be the result of glucose levels that are too high or too low for the patient to tolerate.

Table 32-6 **Risk Factors for Premature Atherosclerosis and Coronary Heart Disease**

Chemistry Test	*Low Risk*	*Moderate Risk*	*High Risk*
Cholesterol	Levels at or below 200 mg/dL	Levels above 200 mg/dL	Levels above 200 mg/dL
HDL	Levels within or above normal range	Levels within or above normal range	Levels below normal range
LDL	Levels within or below normal range	Levels within or below normal range	Levels above normal range
Triglycerides	Levels within or below normal range	Levels within or below normal range	Levels above normal range

Note: Frequently, a patient's chemistry tests will fall into two of the categories so that the patient's risk group is not clearly defined. The physician decides the degree of risk for the patient based on these tests and other risk factors, such as life-style and family history. Normal range will vary by age and sex.

HDL, high-density lipoprotein; LDL, low-density lipoprotein

Table 32-7 **Common Chemistry Panel Tests**

Test	*Function in the Body*	*Normal Values*	*Increases Seen With*	*Decreases Seen With*
Blood urea nitrogen (BUN)	Metabolic by-product	10–20 mg/dL	Kidney disease, kidney obstructions, dehydration	Liver failure, malnutrition
Calcium	Structural element for bones, teeth, and muscles	8.5–10.5 mg/dL	Hyperparathyroidism, hyperthyroidism, Addison's disease, bone cancer, multiple myeloma, other malignancies	Hypoparathyroidism, renal failure
Chloride	Acid–base balance, component of stomach acid	96–110 mEq/L	Dehydration, Cushing's syndrome, hyperventilation	Severe vomiting, severe diarrhea, severe burns, pyloric obstruction, heat exhaustion
Cholesterol	Building block for cell membranes, steroid hormones, and bile acids	120–200 mg/dL	Atherosclerosis, heart disease, certain liver diseases with obstruction, hypothyroidism	Liver disease, hyperthyroidism, malabsorption syndromes
Creatinine	Metabolic by-product	0.6–1.7 mg/dL	Kidney disease, muscle disease	Muscular dystrophy
Glucose	Energy source for body	70–110 mg/dL	Diabetes mellitus, Cushing's syndrome, liver disease	Excess insulin, Addison's disease, bacterial sepsis, hypothyroidism
Phosphorus	Used in bone and endocrine processes	2.5–4.5 mg/dL	Renal disease, hypoparathyroidism, hypocalcemia, Addison's disease	Hyperparathyroidism, bone disease
Potassium	Acid–base balance	3.5–5.0 mEq/L	Kidney disease, cell damage, Addison's disease	Diarrhea, starvation, severe vomiting, severe burns, some forms of liver disease
Sodium	Fluid balance	135–145 mEq/L	Dehydration, Cushing's syndrome, diabetes insipidus	Severe burns, diarrhea, vomiting, Addison's disease
Triglycerides	Energy source, lipid deposits for stored energy and organ support	40–170 mg/dL	Atherosclerosis, liver disease, poorly controlled diabetes, pancreatitis	Malnutrition
Uric acid	Metabolic by-product	Men: 4.0–8.5 mg/dL Women: 2.7–7.3 mg/dL	Renal failure, gout, leukemia, eclampsia	Drug therapy to lower uric acid levels

disease. It is important to remember, however, that these compounds are part of the important building blocks of our bodies and in proper quantities are vital to health maintenance. They are a component of every cell membrane and of the myelin sheath around the nerves. They also cushion and support organs. Testing for these quantities aids the physician in assessing the risk of heart disease and assesses liver function because many of these compounds are formed and stored in the liver.

Cholesterol

Bile acids, formed partially by cholesterol, are produced in the liver and stored in the gallbladder and are then released into the intestine as needed for the digestion of fats. Vitamin D is formed from cholesterol at the skin's surface when exposed to sunlight. Various hormones, such as **cortisol,** testosterone, and estrogen, are synthesized from cholesterol as well. Only in proportions not necessary for cell maintenance and other body functions should cholesterol be considered a health hazard.

Measurement of cholesterol is done on a 12- to 14-hour fasting specimen. The ideal range for cholesterol is 140 to 200 mg/dL (as recommended by the American Heart Association). Anyone with a cholesterol level greater than 200 mg/dL is considered to be at increased risk of developing atherosclerosis.

Low-Density Lipoprotein

Low-density lipoprotein (LDL) is a plasma protein that transports cholesterol, carrying it from the liver and depositing it on the walls of large and medium-sized arteries. Atherosclerotic plaques form, causing the affected vessel to thicken and become more rigid. Circulation is then reduced to the organs and other areas normally supplied by these arteries. Atherosclerosis is the major cause of coronary heart disease, angina pectoris, MIs, and other cardiac disorders. When LDL values are above the normal range, the risk of heart disease is greater.

High-Density Lipoprotein

High-density lipoprotein (HDL) is the protein molecule that carries cholesterol that has been deposited on arterial walls back to the liver. HDL typically exists in lesser quantities than LDL does. Much research has been directed along the lines of increasing HDL because higher levels of this correlate with decreased risk of heart disease. In contrast, decreased HDL levels correlate with increased risk of heart disease.

Triglycerides

Triglycerides are the principal lipids in blood. They also are the lipids in all vegetable and animal fats. Adipose (fatty) tissue is composed almost entirely of triglycerides. The normal range for men is 40 to 160 mg/dL and for women, 35 to 135 mg/dL. Research is implicating triglycerides as a risk factor in heart disease (Table 32-6).

A summary of the common chemistry tests is presented in Table 32-7.

Checkpoint Question

7. *Which lipoprotein is beneficial? Why?*

Answers to Checkpoint Questions

1. *Chemical components tested include ions (K^+, Na^+, C^-), metabolic by-products (urea, creatinine), proteins (albumin, globulin), or hormones (testosterone, thyroid-stimulating hormone).*
2. *Hyponatremia is a sodium deficiency that can be caused by gastrointestinal losses (vomiting, diarrhea), burns, cardiac or renal failure, and hypothyroidism.*
3. *Urea, creatinine, and uric acid are important for assessing renal function.*
4. *Testing of bilirubin levels aids in the diagnosis of liver disease, biliary obstructions, and hemolytic anemias.*
5. *Creatine kinase (CK) can help diagnose myocardial infarction within 3 hours of onset because CK levels increase within 2 to 8 hours of an infarction.*
6. *Hypoglycemia is a syndrome characterized by fasting blood sugar levels below 45 mg/dL. Symptoms include sweating, weakness, dizziness, headache, trembling, lethargy, and other nervous manifestations.*
7. *High-density lipoprotein is beneficial because higher levels of this correlate with a lower risk of heart disease.*

Critical Thinking Challenges

1. A patient with edema is told by her physician to restrict her salt intake. Why may this help improve her condition?
2. A diabetic patient gave herself too much insulin by mistake. Would you expect her glucose to be very high or very low? Why?
3. A patient's amylase level is very high, but her lipase level is in the normal range. What might she have?
4. A medical assistant draws a red top tube for a number of chemistry tests. Unfortunately, the tube is left on the counter for several hours before being centrifuged and refrigerated. Which chemistries may be affected by this? Why?

Suggestions for Further Reading

Bauer, J., & Ackerman, G. (1982). *Clinical Laboratory Methods,* 9th ed. St. Louis: C.V. Mosby.

Bishop, M. L. (Ed.). (1996). *Clinical Chemistry: Principles, Procedures, Correlations,* 3rd ed. Philadelphia: Lippincott-Raven.

Bullock, B. (1996). *Pathophysiology Adaptations and Alterations in Function,* 4th ed. Glenview IL: Scott Foresman.

Fishbach, F. (1996). *A Manual of Laboratory and Diagnostic Tests,* 5th ed. Philadelphia: Lippincott-Raven.

Henry, J. (1991). *Todd-Sanford-Davisohn Clinical Diagnosis and Management by Laboratory Methods,* 18th ed. Philadelphia: W.B. Saunders.

Memmler, R. L., Cohen, B. J., & Wood, D. L. (1996). *The Human Body in Health and Disease,* 8th ed. Philadelphia: Lippincott-Raven.

Porth, C. M. (1998). *Pathophysiology: Concepts of Altered Health States,* 5th ed. Philadelphia: Lippincott Williams & Wilkins.

Rubin, E., & Farber, J. L. (1998). *Pathology,* 3rd ed. Philadelphia: Lippincott-Raven.

Tietz, N. (1990). *Clinical Guide to Laboratory Tests,* 2nd ed. Philadelphia: W.B. Saunders.

Appendix I

Medical Assistant Role Delineation Chart

Administrative

Administrative Procedures

- Perform basic clerical functions
- Schedule, coordinate and, monitor appointments
- Schedule inpatient/outpatient admissions and procedures
- Understand and apply third-party guidelines
- Obtain reimbursement through accurate claims submission
- Monitor third-party reimbursement
- Perform medical transcription
- Understand and adhere to managed care policies and procedures
- * Negotiate managed care contracts (adv)

Practice Finances

- Perform procedural and diagnostic coding
- Apply bookkeeping principles
- Document and maintain accounting and banking records
- Manage accounts receivable
- Manage accounts payable
- Process payroll
- * Develop and maintain fee schedules (adv)
- * Manage renewals of business and professional insurance policies (adv)
- * Manage personnel benefits and maintain records (adv)

Clinical

Fundamental Principles

- Apply principles of aseptic technique and infection control
- Comply with quality assurance practices
- Screen and follow up patient test results

Diagnostic Orders

- Collect and process specimens
- Perform diagnostic tests

Patient Care

- Adhere to established triage procedures
- Obtain patient history and vital signs
- Prepare and maintain examination and treatment areas
- Prepare patient for examinations, procedures, and treatments
- Assist with examinations, procedures, and treatments
- Prepare and administer medications and immunizations
- Maintain medication and immunization records
- Recognize and respond to emergencies
- Coordinate patient care information with other health care providers

General (Transdisciplinary)

Professionalism

- Project a professional manner and image
- Adhere to ethical principles
- Demonstrate initiative and responsibility
- Work as a team member
- Manage time effectively
- Prioritize and perform multiple tasks
- Adapt to change
- Promote the CMA credential
- Enhance skills through continuing education

Communication Skills

- Treat all patients with compassion and empathy
- Recognize and respect cultural diversity
- Adapt communications to individual's ability to understand
- Use professional telephone technique
- Use effective and correct verbal and written communications
- Recognize and respond to verbal and nonverbal communications
- Use medical terminology appropriately
- Receive, organize, prioritize, and transmit information
- Serve as liaison
- Promote the practice through positive public relations

Legal Concepts

- Maintain confidentiality
- Practice within the scope of education, training, and personal capabilities
- Prepare and maintain medical records
- Document accurately
- Use appropriate guidelines when releasing information

**Denotes advanced skills.*

- Follow employer's established policies dealing with the health care contract
- Follow federal, state, and local legal guidelines
- Maintain awareness of federal and state health care legislation and regulations
- Maintain and dispose of regulated substances in compliance with government guidelines
- Comply with established risk management and safety procedures
- Recognize professional credentialing criteria
- Participate in the development and maintenance of personnel, policy, and procedure manuals
- * Develop and maintain personnel, policy, and procedure manuals (adv)

Instruction

- Instruct individuals according to their needs
- Explain office policies and procedures
- Teach methods of health promotion and disease prevention
- Locate community resources and disseminate information
- * Orient and train personnel (adv)
- * Develop educational materials (adv)
- * Conduct continuing education activities (adv)

Operational Functions

- Maintain supply inventory
- Evaluate and recommend equipment and supplies
- Apply computer techniques to support office operations
- * Supervise personnel (adv)
- * Interview and recommend job applicants (adv)
- * Negotiate leases and prices for equipment and supply contracts (adv)

**Denotes advanced skills.*

(Courtesy of American Association of Medical Assistants, Chicago, IL.)

Appendix II Key English-to-Spanish Health Care Phrases

Although English is the major language spoken in North America, a variety of languages are used in certain areas. Prominent among them is Spanish, representing Spain, the Caribbean Islands, Central and South America, and the Philippines. Rapport can be more easily established, and the patient and family will be at ease and feel more relaxed, if someone on the staff speaks their language. Some health care facilities provide interpreters, especially in areas with a large population of Spanish-speaking people . In smaller hospitals or smaller communities this may not be possible.

It is to your advantage to learn the second most prominent language in your community. For this reason, the following table of English-to-Spanish has been prepared. Instructions for using it are simple. Look for the phrase in English in the first column of the table. The second column gives the phrase in Spanish. You can write this or point to it. The third column gives a phonetic pronunciation. The syllable in each word to be accented is printed in italic type. Even if you are not proficient in English-to-Spanish, your Spanish-speaking patients will appreciate your trying to converse in their language. Begin with "Buénos diás. ¿Como se siente?" And remember "por favór."*

Introductory Phrases

Please*	Por favór	Por fah-*vor*
Thank you	Grácias	*Grah*-see-ahs
Good morning	Buénos días	*Bway*-nos *dee*-ahs
Good afternoon	Buénas tárdes	*Bway*-nas *tar*-days
Good evening	Buénas nóches	*Bway*-nas *Noh*-chays
My name is	Mi nómbre es	Me *nohm*-bray ays
Yes/No	Si/No	See/No
What is your name?	¿Cómo se llama?	¿Koh-moh say *jah*-mah?
How old are you?	¿Cuántos años tienes?	¿*Kwan*-tohs ahn-yos tee-*aynj*ays?
Do you understand me?	¿Me entiende?	¿Me ayn-tee-*ayn*-day?
Speak slower	Habla más despacio	*Ah*-blah mahs days-*pah*-see-oh
Say it once again	Repítalo, por favor	Ray-*pee*-tah-loh, por fah-*vor*
How do you feel?	¿Cómo se siente?	¿*Koh*-moh say see-*ayn*-tay?
Good	Bien	Bee-ayn
Bad	Mal	*Mah*l
Physician	Medico	*May*-dee-koh
Hospital	Hospital	*Ooh*-spee-tall
Midwife	Comadre	Koh-*mah*-dray
Native healer	Curandero	Ku-ren-*day*-roh

General

Zero	Cero	*Se*-roh
One	Uno	Oo-noh
Two	Dos	Dohs

**You should begin or end any request with the word PLEASE (POR FAVÓR).*

Three	Tres	Trays
Four	Cuatro	*Kwah*-troh
Five	Cinco	*Sin*-koh
Six	Seis	Says
Seven	Siete	See-*ay*-tay
Eight	Ocho	Oh-choh
Nine	Nueve	New-*ay*-vay
Ten	Diez	*Dee*-ays
Hundred	Ciento, cien	See-*en*-toh, see-*en*
Hundred and one	Ciento uno	See-*en*-toh *oo*-noh
Sunday	Domingo	Doh-*ming*-goh
Monday	Lunes	*Loo*-nays
Tuesday	Martes	*Mar*-tays
Wednesday	Miercoles	Mee-*er*-cohl-ays
Thursday	Jueves	*Hway*-vays
Friday	Viernes	Vee-*ayr*-nays
Saturday	Sabado	*Sah*-bah-doh
Right	Derecha	Day-*ray*-chah
Left	Izqierda	Ees-kee-*ayr*-dah
Early in the morning	Temprano por la mañana	Tehm-*prah*-noh por lah mah-*nyah*-na
In the daytime	En el dia	Ayn el *dee*-ah
At noon	A mediodía	Ah meh-dee-oh-*dee*-ah
At bedtime	Al acostarse	Al ah-kos-*tar*-say
At night	Por la noche	Por la *noh*-chay
Today	Hoy	Oy
Tomorrow	Mañana	Mah-*nyah*-nah
Yesterday	Ayer	Ai-*yer*
Week	Semana	Say-*may*-nah
Month	Mes	Mace

Parts of the body

The head	La cabeza	lah kah-*bay*-sah
The eye	El ojo	El *o*-hoh
The ears	Los oídos	Lohs o-*ee*-dohs
The nose	La nariz	Lah nah-*reez*
The mouth	La boca	Lah *boh*-kah
The tongue	La lengua	La *len*-gwah
The neck	El cuello	El koo-*eh*-joh
The throat	La garganta	Lah gar-*gan*-tah
The skin	La piel	Lah pee-el
The bones	Los huesos	Lohs hoo-*ay*-sos
The muscles	Los músculos	Lohs *moos*-koo-lohs
The nerves	Los nervios	Lohs *nayhr*-vee-ohs
The shoulder blades	Las paletillas	Lahs pah-lay-*tee*-jahs
The arm	El brazo	El *brah*-soh
The elbow	El codo	El *koh*-doh
The wrist	La muñeca	Lah moon-*yeh*-kah
The hand	La mano	Lah *mah*-noh
The chest	El pecho	El *pay*-choh
The lungs	Los pulmones	Lohs *puhl*-moh-nays

The heart	El corazón	El koh-rah-*son*
The ribs	Las costillas	Lahs kohs-*tee*-jahs
The side	El flanco	El *flahn*-koh
The back	La espalda	Lay ays-*pahl*-dah
The abdomen	El abdomen	El *ahb*-doh-men
The stomach	El estómago	El ays-*toh*-mah-goh
The leg	La pierna	Lah pee-ehr-nah
The thigh	El muslo	El *moos*-loh
The ankle	El tobillo	El toh-bee-joh
The foot	El pie	El *pee*-ay
Urine	Urino	U-*re*-noh

Diseases

Allergy	Alergia	Ah-*layr*-hee-ah
Anemia	Anemia	Ah-*nay*-mee-ah
Cancer	Cancer	Kahn-sayr
Chicken pox	Varicela	Vah-ree-*say*-lah
Diabetes	Diabetes	Dee-ah-bay-tees
Diphtheria	Difteria	Deef-*tay*-ree-ah
German measles	Rubéola	Roo-*bay*-oh-lah
Gonorrhea	Gonorrea	Gun-noh-*ree*-ah
Heart disease	Enfermedad del corazón	Ayn-*fayr*-may-*dahd* dayl koh-rah-*sohn*
High blood pressure	Presión alta	Pray-see-*ohn al-ta*
Influenza	Gripe	*Gree*-pay
Lead poisoning	Envenenamiento con plomo	Ayn-vay-nay-nah-mee-*ayn*-toh kohn *ploh*-moh
Liver disease	Enfermedad del hígado	Ayn-*fayr* may-dahd del ee-*gah*-doh
Measles	Sarampion	Sah-rahm-pee-*ohn*
German measles	Rubeola	Roo-be-*oh*-lah
Mumps	Paperas	Pah-*pay*-rahs
Nervous disease	Enfermedades nerviosa	Ayn-fayr-may-*dahd*-days nayr-vee-*oh*-sah
Pleurisy	Pleuresía	Play-oo-ray-*see*-ah
Pneumonia	Pulmonia	Pool-*moh*-nee-ah
Rheumatic fever	Reumatismo (fiebre reumatica)	Ray-oo-mah-*tees*-moh (fee-*ay*-bray ray-oo-*mah*-tee-kah)
Scarlet fever	Escarlatina	Ays-kahr-lah-*tee*-nah
Syphilis	Sifilis	See-fee-lees
Tuberculosis	Tuberculosis	Too-*bayr*-koo-lohs-sees

Signs and Symptoms

Do you have stomach cramps?	¿Tiene calambres en el estómago?	¿Tee-*ay*-nay kah-*lahm*-brays ayn el ays-*toh*-mah-goh?
Chills?	Escalofrios	Ays-kah-loh-*free*-ohs
An attack of fever?	Un ataque de fiebre	Oon ah-*tah*-kay day fee-*ay*-bray
Hemorrhage?	Hemoragia	Ay-moh-*rah*-hee-ah
Nosebleeds?	Hemoragia por la nariz	Ay-moh-*rah*-hee-ah por-lah nah-*rees*
Unusual vaginal bleeding?	Hemoragia vaginal fuera de los periodos	Ay-moh-*rah*-hee-ah *vah*-hee-nahl foo-*ay*-rah day lohs pay-ree-*oh*-dohs
Hoarseness?	Ronquera	Rohn-*kay*-rah

A sore throat?	¿Le duele la garganta?	¿Lay doo-*ay*-lay lah gahr-gahn-tah?
Does it hurt to swallow?	¿Le duele al tragar?	¿Lay doo-ay-lay ahl trah-gar?
Have you any difficulty in breathing?	¿Tiene difficultad al respirar?	¿Tee-*ay*-nay dee-fee-kool-*tahd* ahl rays-*pee*-rahr?
Does it pain you to breathe?	¿Le duele al respirar?	¿Lay doo-*ay*-lay ahl rays-*pee*-rahr?
How does your head feel?	¿Cómo siente la cabeza?	¿*Koh*-moh see-*ayn*-tay lah Kah-*bay*-sah?
Is your memory good?	¿Es buena su memoria?	¿Ays *bway*-nah soo may-moh-*ree*-ah?
Have you any pain in the head?	¿Le duele la cabezo?	¿Lay doo-*ay*-lay lah Kah-*bay*-sah?
Do you feel dizzy?	¿Tiene udsted vértigo?	¿Tee-*ay*-nay ood-*stayd vehr*-tee-goh?
Are you tired?	¿Esté udsted cansado?	¿Ay-*stah* ood-*stayd* kahn-*sah*-doh?
Can you eat?	¿Puede comer?	¿*Pway*-day koh-*mer?*
Have you a good appetite?	¿Tiene udsted buen apetito?	¿Tee-*ay*-nay ood-*stayd* bwayn ah-pay-*tee*-toh?
How are your stools?	¿Cómo son sus heces fecales?	¿*Koh*-moh sohn soos *hay*-says fay-*kal*-ays?
Are they regular?	¿Son regulares?	¿Sohn ray-goo-*lah*-rays?
Are you constipated?	¿Está estreñido?	¿Ay-*stah* ays-trayn-*yee*-do?
Do you have diarrhea?	¿Tiene diarrea?	¿Tee-*ay*-nay dee-ah-*ray*-ah?
Have you any difficulty passing water?	¿Tiene dificultad en orinar?	¿Tee-*ay*-nay dee-fee-kool-*tahd* ayn oh-ree-*nahr?*
Do you pass water involuntarily?	¿Orina sin querer?	¿Oh-*ree*-nah seen kay-rayr?
How long have you felt this way?	¿Desde cuándo se siente asi?	¿*Days*-day *Kwan*-doh say see-*ayn*-tay ah-see?
What diseases have you had?	¿Qué enfermedades ha tenido?	¿Kay ayn-fer-may-*dah*-days hah tay-*nee*-doh?
Do you hear voices?	¿Tiene los voces?	¿Tee-*ay*-nay los *vo*-ses?

Examination

Remove your clothing	Quítese su ropa	*Key*-tay-say soo *roh*-pah
Put on this gown	Pongáse la bata	Pohn-*gah*-say lah *bah*-tah
Need a urine specimen	Es necesário una muéstra de su orina	Ays nay-say-*sar*-ee-oh oo-nah moo-*ay*-strah day oh-*ree*-nah
Be seated	Siéntese	See-*ayn*-tay-say
Recline	Acuestése	Ah-cways-*tay*-say
Sit up	Siéntese	See-*ayn*-tay-say
Stand	Parése	Pah-*ray*-say
Bend your knees	Dóble las rodíllas	*Doh*-blay lahs roh-*dee*-yahs
Relax your muscles	Reláje los músculos	Ray-*lah*-hay lohs *moos*-koo-lohs
Try to	Aténte	Ah-*tayn*-tay
Try again	Aténte ótra vez	Ah-*tayn*-tay *oh*-tra vays
Do not move	No se muéva	Noh say moo-*ay*-vah
Turn on (or to) your left side	Voltése a su ládo izquiérdo	Vohl-*tay*-say ah soo *lah*-doh is-key-*ayr*-doh
Turn on (or to) your right side	Voltése a su ládo derécho	Vohl-*tay*-say ah soo *lah*-doh day-*ray*-choh
Take a deep breath	Respíra profúndo	Ray-*speer*-rah pro-*foon*-doh
Hold your breath	Deténga su respiración	Day-*tayn*-gah soo ray-speer-ah-see-*ohn*
Don't hold your breath	No deténga su respiración	Noh day-*tayn*-gah soo ray-speer-ah-see-*ohn*
Cough	Tosa	*Toh*-sah
Open your mouth	Abra la boca	*Ah*-brah lah *boh*-kah

Show me . . .	Enséñeme . . .	Ayn-*sayn*-yay-may
Here/there	Aquí/allí	Ah-kee/ah-jee
Which side?	¿En qué lado?	Ayn kay *lah*-doh?
Let me see your hand	Enséñeme la mano	Ayn-*sehn*-yah-may lah *mah*-noh
Grasp my hand	Apriete mi mano	Ah-*pree*-it-tay mee *mah*-noh
Raise your arm	Levante el brazo	Lay-*vahn*-tay el *brah*-soh
Raise it more	Más alto	Mahs *ahl*-toh
Now the other	Ahora el otro	Ah-*oh*-rah el *oh*-troh

Treatment

It is necessary	Es necesario	Ays neh-say-*sah*-ree-oh
An operation is necessary	Una operación es necesaria	Oo-nah oh-peh-rah-see-*ohn* ays neh-say-*sah*-ree-ah
A prescription	Una receta	*Oo*-na ray-*say*-tah
Use it regularly	Tómelo con regularidad	*Toh*-may-loh kohn ray-goo-*lah*-ree-dad
Take one teaspoonful three times daily (in water)	Toma una cucharadita tres veces al dia, con agua	*Toh*-may oo-na koo-chah-rah-*dee*-tah trays *vay*-says ahl *dee*-ah, kohn ah-gwah
Gargle	Haga gargaras	*Ah*-gah gar-*gah*-rahs
Use injection	Use una inyección	*Oo*-say *oo*-nah in-*yek*-see-ohn
Oral contraceptives	Una pildora	*Oo*-nah peel-*doh*-rah
A pill	Una pastilla	*Oo*-nah pahs-*tee*-yah
A powder	Un polvo	Oon *pohl*-voh
Before meals	Antes de las comidas	*Ahn*-tays day lahs koh-*mee*-dahs
After meals	Despues de las comidas	*Days*-poo-ehs day lahs koh-mee-dahs
Every day	Todos los dia	*Toh*-dohs lohs *dee*-ah
Every hour	Cada hora	*Kah*-dah *oh*-rah
Breathe slowly—like this (in this manner)	Respire despacio—asi	Rays-*pee*-ray days-*pah*-see-oh—ah-*see*
Remain on a diet	Estar a dieta	Ays-*tar* a dee-*ay*-tah

General

How do you feel?	¿Como se siénte?	¿*Koh*-moh say see-*ayn*-tay?
Do you have pain?	¿Tiéne dolór?	¿Tee-*ay*-nay doh-*lorh?*
Where is the pain?	¿Adónde es el dolór?	¿Ah-*dohn*-day ays ayl doh-*lorh?*
Do you want medication for your pain?	¿Quiére medicación para su dolór?	¿Kay-*ay*-ray may-dee-kah see-*ohn pah*-rah soo doh-*lorh?*
Are you comfortable?	¿Está comfortáble?	¿Ay-*stah* kohn-for-*tah*-blay?
Are you thirsty?	¿Tiéne sed?	¿Tee-*ay*-nay-sayd?
You may not eat/drink	No cóma/béba	Noh *koh*-mah/bay-*bah*
You can only drink water	Solo puéde tomár água	Soh-loh *pway*-day toh-mar *ah*-gwah
Apply bandage to . . .	Ponga una vendaje a . . .	*Pohn*-gah *oo*-nah vehn-*dah*-hay ah . . .
Apply ointment	Aplíquese unguento	Ah-*plee*-kay-say oon-goo-*ayn*-toh
Keep very quiet	Estése muy quieto	Ays-*tay*-say moo-ay key-*ay*-toh
You must not speak	No debe hablar	Noh *day*-bay ha-*blahr*
It will be uncomfortable	Séra incomódo	*Say*-rah een-koh-*moh*-doh
It will sting	Va ardér	Vah ahr-*dayr*
You will feel pressure	Vá a sentír presión	Vah ah sayn-*teer* pray-see-*ohn*
I am going to . . .	Voy a:	Voy ah:

Count (take) your pulse	Tomár su púlso	Toh-*marh* soo *pool*-soh
Take your temperature	Tomár su temperatúra	Toh-*marh* soo taym-pay-rah-*too*-rah
Take your blood pressure	Tomar su presión	Toh-*mahr* soo pray-see-*ohn*
Give you pain medicine	Dárle medicación para dolór	*Dahr*-lay may-dee-kah-see-*ohn* pah-rah doh-*lohr*
You should (try to) . . .	Tráte de:	*Trah*-tay day:
Call for help/assistance	Llamár para asisténcia	Yah-*marh* pah-rah ah-sees-*tayn*-see-ah
Empty your bladder	Orínar	Oh-*ree*-narh
Do you still feel very weak?	¿Se siente muy débil todavía?	Say see-*ayn*-tay moo-ee *day*-beel toh-dah-*vee*-ah
It is important to . . .	Es importánte de:	Ays eem-por-*tahn*-tay day
Walk (ambulate)	Caminár	Kah-mee-*narh*
Drink fluids	Bebér líquidos	Bay-*bayr* *lee*-kay-dohs

(From Rosdahl, C.B. [1995]. Textbook of Basic Nursing, 6th ed. Philadelphia: J.B. Lippincott.)

Appendix III
Abbreviations Commonly Used in Documentation

Abbreviation	*Meaning*	*Abbreviation*	*Meaning*
ā	before	NG	nasogastric
abd	abdomen	NKA	no known allergies
ac	before meals	noc	night
ADL	activities of daily living	NPO	nothing by mouth
ad lib	as needed	os	mouth
adm.	admitted, admission	OOB	out of bed
amp.	ampule	oz	ounce
ant.	anterior	p̄	after
AP	anterior–posterior	p.c.	after meals
ax.	axillary	post	posterior
b.i.d.	twice a day	prep	preparation
BP	blood pressure	prn	when necessary
BR	bed rest	q̄, q	every
BRP	bathroom privileges	q̄ 2 (3, 4, etc.) hours	every 2 (3, 4, etc.) hours
C	Centigrade	qd	every day
c̄	with	qh	every hour
caps	capsule	q.i.d.	four times a day
C.C.	chief complaint	q.o.d.	every other day
cc	cubic centimeter	q.s.	quantity sufficient
	(1 cc =1 mL)	R/O	rule out
CVP	central venous pressure		
c/o	complains of	ROM	range of motion
D/C	discontinue	s̄	without
disch; DC	discharge	SBA	stand by assistance
drsg	dressing	SC	subcutaneous
dr	dram	SL	sublingual
elix	elixir	SOB	shortness of breath
ext	extract or external	sol, soln	solution
F	Fahrenheit	spec	specimen
fx.	fracture, fractional	S/P	status post
gm	gram	sp. gr.	specific gravity
gr	grain	S.S.E.	soapsuds edema
gt/gtt	drop/drops	ss	one-half
"H," SC, or sub q	hypodermic or	stat	immediately
	subcutaneous	tab	tablet
h	hour		
HOB	head of bed	t.i.d.	three times a day
h.s.	bedtime (hour of sleep)		
hx	history	tinct or tr.	tincture
I & O	intake & output	TKO	to keep open
		TPN	total parenteral nutrition
IM	intramuscular		hyperalimentation
		TPR	temperature, pulse,
IV	intravenous		respiration
kg	kilogram	tsp	teaspoon
KVO	keep vein open	TO	telephone order
L	left; liter	TWE	tap water enema
lat	lateral	VO	verbal order

continued

Abbreviation	*Meaning*	*Abbreviation*	*Meaning*
MAE	moves all extremities	VS	vital signs
mg	milligram	VSS	vital signs stable
ml, mL	milliliter (1 mL =1 cc)	W/C	wheelchair
NAD	no apparent distress	WNL	within normal limits
Selected Abbreviations Used for Specific Descriptions			
AKA	above-knee amputation	O.D.	right eye
ASCVD	arteriosclerotic cardiovascular disease	O.S.	left eye
ASHD	arteriosclerotic heart disease	O.U.	each eye
BKA	below-knee amputation	OPD	outpatient department
ca	cancer	ORIF	open reduction internal fixation
chest clear to A & P	chest clear to auscultation &* percussion	Ortho	orthopedics
CMS	circulation movement sensation	OT	occupational therapy
CNS	central nervous system	PE	physical examination
DJD	degenerative joint disease	PERRLA	pupils equal, round, & react to light and accommodation
DOE	dyspnea on exertion	PID	pelvic inflammatory disease
DTs	delirium tremens	PI	present illness
D_5W	5% dextrose in water	PM & R	physical medicine & rehabilitation
FUO	fever of unknown origin	Psych	psychology; psychiatric
GB	gall bladder	PT	physical therapy
GI	gastrointestinal	RL (or LR)	Ringer's lactate; lactated Ringer's
GYN	gynecology	RLE	right lower extremity
H_2O_2	hydrogen peroxide	RLQ	right lower quadrant
HA	hyperalimentation headache	RR, PAR, PACU	recovery room, post-anesthesia room, post-anesthesia care unit
HCVD	hypertensive cardiovascular disease	RUE	right upper extremity
HEENT	head, ear, eye, nose, throat	RUQ	right upper quadrant
HVD	hypertensive vascular disease	Rx	prescription
ICU	intensive care unit	SOB	short of breath
I & D	incision and drainage	STD	sexually transmitted disease
LLE	left lower extremity	STSG	split-thickness skin graft
LLQ	left lower quadrant	Surg	surgery, surgical
LOC	level of consciousness; laxatives of choice	T & A	tonsillectomy & adenoidectomy
LMP	last menstrual period	THR, TJR	total hip replacement; total joint replacement
LUE	left upper extremity	URI	upper respiratory infection
LUQ	left upper quadrant	UTI	urinary tract infection
MI	myocardial infarction	vag	vaginal
Neuro	neurology; neurosurgery	WNWD	well-nourished, well-developed
NS	normal saline		
Nys.	nursery		
NWB	non–weight-bearing		
Selected Abbreviations Related to Common Diagnostic Tests			
BE	barium enema	hct	hematocrit
B.M.R.	basal metabolism rate	hgb	hemoglobin
Ca^{++}	calcium	IVP	intravenous pyelogram
CAT	computed axial tomography	K^+	potassium
CBC	complete blood count	LP	lumbar puncture
Cl^-	chloride	MRI	magnetic resonance imaging

continued

Abbreviation	*Meaning*	*Abbreviation*	*Meaning*
C & S	culture & sensitivity	Na^+	sodium
Dx	diagnosis	RBC	red blood cell
ECG, EKG	electrocardiogram	UGI	upper gastrointestinal x-ray
EEG	electroencephalogram		
FBS	fasting blood sugar	UA	urinalysis
		WBC	white blood cell
Commonly Used Symbols			
>	greater than	@	at
<	less than	+	positive
=	equal to	−	negative
≈	approximately equal to	±	positive or negative
≤	equal to or less than	F_1	first filial generation
≥	equal to or greater than	F_2	second filial generation
↑	increased	PO_2	partial pressure of oxygen
↓	decreased	PCO_2	partial pressure of carbon dioxide
♀	female		
♂	male	:	ratio
°	degree	∴	therefore
#	number or pound	%	percent
×	times	2°	secondary to
		△	change

(From Craven, R.F. & Hirnle, C.J. [1996]. Human Health and Function, 2nd ed. Philadelphia: Lippincott-Raven.)

Appendix IV Metric Measurements

Unit	Abbreviation	Metric Equivalent	U.S. Equivalent
Units of weight			
Kilogram	kg	1000 g	2.2 lb
Gram*	g	1000 mg	0.035 oz.; 28.5 g/oz
Milligram	mg	$\frac{1}{1000}$ g; 0.001 g	
Microgram	μg	$\frac{1}{1000}$ mg; 0.001 mg	
Units of length			
Kilometer	km	1000 meters	0.62 miles; 1.6 km/mile
Meter*	m	100 cm; 1000 mm	39.4 inches; 1.1 yards
Centimeter	cm	$\frac{1}{100}$ m; 0.01 m	0.39 inches; 2.5 cm/inch
Millimeter	mm	$\frac{1}{1000}$ m; 0.001 m	0.039 inches; 25 mm/inch
Micrometer	μm	$\frac{1}{1000}$ mm; 0.001 mm	
Units of volume			
Liter*	L	1000 mL	1.06 qt
Deciliter	dL	$\frac{1}{10}$ L; 0.1 L	
Milliliter	mL	$\frac{1}{1000}$ L; 0.001 L	0.034 oz., 29.4 mL/oz
Microliter	μL	$\frac{1}{1000}$ mL; 0.001 mL	

*Basic unit

(From Memmler, R.L., Cohen, B.J., and Wood, D.L. [1996]. The Human Body in Health and Disease, 8th ed. Philadelphia: Lippincott-Raven.)

Appendix V Celsius–Fahrenheit Temperature Conversion Scale

Celsius to Fahrenheit

Use the following formula to convert Celsius readings to Fahrenheit readings:

°F = 9/5°C + 32

For example, if the Celsius reading is 37°:

°F = (9/5 × 37) +32

= 66.6 + 32

= 98.6°F (normal body temperature)

Fahrenheit to Celsius

Use the following formula to convert Fahrenheit readings to Celsius readings:

°C = 5/9(°F − 32)

For example, if the Fahrenheit reading is 68°:

°C = 5/9(68 − 32)

= 5/9 × 36

= 20°C (a nice spring day)

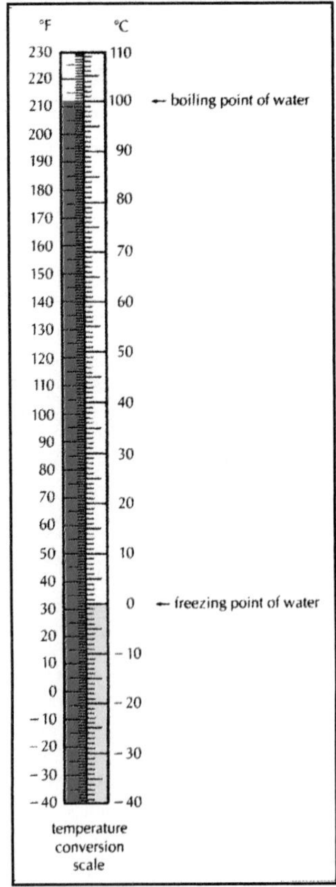

(*From Memmler, R.L., Cohen, B.J., and Wood, D.L. [1996]. The Human Body in Health and Disease, 8th ed. Philadelphia: Lippincott-Raven.*)

Appendix VI Laboratory Tests

Table 1 **Routine Urinalysis**

Test	*Normal Value*	*Clinical Significance*
General characteristics and measurements		
Color	Pale yellow to amber	Color change can be due to concentration or dilution, drugs, metabolic or inflammatory disorders
Odor	Slightly aromatic	Foul odor typical of urinary tract infection, fruity odor in uncontrolled diabetes mellitus
Appearance (clarity)	Clear to slightly hazy	Cloudy urine occurs with infection or after refrigeration; may indicate presence of bacteria, cells, mucus, or crystals
Specific gravity	1.003–1.030 (first morning catch; routine is random)	Decreased in diabetes insipidus, acute renal failure, water intoxication; increased in liver disorders, heart failure, dehydration
pH	4.5–8.0	Acid urine accompanies acidosis, fever, high protein diet; alkaline urine in urinary tract infection, metabolic alkalosis, vegetarian diet
Chemical determinations		
Glucose	Negative	Glucose present in uncontrolled diabetes mellitus, steroid excess
Ketones	Negative	Present in diabetes mellitus and in starvation
Protein	Negative	Present in kidney disorders, such as glomerulonephritis, acute kidney failure
Bilirubin	Negative	Breakdown product of hemoglobin; present in liver disease or in bile blockage
Urobilinogen	0.2–1.0 Ehrlich units/dL	Breakdown product of bilirubin; increased in hemolytic anemias and in liver disease; remains negative in bile obstruction
Blood (occult)	Negative	Detects small amounts of blood cells, hemoglobin, or myoglobin; present in severe trauma, metabolic disorders, bladder infections
Nitrite	Negative	Product of bacterial breakdown of urine; positive result suggests urinary tract infection and needs to be followed up with a culture of the urine.
Microscopic		
Red blood cells	0–3 per high-power field	Increased due to bleeding within the urinary tract from trauma, tumors, inflammation, or damage within the kidney
White blood cells	0–4 per high-power field	Increased in infection of the kidney or bladder
Renal epithelial cells	Occasional	Increased number indicates damage to kidney tubules
Casts	None	Hyaline casts normal; large number of abnormal casts indicates inflammation or a systemic disorder
Crystals	Present	Most are normal; may be acid or alkaline
Bacteria	Few	Increased in infection of urinary tract or contamination from infected genitalia
Others		Any yeasts, parasites, mucus, spermatozoa, or other microscopic findings would be reported here

continued

Table 2 **Complete Blood Count (CBC)**

Test	*Normal Value**	*Clinical Significance*
Red blood cell count (RBC)	Men: 4.2–5.4 million/μL Women: 3.6–5.0 million/μL	Decreased in anemia; increased in dehydration, polycythemia
Hemoglobin (HGB)	Men: 13.5–17.5 g/dL Women: 12–16 g/dL	Decreased in anemia, hemorrhage and hemolytic reactions; increased in dehydration, heart and lung disease
Hematocrit (HCT) or packed cell volume (PCV)	Men: 40%–50% Women: 37%–47%	Decreased in anemia; increased in polycythemia, dehydration
Red blood cell indices (examples)		These values, calculated from the RBC, HGB, and HCT, give information valuable in the diagnosis and classification of anemia
Mean corpuscular volume (MVC)	87–103 μL/red cell	Measures the average size or volume of each red blood cell: Small size (microcytic) in iron-deficiency anemia; large size (macrocytic) typical of pernicious anemia
Mean corpuscular hemoglobin (MCH)	26–34 pg/red cell	Measures the weight of hemoglobin per red blood cell; useful in differentiating types of anemia in a severely anemic patient
Mean corpuscular hemoglobin concentration (MCHC)	31–37 g/dL	Defines the volume of hemoglobin per red blood cell; used to determine the color or concentration of hemoglobin per red cell
White blood count (WBC)	5,000–10,000/μL	Increased in leukemia and in response to infection, inflammation, and dehydration; decreased in bone marrow suppression
Platelets	150,000–350,000/μL	Increased in many malignant disorders; decreased in disseminated intravascular coagulation (DIC) or toxic drug effects; spontaneous bleeding may occur at platelet counts below 20,000
Differential (Peripheral blood smear)		A stained slide of the blood is needed to perform the differential. The percentages of the different white cells are estimated, and the slide is microscopically checked for abnormal characteristics in WBCs, RBCs, and platelets.
White cells		
Segments neutrophils (SEGs, POLYs)	40%–74%	Increased in bacterial infections; low numbers leave person very susceptible to infection
Immature neutrophils (BANDs)	0%–3%	Increase when neutrophil count increases
Lymphocytes (LYMPHs)	20%–40%	Increased in viral infections; low numbers leave a person dangerously susceptible to infection
Monocytes (MONOs)	2%–6%	Increased in specific infections
Eosinophils (EOs)	1%–4%	Increased in allergic disorders
Basophils (BASOs)	0.5%–1%	Increased in allergic disorders

**Values vary depending on instrumentation and type of test.*

Table 3 **Blood Chemistry Tests**

Test	*Normal Value*	*Clinical Significance*
Basic panel: An overview of electrolytes, waste product management, and metabolism		
Blood urea nitrogen (BUN)	7–18 mg/dL	Increased in renal disease and dehydration; decreased in liver damage and malnutrition
Carbon dioxide (CO_2) (includes bicarbonate)	23–30 mmol/L	Useful to evaluate acid–base balance by measuring total carbon dioxide in the blood: Elevated in vomiting and pulmonary disease; decreased in diabetic acidosis, acute renal failure, and hyperventilation
Chloride (Cl)	98–106 mEq/L	Increased in dehydration, hyperventilation, and congestive heart failure; decreased in vomiting, diarrhea, and fever
Creatinine	0.6–1.2 mg/dL	Produced at a constant rate and excreted by the kidney; increased in kidney disease
Glucose	Fasting: 70–110 mg/dL Random: 85–125 mg/dL	Increased in diabetes and severe illness; decreased in insulin overdose or hypoglycemia
Potassium (K)	3.5–5 mEq/L	Increased in renal failure, extensive cell damage and acidosis; decreased in vomiting, diarrhea, and excess administration of diuretics or IV fluids
Sodium (Na)	101–111 mEq/L or 135–148 mEq/L (depending on test)	Increased in dehydration and diabetes insipidus; decreased in overload of IV fluids, burns, diarrhea, or vomiting
Additional blood chemistry tests		
Alanine aminotransferase (ALT)	Men: 7–24 U/L Women: 7–17 U/L	Used to diagnose and monitor treatment of liver disease and to monitor the effects of drugs on the liver, increased in myocardial infarction
Albumin	3.8–5.0 g/dL	Albumin holds water in blood; decreased in liver disease and kidney disease
Albumin–globulin ratio (A/G ratio)	Greater than 1	Low A/G ratio signifies a tendency for edema because globulin is less effective than albumin at holding water in the blood.
Alkaline phosphatase (ALP)	20–70 U/L (varies by method)	Enzyme of bone metabolism; increased in liver disease and metastatic bone disease
Amylase	21–160 U/L	Used to diagnose and monitor treatment of acute pancreatitis and to detect inflammation of the salivary glands
Aspartate aminotransferase (AST)	0–41 U/L (varies)	Enzyme present in tissues with high metabolic activity; increased in myocardial infarction and liver disease
Bilirubin, total	0.2–1.0 mg/dL	Breakdown product of hemoglobin from red blood cells; increased when excessive RBCs are being destroyed or in liver disease
Calcium (Ca)	8.8–10.0 mg/dL	Increased in excess parathyroid hormone production and in cancer; decreased in alkalosis, elevated phosphate in renal failure, and excess IV fluids
Cholesterol	120–220 mg/dL desirable range	Screening test used to evaluate risk of heart disease; levels of 200 or above indicate increased risk of heart disease and warrant further investigation
Creatinine phosphokinase (CPK or CK)	Men: 38–174 U/L Women: 96–140 U/L	Elevated enzyme level indicates myocardial infarction or damage to skeletal muscle. When elevated, specific fractions (isoenzymes) should be tested
Gamma glutamyl transferase (GGT)	Men: 6–26 U/L Women: 4–18 U/L	Used to diagnose liver disease and test for chronic alcoholism
Globulins	2.3–3.5 g/dL	Proteins active in immunity; help albumin keep water in blood
Iron, serum (Fe)	Men: 75–175 μg/dL Women: 65–165 μg/dL	Decreased in iron deficiency and anemia; increased in hemolytic conditions
High-density lipoproteins (HDLs)	Men: 30–70 mg/dL Women: 30–85 mg/dL	Used to evaluate the risk of heart disease

continued

Table 3 Blood Chemistry Tests *(Continued)*

Test	*Normal Value*	*Clinical Significance*
Lactic dehydrogenase (LDH or LD)	95–200 U/L (normal ranges vary greatly)	Enzyme released in many kinds of tissue damage; including myocardial infarction, pulmonary infarction, and liver disease
Lipase	4–24 U/L (varies with test)	Enzyme used to diagnose pancreatitis
Low-density lipoproteins (LDLs)	80–140 mg/dL	Used to evaluate the risk of heart disease
Magnesium (Mg)	1.3–2.1 mEq/L	Vital in neuromuscular function; decreased levels may occur in malnutrition, alcoholism, pancreatitis, diarrhea
Phosphorus (P) (inorganic)	2.7–4.5 mg/dL	Evaluated in response to calcium; main store is in bone: elevated in kidney disease; decreased in excess parathyroid hormone
Protein, total	6–8 g/dL	Increased in dehydration, multiple myeloma; decreased in kidney disease, liver disease, poor nutrition, severe burns, excessive bleeding
Serum glutamic oxalacetic transaminase (SGOT)		See Aspartate aminotransferase (AST)
Serum glutamic pyruvic transaminase (SGPT)		See alanine aminotransferase (ALT)
Thyroxin (T_4)	5–12.5 μg/dL (varies)	Screening test of thyroid function; increased in hyperthyroidism; decreased in myxedema and hypothyroidism
Thyroid stimulating hormone (TSH)	0.5–6 mIU/L	Produced by pituitary to cause thyroid gland to function; elevated when thyroid gland is not functioning
Triiodothyronine (T_3)	120–195 mg/dL	Elevated in specific types of hyperthyroidism
Triglycerides	Men: 40–160 mg/dL Women: 35–135 mg/dL	An indication of ability to metabolism fats; increased triglycerides and cholesterol indicate high risk of atherosclerosis
Uric acid	Men: 3.5–7.2 mg/dL Women: 2.6–6.0 mg/dL	Produced by breakdown of ingested purines in food and nucleic acids; elevated in kidney disease, gout, and leukemia

From Memmler, R.L., Cohen, B.J., and Wood, D.L. [1996]. The Human Body in Health and Disease, 8th ed. Philadelphia: Lippincott-Raven.)

Glossary

abdominal regions divisions of the abdomen into nine regions by two horizontal and two vertical lines; used to identify specific locations

ablation removal or excision of a part; laser ablation is destruction/removal of tissue by use of laser

abortion termination of pregnancy or products of conception prior to fetal viability and/or 20 weeks gestation

abscess an inflamed cavity filled with pus as a result of infection

accounts payable a record of all monies owed

accounts receivable a record of all monies due

acquired immunodeficiency syndrome (AIDS) a cluster of disorders caused by the Human Immunodeficiency Virus (HIV) that specifically destroys cell-mediated immunity

acrosome the superior surface of the head of the spermatozoon

activities of daily living (ADL) activities usually performed in the course of the day, ie, bathing, dressing, feeding oneself

Addison's Disease partial or complete failure of the adrenal cortex functions, causing general physical deterioration

adenosine triphosphate (ATP) the energy currency used by the body; breaking down the phosphate bond of the compound releases high energy potential

adipose of or pertaining to fat

adjustments changes in a posted account

adnexa any part added to a main structure; an accessory part

administrative pertaining to administration (eg, office procedures and nonclinical tasks that a medical assistant will perform)

advance directive a statement of a patient's wishes regarding health care prior to a critical medical event

aerobe microorganism that requires oxygen to live

aerosol suspended particles in gas or air

afferent carrying impulses towards the center

affiliation to connect or associate with, as a medical site would associate with a school to assist in completion of student training

agar a type of seaweed or algae that helps solidify culture media; the media may be referred to as agar

age of majority age at which an individual is considered to be an adult (usually 18–21 years of age)

agglutination clumping of cells due to the presence of antibodies called agglutinins

aging schedule a form used to track outstanding balances

agranulocytes white blood cells that do not contain visible granules when stained

allergen any substance that causes manifestations of an allergy, usually a protein to which the body has built antibodies

allergy an acquired, abnormal response to a substance (allergen) that does not ordinarily cause a reaction

alphabetic filing arranging of names or titles according to the sequence of letters in the alphabet

alphafetoprotein substance produced by the embryonic yolk sac

alveolar-capillary membrane the structure in the lung fields through which oxygen and carbon dioxide diffuse during the respiratory process

amenorrhea condition of not menstruating, without menses

American Medical Technologist Institute for Education (AMTIE) professional organization for medical assistants, medical laboratory technicians, and dental technicians

American Association of Medical Assistants (AAMA) professional organization for medical assistants

Americans With Disabilities Act (ADA) a law designed to meet the needs of people with physical and mental challenges

ammonia a substance produced by decomposition of organic matter containing nitrogen

amniocentesis puncture of the amniotic sac in order to remove fluid for testing

amphiarthroses slightly movable joints

ampule a small glass container that can be sealed and its contents sterilized

anaerobe microorganism that lives without oxygen

anaphylaxis a severe systemic reaction resulting from an allergic reaction

anatomical position a position used for reference in which the subject is standing erect, facing forward, feet are slightly apart and pointing forward, the hands are down at the sides with palms forward and thumbs outward

anatomy the study of the structure of the body

aneurysm a localized dilatation on a vessel wall

angina pectoris paroxysmal chest pain usually caused by myocardial anoxia due to coronary artery occlusion

angiotensin a substance occurring in the blood that works with renin to affect the blood pressure, usually increasing the pressure by vasoconstriction

anisocytosis blood abnormality in which red blood cells are not equal in size (aniso = unequal)

ankylosing spondylitis stiffening of the spine with inflammation

annotation the process of reading, highlighting and summarizing a document for another person

anovulation condition of not ovulating

antagonism mutual opposition or contrary action with something else; opposite of synergism

antagonist any muscle that opposes the action of the prime mover to balance movement. (Example: When the biceps contact and pull the forearm upward, the triceps oppose the motion and relax.)

antecubital space inner surface of the bend of the elbow where the major veins for venipuncture are located

antepartum period of time prior to labor

anthropometric pertaining to measurements of the human body

antibiotic a drug that inhibits or destroys pathogenic microorganisms

antibodies complex glycoproteins produced by B-lymphocytes in response to the presence of an antigen

anticoagulant anything that prevents or delays the clotting of blood

antigens protein markers on cells that cause the formation of antibodies and react specifically with those antibodies

antihistamine medication that opposes the action of a histamine

antiseptic any substance that inhibits the growth of bacteria; used on skin before any procedure that breaks the integumentary barrier

anuria failure of the kidneys to produce urine

appeal process by which a higher court reviews the decision of a lower court

appendicular skeleton the parts of the skeleton added to the axial skeleton, including the shoulder and pelvic girdles and all of the bones of the upper and lower extremities

applicator a device used for making local applications

approximate to bring tissue surfaces together as closely as possible to their original positions

arachnoid web-like membrane covering the brain and spinal cord

arrector pili involuntary muscle attached to the hair follicle that when contracted causes “goose bumps”

arteriole a small arterial branch that joins a capillary to an artery

arthrogram x-ray of a joint

arthroplasty repair of a joint

artifact activity recorded on an electrocardiogram caused by patient movement, loose leads or electrical interference

artifactual something added to a substance or structure, not belonging to it; in medicine, generally implies a negative connotation

artificial insemination the insertion of sperm into a woman’s vagina by artificial means

ascites the accumulation of serous fluid in the peritoneal cavity

asepsis a state of being sterile; a condition free from germs, infection, and any form of life, including spore forms

aspiration drawing in or out by suction; as in breathing objects into the respiratory tract or suctioning substances from a site

assault an attempt or threat to touch another person without his or her consent

assessment the process of gathering information about the patient and the presenting condition

astigmatism unfocused refraction of light rays on the retina

asymmetry lack or absence of symmetry; inequality in size or shape on opposite sides of the body

asymptomatic without any symptoms

atelectasis collapsed lung fields; incomplete expansion of the lungs, either partial or complete

atraumatic without injury; may pertain to treatments or instruments that are not likely to cause further damage

atria (plural) the upper chamber of each half of the heart; the atria receive blood from the great vessels (singular: atrium)

atrioventricular (AV) node located on the floor of the right atrium on or close to the septum; receives the electrical impulse from the SA node after it is transmitted through the upper half of the heart; transmits the impulse to the bundle of His

attenuated diluted or weakened; pertaining to reduced virulence of a pathogenic organism

attribute a characteristic or quality of a person; usually considered a positive feature

audit a review of an account

auscultation the act of listening for sounds within the body, usually with a stethoscope, to evaluate the heart, lungs, pleura, intestines, or fetal heart sounds

autoclave an appliance used to sterilize medical instruments or other objects by steam under pressure

autolet small, sharp, spring-loaded instrument for quick capillary puncture

autonomic self controlling, spontaneous

autonomous existing or functioning independently

axial skeleton the bones forming the main skeleton around which the appendicular skeleton moves, including bones of the head, thorax, and trunk

axon part of the neuron that transmits impulses away from the cell body

Azidothymidine (AZT) a drug used to treat AIDS by blocking the growth of the virus after it enters the T-cell lymphocyte

azotemia from the Latin azote meaning nitrogen plus -emia, meaning blood; the condition of having excessive amounts of nitrogen in the blood

B

B-cells lymphoid stem cells from the bone marrow that migrate to and become mature antigen-specific cells in the spleen and lymph nodes

bacilli rod-shaped or cylindrical organisms

back-up (noun) a duplicate file made to a separate disk to protect information; (verb) to make a duplicate file

bacteriology the science and study of bacteria

balance remainder; amount due

bandage (noun) soft material applied to a body part for treatment purposes; usually a soft, absorbent gauze to hold a dressing, immobilize or support a part, aid in controlling bleeding. (verb) to apply a wrapping material for treatment purposes

Bartholin's glands small mucous glands bilaterally in the vaginal vestibule

basal ganglia pertaining to the gray matter in the cerebral hemispheres

basal metabolic rate the amount of energy used in a unit of time to maintain vital functions by a fasting, resting subject

baseline the original or initial measure by which other judgments will be made

battery actual touching of a person without his or her consent

beliefs ideas that are held to be true

bench trial trial in which the judge hears the case and renders a verdict; no jury is present

benign not cancerous or malignant

bias formation of an opinion without foundation or reason; prejudice

bibulous very absorbent

bicarbonate the dissolved form of carbon dioxide; it combines with water to make carbonic acid, $H2CO_3$. Carbonic acid loses one of its hydrogen (H) ions to then form bicarbonate, HCO_3-.

bile a bitter, yellow-green secretion of the liver stored by the gallbladder; derived from bilirubin, cholesterol, and other substances. Emulsifies fats in the small intestine so they can be further digested and absorbed.

biliary obstruction blockage of one of the bile ducts (the tubes leading from liver and gallbladder into duodenum); common causes include cysts, tumors, and stones

bilirubinuria bilirubin in the urine

bimanual pertaining to the use of both hands; performed by both hands

bioethics moral issues and concerns that affect a person's life

biotransforming conversion of the molecules of a substance from one form to another, as in medications within the body

blister a collection of fluid in or beneath the epidermis; a vesicle

block a type of letter format in which the date, subject line, closing and signatures are to the right margin; all other lines are justified left

body fluids any of the fluids that accumulate in the compartments of the body, such as the blood plasma, and the intracellular and extracellular spaces

boil an abscess of the subcutaneous tissues of the skin; a furuncle

bolus a mobile mass, for instance, a mass of food that passes into the upper gastrointestinal tract in one swallow, or a dose of medication injected intravenously

boot to start up the computer

bradykinesia abnormally slow voluntary movements

Braxton Hicks uterine contractions that occur during pregnancy

bruit an abnormal sound or murmur heard in the blood vessels while auscultating an organ, gland, or blood vessel

budget financial planning tool that helps an organization estimate its anticipated expenditures and revenues

bulla a large blister or vesicle

BUN abbreviation for blood urea nitrogen

bundle of His a band of specialized cardiac muscle fibers that receive the electrical impulse from the AV node and transmit it through right and left branches to the Purkinje fibers

bursae small, pad-like sacs filled with clear synovial fluid that surround some joints

byte a unit of symbolic transfer; each character equals one byte

C

caduceus a symbol using a wand or staff with two serpents coiled around it; sometimes used as the sign of the medical profession (the more appropriate symbol has only one snake)

calibrated measured against a standard

calibrations measurements for size or volume, as in calibrations on a syringe or pipette

callus in the musculoskeletal system, a deposit of new bone tissue that forms between the healing ends of broken bones; in the integumentary system, a thickened area of the epidermis caused by pressure or friction

calyx (pl. calyces) a cup-like collecting structure of the kidney

cancellous porous, spongy bone inside the medulla of the bone, usually filled with marrow

capillary action the raising or lowering of a liquid at the point of contact with a solid; used to pull blood into a capillary tube or small pipette

cardiac cycle the period from the beginning of one heart beat to the beginning of the next; includes the systole and the diastole

cardiac output the amount of blood ejected from either ventricle per minute, either to the pulmonary or to the systemic circulation

cardinal signs usually refers to the vital signs and signifies their importance in the assessment process

cardiogenic shock a type of shock in which the left ventricle fails to adequately pump enough blood for the body to function

carina a ridge-like structure; that part of the trachea that projects from the lower end of the trachea

carrier asymptomatic or unaffected person who can transmit infection to another person

cassette the lightproof holder in which film is exposed

catalyzes increases the rate at which a chemical reaction takes place. Example: Amylase found in saliva catalyzes (speeds up) the rate at which starches are broken down.

cataracts progressive loss of transparency of the lens resulting in opacity and loss of sight

catheterization introducing a tube into the body; urinary catheterization involves the removal of urine from the bladder

cautery a means, device or agent that destroys or coagulates tissue; may be electrical current, freezing or burning agents, or chemical solutions (caustics)

cell the most basic unit of all living organisms

cellular telephone a telephone that works by electronic signals and does not require attachment to a telephone plug

Celsius, centigrade (C) a temperature scale on which 0 degrees is the freezing point of water and 100 degrees is the boiling point of water at sea level

censure a verbal or written reprimand from a professional organization regarding a specific incident

centesis surgical puncture made into a cavity

central processing unit (CPU) circuitry imprinted on a silicon chip that processes information; the "brain" of the computer

centrifugal force a spinning motion to exert force outward, heavier components of a solution are spun downward

cerebellum located in the posterior part of the brain, responsible for balance and muscle coordination

cerebrovascular accident (CVA) ischemia of the brain due to an occlusion of the vessels supplying the brain, resulting in varying degrees of debilitation

cerebrum largest part of the brain, divided into two hemispheres, responsible for thought processes, sensory and motor functions, speech, writing, memory, and emotions

certification voluntary process that involves a testing procedure to prove an individual's baseline competency in a particular area

cerumen the yellowish or brownish waxlike secretion found in the external ear canal; earwax

Chadwick's sign sign of early pregnancy in which the vaginal, cervical, and vulvular tissues develop a bluish-violet color

challenge a method of testing a patient's sensitivity or response to a substance by introducing it into the body and watching its effects

chancre a hard ulcer that appears two to three weeks after exposure to syphilis, near the site of infection

check register place to record checks that have been written

check stub indicates to whom a check was issued, in what amount, and on what date

chemical name the exact chemical structure of a drug

chlamydia a parasitic microorganism with properties common to bacteria but unable to sustain life without a host, in the manner of a virus

chronic obstructive pulmonary disease (COPD) a progressive, irreversible condition with diminished respiratory capacity

chronological order placing in the order of time; usually the most recent is placed foremost

chyle milky, fatty product of digestion absorbed through the small intestines and returned to circulation by the lymphatics

chyme the thick, semi-liquid mass of ingested food mixed with gastric juices as it passes from the stomach

cilia hair-like projections on cells that either propel the cell or objects that come in contact with the cell

circumcision surgical removal of the prepuce

civil law a branch of law that focuses on issues between private citizens

clarification explanation

climacteric period menopause; developmental phase in which a woman's reproductive ability ceases

Clinical Laboratory Improvement Amendments (CLIA) guidelines established by Congress in 1988 to standardize and improve laboratory testing

clinical pertaining to direct patient care (eg, nonadministrative tasks that a medical assistant will perform)

closing a one to two word phrase that precedes the sender's signature and indicates the end of the letter

coagulate to change from a liquid form to a solid or semi-solid mass

coerce to force or compel a person to do something against his or her wishes

collagen protein substance that gives structure to the connective tissue

collection a process of acquiring funds that are due

colpocleisis surgery to occlude the vagina

colporrhaphy suture of the vagina

colposcopy visual examination of the vagina and cervix under magnification

comedo a blackhead

common law traditional laws that were established by the English legal system

comparative negligence a percentage of damage awards based on the contribution of negligence between two parties

complement a group of proteins in the blood that influence the inflammatory process and serve as the primary mediator in the antigen-antibody reactions of the B-cell-mediated response

concussion injury to the brain due to trauma

conference call a telephone call between two or more people that occurs at a designated time and is used for discussing a topic of mutual concern

confidentiality protection of patient data from unauthorized personnel

congenital anomalies abnormalities, either structural or functional, that are present from birth

conjugate joined or paired

consent an agreement between a patient and physician to do a given medical procedure

consideration the exchange of fees for a service

contract an agreement between two or more parties for a given act

contracture abnormal shortening of muscles around a joint caused by atrophy of the muscles and resulting in flexion and fixation

contributory negligence a defense strategy in which the defendant admits to negligence but claims that the plaintiff assisted in promoting the damages

contusion collection of blood in tissues after an injury; also known as a bruise

convoluted tubules the twisted portion of the nephron that connects the glomerulus to the collecting tubules; consists of a proximal and a distal portion connected by the Loop of Henle

convulsion sudden, involuntary muscle contractions of voluntary muscle groups

coping mechanisms unconscious methods of alleviating intense stressors

corpora cavernosa the erectile bodies of the penis or clitoris

corpus spongiosum erectile tissue around the male urethra

corticoid any of the hormonal steroid substances obtained from the adrenal cortex

cortisol a naturally occurring steroidal hormone that regulates metabolism and acts as an anti-inflammatory agent

coumarin an anticoagulant prescribed for persons likely to form blood clots, such as valve replacement recipients; also called Coumadin (trade name) or warfarin

cranium the portion of the skull that encloses the brain

crash "lock up" of the computer central processing unit as a result of a system breakdown

creatine a chemical compound in the body that adds phosphorus to ADP (adenosine diphosphate) to make ATP (adenosine triphosphate) that is the energy currency of the body

creatinine the substance formed when creatine (an important compound in metabolic processes) is used

credit balance in one's favor on an account; promise to pay a bill at a later date

cretinism severe congenital hypothyroidism; signs include dwarfism, low intelligence, puffy features, dry skin, macroglossia, and poor muscle tone

criteria the standard, rule, or test by which something or someone can be judged

cross examination questioning of a witness by the opposing attorney

cross-reference notation in a file telling that a record is stored elsewhere and giving the reference

cul-de-sac blind pouch or cavity, as in the cul-de-sac that lies between the rectum and the posterior uterus

culdocentesis surgical puncture of and aspiration of fluid from the vaginal cul-de-sac for diagnostic/therapeutic purpose

culture a laboratory process whereby microorganisms are grown in a special medium often for the purpose of identifying a causative agent in an infectious disease; also means the way of life, including commonly held beliefs, of a group of people

curettage scraping of a cavity

Current Procedural Terminology (CPT) a comprehensive list of codes used by physicians to bill for procedures and services

cursor flashing line on the monitor indicating where data input will occur

cyanotic a bluish discoloration of the skin due to the lack of oxygen

cyst a sac of fluid or semisolid material under the skin

cystocele herniation of the urinary bladder into the vagina

cystoscopy direct visualization of the bladder for diagnostic purposes

cytology study of cells

D

DACUM a code of educational standards for medical assisting students developed by the American Association of Medical Assistants

damages the resulting injury or suffering that resulted from negligence

data information that is stored and processed by the computer

database accumulation of files on the computer

day sheet/daily journal a daily business record of charges and payments

debit a charge or money owed on an account

decibel (db) a unit for measuring the intensity of sound

deciduous to fall or shed; deciduous teeth: the set of 20 teeth appearing during infancy and shedding during childhood

decongestant substance that reduces congestion or swelling

defamation of character making false or malicious statements about a person's character or reputation

defendant the party that is accused

degenerative joint disease (DJD) also known as osteoarthritis; arthritis characterized by degeneration of the bony structure of the joints, usually noninflammatory

deglutition the act of swallowing

demeanor the way a person looks, behaves, and conducts himself or herself

dementia progressive organic mental deterioration with loss of intellectual function

demographic relating to the statistical characteristics of populations

dendrite part of the neuron that transmits impulses toward the cell body

denial saying that something is not true; refusing to acknowledge

dentin the main component of the tooth structure, surrounds the inner pulp and lies just below the enamel

depolarization progressive wave of stimulation causing contraction of the myocardium

deposition a process in which one party questions another party under oath

dermatitis inflammation of the skin

dermatophytosis a fungus infection of the skin

dermis layer of skin under the epidermis

dextrocardia the condition of having the heart in the right side of the thoracic cavity

diabetes insipidus a disorder of metabolism characterized by polyuria and polydipsia; caused by a deficiency in ADH or an inability of the kidneys to respond to ADH

diagnosis the art of identifying a disease or condition by evaluating physical signs and symptoms, health history, and laboratory tests; the term denoting the name of a disease or condition

Diagnostic Related Group (DRG) categories used to determine hospital and physician reimbursement for Medicare patients' inpatient services

dialysis removal of urine wastes by passing fluid through a semi-permeable barrier that allows normal electrolytes to remain in the general circulation; may be performed either using a machine with circulatory access or by passing a balanced fluid through the peritoneal cavity

diaphragmatic excursion the movement of the diaphragm during respiration

diarthroses freely-movable joints; also called synovial joints

diastole the relaxation phase of the cardiac cycle

diazo a double nitrogen compound that reacts with bilirubin

diction the style of speaking and enunciating words

dideoxycytidine (DDC) a drug used to treat AIDS by blocking the growth of the virus after it enters the T-cell lymphocytes

dideoxyinosine (ddI) a drug used to treat AIDS by blocking the growth of the virus after it enters the T-cell lymphocytes

diencephalon part of the brain lying beneath the hemispheres, containing the thalamus and hypothalamus

digital pertaining to, resembling, or performed with a finger; expressed in digits (0–9)

diluent an agent that dilutes the substance or solution to which it is added

diplococci spherical microorganisms in pairs

diplomacy the art of handling people with tact and genuine concern

direct examination questioning of a witness by the attorney for the individual the witness is representing

directory a "table of contents" of a file system

discrimination making a difference in favor of or against someone

disease a definite pathological process having a descriptive set of symptoms and a general course of progression

disinfectant a chemical that can be applied to objects to destroy microorganisms; will not destroy bacterial spores

disinfection the process of killing or rendering inert most, but not all, pathogenic organisms

disk drive a device that gets information on and off a floppy disk

diuretics substances that promote the formation and excretion of urine

documentation the process of recording patient information

donor one who contributes something to another

dowager's hump exaggerated cervical curve with prominence of the top thoracic vertebrae found in some osteoporotic elderly women; a type of kyphosis

downtime computer malfunction or any time when the machine is not operational

dress to apply a covering to a wound

dressing a covering applied directly to a wound to apply pressure or support, to absorb secretions, to protect from trauma or microorganisms, to stop or slow bleeding, or to hide disfigurement

drug any substance that when taken into the living organism may modify one or more of its functions

due process a formal proceeding in which the accused is considered not guilty until a verdict is reached

dura mater the outer covering of the brain

durable power of attorney a legal document giving another person the authority to act in one's behalf

duress the act of compelling or forcing someone to do something that they do not want to do

dwarfism (endocrine or pituitary) abnormal underdevelopment of the body with extreme shortness but normal proportions; achondroplastic dwarfism is an inherited growth disorder characterized by shortened limbs and a large head but almost normal trunk proportions

dysmenorrhea painful menstruation

dyspareunia painful coitus or sexual intercourse

dysphagia inability or difficulty in swallowing

dysphasia impairment of speech

dyspnea difficulty breathing

E

ecchymosis an accumulation of blood at a bruise site that causes the skin to become black and blue

edema an accumulation of fluid within the tissues

efferent carrying impulses away from the center

elastin protein substance that gives elasticity and flexibility to the connective issues

electrode a medium for conducting or detecting electrical current

electroencephalogram tracing of the electrical activity in the brain

electrolytes certain chemical substances dissolved in the blood and having numerous basic functions such as conducting electrical currents; the principal electrolytes are sodium, potassium, chloride, and bicarbonate

electromyography the process of recording electrical nerve transmission in skeletal muscles

element a substance that cannot be separated or broken down into substances with properties other than its own; a primary substance

ELISA enzyme-linked immunosorbent assay. A test used to screen blood for the antibody to the AIDS virus

elliptocytosis a condition in which all or almost all of the red blood cells are elliptical or oval in shape; typically asymptomatic

emancipated minor a patient under the age of majority but who is legally considered to be an adult

embolus a mass of matter free-floating in the circulatory system, such as a thrombus that has broken free, an air mass, or a fat globule

empathy the ability to understand or to some extent share what someone else is feeling

emulsify to disperse a liquid into another, usually incompatible, liquid

enclosure indication for the reader that an item is accompanying the letter

endemic a disease that occurs continuously in a particular population but has a low mortality; used in contrast to epidemic

endocardium the innermost part of the heart wall; it lines the heart chamber and covers the connective tissue skeleton of the heart valves

endogenous having its origin within an organism

endotracheal tube a large instrument usually inserted through the mouth (may use the nose) and into the trachea to the point of the tracheal division to deliver oxygen under pressure

enumerated counted

enuresis bed wetting

enzyme a protein that begins (catalyzes) a chemical reaction

epicardium the inner or visceral layer of the pericardium that forms the outermost layer of the heart wall

epidermis outer layer of the skin

epiglottis the leaf-like flap that closes down over the glottis during swallowing

epiphyseal end plate a thin layer of cartilage at the end of long bones where new growth takes place

episiotomy incision of the perineum to accommodate vaginal delivery of fetus

Erlich units a unit of measurement for urobilinogen

erythema redness of the skin

erythematous characterized by redness (erythema)

erythropoietin a hormone produced mainly by the kidney in response to lowered oxygen levels; stimulates the production of red blood cells to increase blood oxygen levels

ester compound formed by combining alcohol and acid; fats are esters

esterase an enzyme that splits esters

ethics guidelines for moral behavior that are enforced by peer groups

ethylene oxide a gas used to sterilize surgical instruments and other supplies

etiology cause of disease

eunuchoidism deficient production of male hormone by the testes, resulting in loss of the secondary male characteristics

eustachian tubes a mucous membrane-lined tube between the nasopharynx and the middle ear bilaterally that equalizes the internal and external otic air pressure

euthanasia allowing a patient to die with minimal medical interventions

evaluation the process of indicating how well the patient or person is progressing toward a particular goal; to appraise; to determine the worth or quality of something or someone

exercise performed activity of the muscles, voluntary or otherwise, to maintain fitness

exogenous having its origin outside of the organism; its opposite is endogenous

exophthalmic goiter abnormal protrusion of the eyeballs accompanied by goiter

expected threshold a numerical goal

expert witness a professional who testifies on the standard of care in a trial

expressed consent a statement of approval from the patient for the physician to perform a given procedure after the patient has been educated about the risks and benefits of the particular procedure; also referred to as informed consent

expulsion formal discharge from a professional organization

externship an educational course that allows the student to obtain hands-on experience

extracellular outside of the cell

extraocular pertaining to outside the eye, as in extraocular eye movement

exudate drainage from an inflammatory lesion, such as pus or serum

F

familial a disorder that tends to occur more often in a family than would be anticipated solely by chance

Family and Medical Leave Act a law designed to allow an employee up to 12 weeks of unpaid leave from his or her job to meet family needs

fascia fibrous membrane tissue that covers and supports the muscles and joins the skin with underlying tissue

febrile exhibiting an elevated temperature

fee-splitting sharing of fees between physicians for patient referrals

feedback in communication, the response to input from another

femtoliter one quadrillionth of a liter

file grouping of data that is given a name for easy access

filing system a method for organizing records so that they can be found when needed

film the raw material prior to processing; does not contain a visible image (similar to photographic film)

filtration removal of particles from a solution by passing the solution through a membrane

fissure a groove, cleft, slit or crack-like lesion

fixative a chemical substance used to bind, fix or stabilize specimens of tissue to slides for later examination

flagella hair-like extremity of a bacterium or protozoan; used to facilitate movement

flextime a system of scheduling that allows for a personal choice in hours or days worked

flocculation condition of having a consistency of loose woolly masses

floppy disk thin magnetic film on which to store data

folate a salt of folic acid; it acts to help enzymes that build structures such as blood cells

forceps a surgical instrument used to grasp, handle, compress, pull or join tissues, equipment or supplies

fraud a deceitful act with the intention to conceal the truth

fructose a simple sugar; a monosaccharide

full block a type of letter format in which all letter components are justified left

full-thickness burn a burn that has destroyed all skin layers

G

gait (gat) the manner or style of walking

galactosuria condition in newborns lacking an enzyme that metabolizes galactose; increased levels of galactose appear in the blood and urine (if proper therapy is not initiated, mental retardation and other difficulties will occur).

gastroenteritis inflammation of the gastrointestinal tract caused by bacteria or viruses

gauge a standard of measurement; a device for measuring size, capacity, amount, or power of an object or substance

gel separator a nonreacting substance located in an evacuated tube that forms a physical barrier between the cells and serum or plasma after the specimen has been centrifuged

generic the official name given to a drug that is no longer owned by the company that developed it

germicide a chemical or drug that kills most pathogenic microorganisms

gestation period of time from conception to birth; usually 37–41 weeks

gestational diabetes a disorder characterized by an impaired ability to metabolize carbohydrates, usually due to insulin deficiency occurring in pregnancy and usually disappearing after delivery

gigantism excessive size and stature caused most frequently by hypersecretion of the Human Growth Hormone (HGH)

gingiva the gums; the mucous membrane covered tissues that support the teeth

glaucoma abnormal increase in the fluid within the eye usually as a result of obstructed outflow of aqueous humor resulting in degeneration of the intraocular components

glomerulus a small cluster of blood vessels within the Bowman's Capsule

glucocorticoid an adrenal cortex hormone that increases the conversion of fatty acids and proteins to glucose for energy

glycosuria the presence of glucose in the urine

goiter an enlargement of the thyroid gland

gonads a generic term referring to the sex glands of both sexes, either ovaries or testes

goniometer an instrument used to measure the angle of joints for range of motion. Goniometry is the act of measuring the angle of range of motion

Goodell's sign softening of cervix that occurs in early pregnancy

granulocytes white blood cells that have visible granules when stained

Graves' disease pronounced hyperthyroidism with signs of enlarged thyroid and exophthalmos

gravid pregnant

gravida a pregnant woman

gravidity pregnancy

grief great sadness caused by loss

gross income the amount of money earned by an employee before taxes are withheld

guaiac substance used in laboratory tests for occult blood in the stool

gyri the convolutions of the brain tissue

H

hard copy printed copy on paper

hard drive a place where the computer stores programs and data files

hardware equipment on the computer system, eg, keyboard, disk drive, monitor, printer

HCFA see Health Care Financing Administration

HCPCS see Health Care Financing Administration Common Procedures Coding System

Health Care Financing Administration (HCFA) a federal agency that regulates health care financing and the procedural classification (Volume 3 of the ICD-9-CM coding book)

Health Care Financing Administration Common Procedures Coding System (HCPCS) a numerical system used by HCFA for services not covered by the CPT coding system

healthcare surrogate a patient's representative who makes health care decisions for the patient

heat exhaustion a type of hyperthermia that causes an altered mental status due to inadequate fluid replacement

heat cramps a type of hyperthermia that causes muscle cramping due to high sodium losses

heat stroke the most serious type of hyperthermia in which the body is no longer able to compensate for the elevated temperatures

hematemesis vomiting blood or bloody vomitus

hematocytometer (hemocytometer) device for counting blood cells

hematoma a blood clot at an injury site

hematuria bloody urine

hemoglobin C disease a genetic blood disorder in which the red blood cells contain an abnormal hemoglobin C, which reduces the elasticity of the red cells causing them to hemolyze easily

hemoglobinuria presence of free hemoglobin in urine

hemolysis rupture of erythrocytes with the release of hemoglobin into the plasma or serum causing the specimen to appear pink or red in color

hemolytic anemia a disorder characterized by premature destruction of the red cells; this may be brought on by an infectious process, inherited red cell disorder, or as a response to certain drugs or toxins

hemoptysis coughing up blood from the respiratory tract

hemostat a surgical instrument with slender jaws used for grasping blood vessels

heparin a naturally occurring anticoagulant given to prevent clot formation

hepatomegaly liver enlargement

hepatotoxin a substance that can be damaging to the liver

hereditary traits or disorders that are transmitted from parent to offspring

hernia the protrusion of an organ through the muscle wall of the cavity that normally surrounds it

hiatus an opening or gap; hiatal hernia: a protrusion of part of the stomach upward through the diaphragm

Hippocratic Oath a code of ethics written by Hippocrates

hirsutism abnormal or excessive growth of hair in women

histamine a substance found normally in the body in response to injured cells, resulting in the inflammatory process with dilation of capillaries, increased gastric secretions and contraction of smooth muscles

homeostasis maintaining a constant internal environment by balancing positive and negative feedback

hormone a substance that is produced by an endocrine gland and travels through the blood to a distant organ or gland where it acts to modify the structure or function of that gland or organ

human chorionic gonadotropin (HCG) hormone secreted by the placenta

humidifier appliance that increases the moisture content in the air

hydrogen ion hydrogen that is missing an electron and therefore readily binds with substances having extra electrons; it is an important constituent of acids

hypercalcemia an excessive amount of calcium in the blood

hyperglycemia an increase in blood sugar, as in diabetes mellitus

hyperopia farsightedness

hyperosmolarity a condition of having increased numbers of dissolved substances in the plasma

hyperplasia excessive proliferation of normal cells in the normal tissue arrangement of an organism

hypertension abnormally elevated blood pressure

hyperthermia an elevated body temperature

hypoglycemia deficiency of sugar in the blood

hypothalamus part of the diencephalon; activates and controls the peripheral nervous system, endocrine system, and certain involuntary functions

hypothermia a below-normal body temperature

hypovolemic shock a type of shock caused by fluid loss

hysterosalpingogram radiograph of the uterus and fallopian tubes after injection of contrast media

hysteroscopy visual examination with magnification of the uterus

I

iatrogenic a condition caused by treatment or medical procedures

identification line a series of initials indicating who dictated the letter and who composed it

idiopathic unknown etiology

immune globulins proteins produced by plasma cells in response to foreign antigens; they provide immediate antibody protection, which lasts for a few weeks to a few months

immunization act or process of rendering an individual immune to specific diseases

immunohematology the study of the antigen-antibody reaction including the study of autoimmunity

implementation the process of initiating and carrying out an action such as a teaching plan or patient treatment

implied consent an informal agreement of approval from the patient to perform a given task

impotence inability to achieve or retain an erection

incident report a form used by an organization to document an unusual occurrence to a patient, visitor or employee

incontinence inability to control elimination, either urine or feces or both

indices (sing. index) numbers expressing a property or ratio

infection the presence and multiplication of pathogenic microorganisms leading to tissue damage or a disease process

informed consent a statement of approval from the patient for the physician to perform a given procedure after the patient has been educated about the risks and benefits of the procedure; also referred to as expressed consent

inguinal pertaining to the regions of the groin

inpatient a medical setting in which patients are admitted for diagnostic, radiographic, or treatment purposes

insertion a place of attachment, usually the freely movable portion of a muscle

inspection the act or process of inspecting; visual examination

institutional review board internal committee that reviews ethical issues

instrument a surgical tool or device designed to perform a specific function, such as cutting, dissecting, grasping, holding, retracting, or suturing

insufflator a device for blowing air, gases or powders into a cavity

insula fifth lobe of the cerebrum

insulin dependent diabetes mellitus (IDDM) a deficiency in insulin production that leads to an inability to metabolize carbohydrates

interferon a group of proteins released by white blood cells and fibroblasts when the invading organism is a virus

intermittent occurring at intervals

Internal Revenue Service (IRS) a federal agency that regulates and enforces various taxes

International Classification of Diseases (ICD) a classification system used to assign a numerical code to a disease

interosseous between bones

interstitial the spaces between the cells

intracellular inside of the cell

intraocular pressure pressure within the eyeball

intrauterine pregnancy (IUP) pregnancy located in the uterus

intravascular coagulation clot formation within the vessels; strands of fibrin may form from one wall of the vessel to the other and shear red cells as they pass by

intravenous pyelogram (IVP) an x-ray using contrast medium to evaluate kidney function

intrinsic found within a structure

introitus vaginal orifice

iodine an element that is an essential micronutrient used in the thyroid gland to manufacture its hormones; present in seafood, foods grown in iodized soil, iodized salt and some dairy products

ion an atom or group of atoms that has become electrically charged by the loss or gain of one or more electrons

iontophoresis introducing various chemical ions into the skin by means of electrical current

J

job description a statement that informs an employee about the duties and expectations for a given job

Joint Commission on Accreditation of Health Care Organizations (JCAHO) a voluntary organization that sets and evaluates the standards of care for health care institutions; based on the JCAHO evaluation, an accreditation title will be given to the organization.

K

Kaposi's sarcoma multiple areas of cell proliferation initially in the skin and eventually in other body sites; this condition is frequently related to the immunocompromised state that accompanies AIDS

keratin a tough, insoluble protein substance of the stratum corneum, hair and nails

keratoses (senile) premalignant overgrowth or thickening of the upper layer of epithelium or horny layer of the skin

ketoacidosis acidosis accompanied by an accumulation of ketones in the body

ketones the end products of fat metabolism

kinesics a form of non-verbal communication including gestures, body movements, facial expressions

Krebs cycle a sequence of reactions within cells that metabolizes sugars and other energy sources, such as carbohydrates, proteins and fats, into carbon dioxide, water and ATP

kyphosis abnormally deep dorsal curvature of the thoracic spine; also known as humpback or hunchback

L

labor normal physiological process involving involuntary contractions of the uterine muscle resulting in cervical dilation and effacement (thinning)

laparoscopy process of viewing the internal abdominal cavity and its contents

laparotomy incision of the abdominal cavity

laryngectomy removal of the larynx, either partial or total

laser ablation destruction or removal of tissue by use of laser

lead an electrode or electrical connection attached to the body to record electrical impulses in the body, especially the heart or brain

learning objectives steps that needed to be achieved to accomplish the learning goal

learning goal an agreed upon outcome of the teaching process

ledger card a record of the patient's financial activities

ledger a continuous record of business transactions with debits and credits

lentigines tan or brown macule found on elderly skin after prolonged sun exposure; also known as liver spots

leukocytosis abnormal increase of leukocytes (white blood cells)

libel written statements that defame a person's reputation or character

licensure the strictest form of professional accreditation

ligament a flexible band of tissue that holds joints together

lightening the descent of the fetus further into the pelvis

lipase any of several enzymes that begin the breakdown of fats in the digestive tract

lipids any of the free fatty acids (fats) in the body

lipoproteins a substance made up of a lipid and a protein

lithotripsy crushing a stone

litigation process of filing or contesting a lawsuit

lochia uterine discharge following childbirth, composed of some blood, mucus and tissue

login use of a password to gain access to the computer

loop of henle a portion of the renal tubule, shaped like a U and consisting of a thick ascending and thin descending vessels

lordosis an abnormally deep ventral curve at the lumbar flexure of the spine; also known as swayback

lubricant an agent that reduces friction between parts

Luer adapter a device for connecting a syringe or evacuated holder to the needle to promote a secure fit

lyse to cause disintegration; ie, destruction of adhesions, or the breakdown of red blood cells

M

macrophage a monocyte that has left the circulation and settled and matured in tissue; macrophages process antigens and present them to T-cells, activating the immune specific response

macule small, flat discoloration of the skin

mainframe central computer to which individual computers are connected; used in large institutions

malaise general feeling of illness without specific signs or symptoms

malignant cancerous

malocclusion abnormal contact between the teeth in the upper and lower jaw

malpractice a tort in which the patient is harmed by the actions of a health care worker

manipulation the skillful use of the hands in diagnostic procedures

Mantoux tuberculin skin test using a purified protein derivative (PPD) of tuberculin bacillus given intradermally to establish exposure to tuberculosis

masticate the act of chewing or grinding, as in chewing food

Material Safety Data Sheet (MSDS) a detailed record of all hazardous substances kept within a site

matrix a system for blocking off unavailable patient appointment times

mediastinum the mid-portion of the thoracic cavity containing the heart, the great vessels, the upper esophagus and the trachea

medical history record containing information about a patient's complete past and present health status

medical assistant a multiskilled health professional who performs a variety of clinical and administrative tasks in a medical setting

medical asepsis destruction of organisms after they leave the body

medical setting a place that is designed to meet the health care needs of patients; may be inpatient or outpatient.

medulla oblongata part of the brain that controls breathing, heart rate, and blood pressure

megabyte one million bytes; a way to measure the quantity of computer information that a particular device can hold

megaloblastic anemia a disorder characterized by production of large, dysfunctional erythrocytes; folate deficiency is considered a cause

meiosis the cell division specific to sperm and ova that results in 23 chromosomes rather than 46 (23 pairs)

melanin dark pigment that gives color to the skin, hair and eyes

melanocyte cell that produces melanin

melena black, tarry stools caused by digested blood from the GI tract

memorandum a type of written documentation used for interoffice communication

menarche age at which the first menstruation occurred

meninges membranes of the spinal cord and brain

meningocele meninges protruding through the spinal column

meniscus the curved upper surface of a liquid in a container

menorrhagia excessive or heavy menstruation

menses menstruation; bloody discharge that occurs monthly or cyclically

mensuration the act or process of measuring

message words sent from one person to another; information sent through spoken, written, or body language

metabolic acidosis an acidic condition of the body caused when excess acids are produced in the body's fluids (as in the metabolism of fats instead of glucose) or when the body's natural bicarbonates are lost or diminished

metabolism the total of all chemical processes that result in growth, energy production, elimination of waste and all body functions as digested nutrients are distributed

metrorrhagia irregular uterine bleeding

microbiology the study of microscopic organisms

microfiche sheets of microfilm

microfilm photographs of records in a reduced size

microorganisms microscopic living organisms

microprocessor a chip that allows the computer to function

micturition also known as voiding or urination

midbrain part of the brain stem, responsible for relaying messages

migraine a type of severe headache, usually unilateral, may appear in clusters

mission statement a statement describing the goals of the medical office and those it serves

modem (modulator/demodulator) a communication device that connects a computer to the standard telephone system, allowing information exchange with other computers off site

monitor visual display terminal (VDT) that shows information being input via the keyboard

monosaccharide a simple sugar that cannot be broken down further

mordant a substance used to fix, or bind, dyes or stains

morphology the science and study of structure and form

motherboard fiberglass board that contains the central processing unit (CPU), memory, and other pieces of circuitry

mourning to demonstrate signs of grief; grieving

mouse a device that allows the user to control cursor movement on the monitor

multidisciplinary involving many disciplines; a group of healthcare professionals from various specialties brought together to meet the patient's needs

multimedia various forms of communication available on the computer, eg, stereophonic sound, animation, full-motion video, photographs

multipara woman who has given birth to more than one viable fetus

multiskilled health professional an individual with versatile training in the healthcare field

muscular dystrophies a group of genetically transmitted diseases characterized by progressive atrophy of skeletal muscles

mycology the science and study of fungi

myelofibrosis a disorder in which bone marrow tissue develops in abnormal sites such as the liver and spleen; signs include immature cells in the circulation, anemia, and splenomegaly

myelogram invasive radiologic test in which dye is injected into the spinal fluid

myelomeningocele protrusion of the spinal cord through the spinal defect called a spina bifida

myocardium the middle layer of the walls of the heart, composed of cardiac muscle

myofibrils a slender light/dark strand of muscle tissue in striated muscle

myopia nearsightedness

myxedema the most severe form of hypothyroidism; signs include edema of the extremities and the face

N

nasal septum the wall or partition dividing the nostrils

National Committee for Clinical Laboratory Standards (NCCLS) a committee appointed to establish rules to ensure the safety, standards and integrity of all testing performed on human specimens

nebulizer an instrument for administering a fine spray of medication, usually used in the respiratory tract

needle holder a surgical forceps used to hold and pass a suture through tissue

negative feedback a decrease in function in response to a stimulus

negative stress stress that does not allow for relaxation periods

negligence performance of an act that a reasonable health care worker would not have done or the omission of an act that a reasonable person would have done

neoplasm an abnormal growth of new tissue; a tumor

nephron the portion of the kidney responsible for the production of urine

nephrostomy an opening into the kidney

net pay the amount of money an employee is paid after all taxes are withheld

networking a system of personal and professional relationships through which to share information

neurogenic shock a type of shock caused by a dysfunction of the nervous system

neuron a nerve cell

neurotransmitter chemical needed to transmit a message between synapses

nitrogenous pertaining to or containing nitrogen, usually the end-product of protein metabolism

nitroprusside a nitrogen cyanic compound that reacts with ketones

nocturia excessive urination at night

nodule a small node, mass or swelling

non compos mentis mental incompetence

non–insulin dependent diabetes mellitus (NIDDM) a type of diabetes in which patients do not require insulin to control the blood sugar

noncompliance the patient's inability or refusal to follow prescribed orders

nonlanguage not expressed in spoken language, eg, laughing, sobbing, grunting, sighing

normal value acceptable range as established for an age, a population, or a sex; variations usually indicate a disorder

normal flora organisms normally found in an area; also known as resident or indigenous flora

nosocomial infection infection acquired in a medical setting, generally presumed to be in a hospital setting but may also refer to the medical office

nulligravida woman who has never been pregnant

nullipara woman who has never given birth to a viable fetus

numeric filing arranging files by a numbered order

nutrition the study of food and how it is used for growth, nourishment, and repair

O

obligate to require; a parasite that has no choice but to attach to a living organism

obstipation extreme constipation

obturator a smooth, rounded, removable inner portion of a hollow tube, such as an anoscope, that allows for easier insertion

occult hidden or concealed from observation

olecranon fossa the depression in the posterior surface of the humerus that allows the arm to extend by receiving the olecranon process

olecranon process the proximal end of the ulna that becomes the point of the elbow that fits into the olecranon fossa

oliguria scanty urine formation

on-line direct link to off-site computers

oophorectomy excision of an ovary

operating system the program that tells the computer how to interface with hardware and software

ophthalmoscope lighted instrument to visually examine the inner surfaces of the eye

opportunistic infection infections that result from a defective immune system that cannot defend against pathogens normally found in the environment

optician a trained specialist who grinds lens to fit refraction corrective lens prescriptions written by ophthalmologists and optometrists

optometrist a trained specialist who can measure for errors of refraction and prescribe lens for refraction errors but who cannot treat eye disorders

organ the source or starting point; (muscle) any part that is made up of cells and tissues that cause it to perform its specified function in conjunction with a body system

organizational chart a flow sheet depicting the members of a team in a structured or hierarchical manner

origin the source or starting point; (muscle) the more fixed end of a muscle, usually the proximal end

OSHA Occupational Safety and Health Administration

osteoporosis abnormal porosity of the bone found in the elderly and predisposing the affected bony tissue to fracture

otoscope instrument used to visually examine the ear canal and tympanic membrane

outlier a patient whose hospital stay is longer than allowed by the DRG

outpatient a medical setting in which patients receive care but are not admitted

over-the-counter medications that are available without prescriptions

overdraft protection protection against having insufficient funds to cover checks

ovulation the periodic rupture of the mature ovum from the ovary

ovum (pl. ova) the female reproductive cell; sex cell or egg

P

packing slip a document that accompanies a supply order and lists the enclosed items

Paget's disease degenerative bone disease usually in older persons with bone destruction and poor repair

palliative to relieve or reduce but not to cure

palmar the palm surface of the hand

palpation a technique used in physical examination in which the examiner feels the texture, size, consistency, and location of parts of the body with the hands

pancreatitis an inflammation of the pancreas that may be brought on by alcohol, trauma, infection, or certain drugs

Papanicolaou test or smear (Pap test) a simple smear method of examining tissue cells for cancer, especially of the cervix; named for George N. Papanicolaou, a Greek physician, anatomist, and cytologist in the United States, 1883–1962

papilla (pl. papillae) a small nipple shaped projection

papillae lingua the taste buds

papilloma virus virus that causes papillomas or warts

papilloma a benign form of skin tumor

papule small, red, solid elevation of the skin

paralanguage factors connected with, but not essentially part of language, eg, tone of voice, volume, pitch.

parameters values used to describe or measure a set of data representing a physiologic function or system

parasitology the science and study of parasites

parasympathetic the part of the autonomic nervous system involved in periods free from stress

parity pregnancies that resulted in a viable birth

partial thickness burn a burn that involves the epidermis and varying levels of the dermis

particulate matter a material composed of particles

passive range of motion assisted range-of-motion movements

pathogens disease-causing microorganisms

patient education active participation of the patient in a process that will yield a change in behavior

payroll journal a method for keeping track of payroll data using the pegboard system

payroll the process of calculating employee salary

pediatrician medical doctor who specializes in the care of infants, children, and adolescents

pediatrics specialty of medicine that deals with the care of infants, children and adolescents

pediculosis infestation with lice

percussion the act of striking parts of the body with the hands to evaluate the size, borders, consistency, and presence of fluid in some of the internal organs

pericardium the double-layered serous, membranous sac that encloses the heart and the origins of the great vessels

peripheral pertaining to or situated away from the center

peristalsis rhythmic waves of smooth muscle contractions that force substances to points of elimination

PERRLA abbreviation used in documentation to denote pupils equal, round, reactive to light and accommodation if all findings are normal; refers to the size and shape of the pupils, their reaction to light, and their ability to adjust to distance

pessary device that supports the uterus when inserted into the vagina

petri plate a shallow glass or plastic dish with a lid to hold solid media for cultures

pH abbreviation for potential hydrogen, pH is a scale representing the relative acidity or alkalinity of a substance in which 7.0 is neutral; numbers lower than 7.0 are acid and numbers above 7.0 are basic

phagocyte a cell that has the ability to ingest and destroy particular substances such as bacteria, protozoa, cells and cell debris by ingesting them

phagocytosis the process by which certain cells engulf and dispose of microorganisms; to eat or ingest

pharmacodynamics the study of how drugs act within the body

pharmacokinesis the study of the action of drugs within the body from administration to excretion

pharmacology the study of drugs and their origins, nature, properties, and effects upon living organisms

phimosis narrowing or tightening of the prepuce that prevents retraction over the glans penis

phonophoresis an ultrasound treatment used to force medications into tissues

phosphates a compound containing phosphorus and oxygen; they are very important in living organisms, especially for the transfer of genetic information

physiology the study of the function of the body

pia mater thin vascular covering that adheres to the surface of the brain

plaintiff the party who initiates a lawsuit

planes a point of reference made by a straight cut through the body at any given angle

planning the process of using information gathered during the assessment phase to organize learning or patient care objectives in order to accomplish the specific learning or treatment goal

pleura the serous membrane enclosing the lungs; (visceral pleura: the layer that covers the lungs most closely; parietal pleura: the layer that follows the contours and lines the chest wall, the diaphragm, and the mediastinum)

poikilocytosis abnormal variations in the shapes of red blood cells (poikilo = variation)

policy a statement that reflects the organization's rules on a given topic
polydipsia excessive thirst
polymenorrhea abnormally frequent menstrual periods
polyphagia abnormal hunger
polyuria excessive excretion and elimination of urine
pons part of the brain stem, responsible for communication within the central nervous system
portfolio a portable case containing documents
positive stress stress that allows a person to perform at peak levels and then relax afterward
positive feedback an increase in function in response to a stimulus
positron emission tomography (PET) computerized radiography using radioactive substances to assess metabolic or physiological functions within the body rather than anatomical structures
posting listing financial transactions in a ledger
postural hypotension sudden drop in blood pressure upon standing
potentiation the synergistic action of two substances, such as hormones or drugs, in which the total effects are greater than the sum of the independent effects of the two substances
precedent the use of previous court decisions as a legal foundation
preceptor a teacher; one who gives direction, as in a technical matter
precipitation the settling out of a substance in a solution
prepuce a fold of skin that forms a cover
presbycusis loss of hearing associated with aging
presbyopia vision changes associated with age
preservative a substance that delays decomposition
primary survey an initial assessment of an emergency patient for life-threatening problems
prime mover the muscle most responsible for the desired muscle action or movement
primigravida woman who is pregnant for the first time
printer a device that transfers information on the computer into hard copy
procedure a series of steps required to perform a given task
professional courtesy a discount fee given to healthcare professionals
proofreading a part of editing a document in which the writer reads the draft for accuracy and clarity and corrects errors
proprietary private school with preset curricula
prostate-specific antigen a normal protein produced by the prostate that usually elevates in the presence of cancer
prosthesis any artificial replacement for a missing body part, such as false teeth or an artificial limb
proteinuria the presence of large quantities of protein in the urine; usually a sign of renal dysfunction
proxemic having to do with the degree of physical closeness tolerated by humans
pruritus itching
psychogenic of psychological origin
psychosocial relating to mental and emotional aspects of social encounters
puerperium period of time (about 6 weeks) from childbirth until reproductive structures return to normal
purchase order a document that lists the required items to be purchased
Purkinje fibers extensions of the Bundle of His that branch through the myocardium to end the transmission of the electrical impulse and cause the ventricles to contract
pustules vesicle filled with pus
pyosalpinx pus in the fallopian tube(s)
pyuria pus in the urine

Q

quadrants a division of the abdomen into four equal parts by one horizontal and one vertical line dissecting at the umbilicus
quality assurance an evaluation of health care services as compared to accepted standards
quality control method to evaluate the proper performance of testing procedures, supplies or equipment in a laboratory
quality improvement a plan that allows an organization to scientifically measure the quality of its product and service
quantification the process of ascertaining the amount of something
quantitative the measuring of an amount
Queckenstedt test test to determine the presence of an obstruction in the CSF flow

R

radiograph processed film that contains a visible image
radiographer technical specialist who works to assist the radiologist in the performance of procedures and who is responsible for producing routine examination images for the radiologist to interpret
radiography the art and science of producing diagnostic images to be used in the care of patients
radioimmunoassay (RIA) the introduction of radioactive substances into the body to determine the concentration of a substance in the serum, usually the concentration of antigens, antibodies, or proteins
radiologist a medical doctor who specializes in radiology; performs some procedures and interprets images to provide diagnostic information to physicians
radiology the branch of medicine including diagnostic and therapeutic applications of x-rays and other techniques
radiolucent permitting the passage of x-rays
radionuclide a radioactive material used in small amounts in nuclear medicine studies; has a short life
radiopaque not permeable to the passage of x-rays

random access memory (RAM) temporary memory; data is lost when the computer is turned off if it is not backed up on disk

range of motion (ROM) the range, measured in degrees, through which a joint can be extended and flexed

ratchets notched mechanisms, usually at the handle end of an instrument, that click into position to maintain tension on the opposing blades or tips of the instrument

read only memory (ROM) permanent memory inside the computer

reagent a substance used to react in a certain manner in the presence of specific chemicals to obtain a diagnosis

rectocele herniation of the rectum into the vaginal area

rectovaginal pertaining to the rectum and vagina

reduction correcting a fracture by realigning the bone; may be closed (corrected by manipulation) or open (requires surgery)

reference value a range established for test results assumed to be typical for a population asymptomatic for disease processes

reflux a return or backward flow of fluid

refract, refraction bending the light rays that enter the pupil to reflect exactly on the fovea centralis, the area of greatest visual acuity

remittent fluctuating

renal pelvis the funnel-shaped upper portion of the ureters that collects urine from the kidneys

renal cortex the portion of the kidney that contains the structures that form urine

renal medulla the inner portion of the kidney that contains the collecting structures

renal pyramids situated in the renal medulla, part of the collecting structures

renin enzyme formed in the kidney that works with angiotensin to affect the blood pressure

repolarization the active process of restoring the cardiac fibers to the resting (polarized) state. Re-establishment of the electrical polarized state in a muscle or nerve fiber following contraction or conduction of a nerve impulse

res ipsa loquitur "the thing speaks for itself"

res judicata "the thing has been decided"

Resource-Based Relative Value Scale (RBRVS) a value scale designed to decrease Medicare Part B costs and establish national standards for coding and payment

respiration the exchange of oxygen and carbon dioxide (external respiration: the exchange between the alveoli and the bloodstream; internal respiration: the exchange between the cells and the bloodstream)

respondeat superior "let the master answer"

restrain control or confine movement

resume document summarizing an individual's work experience or professional qualifications

retinal degeneration pathological changes in the cell structure of the retina that impairs or destroys its function (blindness may result)

retrograde pyelogram an x-ray of the urinary tract using contrast medium injected through the bladder and ureters; useful in diagnosing obstructions

retroperitoneal the space behind the peritoneal cavity that contains the kidneys

retrovirus viruses containing reverse transcriptase, which allows the viral cell to replicate its DNA into the DNA of the host cell, thereby taking over the substance of the cell

rickettsia organism that is smaller than bacteria, larger than viruses

ringworm lay term for tinea, a group of fungal diseases

risk factors any issue that possesses a safety or liability concern for an organization

Romberg test inability to maintain body balance when eyes are closed and feet are together, an indication of spinal cord disease

rugae ridges or folds in the skin or mucous membranes that allow for expansion of a part

rule of nines the most common method of determining the extent of burn injury; the body surface is divided into sections of 9% or multiples of 9%

S

salpingectomy excision of the fallopian tube

salpingo-oophorectomy excision of both an ovary and fallopian tube

salutation an introductory phrase that greets the reader of a letter

sanitation the science of maintaining a healthful, disease-free environment

sanitizing the practice of lowering the number of microorganisms on a surface by use of low-level disinfectant practices

scale a thin, dried flake of skin

scalpel a small, pointed knife with a convex blade edge for surgical procedures

scanner a piece of office equipment that transfers a written document into a computer

scissors a sharp instrument composed of two opposing cutting blades, held together by a central pin on which the blades pivot

sclera the white fibrous tissue that covers the eye

scoliosis a lateral curve of the spine, usually in the thoracic area with a corresponding curve in the lumbar region, causing uneven shoulders and hips

screening a preliminary procedure, such as a test or exam, to detect the more characteristic signs of a disorder

sebaceous gland oil gland

seborrhea over-production of sebum with excessive oiliness or dry scales

sebum fatty secretion of the sebaceous gland
secondary survey an assessment of an emergency victim for head to toe injuries
seizure involuntary contractions of voluntary muscles; an abnormal discharge of electrical activity in the brain
semi-block a type of letter format that is styled the same as block, except the first sentence of each paragraph is indented five spaces
sensitivity susceptibility to a certain substance
septic shock a type of shock that is caused by a generalized infection in the body
septicemia presence of pathogenic bacteria in the blood
serology the study of the nature and properties of serum
serrations grooves, either straight or criss-cross, etched or cut into the blades or tips of an instrument to more firmly hold the tissue in its grasp
service charge a charge by a bank for various services
sesamoid resembling the shape of a sesame seed
shock a lack of oxygen to individual cells of the body
sick child visit a pediatric visit for the treatment of illness or injury
sickle cell anemia a condition in which the patient has both copies of the gene for hemoglobin S; the red cells become sickle shaped and non-flexible causing obstruction of small vessels and capillaries. Necrosis due to tissue hypoxia occurs beyond the obstruction. Most commonly seen in African-Americans
signs objective indications of disease or bodily dysfunction
sinoatrial (SA) node considered the pacemaker of the heart, located in the upper portion of the right atrium; a specialized group of cells that initiate the electrical impulse of the heart
slander oral statements that defame a person's reputation or character
smegma a cheesy secretion of the sebaceous glands either in the labia or prepuce
software application programs that direct the hardware to perform given tasks
specific gravity the relative density of a substance (eg, urine)
specificity relating to a definite result
specimen a small portion of anything used to evaluate the nature of the whole
speculum an instrument that enlarges and separates the opening of a cavity to expose its interior for examination
spherocytosis a condition where all or almost all of the red cells are spherocytes; typically asymptomatic
spicules sharp points
spina bifida occulta a congenital defect in the spinal column caused by lack of union of the vertebrae
spinal pertaining to the spine
spirochete long, flexible, motile microorganisms
spore the reproductive stage of certain microorganisms; a thick shell formed by some bacteria during a resting or dormant stage that is very resistant to many forms of disinfection
staff privileges hospital approval for a physician to admit patients for treatment
staghorn stone formation in the renal pelvis that fills the chamber and assumes the shape of the calyces
staphylococci spherical microorganism found in grape-like clusters
Staphylococcus a genus of bacteria, some of which are causative agents for skin infections
stare decisis "the previous decision stands"
status asthmaticus an asthma attack that is not responsive to treatment
statute of limitations a legal time limit; eg, the length of time in which a patient may file a lawsuit
statutes laws that are written by federal, state or local legislators
stereotyping to place in a fixed mold, without consideration of differences
sterile field a specific area, such as within a tray or on a sterile towel, that is considered free of microorganisms
sterilization a process, act or technique for destroying microorganisms using heat, water, chemicals or gases
stoma an opening to the surface; suggests that it is surgically created
stratum corneum outer layer of the epidermis
stratum germinativum innermost layer of the epidermis
streptococci spherical microorganisms clustered in chains
Streptococcus a genus of bacteria that are commonly implicated in diseases of the skin
striated having a striped appearance with alternating light and dark bands
subcutaneous beneath the skin
subject filing arranging files according to their title, grouping similar subjects together
subpoena duces tecum a court order requiring medical records to be submitted to the court at a given date and time
subpoena a court order requiring an individual to appear at court at a given date and time
substrate an underlying layer; a substance acted upon, as by an enzyme or reagent
sudoriferous gland sweat gland
sulci a groove in the brain tissue
sulfosalicylic acid an acid used to test for protein
superbill preprinted patient bill that lists a variety of procedures
superficial burn a burn that is limited to the epidermal layers

surgical asepsis destruction of organisms before they enter the body

surrogate mother a woman who carries a baby to term for another female who is unable to carry a pregnancy to term

suspension temporary removal of privileges

swab (noun) stick topped with cotton or other absorbent man-made fiber for cleaning areas, applying treatments or for obtaining specimens

swab (verb) to wipe with a swab

swaged needle a metal needle fused to a suture material

symmetry equality in size or shape or position of parts on opposite sides of the body

sympathetic the part of the autonomic nervous system involved in stress reaction

sympathy feeling sorry for or pitying someone

symptoms subjective indications of disease or bodily changes as sensed by the patient

synapse the junction of two neurons

synarthroses immovable joints

syncope a sudden fall in blood pressure or cerebral hypoxia resulting in loss of consciousness

synergism the harmonious action of two agents, such as drugs or organs, producing an effect that neither could produce alone or an effect that is greater than the total effects of each agent operating by itself

synergist muscles that work together for more efficient movement

system a collection of organs that perform a certain function

systole the contraction phase of the cardiac cycle

T

T cells lymphoid cells from bone marrow that migrate to the thymus gland where they mature into differentiated lymphocytes that circulate between blood and lymph

tab the projection on a file folder on which the patient name or title is written

tactile pertaining to the sense of touch

task force a group of employees that works together to solve a given problem

tax withholding the amount of tax that is withheld from a paycheck

tendons tough, flexible fibers that bind muscle to bone

tetany severe cramping, convulsions or muscle spasms due to an abnormality of calcium metabolism

thalamus part of the diencephalon, responsible for sorting messages

thalassemia a hemolytic anemia caused by deficient hemoglobin synthesis; more commonly found in those of Mediterranean heritage

therapeutic having to do with treating or curing disease; curative

thoracentesis a surgical puncture into the pleural cavity for aspiration of serous fluid or for the injection of therapeutic medications

thromboplastin a complex substance found in blood and tissues that aids the clotting process

thyrotoxicosis excess quantities of thyroid hormone in the tissues

tickler file a file that provides a reminder to do a given task at a particular date and time

tine test skin test for exposure to tuberculosis, involves pricking the skin with sharp tines coated with the tuberculin bacillus

tinnitus an extraneous noise heard in one or both ears, described as whirring, ringing, whistling, roaring, etc.; may be continuous or intermittent

tissues a group of cells that function together for a specific purpose

titer a measure of the amount of an antibody in serum

tomography procedure in which the x-ray tube and film move in relation to each other during the exposure, blurring out all structures except those in the focal plane; used frequently in excretory urography

tonsils a small mass of lymphoid tissue; includes the palatine, nasopharyngeal and lingual tonsils

tonus the steady, partial contraction of skeletal muscles that allows the body to remain upright

tort the righting of wrongs or injuries suffered by someone because of another person's wrongdoing

toxoid a toxin that has been treated to destroy its toxicity, but is still capable of inducing formation of antibodies on injection

tracheostomy a permanent surgical stoma in the neck with an indwelling tube

tracheotomy incision into the trachea below the larynx to circumvent a blockage superior to this point; suggests an emergency situation and a reversible procedure

trade name the name given to a medication by the company that owns the patent

transient flora organisms that do not normally reside in an area; the presence of transient flora in an area may or may not produce disease

transient ischemic attack (TIA) acute episode of cerebrovascular insufficiency usually as a result of narrowing of an artery by artherosclerotic plaques, emboli, or vasospasm; usually passes quickly but should be considered a warning for predisposition to cerebrovascular accidents

transillumination the passage of light through body tissues for the purpose of examination

transition passing from one place or activity to another

traumatic causing or relating to tissue damage

trigone the triangle formed in the base of the bladder by the entrance of the two ureters and the exit of the urethra

truss a device of pressing against a hernia to keep it in place

turbid cloudy

turbinates mucous membrane-covered conchae, the three scroll-shaped bones that project into the nasal cavity bilaterally from the lateral walls, each covers a sinus meatus

turgor normal tension in a cell or the skin; normal skin turgor resists deformation and will resume its former position after being grasped or pulled

tympanic membrane thin, semitransparent membrane in the middle ear that transmits sound vibrations; also called the eardrum

U

unemployment tax federal tax paid by the employer based on each employee's gross income

unit each part of a name or title that is used in indexing; a quantity of a standard measurement

upcoding billing more for a patient care service than it is worth by selecting a code that is higher on the coding scale; this is an illegal practice

urates a nitrogenous compound derived from protein use and is excreted in the urine

urea the final product of protein metabolism in the body and the main nitrogenous component in the urine

uremic frost a frost-like deposit of uremic compounds on the skin of patients whose kidneys are no longer functional

ureterostomy an opening in a ureter

ureters the pair of tubes designed to carry urine from the kidneys to the bladder

urethra the short tube that carries urine from the bladder to the outside of the body

URI upper respiratory infection

uric acid a by-product of protein metabolism present in the blood and excreted by the kidneys

urinalysis chemical analysis of urine for diagnostic purposes

urinary frequency the urge to urinate occurring more often than is required for normal bladder elimination

urticaria hives

V

vaccine a suspension of infectious agents, or some part of them, given for the purpose of establishing resistance to an infectious disease

values established ideals of life, conduct, customs, etc., of an individual person or members of a society

varicella zoster viral infection manifested by characteristic rash of successive crops of vesicles that scab before resolution; also called chicken pox

vasopressin a hormone formed in the hypothalamus and transported to the posterior lobe of the pituitary through the hypothalamo-hypophyseal tract. It has an antidiuretic and a pressor effect that elevates the blood pressure.

vector (biological) a living, nonhuman carrier of the disease, usually an arthropod; (mechanical) a carrier of disease that does not support growth but will transmit disease; examples include inanimate objects or asymptomatic carriers

ventricle either of the two lower chambers of the heart that when filled with blood contract to propel it into the arteries

venule the small vessel that joins a capillary to a vein

verdict a decision of guilty or not guilty based on evidence presented in a trial

verruca wart

vertigo sensation of whirling of oneself or the environment

vesicle a small sac containing fluid; blister

vial a small bottle for medicines or chemicals

villus (pl. villi) tiny, almost microscopic projections in the mucous membrane of the small intestines

virology the science and study of viruses

virulent highly pathogenic

visualization a relaxation technique that allows the mind to wander and the imagination to run free and focus on positive and relaxing situations

W

wave scheduling a flexible scheduling method that allows time for procedures of varying lengths and the addition of unscheduled patients, as needed

well child (or baby) visit visit for evaluation of growth and development

Western Blot a specific, confirmatory antibody test for the presence of HIV in the blood

wheal small round itchy elevation of the skin with a white center and red border; a hive

whorls a spiral arrangement, as in the ridges on the finger that make up a fingerprint

withdrawing the act of terminating a medical treatment that has already been initiated

withholding not initiating certain medical treatments

Wood's light ultraviolet light used to detect fungal diseases

write off cancellation of an unpaid debt

Y

yolk sac a structure that develops in the inner zygotic cell mass and supplies nourishment for the embryo until the seventh week when the placenta takes over the function

Index

Note: Page numbers in *italics* indicate illustrations; those followed by t indicate tables; those followed by b indicate boxed material; and those followed by p indicate procedures.

C

D

E

H

J

K

L

M

S

T

U

V

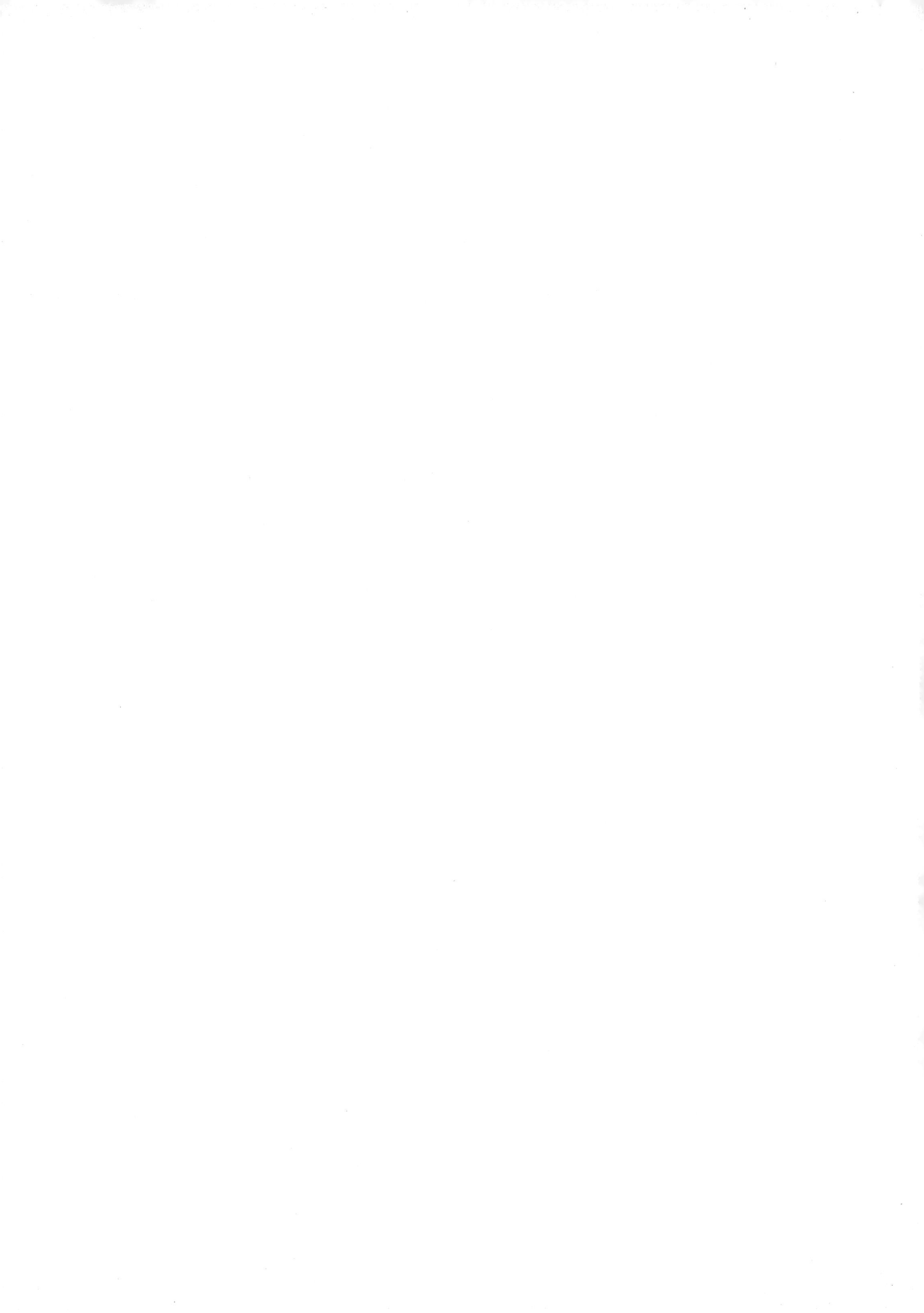

Performance Objectives

Chapter 1

Asepsis and Infection Control 2

1. Perform a medical aseptic handwashing (Procedure 1-1). 17
2. Perform a surgical scrub (Procedure 1-2). 18
3. Put on sterile gloves (Procedure 1-3). 21

Chapter 2

Medical History and Patient Interview 26

1. Interview a patient and correctly complete appropriate sections of the medical history form (Procedure 2-1). 31
2. Demonstrate effective communication techniques during the patient interview process. 30

Chapter 3

Anthropometric Measurements and Vital Signs 42

1. Measure and record a patient's weight (Procedure 3-1). 45
2. Measure and record a patient's height (Procedure 3-2). 46
3. Measure and record a patient's oral temperature using a glass mercury thermometer (Procedure 3-3). 51
4. Measure and record a patient's rectal temperature using a glass mercury thermometer (Procedure 3-4). 53
5. Measure and record a patient's axillary temperature using a glass mercury thermometer (Procedure 3-5). 54
6. Measure and record a patient's temperature using an electronic thermometer (Procedure 3-6). 55
7. Measure and record a patient's temperature using a tympanic thermometer (Procedure 3-7). 57
8. Disinfect a glass thermometer (Procedure 3-8). 58
9. Measure and record a patient's radial pulse (Procedure 3-9). 61
10. Measure and record a patient's apical pulse (Procedure 3-10). 62
11. Count a patient's respirations (Procedure 3-11). 65
12. Measure a patient's blood pressure (Procedure 3-12). 68
13. Auscultate a patient's pedal pulse using a Doppler unit. 63

Chapter 4

Physical Examination 74

1. Assist the physician in all aspects of the physical examination (Procedure 4-1). 86

Chapter 5

Instruments and Equipment 90

1. Sanitize equipment for disinfection or sterilization (Procedure 5-1). 100
2. Properly wrap equipment in preparation for sterilization in an autoclave (Procedure 5-2). 105
3. Operate an autoclave observing protocol for pressure, time, and temperature appropriate for the material to be sterilized (Procedure 5-3). 107

Chapter 6

Assisting With Minor Office Surgery 110

1. Open sterile surgical packs (Procedure 6-1). 115
2. Use sterile transfer forceps (Procedure 6-2). 116
3. Add sterile solution to a sterile field (Procedure 6-3). 117
4. Open sterile packets. 113
5. Add the contents of peel-back packets to the sterile field. 113
6. Perform hair removal and skin preparation (Procedure 6-4). 120
7. Attach a surgical blade to a scalpel handle. 121
8. Remove sutures (Procedure 6-5). 125
9. Remove staples (Procedure 6-6). 127
10. Apply a sterile dressing (Procedure 6-7). 129
11. Change an existing sterile dressing (Procedure 6-8). 131
12. Wrap roller bandages using various techniques. 134
13. Apply tubular gauze bandage (Procedure 6-9). 137
14. Assist with excisional surgery (Procedure 6-10). 140
15. Assist with incision and drainage (Procedure 6-11). 141

Chapter 8

Preparing and Administering Medications 158

1. Administer oral medications (Procedure 8-1). 169
2. Administer sublingual or buccal medications (Procedure 8-2). 171
3. Administer rectal medications. 170
4. Administer vaginal medications. 172
5. Apply transdermal medications (Procedure 8-3). 173
6. Apply topical medications (Procedure 8-4). 174
7. Prepare an injection (Procedure 8-5). 177
8. Administer an intradermal injection (Procedure 8-6). 183
9. Administer and read a tine or Mantoux test (Procedure 8-7). 184
10. Administer a subcutaneous injection (Procedure 8-8). 186
11. Administer an intramuscular injection (Procedure 8-9). 189
12. Administer an intramuscular injection using the Z-track method (Procedure 8-10). 190

Chapter 10

Assisting With Diagnostic and Therapeutic Procedures Associated With the Integumentary System 206

1. Apply cold packs (Procedure 10-1). 223
2. Apply warm or cold compresses (Procedure 10-2). 224
3. Use a hot water bottle or commercial hot pack (Procedure 10-3). 226
4. Assist with therapeutic soaks (Procedure 10-4). 227
5. Obtain a wound culture. 219

Chapter 11

Assisting With Diagnostic and Therapeutic Procedures Associated With the Musculoskeletal System 230

1. Prepare a patient for casting. 247
2. Assist the physician with cast application (Procedure 11-1). 253
3. Apply a triangular arm sling (Procedure 11-2). 254
4. Measure a patient for axillary crutches (Procedure 11-3). 258
5. Instruct a patient in the use of various crutch gaits (Procedure 11-4). 259
6. Transfer a patient to and from a wheelchair (Procedure 11-5). 262

Chapter 12

Assisting With Diagnostic and Therapeutic Procedures Associated With the Neurologic System 266

1. Assist with performance of a lumbar puncture (Procedure 12-1). 283

Chapter 13

Assisting With Diagnostic and Therapeutic Procedures Associated With the Sensory System 288

1. Prepare a diagnostic set for use in the examination of the eye, ear, and nose (Procedure 13-1). 296
2. Measure distance visual acuity with a Snellen chart (Procedure 13-2). 297
3. Measure close (or near) visual acuity with a Jaeger chart (Procedure 13-3). 298
4. Measure color perception with an Ishihara color book (Procedure 13-4). 298
5. Assist with tonometry. 295
6. Instill eye medication (Procedure 13-5). 299
7. Irrigate the eye (Procedure 13-6). 300
8. Assist with corneal lavage (Procedure 13-7). 301
9. Remove a foreign object from the eye (Procedure 13-8). 303
10. Perform audiometry (Procedure 13-9). 308
11. Irrigate the ear (Procedure 13-10). 310
12. Instill ear medication (Procedure 13-11). 311
13. Instill nasal medication (Procedure 13-12). 314